FOUNDATIONS OF ORIENTATION AND MOBILITY

THIRD EDITION

Volume II
INSTRUCTIONAL STRATEGIES
and PRACTICAL APPLICATIONS

WILLIAM R. WIENER, RICHARD L. WELSH, and BRUCE B. BLASCH, Editors

AFB PRESS

American Foundation for the Blind

Printed in the United States of America

Volume II: Instructional Strategies and Practical Applications
ISBN 978-0-89128-461-1

Library of Congress Cataloging-in-Publication Data

Foundations of orientation and mobility / William R. Wiener, Richard L. Welsh, and Bruce B. Blasch, editors. — 3rd ed.
    p. cm.
   "Volume I HISTORY and THEORY."
   Includes bibliographical references and index.
   ISBN 978-0-89128-448-2 (print : alk. paper)—ISBN 978-0-89128-462-8 (asc11 cd)—ISBN 978-0-89128-464-2 (epublication/e-book) 1. People with visual disabilities—Rehabilitation.   2. People with visual disabilities—Orientation and mobility.   3. Blind—Rehabilitation.   4. Blind—Orientation and mobility.   5. Orientation (Psychology) 6. Space perception. I. Wiener, William R.   II. Welsh, Richard L.   III. Blasch, Bruce B.
   HV1626.F68 2010
   362.4'18—dc22
                                                2010018023

The American Foundation for the Blind—the organization to which Helen Keller devoted her life—is a national nonprofit devoted to expanding the possibilities for people with vision loss.

∞

It is the policy of the American Foundation for the Blind to use in the first printing of its books acid-free paper that meets the ANSI Z39.48 Standard. The infinity symbol that appears above indicates that the paper in this printing meets that standard.

The third edition of Foundations of Orientation and Mobility *is dedicated to the memory and the accomplishments of three very significant leaders of the orientation and mobility profession. C. Warren Bledsoe, Russell C. Williams, and Stanley Suterko each played key and complementary roles in the development and progression of the O&M profession. Each has died in the years since the publication of the second edition. It is important that those who open this book for the sake of learning about this profession be reminded of the contributions of these three men.*

C O N T E N T S

vi   Contents

ACKNOWLEDGMENTS

After almost 30 years of working on this textbook, we senior editors find ourselves having committed a substantial portion of our life's work to this textbook and certainly to this third edition. We have witnessed the growth of the profession and have worked to assemble a survey of that knowledge in one place and to keep it up to date. Our work to document this research would not have been possible without the assistance of many colleagues, our family members, and our employers.

William Wiener wishes to acknowledge two special individuals who have contributed significantly to this effort. First and foremost, Peg Bernhard has been generous in sharing the time of her spouse with the coeditors during periodic face-to-face and sometimes weekly teleconference editorial meetings. She has been patient over the past five years as the editors have worked among themselves and with their authors to produce this third edition. She has opened the Wiener home to the editors as they worked to review manuscripts. Most of all, she has served as a major support in between meeting times as drafts were being reviewed.

The production of this textbook would not have been possible without the help of Melody Baker, assistant to Dean Wiener, who offered countless hours of work in helping to track and format the chapters, track permissions, and assemble the 750 individual electronic files that make up this work. Without her help, it would have taken the editors an additional five years to produce this text. The editors also appreciate the support of Marquette University to this endeavor.

Richard Welsh wishes to acknowledge and thank his wife and best friend, Mary Nelle McLennan, for all that she has contributed to this effort. She brought her considerable experience and insight regarding the education of blind children to her role as a sounding board in his consideration of issues that arose during the editing process and especially during the writing of his chapters. She provided technical assistance in the management of the many print and electronic materials that he had to process. She supplied warm and gracious hospitality to the editors as we gathered frequently in the Welsh home during the years of this project. Most of all, her love and support enabled Dr. Welsh to manage and cope with a serious illness that he originally thought would prevent his participation in this project. His work on this book is dedicated to her.

Bruce Blasch wishes to thank his wife, Dr. Barbara Blasch, for her constant support and sacrifice of time while he was working on the book and on conference calls with Rick and Bill. Barbara's encouragement and willingness to listen to problems and serve as a sounding board to solutions has been appreciated. Her long experience and professional background in special education has helped answer many questions that we had as editors. During the course of this project, Bruce and Barbara have retired and made a successful transition from Atlanta, Georgia, to Boise, Idaho.

On the acknowledgments pages of the two prior editions, we speculated about how our nine children, first as elementary schoolchildren and then as college students, felt about our participation in this project. Now we have to wonder about the impact on our nine grandchildren.

It goes without saying that we are most indebted to the many authors who have contributed to this book. They have given freely of their time and their knowledge to provide the most up-to-date information regarding the practice of orientation and mobility. They have studied the most current research, and many have reported on their own research. We are especially appreciative of the efforts of several authors who took on the charge to write about topics that have previously been unavailable in a textbook on orientation and mobility.

No acknowledgment would be complete without recognizing those who built the profes-
sion. Elsewhere in this book is a dedication to Russell Williams, Stanley Suterko, and Warren Bledsoe. These three individuals have passed on since the writing of the second edition of this text. Many of the chapters in this book would not have been possible if not for the pioneering work of these giants. Russell Williams help build the early techniques that have been instrumental in helping people who are blind to travel successfully. Stanley Suterko, one of the original orienters, was instrumental in developing coursework that made up the early university curricula as well as helping to spread this training internationally. Warren Bledsoe not only helped to build a bridge from the early work within the U.S. Army to the Veterans Administration and then to the university, but also helped to create and to preserve the early literature of this field.

Finally, we must recognize the assistance that was provided by the AFB Press and by the peer reviewers that they employed. AFB Press recognized that the knowledge base in the field of orientation and mobility had grown dramatically and permitted the doubling and reorganization of this textbook into a two-volume version. This necessitated a lengthy and comprehensive review process that required additional resources from AFB Press. We are grateful for their support.

CONTRIBUTORS

EDITORS

William R. Wiener, Ph.D., is Vice Provost for Research, Dean of the Graduate School, and Professor in the Department of Counselor Education and Counseling Psychology at Marquette University in Milwaukee, Wisconsin; and Adjunct Professor at the Medical College of Wisconsin. He is a former president of the Association for Education and Rehabilitation of the Blind and Visually Impaired (AER), former chairperson of the Editorial Advisory Board of the *Journal of Visual Impairment & Blindness*, a member of the Board of Directors of the American Foundation for the Blind, and chairperson of the Midwest Association of Graduate Schools. Dr. Wiener is the recipient of AER's Ambrose Shotwell Award as well as the Lawrence E. Blaha Award and Newcomer-Hill Award presented by AER's Division of Orientation and Mobility.

Richard L. Welsh, Ph.D., is retired after more than 40 years of service as an orientation and mobility specialist, university faculty member, and chief executive officer of the Maryland School for the Blind, the Greater Pittsburgh Guild for the Blind, and Pittsburgh Vision Services. He served as the first president of the Association for Education and Rehabilitation of the Blind and Visually Impaired (AER) and has received AER's Ambrose Shotwell and C. Warren Bledsoe Awards and the AER Orientation and Mobility Division's Lawrence E. Blaha Award, as well as the Migel Medal from the American Foundation for the Blind. In 2008, Dr. Welsh was inducted into the Hall of Fame for Leaders and Legends of the Blindness Field.

Bruce B. Blasch, Ph.D., is Chief Executive Officer of Bear Consultants. He is retired after more than 45 years in the field of blindness and orientation and mobility, including 20 years at the Veterans Affairs Rehabilitation Research and Development Center in Decatur, Georgia. Dr. Blasch started the mobility programs at the University of Pittsburgh and the University of Wisconsin and was a faculty member at Western Michigan University. He also served as executive director of the American Association of Workers for the Blind. Dr. Blasch was the recipient of the C. Warren Bledsoe Award from the Association for Education and Rehabilitation of the Blind and Visually Impaired (AER) and the AER Orientation and Mobility Division's Lawrence E. Blaha Award, as well as the international Suterko-Cory Award and the Blinded Veterans Association Award of Appreciation.

CHAPTER AUTHORS

Grace Ambrose-Zaken, Ed.D., is Project Coordinator of Rehabilitation Teaching and Orientation and Mobility Programs, Department of Special Education, at Hunter College of the City University of New York in New York City.

Janet M. Barlow, M.Ed., is President of Accessible Design for the Blind, Asheville, North Carolina.

Billie Louise Bentzen, Ph.D., is Director of Research at Accessible Design for the Blind in Berlin, Massachusetts; and Adjunct Associate Professor, Department of Psychology, at Boston College in Chestnut Hill, Massachusetts.

Eugene A. Bourquin, D.H.A., is a faculty member at AXIA College in Phoenix, Arizona; and Senior Instructor at Helen Keller National Center, Sands Point, New York.

Laura Bozeman, Ph.D., is Associate Professor and Director of Vision Studies at the University of Massachusetts Boston.

Alan Brooks, a certified guide dog mobility instructor and an orientation and mobility instructor, is International Affairs Manager at the Guide Dogs for the Blind Association in Reading, United Kingdom.

Colleen Rae Calhoon, M.Sc., is Orientation and Mobility Supervisor at the Maryland School for the Blind in Baltimore.

Michael P. Corbett, M.A., is an orientation and mobility specialist in private practice and retired from the North Carolina Division of Services for the Blind in 2003.

Julie-Anne Couturier, M.A., M.Sc., is Professor and Program Coordinator, School of Optometry, at the Université de Montréal in Montreal, Quebec, Canada.

James S. Crawford, M.A., is Supervisor of Instruction, at Affiliated Blind of Louisiana, Lafayette.

Bonnie Dodson-Burk, M.A., is Orientation and Mobility Specialist and Teacher of the Visually Impaired in the Hollidaysburg Area School District, Hollidaysburg, Pennsylvania.

Diane L. Fazzi, Ph.D., is Professor and Coordinator of the Orientation and Mobility Specialist Training Program in the Division of Special Education and Counseling, California State University, Los Angeles.

Lukas Franck, M.A., is Supervisor of Community Instruction at The Seeing Eye in Morristown, New Jersey.

Jay Furlong, M.Ed., is a travel instructor and special education teacher, and Adjunct Professor at Widener University, Chester, Pennsylvania.

Duane R. Geruschat, Ph.D., is Research Associate in Ophthalmology at the Johns Hopkins University Wilmer Eye Institute, Baltimore, Maryland, and is editor-in-chief of the *Journal of Visual Impairment & Blindness*.

Nora Griffin-Shirley, Ph.D., is Associate Professor and Director of the Virginia Murray Sowell Center for Research and Education in Visual Impairment and Coordinator of the Orientation and Mobility Program at Texas Tech University, Lubbock.

Rodney Haneline, M.A., is Chief Operating Officer and Vice President at Leader Dogs for the Blind in Rochester, Michigan.

James R. Keim, is an orientation and mobility specialist at the Maryland School for the Blind in Baltimore.

Steven J. LaGrow, Ed.D., is Professor of Rehabilitation and Director of Disability, Health, and Rehabilitation Studies, School of Health Sciences, Massey University in Palmerston North, New Zealand.

Gary D. Lawson, Ph.D., is Coordinator of the Doctor of Audiology Program, Department of

Speech Pathology and Audiology, at Western Michigan University in Kalamazoo.

Dennis Lolli, M.Ed., is Program Coordinator at Perkins International, Perkins School for the Blind in Watertown, Massachusetts.

James Robert Marston, Ph.D., is a research scientist at the Atlanta Vision Loss Center, Atlanta Veterans Medical Center, Decatur, Georgia.

Robert M. McCulley, M.Ed., is Director of the Northeast Regional Center for Vision Education and an employee of the Institute for Community Inclusion in Boston, Massachusetts.

Barbara Minick, Ph.D., is retired after 35 years in the blindness field from her position as Assistant to the Executive Director, Allegheny Intermediate Unit, Pennsylvania Department of Education, Pittsburgh.

Linda Myers, M.A., is an orientation and mobility specialist and teacher of the visually impaired for the Marin County Office of Education, San Rafael, and Lecturer and Supervisor of Student Teachers at San Francisco State University, California.

Brenda J. Naimy, M.A., is a full-time lecturer in the Orientation and Mobility Specialist Training Program in the Division of Special Education and Counseling, California State University, Los Angeles.

Laura Park-Leach, M.Ed., is Vice President of the Personal Adjustment and Rehabilitation Department of the Metrolina Association for the Blind, Charlotte, North Carolina.

William M. Penrod, Ed.D., is Assistant Professor, Department of Teaching and Learning, College of Education and Human Development, University of Louisville, Kentucky.

Agathe Ratelle, M.A., is an orientation and mobility specialist at the Institut Nazareth et Louis-Braille and Associate Professor in Vision Impairment, School of Optometry, at the Université de Montréal in Montreal, Quebec, Canada.

Christine Roman-Lantzy, Ph.D., is an educational consultant and Director of the Pediatric VIEW Program at the Western Pennsylvania Hospital, Pittsburgh, and a private consultant for CVI Resources.

Sandra Rosen, Ph.D., is Coordinator of the Orientation and Mobility Program, San Francisco State University, California.

Wendy K. Sapp, Ph.D., is an orientation and mobility specialist and a consultant for Visual Impairment Education Services, Cohutta, Georgia.

Dona Sauerburger, M.A., is an orientation and mobility specialist in Gambrills, Maryland, and Washington, DC.

Annette C. Skellenger, Ed. D., is Supervising Teacher—Visual Impairment at the Arizona School for the Deaf and Blind in Tucson.

Audrey J. Smith, Ph.D., is Dean and Associate Professor, College of Education and Rehabilitation, Salus University, Elkins Park, Pennsylvania.

Daniel L. Smith, M.A., is Supervisor at the Edward Hines, Jr., Veterans Affairs Hospital, Blind Rehabilitation Center, in Hines, Illinois.

Patricia J. Voorhees, M.Ed., is a travel instructor and special education teacher in Delaware County, Pennsylvania.

IN MEMORIAM

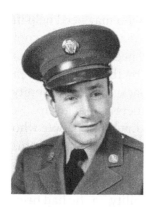

C. Warren Bledsoe, the son of the former superintendent of the Maryland School for the Blind, had been educated as a teacher of the blind and was teaching English and drama at the Maryland School for the Blind before enlisting in the Army during World War II. He was assigned to a special unit for the rehabilitation of blinded military personnel at Valley Forge Army Hospital near Philadelphia. There he worked with Richard Hoover and helped to develop the long-cane method of travel for blind people and to teach it to veterans who were returning from the battlefield with serious eye injuries. Bledsoe tells the entire story of this development and his role in it in Volume 1, Chapter 13.

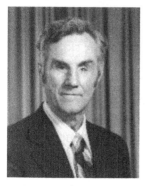

Russell C. Williams was one of the returning soldiers who lost his sight in the battles that followed the D-Day invasion. As a former athlete, teacher, and coach, Williams experienced success with the training he received and was tapped to move into a role as a counselor and teacher at Valley Forge following additional rehabilitation at Avon Old Farms. After returning to Valley Forge as a staff member, Williams added to his mobility techniques while traveling in the Phoenixville community. He refined what he had learned and passed his techniques along to other Valley Forge patients. His story is told as a part of Bledsoe's chapter and in an appendix sidebar published for the first time in this edition.

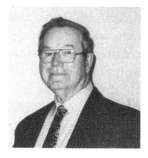

Stanley Suterko was one of the first six "orienters" at the Hines Center, as these mobility specialists were called at that time. Not only did Suterko, himself a World War II veteran who had been trained as a corrective therapist, learn his lessons well, but also he and the other handpicked staff at Hines continued to develop the techniques for independent travel and to establish teaching methods that have served the profession well and have been replicated around the world.

After completing his service with the Army, Bledsoe continued to advocate for the continuation of the training methods initiated at Valley Forge. Working as a private citizen and then as a consultant to the Veterans Administration, Bledsoe was instrumental in persuading the VA to develop a Blind Rehabilitation Center at the Hines VA Hospital in a Chicago suburb. Russell Williams, on the recommendation of Bledsoe, was selected to lead this center and to establish a program that was reflective of his own insight and skill. Bledsoe and Williams, with help from Richard Hoover and Kay Gruber, selected the first group of staff to be trained in the techniques developed by Hoover and Bledsoe at Hines and further enhanced by Williams.

Following his work for the Veterans Administration, Bledsoe moved on to the federal Office of Vocational Rehabilitation in the Department of Medicine and Surgery. There he helped to persuade Mary Switzer of the value of this emerging profession, and soon federal funding was secured to establish university training programs for the education of mobility specialists at the master's degree level. When one of the first programs was established at Western Michigan University in Kalamazoo, Suterko was selected, along with Donald Blasch, to develop the necessary courses and learning experiences to prepare O&M specialists to be of service to all blind and visually impaired people who may need help in learning how to travel independently. This included not only adventitiously blinded adults but also congenitally blind children, as well as seniors who lost their vision as a result of age-related diseases. Suterko helped to develop the course structure for the training program. He was guided by the thinking of an advisory group that had met in 1959 and had suggested the kinds of academic background a mobility specialist should bring to his specialty. Both Bledsoe and Williams had been members of that group.

As the reputation of this profession grew, fed by the practical successes of many blind people who were instructed by the first generation of mobility specialists, the demand for information about this specialty came in from all directions. Suterko was one of the leaders when it came to spreading this profession to other countries and other cultures. He had a major impact in Australia, England, France, Poland, New Zealand, and other countries where he visited. This "St. Peter of Mobility," as he had been dubbed by the Australians, occasionally encountered skeptics. He responded with a gentle but persuasive soft sell that relied on the demonstrated successes of the students whom he taught in those countries. Many were converted by this modern-day apostle because of the effectiveness of the skills taught by this genuinely humble man.

The three men to whom we are dedicating this third edition of *Foundations of Orientation and Mobility* formed the heart, soul, and brains of the profession as it first emerged. They brought it from a practical attempt to help blinded veterans find a way to reclaim their lives to a university-based profession dedicated to assisting every person who is visually impaired, regardless of age, cause, or extent of visual impairment, in learning how to move about his or her own environment or community to the best of his or her ability.

The body of knowledge reflected in the contents of this textbook is the foundation for the training of each mobility specialist. As such, it is the culmination of the work to which Bledsoe, Williams, and Suterko dedicated their lives. When the first edition was published in 1980, Williams wrote its preface, and Suterko wrote a foreword. Bledsoe's unique first-person account of the history of this profession was written for the first edition and has been republished in its original form in each edition since then.

In gratitude for the commitment of Bledsoe, Williams, and Suterko to the establishment of the profession of orientation and mobility and for their success in doing so, the editors humbly and respectfully dedicate our work and that of our authors to these three men who created and promulgated our profession.

INTRODUCTION

The field of orientation and mobility (O&M) continues to expand its knowledge base and adapt its training to meet the needs of the changing population and environment. The evolution of the three editions of *Foundations of Orientation and Mobility* is evidence of this expansion and growth. Within the past two decades, significant environmental changes and an explosion of research and technology have had a major impact on travel without vision. The profession of orientation and mobility has responded to these issues by exploring new strategies for managing the changing environment and by taking advantage of the new technology and other developments emerging from research. This third edition *of Foundations of Orientation and Mobility* incorporates this changing body of knowledge in order to best educate new O&M specialists as well as to update currently practicing O&M specialists and other professionals.

TRENDS AND CHANGES IN THE O&M FIELD

Many sweeping and profound changes have taken place in the field from the original 1980 edition of *Foundations of Orientation and Mobility*

to this third edition. In addition to a dramatic transformation of the built environment, O&M practitioners have witnessed a multitude of changes in the populations with whom they work. Services to children and adults have continued to evolve and change as a result of the changing needs of the client population. In addition to providing instruction to individuals with no useful vision and individuals with low vision, the services have continued to expand to even more individuals, including those with multiple impairments and the elderly. This expansion of practice has necessitated instructors becoming more comfortable with new devices (such as adaptive mobility devices) and other adaptive equipment such as walkers, orthopedic canes, wheelchairs, and other assistive devices. Instruction itself has continued to change and increase its emphasis on meeting both the immediate needs of the student while also teaching generalization to new environments. Instruction also continues to expand to include more emphasis on interventions with infants and toddlers and their parents. It is anticipated that these trends with changing populations will continue to evolve. These ongoing shifts as well as others that have taken place are reflected in both the organization and content emphases selected for this text.

In addition to the needs of changing populations, the environment itself presents new challenges. The Americans with Disabilities Act, through its accessibility guidelines (Americans with Disabilities Act Accessibility Guidelines, or ADAAG), and the Uniform Federal Accessibility Standards from the Architectural Barriers Act (ABA) have designated scoping requirements that serve to make the environment more accessible. The guidelines provide specifications that address features such as protruding objects, headroom, signage, landmarks, stairs, and elevators. The second edition of this text included a discussion of the difficulties presented by semi-actuated and fully actuated traffic signals for many travelers who are blind. In this edition, there is a focus on future concerns. It is already clear that quiet cars are presenting challenges to travelers, as is the growth of roundabouts, channelized intersections, and unusual geometric configurations of intersections. There is a great deal of research centering on each of these changes in the built environment, but there is not yet a consensus on the training options or modifications to provide a solution for individuals who are blind. This text provides a review of the research and attempts to provide some direction for solutions. It will be up to practitioners to continue to follow the research to learn which approaches are best.

At the same time, technology for O&M is flourishing. The history of electronic travel aids (ETAs) is considered in all three editions of *Foundations of Orientation and Mobility*. In general, new ETAs that appear in one edition are generally not available by the publication of the next; however, they are replaced by the next generation of new ETAs. The short-lived sales of these devices are not necessarily due to the quality of the technology but rather the limited demand for the devices and the high price due to the small quantities produced. Electronic orientation aids (EOAs), on the other hand, continue to evolve and to become cheaper, smaller, more user friendly, and more popular. Global positioning systems (GPS) are beginning to provide travelers with a degree of freedom previously unknown. Continued development of these systems will provide a means for O&M specialists to instruct students to expand their horizons and overcome barriers. The future of EOAs looks very promising for individuals with a visual impairment who use canes or dog guides. EOAs also provide new challenges and training opportunities for O&M specialists. The complexity of the environment will require that information already available to people who are sighted be made available to people with vision loss. Accessible pedestrian signals (APS) fill this void and will become more sophisticated and more plentiful in the environment. In this third edition of *Foundations of Orientation and Mobility*, substantially more research is presented regarding the effectiveness and the most appropriate placement of these devices. This information is in some measure due to O&M specialists, consumers, and traffic engineers working together.

FOUNDATIONS OF ORIENTATION AND MOBILITY: THE THIRD EDITION

As the editors of this text undertook its revision, it became clear that this tremendous expansion of knowledge and research and the cumulative impact of the changes seen in recent decades called for an expansion of the text itself. The introduction to Volume 1 explains that it was thus decided to organize the textbook as a two-volume set, with the first volume focusing on history and theory and the second volume focusing on the application of these theories. Although each volume can stand on its own, the two volumes are intended to complement each other, and readers, most especially students, are encouraged to make use of both.

Volume 1 of the text, subtitled *History and Theory*, is divided into three parts: "Human Systems," "Mobility Systems and Adaptations," and "The Profession of O&M and Its Development." The present volume, subtitled *Instructional Strategies and Practical Applications*, is divided into the following four parts: "Sensory Use and Psychosocial Function," "Age-Related Instruction," "Adapted Tools and Complex Environments," and "O&M and Different Disabilities."

The new organization of the text has sometimes resulted in the relocation of certain information that previously appeared in one chapter and now is spread out between two chapters in two separate volumes. Because many of the chapters in the first volume have corresponding chapters in the second, there is cross-referencing between the two volumes as a helpful reminder to readers that additional information is available to them. Readers may also notice that there is redundant information among various chapters. Since the majority of university training programs use chapters in a foundations text independently rather than following the sequence of chapters in the book, it was decided that a certain degree of overlap among chapters was necessary.

Both volumes of *Foundations of Orientation and Mobility* have a common structure that is followed in each chapter. Questions are presented at the beginning of a chapter to promote inquiry-based learning. Following each chapter, implications are provided as a review of important points. Also at the end of the chapter, suggestions for independent learning activities are offered as an opportunity for readers to extend their understanding of the concepts presented. As mentioned at the outset of Volume 1, a word about terminology is in order. The editors have chosen to use consistent terms for people who are blind, visually impaired, and consumers of ser-

vices, using the term *student* to refer to both children and adults.

THE CHAPTERS IN VOLUME 2

Volume 2 complements the first volume by providing more of a focus on the application of many of the principles that were identified in Volume 1. Often the chapters in this volume begin with the terms *improving* or *teaching*. The first group of chapters corresponds to the initial chapters in Volume 1 and focuses on the improvement of the basic sensory systems for the purpose of learning to travel without vision. A second group of chapters focuses on the teaching of O&M to general groups of students, including very young children, school-age children, adults, and seniors. A third group examines the teaching and use of certain tools and elements of the environment. The final group of chapters discusses the teaching of O&M to certain groups of students who have additional disabilities. Some of the chapters in this current volume address issues that have not previously been included in a text on orientation and mobility. For example, for the first time in this text there are chapters dealing with cortical visual impairment, travel in adverse weather, the use of transportation systems, and travel at complex intersections.

Volume 2 of *Foundations of Orientation and Mobility* opens with a chapter by LaGrow that demonstrates how the theories and principles of perception are applied in the fundamental techniques that have been the foundation of the profession. It describes some of the most basic techniques and explains how they are designed to use alternative forms of perception to substitute for vision in providing the basic information that is required for independent travel. The chapter shows how the basic components of the human guide and long-cane techniques that are taught indoors and outdoors are designed to enhance the perception of the environment. Chapter 2 by Bozeman and McCulley continues the discussion of orientation by giving information on how we teach children and adults to establish and maintain their orientation in the environment. Included are strategies to assist with the organization of spatial information, beginning with body awareness and encompassing such areas as spatial relationships, spatial updating, concept formation, exploration, reorientation, integrating sensory and perceptual skills, and teaching learner-based strategies for children and adults.

Geruschat and Smith in Chapter 3 guide the professional who provides instruction to individuals with low vision. It begins with a clinical low vision assessment and continues with a functional assessment before introducing training in visual motor skills, the use of mobility techniques with low vision, and the use of optical devices. Lawson and Wiener in Chapter 4 give instruction on how to develop better orientation through the use of hearing. They include functional hearing assessment; auditory training for O&M in natural settings and with recordings; the use of hearing aids, assistive listening devices, and implants; and the role of the O&M specialist. Rosen in Chapter 5 gives guidance on how to facilitate sensorimotor development and functioning in children and adults. The chapter initially focuses on assessment of sensory functioning, muscle tone, and the integration of neurological reflexes and reactions, and moves into methods of assisting children to develop the necessary building blocks while providing adults with remediation where possible. In Chapter 6, Welsh demonstrates how O&M teaching strategies are used to overcome psychosocial barriers to mobility. These strategies include strengthening the relationship between the student and the instructor, assessing psychosocial functioning, planning, lesson sequencing, involving families, and interacting with the public.

Starting off the second group of chapters focusing on the special needs of general groups of students, Chapter 7 by Skellenger and Sapp provides activities for effective teaching of children in early childhood. They address legislative support, early intervention, developmental stages, the integration of sensory experiences, working with families, working with teams, assessment activities, lesson planning, curriculum content, the use of motivating materials, concept development, ambulatory and nonambulatory children, and children with multiple impairments. Fazzi and Naimy in Chapter 8 provide activities for teaching children of school age. Included in the chapter are planning for programs of excellence, age-appropriate curricular guidelines, individualized assessment and planning, teaching approaches and tools, organizing for delivery of services, and establishing school and family partnerships.

Chapter 9 by Welsh provides information on instruction to adults. This includes characteristics of adults with visual impairment, adjustment to visual loss, approaches to adult learning, assessment and program planning, implementing a training program, vocational rehabilitation, and service delivery options for adults. Chapter 10 by Griffin-Shirley and Welsh provides practical information on working with older adults. Items such as general conditions related to aging; general health status; demographics of aging; strategies for teaching older persons, including andragogy; scheduling issues; the use of memory tools; environmental modifications; avoiding falls; resolving disorientation; O&M outcomes; programming structures; and interacting with the aging system are included.

The next group of chapters focuses on the use of specialized tools and environmental elements that are of use in the teaching of O&M. Chapter 11 by Bentzen and Marston focuses on teaching the use of orientation aids, which includes designing maps, selecting materials for producing maps, teaching map-reading concepts and skills and exploration, route planning, and travel using geographic information system (GIS) and global positioning system devices. Barlow, Bentzen, Sauerburger, and Franck in Chapter 12 cover the essential topics of how to travel at complex intersections. Found within the chapter are changes in infrastructure, street-crossing tasks, problem issues, alignment techniques, medians, channelized turn lanes, roundabouts, ramp and corner configurations, vehicle signalization and phasing plans, and risk assessment. Information is provided on judging traffic gaps, detecting curb ramps, understanding intersection geometry, using techniques for street detection, and crossing at different types of unsignalized and signalized intersections. Chapter 13 by Dodson-Burk, Park-Leach, and Myers is devoted to the use of transportation systems. It gives practical information for cane and dog guide users regarding modes of transportation, components of transit trips, system accessibility, urban bus travel, training of transit personnel, rail travel, paratransit systems, taxi service, air travel, and over-the-road bus service.

Penrod, Smith, Haneline, and Corbett in Chapter 14 provide lesson plans for the use of generic electronic travel aids and GPS orientation aids. The chapter contains instruction on selecting environments, preparing for training, and teaching the use of the devices. Couturier and Ratelle in Chapter 15 provide guidance for travel in adverse weather conditions. They present information on such items as traveling in winter conditions; selecting clothing, footwear, and equipment; scheduling lessons; avoiding slips and falls; selecting canes; traveling in rain, strong winds, and fog; and traveling in extreme heat and hot weather. Chapter 16 by Franck, Haneline, and Brooks gives the orientation and mobility specialist information on how to select and prepare an individual for dog guide training and how to troubleshoot problems after the individual has returned home from the dog guide school. It shares information on acceptance

standards, assessing user potential, preparing the student, the role of the O&M specialist in troubleshooting, and providing orientation assistance.

The final group of chapters in this volume examines the methods and special requirements for teaching students with additional disabilities. Lolli, Sauerburger, and Bourquin in Chapter 17 apply orientation and mobility to working with individuals with vision and hearing loss. Such topics as the deaf-blind population, cultural issues, communication methods, use of interpreting services, modification of the O&M curriculum, street crossings, use of public transportation, use of APS, and use of dog guides are addressed. Chapter 18 by Rosen and Crawford examines how to teach learners with physical and health impairments. It provides a brief overview of common physical and health impairments and presents the use of ambulatory aids and modifications of mobility techniques, including the use of wheelchairs, scooters, canes, crutches, and walkers. Chapter 19 by Ambrose-Zaken, Calhoon, and Keim presents information on how to teach students with cognitive impairments. It presents six classifications of impairment and presents strategies for addressing 10 skill areas: attention, sensory integration, behavior, memory, concept development, generalization, problem solving, social skills, orientation strategies, and mobility techniques. Also included are charts that provide examples of levels of goals for the skill areas.

Chapter 20 by Roman-Lantzy provides information on teaching students with cortical visual impairment (CVI). It presents the visual and behavioral characteristics of students with CVI, assessment and program planning, and instruction strategies based upon cortical visual impairment ranges. Finally, Chapter 21 by Blasch, Wiener, Voorhees, Minick, and Furlong closes the book with a look at the future of travel instruction for persons with disabilities other than blindness. It looks at services that have been provided through schools and agencies and the preparation of instructors through university programs. The chapter looks at similarities and differences between orientation and mobility for students with visual impairment and travel instruction for people with other disabilities. It examines interventions and provides a model for provision of service.

LOOKING AHEAD

As the introduction to Volume 1 pointed out, *Foundations of Orientation and Mobility* is designed to help prepare orientation and mobility special-ists at the university level and to serve as a guide and professional reference for practicing person-nel as well. It is therefore intended to establish the foundational knowledge base for those study-ing to enter the profession but also serves as a resource for those already engaged in service provision. In addition, it provides a body of knowledge for related professionals in disciplines such as psychology, social work, rehabilitation counseling, and traffic engineering. It is the hope of the editors and the authors that this text will play a role in providing the best possible service to people who experience vision loss and require orientation and mobility services.

PART ONE

Sensory Use and Psychosocial Function

CHAPTER 1

Improving Perception for Orientation and Mobility

Steven J. LaGrow

LEARNING QUESTIONS

- How does accuracy in both movement and technique impact perception?
- What role does context have in developing and reinforcing perceptual skill?
- What impact does hand position have on relating objects contacted with the long cane to body plane?
- What role does body alignment play in establishing or maintaining a line of travel?
- What are the different clues utilized to locate streets and stay on track while crossing them?

Orientation and mobility (O&M) refers to the skills and techniques required for independent travel by persons who are blind or visually impaired (LaGrow & Weessies, 1994). Orientation refers to the ability to establish and maintain an awareness of one's position in space (Berube, 1991; LaGrow, 2009), while mobility refers to the act of moving through space in a safe and efficient manner (Berube, 1991; Hill & Ponder, 1976; Jansson, 2000; LaGrow & Weessies, 1994; Long & Hill, 1997). When the two are integrated, the result is purposeful and directed movement

(Darken & Peterson, 2002; Mast & Zaehle, 2008; Thinus-Blanc & Gaunet, 1997). Both are dependent on accurate perception resulting from the successful interpretation of sensory clues into meaningful travel information (Guth & Rieser, 1997; Jansson, 2000; Long & Hill, 1997; Mast & Zaehle, 2008; Rieser, 2008). Teaching people who are blind or visually impaired to attend to and accurately interpret sensory information gained while traveling (perceptual and motor learning) and to use that information along with knowledge of the travel environment (episodic and conceptual knowledge) to direct movement is central to O&M instruction (Hill, Rosen, Correa, & Langley, 1984; see also the section on Perception, Action, and Knowledge in Volume 1, Chapter 1). The purpose of this chapter is to promote enhanced accuracy in perception for orientation and mobility by encouraging care and structure in the introduction to and use of various mobility techniques while illustrating how explicit activities substitute for vision (see Chapter 3 for activities that explicitly utilize low vision for orientation and mobility). The techniques described here are provided for illustration only and are in no way meant to constitute a comprehensive or exhaustive description of the strategies and techniques used in orientation and mobility (for a more complete description of these techniques, see Hill & Ponder, 1976; Jacobson, 1993; LaGrow & Weessies, 1994).

INDOOR ENVIRONMENTS

Instruction usually begins indoors, where the demands imposed by the travel environment (that is, the routes or paths of travel selected) tend to be less complex and easier to control than those imposed by outdoor environments (LaGrow & Weessies, 1994).

Introduction and Use of the Human Guide Techniques

Basic Instructions

Instruction often begins by introducing the student to the human guide (also known as sighted guide) techniques. These techniques are the least threatening form of independent travel and initially require few decisions on the part of the traveler. The guide provides the student with protection from obstacles in the environment and bears the responsibility for orientation, while the student gets used to moving through the environment without fear of injury or incident. The student, in turn, is free to attend to the various sensory clues encountered, including those transmitted by the guide's movements, and learns the environmental and spatial concepts required for establishing orientation and planning routes of travel to various destinations.

Interpreting the environment.   Information about the environment, direction of travel, and terrain is transmitted from the guide's movement through the traveler's hand and arm. Kinesthetic and proprioceptive information is conveyed as the pair move in tandem (see the section on Sources of Perceptual Input in Volume 1, Chapter 1). Thus, the traveler can tell when the guide starts, stops,

and turns; ascends or descends a ramp, step, or flight of stairs; and, in most cases, reaches for a door and pulls or pushes it open or shut. However, the accuracy and degree to which the traveler can gain information from the guide's movements is dependent on both the precision with which the student uses the various techniques required for travel with a human guide and the care with which the guide moves.

The student is one-half step behind the guide. Their shoulders overlap. The relative positions of the guide and traveler are maintained by the positioning of the traveler's arm at her side, the relationship between the traveler's upper arm and forearm (which forms a 90-degree angle at the elbow), and the location of the traveler's grip on the guide's arm. Strict adherence to the position of the arm and grip reduces the degrees of freedom available for variation between the guide and traveler and therefore reduces the chance of both positional and perceptual error (see the section on Motor Learning in Volume 1, Chapter 1). The information obtained from the guide's movement is therefore more precise and, as such, easier for the traveler to interpret than it otherwise would be. Maintaining a consistent 90-degree angle between the traveler's upper arm and forearm while following the guide, for example, makes it possible for the traveler to instantly and unambiguously recognize a change in level when the guide steps up or down to negotiate a step or curb, as this movement forces a change in that angle.

Changing direction.   In addition to the traveler's technique being precise, the guide's movement should be controlled and made only in response to changes in direction dictated by the path of travel, level (curbs, steps or stairways, or terrain), or activity (passing through narrow spaces or doorways), as all of the guide's movement should indicate to the student something about the environment or the path of travel. A backward and forward movement of the guide's arm and trunk, for example, indicates that a door is being pulled open. Use or nonuse of the guiding arm when holding the door open indicates the side the door is on (that is, the guide's side or the traveler's).

Changes in direction should be crisp and made with a definite start and stop in the action to ensure that the student is aware of and able to interpret the degree of change being made. The vestibular sense is the primary source of information about directional change and responds best to clear initiation and cessation in movement (see Chapter 5 and Volume 1, Chapter 5). As a result, a sweeping turn of 90 degrees involving a relatively steady state of motion can be executed without the traveler ever being aware that a change in direction has occurred.

Negotiating a step or stairs.   Stopping or pausing before negotiating a step or stairs is part of the technique for ascending and descending stairs with a guide and should occur at the first and last step to be negotiated in all cases. This indicates that a change is about to occur. The guide's initial movement subsequent to the pause indicates the direction of the stairway (ascending or descending) through a forced change in the angle at the elbow, which remains flexed or extended, respectively, while traversing the stairs in response to the guide's position above or below the traveler. The guide is to pause at the final step before stepping forward onto the landing. Again, the pause alerts the traveler that a change is about to occur and the forced change in angle at the elbow from flexed or extended to the standard 90 degrees as the guide steps out and forward on to the landing informs the traveler that the last step has been reached. Furthermore, if the guide consistently pauses at a curb, step, or beginning of a stairway when it is encountered in such a way that the toes are precisely at the riser or just overlap the top of the stairs before stepping up or down, respectively, the traveler will be aware of the exact distance to the steps to

be negotiated, as this will correspond to the length of the traveler's forearm, as opposed to any characteristic of the guide. This is usually confirmed, initially, by encouraging the student to slide his foot forward to locate the step before the guide continues. Once the student is clear on the distance and confident that it does not vary from situation to situation, this practice is discontinued.

Limiting the degrees of freedom in movement of the limbs by adhering to the prescribed relationship between the upper arm and forearm and the use of the yoke grip (thumb on the outside and fingers on the inside of the guide arm) in the basic human guide technique facilitates the clear transmission of information about the environment to the traveler from the guide's movements. Precise directed movement and good technique make it possible for proximal perception from the hand and elbow to be translated into distal information about the travel environment.

Introducing Sensory Clues and Spatial and Environmental Concepts

The human guide techniques consist of the basic human guide, narrow spaces, changing sides, reversing directions, doorways, stairways, seating, and accepting and refusing aid techniques (see Hill & Ponder, 1976, or LaGrow & Weessies, 1994, for a complete description of each technique). As each is introduced, time for practice is necessary to allow the traveler to get used to the motor responses required and to learn to interpret the information that is conveyed by the guide's movement (see the section on Motor Learning in Volume 1, Chapter 1). The O&M specialist may take advantage of the time needed to ingrain these skills to introduce basic environmental and spatial concepts, establish general orientation skills, and provide the student with opportunities to learn to identify and respond to a range of sensory information encountered while traveling. In time, the traveler may use human guide techniques as a totally independent means of travel, directing the guide through the environment to the destination. To do so, the traveler must learn to focus on and glean meaning from the sensory clues provided by the guide and the environment while following the guide's lead through space.

Beginning formal O&M instruction with the human guide techniques is ideal for introducing the traveler to the use of motor and other sensory clues gained from movement through the environment since these techniques are designed to allow the traveler to gain as much information through the senses as possible. Therefore, as the traveler is being introduced to these mobility techniques, he or she may also be actively taught to be aware of and respond to the guide's body movements, changes in direction, and time and distance traveled (see the section on Skillful Perception and Action: Concepts and Definitions in Volume 1, Chapter 1). In addition, the traveler ought to be instructed to attend to additional sensory information available within the environment in order to be aware of what is happening during the course of travel and to maintain both orientation and a degree of independence in travel (see the section on Walking and Environmental Flow in Volume 1, Chapter 1). This becomes more possible as the traveler gains skill with the techniques introduced and is able to direct attention to the environment itself. Automaticity, or the ingrained used of techniques gained through practice, makes this possible (see the section on Motor Learning in Volume 1, Chapter 1).

Learning to judge distance. Acquiring these skills is facilitated by the control established over travel by the use of human guide techniques and by the O&M specialist's thoughtful selection of objectives set for travel (the purpose or destination to be reached in each phase of travel). For example, learning to judge distance of travel

kinesthetically is based on the time taken to go from point A to point B and is facilitated by consistency, continuity, and repetition. In other words, the starting point and ending point of the route have to be the same, and the route must be traveled at about the same pace without interruption a number of times before the student can be expected to gain a sense of the distance traveled for that particular route (hallway, block, street crossing, corridor or stretch of corridor in a mall, and so on). The human guide techniques, therefore, are particularly useful for introducing this skill, as the guide can control both consistency (speed and starting and ending points) and continuity of movement. Thus, when introducing this skill, the guide ought to travel at a steady pace, minimize interruption in the continuity of travel, and endeavor to start and finish each phase of travel at approximately the same point. Repetition is necessary to ingrain this information into the student's travel repertoire, and to help him develop a point of reference for distance traveled.

As a result, purposefully walking back and forth along a given hallway while the student is introduced to and then practices the basic sighted guide path, narrow spaces, and dynamic changing sides techniques may help the student establish a point of reference for judging distances traveled (that is, the length of that particular hallway). Often, parallel hallways are the same length (for example, in a given building, the north hallway and the south hallway are the same length, as are the east, west, and middle hallways), and therefore once the length of one hallway is established, it may be generalized to others (the north hallway to the south hallway and the east hallway to both the middle and west hallways). Relative length or distance traveled may become important for establishing and maintaining orientation, especially if the lengths of the hallways vary in some systematic way (that is, the north and south hallways are more than twice as long as the east, west, and middle hallways). Thus, spending the time to firmly establish the length of the north hallway through repetition and then comparing it to the south hallway (as the same) and contrasting those with the east, west, and middle hallways (as being much longer than those hallways), for example, may be of benefit later as that information is generalized across all hallways on various floors of a given building. Any exception to that generalization may prove to be of value in identifying a specific location. For example, if the north and south hallways are generally of the same length in all cases except for one floor where one of these hallways is considerably shorter (for example, the north hallway on the sixth floor), then knowledge of that anomaly may serve as an information point for confirming, maintaining, or reestablishing one's orientation (see Volume 1, Chapter 2).

Interpreting context.   Context, therefore, is important, since being able to judge the distance traveled is relevant only in terms of the travel environment and the purpose for this information. If, for example, one of the objectives of a run within a lesson is to have the student identify and locate an intersecting hallway in order to direct the guide to turn and travel to a given destination, then knowing about how far one must go before expecting to find the intersecting hallway (for example, halfway down the north or south hallway) becomes a meaningful skill. This skill allows the student to anticipate the location of the intersection and therefore begin to attend to and look for other sensory clues that may be of use in locating the intersection as well. For example, specific sounds may be associated with different types of intersecting hallways (for example, L- versus T-shaped intersections). The more specific or unique those sounds are (that is, pattern or type of sound and hallway), the more useful they will be for making decisions about travel. In the examples given here, only the middle hallway on each floor con-

tains the building's internal stairwells and elevators. Thus, if the intersecting hallway being sought is the middle hallway, then the traveler may be instructed to tune in to or selectively listen for sounds associated with stairwells and elevators (see Volume 1, Chapter 4). Identification of such sounds would help confirm that it is indeed time to instruct the guide to turn.

Interpreting sensory clues.   The guide points out other sensory clues encountered while traveling and relates them specifically to areas within the environment in terms of function or location. These clues are then used to build up the student's knowledge of the environment and serve as aids to orientation. This process should be very structured so that the knowledge can be absorbed and its significance noted. This is most likely to be accomplished if the student is actively engaged in both purposeful movement (that is, directing the guide's movement through space) and route planning, as these activities require the student to be aware of and purposefully keep track of the distance and direction of travel, as well as any number of specific sensory clues useful for maintaining one's orientation and locating destinations (see the section on Walking and Environmental Flow in Volume 1, Chapter 1). For example, the student may learn to recognize the auditory change in the quality of reflected sound encountered when moving from a wide to a narrower hallway, or when moving from an area with a high ceiling to one with a low ceiling, and relate this auditory clue to the direction of travel in a specific hallway or location within a hallway (Ashmead & Wall, 1999).

However, the student does not learn to recognize these changes by simply having the change pointed out in the course of travel; rather, the student needs to actively practice by looking for and learning to recognize this very subtle change, again through anticipation in terms of knowledge of its location in the environment, feedback, and repetition of the task (Wall Emerson &

Ashmead, 2008). The O&M specialist may choose to introduce this clue and the skill required for its recognition by isolating it from other tasks. The student would be asked to identify any change noticed as the instructor repeatedly guides the student past this environmental feature from varying distances. Feedback is provided to indicate the accuracy of detection. Success would most likely be achieved when approaching this feature as change occurs from wide to narrow or high to low. Thus, the O&M specialist would start from the direction that would afford the best chance for a correct response and repeat the exercise several times until the student could confidently recognize the change. The direction of travel may then be changed, with the pattern repeated to build success and skill from the new direction. Finally, recognition of this sensory clue would be built into the student's repertoire by planning and executing runs from either direction that would involve destinations located near or associated with this change, therefore reinforcing its identification as a useful part of the travel process.

The change or difference encountered here, as with other environmental information gained from the senses, is informative by its uniqueness or context. In other words, it is often the difference from the standard layout that is most informative. If, for example, all hallways have a carpet runner down the middle, the recognition of the texture of the carpet tactilely underfoot tells the traveler only that she is walking down the middle of a hallway, but if the carpet runner is present in only one of a number of hallways, then recognition of the carpet is indicative of that specific hallway. Furthermore, recognition of it may confirm that the student is on course if she is supposed to be traveling along that hallway; update and confirm the traveler's orientation if crossing it is part of the plan; or be used as a clue for reorientation if it is encountered when the traveler is lost or confused. Thus, knowing that a hallway or some feature of it differs from another becomes information that can help with orientation and be used to update one's position in space or confirm when that destination has been reached (see Chapter 2 and Volume 1, Chapter 2). Similarly, if the O&M specialist is attempting to get the student to recognize a wooden floor that corresponds with the location of the foyer of the building, the O&M specialist would point it out and attempt to get the student to recognize the change in floor covering while moving from the tiled hallway to the wood foyer. The pair may walk back and forth along the hallway, with the student responsible for indicating where the change occurs. As with the earlier exercise to recognize the change in the ceiling height or width of the hallway, this could be isolated from other travel tasks and repeated until the student can do this with accuracy and confidence. The O&M specialist could then use the foyer as a destination and incorporate it into the student's knowledge of the building, including the tactile clue corresponding to it that confirms the destination. The more systematically this type of information is developed and used for maintaining orientation during these early lessons, the more likely it will be recognized as being instrumental to successful travel over time.

Interpreting information points and landmarks. Thus, in addition to planning routes of travel to teach basic O&M techniques, the O&M specialist specifically chooses destinations and paths of travel to introduce the student to various information points and landmarks. As mentioned earlier, some floors or hallways may have a different surface (for example, tile as opposed to wood or carpet); some may be lighter or darker or warmer or colder than others (indicating, for example, the presence of windows or external doorways); others may be narrower or have higher ceilings or be busier and therefore sound different; some may be shorter than standard, or have a slope or smell differently. All of these things may prove to be informative in determining one's location and therefore may provide the student with the opportunity to maintain her orientation while being guided, to take over and direct the guide to the desired objective of travel, and even to correct a guide who has taken a wrong turn. Each of these clues may be introduced by the O&M specialist and their recognition ingrained by directed repetition and feedback.

The combination of sensory information and knowledge of the environment provides the traveler with the information necessary to locate destinations, find intersecting paths of travel, and maintain orientation while traveling. However, unless a student has learned to attend to sensory information in some systematic manner, many of these clues may go unnoticed, or if they are noticed, their meaning may not be clear if the student does not have a frame of reference or context with which to interpret them. Therefore, much of the time spent in teaching the human guide techniques may also be used to educate the student to attend to the various sources of information available and to begin to make sense of that information in terms of the environment in which one is traveling. Orientation, like mobility, is a learned skill.

Utilizing repetitive travel. The process of utilizing repetitive travel from one destination to another helps to ingrain motor skills, while the selection of new destinations provides the O&M specialist with a means to expand the travel environment and systematically increase the demands on the student. At the same time, responsibility for locating destinations, maintaining orientation, and planning routes of travel may be progressively shifted from the O&M specialist to the student. This process, as illustrated here with the introduction of the human guide techniques, is repeated as each new mobility technique and travel environment are introduced and, therefore, should be assumed to be utilized throughout the remainder of this chapter without being reiterated in detail.

Long-Cane Techniques

Negotiating the Environment

In travel with a human guide, the guide assumes responsibility for negotiating the environment by establishing a path of travel and avoiding obstacles and surface changes that would interfere with travel. In doing so, the guide ensures the traveler's safety. To progress to independent travel, the student must gain the skills and techniques necessary to take over these functions. The long cane, when used with the appropriate techniques, provides the traveler with the levels of preview necessary to make this possible. The long cane serves to extend the traveler's sense of touch from her finger on the grip through the shaft to the tip, providing the traveler with the opportunity to tactually preview both objects (object preview) in the path of travel and the surface (surface preview) on which she is about to step. The cane, therefore, may be used to identify changes in texture or density of surfaces (see the section on Identifying Surfaces and Materials in Volume 1, Chapter 1), changes in level of the surface plane (see the section on Changes in Elevation: Drop-Offs and Ramps in Volume 1, Chapter 1), and the presence of objects in the path of travel. Therefore, the long cane may be used to acquire the minimal levels of preview necessary for safe, independent travel, depending on the demands of the environment and the technique used (Blasch, LaGrow, & De l'Aune, 1996). The correct technique for use of the cane is fundamental to negotiating the environment for individuals who are blind or visually impaired. See Sidebar 1.1, "Basic Cane Techniques" for basic principles of using a cane properly.

Basic Cane Techniques

THE STANDARD GRIP

The hand is held in much the same way it is when one offers it to shake hands. The index finger is extended and the thumb is up. The grip of the cane is placed along the palm of the hand and the index finger. The index finger is parallel to the cane grip, pointing down the shaft; the remaining fingers are then wrapped around the grip; and the thumb is brought down next to the index finger and placed on top and to the side of the grip.

PROCEDURE: THE DIAGONAL TECHNIQUE USING THE STANDARD GRIP

1. The cane is held using the standard grip. The hand is positioned along the shaft so that when held diagonally across the body, the cane will extend about an inch beyond the body on both sides.

2. The hand is held forward and just to the outside of the hip.

3. The arm is flexed at the shoulder until the hand is approximately at waist height and forward of the body by 10 to 12 inches (25 to 30 cm).

4. The forearm is inwardly rotated until the palm of the hand is facing down.

5. The shaft of the cane is positioned diagonally across the body from the hand grasping the cane to the tip.

6. The tip is positioned forward of the grip and approximately 1 inch (2.5 cm) beyond the outside of the shoulder.

7. The tip of the cane may be raised just above the floor to avoid sticking in carpets or cracks, or kept in contact with the floor and slid along the surface.

8. The cane may be held in either hand depending on the preference of the traveler and expected placement of objects in the path of travel.

PROCEDURE: THE TOUCH TECHNIQUE

1. The cane is held in the standard grip. The top of the cane's grip should come to rest at the top of the palm.

2. The arm is flexed at the shoulder until the hand is at waist height. The arm is fully extended in a firm position, and the elbow is flexed slightly; the upper arm may rest against the body.

3. The hand is positioned at the center of the body.

4. The wrist is outwardly rotated so that the prominent bones at the base of the thumb face upward and the back of the hand faces the side.

5. The cane is moved from side to side by the flexion, extension, and hyperextension of the wrist. This movement describes an arc with the tip, which touches the floor approximately 1 inch (2.5 cm) outside the widest part of the body (that is, the shoulder or hips). The tip is raised slightly as the cane moves from one extreme to the next, touching the floor only at the end of each arc.

6. The cane movement is synchronized with the feet, resulting in an alternating foot-cane pattern. As a result, the cane strikes the floor in front of the foot that is back.

PROCEDURE: THE CONSTANT-CONTACT TECHNIQUE

The constant-contact technique is a variation of the touch technique. The procedures are the same except that the cane is not lifted from the ground at any point within its arc.

Techniques.   The length of the cane and the way it is held and manipulated have an impact on the degree to which the cane's functions are fulfilled. The length of the cane is dictated by the surface preview function and is therefore dependent on the traveler's height, the length of the traveler's stride, and the position of the hand in which the cane is held (LaGrow, Blasch, & De l'Aune, 1997). The technique used dictates the area and amount of surface previewed. The diagonal cane technique, for example, provides preview for only one side of the body, while the touch and constant-contact techniques preview both sides equally. As a result, the use of the diagonal cane technique is limited to controlled, familiar environments, while the touch and constant-contact techniques provide sufficient preview to be of use in uncontrolled and unfamiliar environments as well.

As with the basic human guide technique, the manner in which the cane is held and moved is designed to limit the hand's and arm's degrees of freedom of movement and therefore reduce perceptual error in interpreting information (Guth & Rieser, 1997). When the long cane is used as prescribed, the index finger points directly down the shaft and at the tip and the hand holding the cane is maintained in a constant position, which in the case of the touch and constant-contact techniques corresponds with the midline in both the sagittal and transverse planes of the body (See Volume 1, Chapter 5). With the latter two techniques, movement of the cane is directed by the wrist, and therefore the positions of the tip and shaft are always related to the degree of extension or hyperextension of the wrist and to the constant arm position of the hand holding the cane. In other words, the finger always points at the point of contact and is directed from the middle of the body and corresponds to the way the wrist is turned. If the long cane is used as prescribed, the information gained from the cane's tip and shaft and con-veyed up the shaft to the hand can be easily translated in relation to the position of the hand and thus to the various planes of the body. In the case of the touch and constant-contact techniques, this is directly related to the midline of both the sagittal and transverse planes. If, however, the hand and arm position is allowed to vary, then increased error in that interpretation is likely. The more consistent and precise the technique used, therefore, the better able the traveler is to interpret the information (see the section on Perceiving with a Long Cane in Volume 1, Chapter 1).

Changes in surfaces.   A change in surface texture or density may be picked up by the cane tip and transmitted up the shaft to the hand (see the section on Identifying Surfaces and Materials in Volume 1, Chapter 1). This may be accompanied by a corresponding change in sound. As a result, a light tapping of the cane may be useful when attempting to identify the point at which the change occurs. The greater the change, obviously, the more apparent it is. Sliding the cane tip along the surface to identify textural changes or to detect an edge formed by two surface structures meeting may be very effective. The diagonal and constant-contact techniques naturally do just this and therefore offer some advantage for identifying changes in surface texture over that afforded by the touch technique. The touch-and-slide technique, a variation of the touch technique (see LaGrow & Weessies, 1994), may be used to overcome that limitation when a change in surface texture or level is anticipated. Exploring the surface to identify the point at which a change in texture or density occurs is most efficient if done while maintaining the grip and hand position prescribed for the technique used, as this allows the information to be more accurately translated in relation to body plane than would be the case if the manner in which the search is conducted is less structured.

Drop-offs. Drop-offs are generally identified by the failure of the cane tip to contact the surface at the end of the arc when the tip is brought down to strike the surface while using the touch technique or by having the cane tip drop in level when using the diagonal or constant-contact technique (see the section on Changes in Elevation: Drop-Offs and Ramps in Volume 1, Chapter 1). Thus, a drop-off is recognized as a variation in the position of the wrist as the cane dips in response to a lowering of the surface plane. Reliable recognition of this change has everything to do with the consistency with which the cane is held and the constancy with which it is touched to or held in contact with the surface. Recognition of a drop-off can therefore be very subtle and may be indicated by a small change in the position of the wrist. Obviously, a sloppy, heavy touch or a banging movement of the cane will not facilitate this recognition. Rather, a controlled placement of the tip or light contact with the surface as the cane is pushed forward is most effective. Movement in the wrist or arm will almost certainly reduce one's ability to recognize these changes, especially those that are slight. Recognition of an up curb, or step up in height, is less subtle and is contacted by the cane as though it is an object in the path of travel. In other words, the cane will strike and be stopped by the curb. In all cases, however, consistency of cane use and constancy in the manner in which the cane is held will enhance the traveler's ability to detect changes in the surface or objects in the path.

Reacting to Objects and Drop-offs in the Path of Travel

Determining the location of objects in the path of travel. In the early stages of learning these techniques, the traveler will generally be taught to stop and hold position when any object or change in surface plane has been encountered in the path of travel. This will allow the student the

opportunity to determine the location of that object relative to his body while ensuring that no changes in body position are made in relation to it. This helps reduce localization errors, which may occur if the relative position between the student and the object is altered (see the section on Localization Errors in Volume 1, Chapter 1). In other words, if the student moves before determining the position of the object encountered in the path, then the basis for making that determination would be altered from that when the object was first encountered. Thus, it would be difficult to establish the actual location of the object in relation to the traveler's body plane and line of travel as it was when the object was contacted. It may also be potentially difficult to reestablish the line of travel after contacting the object if movement has occurred, as one of the only indications of the line of travel may be in relation to the traveler's body plane as it was when contact was made. Practically, this means holding the feet in place when travel is interrupted. In this way, the traveler can reestablish the line of travel by realigning body parts and frontal plane to the feet and projecting a straight line of travel off of that plane (see the section on Engaging in Purposeful and Directed Movement later in this chapter). If the object is found to be to the side of the projected path of travel, the traveler may simply keep it to the side and continue traveling. This will be apparent from the position of the wrist as the hand is held in place and the finger points down the shaft to the point of contact, as described earlier. However, if the object is directly in the path of travel, the traveler will have to explore it, determining its dimensions and function to determine how best to deal with it.

Exploring the object. If the traveler wishes to explore the object contacted, it could be done while holding the feet steady, taking care not to turn the feet toward to the point of contact, and thus maintaining a steady focal point to which spatial alignment can be reestablished. To do this, the traveler holds the cane firmly against the object at the point of contact, changes the grip on the cane from a standard grip to a pencil grip (that is, holding the cane so that the grip is held between the finger and thumb as with a pencil), brings the cane to a vertical position, and pushes it forward from the grip to determine the relative height of the object. Held vertically and moved horizontally, the cane can be used to determine the width of the object (see the section on Perceiving the Dimensions of Obstacles and Openings in Volume 1, Chapter 1). The traveler may then conduct further exploration using the hand or even a foot to get a complete picture of the object. In most cases, however, the traveler simply notes the object contacted, seeks and finds a clear space of travel to one side of the object, and continues to move through the environment to the destination. With time and practice, this usually becomes a fluid action followed by a brief pause to allow the traveler to preview the area with a sweep of the cane to locate a clear path of travel. The habit of holding one's position while completing this process is critical to maintaining good orientation.

Determining the location of drop-offs in the path of travel. If the traveler detects a change in surface level, the traveler stops and determines its location (in the path of travel or to the side), as is done with an object in the path of travel. As before, the traveler's finger points down the shaft to the tip. The location of the tip corresponds to the change in surface plane and is therefore related to the traveler's frontal plane through the position of the hand holding the cane (see the section on Changes in Elevation: Drop-Offs and Ramps in Volume 1, Chapter 1). A surface change detected while using the diagonal cane technique is related to the hip opposite the point of contact, as that is where the hand holding the cane is located; however, with the touch and constant-contact techniques, it is located relative to the

midline, as determined by the extension or hyperextension of the wrist.

Exploring the drop-off. If the surface change is in the student's path of travel and therefore is to be traversed, the cane tip is either anchored at the riser (up step) or pulled back against the edge of the drop-off (down step). The grip is changed to a pencil grip, and the cane is brought to vertical and moved to midline. The traveler steps up to the cane so that the toes are to either side of the shaft and therefore positioned at the edge of the step or riser. The traveler may then explore the edge with the cane to establish alignment with it (perpendicular or at an angle). To do this, the cane is held vertically and moved along the edge of the step or drop-off out to arm's length or to the nearest wall on both sides of the body. The cane is changed from hand to hand when passing midline. This process may also be used to establish the traveler's position relative to the nearest handrail and to adjust alignment to the step or stairs to be traversed by squaring the frontal plane off to the arms as they are extended from side to side or adjusting the feet so that the edge of the drop-off is aligned through the soles of the feet (see the section on Engaging in Purposeful and Directed Movement later in this chapter).

If the change in surface plane is found to be a set of stairs, the height of the step and the depth of the tread may be determined through active exploration with the cane tip. For ascending stairs, this is done by lifting the cane vertically along the riser until the tip is no longer in contact with it (determining height) and then moving the cane forward while keeping the shaft vertical until the next riser is contacted (determining tread depth). This same procedure may be followed for descending stairs, except that the tip is lowered vertically along the edge of the riser until the first step is encountered and then out to the edge of that step. In doing this, the traveler may determine whether there is a single step or a series of steps to be traversed, the stair height, and the tread depth. Ensuring that the shaft remains vertical during exploration is necessary to gain an accurate estimation of height and depth. As with all perception gained through motor activity, repetition and precision of movement is required to reliably gain accurate, meaningful information. Having the student do this once will not be sufficient to ensure that accurate information will be gained on subsequent occasions.

Ascending and Descending Stairs

The technique for ascending and descending stairs is a logical extension of the techniques involved in identifying and exploring changes in surface level and step height and tread depth, and is similar to that used with the human guide inasmuch as it focuses on the identification of the first and last steps in the series. With the cane, this is done tactilely and is dependent on the position of the hand and arm and the corresponding location of the tip. The technique is the same regardless of the technique used to locate the stairs (that is, diagonal, touch, or constant-contact technique). When ascending stairs, the hand is moved down the cane onto the shaft, and the tip is held up and forward in such a way that it lightly touches the facing at the edge of the step one or two stairs ahead of the traveler, depending on preference (see Hill & Ponder, 1976, or LaGrow & Weessies, 1994, for a complete description of this procedure). The traveler will be aware that the top has been reached when the cane swings clear at the last step. When descending the stairs, the grip is extended down and out so that the tip is free of and just below the next step or two as the traveler proceeds down the stairs in such a way that the tip will not make contact until the traveler is on the last or next to last step (depending on preference), indicating that the landing has been reached.

Engaging in Purposeful and Directed Movement

Cane techniques are generally introduced in indoor environments, as the vertical planes of the walls keep the student traveler from wandering off the path of travel, as happens on sidewalks and driveways, increasing the opportunity to maintain a straight line of travel and decreasing the risk of becoming too disoriented early in the instructional stage. As with the human guide techniques, the instructional sequence used to introduce the various cane techniques usually begins in a relatively wide, uncluttered hallway. The student is introduced to the cane and the manner in which it is to be held and manipulated, then asked to travel to a specified destination while using the cane to preview the environment. Initially, the student may be asked only to go from one side of a hallway to another, as it is difficult to maintain a straight line of travel for more than a short distance at first. When this task is successfully accomplished, the destination of travel is moved to one end of the hallway. The student is instructed to travel to it and stop when the far wall is reached. The wall itself is used as a destination, as a way of providing the traveler with a tactile indication that the destination has been reached, an opportunity to make planned cane contact with an object in the path of travel, and the chance to continue to develop kinesthetic awareness of the length of the hallways while traveling independently. This process is facilitated by using the same travel environment as that used for teaching the human guide techniques. In this way, environmental and episodic knowledge gained first in learning the human guide techniques, then with the diagonal cane technique, and finally with the touch or constant-contact technique can be continually expanded and reinforced. It also allows the student to concentrate on learning the mechanics of each new technique in relatively familiar and comfortable surroundings.

Walking a Straight Line.   However, this is all dependent on the student being able to maintain a degree of continuity in movement (that is, not continually stopping, readjusting the line of travel, and starting over) while traveling from one point to the next. When the student first begins to travel independently with the long cane, the O&M specialist will generally walk backward in front of traveler, talking to the traveler and commenting on the hand and cane positions. This is done both to give feedback on how the cane is being used and to provide a sound beacon for the student to follow, keeping the student away from the walls and headed down the middle of the hallway. As skill is gained with straight-line travel, these auditory clues are replaced with naturally occurring sound clues (that is, the ambient sound clues that indicate that one is coming close to the wall; see Volume 1, Chapter 2) and tactile clues received if and when the tip strikes the wall. The former is actively taught by the O&M specialist by systematically fading instructor-generated sound clues (talking and comments) and reinforcing each appropriate response to ambient ones. The latter occurs naturally as the student moves down a hallway while using the long cane as a mobility device.

Finding a perpendicular line.   Being able to walk a straight line is largely dependent on establishing the line to be walked in the first place. This is generally done through either perpendicular or parallel alignment with naturally occurring lines in the environment. The object of perpendicular alignment is for the traveler to align his frontal plane with a surface plane perpendicular to the line of intended travel. For example, a student may be asked to travel across a hallway from one door to another directly opposite. The student may initially establish a line for doing so by placing his back against one of the doors in an attempt to align the body with the door so that his frontal plane is aligned with (parallel to) the surface plane of the door. A line projected from

the traveler's frontal plane would then be perpendicular to the surface used for alignment. With perpendicular alignment, the student is taught first to get the back and shoulders flush with the surface, then to bring the head, hips, and feet in line with the trunk. This action relies on proprioceptive awareness and as such takes practice and feedback to be done accurately and skillfully. Once alignment is gained, the student is instructed to mentally project a line from his frontal plane into space and imagine it culminating at the door opposite. The student then travels to the destination and, once at the opposite wall, checks the accuracy of movement in relation to the object reached (that is, tactually investigates the destination to determine whether the student is directly in line with or to either side of the door). This may be done with the cane tip in the same fashion as described for exploring objects in the path of travel or changes in surface plane. This process is repeated using the same starting point and destination a number of times to build the skill and establish relationships of one object to another across open space. With time the distance between targets is increased and the applications made more diverse. At the same time, kinesthetic awareness of the distance traveled is established, allowing the student to adjust his pace and posture to make the encounter with the destination less abrupt and more graceful.

Establishing a line of travel.   A perpendicular line may be acquired from a variety of surfaces, including walls, doors, open doorways, surface change (for example, drop-offs) and even from one's frontal plane relative to a line already traveled. To establish a line in an open doorway, the traveler places the backs of the hands against the door frame on either side of the body and moves the upper body until the frontal plane is aligned between the hands. The head and feet are then moved to align with the frontal plane. With a surface change (for example, a step or edge of a carpet), the traveler may move the feet about on the edge or leading point of the surface change until it feels like the break in the surface runs through the balls of both feet perpendicular to the line of direction; alternatively, the traveler may move the cane vertically along the edge of the step or carpet from midline out to full extension of the arm on each side, as described earlier. The rest of the body is then brought into line with the feet or arms by aligning the knees, the waist, the upper body and then the head with one another. Likewise, the traveler may project a line off of his own frontal plane by using the line already traveled (for example, when moving along the length of a hallway from one intersection to the next) to establish the next line of movement. This needs to be done each time a person is interrupted in travel and must stop. The traveler may then simply hold the line that had been traveled (usually by maintaining the position of the feet) until ready to resume travel. Then, before heading off, the traveler may reestablish alignment by bringing the knees, waist, upper body, and head back into line with the feet, and then project a line off of the body plane to move forward. This may also be done after executing a facing movement of 90 degrees right or left of the line previously traveled, as done when turning into an intersecting hallway. To do this, the traveler must stop, hold position, and then execute an accurate 90-degree turn. A small variation in the execution of this move may result in a large misalignment with the destination, depending on the distance to be traveled without other feedback. As a result, care and precision in maintaining one's alignment and making facing movements ought to be established as being basic to good travel skills. Proper alignment and technique depend on being given the time, experience, and feedback necessary to learn to monitor the alignment and relationship of body parts and planes proprioceptively and the execution of facing movements kinesthetically.

Trailing.   The traveler may establish a line of travel from objects or lines parallel to the path of travel as well. This is done initially with the walls of a hallway and may be accomplished when stationary by placing the cane tip and shoulder or hip against the wall while mentally drawing a line from the shoulder or hip to the point of contact with the cane tip and projecting that line forward. When the traveler is doing this, the hand holding the cane needs to be maintained in the prescribed position in order to give the student an accurate perception of this line. This may also be accomplished while walking by having the student trail the wall for a short distance with the cane tip. As this is done, a straight line may be established as being parallel to the wall trailed and consistent to the one walked. Once this line is established, the student may take a small lateral step away from the surface trailed and continue on.

Trailing is a basic mobility technique that requires the traveler to maintain continual contact with and a constant distance from the line to be followed. Continual contact in the case of the touch or constant-contact technique is, in fact, planned intermittent contact, with the tip striking the line trailed each time it is swept to that side. Continual contact is required to ensure the traveler can (1) maintain a line of travel parallel to that being followed, (2) stay with a line even if it is not straight, and (3) locate destinations along the line in the form of openings (for example, third open door from the corner) or changes in texture, density, or sound (for example, closed doors). Thus, each time contact is broken with the surface, the traveler must immediately check to verify whether the line has ended. If the traveler finds that the line has not ended but rather that the distance between the line and the traveler has changed (the traveler has drifted from the line or the line has diverted away from that being traveled), then the traveler's position needs to be adjusted to reestablish the distance and contact with the line. Both of these requirements (maintaining continual contact with and constant distance from the line trailed) are met by keeping the hand locked in place, keeping the technique used for reaching the surface uniform, and continually adjusting the distance between the self and the trailing surface as necessary. By keeping the hand centered and the technique uniform, the degrees of freedom of movement are restricted and therefore the opportunity for both mechanical (allowing the arm and hand to drift toward the surface trailed) and perceptual error is limited.

When the traveler is trailing a surface, the width of the arc is extended just slightly to the side of the trailing surface only. The amount of this extension should be no more than that needed to keep the body from brushing the trailing surface. Students have a tendency to extend the arc and allow the hand to drift toward the trailing surface while trying to maintain contact with it. This is particularly true when the trailing surface is on the same side as the hand holding the cane while using the touch or constant-contact technique. However, maintaining the position of the hand at midline and keeping the width of the arc uniform is necessary to ensure that the line traveled is indeed parallel to the line trailed. Adjustment of the traveler's positions as opposed to the reach of the cane is necessary to the accuracy and success of this technique.

Establishing parallel and perpendicular alignment. Physically establishing parallel and perpendicular alignment is a fairly simple task. However, the confidence one has in one's ability to establish a line and project it into the environment for travel purposes is dependent on the success experienced in doing so over time (Pereira, 1990). In other words, the traveler establishes a hypothesis concerning the position of one object or plane to another (for example, the door to the stairs), and then tests the validity of that hypothesis through travel. The more often this is

done with success, the more likely the traveler will have confidence in her ability to establish a line and use it. Likewise, the more often this is done accurately, the more likely the traveler will be able to establish precise relationships among objects in the environment. This, of course, is dependent on three things: (1) knowledge of the relationships of objects or environmental features across open space, (2) the ability to establish a line of travel using either perpendicular or parallel alignment techniques, and (3) the ability to move effectively from one place to another by walking a straight line (see Volume 1, Chapter 2).

Interpreting sensory clues, information points, and landmarks. As in the human guide techniques, the travel environment is systematically expanded, sensory clues, information points, and landmarks are pointed out as instruction proceeds, and new skills for independent travel are introduced. Again, this is done under the control of the O&M specialist and facilitated by sending the student to specific destinations and along given routes. However, the responsibility for physically locating the destination is now left to the student. This may be done initially by simply traveling from one end of the hallway to the next, but in order to expand the environment and introduce more complex routes of travel (L-, Z-, U-, and square-shaped routes), more specific destinations are required. These usually are indicated by room number or as a particular door (first, second, or third) from a given corner. To find the destination, the student travels to the intersection, finds the specified corner, and trails to the destination for that run. When doing this, the student is instructed to go to the actual corner of the intersection before beginning to trail to the destination to ensure that no door has been missed in the process.

Locating intersections. Locating the intersecting corner is easily done while trailing. However, trailing is a selective skill, and its use is not encouraged as a primary means of travel, as it results in unnecessary contact with objects in the environment (open doors, hallway furniture, drinking fountains, fire hoses, and so on). Thus, the student is encouraged to travel down the center of the hallway or other path of travel and identify the location of intersecting hallways by other means. This is usually done by combining kinesthetic knowledge of the length of the hallway and the distance traveled with auditory recognition of the presence of an intersection, if no visual information is available to the student. The skill required for the latter is rather subtle and may best be introduced by guiding the student along the hallway and past the intersection while explaining the task at hand (see Chapter 4 and Volume 1, Chapter 4). The human guide techniques are particularly useful for introducing this skill, as the guide can control the distance the student is from the wall and eliminate any contact with it as the intersection is approached. Initially, it helps to be close to the wall, making the difference in sound experienced between walking along a wall and walking past an opening (the intersecting hallway) more distinct (see Chapter 4). The student is initially encouraged to indicate the presence of the intersecting hallway as it is encountered. At first, the student is likely to pass the opening before indicating that it has been encountered. The change in sound is very subtle, and this auditory skill is not normally required of people with vision. Thus, students are generally unsure of just what clues they are looking for or which sounds may indicate that the intersecting hallway has been reached. The instructor provides this information by giving the traveler feedback about the timing of the indication. Initially the student's recognition is often a bit late, that is, a pace or two past the corner, but with subsequent runs it seems that students begin to identify it early, a pace or two before the intersection; this may be due to heightened anticipation and awareness of

lower-frequency sounds that tend to drift around corners. With feedback from the instructor, most students with unimpaired hearing will learn to accurately identify intersecting hallways just as they reach them and even be able to recognize the presence of open or recessed doorways when traveling reasonably close to the wall. As the student gains confidence in recognizing this rather subtle difference, the guide can move the student farther from the wall, making the challenge greater. The student may then be asked to recognize this change while traveling independently with the long cane. It may be helpful at first to isolate this skill, have the student approach the intersection from varying distances until success is achieved, and then incorporate this skill into the travel repertoire. The additional auditory output provided by the tip making contact with the surface of travel (more marked with the touch technique than with the diagonal or constant-contact technique) may be of assistance in this task.

As instruction continues indoors, the O&M specialist continues to expand the environment by having the student travel to more challenging destinations on multiple floors while keeping track of her orientation and planning routes of travel. This pattern continues until the student has gained the perceptual skills and self-confidence required to venture into uncontrolled, outdoor environments.

OUTDOOR ENVIRONMENTS

At this point, nearly all the mobility, orientation, and perceptual skills and techniques needed for independent travel have been introduced. However, outdoor environments of varying complexity pose a unique set of challenges and require some new applications of the skills and techniques learned. Maintaining a straight line of travel, for example, is particularly difficult when traversing open areas. In fact, it appears that veering (deviating from one's intended line of travel) is almost unavoidable in environments where there are no immediately recognizable guidelines to travel along or targets to walk to (Guth, 2008).

Maintaining a Line of Travel

Residential Environments

Cane-tip sticking. Instruction in the residential environment initially begins with straight-line travel, usually from one intersection to the next. However, dealing with the cane tip's sticking in the uneven surface of a sidewalk and simply staying on the footpath while walking down the street may pose problems for the student as the transition is made from indoor to outdoor travel. This is especially true when using the touch technique. As the cane tip comes into contact with the rougher, uneven surface of a sidewalk or the grass edge on either side of it, it tends to stick and break the continuity of travel. At first, the traveler will generally stop and dislodge the cane before continuing on. With time the student should be able to deal with the tendency of the tip to stick in rougher surfaces while maintaining continuous forward movement. This outcome may be facilitated by the use of a light, flexible grip and the development of confidence in the interpretation of the tactile, auditory, and proprioceptive information conveyed by the cane tip. Maintaining the integrity of the technique in terms of hand position, wrist movement, and arc width is particularly important as the demands for accurate perception for successful travel is greater in outdoor environments than in indoor spaces.

Staying on the path of travel. Staying on the path of travel and maintaining a straight line may prove to be more of a challenge, however, as the width of a sidewalk in a residential area is generally narrow and often delineated by no more than a grass border on either side. As a re-

sult, there is no vertical barrier like the walls in an indoor environment to stop the traveler from stepping off the path of travel. The student must therefore learn to stay on the sidewalk by attending to the texture and density of the surface and the feedback provided both tactilely and auditorily by the tip of the cane striking the surface. However, the traveler must also learn to respond to the sensory input from the cane tip and that received through the feet separately, as they may provide different information. For example, it is possible to walk on the sidewalk yet contact the grass verge as the tip strikes the surface just beyond the widest point of the body, as it is designed to do. Doing so simply indicates that the traveler is on the sidewalk and near the edge and, as a result, need not stop or adjust the line of travel. However, it takes some experience to treat this contact as an indication of one's relative position on the sidewalk rather than as an error. Precision in the use of the technique is helpful in developing an accurate perception of one's position in relation to the clues gleaned from the cane. If the traveler's hand moves and the arc is variable, then there can be little confidence in perceiving one's relative distance from the surface contacted.

It also helps if the difference between the surfaces is marked so there is little ambiguity in the information provided. However, in some situations this is simply not the case. A modified touch-and-slide technique (see Hill & Ponder, 1976, or LaGrow & Weessies, 1994, for a complete description of this technique) may be of use in locating the edge of the sidewalk if the difference between the sidewalk and the grass line is not great (for example, if the grass is short or the area next to the sidewalk is hard-packed dirt).

A student who is repeatedly contacting the grass verge with the cane tip while traveling along the sidewalk may be encouraged to take advantage of this situation and purposely trail the grass line for a short distance to establish a parallel line for travel. It is also possible, of course, to establish and project a parallel line while stationary, as described earlier. In both cases, the traveler ought to take a small step to the side once a line of travel has been established to break contact with the grass line. Learning to maintain a straight line of travel, and therefore avoiding having to stop to reestablish alignment, is essential for developing continuity in travel, which in turn is necessary to establish kinesthetic awareness of the distances traveled. Trailing is not encouraged for traveling any longer than necessary (that is, to establish a line, maintain contact with a curving line, or find specific destinations), as it results in excessive and unnecessary contact with obstacles to the side of one's actual path of travel.

Recovering from a veer. Students may veer up a driveway or walk off the sidewalk onto the grass without immediately recognizing the change in texture or sound. When this happens, the traveler will end up on the grass or at a point where the surface changes so that the traveler is standing on the surface of the driveway with a grass line directly in front of him. The student is taught to respond to this situation by stopping and holding his feet steady as he attempts to locate the sidewalk by checking in front and to both sides. If the student finds the sidewalk during this checking process, the student simply steps onto it and continues to travel to the destination. As a general strategy to reestablish orientation if the student does not locate the sidewalk, the student is taught to turn and walk toward the parallel street while looking for the intersecting sidewalk. Thus, it is important to anchor the feet while searching for the sidewalk to ensure that the original line of travel is maintained so that it may be used as a reference when turning to walk to the street. If the sidewalk is located on the way to the parallel street, the student is to turn and continue to the destination. However, if the student gets to the street without locating the sidewalk, the student is taught to

make a 180-degree turn and come back to look for the sidewalk. If this return occurs along a driveway, then the edge of the driveway is trailed while carrying out this recovery procedure (that is, turning and walking to the street, and turning 180 degrees and searching for the sidewalk if the street is found before the sidewalk). Generally, a driveway slopes to the street from the street side of the sidewalk. Thus, it is often possible for the traveler to tell which side of the sidewalk he is on (that is, toward or away from the parallel street) based on the presence or absence of a tilt or incline. Likewise, if crossing a driveway on the street side, the student may be aware of it due to its lateral tilt and may use the tilt to maintain a straight line of travel, keeping the direction of the tilt steady across his feet.

Maintaining orientation. The O&M specialist may aid this process by ensuring that the student is aware of the side of the street being traveled on before leaving for the destination by asking the student to point out the street and indicate whether it is to the right or left. Although this may seem simplistic, it is not uncommon for the student to be so involved in trying to establish the skills necessary for independent travel that he or she simply has not consciously noted this detail. Similarly, the student ought to be encouraged to be aware of the presence of traffic and to listen for it as an indication of the location of the parallel street, an indication of the location of an upcoming perpendicular street, and a general means of updating his progress and maintaining orientation while progressing down the street and making decisions about recovery if required.

Business Environments

Sidewalks in business environments are generally wider than those in residential environments. They often extend from the building line to the curb and have no grass verge to contain the traveler. As such, they pose their own unique problem for maintaining a line when first encountered. In many cases, however, the portion of the sidewalk closest to the street tilts to the curb and therefore provides some indication of the street side of the footpath. As with crossing driveways, the traveler may maintain the line of travel by keeping position on the slope steady when walking along it or by stepping away from it when encountered. It may be possible to follow a line in the texture of the sidewalk formed at the point that the sidewalk tilts toward the street if using the constant-contact technique or a modified touch-and-slide or touch-and-drag technique (the tip of the cane is kept in contact with the surface as it is dragged from one point of contact to a drop-off on the opposite side). Monitoring traffic sounds and maintaining one's distance from the traffic are also helpful in this situation. The traveler may use this information to maintain a straight line or reestablish one if necessary. Building lines may also be followed by maintaining auditory contact with them using ambient sound or the sound reflected from the tap of the cane off the building or from traffic on the parallel street. As a last resort, the building line may be trailed with a cane.

In many business environments, the traveler must maintain a line of travel somewhere near the middle of the sidewalk to avoid parking meters, street furniture, and signs on the street side, and store signs and café tables and chairs on the building side. This is often facilitated by following a rule that states that all objects contacted on the left of the body should remain on the left side and those contacted on the right should remain there. Careful attention to body position when contacting these objects and maintaining precise cane technique are necessary for successful perception of the location of objects when using this technique. As with residential travel, it is important to ensure that arc width is uniform and no wider than prescribed to ensure accurate perception and

avoid contact with objects that are not actually in the line of travel.

The student must also maintain a line of travel when walking L-, Z-, U-, or square-shaped routes. To do so, the student may be required to turn and walk along an intersecting street before or after crossing it. In residential environments, it may be possible to trail the grass line between the street and the intersecting footpath when making a change in direction and, in doing so, establish a new line of travel. However, in business environments, it is more likely that the traveler will have to rely on accurate facing movements (either after the building line or at or after the intersection) to establish the new line to be traveled. In doing so, maintaining the original line of travel is essential, as the accuracy of the line established is based on both the quality of the original line and the accuracy of each subsequent move (that is, either a 90-degree turn when turning up an intersecting street after crossing it or a 180-degree turn followed by a 90-degree turn when turning up an intersecting street if not crossing it). Thus, the student must be careful to hold the line traveled to reach the intersection before making subsequent moves and to execute those with care.

Shopping Malls

The strategy used for maintaining a line of travel in an indoor shopping mall is similar to that used in business environments; however, there is no parallel traffic to rely on, and the storefronts are generally open so that ambient or reflected sounds from a building line are not available. Thus, in this case, the traveler tends to try to stay along one side of the mall during travel and to maintain a degree of contact with displays and other objects along storefronts. If a turn is required, it is usually executed after an intersecting hallway is identified. Once again, it depends on the quality of the line traveled and the accuracy of the facing movement used. Strategies for maintaining a line of travel in the aisles of grocery stores and department stores do not differ greatly from those used when traveling along hallways in indoor environments.

Initial lessons in each area usually start with walking a straight line from one end of the block to the next. This is done to allow the traveler to learn to maintain a line of travel in light of the challenges presented, learn or incorporate recovery techniques, gain an understanding of the distances to be traveled kinesthetically, and get used to the types of sensory clues that may be relied on for maintaining orientation. Subsequent lessons are designed to expand the travel environment by traveling to and locating specific destinations.

Locating Specific Destinations

As in indoor environments, the O&M specialist designates the destination for travel for each run and uses these destinations and the path used to reach them to control the level of the demand posed by the travel environment (sending the student to specific places and avoiding others). Intersections (reached by traveling from one end of the block to the next) are typically used as the first destinations in residential environments, followed by specific houses as designated by the sidewalk or driveway leading up to them. To find the destination, the student needs to travel to the nearest corner and trail the grass line away from the parallel street to locate the designated sidewalk or driveway (for example, second or third from the corner) leading up to the house. Sidewalks leading to houses are not evenly spaced and are often so narrow that they may be contacted only once within a stride. Therefore, the technique must be precise, continual contact maintained, and any change in or loss of contact with the grass line checked immediately.

As instruction moves on to semibusiness and business environments, destinations may more likely be shops or entrances found along building lines. These may be located near a corner, close to a break in the building line, or before or after street furniture or other features in an environment that may be distinctive. Destinations are generally identified as the number of doorways or openings from these distinctive environmental features. In addition, information points are usually provided to verify the location of the destination (that is, the bookshop is the second door on this side of the alley and has a table of books on either side of its entrance; a bakery always gives the fresh smell of baked goods during the day; a playground exhibits sounds of children).

Locating and Crossing Streets

In order to travel in outdoor environments and expand travel environments beyond the initial block used for introducing travel in outdoor environments, students must learn to cross streets. To do this, the student must first locate them.

Locating Intersections

Locating the intersection in a quiet residential setting is generally dependent on recognizing a slight downward movement (drop) in the wrist as an indication (proprioceptive awareness) of a change of surface plane at the curb as the cane tip drops from the surface of the sidewalk to the lower surface of the street. Although this is getting more difficult due to the presence of curb ramps to allow for wheelchair and stroller access, it is assisted by both kinesthetic awareness of the length of the block and a decline in the surface of the sidewalk (through proprioceptive awareness in the ankles), which often occurs prior to the curb or at the curb ramp. Thus, the traveler is able to anticipate and react to the drop-off at the intersection. Tactile clues may be present as well, while auditory information is likely to be available in busier environments, where both automobile and pedestrian traffic may alert the traveler to the presence of the intersections. Likewise, in business environments, the end of the building line prior to the intersection often results in a change of sound, temperature, light, and breeze, all of which may alert the traveler to the fact that she is approaching an intersection. Once the intersection has been located, the student may sweep the surface ahead to confirm that she is indeed at a curb. The cane tip may be moved 90 degrees or more to each side to ensure that the student is in fact standing at a curb.

Crossing the Intersection

Street crossings are initially taught in quiet residential environments; busier and more complex intersections are introduced as the student moves into semibusiness and business travel. Once the curb is located, the student establishes a line to cross the street using any number of methods (for example, parallel alignment with the grass line or parallel traffic, perpendicular alignment with the curb or off the body plane following a straight line of travel). In general, once a student establishes some consistency with straight-line travel in the block preceding the crossing, the method of choice is maintaining a line of direction with verification from parallel traffic sounds (see the section on Crossing Streets without Vision in Volume 1, Chapter 1). Establishing or verifying a parallel or perpendicular line auditorily is an extension of basic direction-taking skills and is introduced as soon as possible in outdoor travel (see Chapter 4). It is also possible to establish perpendicular alignment from traffic sounds by listening to traffic pass along a road in front of the traveler and identifying the position where the sound of traffic appears to move from one side of the face to the other or past the nose; this is aided by moving the head back and forth to sample the sound. However, sufficient traffic for this procedure is not usually present until the traveler has moved on to a busier environment.

The student is introduced to street crossings using human guide techniques initially to pro-

vide the student with a kinesthetic understanding of the width of the street to be crossed and to be introduced to the camber in the middle of the street. The camber is designed to allow rain to run off the street and presents itself proprioceptively to the crossing traveler as an initial incline, a leveling off, and an eventual decline. The camber provides the traveler with a means to monitor progress when crossing and to check whether the crossing is straight (that is, results in the expected pattern). The student is then encouraged to cross the street when there is no traffic coming from either direction. The O&M specialist initially verifies the decision for the student and gradually allows the timing of the crossing to become the student's alone. With time, the student will learn to time a crossing with passing parallel traffic if no traffic is present on the perpendicular street and the traffic on the parallel street is deemed to be moving too fast to turn into the perpendicular street. However, the traveler is usually limited to crossing busier perpendicular streets at controlled intersections.

Determining when to cross is dependent on both traffic flow and the system in place to control the traffic (see the section on Initiating the Crossing in Volume 1, Chapter 1). As before, the student will be introduced to crossing light-controlled intersections with a human guide. In this case the student and instructor will cross together a number of times to allow the student to get a good idea of the distance to cross, the feel of the camber, and the length of the light cycle. Initially the instructor will determine when to cross, then later will cross at the student's instruction. The student will then be asked to cross independently but with the instructor verifying the student's decision as to when to cross with the instructor intervening only if necessary. In following this pattern, the student will get used to crossing streets with the parallel traffic (1) going in the same direction as the traveler (2) in the lane closest, going the same way but with the traffic farther away, (3) going against and in the closest lane, and (4) going against farther away. Students will first be introduced to simple plus-shaped (+) intersections with traffic starting in response to the changing of the light and then to more complex intersections with turning lanes and other timed patterns (see Chapter 12). Crossing streets safely is dependent on the ability to interpret traffic patterns auditorily. For a complete discussion of traffic-control devices and decision-making practices, see Barlow, Bentzen, & Bond (2005); Barlow & Franck (2005); Long (2008); and Long, Guth, Ashmead, Wall Emerson, & Ponchillia (2005). For alternatives for crossing streets with no traffic controls, see Sauerburger (2005, 2006).

Veering

The student may veer into either the perpendicular or the parallel street when crossing intersections. Veers into the parallel street (that is, toward traffic) are usually recognized kinesthetically; travelers simply feel that they have traveled too far for a standard street crossing. They may also note that the expected incline, leveling off, and decline of the camber are replaced by a lateral tilt or a prolonged leveling of the surface traveled. In busier environments, they may notice that the traffic on the parallel street sounds too close. Veers into the perpendicular street (that is, away from traffic) become obvious when the sidewalk is not located over the curb or when parked traffic is encountered along the curb, and in busier environments, when cars stopped at the light are encountered.

The instructor needs to be aware of the direction of veers as they occur over time in order to know where to intervene. If the student is consistently veering in one direction regardless of the location of the parallel street, for example, it is probably due to a technical or perceptual problem (for example, the student may not be aligning the feet and trunk with the head or may not be shifting the center of gravity for-

ward before stepping out). However, if the veer is consistently away from or toward the parallel street regardless of the side that street is on, it is probably due to either a desire to avoid traffic or a misunderstanding of when and how to obtain alignment using parallel traffic sounds (that is, the student may not be listening to traffic long enough before deciding it is parallel). Students are often intimidated by busy streets when first encountering them. However, the traveler soon finds that a wealth of auditory information is provided by high traffic volume. Experienced travelers often plan their route of travel along busy streets, avoiding quiet ones. See Guth (2008) for a complete discussion of veering.

CONCLUSION

O&M skills and techniques are continuously built one upon the other as the instructional sequence moves from indoor to outdoor environments and the student progresses from walking with a guide to independent, self-directed travel. The techniques required for this transition are designed to provide accurate perception of motor and sensory information. This information, along with knowledge of the layout and structure of the travel environments, is necessary to establish meaningful and directed movement. The more care taken in the introduction to and the use of these various techniques, the more likely success will be achieved. The purpose of this chapter is to illustrate how this may be done while focusing on a number of explicit perceptual activities that substitute for vision and emphasizing the importance of precision in their use to improve perception in orientation and mobility. The O&M specialist not only is teaching mobility techniques and orientation procedures but is also teaching students with visual impairments how to use perceptual skills to understand the environment when vision is not available.

IMPLICATIONS FOR O&M PRACTICE

1. Limiting the degrees of freedom in movement of the limbs by adhering to the prescribed relationship between the upper arm and forearm and the use of the yoke grip in the basic human guide technique facilitates the clear transmission of information about the environment to the traveler from the guide's movements. Precise directed movement and good technique make it possible for proximal perception from the hand and elbow to be translated into distal information about the travel environment.

2. The combination of sensory information with knowledge of the environment provides the traveler with the information necessary to locate destinations, find intersecting paths of travel, and maintain orientation while traveling. However, unless a student has learned to attend to sensory information in some systematic manner, many of these clues may go unnoticed, or if they are noticed, their meaning may not be clear if the student does not have a frame of reference or context with which to interpret them.

3. The long cane serves to extend the traveler's sense of touch from the finger on the grip, through the shaft, to the tip, providing the traveler with the opportunity to tactually preview both objects (object preview) in the path of travel and the surface (surface preview) upon which she is about to step. The cane, therefore, may be used to identify changes in texture or density of surfaces, changes in level of the surface plane, and objects in the path of travel. As a result, the long cane may be used to acquire the minimal levels of preview necessary for safe, independent travel, depending on the demands of the environment and the technique used.

4. The technique used for ascending and descending stairs is a logical extension of the techniques involved in identifying and exploring changes in surface level, step height, and tread depth, and is similar to that used with the human guide inasmuch as it focuses on the identification of the first and last steps in the series. With the cane, this is done tactually and is dependent on the position of the hand and arm and the corresponding location of the tip.

5. Trailing is a basic mobility technique that requires the traveler to maintain continual contact with and a constant distance from the line to be followed. Continual contact in the case of the touch or constant-contact technique is, in fact, planned intermittent contact, with the tip striking the line trailed each time it is swept to that side. Continual contact is required to ensure the traveler can (1) maintain a line of travel parallel to that being followed, (2) stay with a line even if it is not straight, and (3) locate destinations along the line in the form of openings (for example, the third open door from the corner) or changes in texture, density, or sound (for example, closed doors).

6. Maintaining the integrity of the technique in terms of hand position, wrist movement, and arc width is particularly important as the demands for accurate perception for successful travel are even greater in outdoor environments than in indoor spaces.

7. Learning to maintain a straight line of travel, and therefore avoiding having to stop to re-establish alignment, is essential for developing continuity in travel, which in turn is necessary to establish kinesthetic awareness of the distances traveled.

8. Veers into the parallel street (that is, toward traffic) are usually recognized kinesthetically; travelers simply feel that they have traveled too far for a standard street crossing.

They may also note that the expected incline, leveling off, and decline of the camber are replaced with a lateral tilt or a prolonged leveling of the surface traveled. In busier environments, they may notice that the traffic on the parallel street sounds too close.

LEARNING ACTIVITIES

1. Demonstrate ways in which varying degrees of precision in both movement and technique impact on accuracy in perception using at least one human guide technique, cane technique, and alignment procedure.

2. Identify the various demands imposed on a traveler by the environment, and illustrate how the O&M specialist can control these demands through the selection of destinations for travel.

3. Trail a curving pathway through the environment while scrupulously maintaining both hand position and arc to illustrate the impact of using good technique to limit degrees of freedom of movement and therefore reduce perceptual error while traveling.

4. Teach a fellow student to recognize a subtle environmental change (such as a change in height of an overhead or a hanging sign the student must pass under) by isolating the task of recognition and using repetition and feedback to acquire accuracy and consistency in its identification.

5. Identify various (1) auditory, (2) kinesthetic, and (3) proprioceptive clues relied on for determining the accuracy of one's line while crossing a street, and illustrate the role movement may have on the accurate perception of each.

CHAPTER 2

Improving Orientation for Students with Vision Loss

Laura Bozeman and Robert M. McCulley

LEARNING QUESTIONS

- What is orientation, and how are the many facets of this skill individualized across the life span?

- How do the concepts of *simple to complex* and *concrete to abstract* relate to teaching orientation?

- All people become disoriented at times. What are the components of reorientation for the student with visual impairment?

- How does the orientation and mobility (O&M) specialist help shape the student's cognitive map through *self-talk* and *parallel talk*?

- What is the "passive passenger," and how is this related to teaching orientation?

Orientation and mobility are interrelated components of teaching purposeful travel to an individual who is visually impaired. In the profession of orientation and mobility, orientation is defined as the process of using information received through the senses to know one's location and one's destination in relation to significant objects in the environment (Blasch, Wiener, & Welsh, 1997). A related component is spatial updating, or the ability to keep track of these spatial relationships while moving (Blasch et al., 1997; Hill & Ponder, 1976; Jacobson, 1993; LaGrow & Weessies, 1994). Mobility may be defined as getting from one's present location (point A) to the desired destination (point B) safely, efficiently, and as independently as possible (Blasch et al., 1997; Jacobson, 1993; LaGrow & Weessies, 1994). The terms can be defined separately; however, orientation and mobility form a concept that is integrated and more than the sum of its parts.

Orientation, a critical aspect of safe and purposeful movement for people who are visually impaired, has received little attention in the literature. Much of the knowledge base in teaching orientation is derived from generalized research. However, in Volume 1, Chapter 2, of this text, Long and Giudice note emerging research on the theories of orientation in recent years (Guth &

Rieser, 1997; Long & Hill, 1997; see Volume 1, Chapter 2). While theoretical attention to this important component of safe and efficient travel is a positive step, still neglected is the practical discussion of how O&M specialists teach people with vision loss to establish, maintain, and integrate orientation strategies. There is a great need for additional research, with particular attention to the onset of visual impairment as related to the understanding of spatial relationships, including individual learning styles and cognition, memory, cognitive mapping, and spatial updating; and the ability to integrate perceptual motor information.

For the person who is blind or visually impaired, common questions related to practical orientation are: Where am I located within this environment? What is around me? Where is my destination? What environmental features and clues can I access that will provide information? What is my plan to obtain the necessary information and safely reach my destination? If I become lost, how will I access the needed information to reorient and continue my route? Methods to obtain the essential pieces of the puzzle and hypothesis testing to apply the information effectively are key points of this chapter about teaching orientation skills to people with visual impairments.

This chapter examines instructional strategies across each of the primary orientation components, including spatial concepts, cognition, and the impact of perceptual motor information. Strategies are presented to assist the cognitive organization of spatial information with emphases on sequenced content and environmental and instructional support. This chapter also addresses instructional strategies specific to individuals across the life span and people who have visual impairments as well as additional disabilities. Further information about specific populations may be found in various chapters in this text.

GUIDING PRINCIPLES

In light of the limited research available to inform instructional practice, it is helpful to identify areas of consensus within the field of O&M instruction (Wall Emerson & Corn, 2006). Overarching practices that form the basis for advocacy and support of instructional intervention are that safety and well-being are enhanced by improved orientation (Blasch et al., 1997) and that all individuals with visual impairments must have access to the supports needed to maximize safety and independence (Crouse & Bina, 1997).

Skilled attention to the environment is useful for all people but essential for those who have sensory impairments. Individuals with visual impairments, supported through instruction in cognitive and perceptual information-processing skills, benefit from effective, safer travel. Also, a person's ability to maximize her own safety and independence should not be limited. Regardless of the individual's age, cognition, learning style, or ability to ambulate, safety and well-being are fostered when the individual is familiar with her surroundings. Each individual has the right to highly qualified supports and instruction to attain the greatest level of safety through awareness of where she is, where she is going, what is around her, and how the relationships between the individual and objects change as she moves to her destination.

Some of the guiding principles in O&M instruction are as follows:

- *Orientation, as with many aspects of O&M instruction, is individualized.*

  Everyone possesses a level of spatial orientation, along a continuum from a concrete, person-centered knowledge to a more abstract understanding of space, or a combination of both. The O&M specialist's goal is to teach and support each person to advance along the continuum in relation to the individual's experiences, goals, interests, and abilities (Wall Emerson & Corn, 2006). Since O&M instruction is individualized, the person's understanding and use of space may be expanded by careful assessment of his current level of functioning and planned experiential opportunities. For the O&M specialist, a positive relationship with the student may be the first step in effective instruction. Such a relationship requires a respect for diversity and is important in all forms of teaching and student interaction.

To build a rapport, the O&M specialist must understand the student's values, priorities, and perspective as well as the instructor's own personal biases. Hatton, McWilliam, and Winton (2003a) referred to *cultural reframing*, defined as an attempt to understand a situation from another's perspective, as an initial step to honor diversity. For any student to progress, the instructor must know the student and the experiences that shaped him.

Progress may also be affected by cognitive abilities or by a lack of instruction, motivation, time, or practical need. As in all functional skill instruction, the goal is to sequence activities from simple to complex and concrete to abstract in order to provide scaffolding, or temporary supports, and to challenge the individual to improve his current skill level. A gradual increase in complex experiences designed to expand understanding will support progress toward a more abstract understanding of space.

Each person will not achieve or need the same level of orientation. A student with developmental disabilities may be most effectively supported through a concrete, structured, and familiar route. The advanced spatial organizer, however, is able to generalize the layout within the environment and gather in-formation needed to reestablish orientation if he veers from the desired line of travel (LaGrow & Weessies, 1994; Long & Hill, 1997). With appropriate intervention, both types of students can be taught to achieve their highest level of independence and safety.

- *Orientation is an integration of cognitive and perceptual learning.*

   The student with visual impairment must learn to gather sensory information, determine what is relevant, and create a plan that effectively incorporates all of these elements. The student then tests that plan in relation to the continual influx of new information. For the student to move purposefully to the desired destination requires a cognitive understanding of the area and effective use of kinesthetic and proprioceptive information received through the muscles, bones, and joints related to the presence of environmental changes such as inclines, declines, and curb cuts. Awareness and integration of information from other remaining senses (for example, vision for signs and building and architectural clues; hearing for traffic and pedestrian sounds, and echoes in stairwells and bathrooms; and tactual clues about the walking surface) may affect orientation as well (see Chapter 1).

- *The person's level of attained orientation skills is influenced by the person's life stage and environment.*

   Young children who are visually impaired need to move in order to learn, to develop body concepts, and to generally explore the environment. Anthony, Lowry, Brown, and Hatton (2004) stated that young children with visual impairments do not reach or move independently toward objects until they achieve the conceptual understanding of people and objects in the environment. Therefore, developmental readiness is an essential factor that must be considered for a child's instruction while ensuring the age-appropriate components of orientation (Pogrund, 2002). On the other end of the life spectrum, a person who lives in an extended-care facility and who has limited control over his surroundings may have little opportunity to use generalized skills. Further, people of any age may possess additional disabilities that impede the physical ability to move; however, environmental understanding should be taught even to the person who is not ambulatory to prevent further isolation and to foster control of his personal area (Blasch et al., 1997). Thus, spatial awareness and the ability to exercise some understanding of the environment are essential elements for all individuals with vision loss.

The student's learning style and part-to-whole or whole-to-part approach to information processing are major components of learning effective orientation strategies. Generally speaking, a person with congenital blindness or vision loss that occurs before visual memory is established learns new concepts by first understanding the individual parts and may have difficulty conceptualizing the whole or gestalt concept. The person who has an adventitious vision loss will often have the benefit of the entire picture and is able to concentrate on the subparts that comprise the whole idea.

- *Orientation should be integrated into the overall O&M instruction.*

    Orientation begins at birth and is a continuous cognitive process exercised throughout life. "Orientation should be incorporated into mobility training from the beginning. Ideally, a student should progress from concrete understanding of orientation principles to a functional level, and finally into an abstract level" (Hill & Ponder, 1976, p. 1). For individuals with visual impairment who receive instructional support, orientation is incorporated into every lesson, expanding the

student's functional understanding of the environment and advancing that understanding to travel safely and conceptualize more broadly across increasingly complex environments. As Jacobson wrote, "The teaching of O&M skills is as much an art as it is a science. Knowing how and when to combine teaching orientation skills and mobility skills is the core of the process" (Jacobson, 1993, p. 4). Orientation must be functionally integrated into the sequence of mobility skills and techniques, each lesson containing some component of orientation, resulting in purposeful movement (see Chapter 1).

An example is the introduction of a new technique, such as the touch technique with the long cane. The O&M specialist will choose a quiet, indoor environment to first teach the technique. Initially, the student may be released from the responsibility of orientation in order to learn and apply the steps that comprise the cane technique. After the student achieves a level of competency with the touch technique, the O&M specialist gradually integrates orientation back into the lesson, combining the motor skills with an increased cognitive responsibility for the student to attend to her location and the surrounding environment.

- *Orientation skills are integrated into a success-oriented continuum of instruction that requires consistent reinforcement across all levels of learning.*

    From the body awareness of the youngest child to the cognitive mapping of the health care facility for the elderly resident, orientation skills are taught across the continuum and the life span. The effective program of study is person centered and sustained by the student's individual support system. Family, friends, educators, and team members can promote much more integrated learning, supporting and providing carryover, than an individual instructor in isolated lessons. O&M instruction should be designed to maximize the integration of all available support systems.

- *Understanding must be demonstrated.*

  As with all functional skills, a verbal description is not sufficient for the student to display understanding or competence. Orientation skills must be demonstrated for the student to show his comprehension. The O&M specialist looks for evidence that the student is able to integrate the instruction and apply the knowledge to the current environment. The O&M specialist may ask the student to "point to various landmarks in the area" to demonstrate body-to-object awareness. Similarly, the O&M specialist may expect the student to display object-to-object relationships using a map or model.

INSTRUCTIONAL FOUNDATIONS: SPATIAL UNDERSTANDING

Essential aspects of orientation skill building are the fundamental spatial concepts required for individuals of all ages who have visual impairments. These fundamental concepts, defined by Skellenger and Sapp in Chapter 7, as mental representations or ideas of what something should be, include body awareness, body-part relationships, and body-to-object and object-to-object relationships (Hill & Blasch, 1980; Long & Hill, 1997). Skellenger and Sapp use the term *O&M development* to describe the skills and concepts necessary for the young child to build future O&M skills. Development of this foundational knowledge supports more advanced cognitive skills of mapping and spatial updating. This process begins with the child and her ability to organize information relating to her body, the knowledge that she has body parts, also called *body awareness*, the relationship of body parts to one another, and how those parts make up a whole (Anthony et al., 2004).

Body Awareness

For a child, understanding spatial concepts begins with a focus on body awareness as a foundation to near, far, and remote spatial relationships. Body awareness emerges as the child understands his body parts and the names of those parts. Parents, family, and caregivers begin to teach body awareness, naturally, from the moment the newborn child comes home. Daily routines and activities of bathing, dressing, and wiping the child's face and hands are the first lessons about the parts of the body (Anthony et al., 2004). Labeling of the body parts provides the child with the tactile and auditory information to link the body part with its name. Examples include "Let me clean your toes" and "Let's wash your hands." Family members and caregivers may use a game like This Little Piggy to bring the child's attention to his toes or Patty-Cake to focus on his hands. Learning follows in a simple-to-complex fashion, with eyes, nose, hands, and feet as examples of the gross parts that are first learned. As the sighted child grows, vision and incidental learning take over, and he learns more specific body parts, such as elbow, wrist, and calf. For the child with visual impairment, other senses must be used and the process of pairing sensory information continues until the child understands the whole body and all of the parts.

As the child matures, games and songs increase body awareness. The game of Head, Shoulders, Knees, and Toes is a fun way to identify body parts and their locations. Simon Says is a game that can be simple—"Simon says to blink your eyes" or "Simon says to open your mouth"—or more complex in order to practice the next stage of body-part relationships.

Body-Part Relationships

The next step in acquiring spatial concepts is the knowledge of body-part relationships. Understanding the relationship between body parts is a natural progression from body awareness and includes positional concepts, including laterality. *Laterality* is, from the egocentric perspective, the awareness that the body has two sides, right and left (Blasch et al., 1997).

The student can demonstrate his understanding of body-part relationships by touching his head with a hand or clapping two hands together, upon request. A more complex aspect of body-part relationships is for the student to exhibit laterality and place his right hand on his left knee when asked.

Understanding spatial relationships between body parts may also occur incidentally and can be encouraged by the family by labeling the action. An example is to say "Cover your mouth when you cough" and demonstrate that the hand goes over the mouth by supporting the child's hand to cover his mouth.

The Hill Performance Test of Selected Positional Concepts (Hill, 1981) served as a primary tool that inspired additional resources to assess and support instructional intervention in this area (Pogrund et al., 1995). Again, the game "Simon Says" can be employed to assist the child to identify positional relationships of body parts through the list provided: "Touch the top of your head, front of your leg, right eye, back of your neck, bottom of your foot, left side of your body, center of your face, right hand, part of your body nearest to your toes, touch your nose with your middle finger, left leg" (Hill, 1981, p. 19).

There is a natural progression from positional body concepts to functional applications in orientation and mobility. The student's spatial understanding in relation to positional concepts naturally proceeds from his knowledge of body parts to the ability to move his body parts in relationship to each other (Hill, 1981). Examples include "Turn your body so that your heels are higher than your toes; center your cane hand, and turn your palm away from you."

Body-to-Object Relationships

The student's understanding of spatial relationships develops from internal to external space. One example, directionality, is an extension of laterality. Directionality is defined by Fazzi and Petersmeyer (2001) as "understanding of the points or lines toward which something faces or moves . . . [a concept] even more important to visually impaired individuals' orientation while traveling" (p. 95). This transition is a big jump, as the relationships involve people and objects outside of the student's body. Once objects are understood to be permanent, the expanded spatial relationships that were intrinsically linked to the body are transitioned outward with the student as the center. This body-to-object understanding is also called an *egocentric frame of reference*. Long and Giudice (Volume 1, Chapter 2) describe an egocentric frame of reference as one in which "information is perceived, remembered, and acted on from the perspective of the individual's current location. That is, a person using only an egocentric frame of reference does not imagine the spatial relations among places from perspectives other than his current perspective." Blasch et al. (1997) noted the importance of body-to-object understanding in the very definition of orientation, as the "knowledge of one's distance and direction relative to things observed or remembered in the surroundings and keeping track of these spatial relationships as they change during locomotion" (p. 750).

Body-to-object relationships are more easily organized cognitively from a single, fixed location. Applying the principles of sequenced learning strategy, the O&M specialist supports the student by addressing proximal or closer objects before advancing to distal or distant objects. The O&M specialist chooses an indoor, quiet location with few barriers and places a chair, for example, representing home base (the chair becomes a landmark, anchored in space), facing forward, with three additional, distinctly different chairs (small, medium, large) in front of the student to facilitate direct, forward relationships. One chair is centered, one is located to the right of center, and one is to the left. The student is directed forward to find the centered chair, walk back to the home-base chair, and then point to the location of the first, centered chair. The O&M specialist introduces the other two, off-center, chairs and repeats the exercise until each of the three chairs is accurately represented, cognitively, in relation to the student's home-base chair. The student demonstrates his knowledge by pointing and walking directly to each of the three chairs. The O&M specialist may then change the distances and locations of the chairs, which increases the level of difficulty and requires the student to spatially update the cognitive representation of the rearranged items in the environment.

To further challenge a student to cognitively represent body-to-object relationships in an abstract way, the O&M specialist will often "draw" on the student's back, demonstrating the relationship between the student's location and locations within the current environment. The back is a good mapping surface, as it maintains orientation with the direction the student faces. If the O&M specialist draws the map on the student's hand, orientation is difficult to maintain, as the orientation of the hand can be separated from the direction the student faces and changes easily. An example of the back-mapping strategy is described in Sidebar 2.1.

Spatial Updating

Spatial updating requires the student to know the location of objects in the environment *and* accurately monitor the changing relationships between the student and the surrounding objects in the area. Initially, the student demonstrates orientation while walking from the home base to multiple objects around that point. Repositioning the home base exercises the student's ability to redesign that representation from another fixed point. The ability to travel through an area and accurately alter the cognitive representation of objects within the area is the skill of spatial updating (see Volume 1, Chapter 2). The ability to process a wider range of perceptual information is critical to updating the mental map and understanding relationships between objects.

Use of the Student's Back as a Mapping Strategy

To give the overall layout of a mall, the O&M specialist guides the student to a central place and uses the student's back as a mapping surface. The O&M specialist then "draws" the locations of the anchor stores and landmarks as they relate to the student's body position. If the student is facing north, and Macy's is located at the north end of the hall and Sears is at the south end, the O&M specialist "draws" the location of Macy's by the student's neck and the location of Sears lower on the student's back, closer to her waist. This tactile map also reinforces the body-to-object relationship, with the map on the student's back "oriented" to the area and the way she is facing. For the student to accurately update her cognitive map, she must understand the spatial relationships between her body and the objects and people in the environment.

Object-to-Object Relationships

Sequentially, spatial understanding progresses from an egocentric to an *allocentric frame of reference*, in which a traveler relates the locations of objects or places to one another, *independent* of her current location in space (see Volume 1, Chapter 2). An allocentric understanding allows the student to imagine the environment from a serial or global-map perspective. The object-to-object relationships do not change as the student moves through the environment.

To advance spatial understanding of allocentric relationships, Blasch, Welsh, and Davidson (1973) identified reference systems that describe types of information available in object-to-object understanding. *Topocentric* information includes landmarks or unique environmental features; *polarcentric* information includes cardinal directions and the use of compass directions; *cartographic* information includes patterns and shapes, such as squares, rectangles, grid patterns, or numbering systems. This understanding is important to route planning and orientation in general (see Volume 1, Chapter 2).

To foster object-to-object expertise, the O&M specialist chooses a familiar indoor environment and, beginning with a small, well-defined area, asks the student to initially explore the relationships of three familiar, unique, objects that form a natural geographic pattern. This strategy allows the student to venture out and examine the relationships and distances between the objects. Physically walking between objects allows the student to experientially learn distances and object-to-object relationships needed to support the cognitive representation of how the objects relate to the student as well as to each other; that is, the desk is to the right of the door; the bathroom is across the hall from the office. The O&M specialist may then ask the student to verbalize those relationships and critically think about the fact that object-to-object relationships do not change as the student moves through the

area. The O&M specialist may use the classroom as a natural, familiar environment and choose three or more distinct items that have relevance for the student, for example, the door to the classroom, the teacher's desk, and the student's desk. The student can demonstrate her own perceptions of the object-to-object relationships via tactile maps or models and further advance accurate conceptualization of the space (see Chapter 11). Utilizing spatial foundations, the O&M specialist then teaches the student using instructional strategies appropriate for the situation.

INSTRUCTIONAL STRATEGIES: COGNITIVE AND PERCEPTUAL REPRESENTATION OF SPACE

As previously emphasized, spatial cognition and attention to sensory information are essentially linked to improved orientation, independence, and safety. For the student to develop orientation skills, he must first have the foundational knowledge of concepts.

Understanding Concepts

An essential aspect of orientation is *fundamental concept* knowledge. A conceptual understanding of objects is important to orientation in that objects have size, shape, and mass that occupy space. Objects may also be associated with other perceptual information that cannot be used unless understood. Knowing the characteristics of object (their similarities and differences of design and function) becomes important to orientation as the student contacts and safely negotiates various objects in the area. Cars, trains, and buses are examples of well-known objects in the environment that also provide a wide range of perceptual data to the student. The electric car, with quieter engine sounds, and the Segway (a battery-operated, self-balancing personal transportation device with two wheels) are new objects that may not be familiar to the student. The O&M specialist must link these concepts for the student to understand how these objects impact the perceptual environment.

Similarly, environments have distinctive, defining features, and knowledge of these features maximizes the student's spatial abilities. Indoor environments are defined by the nature of being enclosed (for example, rooms, defined by walls). Residential environments are characterized by streets, blocks, and sidewalks, while urban environments are represented by multiple businesses, more pedestrians, and increased vehicle congestion. Some areas have even more advanced concepts that include courtyards, atriums, revolving restaurants, and moving sidewalks. Spatial concepts of size, position, planes, and directionality are essential components of space, intentional movement, and organization. The foundational basis of this knowledge is addressed earlier in the chapter and forms the groundwork for environmental exploration.

Cognitive Process

In the absence of visual cues, audition becomes the primary distance sense and, with the remaining senses, becomes critical to perceiving and substantiating cognitive representations. The ability to cognitively represent spatial relationships must remain fluid and must be updated by the continuous sensory information that supports the mental image. Overreliance on a mental map, to the exclusion of current sensory information, is frequently observed when the student veers toward a wall, takes two steps sideways, and walks directly toward the wall again. It is not at all unusual for a student to do this many times before the realization that the perceptual information is not matching the cognitive representation and that the cognitive map must be revised.

An essential strategy is to guide the student to use a full sensory approach to gather the in-

formation critical to problem solving. The cognitive problem-solving process demonstrates the integration of perceptual information to establish an accurate cognitive map. The process is also a good strategy for reorientation. Hill and Ponder (1976) described the cognitive process as follows:

1. Gather all available sensory information while stationary, such as odors and sounds.

2. Analyze all recognized sensory information, such as familiar voices, traffic sounds, and tactile information that may indicate an incline or decline.

3. Select the information that best fulfills the orientation need based on relevance or importance to the task.

4. Establish a hypothesis based on the gathered information and form a plan of action.

5. Test the hypothesis by executing the plan.

The student continually receives more sensory information, and the process is ongoing. Figure 2.1 depicts the integrated steps that develop orientation and lead to purposeful movement.

Structured Opportunities for Reorientation

All people become disoriented at times. The O&M specialist may utilize reorientation strategies for the student to efficiently resume travel. As described by Long and Hill (1997) and Long and Giudice (Volume 1, Chapter 2), the drop-off lesson builds problem-solving skills as reorientation strategies. The O&M specialist provides planned, structured, educational opportunities for a student to utilize the steps of the cognitive process, to plant his feet; perceive, analyze, and select information; develop a hypothesis; and execute the plan as essential skills to establish and reestablish orientation as necessary.

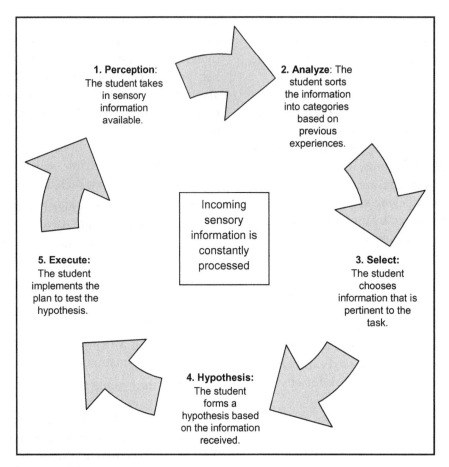

Figure 2.1. The Cognitive Process

There are many forms of drop-off lessons. The drop-off lesson is a situation in which the student knows the destination but is not sure of his current location. In a familiar area, the O&M specialist may "disorient" the student purposefully and assign the student to locate a destination to facilitate opportunities for exploration and confidence building. The student knows point B (destination), but does not know point A (current location). The strategy is to use the cognitive process to gather, interpret, and apply information to move safely until the student encounters a landmark or any information that gives specifics about his location. A situational example of problem solving using this process can be found in Sidebar 2.2, with an illustration provided by Figure 2.2.

This technique can be integrated across a series of increasingly complex environments. The drop-off lesson may be exercised at the completion of each new area where instruction has occurred: a building, campus, residential, or advanced urban environment, or a combination of environments along a route.

Monitoring the Learning

The cognitive process involves using available perceptual information and integrating that information into a plan. The O&M specialist can

Problem Solving in Orientation

Problem solving in orientation includes four stages:

(1) Identifying that a problem exists

(2) Identifying alternative strategies for solving the problem

(3) Selecting a hypothesis from the available alternatives

(4) Evaluating the effectiveness of the selected hypothesis

A traveler using a long cane lives in a city neighborhood that is mostly residential in character but is adjacent to a small-business area and has access to bus transportation.

The 11-square-block area that is the focus of this example of problem solving in orientation is represented by Figure 2.2.

Walnut Street forms the north border of the area used for this example. It is a commercial street with many shops and restaurants. Going south from Walnut, the parallel east-west streets are Virginia Street, Kentucky Street, Tennessee Street, and Fifth Avenue (a busy four-lane street with fast-moving traffic). The block from Tennessee Street to Fifth Avenue is uphill going toward Fifth.

The north-south streets in the area, starting from the easternmost and going toward the west, are Negley Avenue, Ivy Avenue, Maple Avenue, Oak Avenue, Locust Avenue, and Aiken Avenue. Negley and Aiken are busy two-lane streets that also carry bus traffic.

Except for the perimeter streets, all of the streets within the model area are quiet and tree-lined. They usually carry modest amounts of vehicle and pedestrian traffic.

Mike, who travels with a long cane, lives on the west side of Oak Avenue between Kentucky and Tennessee streets. His destination this morning is the Starbucks coffee shop on the

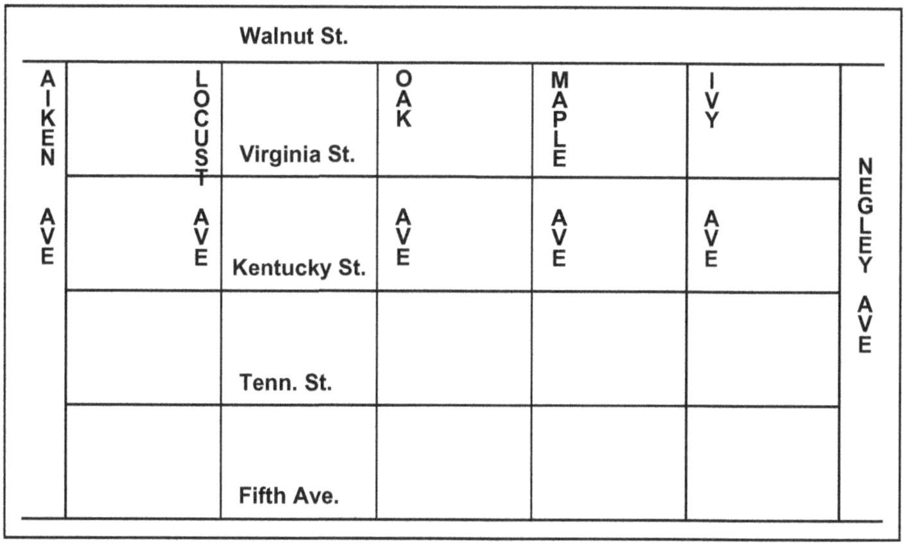

	Walnut St.				
AIKEN AVE	LOCUST AVE	Virginia St. OAK AVE	MAPLE AVE	IVY AVE	NEGLEY AVE
		Kentucky St.			
		Tenn. St.			
		Fifth Ave.			

Figure 2.2. Grid for Problem-Solving Example

(continued on next page)

south side of Walnut Street between Oak and Maple avenues. He routinely enjoys coffee and pastry and boards a bus at the shelter that is just west of the Starbucks.

This morning, Mike had a lot on his mind. As he traveled north on Oak Avenue and approached Kentucky Street, his cane stuck briefly in a crack just before he got to the curb and affected his line of direction. Since there was not much traffic along these two streets to verify his line of direction, he trusted that he was okay and inadvertently made a diagonal crossing. As he stepped up on the curb, a car passed and Mike adjusted his line to have the traffic on his right and continued. As a result of the diagonal crossing, Mike was now heading east along Kentucky Street instead of north along Oak Avenue.

Just before coming to the end of the block, Mike noticed a large shrub covering part of the sidewalk. In all of his trips along Oak Avenue, he had never noticed this shrub before. It also seemed to him that the block was slightly longer than the block along Oak Avenue between Kentucky and Virginia streets. Now he began to worry about that last crossing he made. He did seem to be out in the street a little longer than usual.

When he arrived at Maple Avenue, he could not tell for sure whether he was at the southwest corner of Oak and Virginia (location A) as planned or whether he had made a diagonal crossing and was now at the northwest corner of Kentucky and Maple (location B). The combination of the protruding shrub and the slightly longer block suggested to Mike that he might not be at the intended corner. But the sound of this intersection was no different from the sound of the intersection he was intending to reach. Had the sun been shining that morning, its location relative to his facing

position could have confirmed to him that he was facing east instead of north. But it was a cloudy day. He suspected that he had an orientation problem.

As Mike considered his options, he concluded that he could go one of four ways. (1) He could turn around and retrace his steps. Regardless of whether he was at the corner of Oak and Virginia or at the corner of Kentucky and Maple, if he retraced his steps he would arrive at a quiet intersection. Neither of these would provide any distinctive information to verify his location. (2) He could turn right, cross the street that was on his right, and walk a block in that direction. Once again, this choice, whether he was at location A or location B, would bring him to a quiet intersection that would not solve the problem. (3) Mike could turn left and walk another block. Once again, in neither case would he come to an intersection that would give him information to solve his location and facing problems. (4) He could cross the street in front of him and walk another block. If he was at location A, facing north at Oak and Virginia, one more block north would bring him to Walnut and Oak. He would recognize the sound of pedestrian and vehicle traffic. This would confirm that he had not made a mistake and he could continue to his destination. If, however, he was facing east at location B, another block in that direction would bring him to another quiet intersection. In this case, he could then conclude that he was at the corner of Kentucky and Ivy facing east. Once his location and facing direction had been confirmed, he could then plan his new route to the coffee shop.

Faced with these options, Mike decided to select option 4, cross the street in front of him and proceed in the direction he was facing. After walking one block, he came to a quiet

(continued on next page)

intersection and concluded that he was now at the corner of Kentucky and Ivy facing east. With this confirmation, Mike decided that he would turn left and walk two blocks to get to Walnut Street. Hearing the pedestrian and commercial traffic along Walnut confirmed that his decision was correct. At that point, he turned west, walked along Walnut Street, came to and crossed Maple Avenue, and then located the coffee shop.

Mike also had realized that the process of finding the coffee shop would have to change

a little. Normally, as he walked east along Walnut, he would notice the bus shelter on his left, and the door to the coffee shop would be the next door on his right. Coming from the east, Mike had to walk to the point where he heard the bus shelter on his right. Then he traced his steps backward to the first door to find the coffee shop. Arriving at the coffee shop was the ultimate verification that his problem-solving process had been effective.

use this strategy to help the student work through the process, reconstruct the mental map, and improve his overall orientation.

Self-Talk

Since the cognitive map is the mental image or perception in the student's mind, the O&M specialist may employ several approaches to help shape an accurate cognitive map. The O&M specialist may use the strategy of *self-talk* and ask the student to verbalize what he is thinking and doing while traveling and making decisions.

The concept of self-talk or inner speech emerged from L. S. Vygotsky's work, published in 1987. Vygotsky determined that self-talk proved useful in enhancing one's memory and ability to problem solve. The O&M specialist is able to listen and understand what might appear to be decisions made without logic. Verbalizing the thought process becomes a powerful tool for the O&M specialist to recognize what is not working well or aspects that may be misunderstood by the student (Schickedanz, Schickedanz, Forsyth, & Forsyth, 1998; Vygotsky, 1987).

Parallel Talk

A related tool is *parallel talk*. With this strategy, the O&M specialist verbalizes the actions of the

student as she moves and interacts with the environment. Parallel talk is beneficial if the student is unaware of her movements and body language. This strategy may be more useful for children (Baumgart et al., 1982) and students with cognitive challenges.

Systematic and Structured Exploration

O&M specialists utilize systematic, structured exploration as an instructional technique to assist students with information gathering and organization of spatial information. This strategy serves to support skills in building an allocentric representation and using cognitive mapping and spatial updating to advance a student's ability to conceptualize environments, routes, or areas. Room *familiarization* is an example of applying systematic exploration to advance cognitive mapping of individual routes that can be connected and spatially updated to define an area.

The O&M specialist assists the student to select a permanent and unique landmark to distinguish the home base (for example, a doorway entering the room) and aid future recognition of the starting point once the exploration begins. Next, the student is instructed to complete a *perimeter walk* from home base, following the walls of the room, and return. Back at home base, the student is queried about the size and shape of the room, number of walls, and major distinguishing objects that she can recall along each border. The student then is asked to cognitively and experientially establish a direct relationship from the home base to the information points on each wall. With accuracy established through repetition, the cognitive map becomes "one" with the physical environment, all from a single point of reference—home base. As she walks from the home base to critical objects on each wall, the student uses a grid-pattern approach to systematically explore the interior of the room to familiarize herself with the contents.

The final process of this instructional strategy is to switch the location of the home base and repeat the experiential component of walking from the new home base to each major landmark on each wall. Changing the home base and repeating the purposeful movement to each identified object perfects the spatial relationships in the mental map and supports the student's ability to spatially update from a new perspective within the room. The O&M specialist can increase the complexity further by expecting the student to travel through the established area, remember the interior objects previously encountered, and intentionally move around them without contact. The ability of the student to demonstrate this level of skill is strong evidence of advanced spatial cognition. This familiarization technique is a powerful strategy to expand spatial cognition and orientation competency across diverse environments.

In larger areas, it may not be feasible to complete a perimeter walk. The O&M specialist may explore the hallway with the student, providing a descriptive reference to the shape and the characteristics of the landmarks along the walls, connecting the student spatially by having the student point to the landmark or home base from different positions in the area. By expanding instructional strategies and advancing the student's full perceptual abilities with the richness of available sensory information, the O&M specialist helps students with visual impairments to remain oriented to larger, more diverse environments.

Integrating Sensory and Perceptual Skills

Another instructional strategy to assist perception and spatial orientation is the utilization of a *human guide*. The O&M specialist may guide the traveler to an area and ask him to use the cognitive process to isolate sensory information and select what is useful to the task. The O&M specialist, as the guide, may take the student directly to critical landmarks to help the student mentally map the area. Using a guide may facilitate a greater level of focus and the freedom to concentrate on the task at hand.

As mentioned, isolating the task frees the student to apply perceptual information and give attention to the orientation components of the environment. The O&M specialist is also better able to structure the environment with the use of human guide techniques, guiding the student to areas where sensory information is readily available. An example of this process can be found in Sidebar 2.3.

Straight-line travel is important both to the mental map and to orientation in general. The ability to maintain a straight line of travel is not easily done without perceptual support and guidance. For the person without vision, diverting from an intended straight line of travel, called *veer*, can occur in the absence of tactile or auditory information or if the student fails to interpret that information correctly.

Straight-line travel is often related to body posture and gait; when postural or gait abnormalities significantly affect straight travel, the

SIDEBAR 2.3

Using a Human Guide to Structure the Lesson

The O&M specialist wants the student to be aware of the intersecting, main hallway in his building. This particular hallway has double doors on the north end, and there is usually a breeze from that area. Since it is a main hallway, there is a more "open" sound at that intersection. By serving as the guide, the O&M specialist provides protection and the student is able to take in the perceptual information available as the pair moves through the area. By isolating the task, the O&M specialist enables the student to give his full attention to the information available. Later, the student can integrate his mobility skills with the perceptual and spatial information in his mental map, then implement the strategies to maintain that map.

student may deviate from his intended path. Since the student is usually unaware of the veer (Guth, 2008), he may also inaccurately reorganize his cognitive map, further affecting his orientation.

O&M specialists traditionally emphasize recovery techniques to address veering problems, such as the recovery procedure after veering into the parallel street (LaGrow & Weesies, 1994). The first step to prevent the problem is for the student to recognize that he is veering.

One cause for veer may be a cane arc that is not balanced or equal on both sides. An uneven cane arc may pull the student toward the side with the greater arc. The O&M specialist may prompt the student to recognize the uneven arc and the veer through muscle and skeletal input as well as the results of the veer.

While a certain degree of asymmetry in leg length is normal, a significant difference may affect the person's gait (Guth, 2008; Children's Hospital Boston, n.d.). The O&M specialist needs to be aware of this possibility. Similarly, if the student has other orthopedic concerns, such as arthritis, joint replacement, or scoliosis, gait may be affected.

The student may not have his "nose over his toes." If the student's nose or face is turned to the right or left, he may veer to that side. If the heels of the student's shoes are unevenly worn, this may also reflect a gait problem (Gikling, 1949; Rossi, 2007). Often students carry a heavy backpack on one shoulder rather than squarely across the back. This practice may disrupt straight line of travel and is detrimental to the spine and posture as well (Chow et al., 2005).

The ability to make accurate turns is a perceptual motor skill that plays an important role in maintaining an accurate representation of spatial relationships and subsequent orientation. The O&M specialist may ask the student to make a 90-degree turn. Accurate turns without visual input may be difficult. The student must understand how it feels to make a good turn and create the muscle memory associated with the correct position of the muscles, bones, and joints. Instructional strategies to improve turn accuracy include physical contact with the environment, for example, squaring off or taking a line of direction to monitor positioning. Examples include "Put the wall behind you" and "Put the wall to your side." Strategies include verbal feedback about the turns—overturning or underturning—and practicing military turns, in which the student places the heel of one foot so that it touches the heel of the other foot to form a 90-degree angle. Subsequent practice is important so turns do not continue to be so regimented. Often, this concrete method improves the student's ability to make accurate turns.

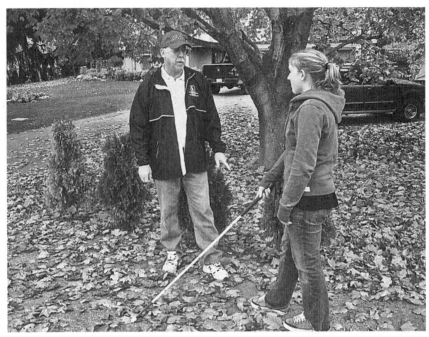

Lynn Langille

An O&M specialist talks with a teenage girl about the importance of maintaining an equal cane arc to maintain a straight line of travel.

Another skill involving muscle memory is accurate time and distance awareness. Time and distance estimation is a technique that the O&M specialist must consider for the student who has difficulty maintaining orientation. Students who are unable to correctly determine distances may attempt a turn too early or too late. Crossing a street, anticipating a veer into the parallel street, and turning toward the curb too early is an example of a time and distance error. Time and distance errors can cause disorientation and the need to continuously problem solve after disorientation has been noticed. Methods to teach time and distance judgment generally include repetition and experience.

Practice may begin indoors, with the student walking the length of a hallway, then attempting to walk it again and stop halfway. In this exercise, the O&M specialist isolates the variables by ensuring that no other clues indicate the halfway point, for example, specific sounds or clues

underfoot. Similarly, the student may walk the length of a residential block, then return and attempt to locate the halfway point. The O&M specialist may initially help the student know when he is halfway or three-quarters of the way to the end by providing verbal information. The student then relates this information to his muscle and motor memory.

Attention to the sounds of the intersection as the student approaches can confirm time and distance awareness by pairing auditory sounds with muscle memory as the student walks the length of the block. Critical attention to the skill can be fostered through experiential learning by selecting a rectangular-shaped block or floor in a building and supporting the student's critical analysis of the time required to walk each leg of the route. While many creative approaches can be utilized, accurate perception of time and distance and the ability to walk a straight line are essential aspects of orientation.

Orientation Aids to Teach Cognitive Mapping

Orientation aids support cognitive route mapping, spatial representation, and long-term recall of spatial relationships. Bentzen (1997) identified five spatial and map concepts that should be considered when incorporating orientation aids into the instructional process. Bentzen reports that effective use of orientation aids requires the knowledge that "1) symbols represent real objects, 2) location of symbols on the map represents the location of these objects in the mapped space, 3) directions on the map correspond to the directions in the mapped space, 4) maps are like a bird's eye view, and 5) shapes shown on the map represent shapes of objects or areas in the mapped space" (Bentzen, 1997, p. 286). Bentzen further suggests the use of three-dimensional models, tactile, and visual maps, and verbal aids (see Chapter 11).

The advantage of models to teach spatial orientation is the three-dimensional quality they possess. A model of a building contains conceptual representations: multiple floors that are parallel and positioned on top of one another, the spatial relationship of the roof to the foundation, the perpendicular driveway and walkway to the door. Another useful model is that of an intersection with curbs, sidewalks, grass lines, and street furniture. Toy cars with wheels that spin, integrated within the model intersection, comprise a rich conceptual environment to explore traffic patterns.

Tactile maps and visual maps are extremely useful to convey unique or easily recognized landmarks and specific content or routes within both large and small areas. The O&M specialist may provide orientation to a specific travel route and use tactile maps to convey route shapes, landmarks, and spatial relationships between and among landmarks along the travel route. The map may represent any area of particular interest, such as a lobby, a group of related hallways, or a train station. In large areas, such as residential or business areas, maps can be used for planning multiple routes to the same destination. Other uses of tactile maps and visual maps include simple or complex intersections, unique areas such as airports, college campuses, or grocery stores, or larger geographies such as cities, states, or continents.

The Picture Maker Wheatley Tactile Diagramming Kit and Chang Tactual Diagram Kit are available from the American Printing House. They are easy to manipulate and are designed for intersection, street, and traffic representations (Bentzen, 1997). The Tactile Image Enhancer creates tactile images from a pencil drawing. Low-tech options, including magnetic boards and Wikki Stix, provide quick, portable methods to tactually depict a map. The keys to constructing such maps are to focus on the purpose and limit the content, omitting unnecessary information or clutter that is unrelated to the intended purpose. Tactile maps are frequently used to represent spaces that are larger than one can physically experience through exploration alone.

Prerecorded auditory orientation devices or brailled or print instructions provide a serial map, an option that is many times overlooked. Sighted individuals frequently write down directions as a memory aid. Given the complex skills required to attend to multiple sensory data and the ongoing immediate orientation demands, the potential to lose track of extended directions is likely. A serial map that is recorded, brailled, or printed in large print offers a memory aid that is helpful and may be a necessary support for orientation.

Global Positioning Systems

The advancement of real-time auditory support through global positioning systems, used to identify a traveler's current position in relationship to her destination, has revolutionized the field of orientation and mobility and will continue to do so. The rich opportunity to solicit data in real time without reliance on the availability of the general public is an improvement that fosters increased independence for the student. The technology continues to drive the professional field of orientation and mobility to rethink and reorganize instructional processes and methods to incorporate new technology. The O&M specialist seeks to expand the student's ability to cognitively map increasingly complex and dynamic areas, resulting in more options for route planning and safer travel. On-demand data to assist spatial updating greatly expands the resources available to the O&M specialist and to the student who is blind or visually impaired (see Chapters 11 and 14 and Volume 1, Chapters 8 and 10).

Environmental Patterns

Planned environments, both indoor and outdoor, have regular and predictable patterns that can aid the student's orientation. Examples of useful patterns include numbering systems, the consistent location of bathrooms and water fountains near elevators, and floors that generalize or mirror one another in design. The knowledge of *patterns* is powerful in data organization, cognitive mapping, and use as a memory tool.

Typical organizational patterns are seen in numbering systems, for example, odd numbers on one side of a hallway or street and even numbers on the other side. There is usually a starting point, or home base, where the numbering begins—often by the elevators or the entrance to the building. An O&M specialist who is teaching numbering systems may ask the student to explore the hallway and solicit assistance to learn the room numbers of two consecutive rooms on the same side of the hall. These two pieces of information often provide clues to the numbering pattern within the building. Predictable patterns exist in larger areas as well.

Urban planners frequently design a central location within a major city. This central point, typically downtown, may serve as a reference point for the rest of the city. Streets located near the downtown center usually have the lowest numbers, and street numbers increase with the distance away from downtown. In Boston, the center is downtown and trains are described as inbound, toward the center of the city, or outbound, away from the center. An O&M specialist in New York City would explain to the student that the borough of Manhattan is comprised of quadrants, upper and lower east and west areas. Each section, for example, the Lower East Side, provides a clear cognitive representation that aids orientation. Further, avenues run north and south and streets run east and west, with Fifth Avenue as the east-west divider. Both avenues and streets are designated by numbers, with 50th Street as the north-south division. This information gives further shape to the cognitive picture of the city. The sensory environment that initially appears overwhelming is actually a rich perceptual training site with predictable and useful patterns.

Other patterns that support orientation include typical shapes as schematic representations of routes, areas, and intersections. The O&M specialist may describe routes as L-shaped and Z-shaped or intersections as T-shaped or plus (+)-shaped. If the student has a conceptual understanding that these shapes represent a picture of the area, this mental map may be helpful to his orientation.

LEARNER-BASED STRATEGIES

Many instructional techniques are applicable to most students; however, some strategies are tailored to specific populations for optimal results. Orientation approaches for children, individuals in assisted-living or extended-care settings, and individuals with additional disabilities are presented in this section.

Orientation Strategies for the Young Child

The content knowledge and skills required for orientation instruction are similar for all individuals with vision impairment. However, since the young child is developing and still a work in progress, the approach to instruction differs. The traditional definition of orientation must be expanded to include motor, cognitive, and perceptual development (Anthony et al., 2004). "With very young children, orientation can be directly tied to the cognitive mastery of concepts of body image, spatial constructs, causality, means and ends, and object permanence" (Anthony, Bleier, Fazzi, Kish, & Pogrund, 2002, p. 328). The overall process for the very young child involves developing the initial concepts and the access to sensory information that must be integrated into the child's overall development. This O&M developmental process prepares the child to understand and learn the O&M techniques that are provided when she is developmentally, cognitively, and perceptually ready (see Chapter 7).

Early intervention provides the basis for future O&M instruction and is important for children who may experience developmental delays due to vision impairment. The O&M specialist may provide opportunities and incentives for exploration, creating the desire in the student to move and further expand her world. Movement and exploration help the young child interact with the environment, using sensory information to create knowledge of the environment and the concepts within. Pogrund's (2002) discussion of the impact of vision loss on learning is shown in Sidebar 2.4.

Intervention and guiding the child to explore objects is often approached in a hand-over-hand method, with the instructor or parent guiding the child's hand in a directed way (Story, 1998). Lilli Nielsen, among others, noted that a hand-under-hand approach may better develop

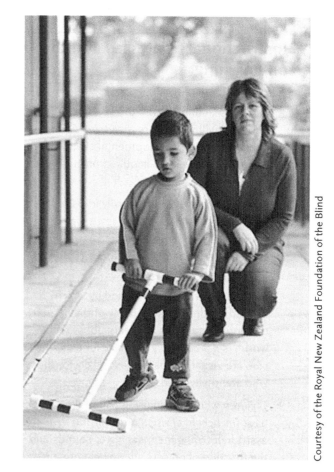

An O&M specialist watches as a young boy explores the environment using an adapted mobility device.

independence in learning, as the child is not guided but is supported to explore. Nielsen reported a decrease in tactile defensiveness and increased initiation of movement and exploration, as well as better grasp and use of the hands with this technique (Nielsen, 1992).

Often, instructional strategies take the form of play. Songs and rhymes are fun and often help the child remember the concepts and ideas presented. The O&M specialist may use routines to present tasks and instruction as natural and effective methods for incorporating O&M instruction into daily activities, utilizing the natural environments in which the tasks occur.

SIDEBAR 2.4

Instructional Strategies and the Unique Impact of Vision Loss on Learning

- In general, children who are visually impaired will need *more time* than sighted peers to acquire developmental skills, especially those skills acquired primarily through vision.

- Young children who are visually impaired may demonstrate a *different sequence of acquisition* than sighted children in reaching certain developmental milestones (Ferrell, 2000).

- *Incidental learning*, the method by which sighted children achieve many of their developmental skills and learn about their world, is *not as readily available* for children who are visually impaired, especially for those who are totally blind.

- Children who are visually impaired do not have *the benefit of vision as a unifying sense* to assist in learning the meaning of sounds and the function of objects and to help organize their world.

- Some *concepts may be fragmented* for children who are visually impaired, as touch and sound may provide only partial understanding without guided exploration and verbal explanations.

- Use of *real objects and experiences* during intervention increases tactile, auditory, and visual comprehension for children who are visually impaired.

- *Active involvement and participation in exploring the world* help to optimize the motor and cognitive development of young children who are visually impaired.

- Children who are visually impaired and their families need *specialized instruction and educational guidance from professionals* who have expertise in addressing their disability-specific needs. These educational vision specialists should be involved in all phases of the planning and implementation of the educational program of young children who are visually impaired.

Source: Reprinted with permission from Rona L. Pogrund, "Refocus: Setting the Stage for Working with Young Children Who Are Blind or Visually Impaired," in Rona L. Pogrund and Diane L. Fazzi, Eds., *Early Focus: Working with Young Children Who Are Blind or Visually Impaired and Their Families, 2nd ed.* (New York: AFB Press, 2002), p. 6; italics added.

Supporting orientation for the young child requires sensitivity to her maturity and experiences. The student's developmental readiness is critical to the success of the instruction. Fazzi and Naimy (Chapter 8) present a chart to guide instructional expectations and related ages. Among other orientation strategies, Fazzi and Naimy note that many children in kindergarten through third grade are able to understand the characteristics of landmarks, maintain orienta-

tion on simple routes, use problem-solving strategies, and construct simple maps and models. For in-depth information about orientation and mobility for children, see Chapter 7.

Strategies for Individuals in Extended-Care Facilities

Specialized populations, in general, require increased creativity and attention to individual circumstances. Expanding a student's knowledge and ability to organize and relate to the space around him has a positive impact in the individual's quality of life and essential sense of control.

O&M instruction for the individual in an extended-care setting is often overlooked. Orientation instruction is essential whether the person is physically active and mobile or has limited capacity for movement. People with visual impairments who also have limited ambulation skills may have reduced travel opportunities and are usually assisted with even short routes, for example, routes from the room or apartment to the dining room or activity area. This increased sense of isolation, loss of control, and decreased

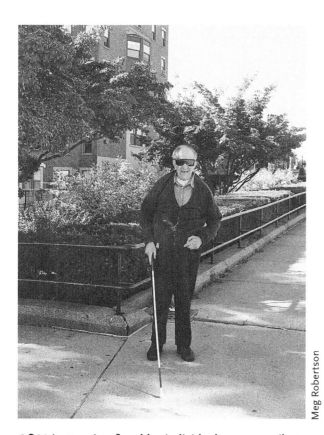

Meg Robertson

O&M instruction for older individuals can contribute to their overall well-being through improved orientation and sense of control over their environment.

opportunity for engagement can easily lead to depression (Blasch et al., 1997). Orientation and mobility instruction for these particular students is essential. Realistically high expectations for the student contribute positively to orientation and overall well-being through a sense of environmental control.

A modified individualized approach to room familiarization is an example of one strategy for the student with visual and physical challenges. The O&M specialist facilitates the cognitive map of the room by using the student's location (chair or bed) as the home base. While the student may not be able to physically walk the perimeter of the area, the essential components of gathering the information remain the same. Cognitive attention may be problematic; therefore, it is helpful to limit the demand on the student by focusing on a limited number of primary points of reference that have particular significance. For the student sitting in a chair, ambulatory or not, these points may be the door to the bedroom, the entrance to the bathroom, and one other point of reference such as a window or closet. The O&M specialist can prompt attention to each of these landmarks by going to each location, and, through auditory cueing, ask the student to point to the O&M specialist's location paired with the landmark. The O&M specialist may then gradually remove the auditory prompts so that the student sustains the cognitive map required to remember the locations. With practice and success, the student can learn the additional details of the perimeter with confidence. As in all sequenced learning, the O&M specialist can increase the level of cognitive demand through higher-level tasks. The transition moves from "I am standing at the entrance to the bathroom door; point to me" to "I am sitting on the bed; point to the entrance to the room" to "I am standing by the window; tell me how to get to the bathroom," demonstrating object-to-object spatial understanding. Whether or not the student is able to physically move to each of these locations, the primary issues of quality of life and well-being are addressed through awareness of the surroundings and a sense of control over the environment.

Beyond room familiarization, the O&M specialist plays a critical role and advocates for the student's right to socialization rather than isolation. The student may not be interested in exploration unless he knows what is outside of his room. The O&M specialist can facilitate that interest by choosing destinations of significance and supporting exploration and familiarity regardless of the student's ambulation abilities.

Strategies for People in Wheelchairs

The population of people with visual impairments who also use a wheelchair is significant enough to warrant mention (see Chapters 5 and 18). Some individuals are unable to bear weight and must use a wheelchair for all mobility. Others may need the wheelchair only due to stamina concerns and may use it occasionally. In either case, orientation instruction is still important and useful for the student to engage more fully with the environment and extend her independence beyond her physical capacity, thus opening opportunities for additional orientation.

For the person who uses any support device, other professionals (for example, physical or occupational therapists) are often members of the service-delivery team. A unified approach, understanding and respecting each professional's goals and methods, results in a collaborative effort to maximize the student's physical and cognitive abilities and resulting outcomes. The student's ability to control and expand her environment is quite possible using the wheelchair as a mobility device.

Orientation information should be taught to the student using a wheelchair, not only for environmental control, but also to avoid the "passive passenger" situation. Held and Hein (1963) conducted landmark research linking experience, action, and perception to self-initiated move-

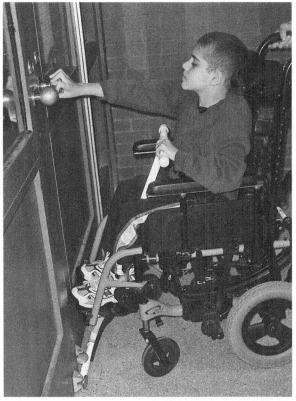

Taan Shapiro

A boy who uses a wheelchair also uses an adaptive mobility device to explore the environment and locate the door.

ment. Similar to a person who rides in a car as a passenger and does not learn the directions to an often-visited destination, the passive passenger may not interact fully with the environment. If the student knows the directions or is oriented to the area, she can direct the driver or person pushing the wheelchair and can participate in the experience, increasing her knowledge (Gregory, 1995).

Thus, cognitive mapping for the student who uses a wheelchair can be addressed regardless of the student's ability to self-propel through the environment. The O&M specialist may provide the momentum and push the wheelchair during the process of exploration, much like serving as a human guide. An example of this instruction uses the floor plan of an extended-care facility as the environmental area that is represented via a map or model containing the information tailored to the student's needs. The O&M specialist establishes time and distance awareness by moving with the student through the route to reinforce the shape of the hallway. The two travel together from one end to the other, focusing on the main hallway first, end to end, generally with an I-shaped route. Whether the O&M specialist concentrates on the entire area or the detail contained within the main hallway depends on the abilities and needs of the student and her overall, practical use of the environment.

A socially engaging opportunity that "personalizes" the landmarks is to introduce the student to the people who live at either end of the hall. This functional integration has practical application—the potential for social interaction and a possible motivation that aids cognitive mapping—by making the end of the hallway the location of Helen's room on the east end and the location of Edward's room on the west end.

It is important to expand perceptual skills in order to maintain orientation established by information points. The O&M specialist may propel the wheelchair and, maintaining orientation, support the student's attention to perceptual information: "What do you hear, see, smell?" (perception and analysis) and "What is useful information for what you want to do?" (hypothesis and plan). Guiding the student through the environment, providing the opportunity to perceive and process perceptual information and test the hypothesis, readies her for problem solving when she becomes disoriented. Providing she achieves success with each of the activities described, the student is likely well oriented to the area and ready for orientation to specific routes of interest. To complete the training, the O&M specialist may test problem solving by using a drop-off lesson anywhere in the learned area.

For the nonambulatory student who knows the environment, informed choices are possible about where she prefers to be—in her room or elsewhere. When transported to other areas, the student can be in control of the environment and exercise cognitive attention by directing the way. Once the student has that feeling of security—knowing where she is and what is around her—the student may have increased confidence and a feeling of safety.

Cognitive Challenges

"Learning to move about the environment with purpose may not come automatically to students who have visual impairments with other disabilities. Effective instructional programs make full use of natural opportunities for movement at home, in school, and within community environments" (Fazzi, 1998, p. 454). As the O&M specialist develops a rapport and gains expertise in reading the student's body language and communication abilities, travel may be better supported and guided through instruction (Sauerburger, Sifferman, & Rosen, 2006).

Orientation for the person with cognitive challenges is modified, mainly, in the approach to teaching. Routes that occur frequently in the student's daily routine should contain obvious landmarks that occur in natural environments. Selecting clear, tangible, and appropriate landmarks that are relevant and interesting to the student helps promote success and creates continued interest in the training.

Students with limited abilities to organize multiple landmarks and sensory clues are frequently assisted by organizing spatial relationships in a concrete, linear fashion. The process is that each landmark triggers an anticipated next landmark, so, for example, landmark A triggers landmark B, B triggers C, and C triggers D. When that sequence is interrupted, for example, when A is followed by B and then D, the missing, yet anticipated, C can be confusing for the student. One strategy to support spatial progression is to encourage, through practice, for the student at point A not only to anticipate B, but also to anticipate that C and D will follow. Then, if the student misses B and ends up at C, the student can problem solve that B was missed and that D is next. This strategy is designed to promote cognitive representation of the route with a starting point, an ending point, and sequential landmarks along the way.

Critical observation helps the O&M specialist determine the student's current spatial organizational skills. How does the student organize spatial information? A student with cognitive impairments may travel from landmark to landmark in a chained fashion with continued contact with the environment. When asked how to get from one place to another, the student might describe a series of continuous landmarks

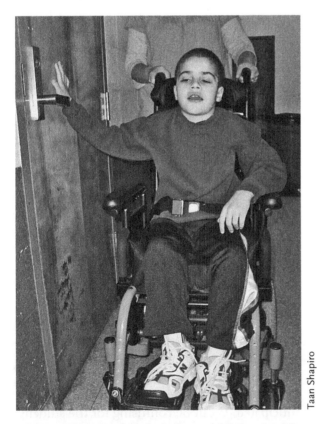

Taan Shapiro

A boy trails the wall to find the next landmark while being pushed in his wheelchair.

that connect to each other, much like a grass line from the fence to the side of the building.

For many students with cognitive disabilities, mobility may appear random. The student may demonstrate little attention to appropriate landmarks that are important to his orientation, yet attend to more temporary objects. Does the student appear to be making meaningful or purposeful movements with any consistency? What perceptual information is available? Is the student responding to the information, or is he missing significant clues?

The O&M specialist may begin the assessment at home, as it provides a familiar environment where the student has accumulated substantial practice and experience. Strategies established at home may be clear indicators of the student's current skills and capacity in new, unfamiliar areas.

Functional routes to the bathroom and various destinations within the home are often the focus of initial lessons. More complex routes (for example, bus travel) are possible with support and modified instructional strategies. One strategy, *task analysis*, involves dividing the overall route into smaller segments and supports the student's ability to complete a part of the route, facilitating confidence. While instruction centers on the smaller pieces, the entire route should be traveled with whatever supports are necessary, so that the order and parts make up the whole (see Volume 1, Chapter 7). A variation of task analysis is *backward chaining* (see Chapters 8 and 19), with instruction beginning with the final portion of the route that leads to the destination. An example is the route from a student's home to the convenience store located on the corner of his block, just down the street. The O&M specialist may divide the route into sections as follows:

- From the student's front door, walk down the front walk to the sidewalk.

- Turn right, and walk to the end of the block, locating the street.

• Walk from the street back to the store, and locate the door.

With backward chaining, the initial lesson emphasizes the route from the street to the store-front and locating the door. The next focus is from the end of the student's front walk to the end of the block, and finding the street. The O&M specialist integrates the segments by supporting the student as he walks each piece, gradually stringing the pieces together to form the entire route from his front door to the store.

Students with developmental disabilities may have difficulty generalizing spatial relationships necessary for cognitive mapping. The O&M specialist can assist purposeful movement by introducing concrete relationships between physical objects in a natural setting that may be used as consecutive landmarks leading to a desired location. This concrete route instruction occurs within practical and functional routines, which makes attention to the task meaningful. The direct link of one landmark to the next is made from the starting point to the destination. Specific sensory support can further sustain this student's travel.

Additional concrete support can be established by introducing auditory landmarks that can be unobtrusively added to the area. One example in a home or work area is to have music in the kitchen playing from a source above the refrigerator. The additional perceptual information provides a rich resource for establishing relationships between the student's location and the kitchen and, specifically, the refrigerator. Having the student locate the refrigerator and remove a sack lunch makes the cognitive effort meaningful and practical. For more complicated routes, verbal and physical prompts provided along the route facilitate success-based repetition and experiential learning. In summary, the O&M specialist needs a variety of tools to construct creative approaches for instruction. Sidebar 2.5 contains Joffee and Ehresman's (1997) special-ized instructional strategies for students with vision loss and developmental disabilities to assist the O&M specialist to construct an effective plan.

CONCLUSION

This chapter presents orientation as an integral part of O&M instruction to enable the student to access and integrate information from the environment. Among the strategies used by the O&M specialist, creativity, simple-to-complex scaffolding, and the goal to teach to the highest level for each student are all part of a successful, individualized plan for the student. Furthermore, a full sensory and discovery learning approach, to "learn by doing," is an effective method for the student to be able to problem solve when traveling and to make sense of an area. Techniques to promote the cognitive organization of spatial information with emphases on sequenced content and the impact of perceptual motor components are keys to a better understanding of orientation and better outcomes for all students.

IMPLICATIONS FOR O&M PRACTICE

1. Orientation is individualized, depending on the goals, interests, and experiences of the student.

2. Infusing orientation into the overall O&M instruction optimizes the teachable moment and can tailor lessons to the student's interests; however, occasionally, orientation may be taught separately from mobility, then integrated within the instruction for generalization and applicability.

3. Orientation strategies may be taught across a continuum, from a simple, concrete, area such as a room or a hall to an abstract environment, such as an entire city grid.

SIDEBAR 2.5

Specialized Instructional Strategies for People with Vision Loss and Developmental Disabilities

- Utilizing hand-over-hand instruction and physical positioning to introduce and monitor indoor mobility and cane techniques, gradually fading this support as learners progress

- Creating a system of prompts, with time frames and milestones for fading prompts

- Providing instruction using communication strategies (verbal and/or non-verbal) that are appropriate for the student's learning needs

- Providing abundant opportunities for repetition and successful experiences during lessons, and opportunities to practice and utilize skills between lessons

- Providing several shortened periods of instruction throughout the school day

- Providing O&M instruction in a natural setting at the time when movement skills are utilized

- Breaking down instructional activities related to teaching travel routes using a task analysis approach

- Participating with the learner in the activity just prior to and immediately following an O&M lesson, to help the learner make the transition to and from an O&M lesson that is integrated in daily routines

- Beginning O&M lessons at a learner's favorite place or in a very familiar location and building to lessons that address travel needs in other locations

- Breaking a long daily travel route into segments and introducing learners to portion of the route, gradually piecing together the full route

- Introducing new O&M skills with the cooperation of a significant person in the learner's life, who has a good rapport with the student

Source: Reprinted with permission from Elga Joffee and Paul Ehresman, "Learners with Visual and Cognitive Impairments," in Bruce B. Blasch, William R. Wiener, and Richard L. Welsh, Eds., *Foundations of Orientation and Mobility, 2nd ed.* (New York: American Foundation for the Blind, 1997), pp. 490–492.

4. Spatial concepts are critical foundations to effective orientation and can be assessed prior to and during the instructional sequence.

5. The O&M specialist expects the student to functionally demonstrate her understanding of a particular concept, route, or spatial relationship rather than rely on verbal explanations that may not actually reflect the student's skill and understanding.

6. Spatial updating is egocentric and assists the student to understand the changing relationships between herself and people or objects in the environment as she moves through an area.

7. The O&M specialist can utilize the drop-off lesson as an amazing tool to teach the student problem-solving skills in order to reestablish orientation and may be used in any area once the student has some familiarization with the surroundings.

8. As with any instruction, creativity can help the O&M specialist to individualize teaching and improve the outcomes for the student.

LEARNING ACTIVITIES

1. Discuss the four areas of spatial development and provide some examples of their application to orientation.

2. List some causes of veering and how the O&M specialist can teach the student to improve straight line of travel.

3. Discuss two learning strategies used to break a route into smaller, more attainable segments.

4. What is the concept of the "passive passenger," and how does it relate to orientation and mobility?

5. How would an O&M specialist use the strategies of self-talk and parallel talk to teach orientation?

Improving the Use of Low Vision for Orientation and Mobility

Duane R. Geruschat and Audrey J. Smith

LEARNING QUESTIONS

- What are the major components to a comprehensive functional low vision mobility assessment?

- How does the environment affect visual ability when walking?

- Why is it important to develop good visual skills prior to the introduction of optical devices?

- Why is the power of a telescope a critical issue during the teaching process?

- Can a person with less than full vision drive a car safely?

Chapter 3 of Volume 1, "Low Vision for Orientation and Mobility," presents the key concepts and background information that should be considered when providing orientation and mobility (O&M) services to students with low vision. For the purposes of this chapter, low vision

is defined as usable vision, not fully correctable by conventional eyeglasses, which results in difficulty with the visual tasks of mobility. The most common functional low vision mobility problems (glare, lighting, light adaptation; changes in terrain and elevation; unwanted contacts; crossing streets) are described in Volume 1, Chapter 3. In addition, differences between various groupings of eye pathologies are highlighted, with central vision loss (for example, macular degeneration) resulting in a different type of mobility problem from that caused by peripheral vision loss (for example, advanced glaucoma or retinitis pigmentosa). This chapter presents methods for assessing low vision mobility followed by strategies for teaching low vision mobility without optical devices, and then strategies for teaching low vision mobility with optical devices. The chapter also addresses the effects of congenital onset versus adventitious loss of vision, and the differences in some of the teaching approaches caused by the dissimilar life experiences and the different needs resulting from the time of onset of low vision.

In preparation for the mobility assessment, background information should be obtained from a clinical low vision eye exam, and an interview should be completed with the student who will be receiving O&M services. This information will help the O&M specialist to tailor the assessment to more efficiently identify mobility problems. For example, obtaining the visual acuity, visual field, and pathology from the clinical eye report, knowing from the interview with the student that independent travel to the house of worship, bank, medical care, and grocery is the reason to seek mobility instruction, and learning that these locations are in the immediate area of five blocks from the home the student has lived in for 20 years facilitates the tailoring of the assessment to identify the types of abilities and challenges that will need to be addressed when planning the instructional program.

CLINICAL LOW VISION ASSESSMENT

The clinical low vision examination varies in scope depending on the provider but usually contains the following primary components:

1. Visual acuity
2. Visual field
3. Refractive error
4. Ocular health
5. Response to optical devices
6. Specialized testing

One of the primary goals of the clinical low vision exam is to document what the student can see under ideal viewing conditions. Ideally, the clinical low vision examination is completed by a qualified ophthalmologist or optometrist either prior to the O&M specialist's provision of service or shortly after the O&M specialist has begun the O&M assessment. Although additional certification as a low vision specialist is not a requirement, the professional organizations representing the different eye care specialists have diplomate programs that offer this specialty. The examiner attempts to control the major visual factors (lighting, contrast, size, and so forth) that provide the student with optimal vision.

Visual Acuity

Measurement of visual acuity defines the smallest size print or target the student can accurately identify at a certain distance. Figure 3.1 is one example of a visual acuity chart. The result is reported as a fraction and provides a general sense of the amount of clarity the student possesses when looking at objects. In the visual acuity fraction, the numerator represents the viewing distance from the measuring chart and the denominator represents the size of the smallest letter that can be correctly identified. For example, a visual acuity of 20/200 (6/60) indicates that the testing occurred at 20 feet (6 m) with a 200 (60) size letter being correctly identified. In more functional language, a student with 20/200 visual acuity will see at 20 feet what someone with 20/20 (6/6) vision can see from 200 feet (60 m). Because clinical visual acuity is tested with a standardized chart with consistent illumination, the results are expected to be repeatable. By comparison, the natural environment can introduce many other factors that affect functional visual acuity. For example, when looking at a street sign, what is the background, contrast, and angle of viewing? Acknowledging the measure of clinical visual acuity does not predict mobility performance; it does increase the O&M specialist's ability to anticipate the ability of a student to accomplish various tasks (for example, read street signs or bus numbers).

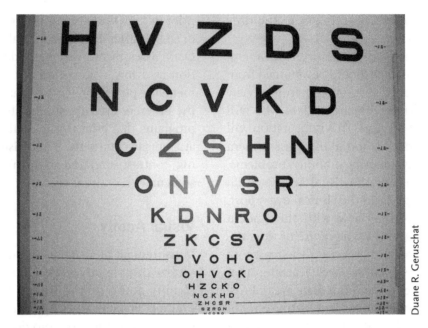

Duane R. Geruschat

Figure 3.1.
Visual acuity can be tested by using specially designed charts that allow finer discriminations in acuity levels for people with low vision.

Visual Field

Mapping the visual field is especially important and useful for designing a program of mobility instruction. Unfortunately visual fields can be difficult and time-consuming to obtain, so a low vision clinic may not always provide a clinical visual field. Four different clinical visual field tests can be administered: (1) confrontation; (2) Amsler grid; (3) tangent screen; and (4) perimetry. *Confrontation* visual field testing is a screening procedure involving lights or objects that are presented from the periphery and gradually moved in from various angles toward the central field. This test yields functional information rather than a precise clinical measurement. It provides a general estimate of the size and location of peripheral field losses. For the O&M specialist, this screening is especially valuable since it is easily administered, requires little equipment, and evaluates the peripheral visual field, which is of particular importance to mo-

bility. This approach is also useful with young children and students with severe multiple impairments as a quick screening for use at school or home.

The *Amsler grid* is a clinical assessment of the central 10 degrees of the visual field. It is useful for identifying the size and location of a small central scotoma caused by maculopathy—pathologies such as age-related macular degeneration (AMD) or Stargardt disease. The Amsler grid shown in Figure 3.2 provides findings that can be useful for understanding how a student uses vision for activities related to fine detail, such as reading a bus schedule or using a telescope to read a street sign.

The *tangent screen* shown in Figure 3.3 is another type of clinical field assessment for low vision, testing the central 25–30 degrees of the visual field. Because it describes both the central and midperipheral visual fields, the tangent screen results can address both near-point and mobility activities.

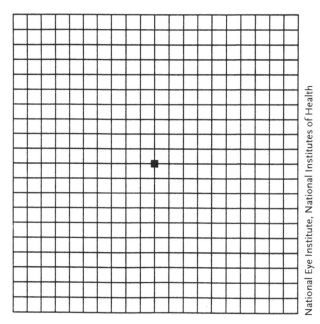

National Eye Institute, National Institutes of Health

Figure 3.2.
The Amsler grid is a tool used to test the area of central vision.

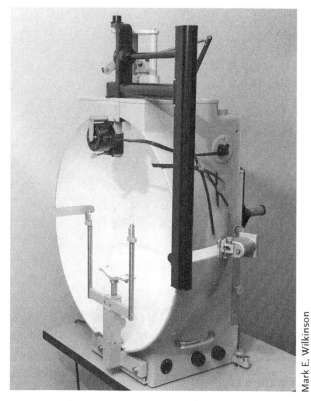

Mark E. Wilkinson

Figure 3.4.
The Goldmann perimeter (arc perimeter) is used to evaluate the entire visual field and identify significant vision losses.

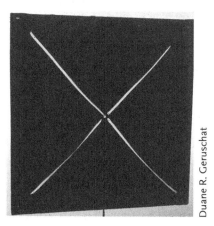

Duane R. Geruschat

Figure 3.3.
The tangent screen is used to test the visual field within 25–30 degrees of fixation.

The *Goldmann perimeter* shown in Figure 3.4 evaluates the entire visual field. This test is useful for mobility instruction as its results often identify areas of significant field loss, such as

hemianopsia, and restricted fields due to advanced glaucoma or retinitis pigmentosa.

Computerized visual field assessment is the most common assessment in eye clinics (see Figure 3.5). The advantage of the computerized assessment is that it is standardized and does not require a skilled perimetrist to administer the test. The disadvantages for a low vision clinic are that it has a limited range of target size and brightness, with many students with low vision not having enough vision to see the target.

Identifying the location of field losses helps to explain travel difficulties, which is especially important information for the O&M specialist. One challenge for the O&M specialist is to understand which field test to consider. The different

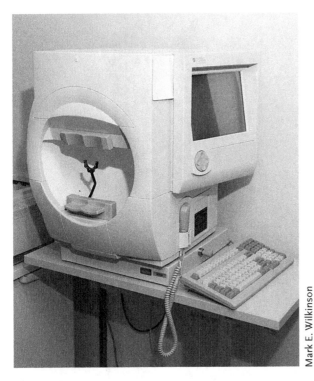

Mark E. Wilkinson

Figure 3.5.
The Humphrey automated perimeter, a computerized visual field assessment.

visual field assessments can be remembered through a common example of route planning. The use of road maps to help plan before and navigate during a trip is analogous to the use of field tests to help plan for understanding potential mobility performance. For example, when planning to travel from Chicago to Washington, D.C., one would begin by looking at a map of the United States (arc perimeter). This map would allow one to determine the interstate roads between Illinois and Washington. To identify the specific road for entering Washington, D.C., one would need a map of Virginia, Maryland, and the District of Columbia (tangent screen). The exact roads for entering Washington, D.C., and the location of the Capitol would require a detailed map of the District of Columbia (Amsler grid). Which map one chooses involves identifying the question one wants to answer. Similarly, which

field test the O&M specialist chooses involves determining what area of the visual field is required to complete the functional task. For example, reading a street map or train schedule involves the central visual field, which is best described by the Amsler grid or tangent screen, while walking on the sidewalk is a general task involving the entire visual field, which is best evaluated by a full perimetry field test. Just as a map of the District of Columbia will not answer the question of how to travel from Chicago to Washington, D.C., the Amsler grid will not answer the question of why someone is consistently bumping into objects on the left side.

Refractive Error

Refractive error determines whether the eye has too much or not enough bending power, and what type and amount of prescription eyeglasses will correct this condition. There are three primary types of refractive error: hyperopia, myopia, and astigmatism. A schematic drawing of refractive errors is provided in Figure 3.6.

Briefly, *hyperopia*, or farsightedness, is when a distant image focuses at a point behind the retina, requiring a plus (+) or convex-shaped lens to bring the image forward to focus it onto the retina. Functionally, the student with hyperopia experiences difficulty clearly seeing objects up close, such as when reading a bus schedule. *Myopia*, or nearsightededness, is when a distant image focuses at a point in front of the retina, requiring a minus (–) or concave-shaped lens to bring the image to focus farther back onto the retina. Functionally the student with myopia experiences difficulty seeing objects or reading signs in the distance, such as when reading a street sign. Both hyperopia and myopia are corrected with a spherical lens, offering the necessary plus or minus correction in all planes of the lens. *Astigmatism* is an irregular or uneven shape of the cornea, lens, or both. This irregularity is similar to looking through a windowpane of

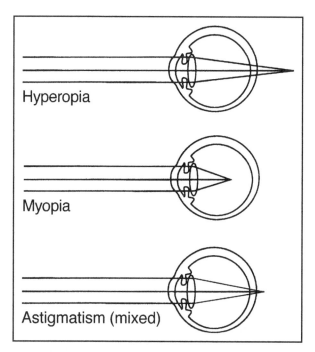

Figure 3.6.
The three most common types of refractive error: hyperopia, myopia, and astigmatism.

very old glass. As one scans through the glass, a thin line of irregularity may appear. This irregularity in the window is similar to the problem of astigmatism. It is corrected with a cylindrical lens that offers correction in only one plane of the lens (known as the axis of astigmatism), corresponding to the identified plane of irregularity. Comprehensive and functional explanations of refractive errors are available in Smith and Cote (2001), Jose (1983), or Chalkley (2000).

For the O&M specialist, it is important to understand the difference between eyeglasses that correct for refractive error and eyeglasses that are prescribed for assisting with magnification. Eyeglasses that correct for refractive error can be worn for most mobility activities, while eyeglasses for magnification (microscopic spectacles) are worn only to see print or objects at a close distance when the student is stationary.

Ocular Health

The basic examination procedures for ocular health are the same for students with low vision as they are for the general public. More extensive examinations may occur if there is concern about a specific pathology. This component of the eye exam begins with analysis of the external eye. Examinations of the eyelids, eye alignment, and response of the pupils to light are the most common elements. Next is the examination of the internal structures of the eye. The cornea, aqueous, and front portion of the lens are evaluated with a biomicroscope, also known as a slit lamp (see Figure 3.7a). Examination of the retina is the final step. With the pupil dilated, the direct ophthalmoscope (Figure 3.7b) or the indirect ophthalmoscope (Figure 3.7c) can be used to perform a comprehensive examination of the retina (Riordan-Eva, Asbury, & Whitcher, 2008).

The clinical low vision assessment provides the O&M specialist with a baseline of the student's visual status. By obtaining clinical information under ideal viewing conditions, in which all visual factors that often degrade functional vision are controlled, the eye care specialist serves a valuable role in describing the visual status of the student. Measures of visual acuity, visual field, refractive error, the health status of the eye, and the student's response to optical devices are useful precursors to effective education or rehabilitation intervention.

Response to Optical Devices

The one aspect of the eye exam that is unique to low vision is response to optical devices. During this part of the examination, the student is presented with a variety of optical devices to determine how visual acuity changes while the student is looking through the device. The working assumption is that acuity will improve, but the issue is whether it will improve as much as expected. For example, when the student is

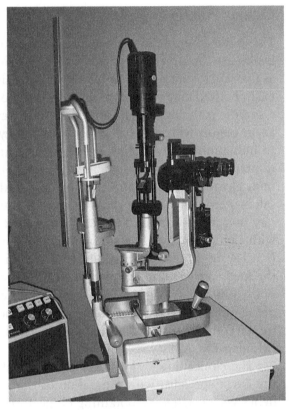

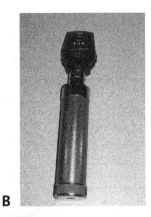

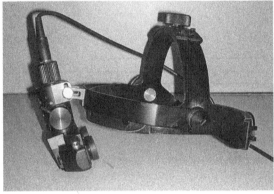

Duane R. Geruschat

Figures 3.7.
The three most commonly used instruments in a general eye examination are the (A) biomicroscope or slit lamp, (B) direct ophthalmoscope, and (C) indirect ophthalmoscope.

presented with a 4× telescope, visual acuity is expected to improve by approximately 4 times such that a student with 20/120 (6/36) visual acuity will have approximately 20/30 (6/9) visual acuity when viewing through the 4× telescope (120 divided by 4 equals 30). If the acuity does not improve, the student's response may be due to a variety of issues that will need to be explored by the eye care specialist.

Specialized Testing

Binocularity

Binocularity is the ability of the two eyes to work together. Functionally, this allows the brain to

fuse the information from the two eyes into one image, providing depth perception. Binocularity primarily involves the central vision of both eyes, which is usually reduced in students seen by a mobility specialist. As a general statement, the majority of students receiving mobility instruction have unequal acuity, or have a significant eye turn (for example, esotropia, exotropia) that precludes any possibility for the eyes to work together in a binocular fashion.

Many students have remaining vision in both eyes but with unequal acuity such that the brain cannot merge the two images into one. These individuals are biocular. Though both eyes work, they do not work together to form one image. In mobility, the peripheral vision of both eyes will provide critical information regardless of whether the student is biocular or binocular. If there is a question as to whether someone is binocular, the eye care specialist can perform a variety of tests specifically designed to make this determination.

Color Vision Testing

Color vision screening is accomplished with iso-chromatic plates. In this screening the student is required to look at a card containing small circles of various colors. In the center of the card is either a number or a letter that can be seen if the student sees the specific color. The complete screening involves a series of plates with varying colors. If the letters or numbers cannot be distinguished, then a comprehensive vision test may be ordered. The comprehensive color vision test is called the Farnsworth D15 test of color vision. This test requires the student to sequence various shadings of one area of the color spectrum. The sequence is recorded on a score sheet, which provides an analysis of any color deficit. The time required to complete this test limits its use with students who have low vision. In a mobility context, color identification and color cues are useful to identify landmarks as well as landmark functions. For example, an object near the street corner that is slightly higher than head height and is seen as red, even if the shape and letters cannot be identified, is usually a stop sign.

Contrast Sensitivity Function

Contrast sensitivity function measures the ability to discriminate various shades of gray. This test, shown in Figure 3.8, involves identifying letters that begin as high-contrast black letters on a white background and gradually are reduced in contrast. The requirement is to read the lightest shade of letters possible. This is an estimate of the student's peak contrast sensitivity. If color vision is impaired, contrast is quite useful in mobility, as environmental details such as curbs or

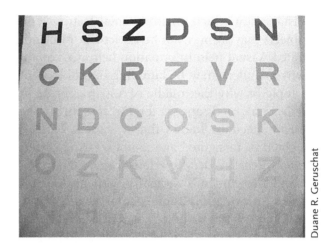

Duane R. Geruschat

Figure 3.8.
A chart used to test contrast sensitivity.

outdoor stairs may then consist only of shades of gray. This type of testing has been shown to be highly predictive of mobility performance.

FUNCTIONAL LOW VISION MOBILITY ASSESSMENT

There are five components to a low vision mobility assessment: (1) review of information from the clinical low vision examination; (2) interview; (3) assessment of functional vision; (4) assessment of the student's mobility in different travel environments (critical incidents assessment); and (5) assessment of the travel environment. Each component of the assessment contributes a piece of the puzzle that ultimately forms a comprehensive understanding of the student's low vision mobility needs and abilities.

Review of Clinical Examination Information

As discussed previously, a review of the findings from the clinical examination helps the O&M specialist to anticipate specific mobility difficulties. For example, visual acuity information can help the O&M instructor to anticipate the distances at which environmental features and objects may or may not be noticed or discriminated. Visual field information helps to explain why a student may be bumping into objects or people or why the middle of a map appears to fade away or disappear for the student. If the O&M specialist knows that a student is near-sighted or farsighted and is not wearing corrective lenses, the O&M specialist can better understand the student's difficulty with near or far tasks. Information about ocular health, especially the ocular pathology, can be a critical tool for the mobility specialist. Knowing that a student has high ocular pressure, or is prone to retinal detachment, or has diabetic low blood sugar periods, helps the mobility specialist to anticipate the mobility challenges the various pathologies could present. Information about contrast sensitivity and color vision provides details about whether or not objects under varying contrast conditions such as curbs and stairs, or the color of a light at a street crossing, may or may not be seen.

Although clinical information is a valuable resource, the student's performance in real-world mobility situations cannot be predicted from it. Clinical reports assist the O&M specialist in quantifying the level of visual functioning under static conditions using standardized charts and stimuli. What remains to be determined is the functional level of vision under everyday dynamic situations, under varying lighting conditions, and with real-world objects of various sizes and contrast. Careful observation of how these factors impact a student's mobility performance in different environments is central to what the O&M specialist needs to assess.

Low Vision Mobility Interview

Depending on the style and personality of the O&M specialist and the student, the interview can occur in a variety of ways (structured questionnaire, open-ended conversation). After some experience with clients, O&M instructors find that an open-ended discussion is usually preferred, with the interviewer guiding and monitoring the process to obtain the necessary information, while remaining sensitive to the student's unique needs and concerns.

Basic levels of information that are important to obtain in the functional assessment and instructional process include the following:

- *Student needs, concerns, and goals.* The O&M specialist ought to ask the student to describe his or her mobility goals and desired level of independence. If the student is unsure or not very specific, the O&M specialist can prompt the student's thinking by exploring school, employment, recreation, and other areas where the student may have mobility needs and concerns.

- *Demographic information and emergency contacts.* The O&M specialist should obtain the necessary demographic and contact information for emergency situations.

- *Diagnostic information, including visual and medical diagnoses, as well as medications and their systemic and visual side effects.* This information is necessary for anticipating visual and physical limitations and for planning for weather conditions and times of the day for mobility lessons.

- *Previous mobility instruction.* It is helpful for the O&M specialist to ask about the time and duration of previous instruction and whether any periodic follow-up was provided. If possible, the O&M specialist should review records and contact previous instructors for additional information and suggestions.

- *Self-reported areas of proficiency and problems regarding vision and mobility performance.* The O&M specialist ought to ask what the student perceives as her own areas of proficiency or strength in mobility. Is the student currently traveling independently? What does the student perceive as difficult to do or as requiring assistance? Explore how the student perceives vision in the context of mobility. Is independent mobility limited or avoided because of visual status? Is there a fear of independent travel? What was the level of independent travel prior to the loss of vision? What does the student feel are the most significant mobility issues or problems? A listing of common self-reported problems with mobility can be found in Turano, Geruschat, Massof, and Stahl (1999) and Smith, De l'Aune, and Geruschat (1992).

- *Use of assistive devices—cane; dog guide; optical, nonoptical, and electronic travel aids.* The O&M specialist ought to ask whether any visual or mobility devices have been prescribed to assist in functional vision or mobility. Is the student using them and at what level or frequency? Does the student find them to be helpful? Why or why not?

- *Questions and comments.* It is important that the O&M specialist allow time for any questions the student may have about the specialist's role, what to expect regarding lessons and time together, and the like. It is helpful for the specialist to clarify expectations and offer assurances that the O&M specialist is planning *with* and not *for* the student and that instruction will emphasize the specific needs and goals of the student.

Assessment of Functional Vision

Functional Visual Acuity

Clinical measures of visual acuity are obtained in a static, controlled environment. By design, functional acuity is obtained in the uncontrolled environment, which is affected by a wide range of visual factors. For example, during the course of a typical walk, functional vision may fluctuate because of variations in the size of objects, changes in illumination, and complexity of the environment (frequency of stairs, lighting, volume of other pedestrians, and so on). The combination of low vision and environmental variation often results in a range of functional visual ability from no measurable acuity (functioning as totally blind) to the ability to see small cracks in the sidewalk and the change of a traffic light from red to green, and to identify people moving at distances greater than 100 feet (30 m). These differences may all be caused by changes in contrast and illumination and by the effects of glare.

Because functional visual performance fluctuates, it is important to determine functional vision acuities in a variety of environments and under a variety of lighting conditions. Different approaches can be effective. Ludt and Goodrich (2002) and Goodrich and Ludt (2003) described an approach to functional vision assessment known as Dynamic Visual Assessment and Training. Their research shows that pre-test functional assessment is a good predictor of postinstruction performance.

There are other approaches to the assessment of functional visual acuities. For example, functional visual acuity can be divided into three types:

- *Awareness acuity*—the farthest possible distance at which the presence of any form is *first* detected yet not able to be identified. This is determined by asking the student to look as far away as possible and indicate when the presence of any form is *first* detected. Examples may include building shapes contrasted against the sky, blobs or blurs of colors, and indistinguishable objects, shapes, and contrasts.

- *Identification acuity*—the farthest possible distance at which a detected form is *first* correctly identified. The O&M specialist can ask the student to slowly move forward after awareness is obtained to identify the same detected form from the farthest possible distance. As an example, the student might say, "That red blob is beginning to look like a car."

- *Preferred viewing distance*—the most comfortable distance for identifying a detected form. The O&M specialist can ask the student to continue to move forward until she is at a distance comfortable enough to provide sure identification (for example, "I'm definitely sure now that it's a car").

Everyone who has vision, whether fully or partially sighted, can detect and identify the presence of objects at greater distances, yet feels more comfortable working at shorter, preferred distances. The exception may be those with severely constricted visual fields who prefer a greater viewing distance to fit more detail into their narrow field of view.

One of the great benefits of vision is that it allows us to function at a variety of distances that are dependent on the acuity that is required to complete the task. When selecting tasks for the assessment of functional acuity, the O&M specialist needs to choose tasks that require different distances and ought to use objects of various sizes for the purpose of gaining a fuller understanding of their effect on awareness, identification, and preferred viewing distance acuity. For example, activities that are typically completed at near and intermediate ranges, such as reading a bus schedule, building directories, or menus in fast-food restaurants, can be introduced along with those involving the detection and identification of traffic lights, people, cars, and the like at greater distances.

This portion of the assessment should be conducted in familiar and unfamiliar environments, and under different real-world lighting conditions. A comprehensive functional acuity assessment necessitates repeated measures at different times on different days, in both indoor and outdoor environments. In essence, the O&M specialist takes advantage of the naturally occur-

ring variation of the environment: different settings, cloudy and sunny conditions, bright and dim lighting. The pieces of the puzzle are gradually assembled to create an understanding of the range of functional visual acuity, and the factors that facilitate or hinder functional acuity. An example of an excerpt from a low vision mobility assessment report describing a student's functional vision acuity might read as follows:

Optimum visual acuity occurs on cloudy days, when Stephanie is first able to detect the presence of cars, trees, and larger objects at distances of 80–100 feet (24–30 m). She first correctly identifies these objects at 50–60 feet (15–18 m) but feels most comfortable identifying them at approximately 20 feet (6 m). On sunny days, Stephanie's functional acuity is reduced to 40 feet (12 m) for awareness of these large objects and to 15 feet (4.5 m) before they are first correctly identified. The presence of glare, directly from the sun or indirectly from reflective surfaces, further reduces her functional acuity to a range of 1–5 feet (30 cm to 1.5 m), depending on the size and contrast of the object being viewed (bold contrast increases her distance identification). Indoors, under overhead fluorescent lighting, Stephanie is aware of the presence of another student at 35 feet (10 m) and identifies him by facial detail at 6–8 feet (1.8–2.4 m). She identifies a posted bus schedule in the main terminal from 6 feet (1.8 m) and reads it with a 4× short-focus telescope from 2.5 feet (75 cm). Stephanie demonstrates significant reduction in acuity when adapting to lighting changes—outdoors to indoors (30 seconds to 1 minute) and indoors to outdoors (1 to 2 minutes)—before her acuity stabilizes.

Functional Visual Fields

Similar to the clinical testing of visual acuity, the clinical assessment of the visual field occurs in a setting that controls for illumination, the size of the target, and the distance at which the test is administered. By comparison, assessment of the functional visual field occurs in a variety of environments and lighting conditions. This occurs by applying the same principles of assessing visual acuity to the assessment of the visual field. For example, illumination was mentioned as an important factor to vary during the evaluation because of its effect on acuity. It is also important to vary illumination during the assessment of functional visual fields since reduction in lighting often results in a reduction of the functional field. Functional field assessment uses real-world settings with everyday objects such as people, cars, signs, and objects in a variety of sizes. To measure a functional visual field, the O&M specialist needs to assess the following features.

Static visual field. This measure of the outermost boundaries of the visual field is performed in the natural environment, with the student in a static position, keeping head and eyes still.

Standing still, keeping the head and eyes still, the student is asked to fixate straight ahead on a stationary object in the distance (the distance depends on the purpose of the assessment). For example, when the assessment is conducted outside, the student is asked to fixate on something down the block. The student describes what can be seen at the highest, lowest, and farthest boundaries to the left and right. This provides an estimate of the student's far distance field of view. The O&M specialist might also want to get a sense of the student's field of view while viewing a map or page of print. In this case, the target may be within 6 inches (15 cm). Examples of excerpts from a report describing a student's static visual field might read as follows:

Tony appears to have relatively full visual fields. He noted the edge of the rug directly in front of his feet, the ceiling fan hanging from the 8-foot (2.4 m)-high ceiling, as well as posters on both sides of the 6-foot (1.8 m)-wide hall and 4 feet (1.2 m) in front.

When Mary is looking at a page of print from 6 inches (15 cm), she has a 4-inch (10 cm) field of view. All other words are not visible in her field unless she moves her head to see them.

Depending on what the O&M specialist wants to learn about the visual field, it may be helpful to obtain functional field measures at near, intermediate, and distance points, especially to show the effect of different distances on the diameter of functional field (that is, the closer one is to the target, the smaller the functional field of view, and as the distance from the target increases, the larger the apparent functional field). Sometimes when the student is moving around, less functional field may be noticed, as concentration may be focused in only select areas of the field.

Preferred visual field. This dynamic measure of a student's regular pattern of viewing in everyday environments places no limitations on head or eye movement, and emphasis is on the areas of the visual field where information is most often obtained.

The student walks and tells the O&M specialist everything seen. The specialist tells the student to look around normally, without placing limitations on head or eye movements. The O&M specialist observes the student's regular pattern of viewing (for example, frequent scanning, consistently gazes downward, and so on), and where visual information about the environment is obtained (for example, notices only objects on the right side). Using a chart like the ones in Figure 3.9, with the center point representing the student's straight-ahead view, the O&M specialist places a mark corresponding to where the student describes each object or student. By the end of the session, a pattern will emerge that describes the preferred visual field.

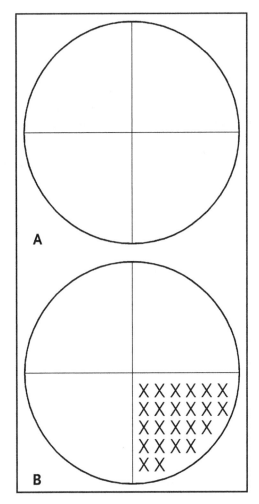

Figure 3.9.
Examples of a (A) blank and a (B) completed chart on which a student's preferred vision field is plotted.

An example of an excerpt from a sample report describing a student's preferred visual field might read as follows:

> Ryan consistently gazed downward and ahead. He noted most objects in the lower field of view and within 3–6 feet (90 cm–1.8 m) ahead. Some objects were noted infrequently on the lower right side, but no objects were noted on his left side.

Once the assessment data have been collected, it is useful to compare the findings. For example, the static assessment provides the area of visual field available to the student. The preferred field assessment tells the O&M specialist what area of existing field the student is actually using, given a dynamic situation, with no restrictions on how or where looking occurs. The findings from these two types of visual fields are often very different. Conducting a preferred visual field assessment yields the most significant information for the O&M specialist, as it more accurately reflects how the student uses his or her field of view for mobility purposes. The static visual field is important because it suggests how much potential exists for changing and improving scanning ability.

A final functional field assessment is recommended for students with known or suspected constricted fields. It is particularly helpful for determining how a field loss might affect early detection of objects or people at the sides.

Peripheral constriction or early warning field. This measure of peripheral, or side, visual field is performed in everyday environments, with the student in a static position, keeping the head and eyes still and centered.

The student stands still, fixating straight ahead on a distant object. Standing next to the student's shoulder, the O&M specialist walks a straight line that is parallel to the student's line of sight; the student indicates when any part of the O&M specialist is first visually detected. This same procedure is repeated on the other side. This assessment provides information on the amount of field restriction on each side and estimates the extent of the functional field loss. An example of an excerpt from a sample report describing a student's peripheral constriction or early warning field might read as follows:

> Lisa was visually aware of my passing by her right side when I was approximately 3 feet (90 cm) away. After 3 feet (90 cm), she had consistent visual awareness along her entire right

side. On the left side, she demonstrated less field awareness, and was not able to detect me passing by until I was 6–8 feet (1.8–2.4 m) away. This may help to explain her frequent bumping into objects, especially on her left side. If she is looking straight ahead, she will not detect objects or people on her left side within 6 feet (1.8 m) from her, unless she turns her head to scan.

Review of clinical findings and completion of functional acuity and field assessments provide the O&M specialist with an understanding of the student's functional use of vision and insights into the potential to enhance mobility through instruction in the use of vision. This information, obtained in various settings and under different lighting conditions, enables the O&M specialist and the student being assessed to explain and predict visual functioning. In addition, the O&M specialist is now better able to assist the student in understanding what frequently has seemed a puzzling, inconsistent visual picture, while teaching the student to know when vision may or may not be relied on and when other sensory information or mobility devices will be of benefit for safe travel. O&M instruction for low vision is philosophically designed to teach the student to become proactive with visual abilities for increased safety and mobility efficiency.

If the student is currently using optical devices, these devices should be included in the functional evaluation. If the student does not use optical devices, he or she should be informed of the options and potential benefits of a complete evaluation and the possible use of both optical and nonoptical devices to enhance visual functioning.

Other mobility devices, such as a long cane, dog guide, and electronic travel devices, can also be included in the dynamic assessment. A great deal can be learned by comparing visual behavior with and without assistive mobility devices.

Many students do not realize the increase in visual functioning that can come from using devices. For instance, when a cane is used to detect changes in elevation such as curbs and stairs, vision is freed for object identification, orientation purposes, and viewing at greater distances, both with and without devices such as telescopes.

Critical Incidents Assessment

A comprehensive mobility assessment is accomplished over a number of hours on different days. It involves assessment in both familiar and unfamiliar areas, in indoor and outdoor settings, under varying lighting conditions, and at different times of the day.

Whether the O&M specialist has the time to complete a comprehensive or only a brief assessment, the use of the critical incidents approach is helpful in determining areas of mobility proficiency and difficulty. The critical incidents assessment focuses on observing independent travel and identifying mobility problems as they naturally occur. These problems or incidents are behaviors not normally observed in students with full vision, such as bumping and tripping, and include behavioral changes such as head or postural changes, and signs of tension such as clenched fists or slow gait. Acknowledging the more common approaches to assessment involving the completion of a prearranged form that directs the O&M specialist's attention toward collating information for prescribed assessment items, we strongly encourage the instructor to try the critical incidents approach because it individualizes the assessment. Attention is directed to observation of the student rather than completion of a prescribed form, and there are no predetermined areas to fit the student into.

When conducting a critical incidents assessment, the O&M specialist observes the student's mobility performance, noting mobility problems (critical incidents) in the order they naturally occur. At the completion of a route, the O&M specialist can group and tally critical incidents (for example, bumping into an object, missing a step or curb, shuffling feet, underreaching, considerably slowing pace, misjudging a street crossing, becoming disoriented, clenching fists, tightening shoulders). An example of an excerpt from a sample report describing the assessment of a student's critical incidents might read as follows:

> Bill decreases his pace and moves with hesitation in the brightly lit bus terminal. He frequently scans from side to side, and demonstrates no reciprocal arm and leg swing. Bill experiences problems reading the information board due to an insufficient amount of light on the board. Natural sunlight is preferred, while fluorescent lights cause visual discomfort. Moving into the bus terminal, he experienced approximately 30 seconds of decreased vision. In response to this, Bill stood to the side until his eyes adapted to the new light level. He avoided objects on his right side but periodically bumped into people passing on his left side. In the terminal's fast-food restaurant, he experienced difficulty reading the overhead food menu because of glare reflecting from fluorescent lights. Bill was able to locate the first and last steps to the train platform with the help of high-contrast colored strips on the steps (normally he experiences difficulty identifying the first step, consequently shuffling his feet to detect the edge of the step).

Where possible, a description of the incident is followed by more detailed information, such as the following:

> Bill bumped into a shoulder-high object on the right side, tripped down a 6-inch (15 cm) curb, and did not see a turning car from the left before stepping into the street (no side-to-side scanning).

In addition, the environmental conditions should be described. For example, lighting, contrast, glare, pedestrian volume, and complexity of the environment can be important environmental features, and a student can be expected to exhibit different abilities to negotiate the same mobility routes at different times of the day or under different lighting conditions.

What emerges are clusters of the most frequently occurring critical incidents or mobility problems unique to each student, as well as student behaviors and environmental variables that contribute to them. An individualized plan of instruction can then be developed, plotting the goals and instructional objectives that guide the direction of intervention.

Environmental Assessment

Systematic analysis of environmental factors is a reflection of the importance attributed to the effects of the environment on functional vision. Teaching students about the effects of the environment can improve their understanding of how environmental changes affect their visual ability. They, in turn, can use this information to become better consumers and increase their independence.

Everyone who has functional vision has experienced situations where vision is not optimal for completing a task. Two examples are moving about in a dark bedroom to locate the bathroom and walking into a dimly lit movie theater on a sunny afternoon. In both situations, even marginal amounts of vision can have positive effects on mobility. For example, the glow of a streetlight or the moon through a window may provide enough ambient vision to locate the edge of the bathroom door. In the movie theater, standing at the back of the theater for 30 seconds may provide sufficient time to adapt to the low level of illumination, allowing one to become oriented to the seating layout and to walk to an empty seat. With an understanding that the environment plays a critical role in how one uses one's vision, a comprehensive functional low vision mobility assessment must consider the environment in which the assessment is occurring, as the student does not function in a static setting with environmental variables controlled.

Independence in the context of mobility depends on two main factors: the ability of the student and the demands of the environment and task. As long as the student's ability is equal to or exceeds the demands of the task, independence can be maintained. Problems occur when the demands of the environment and task exceed the student's abilities. This relationship is dynamic and will change as the environment or the student's vision or skills change.

Determining the impact of the environment on mobility involves analysis of several environmental characteristics, such as space layout, movement patterns, and objects in the environment. Mobility lessons are contingent on the specific environment in which the student is traveling. For example, lessons are sequenced from indoors to outdoors, residential to small business, and quiet areas to crowded city centers. These sequences recognize the effects of changes in pedestrian and vehicular traffic, weather, and so on. Lessons are specifically sequenced to gradually increase the number and complexity of environmental characteristics. The O&M specialist is constantly analyzing the environment to determine the cause of, and solutions to, problems. For example, after accurately crossing a series of streets, the student may become confused because of an offset intersection (where the center line of a road is shifted laterally on the opposite side of the intersection; see Chapter 12). In this example, the O&M specialist attributes the problem to the uniqueness of the intersection, not a specific deficit in the student's travel skills. This type of environmental analysis is an important component of all mobility instruction, whether the student has low vision, is totally blind, or is fully sighted (see Chapter 21).

When considering the environment to be used by a student with low vision, special emphasis is placed on significant visual environmental characteristics, such as illumination, color, and contrast. The factors of specific importance are shown in Sidebar 3.1, "Environmental Factors to Consider for Students with Low Vision."

Combining Assessment Findings

Comparing and integrating the assessment findings provides insights that are useful when developing a program of intervention. For example, the clinical record shows: "Albinism, visual acuity of 20/400 (6/120) without lenses, 20/120 (6/36) OU (both eyes) with corrective lenses, refractive error of $+6.50 - 4.75 \times 120$ OU." The mobility assessment indicated that this student's functional visual acuity was better with prescription lenses, that functional visual fields were full, and that the biggest problem was traveling in brightly lit areas, specifically outdoors on a sunny day. A review of Table 3.1 in Volume 1, Chapter 3, provides the information that students with albinism have problems with glare and often have a significant refractive error. These characteristics have been confirmed in the functional assessment and indicate the importance of working with the student to cope with the issue of lighting, as well as the benefits of wearing corrective lenses to achieve the best visual acuity.

A second example is the student with a diagnosed retinal detachment. The clinical exam reports the following: "The student had a visual acuity of 10/100 (3/30) OU, and an inferior temporal field loss OD (right eye) with no significant refractive error. During the mobility assessment, unwanted contact with garbage cans, bicycles, and low-lying shrubs on the right side incur the highest number of critical incidents, confirming the presence of a loss of visual field in the lower part of the right eye."

Environmental Factors to Consider for Students with Low Vision

- Amount of light. This includes analysis of the following:
  - Overall lighting in the area (for example, bus terminal)
  - Lighting on the specific task area (for example, schedule information board)
- Type of light. This includes identification of the following:
  - Different light sources such as natural, incandescent, or fluorescent
  - Type of light source student prefers and types that hinder performance
- Light angle and location. This includes descriptions of the following:
  - Relationship of natural and artificial light sources
  - Effect of different light positions on mobility performance
- Light adaptation. This includes evaluating the following:
  - Changes in functional vision from indoors to outdoors and vice versa

- Changes in functional vision from one level of lighting to another (for example, shade to sun, hallway to classroom)
- Amount of time student needs to adapt to the various lighting changes
- Glare. This includes determination of the following:
  - Sources of glare (for example, reflections off windows, shiny walls, floors, or puddles of water)
  - Effect of sun wear and other eyeshades, such as hats and visors, on functional vision performance
- Color or contrast. This includes identification of the following:
  - Color and contrast cues available to assist orientation (for example, crosswalk lines, church steeples)
  - Changes in terrain color and contrast (for example, broken sidewalks, puddles, curbs, stairs, potholes)

Both of these examples illustrate how the clinical and functional assessments can be combined to confirm the functional characteristics of the clinical findings. In addition, the clinical findings offer the O&M specialist insights into the types of problems the student may experience, allowing for the individualization of the functional assessment to specifically evaluate the anticipated areas of concern.

Combining assessment of the student (clinical assessment of vision, functional assessment of vision, critical incidents) with assessment of the visual demands of the environment and the student's functioning in the environment provides the O&M specialist with the quantity and quality of information that can be used to develop an instructional program. Comprehensive assessment is a prerequisite to the provision of quality services in low vision mobility.

IMPROVING FUNCTIONAL USE OF VISION

As a general statement professionals perform assessments to understand the student's ability and to identify challenges or deficits in skills. With this information an instructional program can be developed to improve the functional use of vision.

Congenital versus Adventitious Vision Loss

Whether the student is born with low vision or acquires low vision later in life is significant with regard to the need for, as well as the type and extent of, visual stimulation and efficiency instruction. Children born with low vision have differing levels of visual memory, ranging from very little to significant amounts. By comparison, students who experience a loss of vision as adolescents or adults have developed and maintain unimpaired visual concepts and visual memory. The time when vision loss occurs has a major impact on the types of instruction that will be required to address mobility, and this must be taken into account when tailoring programs for improving functional vision.

Although many functional vision enhancement techniques are similar for both populations, students with congenital low vision usually require considerably more time and effort if they are to form and understand visual language and memory. A common mistake is the assumption that children with severely reduced visual acuity, because they cannot see clearly, lack the potential to more effectively and efficiently interpret visual cues for mobility or other purposes. Equally common is the assumption that students with higher levels of visual acuity do not necessarily need mobility instruction because they *appear* to be moving about with relatively few problems in familiar areas.

Both of these examples result in students who may fall through the cracks due to assumptions on the part of the O&M specialist. Many students with adventitious vision loss at low and high extremes frequently fall through the same cracks in rehabilitation service-delivery systems.

An advisable rule of thumb is to assess all students for visual and mobility proficiency and problems and to plan a range of low vision mobility instruction from basic to advanced, depending on the student's assessed needs.

In the example of the student with congenital low vision, an early intervention program of vision stimulation is recommended. Absent structured learning, many students may not acquire the basic skills to interpret visual stimuli and make the necessary discriminations and judgments about visual information that is available to them. A vision stimulation program helps the student learn about and develop labels for critical visual features such as lines, angles, curves, and colors; how to identify them separately and as parts of common shapes and objects; and how to piece together missing details from what is seen, to better interpret an incomplete visual picture of the environment. Barraga and Morris (1980), Erin (1996), Erin and Paul (1996), Levack (1991), Lueck and Heinze (2004), Smith and Cote (2001), and Smith and O'Donnell (2001) are but a few of the references available to assist in the implementation of a sequential vision stimulation and vision enhancement program that incorporates the use of vision in different environments. Just as rolling and crawling are precursors to walking, the ability to learn critical visual features is a precursor to the use of vision while mobile. Combining these basic visual skills with a systematic exposure to environmental concepts used to develop orientation ensures a comprehensive approach to mobility instruction.

Visual Efficiency without Optical Devices

The O&M specialist assists the student in visual interpretation and movement through the environment. This is accomplished through lessons geared toward maximizing visual efficiency, in conjunction with instruction in other sensory training and mobility tools such as long canes and electronic travel aids, and travel techniques that maximize safety and efficiency of movement.

A starting point for maximizing visual efficiency is a discussion with the student about his visual condition and the functional implications of the condition. This conversation necessitates a familiarization with the student's record, including the results of the clinical low vision examination. The O&M specialist ought not to be surprised if the student is either unaware of, or confused about, his or her visual condition and its effect on functional vision. Either the student was never provided with this type of information, or it was provided using technical language. Remember that both internal and external factors affect functional vision from day to day and, in some cases, from one minute to the next. The O&M specialist's role is to assist the student in understanding this visual information and to teach when vision can or cannot be relied on for decision making while mobile.

As the discussion of the functional implications of visual impairment occurs, the O&M specialist needs to be aware of the effect that medical terminology can have so that the student is not bombarded or overwhelmed with information. Many students with low vision lack an understanding of their vision because no one has taken the time to provide them with a meaningful description of their condition and its effect on their ability to do visual tasks. Explaining how the eye works, which part of the eye is affected, and how this, in turn, effects their functional vision (for example, a sensitivity to light, the need to wear eyeglasses, bumping into objects on the side) can help students understand what they are experiencing. Erin and Corn (1994) reported on children's first understanding of being visually impaired. Their findings indicate that, for children, low vision is a more complex concept than blindness. Detailed ex-

planations, at a pace and level students (children or adults) can understand, that describes the functional implications of their eye conditions and how they affect mobility performance, are beneficial. It is also recommended that students keep a mobility diary or journal, which can include, but is not limited to the following:

- a description of eye conditions and functional effects
- best and worst times of day and weather conditions affecting visual performance
- best and worst environmental conditions, with emphasis on lighting conditions (indoor and outdoor)
- medications and any visual side effects of them
- most common mobility problems that can or cannot be managed solely through visual input
- optical and nonoptical devices for mobility
- visual and mobility skills, and techniques, concepts, and routes mastered
- tips for upkeep of skills

Whether it is for a child or an adult, this journal provides the student with an opportunity to increase understanding of the patterns of problems and opportunities that exist when the student uses functional vision, and the internal and external factors that affect day-to-day mobility. A journal can also serve as a monitor of progress. Reading the journal at the end of a semester or school year, or at the completion of a rehabilitation training program, provides a wonderful opportunity to reflect on the concepts that were learned, the techniques that were mastered (both visual and nonvisual), trips that were taken, and orientation skills that were developed.

For those with adventitious low vision (usually adults and elderly individuals), the O&M

specialist can provide educational support for the purpose of understanding the visual *changes* they experience, as compared to their prior experiences with full vision. For example, unfortunately too many students do not understand their eye pathology, its effect on their vision, and the internal and external factors that can be expected to affect visual performance. They may be confused by the decision-making process for when they can or cannot rely solely or primarily on visual information when mobile. Most students with adventitious loss of vision will benefit from instruction for new ways of using their vision, such as eccentric viewing for those with age-related maculopathy, or new scanning techniques for those with advanced glaucoma or retinitis pigmentosa.

The timing and sequencing of the presentation of this material is important. For example, a student may be experiencing a very difficult adjustment to the loss of vision and as a result may be resistant to the idea of mobility instruction. A comprehensive analysis of each student's situation (student confidentiality factors, vision status, family support, and so forth) will provide insights that can enable the instructor to determine the best timing and sequencing for this information.

VISUAL SKILLS AND MOBILITY

Visual Motor Skills

Some visual skills can be described as the fundamentals of functional vision. Whether the student has congenital or adventitious low vision, and irrespective of the cause of the vision impairment, these visual skills form the basis on which instruction in the use of vision for mobility is built. The student must have or develop these skills to maximize the use of functional vision. The initial skills that fit this description are tracing, scanning, and tracking. Excellent re-

sources are available for lesson plans and curricula to teach these skills (Barraga & Morris, 1980; Smith & Cote, 2001; Smith & O'Donnell, 2001). In this chapter we concentrate on their introduction in the context of mobility.

Tracing, or visually following a stationary line, is particularly useful for orientation purposes. In effect, it is the visual counterpart of trailing with one's hand or cane. Compared to tactile methods, visual tracing provides greater distance because vision allows for projection into space. It is important to evaluate, and useful to practice, tracing a variety of environmental lines, such as grass lines, hedge lines, and baseboards. Perhaps a student can discern only contrast and can trace along a baseboard edge contrasted to the floor coloring. Even this limited ability might allow the student to know that an office is located at the fourth break in the baseboard, with the fifth break indicating the location of the door to the library. Another student with very low vision can trace along and count six breaks in the hedge line, signaling the path to the house of a best friend. A student may have only light projection, yet could use this vision to trace a line of fluorescent lights along the ceiling to maintain a straight line of direction, with the last set of lights indicating an intersecting hallway.

While these basic visual skills are necessary, the approach that the O&M specialist takes for providing instruction will vary a great deal, depending on the age of the student, whether the vision loss is congenital or adventitious, and the amount of vision impairment that is present. For example, with some younger students, placing objects at the end of short lines, then gradually lengthening lines, of brightly colored yarn or string assists in teaching the skill of tracing. This helps to establish head and eye movement patterns. Gradually increasing the length of the yarn and the complexity of the surrounding environment teaches the student to search ahead for environmental lines of borders, lights, contrast, and so on, which assist in orientation and maintaining a desired line of travel. If the O&M specialist is working with an elderly student who is having difficulty because of multiple scotomas, the O&M specialist would use age-appropriate activities such as tracing the outline of a flower garden in the backyard.

Tracking, or visually following a moving target, can be a particularly helpful skill for both maintaining orientation and locating targets. The O&M specialist should teach students to follow the shoulder of a person walking in front of them, and watch for a raising or lowering of the person's shoulder. This might indicate up or down steps, or any change in the level of the terrain, such as a raised sidewalk or a hole in the ground. When going out to a dimly lit restaurant, the student could ask her companion to wear a light or bright shirt, blouse, or jacket, increasing the contrast to make tracking the companion walking through the restaurant a bit easier. By walking slightly ahead of the student and wearing a distinctive piece of clothing, the companion serves as an orientation cue that the student can use to track a path through the dimly lit area.

Perhaps one of the more common uses of tracking is at street crossings or corners while waiting for a bus. The student may begin by practicing tracking cars through busy intersections. The O&M specialist needs to determine whether the student can follow movement and discern turning cars from those continuing through the intersection. Good tracking skills can significantly augment safety and decision making when crossing streets, and combining this with auditory cues can result in greater efficiency.

If the O&M specialist determines that the student needs instruction to improve tracking skills, the sequence should begin with head and eye tracking and progress to refining eye-only tracking as the student's skills improve. The O&M specialist might begin with the student seated while following moving targets

such as people walking through a cafeteria. Then the O&M specialist might have the student begin to walk and look for moving targets, gradually increasing the complexity of the task until the student is able to follow other pedestrians in crowded situations, such as moving through congested stores.

This combination of systematic tracing and tracking skills contributes to the proactive use of vision, as opposed to simply moving without using vision to acquire information that can be used for travel. As discussed in Chapter 1, there are opportunities that vision provides, and these visual skills allow the student to quickly access information from greater distances and can enhance problem solving through finding and using visual cues for safety and orientation purposes.

Scanning is the systematic use of head and eye movement to search for targets. This skill can be used for a variety of purposes, including locating targets, establishing and reestablishing lines of direction, and finding landmarks. The O&M specialist's role is to help the student who exhibits erratic or random patterns to change this approach into systematic and goal-specific visual scanning behavior. Random scanning patterns can be observed regardless of age, amount of vision loss, or cognitive ability. The example that follows briefly describes a teaching approach.

Initially, the O&M specialist asks the student to visually locate a number of different targets or landmarks in indoor and outdoor environments. The O&M specialist will observe the student's visual behavior to determine whether a systematic search pattern is being used. Does the scanning miss some areas completely while others are repeatedly checked? Is the scanning too slow or time-consuming and inefficient? If the answer to either question is yes, then the student would benefit from basic instruction in patterned scanning. The O&M specialist can ask the student to search a wall or any large surface for a specific element such as a sign or clock. If necessary, the student is instructed to direct head and eyes to the top left corner of the wall. Then the O&M specialist has the student begin to trace from the left to the right corner, then lower the head slightly and trace back to the left side, again lowering the head and tracing to the right side, continuing this pattern until the target is located. The O&M specialist can point out how this systematic approach ensures that areas are not missed or repeated, because of the nature of the scanning pattern (Figure 3.10). This skill would then be generalized to more functional settings and activities. For example, this pattern can be used in stores when scanning for overhead signs or when attempting to locate specific food items.

If objects are typically located around the borders of a wall, then a perimeter scanning pattern along the edge of the wall is more effective. Objects in the upper visual field, such as hanging plants, require upper-field scanning, whereas a floor pillow against the wall is more quickly lo-

cated by a lower-field perimeter-scanning pattern. Many students with congenital visual impairment benefit from systematic instruction in the common positional locations of different environmental objects, though it should not be assumed that students will automatically know where and how to look for targets. This is also why an initial evaluation is helpful in planning instruction.

One general rule to emphasize for scanning to increase the chances of quickly finding the target is that when students are looking for vertical targets, they should scan horizontally, and when they are looking for horizontal targets, they should scan vertically. For example, when looking for a street sign, scanning will be horizontal, along the curb or sidewalk border, to locate the bottom of the intersecting vertical pole. Then scanning will switch to vertical, up the pole, to locate the intersecting horizontal street sign. This increases the chance of locating the target quickly and efficiently.

Students should also learn and practice the concept that a combination of scanning techniques can be useful. A good example of this is scanning to locate a house address. Some are on the mailbox or beside the front door or on the step, while other addresses are painted on the front curbs. Systematic use of visual scanning saves time and contributes to more proactive and efficient mobility.

Other mobility activities that lend themselves to the opportunity for scanning instruction are general orientation, street crossings, and maintaining and reestablishing a line of direction. For example, for the use of scanning for general orientation, the student can be taught to scan for a series of visual landmarks along a new route. Then the student can develop a record of the landmarks and their positional location (for example, "fire hydrant, lower left side") and use this list to assist in recalling the scanning sequence until the landmarks are committed to memory. This type of activity can also be generalized through route reversal, with a reverse chaining sequence of

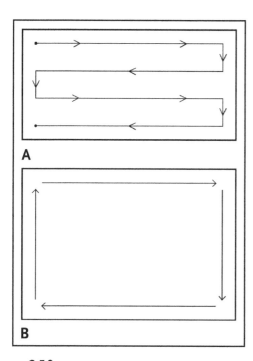

Figure 3.10.
(A) Gridline scanning pattern; (B) perimeter scanning pattern.

landmarks on the opposite side. At street crossings, the student can scan for vehicles and other pedestrians to help identify the approximate location of the curb. Scanning for traffic lights and Walk / Don't Walk signs is an excellent time to teach the concept of horizontal scanning to locate a vertical traffic light or street-name pole and vertical scanning to locate the traffic light or the name of the street, respectively. As the street crossing begins, scanning to the near side for turning cars on the parallel street addresses the immediate danger posed by moving vehicles. Intersections are dynamic—crossing the street can be one of the most dangerous mobility activities—and systematic scanning will significantly enhance safety at busy intersections. Unfortunately, many students do not use scanning at intersections beyond looking for traffic lights. Some may scan for vehicles only before crossing, and discontinue once they step off the curb. For younger students, lessons in the concept of traffic and intersections may be necessary first, whereas for older students, reminders of the safety hazards and the need for more effective and systematic scanning may need to be reemphasized.

Scanning for establishing and reestablishing a line of direction can be used when traveling to a new location. The student can be taught to scan down the street as far as possible to look for a distinctive landmark (for example, the blue mailbox or the colorful bed of flowers up ahead on the right), and then to visually maintain the same line of direction toward the landmark. This reduces the chances of veering into a driveway. If veering does occur, the student can scan to reestablish the location of the landmark, after exiting the driveway. Although some of us automatically employ scanning for landmarks (for example, the red floor in a parking garage, or the third car after the "green 2A" sign in the mall parking lot), many students with low vision may require instruction in systematic scanning to first establish, then reestablish orientation cues.

Eye-hand and eye-foot coordination are frequently lacking in students with low vision. It is not unusual for students to misjudge distances of objects by over- or underreaching and groping with their hands to locate objects, or to misjudge steps and shuffle their feet to locate the first step. This is because the eyes and hands (or eyes and feet) are functioning independently of each other. For instance, the object or target may first be located visually, then identified tactually, independent of vision. Through instruction and practice of reaching for objects while keeping the hand in view, this problem can be minimized. For example, the O&M specialist might ask the student to visually locate a series of doorknobs, then ask the student to place his hand between his eyes and the doorknob, and watch the hand as it approaches the doorknob. This should reduce groping and enable the student to achieve greater accuracy when reaching for targets. Students should also be instructed to watch their feet as they approach stairs to enable them to more accurately judge the location of the first step.

Eccentric viewing is the use of the off-center or paramacular (*para* meaning "near" or "beside") area of vision for a clearer view. Children with a loss of central vision, due to Best or Stargardt disease or any condition that results in a central scotoma or blind spot, typically develop eccentric viewing postures automatically. This involves a tilt of the head or a turning of the eye to one side or a combination of both to view around the scotoma. Adults who lose their central vision to age-related maculopathy may need instruction in locating and maintaining the best eccentric area for fixating and viewing, as it may be difficult to automatically change long-established patterns of looking directly at objects to best see them.

The clinical report may provide information as to how the student eccentrically views. If this information is not available, one method for establishing the best viewing position is for the O&M specialist to ask the student to look directly at her face and describe the details of the specialist's face. The O&M specialist should have the student shift the eyes up, down, to the right, and to the left and describe the effect of changing eye position on the ability to describe the O&M specialist's facial features. As the student begins to appreciate that changing eye position also changes clarity, this process can be refined to determine the best angle of viewing. Viewing a clock on the wall is another way of demonstrating and locating an eccentric viewing position. If the student with a central scotoma looks straight ahead at the clock, the middle section will appear to be missing. The student can then experiment with different head and eye positions, experiencing how these positions improve or degrade visual acuity, with the goal of determining the position in which the face of the clock is the clearest. Once this position is learned (for example, moving the eye to the nine o'clock position for clearest view), the student can use it for short-term tasks such as reading signs with or without telescopes, or long-term viewing such as watching television.

The Long Cane as a Complement to Vision and Mobility

The long cane can be one of the most important tools for enhancing visual efficiency. If the student trusts the information provided by the cane for detecting changes in elevation (stairs and curbs, for instance), then vision can be used for more detailed viewing of the general environment for orientation and safety cues. Students who may need the long cane but do not use it correctly tend to spend a considerable amount of time looking down to detect or confirm the cane's detection of changes in elevation. The student then uses vision primarily for safety and rechecking the cane's feedback, compromising its use for orientation, which is one of the greatest advantages of vision. If the long cane can address the safety issue, then vision can be used

more effectively to detect the whole range of visual cues that are available in the environment.

The authors feel that while consistent use of a long cane complements safe and efficient travel and enhances the use of vision for mobility purposes, there may be instances in which a student with sufficient vision decides that the constant use of a long cane is not necessary. For example, in daylight or well-lit conditions, traveling a familiar indoor or outdoor route during the middle of the day when there are few pedestrians and vehicles, the student may choose not to use a long cane. However, this same route traveled in the winter during the late afternoon when it is getting dark and the sidewalks and streets are busy with commuters may present a very different challenge because of the environmental changes. In addition, unexpected obstacles such as construction areas pose a greater danger to the student not using a long cane. One of the most important aspects of instruction in low vision mobility is teaching the student the critical variables to assess when making the decision about the use of the long cane. Just as learning to use one's vision more efficiently is important to mobility, learning when vision is not effective for travel decisions is equally important. At these times the use of the long cane in combination with other sensory cues enhances travel safety and efficiency.

Depth-Perception Cues

Locating and judging changes in elevation, which we refer to as a problem with depth perception, are, along with the challenge of illumination, universal problems for students with low vision. This problem can be especially challenging in environments with minimal visual cues, such as low-contrast steps or curbs. Although people in general look down when they sense the presence of stairs, there are a number of other visual cues that can be used to identify the location of changes in elevation. Cues that could assist in locating stairs include the following:

- the *slope of a railing*, indicating whether the stairs are going up or down
- the *height change of people* in front, slowly rising or descending in the visual field, indicating up or down stairs
- the *blocking of students' feet or lower body* when approaching downward steps; for example, the student may see only the upper body of a student coming up those same stairs
- *jagged or broken edged shadows*, often indicating the presence of steps
- *right angles or triangular shapes* along the side border where the riser and adjoining step meet, indicating steps, with a long succession of these angles indicating a long flight of steps
- *contrasting strips at the edges of steps*, which can enhance detection of first and last steps

In addition, sounds emanating from above or below, such as voices or footsteps, can indicate the presence of steps. Designing lessons that allow students to practice integrating visual and auditory cues helps them to become more proactive, especially in potentially dangerous situations.

Examples of visual cues and landmarks that assist in locating curbs include the following:

- *Crosswalk lines contrasting with the street* can provide cues to the location of curbs and can be used to maintain a straight line of direction for crossing streets.
- *Vehicles (parked or moving) on a nearby perpendicular street* indicate an upcoming intersection.
- *Visual contrast of street to sidewalk pavement and/ or curb* helps to anticipate an upcoming street problem.
- *The end of a building, grass line, or other continuous shoreline* indicates the presence of an intersecting sidewalk and potential intersecting street.

- *Curbs painted in contrasting colors* (for example, yellow and blue) help to locate the curb of the upcoming street.
- *Broken shadows at the curb* from light poles or other objects near the corner help to determine the location and depth of curbs. The greater the displacement of the broken shadow, the deeper the curb.

In addition, pedestrians suddenly stopping or congregating at a corner, as well as the presence of various objects, such as newspaper stands, traffic light control boxes, and so on, at corners, indicate oncoming intersections. The sounds of cars traveling perpendicular to the student's line of travel, even before they can be seen, provide another sensory cue for detecting an oncoming curb area.

The long cane represents one of the best tools for detecting changes in elevation. Its use, in combination with visual scanning, affords the student with low vision with the greatest level of safety and efficiency when traveling. Although visual cues alone may enable the student to detect the presence of stairs and curbs, the exact amount of depth is frequently difficult to judge without the use of a cane. One visual cue that does assist in judging the height of curbs involves scanning for the tires of parked cars (see Figure 3.11). By estimating how much of the bottom of the tire is blocked or obscured by the curb, the student can establish a relatively accurate estimation of the height of the curb.

Terrain Changes

An unanticipated change of terrain is one of the most difficult areas for the student with low vision. For those with sufficient vision, the following cues may prove helpful:

- For detecting *missing slabs of sidewalk*, a change in color from light to dark or vice versa, as

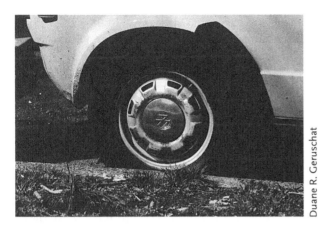

Duane R. Geruschat

Figure 3.11.
The depth of a curb can be determined by observing the extent to which the curb obscures the bottom of a car's tires.

well as the presence of dirt that gives a granular or bumpy appearance, may be useful cues.

- For detecting *puddles*, reflections on the ground or a broken or ripple effect from raindrops may be helpful.
- *Wet cement* may be detected by noticing a darker shade underfoot or the presence of construction, indicated by contrasting orange or yellow tape strips or ropes sectioning off newly finished areas.
- *Raised slabs of cement* may be detected by darkly lined, uneven, or thick sections of sidewalk, which indicate the raised section or slab .
- *Broken sidewalks* are indicated by color or shading changes in the broken areas, as well as by additional lines bordering the broken areas.

Visual Landmarks

Orientation can be greatly facilitated by the use of visual landmarks. The following represent a few of the many landmarks and techniques that can assist a student with low vision to use vision more effectively while traveling:

- *distinctive shapes* such as McDonald's arches, a steeply sloped roof along a street with flat-roofed buildings, or an oddly shaped lawn sculpture, which if scanned for, can reduce the amount of time it takes to locate objectives or areas near them
- *distinctive color*, such as a bright-red door, the color yellow along a row of condiments to signal mustard, the color purple to signal cabbage in the vegetable section of a store, or the blue arrow line along the floor to signal the route through a cafeteria
- *scanning the upper field of view* for landmarks, such as different heights of buildings or church steeples, or the top of a silo, to establish or re-establish one's direction
- remembering *forward and reverse sequencing of visual landmarks*, along with the ability to recall which visual cue is next, to facilitate learning routes and maintaining orientation

The careful selection of distinctive visual landmarks will enhance the proactive use of vision, as opposed to a random approach of simply reacting to whatever visual stimuli are stumbled on, which will minimize the benefits of functional vision. Active looking and the use of visual landmarks enhance mobility skills, especially as they relate to orientation.

Glare and Light Adaptation

Lighting (for example, glare, light adaptation, low illumination) represents the single most critical problem for students with low vision. The following strategies will assist the student who experiences these problems:

- Wear appropriate *absorptive sun filters* to shield the eyes from glare. A sun-lens evaluation should include experiences with different color tints and light transmission levels, to determine which provide the most comfort from glare and maximize visual acuity. Lenses with top and side filters are especially effective for protection from glare.

- With or without sun lenses, *visors or wide-brimmed or billed hats*, such as baseball caps, can be worn to eliminate glare from above and improve visual acuity.

- Movement can minimize the harsh effects of glare. For example, *changing the angle of viewing* when trying to read the name on a street sign can reduce or eliminate the effect of harsh light and improve readability. Another example is the challenge of identifying the color of a traffic light. These lights are usually placed up high, with the sky as a background, causing glare. It may be possible to reduce the glare by *turning to view the opposing traffic light.*

- For students who have difficulty under low light (dusk) or are night-blind, the use of *night vision technology* may be of benefit (Bradette, Couturier, & Rousseau, 2005; Mancil et al., 2005).

- *Conducting mobility lessons in low light and nighttime conditions* when mobility can be severely affected can be beneficial. Additional training in the use of the long cane may be necessary, especially as many students experience significantly decreased or even a total loss of visual cues under these conditions.

- *Evaluating light adaptation times* from indoors to outdoors and vice versa can help the student negotiate these problems. Document how long and to what degree visual functioning is affected by changes in illumination. Some students need a few seconds to adjust, others a few minutes, and others longer still. Some students may experience periods of no functional vision and may need to step aside and wait, use a guide, or use a folding cane to maneuver safely.

The O&M specialist can help students to understand the conditions under which these changes occur, their effects on functional vision, and different strategies to cope with these problems.

Ideally O&M lessons will occur with these types of lighting changes. However, sometimes schedules do not permit this. One option is to use sun lenses of different transmissions to simulate dim or nighttime conditions However, this is a significant compromise and should be considered only if it is not possible to have these lighting conditions at the time of the evaluation.

O&M specialists can also assess the effectiveness of different light sources (for example, fluorescent, incandescent, halogen, and natural light) for near tasks, such as reading maps, bus schedules, or menus. The student can be advised to carry a small, portable flashlight in addition to portable magnifying devices such as microscopic reading eyeglasses or hand or stand magnifiers.

It is important to keep in mind that students are constantly dealing with the changing effects of a variety of everyday lighting situations and require different strategies for varying conditions, including the use of nonvisual cues when vision is not effective enough for making sound mobility decisions.

A number of references provide more extensive coverage of low vision mobility, both with and without optical devices. For example, Smith and Geruschat (1996) overview low vision mobility with suggestions for functional assessment and instructional strategies. Cowen and Shepler (2000) provide activities and games for teaching children how to use monocular telescopes and magnifiers. "A Curriculum for Teaching Clients to Use Landmarks while Traveling" by Mac-William (1980) provides instruction in the use of landmarks. Beliveau and Smith (1980) offer techniques for enhancement of unaided vision, instruction with telescopes, and environmental modifications to increase visual efficiency. *Beyond Arm's Reach* (Smith & O'Donnell, 2001) offers a sequential curriculum for enhancing distance visual efficiency, with an emphasis on outdoor environments. Cowen and Shepler (2000), Geruschat (1980), Wiener and Vopata (1980), and Berg, Jose, and Carter (1983) present instructional strategies for introducing handheld telescopes for mobility.

Whether the students are children or adults, or are at varying levels of visual acuity or fields of view, the O&M specialist provides tools to enhance mobility performance by concentrating on their visual capabilities and incorporating their visual skills within the broader array of nonvisual techniques, including the use of other senses and assistive devices such as the long cane and electronic travel devices. This combination of visual and nonvisual information affords the student the greatest opportunity for comfortable, efficient, pleasurable, and safe mobility.

INSTRUCTIONAL CONSIDERATIONS FOR LOW VISION MOBILITY WITH OPTICAL DEVICES

In Chapter 3, Volume 1, we presented the advantages that vision offers for mobility with one of the main advantages being the ability to acquire information in the far distance. Of course the person with low vision experiences a reduction of distance vision that can be improved through the use of telescopes. O&M specialists are well positioned to teach the use of telescopes for distance viewing in the context of mobility instruction.

Basic Introduction to Teaching the Use of Telescopes

In comparison to optical devices for reading, the telescope, whether handheld or spectacle mounted, is relatively simple to teach. This is because of the optical characteristics of telescopes, particularly the ease of maintaining and changing focus, and because many students have prior experiences with binoculars. Additionally, as young children many of us took the paper towel tube and "played pirate," experiencing one of the primary functional characteristics of telescopes, a reduced visual field.

Instruction with telescopes involves six basic steps: (1) familiarization, (2) localization, (3) focusing, (4) scanning, (5) tracing, and (6) tracking.

The purpose of instruction with a telescope is to familiarize the student with its structure and focusing mechanism, offer tips on the five skills (localization, focusing, scanning, tracing, and tracking), and suggest a few strategies for increasing ease of use of problem-solving strategies when problems arise. Many adults may already be familiar with telescopes and require little to no instruction. The following section is designed for those unfamiliar with telescopes, particularly children.

Familiarization

The development of a common nomenclature is critical. The student should be able to identify various parts of the telescope so that a common language can be used. The O&M specialist begins with the student visually and tactually identifying the *ocular* (closest to the eye) and *objective* (closest to the target) lenses. Without looking through the telescope, the student should demonstrate the full range of the focusing mechanism. This approach has two key points. First, it is difficult for a student to view through the telescope while listening to the O&M specialist's instructions. From the student's point of view, the magnified image may be more interesting than the O&M specialist's instruction. Initially, talking should occur only when the telescope is away from the student's eye. Second, when the student is holding the telescope to his eye, it is usually difficult to turn the focusing mechanism through its full range. Introducing the motor skills of focusing when the student is not looking though the telescope can facilitate the transition to focusing while viewing through the telescope. This approach allows the student to experience the full range of turning the focusing mechanism from far left to far right both with and without viewing through the telescope.

Localization and Stabilization

Localization involves alignment of the eye, telescope, and object. The first concept to teach is the importance of localizing without looking through the telescope. The magnified image and restricted visual field of the telescope can make finding the object more difficult. Even though the object will not be seen clearly when localizing without the telescope, successful users of telescopes will always attempt to identify at least the approximate location of an object prior to viewing through the telescope. This is an important concept that should be emphasized and practiced. Some students begin to localize an object by immediately looking through the telescope. The O&M specialist needs to teach the student to look for the object without the telescope. Once the object, or an area where it is most likely situated, has been grossly identified, the telescope can be placed in front of the eye for positive and clearer identification. If localization is a problem, it is typically because of one of three reasons:

1. The student cannot find or maintain a straight line between the eye, the telescope, and the target.

2. The student's motor difficulties impair the ability to control the telescope.

3. A large central scotoma is present and the student is not eccentrically viewing.

If the student experiences difficulty with alignment, television viewing can serve as a good activity. While the student holds the telescope to her eye, the O&M specialist may be able to see the reflection of the television on the student's cornea and to assist the student by describing how the angle of the telescope needs to be adjusted to see the television. If that is not successful, the O&M specialist can try shining a penlight toward the student from a distance to provide a brighter target, or directing the student to find a light source (for example, window, overhead fluorescent light). Then the student holds the telescope toward the light but places the ocular lens about 12 inches away from the eye. The student will see a small circle of light. Then the student gradually moves the ocular lens directly in front of the eye, and localization through the telescope will be facilitated.

Stabilization is critical, especially for students with motor impairment. Stabilization requires the student to maintain a steady balance and consistent grip, which may require the student to rest her elbows on a hard surface or hold the telescope with both hands. Stability provides the student with the best visual acuity and the greatest opportunity to see the target. Larger telescopes, and those with grooved surfaces, also make it easier for those experiencing difficulty gripping the telescope.

For students experiencing problems caused by a central scotoma, one option is to begin instruction with a reduced-power telescope to provide a wider field of view. As eccentric viewing through the telescope improves, magnification is gradually increased.

Focusing

During initial instruction with the telescope the O&M specialist should focus the telescope prior to giving it to the student so the image will be clear or only slightly blurry. Once the student is successful with localization, the technique for obtaining the best focus can be introduced. Teaching the student to focus begins with a brief review of the motor skill required to focus the telescope. Looking through the telescope, once an object is successfully localized, the student turns the focusing mechanism a quarter turn to the right to determine whether the image has increased or decreased in clarity. If the image has increased in clarity, the student continues with another quarter turn to the right. The student continues this pattern until the image clarity decreases. Then the O&M specialist instructs the student to turn the focusing mechanism a quarter turn to the left, which is, in fact, returning to the previous focus. The general concept taught here is that the identification of best focus is achieved by turning the focusing mechanism in the direction that improves the image. Once the image starts to blur, the focusing mechanism is rotated to return to the prior focus, which provides the sharpest image. A good analogy is the tuning of an analog radio: Most people tune a station by passing the best reception, then returning to the strongest signal. This is also a method of self-checking that helps students to assure themselves and the instructor that the best focus has been obtained. In addition, if the O&M specialist and the student do not have a refractive error, the O&M specialist may focus the telescope since the focusing will be the same for both the student and the O&M specialist. This is possible because focusing depends on refractive error and target distance. If both the O&M specialist and the student have the proper refractive correction and are viewing the same target, then the focus will be the same.

The second concept is the relationship of the target distance to the length of the telescope. The student is taught that objects far away are viewed through a telescope at a short length, while objects that are close require the telescope to be extended to a longer length to attain best focus. The short-focus telescope can vary its length by a factor of approximately 2. For example, a 3-inch (7.5 cm) short-focus telescope can increase its length to approximately 6 inches (15 cm). Therefore, when using this telescope, viewing an object at a short distance would require the telescope to be longer, for example, 5–6 inches (13–15 cm) long, while viewing an object far away, such as a street sign, would require the telescope to be 3–4 inches (7.5–10 cm) in length. Once the target is localized, the focus can be refined.

Scanning

The key concept for successful scanning is the importance of being *systematic*. The second concept for improving scanning skills is the development and selection of different scanning patterns, which will be based on the location and orientation of the target. For example, the pole that holds a street sign has a primarily vertical orientation. Horizontal scanning will provide the quickest approach to locating the pole. The opposite is also true: if the student is looking for the name of a business along a building line, vertical scanning will allow the quickest approach to *locating* signs, while scanning horizontally facilitates *reading* each sign. The reader can review scanning techniques in the previous section on basic visual motor skills for more instructional tips that can be utilized with or without telescopes.

Tracing

Visual tracing involves following stationary lines in the environment. It is a precursor to tracking people or vehicles that are moving. Students are asked to view through the telescope while moving their heads to trace along lines such as baseboards, grass lines, and so on. Students can also trace along the outlines of houses, furniture, and storefronts.

Tracking

Tracking involves maintaining a consistent alignment of the eye, the telescope, and the object being viewed while the object is moving. Tracking is easiest when looking at objects at a far distance. The closer the object is to the student, the more challenging the tracking task. This is because of the relationship between the functional visual field and distance. When viewed through a telescope, objects are magnified, resulting in a limited field of view. The greater the distance between the student and the object being viewed, the larger the functional field of view will be. As an object gets closer, the acuity will increase, while the functional field of view (amount of the object seen) will decrease.

If the student has difficulty tracking objects while looking through the telescope, instruction can begin with the student seated and visually following people who are moving slowly in the distance. As the student demonstrates improvement, the goal is to gradually increase the speed of the targets. For example, with the O&M specialist as the target and standing 40 feet (12 m) away from the student, the specialist walks to the left, then right. The specialist gradually increases walking speed while maintaining the same distance. Then the specialist gradually decreases the distance. It is important to recognize that getting closer makes the task more challenging because the functional field of view is changing. As the student gains the ability to track, the O&M specialist asks the student to stand and repeat the same series of activities. Outdoors, the specialist can have the student practice tracking pedestrians and cars. The O&M specialist should try to choose activities and targets of interest to the student. The student may prefer people watching, or sporting events, or concerts, or television viewing. Practice with these activities can be more motivating for quickly achieving the goals of instruction.

Environmental Sequencing and Instructional Considerations

Teaching a student to use a telescope involves five basic skills and the appropriate sequencing of the environment. Teaching the use of a telescope is similar to teaching the touch technique with the long cane. For example, when teaching the basic skill of the touch technique, a common approach is to isolate the skill and practice until a basic level of competence is achieved. The skill of touch technique is then applied to indoor and outdoor, and residential and small and large business environments. This same approach works well when introducing telescopes. For example, the O&M specialist begins teaching the use of the telescope indoors, with the skills isolated. As skills are demonstrated, the student moves to an outdoor residential and then a business environment.

Target selection is critical to the successful development of these skills. Three variables should be considered when selecting targets: (1) size, (2) distance, and (3) contrast. The importance of *size* is self-evident. In general, the larger the target, the easier it is to locate and read unless the student has a severely constricted visual field. There is a constant inverse relationship between size and *distance*. As distance decreases, relative size increases. As distance increases, relative size decreases. Therefore, size and viewing distance are both considered when selecting targets. The third variable, *contrast*, can be more important than size. For example, with camouflage (which is a form of low contrast) it is possible to hide large objects, while a single candle on an overcast night (high contrast) can be seen from great distances. The higher the contrast, the more quickly the target will be located and identified. Therefore, when selecting targets, attention should be given to the contrast of a target and the effect of the figure-ground relationship on target visibility.

The eye care specialist will typically prescribe a telescope that achieves 20/20 (6/6) to 20/40 (6/12) visual acuity. This is the amount of clarity required to view most street signs and bus numbers from a distance. At times, the beginner may have difficulty localizing a target because the eye care specialist prescribed a high-powered telescope to achieve the recommended visual acuity. The problem is that the visual field of the higher-power telescopes will be too restrictive for the beginner to even localize a target. While the acuity requirement is met by the telescope, the functional skills of the student are not sufficiently developed for the telescope to be of much use. This student will have difficulty finding things and maintaining fixation on targets. The eye care specialist's role is to provide the necessary magnification for the student to see signs. It is the O&M specialist's job to teach the skills necessary for the student to find the sign. Some students will simply not be able to localize a sign with a 6× or more powerful telescope. In this situation, the O&M specialist should consider reducing the power of the telescope for the purpose of instruction. For example, working with a 2.8× or 4× telescope will give the student a larger field of view and more illumination, making localization, tracing, tracking, and scanning easier to accomplish, though the target will not be as clear. This is analogous to lifting weights: if a student cannot lift 100 pounds (45 kg), the teacher will begin with 25 pounds (11 kg) and work toward a goal of 100 pounds. The same concept applies with telescopes. Selecting a lower-power telescope and working to the higher-power telescope develops the prerequisite skills and provides the foundation for a successful experience. Always remember that a low-power telescope reduces visual acuity; therefore, larger targets need to be selected or the student must be closer to the target if the student wants to resolve images.

Many people, including those with low vision, wear prescriptive lenses. When a student tries to look through a telescope while wearing prescriptive lenses, two problems often occur. First is the absence of tactual information that is received when the telescope is placed directly against the cheek and skin that surrounds the eye. Second is the reduced field of view that re-

sults from the increased distance between the eye and the telescope. Students will often independently solve this problem by simply removing their eyeglasses, increasing the tactual information and, because the telescope is closer to the eye, increasing the functional visual field. If the student is hyperopic (farsighted), the focusing mechanism may need to be changed (focused outward) to accommodate for the uncorrected refractive error. If the student is myopic (nearsighted), the focusing mechanism may need to be changed (focused inward) to accommodate for the uncorrected refractive error. If the student has significant myopia, he or she will have to function with a blurry image because handheld telescopes do not have the capacity to correct for large amounts of myopia.

Bioptic Telescopes—Additional Considerations

Instruction with bioptic, or head-mounted, telescopes (see Figure 3.12), involves working with either monocular or binocular units mounted on spectacles and offers a hands-free approach to intermediate and distance magnification (Greene et al., 1991).

Since the hands are not involved in holding the telescope, proper alignment with the bioptic telescope is affected only by the mounting and fitting of the telescopes. If the alignment and

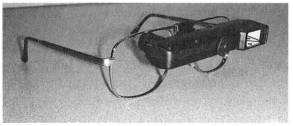

Figure 3.12.
A bioptic telescope system, consisting of telescopes mounted on spectacles, allows some people with low vision to drive.

fitting are poor, the student will have difficulty viewing through the center of one or both telescopes. The student may report a dark portion of the lens, a border on the image, or double vision. Consultation with the eye care specialist may be needed in this situation to make adjustments to the eyeglasses. Velcro straps on the temples of the eyeglasses are also helpful for holding the eyeglasses in place. The technique for localizing through a head-mounted telescope is to have the student tilt the head up and look under the telescopes to begin to localize the target. Once the target is localized, the student tilts the head downward while the eyes move up into alignment with the telescopes. The student continues guided practice until this movement becomes fluid.

Focusing systems vary and include autofocusing; manual focus by pulling the scope outward for intermediate distances and inward for close work; or manual focus by turning a focusing ring at the end of the objective lens. Some systems have a ridged focusing bar atop the bridge of the lenses, which is turned to focus the telescopic system without changing the apparent length. For most other bioptic telescopes, the same principles apply that were presented with handheld telescopes—specifically, the concept that the telescope will focus out (become longer) the closer the target, and focus in (become shorter) the farther away the target. This concept is important since, with practice, the student can begin to approximate the length of the telescope that will be required to focus on a target.

Instructional techniques with bioptic telescopes for localizing and following targets through scanning, tracing, and tracking are the same as the strategies for handheld telescopes. Just as with handheld telescopes, to obtain mastery with bioptics, mastery of the four basic skills, followed by increasing the speed and complexity of the tasks, is the best instructional approach.

Basic Introduction to Teaching the Use of Visual-Field Enhancement Systems

Students with good visual acuity but severely constricted peripheral visual fields (less than 10 degrees) usually experience serious problems with mobility. The problem is the amount of time required to turn the eyes or head to obtain the information needed for safe travel. For example, when a student with severely restricted visual fields is looking left, the student cannot obtain information from straight ahead or to the right, such as objects to the right or straight ahead or people passing in front of or by the student's right side. Thus, significant pieces of critical information needed for safe mobility are missing. As discussed in Volume 1, Chapter 3, there are a number of devices to assist in visual-field enhancement for these individuals, though they are infrequently prescribed compared to magnification systems that improve the clarity of images for students with low vision. Some instructional considerations follow.

Fresnel Prisms

Fresnel prisms are a series of prisms compressed into a flat plastic membrane that can be affixed to a student's eyeglasses at different locations corresponding to the area of field loss (see Figure 3.13). The base of the Fresnel prism faces the field loss. Since light passing through a prism is deflected toward its base, the student who is looking through the prism area experiences images displaced into the viable field of view. Fresnel prisms help specifically to address the problem of eye scanning by assisting the student in obtaining information from a much larger area of the visual field with only a slight increase in eye movement toward the prism area. The Fresnel prism provides a functional view of objects off to the side in the 80–90-degree area for a potential total field awareness of approximately 160 degrees, if the prisms are worn bilaterally on the peripheral edges of the eye. Fresnel prisms, therefore, enable the student to obtain significantly more peripheral information quickly and efficiently than eyeglasses alone (Geruschat & Turano, 2002; Peli, 2000; Rossi, Kheyfets, & Reding, 1990; Smith & Geruschat, 1983; Szlyk, Seiple, Stelmack, & McMahon, 2005).

The keys to success with Fresnel prisms include:

1. a highly motivated student who experiences problems with bumping into objects and people because of peripheral visual field constriction;

2. fairly good visual acuity (20/20 to 20/200, or 6/6 to 6/60) and severely constricted visual field (less than 10 degrees);

3. accurate placement of the prism that accounts for the natural eye scanning patterns of the student;

4. sequential instruction for adapting to the displacement of objects that occurs when viewed through the prism; and

5. sequential exposure to increasingly complex and crowded travel environments.

The instructional program involves establishing a baseline of natural eye and head scanning

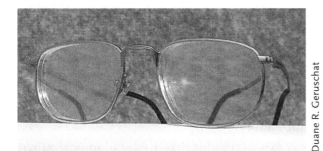

Duane R. Geruschat

Figure 3.13.
A Fresnel prism is a series of plastic prisms applied to regular eyeglasses to help correct the wearer's peripheral vision loss.

so the prism can be placed on the lens temporally enough to be outside of the student's natural eye scanning. This approach enhances the student's natural scanning ability by encouraging scanning to view through the prism. It also allows the student to control viewing through the prism. The only time the student will see objects through the prism is when a definite increase in scanning to the side occurs. This reduces visual confusion and problems with double vision.

As with all mobility instruction, sequencing of the presentation of the environment is critical to a positive experience and ultimately a successful outcome. The sequence begins with seated indoor activities that introduce the student to the effects of the displacement of objects while looking through the prism. As the student becomes more accurate touching objects while viewing through the prism, movement can be introduced. Beginning in quiet hallways and gradually working toward shopping malls increases complexity. These indoor experiences will involve frequent viewing through the prism and touching objects to connect the apparent visual location of objects with their actual location. As the student demonstrates successful adaptation to the effect of displacement, outdoor travel in increasingly complex areas can be introduced. Through frequent comparisons of both straight-ahead and prism vision and, when possible, touching to confirm the location of objects, the student can gradually adapt to the effects of displacement. Ultimately, improved mobility will be demonstrated as the student is capable of efficiently looking for information in the far periphery with a simple eye scan. Evaluation and instructional lesson plans for Fresnel prism use are detailed by Smith and Geruschat (1983).

Minification Systems

Case studies have reported on the use of a minifying system. Minification occurs by looking through a reverse telescope, which is nothing more than looking through the objective versus the ocular lens of the same telescope that is used to magnify. Looking through the fish-eye lens of a hotel door is an example of a reverse telescope. The student on the other side of the door may be a distance of only 2 feet (60 cm) away but one will be able to see the student's entire body. This enhanced field, where objects appear smaller and farther away than they really are, occurs through minification. The amount of minification is equivalent to the amount of magnification, so, for example, if a student views through a 4× telescope, objects will appear four times larger and four times closer, while a 6× telescope makes objects appear six times larger and six times closer. When viewed through the objective lens of a 4× telescope, objects will appear four times smaller and four times farther away, resulting in four times as much information fitting into the visual field.

It is helpful for instruction to take place in areas the student frequents. For instance, in school, the student can practice finding an empty seat in an auditorium or looking into a classroom before entering to locate bookshelves, other students, or the teacher. Without the reversed telescope, the student may need to do excessive head scanning to locate the same things or students, whereas a quick look through the reversed telescope accomplishes this task in a more efficient manner.

This also holds true for a handheld minification system. A handheld minifier is a minus lens in a handheld form that is used at near, as opposed to distance viewing. It is analogous to a handheld magnifier, except for the fact that a minus lens minifies, as opposed to magnifies, objects, thus allowing more of the image to fit into the student's field of view. The student simply holds the minifier in front of the material and views a wider circle of detail, as objects and words are smaller, and the view thus encompasses a larger field of information.

Driving with Low Vision

Driving with low vision is now legal in many states. Laws and requirements vary but most states require some type of instruction prior to taking the driving test. In states where bioptic telescopes can be used to drive, instruction with the telescope can be offered by the O&M specialist before the person obtains driver training. The driver with low vision uses the bioptic for brief periods (approximately 5 percent) of time to identify traffic controls, street signs, other aids to orientation, and unexpected events such as something moving across the street in the path of the vehicle. A paramount goal of bioptic instruction for driving is to develop the skill of quickly locating and viewing through the bioptic, then viewing out of the bioptic while in a dynamic driving environment. The instructional sequence begins with the same set of required skills for the use of a handheld telescope: localize, focus, scan, trace, and track. Once these skills are developed, movement can be introduced through slow walking while looking through the bioptic telescope. Walking while looking through the telescope for extended periods of time is not a safe activity because of the restricted field of view of the telescope. Therefore, attention must be paid to the student's safety during this activity. As the student's ability to walk while viewing into and out of the telescope improves, riding a bicycle and riding as the passenger in a vehicle will continue to improve these skills. Riding as the passenger in a vehicle is especially effective for simulating the technique that is required once the student gets behind the wheel. A comprehensive review of the literature on driving with low vision can be found in Strong, Jutai, Russell-Minda, and Evans (2008a, 2008b).

Registering for driver education is required in some states (Marta & Geruschat, 2004). Even in the states where this is not required, driver education is definitely recommended; it has a positive effect on the student's overall driving performance and provides more time for the integration of the bioptic telescope.

SUMMARY

This chapter describes the components of a comprehensive assessment of mobility and strategies for improving the use of low vision for mobility. The components include a review and interpretation of the eye exam, the acquisition of functional visual acuities and functional visual fields, and the major features of the environment that impact on mobility. Methods for enhancing functional visual performance both without and with optical devices are introduced. Emphasis is placed on the importance of developing good visual skills prior to the introduction of optical devices. The chapter concludes with specialized instruction with Fresnel prisms for severely constricted visual fields and driving with low vision and bioptic telescopes.

IMPLICATIONS FOR O&M PRACTICE

1. The clinical low vision assessment can offer important information for the O&M specialist when working with a student who has low vision. Visual acuity, visual fields, pathology, and refractive error are all important pieces of information for understanding the visual performance of the mobility student.

2. Eyeglasses can serve two very different purposes: to correct for refractive error or to assist in clarifying a magnified image. It is important for the O&M specialist to know why eyeglasses have been prescribed and for what purpose, as magnifying eyeglasses can be worn only when seated and are for looking at very close distances.

3. The functional low vision mobility assessment begins with an interview. This interview establishes the student's needs and goals, identifies areas of self-reported problems and proficiency, and describes any previous O&M instruction.

4. Functional visual acuities and visual fields offer the O&M specialist insights into how the student is using remaining vision.

5. The environment plays a significant role in the student's ability to use remaining vision. Assessing the environment is therefore critical for the O&M specialist to understand and anticipate the student's performance.

6. The student with congenital low vision does not have the visual memory and many visual concepts that the student with adventitious vision loss maintains. The O&M specialist may need to teach basic visual concepts and skills to the student with congenital low vision who has had no previous instruction.

7. Visual strategies such as eccentric viewing and monocular depth perception cues are useful skills for the student with low vision. The O&M specialist can teach these skills in a systematic method to improve the student's mobility performance.

LEARNING ACTIVITIES

1. Ask a colleague to wear visual distorters (vision simulators) for visual acuity or visual field. Using indoor and outdoor environments, obtain distances for the three types of visual acuity (awareness, identification, preferred) and estimates for the three types of visual field (static, preferred, early warning).

2. Walking a mobility route, evaluate the types and amount of variation in illumination that occur. Make note of shadows from buildings, the location of the sun, and the effect of shiny surfaces.

3. Using telescopes that vary in magnification, watch a live sporting event. Notice the effect

of the different amounts of magnification on your ability to keep up with the action. Next, change your seat to increase and decrease your viewing distance. What effect does this have on your viewing ability?

4. Driving at low levels of light or at night, estimate how often you need 20/20 (6/6) visual acuity. For example, do you need 20/20 visual acuity for changing lanes, accelerating and decelerating, seeing the brake lights of the vehicle in front, and monitoring pedestrians as they cross the street?

5. Wearing visual distorters, and being monitored by a colleague, cross at a variety of residential and business intersections. When signals were present (traffic lights, Walk / Don't Walk signals), did you use this information, or did you primarily attend to vehicles?

CHAPTER 4

Improving the Use of Hearing for Orientation and Mobility

Gary D. Lawson and William R. Wiener

LEARNING QUESTIONS

- How can orientation and mobility (O&M) specialists estimate the adult student's hearing without the use of an audiometer?

- How can auditory training be implemented in natural settings or with recorded sound, and what important skills should be learned?

- What are the basic components of a simple hearing aid, what are their functions, and what distinguishes linear from compression amplification?

- What persons should the O&M specialist consider for referral to an audiologist?

- How can traditional hearing aids, implants, and other options be useful to persons who are blind and have hearing loss?

INTRODUCTION

Chapter 4 in Volume 1 of this text describes the physical and biological basis for hearing, the methods for identifying, quantifying, and classifying hearing loss, and the specific auditory skills used by people who are visually impaired. These areas provide a foundation for the use of hearing for effective orientation and mobility. As a complement to those foundational concepts, this chapter discusses how to facilitate and improve the use of audition in the rehabilitation of people who are visually impaired. The chapter begins with a discussion of methods for evaluation of hearing function that do not depend on sophisticated instrumentation. It continues first with a discussion of hearing training activities and then with a description of the various types of hearing aids and their uses. The chapter concludes with the latest advancements in hearing rehabilitation.

FUNCTIONAL HEARING ASSESSMENT

The O&M specialist should be constantly alert to the possibility of hearing problems, particularly among older adults with vision problems.

Observation of a student's use of hearing during travel is a good method for determining whether difficulties exist. A self-report questionnaire may also be useful. Weinstein (2009, pp. 720–721) noted that as of January 1, 2005, Medicare guidelines encourage physicians and nonphysicians to use self-report questionnaires to review the functional ability and level of safety of new Medicare Part B beneficiaries in several areas, including hearing. Furthermore, the guidelines indicate that those who do not pass the screenings must be offered education, counseling, and referral. Although self-report questionnaires are imperfect instruments, they may be useful as an aid in determining when to refer the student for audiologic and medical evaluation. It is beyond the scope of this chapter to describe all self-assessment questionnaires. Some self-report screening measures, however, do appear to show promise or have substantial acceptance.

Hearing Handicap Index for the Elderly

There are several variants of the Hearing Handicap Index for the Elderly (HHI-E), which was introduced by Ventry and Weinstein (1982). The 10-item Hearing Handicap Inventory for Screening (HHIE-S; Weinstein, 1986) requires less administration time than does the 25-item HHI-E. Newman and Weinstein (1988) introduced the Hearing Handicap Inventory for Spouses to compare perceptions of handicap by veterans and their spouses. Newman, Weinstein, Jacobson, and Hug (1990) introduced the Hearing Handicap Inventory for Adults (HHI-A) for use with adults less than 65 years of age. It differs very little from the HHI-E.

The most widely used variant of the HHI-E appears to be the 10-item HHIE-S, a screening version introduced by Weinstein (1986). According to Kotchkin (2005), the National Institutes of Health has endorsed the use of the HHIE-S. The HHIE-S is a 10-item version of the 25-item HHI-E, which can be found in use in a variety of places on the Internet. The scoring procedure is the same for the HHI-E and the HHIE-S. Each item is scored 0 for a "no" response, 2 for a "sometimes" response, and 4 for a "yes" response. When points are summed, total scores range from 0 to 40. Weinstein (2000) recommended that those who obtain scores of greater than 10 on the HHIE-S be referred to an audiologist. Lichtenstein, Bess, and Logan (1988) found that HHIE-S scores of 10–24 showed a 50 percent probability of hearing impairment and that HHIE-S scores of 26–40 showed an 84 percent probability of hearing impairment. The screening criteria for hearing impairment was a 40 decibel (dB) hearing loss in both ears at 1,000 or 2,000 hertz (Hz) or a 40 dB hearing loss in either ear for 1,000 and 2,000 Hz.

Although the results from the HHI-E have proven to be reliable, one must recognize that the HHI-E is an indication of one's self-perception of hearing and hearing loss as well as an indication of hearing function. In a study of the effects of age on self-perceived hearing disability as measured on the HHI-A and the HHI-E, Gordon-Salant, Lantz, and Fitzgibbons (1994) found an age effect that was not attributed to differences in degree of hearing loss between young and elderly persons with hearing loss. Younger subjects reported greater handicapping effects of hearing loss than did elderly subjects.

Questionnaires for Detecting or Assessing Hearing Loss

If the primary interest is in predicting hearing loss without using an audiometer, one can consider the use of questionnaires to make gross distinctions between those with unimpaired hearing and those with hearing loss. Examples are discussed here to illustrate the use of questionnaires.

Figure 4.1 shows the 12-item Hearing Screening Inventory (HSI) developed by Coren and Hakstian (1992). According to Coren and Hakstian (1992), HSI scores correlate highly with

HEARING SCREENING INVENTORY

Instructions:

This questionnaire deals with a number of common situations. For each question you should select the response that describes *you* and your behaviors best. You can select from among the following response alternatives:

Never (or almost never),   Seldom,   Occasionally,

Frequently,   Always (or almost always)

Simply circle the letter that corresponds to the first letter of your choice. (If you normally use a hearing aid, answer as if you were not wearing it.)

1) Are you ever bothered by feelings that your hearing is poor?
.... N S O F A

2) Is your reading or studying easily interrupted by noises in nearby rooms?
.... N S O F A

3) Can you hear the telephone ring when you are in the same room in which it is located?
.... N S O F A

4) Can you hear the telephone ring when you are in the room next door?
.... N S O F A

5) Do you find it difficult to make out the words in recordings of popular songs?
.... N S O F A

6) When several people are talking in a room, do you have difficulty hearing an
individual conversation .... N S O F A

7) Can you hear the water boiling in a pot when you are in the kitchen?
.... N S O F A

8) Can you follow the conversation when you are at a large dinner table?
.... N S O F A

Answer these questions using

Good,   Average,   Slightly below average,   Poor,   Very poor

(Circle the first letter corresponding to your choice)

9) Overall I would judge my hearing in my RIGHT ear to be
.... G A S P V

10) Overall I would judge my hearing in my LEFT ear to be
.... G A S P V

11) Overall I would judge my ability to make out speech or conversations to be
.... G A S P V

12) Overall I would judge my ability to judge the location of things by the sound
they are making alone to be .... G A S P V

Scoring instructions:

Responses are scored 1 for "Never," 2 for "Seldom," 3 for "Occasionally," 4 for "Frequently," and 5 for "Always" (or "Good" = 1 to "Very Poor" = 5). The total score is simply the sum of the 12 responses. (Items 2, 3, 4, 7, and 8 are reverse scored.)

Figure 4.1. Hearing Screening Inventory

Source: Reprinted with permission from S. Coren and A. R. Hakstian. "The development and cross validation of a self-report inventory to assess pure-tone threshold hearing sensitivity," *Journal of Speech and Hearing Research, 35*, 921-928. Copyright © 1992 by American Speech-Language-Hearing Association. All rights reserved.

pure-tone thresholds, yielding validity coefficients of approximately 0.80 for the better ear. The high correlation made it possible for Coren and Hakstian to produce a regression-based estimate of an old American Medical Association formula-based average threshold using the frequencies 0.5, 1, 2, and 4 kilohertz (kHz; American Medical Association, 1947). On the basis of effects on speech intelligibility, the American Academy of Ophthalmology and Otolaryngology (1969) established 25 dB hearing level (HL) as the border between "no hearing handicap" and "slight hearing handicap" and established 55 dB HL as the border between "mild hearing handicap" and "marked hearing handicap." Coren and Hakstian determined that an HSI score of 27 (estimated equivalent of 25 dB HL) indicates "mild" hearing loss and an HSI score of 37 (estimated equivalent of 55 dB HL) or greater indicates "marked" hearing loss. Using these criteria, they found that the misclassification rate across 806 subjects was only 7.9 percent for mild losses and 6.6 percent for marked losses.

A study by Choi et al. (2006) examined the sensitivity and specificity of three simple questionnaires that were developed and implemented in the National Health Interview Survey (Ries, 1994; Schein, Gentie, & Haase, 1970): the hearing screening questions, the Rating Scale for Each Ear (RSEE), and the Health, Education and Welfare Expanded Hearing Ability Scale (HEW-EHAS). Their subjects were Iowa farmers. The number of questions was four for the Screening Questions, two for the Rating Scale for Each Ear, and four for the Health, Education and Welfare Expanded Hearing Ability Scale. Choi et al. (2006) examined the sensitivity and specificity of these measures, using bilateral pure-tone threshold average (PTA) for 1,000, 2,000, 3,000, and 4,000 Hz as the standard for hearing loss. In other words, the PTA was based on eight frequencies, four in each ear. Hearing loss was indicated by a PTA greater than 25 dB HL. Sensitivity is the proportion of those testing positive who actually have

hearing loss. Specificity is the proportion of those testing negative who actually do not have hearing loss. Sensitivity and specificity for each of the three screening approaches were reported for two age-groups and for all subjects. The PTA showed a higher prevalence of hearing loss than did the questionnaires for the older subjects, but the PTA showed a lower prevalence of hearing loss than did the questionnaires for the younger subjects. Overall, the screening questions had the highest sensitivity (73 percent), and all three approaches had similar specificity (81.4–84.8 percent).

Limitations and the Need for Collaboration in Functional Hearing Assessment

Ideally, all persons with blindness or low vision should have an audiologic evaluation. In the absence of full assessment or screening by an audiologist, questionnaires may be helpful in learning about self-perception of hearing loss or in identifying hearing loss. The HSI appears be an interesting option for identifying hearing loss. If a hearing loss is suspected, the student should be referred to an audiologist or physician without having to undergo a hearing screening. Hearing threshold levels are a measure of audibility across frequencies and can influence one's ability to travel independently. Statistical results from studies using questionnaires tend to be based on a limited portion of the test frequency range, one that was chosen because of its relation to speech communication rather than orientation.

When referral to an audiologist leads to the discovery of a hearing loss, the O&M specialist is in a position to work with the audiologist to describe functional difficulties and acquaint the audiologist with the special auditory needs of the individual who is blind. The audiologist and the O&M specialist can then work together to follow the hearing aid fitting with an appraisal of the individual's functioning with the aid, in both communication and orientation. Together the O&M specialist and the audiologist can help the person with visual and hearing impairments to achieve a higher level of rehabilitation.

FUNCTIONAL BALANCE ASSESSMENT

Although our primary interest in this chapter is the use of hearing, it may be useful to know that Jacobson and Newman (1990) introduced the Dizziness Handicap Inventory (DHI) and found it to be a potentially useful instrument. Jacobson and Calder (1998) developed a 10-item screening version of the DHI and found results from the DHI and the screening version to be highly correlated ($r = 0.86$, $p = 0.001$). In addition to endorsing the use of the HHIE for screening, the National Institutes of Health has, according to Kotchkin (2005), endorsed the use of the DHI for screening. As noted above, as of January 1, 2005, Medicare guidelines encourage physicians and nonphysicians to use self-report questionnaires to review the functional ability and level of safety of new Medicare Part B beneficiaries in several areas, and these areas include balance function (Weinstein, 2009, pp. 720–721).

OPTIMIZATION OF AUDITION

Development of Auditory Skills for Orientation and Mobility

Effective use of sound is essential if an individual with visual impairment is to become a well-oriented and successful traveler. This is why O&M specialists include a form of auditory training as part of their plan for developing auditory skills for orientation and mobility. Carhart (1960), sometimes called the father of audiology, described auditory training as a process for teaching children or adults with a hearing impairment to take full advantage of auditory cues and

recommended emphasis on developing awareness of sound, gross discrimination of nonverbal stimuli, and gross and fine discrimination of speech (Nerbonne & Schow, 2007). The audiologist may include auditory training as one part of a broader concept called *aural habilitation*, *aural rehabilitation*, or *audiologic treatment of hearing loss*, in which improvement of communication skills is a primary goal. The O&M specialist, however, provides a different type of auditory training that focuses on the auditory skills necessary for independent movement.

The earliest and most widely used approach to auditory training for orientation and mobility has typically occurred in natural settings. Since it is generally recognized that actual experience coupled with immediate feedback is the most effective method for improving auditory functioning, O&M specialists have developed training procedures that use real environments and actual sounds. Two approaches to this type of training have evolved. The O&M specialist may provide auditory training using (1) one-to-one student-teacher interactions to provide auditory training as part of active travel lessons or (2) auditory training that is separate from the active travel lessons. The first approach is conducted with a one-to-one student-teacher ratio to ensure safety, while the second approach can be conducted with an individual or with a group of individuals. Both approaches have advantages and disadvantages.

In the first approach, exercises are given to teach the student to use specific auditory skills that relate directly to travel situations. Usually the use of an auditory skill and the actual travel procedure are taught together, which has the advantage of illustrating to the student in the most direct way how auditory skills can be used. This procedure may increase motivation by showing the relevance of the auditory skill. In addition, working one-to-one, the O&M specialist is able to individualize training, taking into consideration the abilities and needs of each student.

The second approach separates auditory training from the actual travel lesson. This approach allows the student to concentrate fully on the sounds without worrying about related wayfinding skills or being inhibited by a fear of dangerous situations. Another advantage is that auditory training can precede formal travel lessons and prepare the individual for travel before actually taking part in a travel program. This allows the building of essential skills in young children before teaching wayfinding. It also permits group lessons, which can have the effect of building self-efficacy through observation and interaction with other successful learners (Volume 1, Chapter 6).

Part of the role of the O&M specialist or his or her assistant is to provide practice in using auditory information (Wiener et al., 1990; see Volume 1, Chapter 14, for information on the growth of this profession). In this model the instructor uses human guide techniques to guide the student through the environment while monitoring the student's ability to interpret pertinent auditory information.

Training in Natural Settings

Auditory training skills can be practiced with students who are totally blind or, when appropriate, with students with low vision. The question always arises as to whether or not it would be beneficial to blindfold those with low vision to assist them in learning to use their hearing more effectively. The Orientation and Mobility Division of AER in its position paper indicates that unless vision is all but unusable, it is best not to blindfold and instead best to teach the student how to use hearing to interact with residual vision (http://oandm.aerbvi.org/position_papers.htm). When vision interferes or when there is the prognosis of continued reduction in vision, it may be helpful to blindfold. Intermittent use of a blindfold may be useful in situations where the student with low

vision needs to learn how to integrate auditory skills with remaining vision. Sidebar 4.1 outlines several approaches to developing auditory skills in natural settings for use in independent travel.

Training with Recorded Sounds

A less widely used approach to auditory training involves the use of recorded sounds for improving auditory skills. Training with recorded sounds could alternate with training in the natural environment. It is a supplement not meant to replace on-the-street instruction. Training may be done with binaural recordings using headphones or monaural recordings played through speakers in a controlled sound field, or both. The procedure used for binaural training is to record environmental sounds on a multitrack recorder, with each track recording the sound received at ear level for the respective ear. The recording microphones are placed in positions that correspond to each ear. They may either be implanted in an artificial head at ear position or worn at ear level by a person. The separation of the microphones coupled with the head-shadow effect combine to create authentic recordings for practice in localization of sounds. With high-quality equipment having a wide-frequency response, fidelity approaches realistic levels. Reproduction is accomplished by amplifying the sounds and playing them back over headphones.

There are many advantages to such a system. Recordings provide sounds of the environment without the fear usually associated with traffic and other hazardous situations. Recordings also allow better control of environmental sounds for training situations. Instead of random experiences that are often encountered in on-the-spot training procedures, recordings permit planned sequencing of principles in an order that will facilitate learning. Also, recordings can be replayed for repeated study and can be used as a supplement to the actual travel-training on the street.

Practice Activities for the Use of Audition for Independent Travel in Natural Settings

The following outline includes possible methods for teaching many skills helpful to independent travel. It is not meant to be an exhaustive list of procedures to be followed, but suggested activities on which practitioners can expand. The tasks are based on the perceptual skills necessary for effective interpretation of auditory information and may be taught as part of travel instruction or separately.

I. Use of sound coming directly from a sound source to the listener

    A. Training in sound localization

        1. In a large room

            a) The student stands in the center of the room.

            b) The O&M specialist moves around the student and claps from different positions.

            c) The student turns and points to the O&M specialist each time the O&M specialist claps.

            d) The student walks to the O&M specialist each time the O&M specialist claps.

            e) The O&M specialist moves around the student, stopping in different locations, and the student must localize the point at which the O&M specialist's footsteps stopped.

            f) The student, using self-protective techniques, finds the way out of the room by localizing the sound coming through the doorway.

            g) The student repeats Step f in different rooms.

        2. In a large open area with an audible ball (a bell embedded in a ball)

            a) The student stands in the center of the area.

            b) The O&M specialist rolls the audible ball toward the student.

            c) The student must turn toward the ball, judge when the ball is nearby, then bend and pick it up.

        3. In a space with a hard floor (Coin localization can be taught in conjunction with the basic skills used in picking up dropped objects.)

            a) The O&M specialist throws a coin into the air.

            b) The student localizes the sound as the coin hits the floor.

            c) The student must point to the coin and walk toward it, using proper techniques to pick it up.

            d) The student repeats the procedure many times with up to as many as three coins dropped at the same time.

        4. In a variety of locations

            a) The student continues to practice sound localization.

            b) Localization is incorporated with training in sound identification as described in the next section.

    B. Training in sound identification

        1. In a building

            a) The O&M specialist takes the student through the building and asks the student to identify and localize varying sounds while passing through the halls and into some rooms.

            b) The O&M specialist can consider including sounds such as people keyboarding, phones ringing, doors opening, people walking, people writing, elevator doors opening, and so forth.

(continued on next page)

2. In a room

   a) The O&M specialist tells the student that by listening to the sounds of maneuvers made by others, much can be discovered about what a person is doing and about what is in a room.

   b) The O&M specialist asks the student to be seated and to listen to what the O&M specialist does between the time the O&M specialist enters the room and the time he or she leaves the room.

   c) The O&M specialist has the student later tell the O&M specialist what the specialist did on his or her maneuvers.

   d) The O&M specialist goes to different parts of the room on different maneuvers and uses different equipment. For example, the O&M specialist may enter the room, pull out a chair, sit at a desk, open a drawer, take out paper, write a few sentences, stand up, walk to a filing box, and file the paper.

3. In a residential neighborhood

   a) Using human guide techniques, the O&M specialist takes the student through a residential neighborhood to identify and localize sounds.

   b) The O&M specialist emphasizes determining the width of the street and the number of pedestrians in a group, and identifying car sounds, lawnmowers, and other sound-producing objects.

4. In a semibusiness area

   a) The O&M specialist takes the student through a semibusiness area to identify and localize sounds

of buses, trucks, cars, motorcycles, people entering cars, cars pulling away from traffic lights, cars slowing down, and other contextual sounds.

   b) The O&M specialist has the student estimate his or her distance from the corner by listening to cars going by on the perpendicular street.

   c) The O&M specialist has the student identify the characteristics of the street by listening to traffic. Is it one-way or two-way? Does it have heavy or light traffic? Is it straight or does it curve? What type of traffic control does it have? At signalized intersections, is there actuated, semi-actuated, or traditional timing?

   d) The O&M specialist has the student estimate the distance to the corner by listening to the cars stopping at the corner.

   e) The O&M specialist takes the student into different stores to identify the type of store by the sounds made.

5. Sound identification with the cane (Many common objects that the cane will strike have identifiable sounds. Learning to identify these sounds will aid in orientation.)

   a) The O&M specialist has the student strike a long cane against common objects outdoors to teach identification of objects by their sounds.

   b) The O&M specialist can include the following objects: automobile fenders, automobile bumpers, mailboxes, wooden poles, and other obstacles.

(continued on next page)

C. Training in discrimination between varying sounds

1. Sound-producing objects

a) The O&M specialist uses varying sound-producing objects such as bells or rattles with different pitches.

b) The student distinguishes between different sound-producing objects and pairs or matches those that sound alike.

2. Coin sounds

a) The O&M specialist drops a penny, nickel, dime, and quarter on the floor and asks the student to memorize the sound of each coin.

b) The O&M specialist drops each coin and has the student identify the order in which the coins were dropped.

3. Environment sounds

a) The O&M specialist plans routes through environments that expose the student to similar sounds, and has the student differentiate between those sounds.

b) The O&M specialist asks the student to localize and point at different objects.

4. Automobile sounds

a) At a signalized intersection, the O&M specialist teaches the student to differentiate between cars pulling away and cars idling in accordance with the changing traffic light.

b) The O&M specialist and student go to different intersections, and the student tells the O&M specialist when to cross the street by listening to traffic sounds.

c) The O&M specialist has the student identify the sounds of cars backing out of driveways.

d) The O&M specialist has the student identify both traditional and quieter hybrid vehicles.

D. Training in the use of sound shadow (A visual shadow is created when an object is between a light source and an observer. The object blocks out light that would ordinarily fall on the observer. A sound shadow is similar to a visual shadow except that sound is substituted for light. An object between a sound source and an observer blocks or muffles sound. The sound bending around the object and reaching the observer's ears will be of lower intensity and will lack the high-frequency components.)

1. Purpose: Sound shadow enables the student to become aware of an object between the student and a sound source. A student can use sound shadow to identify poles and parked cars along a street or at a corner.

2. Methods

a) The O&M specialist takes the student outdoors in a semibusiness area and places the student facing the street in front of a large object such as a truck or car.

b) The O&M specialist teaches the student to listen for the blocking out of sound as other motor vehicles pass the truck or car.

c) The O&M specialist places the student in front of a space where a large object may be present and has the student indicate whether something is present by listening to passing vehicles.

d) The process is repeated until the student is able to hear the sound shadow.

(*continued on next page*)

e) These procedures are repeated, using first wide poles and then thinner poles.

3. Reinforcement

a) The O&M specialist takes the student to different intersections and has the student indicate whether poles or parked cars are present.

b) The O&M specialist has the student walk along the street with the O&M specialist, telling the O&M specialist when he or she passes poles, parked cars, and bus shelters.

E. Training in the use of sound tracking or taking direction from a sound (Sound tracking is the process of listening and mentally tracing the paths of moving vehicles as they pass by.)

1. This technique may be used to place oneself parallel to the traffic before crossing a street, to enable one to walk straight across the street, to avoid walking near moving traffic on one side or into automobiles behind the crosswalk on the other side, or to determine one's position while walking along a sidewalk.

2. The O&M specialist reviews the possible paths of moving vehicles with the student.

3. As a prerequisite skill, the O&M specialist asks the student to track the movements of the O&M specialist.

a) The O&M specialist places the student in the center of a large room.

b) The O&M specialist explains the plan to stand to the right and in front of the student and walk parallel to the side of the student's body to represent an automobile moving toward, alongside, and past the student. (A path parallel to the student means that a passing object will be the same distance to the side when it starts moving, when it is alongside, and when it has passed. In other words, the paths of the student and object will never meet.)

c) The O&M specialist has the student listen to the O&M specialist, who will clap hands and walk alongside the student.

d) This time, as the O&M specialist walks the same route, clapping hands, the O&M specialist has the student trace the O&M specialist's path, pointing to the specialist while he or she is walking along the route.

e) The O&M specialist should walk several routes, some parallel and some not parallel to the student. After each walk, the O&M specialist has the student tell whether the route was parallel or not.

f) The O&M specialist has the student demonstrate whether the next route is parallel to him or her. If it is not, the O&M specialist has the student turn and make his or her projected path parallel to the O&M specialist's path. This exercise is repeated until the student performs satisfactorily.

g) Steps a through f are repeated, with the O&M specialist starting on the right side and behind the student and walking to a position ahead of the student.

h) Steps a through f are repeated, with the O&M specialist starting on the left side and in front of the student and walking to a position behind the student.

i) Steps a through f are repeated, with the O&M specialist starting on the left side and behind the student and

(*continued on next page*)

walking to a position in front of the student.

   j) Steps a through f are repeated, with the student trying to stand perpendicular to the path the O&M specialist walks.

4. Intersections

   a) At an intersection the O&M specialist has the student track traffic and line up with both parallel and perpendicular traffic. It should be noted that alignment to perpendicular traffic should be used only when the student is sure he or she is at a right-angle intersection.

   b) The O&M specialist guides the student across the street based on the way the student is facing. This provides immediate feedback and should help to improve sound tracking.

   c) Steps a and b are repeated until the student's performance is satisfactory.

II. Use of reflected sound

A. Training to use spatial hearing and echolocation

1. Determine room characteristics by use of reflected, refracted, and absorbed sound (The sound in a room may provide clues to the furnishing due to the reflection, refraction, or absorption of sound by the room's contents.)

   a) The O&M specialist takes the student into rooms containing sound-altering objects and acquaints the student with the sound quality present.

   b) The O&M specialist takes the student into rooms with varying furnishings and has the student identify those rooms that contain soft objects that refract and absorb sound, such as drapes, cloth chairs, or thick carpets.

   c) The O&M specialist takes the student into rooms that have furnishings that reflect sound and provide a harsh sound.

2. Use of a large board with the student in a stationary position

   a) With a large board in hand, the O&M specialist stands in front of the student, who is sitting down.

   b) The O&M specialist moves the board toward the student until the student becomes aware of it by utilizing ambient reflected sound. Next the O&M specialist moves the board back until it becomes imperceptible.

   c) This process is repeated until the student is able to detect the board effectively.

   d) The O&M specialist holds the board parallel to the front of the student's face, then tilts the board to the right or to the left and has the student identify the direction to which the board was tilted.

3. Echolocation combined with movement

   a) The O&M specialist holds a board at eye level while the student is at the other end of a hall. While using a modified upper hand and forearm technique, the O&M specialist has the student walk forward and try to stop before touching the board.

   b) This process is repeated until the student can stop before touching the board.

   c) When the student can repeatedly identify the presence of the board, the O&M specialist has the

(*continued on next page*)

student continue walking, getting as close as possible to the board without touching it.

d) Next, the O&M specialist has the student walk toward a wall, using self-protective techniques, and stop within 1 foot (30 cm) of the wall by listening to the ambient sound of his or her footsteps as he or she approaches it.

e) This process is repeated until the student is able to stop very close to the wall.

f) Steps e and f are repeated with the student's shoes off. Instead of using the sound of footsteps, the student should now rely on ambient sound in the hall.

g) The O&M specialist stands between the student and the end of a long hall. The O&M specialist instructs the student to walk through the hall and use the upper hand and forearm technique upon feeling that an object is in front of him or her.

h) This process is repeated until the student begins using the upper hand and forearm technique early enough to protect him- or herself.

B. Training to use ambient reflected sound to identify the presence or absence of walls on the side of the path of travel

1. Indoors

   a) Using the human guide techniques, the O&M specialist walks down a hall toward an intersecting corridor.

   b) The O&M specialist walks at a brisk speed, with the student close to the wall.

   c) The O&M specialist has the student use the change in sound to identify

the point at which the wall ends at the intersecting corridor.

d) Steps a through c are repeated until the student locates the opening consistently.

e) Next, using human guide techniques, the O&M specialist walks with the student past several open doorways, with the student close to the wall, and has the student identify openings as they are passed.

f) Next, the O&M specialist has the student travel down the hall independently, listening for the intersecting corridor.

g) After this is done with consistency, the O&M specialist has the student travel down the hall and count all open doorways.

h) The O&M specialist then has the student, using self-protective techniques, practice making turns in the halls without touching the walls.

2. Outdoors

   a) Using human guide techniques, the O&M specialist walks with the student along a street with many buildings that are close to the sidewalk and that have occasional alleyways between the buildings. The O&M specialist and student start at the corner and the O&M specialist has the student determine when the building line begins and has the student indicate the presence of alleys that are being passed.

   b) After the student has mastered these tasks, the O&M specialist has the student locate recesses or open doorways while walking along other streets.

There are also disadvantages to the use of recorded training materials. When used as a substitute for practice with actual environmental sounds, recordings deprive the student of necessary experience with using sound cues during actual travel. Another drawback concerns problems with front-rear localization, which seems to be inherent in such prerecorded stimuli. Many students undergoing such training have reported that although they could easily distinguish between sounds coming from the left and those coming from the right, they had difficulty determining whether some sounds originated from the front or the rear. This difficulty occurs often enough to be considered a serious problem. Because localization is due to differences in the time of arrival, phase, intensity, and spectral components between the two ears, sounds coming directly from either the front or rear are easily confused in a live listening situation until the head is moved slightly. Head movement changes these interaural differences enough to permit accurate localization. In a taped situation using headphones, turning the head does not change the signals at the two ears and does not resolve localization problems. Instead, the auditory environment turns with the head through the headphones. Some individuals rely more heavily on head movements to localize sound than others. Those who are more dependent on such movement find difficulty in localization with recordings. They report hearing all sounds as coming either from the front or from the rear. Recent advancements that utilize head-related transfer functions in the recording of auditory environmental information hold the promise of overcoming these deficits by linking head movements to the changes in sound that result with such motion.

HEARING AIDS

Chapter 4 in Volume 1 of this text considered the basic components of hearing aids, electroacoustic characteristics of hearing aids, and traditional hearing aids versus signal-processing aids. In this section we begin with a discussion of hearing aid candidacy and end with hearing aid amplification as a rehabilitation tool. It does not take long to discover that there is much to be learned about how best to help people with hearing aids and that much of what we know has not been considered with regard to persons who are blind.

Hearing Aid Candidates

Being a hearing aid candidate means that one should be evaluated to assess the need for and potential benefits from amplification. Hearing aid candidacy is typically based on audiometric and motivational factors.

Audiometric factors include the type and degree of loss shown on pure-tone tests, speech-recognition thresholds, the percent-correct speech-recognition scores, and the dynamic range or range of usable hearing. Most hearing aid users have sensorineural hearing loss, and relatively few have conductive loss, since most conductive losses can be remediated medically. High speech recognition scores and wide dynamic ranges suggest more benefits from amplification; low speech recognition scores and narrow dynamic ranges suggest less benefit. A variety of rules have been proposed for deciding what degree of hearing loss indicates a need for amplification. For example, it has sometimes been said that anyone whose average hearing loss or speech recognition threshold (SRT) is worse than 25 dB HL in the better ear is a candidate for a hearing aid. *Simply put, however, anyone who has difficulty with speech communication due to a hearing problem should be considered a candidate for hearing aid use.* Even those with unilateral losses or very severe bilateral losses should be considered as candidates. Hearing aids may make listening and localization easier even for persons with mild impairments; they may improve sound detection and speech reading (lipreading) even for those whose hearing loss is so severe (greater than 85 dB HL) that their speech recognition scores are not improved with amplification. Perhaps in situations with persons who are blind, anyone whose hearing problem causes difficulty with the use of auditory cues in orientation and mobility should also be considered a candidate for hearing aid use.

Motivational factors are represented by one's desire to alleviate a hearing disability, that is, by the impact of one's impairment or deviation from unimpaired hearing on the ability to communicate and participate in other desired activities (for example, independent travel). Although audiometric factors may suggest possible benefit from hearing aid use, one must be or become somewhat motivated in order to use amplification successfully.

Individuals with profound hearing loss who do not receive adequate assistance from the use of conventional amplification may be candidates for using vibrotactile aids. These devices provide limited information about speech and have been used primarily as aids to speech reading (Hnath-Chisolm, 1994).

Types of Hearing Aids

A variety of hearing aid types are shown in Figure 4.2. According to Kirkwood (1990) the three most common types of hearing aids, based on percentage of sales, are the in-the-ear (ITE) aids at 47.2 percent, in-the-canal (ITC) aids at 31.2 percent, and behind-the-ear (BTE) aids at 21.1 percent, while both body-worn and eyeglass aids combined represent less than 1 percent of sales. According to Strom (2006), the types of aids most often sold in 2005 were the ITE aids (37.12 percent) and the BTE aids (32.64 percent), with sales of ITC and completely in-the-canal (CIC) aids

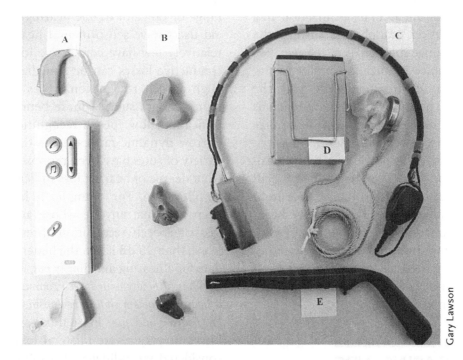

Gary Lawson

Figure 4.2.

Types of hearing aids: (A) Two behind-the-ear aids separated by a remote control; (B) in-the-ear, in-the-canal, and completely in-the-canal aids; (C) head-worn bone conduction hearing aid; (D) body aid with external air conduction receiver; (E) temple of eyeglasses aid.

representing 18.22 and 11.97 percent, respectively. Strom noted that sales of BTE aids clearly surged from 2004 to 2005 and that the increase in sales of BTE aids came mostly at the expense of sales of ITE aids. He also noted that in 2005, digital signal processing aids represented 89.08 percent of the market, while analog processing aids represented 10.92 percent and that, when compared to 2004 sales, the data show a clear decrease in the sale of traditional analog technology in favor of digital technology.

In-the-Ear and In-the-Canal Devices

Most ITE aids and ITC aids (Figure 4.2B) are of the custom variety, in which electronic components are built into an acrylic shell made by the manufacturer from the audiologist's impression of the user's ear. The ITE shell fits into the ear canal and the concha. ITE aids are called full-concha, low-profile, or half-concha instruments, depending on the degree to which they fill and protrude from the concha. ITC aids are located mostly or entirely within the external ear canal; CIC aids have recently achieved considerable popularity. While most CIC aids require screwdriver adjustment of the gain control, persons who are visually impaired may find remote control to be more satisfactory. The probability for successful use of ITE aids is reduced for average hearing losses (500, 1,000, or 2,000 Hz) of less than 35 dB HL (Staab & Lybarger, 1994) or greater than 70 dB HL (Wernick, 1985). Similar results are likely for ITC aids. Nevertheless, there are successful ITE and ITC hearing aid users whose hearing loss falls outside the 35–70 dB HL range.

Behind-the-Ear Aids

The postaural, or BTE, aid is contoured to fit behind the ear (Figure 4.2A). All components are typically contained within the unit behind the pinna, and amplification is sent from an air-conduction receiver through tubing to an ear mold. When two aids are used together to fit symmetrical losses, true binaural amplification can be attained, permitting accurate localization in many instances. Ample space is available on BTE aids for a variety of controls; a variety of appropriate frequency response, gain, and output characteristics are available in BTE aids for fitting a variety of hearing losses that range from mild to profound. Based on the sales statistics reported above, those with hearing loss appear to be developing greater acceptance of BTE hearing aids.

Eyeglass Aids

The eyeglass aid (Figure 4.2E) is similar in design to the BTE aid. The components of the aid are enclosed within the temple of the eyeglasses and can be installed in any pair of eyeglasses with a five- or seven-barrel bridge. Assuming similar microphone locations, the advantages of the BTE aid are also applicable for the eyeglass aid. Eyeglass aids may be more comfortable than BTE aids for the individual who is visually impaired who must wear eyeglasses and a hearing aid. This issue can typically be avoided, however, by careful selection of a BTE with a small case and templates (that is, a BTE that does not require a large space); if appropriate, this issue could also be avoided by using an ITE or ITC aid. Eyeglass aids have a disadvantage: The user may need an extra pair of eyeglasses for times when the hearing aid is being repaired. Eyeglass aids are rarely manufactured today (Staab, 2002).

Contralateral-Routing-of-Sound Aids

Staab (2002) describes, via narrative and figures including audiograms, several variations of contralateral-routing-of-sound aids. Only the classic contralateral-routing-of-sound (CROS) aid (Harford & Barry, 1965) and the bilateral-contralateral-routing-of-sound (BICROS) aid are described here. These aids can transmit the signal from a nonhearing ear on one side of the head to a better hearing ear on the other side by a wire, but radio-frequency transmission appears be the more commonly used method. The classic CROS aid consists of the components for a complete hearing aid housed in two hearing aid cases; one case contains the amplifier and receiver, and the other contains the microphone. This device picks up sound with a microphone at a nonhearing ear and routes it to an amplifier and receiver at a nearly unimpaired ear. The nearly unimpaired ear is fit with a tube or a nonoccluding ear mold to keep the ear open to environmental sound. This arrangement eliminates head shadow on the hearing side when the sound source is on the nonhearing side and can improve sound localization. The bilateral-contralateral-routing-of-sound (BICROS) aid also consists of two hearing aid cases, one containing a complete hearing aid coupled to an occluding ear mold and the other containing only a microphone with an on-off switch. The BICROS aid can be fitted for a bilateral hearing loss in which one ear is functional and the other is not. The complete hearing aid is fit to the hearing side and the microphone to the nonhearing side to eliminate head shadow. The fitting of CROS aids should be considered for persons who are blind since they can have an enhancing effect on sound localization; however, the BICROS aid may actually decrease sound-localization ability.

Body Aids

The microphone and amplifier of the body aid are contained in a case that is placed in a pocket, clipped to the user's clothing, or worn in a harness on the torso; the external receiver is connected to the amplifier in the case by a wire and snapped to the ear mold (Figure 4.2D). The location of the microphone in a case worn on the body makes it susceptible to clothing noise and body baffle and shadow effects that are more undesirable than those associated with ear-level aids. Furthermore, even when two aids are used and placed far apart on the body, true binaural amplification is not obtained because the micro-

phones are not at ear level. The relatively large external receivers used with body aids typically have a poorer high-frequency response range than do smaller receivers in ear-level aids. Today, such aids are rarely used, and few manufacturers still make them (Staab, 2002). Their advantages over aids worn at the ear may include increased gain with less chance of acoustic feedback, larger controls and batteries, room for more controls, and better ruggedness and durability. They may occasionally be recommended for geriatric persons with poor manual dexterity or very young, active children who have a hearing loss of 85 to 100 dB HL.

Hearing Aids with Bone-Conduction Receivers

Although the vast majority of hearing aids (described previously) amplify by an air-conduction receiver, a small number do so by a bone-conduction receiver (see, for example, Figure 4.2C). Bone-conduction receivers are typically used in rare situations when an ITE aid or an ear mold cannot be put into the ear canal for medical reasons or when a large conductive component to a hearing loss exists. For BTE and body aids, the bone-conduction receiver is attached to a headband placed on the mastoid on the opposite side of the head from the other components; the receiver is connected to the hearing aid case by a wire. For an eyeglass aid, the bone-conduction vibrator is part of the eyeglass template that fits behind the pinna, and the remaining components are located in the template on the opposite side of the head; the wire connecting the receiver to the amplifier can be very conveniently routed through the frame of the eyeglasses. Generally speaking, a significant amount of force must be amplified to the vibrator; because this force is more easily applied by a headband than by spring-loaded eyeglass templates, eyeglass aids tend to have lower vibrator outputs than do BTE aids (Staab & Lybarger, 1994). A recent variation of bone-conduction hearing aids transposes signals into audible ultrasound (30 to 40 kHz) before directing them to the skull via a bone-conduction vibrator (Staab et al., 1998).

Recommendation of Hearing Aid Types

The fitting of special types of hearing aids may be particularly challenging for some dispensers because of infrequent experience with such aids. In general, the smaller aids (ITC and ITE) have less electronic flexibility, require smaller controls, can accommodate fewer controls, allow fewer modifications, and require a smaller battery than do larger aids. Nevertheless, they are often adequately adjustable; they require less power than larger aids for achieving a given result because the internal receiver is located relatively close to the tympanic membrane; their use provides possible benefits from the natural resonances of the external ear; they facilitate localization; they are typically easier to insert and remove; and, cosmetically speaking, they are typically more appealing than larger aids. Although cosmetic judgments are an individual matter, it is not surprising that collectively ITE and ITC aids represent more than 75 percent of hearing aid sales. Although small hearing aids are often the instruments of choice, when selecting the type of device, hearing aid users and fitters should carefully consider the individual's needs.

Hearing Aids as a Rehabilitation Tool

The hearing aid industry is largely market driven. Manufacturers would like to sell products that are in demand, and most hearing aid dispensers would like to fit reasonably priced products that are beneficial and in demand. Nevertheless, the selection and fitting of hearing aids is not an exact science, and manufacturers must deal with the challenge of providing the best technology at a marketable price. The nature of the tools available for aural rehabilitation is determined to some extent by market forces.

Traditionally, most hearing aids have been fixed-frequency response devices that limit their maximum output by distortion-causing peak clipping. Typically they have been built to function within a limited frequency range of about 400 to 4,000 Hz, and fitting trends have emphasized amplification for frequencies of approximately 1,000 to 4,000 Hz, a range that is particularly important to the intelligibility of speech. Frequencies beyond this range could, in theory, contribute additional cues for speech intelligibility and for orientation and mobility. However, lower frequencies, which contain more noise, are generally not amplified as much as the higher frequencies because enhancing them generally can make sound uncomfortable and communication difficult. However, gain in the lower frequencies may be useful for the traveler who requires low frequencies to identify openings in a wall or building line. The use of programmable hearing aids that can be switched to amplify low frequencies in those instances may be useful for this individual.

More gain may be needed for greater hearing loss, and hearing loss tends to be greater at higher frequencies. The increase of gain at high frequencies (even at 4,000 Hz) is sometimes limited by problems with *feedback*, a squealing sound produced by the reamplification of sound leaking from the system. In other words, there is a limit to the amount of gain possible before feedback. The amount of gain possible at a given frequency is also limited by the difference between the level of the input signal to the hearing aid and the user's loudness discomfort level, both of which can vary with frequency. It is important to note that output equals input plus gain and that output should not equal or exceed the loudness discomfort level. Less gain can be added to high input levels than to low input levels before reaching a given loudness discomfort level. Because of physical and physiological limitations, it may be impossible, particularly with traditional technology, to provide all of the perceptual cues above the threshold level that ordinarily is necessary for understanding speech or for orientation and mobility.

In spite of their limitations, hearing aids have great potential as a rehabilitation tool for the traveler who is blind and hearing impaired. Rehabilitation should include improvement of O&M skills as well as communication skills. Although traditional hearing aid technology provides significant benefits for many hearing impaired users, newer technologies also should be considered as options. Advantages of newer digital technology include greater precision and flexibility in adjusting the aid's amplification. These aids are capable of fitting a wide range of hearing losses. Although they are often the most expensive hearing aids on the market today, their popularity, sophistication, and benefits still make them the highest percentage of hearing aids sold.

Amplification of Traffic Sounds

A spectral analysis of traffic sounds (Wiener & Goldstein, 1977; Wiener et al., 1997) found the greatest absolute intensity to be in the lower frequencies. When the sensitivity of the human ear to different frequencies is considered, it becomes evident that the greatest traffic-sound intensity available to the individual is between 500 and 4,000 Hz. Although these mid- to upper-frequencies play the greatest role in the audibility of traffic sounds, frequencies between 125 and 500 Hz also contain energy that is sufficiently audible for use in orientation and mobility. Most individuals who are hearing impaired have better hearing for low frequencies than for high frequencies. Therefore, a hearing aid that emphasizes only frequencies above 1,000 Hz may fail to provide some useful information for interpretation of traffic sounds. If a traveler in an outdoor area near traffic would like to optimize reception of low-frequency cues, a programmable

hearing aid could allow the traveler to select a predominantly low-frequency response or a broad-frequency response. The result should be better reception of low-frequency traffic cues. This could be accomplished by using a programmable aid that has base increase at low levels (see Volume 1, Chapter 4). Now assume that the traveler reaches his or her desk in a quiet office environment and wishes to eliminate low-frequency noise and maximize reception of speech cues. The traveler could now select a predominantly high-frequency response. The flexibility offered by programmable hearing aids may be important to visually and hearing impaired travelers.

Sound localization has been shown to be more accurate in both the lower and higher frequencies than in the middle frequencies. Given that the ability to localize sound is critical for acquisition of good mobility skills, it is important that hearing aids have the capability of amplifying both lower and higher frequencies.

According to De l'Aune, Lewis, Dolan, Grimmelsman, and Needham (1976), the ability to judge the distance of a sound-emitting object may be impaired by some hearing aids. They explain that environmental sounds that are closer to the individual have higher-frequency components than sounds that are farther away. The more distant sounds lose high frequencies as they travel through the air. Hearing aids that do not have a sufficient high-frequency response may not allow the individual to receive the high frequencies necessary for distance judgment. De l'Aune et al. also stated that hearing aids that are designed to limit gain in response to loud sounds may also make distance judgment difficult. Although this usually is not the case, an automatic volume control in a hearing aid may reduce the intensity differences between the near and far sounds while preventing user discomfort from overamplification. For those who need large amounts of amplification and have a narrow range of usable hearing, hearing aids may be specifically designed to greatly limit gain at high input levels. Therefore, intense sounds from objects nearby may be transmitted at a softer level and judged by the individual as being farther away than they really are. In the case of a fast-moving automobile, this could be a dangerous situation. Automatic-volume-control or compression hearing aids have traditionally limited hearing aid output across the frequency range by adding progressively less gain to the input as input levels increase. Today, some multichannel hearing aids are capable of using this technique to differentially limit output in particular frequency bands. Such aids might retain some of the frequency cues that would assist in distance judgment. De l'Aune et al. recommended that hearing aids have an automatic-volume-control switch that would permit turning off output limitation circuitry during travel times. Although such hearing aids are currently possible, user-operated output controls are not common.

Unilateral versus Bilateral Loss

Hearing aids should help persons who are hearing impaired improve their sound localization. Unilateral hearing loss disrupts the natural balance of acoustic cues arriving at the two ears. As reported by Bergman (1957), when sound levels reach the threshold of the ear with a greater hearing loss, the ability to determine the direction of the sound is greatly improved. The closer the sensitivity of the two ears, the better the localization will be. Therefore, a hearing aid that provides more intensity to the ear with a greater hearing loss should help to improve localization.

Whenever bilateral hearing loss is a factor, binaural hearing aids should be used when possible to balance the hearing sensitivity of the two ears. Although binaural amplification helps one to determine whether a sound is coming from the right or left, front-rear reversals can still be a problem. As noted by Yost (2000, pp. 183–184), there are a number of directional sound locations that would produce the same interaural

time and intensity differences. One example would be sound locations directly in front of and behind the listener; this is why a sound from the front is sometimes thought to be coming from the rear. Without head movement and the spectral and phase differences associated with the effects of anatomical transfer functions on complex signals (Hartmann, 1999), only pinna effects differentiate sound from the front and rear. Reversals are not a severe problem for people with unimpaired vision because vision is used to verify sound origin. The traveler who is blind, however, cannot use sight to help localize the sound when experiencing reversals.

Keane (1965) suggested that these reversals might be due to the location of the microphone port in most BTE hearing devices. During one period of time, the microphone port was behind or above the pinna of the ear and was not shadowed from the rear by the pinna. Today, the microphone is typically covered by a windscreen and located above the ear. ITE or ITC hearing aids might solve any problems associated with the location of microphone ports.

Because of sound-localizing difficulties with hearing aids, De l'Aune et al. (1976) suggested that individuals with visual impairment and with mild hearing losses who experience localization difficulties while using their hearing aids might do better to remove their aids for travel purposes. They cautioned, however, that such a decision be made only in collaboration with an audiologist. Presumably, those with more severe losses would have to depend on hearing aids. Ericson and Staley (2003) presented noise to six subjects in order to study the effects of noise-induced hearing loss and head motion on the listeners' ability to localize sound. They found that when allowed to move their heads, the subjects with unimpaired hearing and the subjects with mild hearing loss showed improved acuity for azimuth and greatly reduced front-to-back reversal rates. In contrast, they found that when allowed to move their heads, the subjects with moderate hearing impairment showed poorer acuity for azimuth and elevation and had higher front-to-back reversal rates.

When hearing aids are worn for localization, every attempt should be made to provide localization training coupled with immediate feedback to improve accuracy. Often, when inaccuracies are found in distinguishing sounds coming from the right or left, the difficulty can be overcome by adjusting the gain control of the hearing aid. A simple "fusion test" can help a person to adjust the gain control or other controls to equalize the sensitivity of the two ears more closely and thus improve localization (Keane, 1965). The O&M specialist should stand directly in front of the student and instruct the student to adjust the gain control on the aid or aids until the specialist's voice sounds as though it is coming from directly ahead. Noting the control position at this point will facilitate returning to it when necessary.

A person with one near-normal ear and one totally deaf ear may have trouble localizing sound accurately. If so, localization can often be greatly improved with a CROS hearing aid. Successful use of this aid for independent travel has been documented (Rintelmann, Harford, & Burchfield, 1970). The reality is that some audiologists see very few people who are blind and may not be immediately aware of a given blind person's auditory needs. The audiologist who is concerned only with helping someone understand speech in particular settings may not consider all the options for amplification. The use of the CROS aid, for example, might not be seriously considered. Interpreting information with CROS aids takes practice. The necessity for a blind person to be able to localize traffic and other environmental sounds, however, may make the extra time needed to learn to use a CROS aid well worthwhile. In contrast, some feel that a BICROS aid reduces directional information, makes localization more difficult, and should not be recommended for people who are blind.

A Commentary on the Use of Hearing Aids

Flamme (2002) described a variety of issues on localization, hearing loss, and hearing aids. These descriptions provide the basis for thinking and commentary about what one might expect of those who use hearing aids in localization tasks.

Some broad generalizations can be made. Binaural cues are important to localization, and binaural hearing aid fittings should be most useful in cases where they are appropriately fit. Since localization in a vertical plane is dependent largely on high-frequency cues, it will be more difficult than localization in a horizontal plane. For average hearing losses, greater than approximately 50 dB HL, hearing aids may, within limits, improve sound localization in the horizontal plane. In general, benefits of hearing aid use are more easily recognized when hearing loss is approximately 55 dB HL or greater. It seems likely that localization, and audition in general, will be challenged further by the most severe losses.

For less severe hearing losses with relatively good low-frequency hearing, hearing aids may make localization poorer, particularly if the ear canal is completely plugged. Simply plugging the ear with a hearing aid or an ear mold can reduce low-frequency cues (for example, interaural time differences) and eliminate concha resonance. When fitting mild to moderate hearing losses, it may be advisable whenever possible to use relatively open fittings and place the microphone inside the entrance to the ear canal. Such fittings allow low-frequency localization cues to enter the ear canal and may allow retention of the concha resonance that enhances high-frequency cues. Vented CIC hearing aids and BTE aids with thin tubes and relatively open earmold systems may accomplish this goal. Acoustically speaking, such fittings may facilitate the transition from unaided to aided localization.

Since directional hearing aids tend to improve the audibility of sounds coming directly from in front of the listener and to reduce audibility of sounds from other directions, they may improve the listener's ability to understand speech in background noise but reduce the user's ability to detect localization cues. However, aids with directional microphones are not completely effective and do not eliminate localization cues altogether. Again, where appropriate, ear-mold and vent systems that allow low-frequency cues to enter the ear canal may help the individual to overcome the loss of some directional cues. Directional microphones that can be switched on and off may be preferred over those that cannot be.

Compression hearing aids that do not have high compression thresholds and therefore apply compression at relatively low stimulus levels may complicate localization. Consider how identical binaural hearing aids might respond to three different stimulus levels. For example, a low stimulus level might not result in compression in either aid. A little higher stimulus level might result in compression at the near aid but not at the far aid. A higher stimulus level might result in compression in both aids. Such situations might greatly complicate the judgment of distance and confound the use of overall intensity and spectral cues in localization. The use of relatively high compression thresholds may, in some instances, help to avoid degradation of localization by retaining linear amplification over most of the useful range of amplification.

The fitting of hearing aids involves art as well as science. Hearing aids do not solve all hearing problems under the best of circumstances. Fitting aids for optimal reception of speech may, in some instances, not lead to optimal reception of localization cues. The optimal fitting for one person will not be the optimal fitting for all, and some desired results may not be possible for those with the most severe hearing losses. Programmable hearing aids with multiple memories, whether their processing is analog or digital, can provide alternative responses that may

be particularly useful to the traveler who is visually impaired. Such aids allow the user to choose a different frequency response for different listening situations. For some these aids may simply complicate the user's use of auditory cues for independent travel.

ALTERNATIVE APPROACHES: ASSISTIVE LISTENING DEVICES AND IMPLANTS

Alternative hearing aids, such as cochlear implants and tactile devices, pick up acoustic signals and amplify or process them for transmission to the patient in some nonacoustic manner. Some devices (for example, cochlear implants) are typically used only by those with severe to profound hearing loss, whereas others (for example, sound-field listening devices) may be helpful to those with little or no hearing loss. Assistive devices or systems may pick up information other than oral speech and send it to one or more of the sensory systems. For example, an alarm clock might signal the user with a flashing light or a vibratory stimulus. Those with profound hearing loss who do not receive adequate assistance from the use of conventional amplification may be candidates for using vibrotactile aids. These devices provide limited information about speech and have been used primarily as aids to speech reading (Hnath-Chisolm, 1994). Following are four categories of assistive listening devices and the basic functions of four categories of surgical implants.

Assistive Listening Devices

Assistive listening devices (ALDs) may be categorized as personal and group amplification systems, television amplification systems, telephone systems, and signaling devices (Mueller & Carter, 2002). Personal and group amplification systems include hardwired systems, induction loop systems, infrared systems, and FM systems. Television amplification systems include the systems listed under personal and group amplification systems in conjunction with television. Telephone devices include telephone amplifiers, telecoils on hearing aids, and telecommunication devices for the deaf. Signaling devices are designed to monitor the output from such sources as an alarm clock, a doorbell, a smoke alarm, or a baby's cry. Although detailed description of these ALDs is beyond the scope of this chapter, additional information on ALDs is available in Mueller, Johnson, and Carter (2007); Mueller and Carter (2002); and Tyler and Schum (1995).

Surgical Implants

As noted by Weber (2002), there are currently four categories of surgically implanted hearing prosthetic devices: bone-anchored hearing aids (that is, the Baha), middle-ear implants, cochlear implants, and auditory brain-stem implants. Each of the four categories of implants is described in the following sections. A summary of information about implants and their role in sound localization follows the four descriptions.

Bone-Anchored Hearing Aid

Figure 4.3 shows the Baha components (Figures 4.3A and B) and the appearance of the Baha as worn (Figure 4.3C). Surgery for the Baha involves implantation of a titanium screw into the skull's temporal bone, typically posterior to the pinna and at a level just above the top of the pinna (Figure 4.3A). The implant connects to an abutment that connects to the sound processor (that is, the housing containing the microphone, battery, and the components for processing sound) (Figure 4.3B). One's appearance when wearing the device (Figure 4.3 C) can vary on an individual basis.

The Baha's sound processor sends sound vibrations directly to the inner ear via bone conduction without going through the skin first. Some think of it as a replacement for a traditional bone-conduction hearing aid (for example, Mueller & Carter, 2002). Sound picked up by the microphone in the sound processor is transmitted equally well via bone conduction to both cochleae. The Baha is designed for those with moderate to severe unilateral or bilateral conductive or mixed hearing loss, or both, or for those with profound unilateral sensorineural hearing loss (Weber, 2002). Examples of those who might

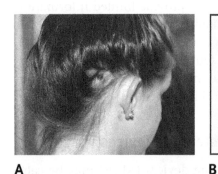
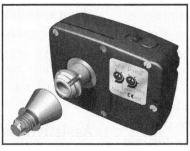
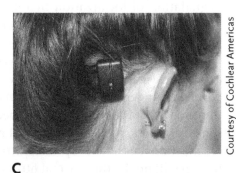

A   B   C

Courtesy of Cochlear Americas

Figure 4.3. The Baha System
(A) The titanium implant following surgery and healing. (B) The three parts of the Baha system: an implant connected to an abutment and the detachable sound processor. (C) The processor in place. When the hair is worn down, it hides the processor.

benefit from this type of aid are those with chronic infection of the ear canal, those with congenital malformations resulting in a narrowing or absence of the ear canal, those with middle ear disease, or those who have lost their hearing on one side due to surgery for a tumor on CN VIII. In other words, the Baha may be an option for those who have conditions that may preclude the use of a traditional hearing aid.

Middle Ear Implants

Over the past several years, a number of developments in middle ear implantable hearing devices occurred to some degree using a variety of approaches, but, apparently, few received any form of FDA approval (Ross and Levitt, 2000; Weber, 2002). A common aspect of most approaches is the placement of a receiver on the ossicular chain in the middle ear in order to directly vibrate the ossicles, sending vibrations into the cochlea. Developments include external and internal components. External components include a behind-the-ear or in-the-ear sound processor (microphone, battery, processing circuitry, and electromagnetic coil), and the internal component is a receiver magnet implanted in the middle ear on the stapes. At least one device is designed to place all components in the middle ear (Ross and Levitt, 2000; Weber, 2002). Middle ear implants can be used by adults who have moderately severe sensorineural hearing loss and word-recognition scores of at least 60 percent (Weber, 2002).

Cochlear Implants

A cochlear implant is essentially a system that converts sound to electrical signals, applies a special coding strategy to the signals, and then uses the coded signals to stimulate auditory nerve fibers. The goal is to provide acoustic information to persons who have a severely damaged or poorly developed cochlea and adequately functioning auditory neurons.

A cochlear implant consists of three major externally worn components and two major internal, that is, implanted, components. The *three external components* consist of a microphone, a speech processor, and an external transmitter. In older implant systems, the microphone is worn in a case that looks like a behind-the-ear hearing aid, and the speech processor is worn, often on the belt, in a case that looks like a body hearing aid. In newer implant systems (Figure 4.4) the microphone and the speech processor (now smaller) are both worn in the same case, which looks like a behind-the-ear hearing aid. The *two internal components* consist of a receiver implanted in the mastoid bone and an electrode array implanted in the cochlea.

So, how does the system work? The microphone, an input transducer, converts sound into electrical signals and sends them to the speech processor over a wire. The speech processor, a coding device, applies a device-specific coding strategy to the incoming electrical signal and then sends the coded electrical signal over a wire to the external transmitter. The transmitter, a coil held in place by a magnet attached to the receiver, sends the coded signal through the skin to the receiver (implanted in the mastoid bone) via FM radio waves. The receiver, an output transducer-stimulator, converts the FM waves to electrical signals and sends them to an array of electrodes implanted in the cochlea. Although separated from the auditory neurons by bone, the electrode array is in close proximity to the neurons and is able to stimulate functioning nerve fibers electrically. These neurons are then able to carry information to the brain.

Historically, candidates for cochlear implants often had pure-tone thresholds in the 90–109 dB HL range, no open-set word recognition with appropriately fitted hearing aids, and no apparent physical or mental contraindications for having the surgery and benefiting from the results (Hnath-Chisolm, 1994). Candidacy criteria have

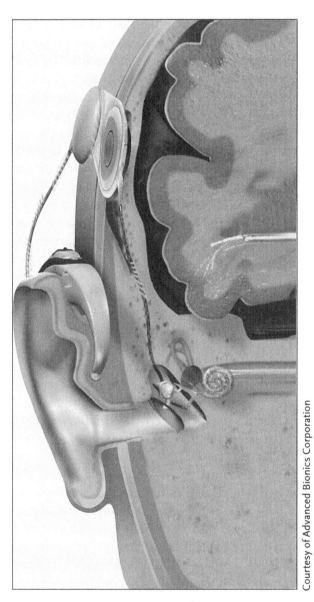

Courtesy of Advanced Bionics Corporation

Figure 4.4.
A recent cochlear implant system as might be worn on a cross-section of a model head.

changed over time. Current implantation criteria for children and adults, information about insurance coverage, and other information can often be found on the web sites of reputable organizations and implant centers (see the Resources section and the list of web sites in the Learning Ac-

tivities at the end of this chapter). Some successful implant users are able to use timing and voice cues to aid speech reading and may even have some limited success in telephone listening. At the very least, implant users usually benefit from an awareness of sound. According to Hnath-Chisolm (1994), improvements in speech production are greater for children who undergo implantation during early childhood.

Auditory Brain Stem Implant

An auditory brain stem implant (ABI) is a system that takes the place of a defective cochlea and a defective auditory nerve. The ABI was developed to help patients who have neurofibromatosis type 2 and have lost auditory nerve function due to tumors on their vestibulocochlear nerves. However, the system may be helpful to others as well, for example, those with other bilateral eighth-nerve dysfunction, those with bilateral temporal bone fractures, or those with bilateral failure of cochlear and auditory nerve development (Weber, 2002). The ABI is based largely on concepts used in cochlear implants. The system is able to pick up sound at a location on the outer ear and to transmit information about that sound directly to an electrode array at the cochlear nuclei in the brainstem. Thus, the system enables transfer of auditory information from the outer ear to the central auditory pathways in the brain, while bypassing the cochlea and auditory nerve.

The ABI system consists of external (worn) and internal (implanted) parts similar to those used in cochlear implants. The external parts consist of a microphone, speech processor, and transmitter. The internal parts consist of a receiver-stimulator implanted in the mastoid bone behind the ear, an electrode array implanted in the brain stem, and a wire connecting the receiver-stimulator to the electrode array. The microphone converts sounds into electrical signals and sends them to the speech processor over a wire. The speech processor applies a coding strategy to the incoming electrical signal, and then sends the coded electrical signal over a wire to the external transmitter. The external transmitter, a coil held in place on the mastoid by a magnet attached to a receiver implanted in the mastoid bone, sends the coded signal through the skin to a receiver via FM radio waves. The receiver-stimulator converts the FM waves to electrical signals and sends them past the defective cochlea and auditory nerve to an array of electrodes implanted on or in the brain stem, near the cochlear nucleus. The electrode array electrically stimulates functioning auditory pathways in the brain stem, allowing the transfer of auditory information throughout the central auditory pathways.

Implants: Localization and Research

It is well established that cochlear implants provide substantial benefit to speech perception and to language development, particularly when implantation occurs at an early age. Are cochlear implants useful in sound localization? That appears to be the case. Schoen, Mueller, and Helms (1999) found that their bilaterally implanted subjects could achieve a minimum audible angle of 5 degrees in the frontal horizontal plane. In a study of five bilateral implant users, Van Hoesel and Tyler (2003) concluded that accuracy of sound localization in quiet environments is significantly improved by the use of two implants rather than one. Nopp, Schleich, and D'Haese (2004) studied sound localization with bilateral and unilateral implants in 18 adults deafened after 5 or 6 years of age and in two adults who became deaf before 6 years of age. They found substantial benefit for bilateral implants in the adults who experienced deafness late in life. Recognizing the limited data on two subjects, they speculated that subjects who experienced deafness early in life and received implants late in life may not localize sound well and that ear-

lier implantation might lead to improved localization. Seebar, Baumann, and Fasti (2004) studied localization in subjects using a cochlear implant on one ear and a hearing aid on the other and in subjects with bilateral implants. They found successful localization in either arrangement, as long as the bimodal subjects had sufficient residual hearing in one ear. In considering the possible benefits from implantations and other forms of remediation, one must always be aware that individual results may vary from what might reasonably be expected. In a preliminary study of mobility functioning of two individuals with vision loss who had received cochlear implants, it was found that both individuals achieved some level of success with localization and alignment with parallel traffic (Ratelle & Dufour, 2006).

Although research on localization via the use of Baha, middle ear implants, and ABI devices is not readily available, it seems reasonable, assuming that binaural audibility is improved, that localization might also be improved, at least to some extent. Such improvements do, however, need to be demonstrated, and it is likely that they will not always be forthcoming.

THE O&M SPECIALIST'S ROLE

In order to prepare students for independent travel, the O&M specialist needs to have a realistic understanding of the auditory functioning of each individual. The specialist should ensure that in addition to a battery of social, medical, and ophthalmologic information, each student's file includes valid audiometric information. The specialist should be sufficiently skilled in the interpretation of audiograms to evaluate general auditory function as a starting point in communication with the student. Audiometric data are useful but must be combined with observation of auditory functioning in natural environments because people with very similar audiograms can function very differently. It is a known fact that some learn to use hearing more effectively than others; therefore, actual observation is necessary. Speech-recognition scores can be a useful supplementary tool for assessing speech comprehension. Pathology and type of hearing loss may give the O&M specialist a rough idea about functional expectations. For example, conductive losses are relatively free from distortion. Sensorineural losses, on the other hand, are prone to distortion even with hearing aids. Together, the O&M specialist and the audiologist can help the person who is visually and hearing impaired to achieve a higher level of rehabilitation.

The O&M specialist is responsible for developing a training program to teach the necessary auditory skills for independent travel. As indicated earlier, the auditory skills program may be implemented before formal training in travel techniques, concurrently with but separate from such training, or as an integral part of it. The training may be provided in natural settings or in a combination of natural settings and recorded-sound settings. The O&M specialist is often in a position to consult with family and teachers on auditory training activities. Explaining to family members the necessity for stimulating the child with auditory toys and games to initiate ear-hand coordination, exploration of the environment, and auditory development is most helpful. Providing auditory training suggestions to the classroom teacher is also beneficial. All in all, the O&M specialist should function as a member of the auditory rehabilitation team, working alongside the otolaryngologist, audiologist, and family.

IMPLICATIONS FOR O&M PRACTICE

1. Adults typically develop auditory skills during active travel instruction in orientation and mobility, but some develop skills through sensory training classes. Children often learn these skills through play, incidental learning, and structured learning experiences.

2. Hearing aid fittings attempt to selectively amplify frequencies enough to make speech intelligible, but not uncomfortably loud.

3. In order to prevent amplification from reaching the level of discomfort, linear hearing aids use a peak clipping approach to limit the output of the aid, while signal-processing aids limit output by compression.

4. Digitally programmable signal processing hearing aids may allow users who are blind to select characteristics that are likely to meet both communication and travel needs.

5. Most persons who are hearing impaired will use hearing aids, but ALDs and surgically implanted devices represent important alternatives in some cases.

6. ALDs may be categorized as personal and group amplification systems, television amplification systems, telephone systems, and signaling devices. Information about these devices is typically available in books on audiologic treatment of hearing loss.

7. The four main categories of surgically implanted hearing prosthetic devices are bone-anchored hearing aids, middle ear implants, cochlear implants, and auditory brain-stem implants. A middle ear implant is placed in a malfunctioning middle ear. A cochlear implant is a system that can provide acoustic information to persons who have a severely damaged or poorly developed cochlea and adequately functioning auditory neurons. An auditory brain stem implant replaces a poorly functioning or nonfunctioning cochlea and a poorly functioning or nonfunctioning auditory nerve.

8. Although research has demonstrated improved sound localization with cochlear implants, more research is needed to study sound localization with middle ear implants and with auditory brain stem implants.

9. The O&M specialist should understand an individual's auditory function well enough to teach the auditory skills needed for independent travel and serve on the auditory rehabilitation team, working in consultation with the otolaryngologist, audiologist, and student's family.

LEARNING ACTIVITIES

1. Visit a center for assistive listening devices to see what is available for those who have hearing impairments and what may be appropriate for those with both visual and hearing impairments.

2. Explore web sites on surgical implants to learn more about implants, to see images of FDA-approved hardware, and to see the latest criteria for implantation of children and adults. To begin, try the following sites:

- American Academy of Audiology: www .audiology.org/
- American Speech-Language-Hearing Association: http://www.asha.org/default.htm
- University of Michigan Medical Center: www.med.umich.edu/oto/ci/implant .htm
- University of Miami School of Medicine: http://cochlearimplants.med.miami.edu/ patients/01_Criteria%20for%20Cochlear %20Implantation.asp
- The Otology Group at Vanderbilt University Medical Center: www.mc.vanderbilt .edu/root/vumc.php?site=otology&doc= 5003
- Manufacturers of surgical implant devices:
  - Vibrant Soundbridge (MED-EL): www .symphonix.com/archive/layout/ splash.asp
  - Cochlear Americas: www.cochlear americas.com/
  - Advanced Bionics: www.advancedbi onics.com/
  - MED-EL Cochlear Implants: www.me del.com/

CHAPTER 5

Improving Sensorimotor Functioning for Orientation and Mobility

Sandra Rosen

LEARNING QUESTIONS

- What is the role of the orientation and mobility (O&M) specialist in facilitating sensorimotor development and functioning?

- What types of activities can facilitate development of each of the following sensory systems: proprioception, vestibular, tactile?

- How can the influence of primitive neurological reactions on O&M skills be addressed?

- What strategies can be used to address stereotypies in children?

- What special considerations do elderly travelers present with regard to gait and balance?

Chapter 5 in Volume 1 provides an overview and analysis of the components and building blocks of sensorimotor functioning that underlie the poor performance of many of the common motor skills needed for mobility. Sensorimotor functioning involves the awareness and interpretation of sensory information and its integration with motor skills to perform activities in an effective and efficient manner. Very little research has been done in the area of activities to facilitate sensorimotor development and functioning in children and adults with visual impairments. Much of what is known in the field is from observation and anecdotal data. Still, this information is valuable and enables us to consider a systematic approach to addressing the types of sensorimotor problems commonly seen in students with visual impairments.

Most of the information in this chapter concerns working with children. The sensorimotor problems seen in children (excluding those who have physical or other health impairments) are due to a lack of sensorimotor development and integration. The underlying neurological structure is sufficiently intact and healthy, and so facilitation activities can often be effective. This is not the case when working with students who are elderly.

While many similar sensorimotor problems are seen in young children with visual impairments and in elderly persons (see Volume 1, Chapter 5), the underlying causes are quite different. The sensorimotor problems seen in the elderly population are not due to a lack of stimulation of an otherwise basically healthy neurological system; instead, the problems are compensations for the physical decline in neurological and physical abilities secondary to the aging process.

While some activities discussed in this chapter have been shown to be helpful in slowing a decline in physical functioning, a concerted program in sensorimotor facilitation is generally not as effective in improving motor performance for travel needs with elderly individuals as it is with children.

Last, as was seen in Volume 1, Chapter 5, many of the underlying sensorimotor skills develop during the early years and have already developed in adults. For this reason, activities that focus on such things as the development of neurological reactions, learning basic motor activities from crawling to walking, are not relevant when working with adults. Other areas of sensorimotor functioning, such as posture and gait development, tend to stabilize at certain ages and can be difficult to change in later years. Sensorimotor activities that focus on improving posture and gait, therefore, generally do not have a major impact on the travel skills of adults. When activities can be effectively used with adults as well as with children, this is noted in the chapter.

Some of the most common sensorimotor performance issues that affect mobility include veering, poor cane technique (for example, arc too high, arc too wide, hand position not centered; see Chapter 1, for more information on long-cane techniques), poor arm positioning in such noncane techniques as upper hand and forearm, immature gait pattern, poor posture, poor balance, and poor skill at performing physical activities such as jumping, hopping, and skipping. These issues are most notably seen in people who are congenitally blind. Additional issues of concern include the presence of stereotypies and tactile defensiveness in some young children.

Many O&M specialists recommend a direct approach to dealing with motor problems that emphasizes feedback and modeling. In this approach, if students demonstrate an immature gait pattern, for example, the O&M specialist makes sure the students are aware of what changes they need to make to their gait pattern and provides feedback and opportunities for the students to practice the target skill. Such efforts can be highly successful with some students. For others, such feedback and practice do not result in long-term or generalized improvement. In such cases, it may be necessary to help students develop motor skills by first developing the most basic sensorimotor components that support performance of that skill. This chapter will focuses on the latter approach, not only because of its effectiveness in addressing complex sensorimotor problems, but also because of the anecdotal evidence available to support its effectiveness, especially when working with children who are congenitally blind. While some suggested activities are given to facilitate specific sensorimotor skills, the purpose of this chapter is not to provide a comprehensive list of activities, but rather to provide guidelines and a systematic approach for evaluating the building blocks that are present or are not fully developed in students' movement and for formulating a plan for facilitating sensorimotor development through activities that can be meaningfully incorporated into O&M instruction. It must be emphasized, however, that the activities in this chapter are intended for use *only* with students who do not have orthopedic, neurological, or health impairments (see Chapter 18). The reason for this caution is that while the activities described in this chapter can be very effective when used with students who do not have other health issues, some activities can actually exacerbate motor difficulties in students who do have other health problems. For example, activities to increase muscle tone in children with hypotonia can actually aggravate the hypertonus common in some forms of cerebral palsy. The O&M specialist is encouraged to work with health professionals such as physical therapists or occupational therapists, or with other professionals such as adapted physical education teachers and recreational therapists, to learn how to safely and appropriately modify activities for use with such students. In turn, such teaming also allows the O&M specialist to teach other professionals about the motor skills used in orientation and mobility and the impact of visual impairment on motor development and functioning.

THE FIRST STEP

When working with students who have visual impairments, it is important to begin with a comprehensive assessment and a well-developed plan. In order to address the development of specific motor skills, it is necessary to look first at the specific building blocks of sensorimotor functioning, including selected areas of sensory functioning, development of muscle tone, and integration of neurological reflexes and reactions.

Sensory Functioning

The efficient use of sensory information is fundamental to development and learning. It is the interaction between the proprioceptive, vestibular, and tactile systems that, along with vision, provides the foundation for functional movement (See Volume 1, Chapter 5).

Proprioceptive Awareness

While poor development of proprioceptive awareness (awareness of body position) can be seen in many students with congenital visual impairment, it is most commonly seen in those who have no functional vision and in those with low muscle tone. Some students lack proprioceptive awareness throughout their bodies, others only at selected joints. Professionals such as biomechanists, kinesiologists, and physical and occupa-

tional therapists can perform detailed assessments to identify in which joints, and when performing which motions, a student lacks proprioceptive awareness.

One of the best pieces of news is that unlike some motor skills that develop best during limited windows of development, proprioception can often be improved at almost any age. When decreased proprioceptive awareness is an issue, there are some basic strategies that the O&M specialist can use to facilitate improved awareness. Two of these strategies are resistance and joint compression, and these work especially well with older children and adults. Resistance involves moving the body part against more than gravity. A heavier cane, or adding weights to a cane, for example, provides resistance by making the arm muscles contract more strongly than they do when using a lighter-weight cane. This is why some students who have decreased proprioception perform better when using a heavier cane. (A caution must be added here: If weights are added to a cane, it is important that they not significantly alter the balance of the cane, negatively impacting the student's cane technique.) Once proprioceptive awareness is developed, the added weights can be removed. Gymnastics and wrestling provide excellent proprioceptive input for students old enough to participate in such activities. Small children, in turn, can engage in turn taking and other games that incorporate resistance by pushing each other in carts, playing tug-of-war and wheelbarrow games, swimming, climbing on playground equipment, and other such activities. Joint compression can be provided for young children through age-appropriate activities that involve firm touch; weight bearing on the hands, knees, and feet; and other activities in which the ends of the long bones are stimulated. These activities can include crawling, wheelbarrow games, jumping, hopping, stamping, marching, and more. Facilitating proprioceptive awareness is, in fact, one of the most fundamental ways to help students learn to perform specific motions and to improve coordination throughout the body.

Vestibular Input

Vestibular input plays an important role in the regulation of muscle tone and coordination, balance and equilibrium, arousal, and attending state and works in conjunction with proprioceptive and visual sensory input to enable people to move with efficiency and coordination (Kasai, 1991). Poor development of vestibular awareness often manifests itself in such things as poor equilibrium and especially in a lack of protective extension reactions. (See Volume 1, Chapter 5, for an overview of protective extension reactions.)

Activities that provide age-appropriate vestibular experience such as gymnastics, wrestling, rocking, swinging, roughhousing, and riding merry-go-rounds facilitate the development of the vestibular system. Studies of children with Down syndrome and other developmental delays have shown that brief periods of vestibular stimulation also positively affect muscle tone, gross-motor skills, fine-motor skills, and reflexive behavior (Humphries, Snider, & McDougall, 1993; Kantner, Clark, Allen, & Chase, 1976; MacLean & Baumeister, 1982). Anecdotal evidence in working with preschool-aged children who are blind has also shown that for children who have vestibular-based stereotypies (self-stimulatory behaviors or mannerisms) such as rocking, the frequency and intensity of such stereotypies can often be reduced or eliminated by giving the child adequate experiences in activities that stimulate the vestibular sense.

Stereotypies

There are many approaches to decreasing stereotypies (also called stereotypic behaviors) in people. These approaches include providing them with prompts or reminders to cease the specific behavior whenever they are found to be engaging in stereotypies. Others focus on teaching children incompatible activities (for example, if a child needs to decrease hand flapping, he is taught to do a task that requires his hands to be engaged in a specific activity) or using positive reinforcement (for example, praising the student) each time the child self-corrects or refrains from engaging in stereotypies.

Another approach, equally effective with children, is to provide alternative stimulation to the sensory system that is being targeted by the stereotypy. One of the most intriguing theories as to the cause of stereotypies is poor sensory integration (See Volume 1, Chapter 5). Because such stereotypies as rocking, spinning, and hand flapping are so obviously tied to vestibular and proprioceptive input, it is easy to see how this interaction with the environment may be the way in which children provide the sensory input that they need. Studies have shown that providing opportunities for physical activities and age-appropriate and socially appropriate means of acquiring needed sensory stimulation can reduce some stereotypies (McHugh & Pyfer, 1999). For example, in their in-depth research study involving children aged 10–13 who were blind, the researchers found that the child who had the most opportunities for vigorous physical activity at home (and who was, incidentally, the only one in the study who received consistent, long-term adapted physical education) was the one who demonstrated the most control over her stereotypy of rocking. This finding, along with evidence from the literature (Bachman & Sluyter, 1988; Ellis, MacLean, & Gazdag, 1990; Kern, Koegel, Dyer, Blew, & Fenton, 1982; Kern, Koegel, & Dunlap, 1984; Ohlsen, 1978; Powers, Thibadeau, & Rose, 1992, cited in McHugh & Pyfer, 1999), supports the notion that vigorous physical activity can reduce the incidence of stereotypies. Another study (Ohlsen, 1978) similarly showed that the duration of rocking in participants who were blind could be reduced using an apparatus called a Slim Gym. Additional studies (Bachman & Fuqua, 1983; Bachman & Sluyter, 1988; Ellis et al., 1990; Kern et al., 1982; Kern, Koegel, & Dunlap, 1984; Levinson & Reid, 1993; Powers et al., 1992) that involved exercise interventions with people who have autism, mental retardation, or multiple disabilities also revealed similarly positive outcomes.

Tactile Input

Tactile input provides information about objects and the environment, and is used in all aspects of daily life. Tactile and haptic awareness, discrimination, and the ability to use such information accurately and efficiently are critical to the optimum functioning of people who are visually impaired. Touch is used to identify objects encountered during travel and to recognize familiar landmarks. It facilitates the development of concepts about objects and the environment, systematic search and exploration skills, reading maps, and orientation.

Efficient use of tactile information does not necessarily develop automatically in people who have significant visual impairments. It is therefore important that early instruction in orientation and mobility facilitate tactile awareness and the use of tactile information, especially with young children. This need is just as important as facilitating the use of residual vision, and of proprioceptive and vestibular functioning. Activities to develop optimum use of tactile information generally emphasize two functions—discrimination and tolerance.

Discrimination. The first of these, discrimination, needs to cover all aspects of touch—deep touch and haptic awareness, light touch for identifying textures (for example, rough, smooth, soft, hard), and awareness of temperature differences. Games, activities, and involvement in everyday household activities, can encourage tactile exploration. O&M lessons can involve toys and materials that offer decreasingly discernible textures, shapes, weights, temperatures, manipulative features, and functions. When working with young children, the O&M specialist can play with and use a variety of safe household objects such as washcloths, hairbrushes, paper, spoons, and bowls. Children can practice retrieving items buried in sand, rice, beans, or other highly tactile substances. Older children and adults can explore objects in whichever environments they are traveling. Doing so not only can help to develop tactile discrimination skills, but, when working with children, it can also teach concepts about the environment and age-appropriate self-help skills.

Tolerance. With regard to developing the second aspect of tactile functioning, that of tolerance, it is important to provide tactile opportunities, but when working with children, the O&M specialist ought to allow the child to initiate and withdraw as necessary. The key here is gradual exposure, as tolerated. Forcing tactile experiences on children can lead to withdrawal and resistance to tactile exploration in some children. Furthermore, some children with visual impairments, especially those with sensorimotor integration problems, can have tactilely defensive behaviors. Tactile defensiveness refers to a strong aversive reaction to ordinary tactile information (Ayres, 1979; Colby Trott, Laurel, & Windeck, 1993). It has been described as being in a state of "red alert" (Colby Trott et al., 1993, p. 4) with regard to tactile input. For children who are tactilely defensive, sensations that others find innocuous elicit feelings of irritation and discomfort. For these children, light touch is often the most unpleasant of the tactile sensations. Common irritants include certain textures of clothing, grass or sand against bare skin, and the light touch of another person (Parham & Mailloux, 1996). Young children might respond to such sensations with crying, fear, withdrawal, and various expressions of emotional distress (Parham & Mailloux, 1996). For children who are truly tactilely defensive, working with an occupational therapist who holds sensory integration certification can often be beneficial. Using such treatments as sensory integration therapy (an approach to assisting the central nervous system to meaningfully integrate sensory information by providing systematic, targeted sensory stimulation), the occupational therapist can often help children to integrate the tactile sensation at a neurological level, enabling them to tolerate and use tactile information more effectively.

Outside of true tactile defensiveness, however, some children with visual impairments may simply be reluctant to touch new textures or materials. Mamer (1995) suggested that this response might be more appropriately described as "tactile selectivity." For some children, this is a natural response to new experiences, and for others it is directly due to the impact of not having vision to allow them to anticipate what is going to happen. In this latter situation, the protective system may be activated and sudden touch may be perceived as a threat (Anthony & Lowry, 2004). For this reason, it is always critical to inform children and adults when they are about to be touched (and to ask for permission to do so when appropriate). Effective ways to encourage tactile exploration without eliciting a protective or withdrawal response in which the student pulls her hand away is to always tell the student where her hand is about to be directed. Furthermore, using a hand-under-hand approach in which the O&M specialist places her hand under the student's hand when guiding it toward an object (see Figure 5.1), rather than simply grasping the student's hand, can help to avoid a withdrawal response. A hand-under-hand approach also enables the student to more actively participate in the guidance or mutual tactile exploration of an object. Lastly, a hand-under-hand approach addresses the concern that grasping, when done routinely, may condition the

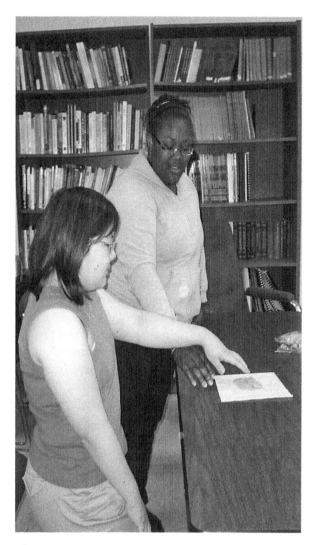

Figure 5.1.
Demonstrating the hand-under-hand technique.

hands of children to be passive and to wait for direction from others rather than reaching out by themselves to explore (Miles, 2003).

Motor Planning and Sensory Integration

Children with congenital visual impairments frequently exhibit difficulties in motor planning. A visual impairment can obviously affect motor planning due to the impact of decreased sensory awareness, low muscle tone, issues of neurological integration, and lack of movement experience, discussed earlier (see Volume 1, Chapter 5). Suggested activities to facilitate motor planning are listed in Sidebar 5.1.

For some children, however, a motor-planning problem might be present due to broader sensory integrative deficits. Such children might develop nonpurposeful, idiosyncratic movement patterns, demonstrate hypersensitivity to auditory and tactile stimuli, and resist noisy or crowded environments. Problems with sensory integration can also negatively impact the development of such things as spatial awareness and organizational

---

SIDEBAR 5.1

Suggested Activities for Motor Planning

Motor planning refers to the ability to develop a mental strategy to carry out a movement or an action. This includes the sequencing of movements, coordinating movement of the body and limbs, matching the amount of speed or strength needed for the task at hand, and sequencing the necessary steps needed to achieve a specific goal. At a higher level, motor planning includes self-assessment of motion and errors in movement, and planning and carrying out corrective motions. These actions involve attention and concentration.

To assist students to coordinate movement, the following steps are suggested:

- It is often helpful to physically and visually demonstrate new skills as you describe them.
- Use rhythm activities (for example, music) to increase awareness of movement and speed.
- Physically help children inhibit unnecessary (overflow) movements while they are moving.
- Incorporate activities that develop muscle tone, proprioception, and balance—these play key roles in motor planning.
- Provide opportunities for repeated practice, and gradually increase the difficulty of the activities, linking them to functional daily tasks.

To increase students' awareness of movement and to assist students to self-monitor

movement, the following activities are suggested.

- Use movement exploration to increase children's awareness of individual movements and of movement pairs (for example, "bend forward; then bend to the side"; "bend forward at the waist while reaching toward the table").
- Have children describe their movements; have children describe the movements of others.
- For children who can see their reflection in a mirror, practicing motions in a mirror can provide valuable feedback.

To assist students to develop a mental strategy and sequence for a movement or activity, the following steps are recommended:

- Break down directions into simple, one- or two-step segments.
- Give children time to process directions and plan their movements.
- Stress "sequence" words (for example, first, last, next, before, after) to help children organize and plan their movements.
- Have students repeat directions before they begin to move.

skills, with resultant long-term implications that can affect movement patterns and future learning opportunities. With appropriate early intervention, however, many of these sensory problems can be effectively addressed.

Sensory integration is defined as "the neurological process that organizes sensation from one's own body and from the environment and makes it possible to use the body effectively within the environment. The spatial and temporal aspects of inputs from different sensory modalities are interpreted, associated, and unified" (Ayres, 1989, p. 11). Sensory integration therapy is based on the premise that optimal motor and cognitive development depend on the functioning of the basic sensory systems. It is also based on the premise that providing systematic targeted sensory stimulation can assist the central nervous system to meaningfully integrate information received from those systems. Sensory integration therapy begins by conducting an evaluation of how the sensory systems are currently influencing development (Ayres, 1989). An intervention plan is then formulated to provide needed input. Sensory integration theory suggests that as the central nervous system is forced to process increased sensory input, it becomes more efficient, resulting in more efficient motor output and indirectly facilitating cognitive development. Sensory integration therapy is being discussed more and more as an avenue of assisting children who have visual impairments to develop improved sensorimotor skills. As mentioned earlier, occupational therapists are excellent resources for more information on sensory integration therapy.

Muscle Tone

Low muscle tone is responsible for many of the posture, gait, balance, and coordination difficulties exhibited by children with visual impairments (See Volume 1, Chapter 5). The key to improving muscle tone is simple—activity. That is why it is so important to facilitate active move-

ment in children with visual impairments who have low tone. Rather than placing very young children in position for an activity (for example, picking them up from supine and placing them in a sitting position), the O&M specialist should encourage children to move into sitting on their own. When sitting on the O&M specialist's lap, infants should be encouraged to hold their own head and trunk upright, if they are able to do so. By not providing unneeded trunk and head support, it is possible to enhance the development of muscle tone in the trunk muscles, which will be important in the later development of good posture. For older children and adults, muscle tone can best be improved through more demanding physical activity, especially that performed against resistance. Sample activities include those that involve weight bearing on the arms and legs and activities in which the muscles move against resistance, such as tug-of-war, swimming, wrestling, using a scooter board—even doing chores around the house that require physical exertion can help develop muscle tone. As a point of interest, low muscle tone is often correlated with decreased proprioception. For this reason, the same resistive activities that stimulated the proprioceptive sense will often facilitate the development of more normal muscle tone. Similarly, when muscle tone improves, proprioceptive awareness also improves.

A reminder: Some students who have cerebral palsy will have muscle tone that is too high and interferes with coordinated movement. When this is the case, resistive exercises can be done only in consultation with a physical therapist or occupational therapist. For this population, resistive exercises need to be modified in a way specific to each student's muscle tone in order to avoid exacerbating problems with hypertonus.

Reflexes and Reactions

Many of the motor difficulties exhibited by children and adults with congenital blindness have their origin in incomplete integration of neurological reflexes and reactions, which normally happens in the first few years life. For this reason, it is important to begin work in these areas while children are very young, even in infancy. The major reflexes and reactions that impact orientation and mobility are reviewed here with suggestions for facilitating their development in young children.

Reflexes

The key to integrating primitive reflexes when they are retained beyond the typical age is to encourage children to perform activities "out of pattern." For example, the asymmetrical nature of the asymmetrical tonic neck reflex (ATNR) is often a factor in the difficulty some children have maintaining the cane hand in a midline position when performing the touch technique. By incorporating a midline element into the task, it is sometimes possible to help inhibit the strength of, and sometimes possible to help to integrate, the ATNR. For example, having students hold the wrist of the cane hand with the free hand can help to decrease the influence of the ATNR in learning the centered hand position. Other ways to inhibit the influence of the ATNR include handing objects to students at midline, encouraging bilateral activities (for example, introduce items that require both hands to hold or manipulate), or even having students place one hand in midline while performing a task with the other hand. Another way to minimize the influence of the ATNR is to have students anchor the elbow of the cane arm against the side and to hold the cane arm with a small degree of flexion at the elbow (see the glossary or Table 5.1 in Chapter 5, Volume 1, for definitions of kinesiological terms). By incorporating elbow flexion into the technique, the ATNR pattern can often be inhibited.

Another reflex that may be seen is the symmetrical tonic neck reflex, which links neck flexion with arm flexion and leg extension. Activities such as crawling, climbing, and moving forward and backward on a scooter board (in which the child must hold his head up while propelling with his limbs) can help to integrate the symmetrical tonic neck reflex.

A reminder: Primitive reflexes are often retained in the presence of some forms of cerebral palsy. When this is the case, activities to integrate reflexes and facilitate reactions should be done only in consultation with a physical therapist or an occupational therapist.

Reactions

With regard to neurological reactions, the key to facilitating mature reactions is practice, practice, practice. Sample activities are given below for the main neurological reactions that are most critical to orientation and mobility.

Head-righting reaction. It has often been noted that visual impairments may result in a decrease in head-righting responses, in which infants align the head vertically in relation to gravity (Adelson & Fraiberg, 1974; Brown & Bour, 1986; Hart, 1984; Tröster & Brambring, 1993). When working with infants, it is often helpful to hold them in positions that vary the vestibular input and provide opportunities for independent head righting through providing visual, tactile, and auditory encouragement and rewards when they move their head into an erect position.

Neck-righting and body-on-body-righting reactions. Poor integration of the neck-righting and body-on-body-righting reactions has been shown to negatively impact the development of the ability to cross midline, employ bilateral hand use, and move in and out of positions easily. A lack of head turning also decreases vestibular input, further impacting motor development in general.

Activities to develop and integrate neck-righting and body-on-body-righting responses include those that involve "segmental" rolling (rotating first the head, followed by the shoulders, and then the hips, or vice versa)—on level ground, or up or down slight inclines. Age-appropriate activities to help integrate it include those that encourage head and trunk rotation. Such activities, depending on the student's age, might include games where children look for and then reach for objects on their side or pass a ball to a person at their side, crawling up and down stairs (the student crawls backward down the stairs for safety), crawling through obstacle courses, and so on. For other students, gymnastics, dance, and even wrestling and other sports can be effective ways of providing experiences with physical activities that involve head and trunk rotation.

Landau reaction.   The Landau reaction is a prime facilitator of extensor muscle tone in the trunk, which in turn supports the development of erect posture. It can be stimulated by activities that support the student at the shoulders and trunk and yet allow free movement of the head, arms, and legs. This stimulation of the trunk muscles is critical to facilitate a more erect trunk posture as children develop. Parents often stimulate this reaction when they play Airplane with their infants. When working with older children, this reaction comes into play when doing such things as playing games or performing activities while lying prone on a large ball or scooter board (with the head held up). Of note, however, is that as children age and their limbs become larger and heavier, their legs will often not rise in the air, but extension of the trunk and neck will be evident.

Protective extension reaction.   Protective extension reactions stimulate the arms and legs to extend in reaching out to break a fall. In young children the protective extension reactions develop first in the forward direction, next to the side, and last to the rear.

With young children, activities using a big ball can be effective ways in which to stimulate these reactions. For example, the child can lie on the ball in a prone position while the O&M specialist rolls the ball forward, backward, or to the side, encouraging the child to "reach out" and touch the ground. The ball must be small enough to enable the child to reach the ground without being rolled so far forward or to the side that the child cannot remain supported on the ball. If a larger ball is needed to support the weight of the child, place a low, stable chair near the ball and have the child reach for the chair, supporting his or her weight on it. This is done slowly at first, with encouragement and prior warning that the ball is about to roll, gradually reducing the warning and increasing the speed at which the ball is rotated to simulate the speed of an actual loss of balance to elicit the reaction automatically. In doing this activity, it is critical to never let the child fall off of the ball or feel threatened. To stimulate protective extension reactions in the legs, the child can also sit on the ball while it is rolled in various directions. For older children, activities that can further stimulate the reaction in the legs include those that involve jumping, hopping, using a trampoline, and various gymnastics.

Equilibrium reactions.   Equilibrium reactions are the most advanced of all of the neurological reactions. As such, they depend on the optimum development of the earlier righting reactions, muscle tone, and proprioception for their development. As is the case with the protective extension reactions, equilibrium reactions develop in a specific sequence—in supine, then long sitting, then on all fours, then kneeling, then standing. To facilitate improved development of equilibrium reactions, some of the most effective activities to do with young children are those that require the student to react to slow, subtle changes in the supporting surface. Such activities might include playing on a rocker board or a T-stool (see Figure 5.2) or engaging in other activities

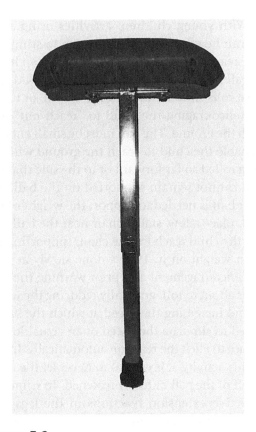

Figure 5.2.
Playing on a T-stool can reinforce equilibrium reactions.

such as bicycling and horseback riding. Walking on a balance beam can also reinforce equilibrium reactions, but only if reactions on the rocker board are already developed at the supine through standing levels. Other activities that reinforce equilibrium reactions include dance, tai chi, yoga, wrestling, running, gymnastics, and most sports.

Sensorimotor Development of Infants and Toddlers Who Have Visual Impairments

Motor skills are ideally developed in sequence. Missed stages can lead to the development of splinter skills and to poor motor functioning later on (See Volume 1, Chapter 5).

Activities in Prone Position

Infants who are visually impaired typically dislike being in the prone position. Until they begin to crawl, however, it is important to encourage the infant to spend time doing activities in the prone position. Placing the infant on a knee or on a wedge or placing a rolled towel under the infant's chest can help to elevate the upper chest, making it easier for the child to breath and placing the arms in position to bear weight or reach. Playing with toys or interacting with an adult while in the prone position should emphasize weight bearing on the arms and reaching.

Crawling

It is an established fact that many children who are born with visual impairments either show delays in crawling or skip that stage of independent movement completely (Rosen, 1997; Tröster, Hecker, & Brambring, 1994). For some children, it might be due to a lack of visual modeling combined with the effects of low muscle tone and consequent instability at the shoulder girdle that make crawling difficult. In place of crawling, some children prefer to scoot along the floor on their bottoms to protect their heads from bumping into objects in the environment. Consequences of not crawling include decreased upper-body strength, decreased trunk rotation, and decreased joint stability in the shoulder girdle.

Early intervention is critical with regard to facilitating crawling in children who have visual impairments. Playing in an all-fours position, especially shifting weight from side to side, also helps to develop the muscle tone and stability in the shoulder girdle that is needed to free one hand to reach for objects and to move forward. In addition, practicing movement transitions from sitting to all fours, as well as earlier transitions (prone to supine, supine to sit), will help greatly to develop the underlying components of movement needed for crawling. Reaching, and moving to and from the sitting position are, in fact, considered to be the most critical precursors to actual crawling (Maida & McCune, 1996).

Young children who have visual impairments can benefit from age-appropriate activities involving crawling even after they begin to walk independently. Toddlers, for example, might play games that involve crawling up and down ramps and stairs (crawling backward down stairs for safety). These experiences help build a foundation of upper-body strength, reciprocal movement of the arms and legs, and trunk and pelvic rotation, and may even stimulate some tactile discrimination. Age-appropriate activities for older children might include obstacle courses, races, and using playground equipment.

Cruising

As children move from crawling to unsupported walking, they often engage in an intermediate activity called "cruising." Cruising refers to the act of walking sideways along furniture, a wall, or even kitchen cabinets, using both hands to support oneself on the surface. Cruising serves many functional purposes (Lowry & Hatton, 2002), including:

- Providing repeated experience with common objects, landmarks, and surfaces. This experience may help to develop broader environmental concepts, a reinforced understanding of object permanence, and goal-directed movement.

- Providing beginning opportunities to develop a mental map of an area. It is felt that this, in turn, leads to greater confidence and incentives for movement as independent walking emerges.

- Preparing the child for trailing at a later point in time.

It is therefore important to encourage children to experience cruising as they prepare to walk. A common strategy for doing this and for assisting the transition to unsupported walking

is to place pieces of furniture close together to provide an environment suitable for cruising. Placing toys or other items of interest at intervals along the surface or using some sort of reward system can encourage cruising. The distance between the pieces of furniture can gradually be increased, encouraging children to experience moments of unsupported walking as they move between supporting surfaces.

Walking

Studies have shown that in general, children who are blind may stand alone, or even take steps holding someone's hand at around 1 year of age, but that unsupported walking (a distance of 10 feet [3 m]) often does not occur until around 18 months of age (Adelson & Fraiberg, 1974; Ferrell, 1998; Tröster et al., 1994), several months after children with unimpaired vision typically begin to walk (See Volume 1, Chapter 5).

Walking without vision requires greater concentration on balance, heightened postural awareness, and attention to personal safety. Walking can be made less stressful and more enticing to children when furniture and items in the house are kept in predictable positions and when favorite objects are placed strategically in the environment to encourage movement.

There are many devices, both produced commercially and homemade, that purport to "help a child walk." The use of these devices with children who have visual impairments, however, must be done with caution, and with clear goals in mind. Many commercial "baby walkers," for example, position a child's legs in such a way as to interfere with a normal gait pattern. In addition, while support walkers provide invaluable assistance for children who have orthopedic or neurological conditions, they can negatively alter the developing gait pattern of children who are visually impaired, as they change the center of gravity and thereby impact the development of balance reactions. Lastly, long canes, push toys, and adaptive mobility devices are not recommended as a means of encouraging children to develop walking. These devices do provide some protection and object detection and are excellent means of encouraging children who can already walk to move into the environment. These devices, however, require a degree of postural control in order to push easily and safely. Introducing these devices before a child has developed the ability to walk unsupported may interfere with the development of gait patterns, balance, weight shift, and protective reactions. These devices, therefore, need to be used only with children who can already walk unsupported with their hands in the low-guard position, and then just used as bumpers or for social play activities.

What is most important is not the age at which the child begins walking, but that the underlying sensorimotor components be developed as much as possible and that this development effort continue beyond the point at which the child starts walking in order to facilitate a mature gait pattern and more efficient travel skills down the road.

This leads us to consider the specific roles of posture, gait, and balance in the motor development of children with visual impairments.

Sensorimotor Functioning in Older Children, Adolescents, and Young Adults Who Have Visual Impairments

Posture

Throughout the years many researchers and authors have emphasized the importance of good posture for people who are visually impaired (as for all people; Rosen, 1997; Wall Emerson & Corn, 2006). Good posture has been correlated both scientifically and anecdotally with improved health and physical functioning as well as positive social experiences.

As is true of many motor skills, it is generally easier to modify posture when children are younger, before they have completed growing. However, when highly motivated, people can improve their posture at any age, limited only by any structural changes, such as joint stiffness, or lordosis, scoliosis, or kyphosis of the spine, that may have already set in. Since muscle tone and proprioception are key elements in posture, activities that emphasize development and functioning in these areas are of great potential value in facilitating improved posture. Chapter 5 in Volume 1 provides a description of the ideal positioning of body segments in proper posture.

As a special note about posture, O&M specialists, other professionals, and even family and friends often encourage students who typically hold their heads down to hold them erect. The potential and real benefits of this small postural change are evident for both physical and social reasons. Children can be encouraged to maintain the head in an erect position through the use of age-appropriate means of social reinforcement. In addition, there are some devices on the market designed to provide auditory feedback when students successfully hold the head erect, and other devices that do so when students fail to hold the head erect. Such devices can be used successfully with students who desire an inconspicuous way of obtaining self-feedback on their head position. Anecdotal evidence supports the effectiveness of this feedback in classroom and nonmobility situations when used with motivated students.

However, because the head-down position is also correlated with a sensation of increased equilibrium, even if only at a subliminal level, the answer is unclear as to whether or not the head-down position should be allowed, or whether an extensive effort should be made to alter it, during travel, since equilibrium is such a crucial element in walking. Similar arguments can be made for increased knee flexion and other aspects of poor posture seen in some people, whether they are young or old. While good posture has obvious social and health benefits, the decision as to whether or not effort should be made to alter a postural feature while walking needs to be made on an individual basis depending on a student's ability, need, and motivation, and the effect of the postural change on balance. Research in this area is needed to identify any true causal relationships between better posture and safe, efficient mobility and to evaluate the effectiveness of postural remediation on independent travel.

Balance

It is perhaps the lack of development of equilibrium reactions that most notably impacts independent travel due to equilibrium's role in supporting a mature gait pattern and the student's corresponding ability for straight-line travel (Rosen, 1989). Since equilibrium reactions depend on well-developed proprioceptive awareness and muscle tone for their optimum development, activities to facilitate improved balance must begin there. In addition, activities that naturally call on equilibrium reactions are excellent ways to help stimulate their development. Sample age-appropriate activities for older children, adolescents, and adults might include such things as skiing, bicycling or tandem bicycling, boating, horseback riding, skating, dance, walking or hiking on uneven terrain, and tai chi.

Gait

The development and retention of mature gait patterns is important in several ways. Immature gait patterns have been shown to negatively impact mobility. Evidence indicates that as speed is decreased and out-toeing occurs, there is an increase in the tendency to veer from a straight line of travel (Rosen, 1989). Also, anecdotal evidence suggests that immature gait patterns are associated with decreased endurance in travel (logically, due to the higher energy demands of less efficient motor performance).

As in the case of posture, a person who is highly motivated can often develop more mature gait patterns at almost any age, assuming that the physical prerequisites of muscle tone, proprioception, and balance are present to support the change. However, it must be remembered that since gait patterns tend to stabilize at around 6–7 years of age, the optimum time to begin activities designed to facilitate the development of a mature gait pattern is during the preschool years. In planning such activities, the key is to develop the fundamental supports of a mature gait pattern: muscle tone, proprioception, and equilibrium reactions. Anecdotal observations have also shown that activities such as walking faster than usual (guided, or using a cane or other mobility device, or even using push toys for very young children) can help promote more mature gait patterns. The observations have tended to show a marked improvement in gait patterns while engaging in such supported fast walking, but without generalization to walking in everyday travel. Perhaps such activities, coupled with activities to develop the proprioceptive, equilibrium, and muscle tone supports of gait as well as consistent and meaningful feedback on mature gait patterns, are the best way to help children develop the gait patterns that will support straight-line travel and efficient mobility skills as they grow. This is an area of needed research in the field of orientation and mobility.

Sensorimotor Functioning in Senior Citizens Who Have Visual Impairments

Much has been said about activities to develop sensorimotor skills in infants, children, adolescents, and even young adults. Many healthy senior citizens can also benefit from physical and motor activities such as dance or other forms of mild to moderate exercise, although generalization of such improvements to mobility performance has not been established scientifically. Some studies have shown that tai chi practice can help to maintain joint flexibility and muscle strength, improve balance, increase aerobic capacity, enhance postural stability, and lower blood pressure in older adults (Hartman et al., 2000; Husted, Pham, Hekking, & Niederman, 1999; Lan, Lai, Chen, & Wong, 1998; Ray, Horvat, Keen, & Blasch, 2005; Wang, Lan, Chen, & Wong, 2002; Wolf et al., 1996; Young, Appel, Jee, & Miller, 1999). Other studies have reported a decrease in the fear of falling after regular tai chi practice (Kutner, Barnhart, Wolf, McNeeley, & Xu, 1997). The Atlanta Frailty and Injuries: Cooperative Studies of Intervention Techniques trial demonstrated that tai chi practice can reduce the risk of falls by 47.5 percent in older adults (Wolf et al., 1996). Furthermore, a pilot study conducted by Miszko, Ramsey, and Blasch (2004a), involving adults aged 36–77 years who have visual impairments, suggested that participants were more confident in their mobility-related abilities and engaged in social activities more frequently and considered tai chi to be an effective means of improving balance, strength, and quality of life for individuals with visual impairments. For people who are physically able, physical activity is an important part of staying in shape and maintaining physical functioning.

It is the frail elderly population, however, in which posture, balance, and gait problems become most notable. With regard to improving the motor functioning of this population, the value and appropriateness of movement activities have to be weighed carefully. One of the most important distinctions to be made in determining whether or not to modify a person's posture or gait pattern has to do with the person's age and the reasons for any deviations. Although many of the changes in gait mimic those

seen in congenitally blind children (for example, small step length, decreased reciprocal arm swing) these changes to gait seen in frail elderly persons generally occur as a means of compensating for the decline in muscle strength, speed, and reliability of neurological reactions including equilibrium rather than from a lack of development of these skills in the presence of an intact neuromotor system. For this reason, efforts to modify gait problems in elderly persons may not yield significant results and may, in effect, be counterproductive to the person's functioning in mobility. However, if the student is motivated and physically able to participate in an exercise program to address the decline in muscle strength and equilibrium, there is theoretically the potential for improved physical functioning and mobility. When working with students who are elderly, however, collaboration with physicians and physical therapists or certified exercise therapists is crucial before engaging in any attempts to improve motor functioning. Due to the potential for complications from additional health conditions (for example, osteoporosis, neurological or cardiac conditions), any motor or movement facilitation activities should first be medically approved.

Key Principles of Sensorimotor Development and Functioning

Up to this point, we have focused on the components of sensorimotor development and functioning one by one, looking at each in some degree of detail. Putting them all together in a coordinated program of development involves a thorough understanding of each, but also attention to some key principles of motor development.

Predictability

Predictability comes into play at both personal and environmental levels. At the personal level, vision serves an important function of preparing one for changes in sensory or motor input. As mentioned earlier, if one touches young children with visual impairments and the children are not prepared for the contact, they may demonstrate protective responses such as startling, pulling away, or crying. This hypersensitivity may reflect the inability, due to lack of visual information, to anticipate touch and is a variant of the startle response that an adult or a sighted person of any age might have if touched unexpectedly. Hands-on demonstration and facilitation are a normal and necessary part of teaching sensorimotor skills. Letting students know what you are going to do or what is going to happen first is an important strategy to prepare them for an activity without eliciting a protective response.

At the environmental level, some people may hesitate to move freely within the environment due to fear of the unknown and an inability to monitor changes in the environment. Parents can provide a safe home environment in which young children can explore and learn not only to move freely but also to enjoy movement. Parents can provide visual, tactile, and auditory clues for safety and mental organization of the space while providing opportunities for children to experience movement within that space. For people of all ages, allowing time to familiarize to new spaces as well as teaching safe mobility skills can help to minimize fear of movement in unfamiliar spaces and to encourage people to practice new movement skills and to move confidently in any environment.

For seniors who are at risk for falling, the value of environmental modifications cannot be overstressed. Some helpful suggestions are to make sure that floors and stairs are free of clutter and to mark the edges of stairs in a contrasting color when necessary. Good lighting can help minimize falls. It may be necessary to work with local city offices to have outdoor hazards addressed such as uneven sidewalks and traffic

lights at which the walking interval is too short to allow people who walk slowly to cross the street safely before traffic begins to move.

Sequencing

Motor development is sequential (children must sit before they can walk), and visual impairment affects the development of most motor skills, including those that we most readily associate with successful travel—posture, gait, and balance. The optimal performance of sensorimotor skills relies not only on the previous development of lower level skills, but also on the adequate development of fundamental sensorimotor elements—sensory awareness, muscle tone, and coordination. Therefore, when choosing and designing sensorimotor activities for students who are visually impaired, it is important for the O&M specialist to consider what functional skills the students need and what prerequisite abilities they must have, and to choose activities that facilitate normal muscle tone, sensory development, the integration of primitive reflexes, and the fine-tuning of equilibrium and other mature neurological reactions as appropriate.

Active Movement

Purposeful, self-initiated movement, not passive movement, is essential for developing motor skills. Only through active movement can people develop muscle tone, proprioceptive awareness, and coordination. Only through active interaction with the environment can people learn how to function within it. Although some students may fear moving in the environment due to the potential for injury (Sleeuwenhoek & Boter, 1995), it is through movement experience that they are able to decrease this anxiety. Increasingly, O&M specialists advocate teaching young children to use a cane or an adaptive mobility device during the preschool years in order to reduce the development of any movement apprehension and enable the children to feel protected while moving.

Quality of Movement

For people with visual impairments, quality is as important as function. True, there may be times when the need for function outweighs the need for quality in performing a task. For example, a student may need to learn a route or how to perform a self-help task immediately, whether or not it is done with the highest level of grace or coordination. However, in the area of sensorimotor development and functioning, quality cannot always be ignored in a rush for function. Because the acquisition of higher-level motor skills relies so heavily on the development of lower-level skills and abilities, it is important to weigh immediate need against the long-term benefit of emphasizing quality in movement. For example, a child may be delayed in walking. Rather than just having the child practice how to walk, however, it may be more effective to address proprioceptive, muscle tone, and balance needs and to encourage the child to crawl on all fours (if age appropriate) first in order to develop trunk rotation and other prerequisites for the development of mature, efficient gait patterns. These more mature gait patterns, in turn, will facilitate greater straight-line travel ability later on.

It is also important to consider the impact of any additional disabilities. Cognitive impairments, for example, may limit the potential of some students to learn some skills precisely. In this case it may be more important to achieve any level of skill performance quickly, regardless of quality, in order to allow the children to go on to learn other things. Working closely with professionals who serve these students (for example, teachers of children who have severe disabilities) is important in determining goals for students with significant cognitive impairments. Similarly, some physical disabilities may limit the ability of some students to develop the

same level of quality in movement as their peers. When working with students who have physical impairments, it is important to consult a physical or occupational therapist, or both, before engaging in motor development activities. The therapist can determine the best motor activities for the students as well as provide information on which activities to avoid in the presence of specific physical impairments or health conditions.

Timing of Movement

Specific skills are learned best during their "critical periods," when the appropriate sensory and motor inputs are coming together (Langley, 1980). Greenough, Black, & Wallace (1987) proposed a neurophysiological mechanism to explain the role of what they termed "sensitive periods" for the development of certain types of abilities. They organized their model around the concept of experience-expectancy. They proposed that during such periods, an excess number of synaptic connections among brain neurons generates. As children develop, those synapses that are activated by sensory or motor experiences survive; the rest are lost through disuse. If it takes longer to acquire a certain skill, or if the acquisition of a skill begins after the "critical period," higher-level skills based on that first skill will be delayed even further. Furthermore, if these critical periods are missed, some skills might never be learned, or if they are learned out of sequence, higher-level skills may rest on a faulty foundation (Langley, 1980; Moore, 1984; Scott, 1962). The consequences of missing such periods can be seen in children with visual impairments who skip the stage of crawling on all fours, for example, and therefore do not have the opportunity to practice weight shifting, reciprocal balance, and hip and trunk rotation. As a result, their gait often lacks fluidity, and they may walk stiff legged, shifting weight from one leg to the other with feet spread wide apart (Ferrell, 1985).

In planning motor and mobility goals for young children with visual impairments, it is vital to encourage the sequential development of sensorimotor skills at normal developmental ages. By continually emphasizing age-appropriate sensorimotor functioning throughout O&M instruction with infants, toddlers, preschoolers, and young school-age children, one can build foundations to support the development of effective functional motor and mobility skills later on.

Integration of Movement

In addition to sensorimotor activities done in the context of an O&M lesson, it is important to integrate new sensorimotor activities into students' everyday lives when possible. With the O&M specialist working with parents, family members, and other members of the students' educational or rehabilitation team, motor activities can be taught, practiced, and easily incorporated into all aspects of life. For example, activities and games that incorporate coordination, proprioception, and muscle tone development, such as swinging, climbing, riding a tricycle, using playground equipment, running relay races, going through obstacle courses, and orienteering, can be part of children's activities done on family and school outings. In addition to providing sensorimotor stimulation, these activities also provide a common ground for interacting with one's peers and for developing social skills. For adolescents and adults, activities such as orienteering, hiking, rock climbing, wrestling, gymnastics, dance, tai chi, horseback riding, and swimming provide recreation and social opportunities and can contribute to one's quality of life while facilitating sensorimotor functioning.

The Role of the O&M Specialist and the Team in Sensorimotor Facilitation

O&M specialists play a vital role in facilitating sensorimotor functioning of people with visual impairments. This is true whether it involves teaching new motor skills (such as how to use a long cane) to adults or giving people who are elderly the skills to travel independently and thereby remain active and more physically fit. It is most notably true in the sensorimotor development of children. In fact, the role of the O&M specialist begins in a student's infancy, when early intervention can do much to minimize sensorimotor delays and alleviate their impact on other areas of development. Given the impact of neuromotor development in the first few years of life on sensorimotor functioning throughout life, the importance of early intervention cannot be overstated. Yet, at all ages, well-developed sensorimotor skills are a critical element of effective mobility, and working with family members and other professionals such as adapted physical education specialists, physical therapists and occupational therapists, teachers of the visually impaired, other special educators, regular education professionals, or rehabilitation counselors, is essential. Occupational and physical therapists, for example, can provide unique knowledge of sensorimotor development patterns, activities, and modifications of activities for children and adults who may have multiple disabilities or health conditions that impact motor performance. Therapists can also observe a person's movement, analyze and assess atypical movement, and suggest individualized strategies to facilitate sensorimotor functioning. Such input is critical when sensorimotor functioning is compromised by neurological or orthopedic impairments. In turn, the O&M specialist brings to the table a unique understanding of the impact of blindness on the developing sensory systems of children who are visually impaired and the importance of highly developed sensorimotor skills in independent mobility. O&M specialists encourage meaningful movement by demonstrating skills using kinesthetic and visual modeling and by providing structured sensorimotor development activities that emphasize auditory, olfactory, tactile, vestibular, and other sensory inputs while assisting children to perform motor skills and to incorporate them into independent travel and functioning in the environment. The value of such a contribution cannot be overemphasized. Similarly, working together with regular and special education teachers, O&M specialists can integrate sensorimotor activities into both O&M lessons and classroom learning to facilitate sensorimotor skill development and the subsequent benefit to learning that good sensorimotor skills provide.

Addressing the sensorimotor development and functioning of people with visual impairments is a team activity, and the benefits of including sensorimotor considerations in O&M services are well worth the effort.

IMPLICATIONS FOR O&M PRACTICE

1. When choosing and designing sensorimotor activities for children who are visually impaired, it is important to consider activities that facilitate:

   a. sensory development

   b. normal muscle tone in children who are hypotonic

   c. integration of primitive reflexes

   d. fine-tuning of balance and other mature neurologic reactions

2. Research has shown that falls in the elderly population are associated with poor visual acuity and contrast sensitivity. For minimizing the potential for falls among elderly individuals, good mobility skills, elimination of household hazards, and good illumination are important.

3. Good posture has been correlated both scientifically and anecdotally with improved health and physical functioning as well as positive social experiences.

4. In some travelers, the head-down position may be correlated with a sense of improved balance. Decisions about which postural problems to focus on for correction and in which circumstances they should be corrected must be made on an individual basis, weighing both social appropriateness and function.

5. In order to be effective, individual sensorimotor development activities must address the basic components of sensorimotor functioning: sensory awareness, muscle tone, and neurological integration. In addition, there are general key principles that must be considered when developing comprehensive, integrated sensorimotor programs:

   a. predictability

   b. sequencing

   c. active movement

   d. quality of movement

   e. timing of movement

   f. integration of movement

6. Opportunities for movement and exploration not only facilitate sensorimotor skills but also are critical to the optimum development of mobility, cognitive, and other skills as well.

7. Sensorimotor activities are best done not in isolation, but when they are incorporated into functional activities. Whenever possible, the O&M specialist should integrate activities into daily tasks, play with peers, and a variety of home and school experiences.

LEARNING ACTIVITIES

1. Observe physical therapists and occupational therapists working with children who have visual impairments or neurological disorders. Note what activities they use to develop basic sensorimotor skills, and ask how they can be

used or modified for use with specific children who have visual impairments.

2. Practice age-appropriate sensorimotor development activities with nondisabled children. Watch how they respond during activities. Next, try the same activities, when appropriate, with children who have visual impairments and who show sensorimotor delays.

3. Work with other professionals and team members such as adapted physical education professionals, physical and occupational therapists, early childhood educators, families,

and students themselves to identify fun and effective activities that facilitate sensorimotor functioning. Consider activities that can be done individually, in groups, and as part of family or other social activities for all ages—children, adults, and seniors.

4. Do an Internet search for recreation organizations and organizations serving people with disabilities in your area. What activities do they offer that might address sensorimotor functioning needs or recreational interests, or both?

Improving Psychosocial Functioning for Orientation and Mobility

Richard L. Welsh

LEARNING QUESTIONS

- How do the teaching approaches that facilitate the development of psychosocial factors in orientation and mobility relate to the origins of this profession?

- What is a "helping relationship," and why is it important to orientation and mobility (O&M) instruction?

- How are the psychosocial factors that affect an individual student assessed?

- What are some of the objections that families may have to O&M training, and how can they be effectively addressed?

- How do interactions with the public have an impact on independent travel both positively and negatively?

Chapter 6 in Volume 1 reviewed personality theories and theories related to the adjustment to vision loss and discussed how these theories have an impact on orientation and independent mobility without vision. The current chapter demonstrates how this information can help

mobility specialists develop approaches to individual students to help them overcome psychosocial barriers to independent travel and harness positive forces that promote independence and self-efficacy. The history of the success of this profession provides many practical reasons to believe that these approaches are successful. However, orientation and mobility, like many practice professions, faces the challenge of documenting its successes and a better understanding of how each aspect of mobility training impacts students with different patterns of psychosocial variables.

Practically every human behavior, especially the complex behavior related to traveling through the environment, is affected by sensory, motor, intellectual, psychological, and social aspects of the person performing the behavior. Some of these aspects interact so closely and in such a complex manner that it is difficult to think of them and to talk about them separately. This is certainly true for the interactions among intellectual, psychological, and social factors. For this reason, this chapter and the corresponding chapter in Volume 1 discuss these factors as they interact and refer to them as *psychosocial factors*.

Such factors include motivation, self-concept, anxiety, attitudes, family dynamics, and stigmatization, to name a few.

PERSON-ORIENTED, PRACTICAL, AND INTERACTIVE

From its origin in the war blind program at Valley Forge Army General Hospital during World War II (see Volume 1, Chapter 13), the practice of helping people with vision loss learn to get around their various environments had a very concrete focus. It was based not on a priori theory but on common sense and practical results. Those who were assigned to help blinded veterans learn to travel did not bring preconceived notions to the challenge. They tried tools and techniques developed with blinded military personnel until they found methods that worked. Given the nature of the clientele who had lost their vision in service to their country and the trauma that they had experienced, special attention was given to the emotional and social aspects of their rehabilitation.

These first approaches to teaching independent travel reflected a strong orientation of "putting the person first." This characterized the origin of mobility instruction at Valley Forge Hospital and then at the Hines Veterans Administration Hospital. In doing so, these methods effectively addressed many of the psychological and social barriers that inhibit independent mobility for some people who are blind and harnessed a number of positive factors that facilitate travel.

As discussed by Richard Welsh (Volume 1, Chapter 6), the research of Albert Bandura (1986) provided theoretical underpinning after the fact for the success of the work of the Valley Forge and Hines programs. Bandura's work integrates cognitive and other personal factors with the role of social and environmental influences in efforts to explain, predict, and change behavior. Central to Bandura's *social cognitive theory* is the concept that

personality develops through a process of "reciprocal determinism," which refers to the continuous interaction of personal and environmental factors and the person's own behavior.

In Bandura's three-sided model (Figure 6.1), an individual's behavior is influenced by personal factors such as anxiety or self-confidence, just as these personal factors are influenced by the individual's behavior. In addition, the environment, especially the social environment, influences behavior, and the environment changes as a result of a person's behavior. To complete the third dimension of the model, the social environment can impact an individual's personal factors and can be influenced by an individual's personal factors as well.

The interactions that link successful orientation and mobility with one's self-concept, the motivation for rehabilitation, the attitudes of the family, and the ability to cope effectively with people on the street are continuous and reciprocal. A positive self-concept can be both a cause and an effect of success in mobility. In contrast, a negative self-image can result from a lack of independent mobility or can make progress toward independent functioning more difficult.

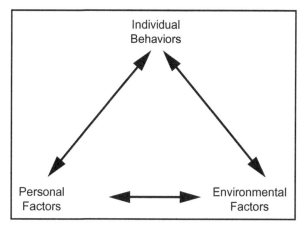

Figure 6.1. Bandura's (1986) Three-Sided Model of Reciprocal Determinism
Source: Adapted from A. Bandura, *Social Foundations of Thought and Action: A Social Cognitive Theory* (Englewood Cliffs, NJ: Prentice Hall, 1986).

Bandura (1986) pointed out that researching how the three-way interactions among the elements of social cognitive theory operate is very difficult. "This is a formidable task not only because the triadic systems are interactive, but because each subsystem itself contains multiple reciprocal processes" (Bandura, 1986, p. 28). Many factors working together in different blends influence particular behaviors in each situation. This is the practice challenge facing the O&M specialist. How can the specialist most effectively help a specific person who is visually impaired cope with a particular situation in which multiple psychosocial and environmental factors are operating?

In order to address as many of the factors as possible that may impact a specific individual learning to travel, the Valley Forge and Hines traditions offered training to one student at a time in actual hospital or community environments. This was unlike the tradition of other more medical-based therapies that function almost entirely within the clinical environment of a hospital or medical facility. The teaching of orientation and mobility in real travel environments enables the student to experience the many emotional and social factors associated with independent travel. The tradition of one-to-one instruction permits the mobility specialist to identify and address the specific psychosocial variables affecting each student in a manner that reflects what each student needs at each point in the training.

THE RELATIONSHIP BETWEEN THE O&M SPECIALIST AND THE STUDENT

The Teaching Relationship

Because orientation and mobility is taught using a one-on-one teaching approach and the process frequently involves the confronting of various psychosocial barriers and significant personal challenges by the student, the relationship that develops between the student and the instructor is especially important. This factor was recognized by the pioneers of mobility training. Warren Bledsoe (in Volume 1, Chapter 13) quotes from an unpublished paper by Richard Hoover in which Hoover's concept of the appropriate relationship between the student and the instructor reflects the need for collaboration between the two, each learning from the other. He also stressed the need to accept the student and his feelings, to communicate genuine caring for him, and to speak the truth, especially with regard to the student's actual ability and potential for independent travel.

These expectations of the relationship that should exist between the O&M specialist and the student were inculcated in the early instructors at Hines by Bledsoe and Williams (Welsh, 2005). They represent the basis for the teaching methodology that emanated from Hines and have become the psychosocial foundation of professional O&M instruction. The type of instructor-student relationship described by Hoover is very similar to the client-centered approach to counseling developed by Rogers (1951) and refined for the use of teachers, rehabilitation specialists, and other helpers by Carkhuff (1969, 2000). This approach was specifically suggested for teachers of the visually impaired by Welsh (1972) and Tuttle (1987).

According to this approach, the O&M specialist must be honest and genuine with the student. At some point, it may be necessary for the student to place his trust in the specialist at a time of high anxiety. When that happens, the student should have no reason to doubt that the O&M specialist is trustworthy. The specialist should share openly with the student where she will be during the lesson and whether or not she will be in a position to intervene to prevent injury or embarrassment. The student should know when he is being observed and when he is functioning on his own. The O&M specialist must communicate a positive acceptance of the student, regardless of success or failure, and a respect for the student's right to be involved in planning and decision making about his own program of instruction.

Listening Skills

A positive and trusting relationship is also an important tool in the mobility specialist's effort to learn as much as possible about the psychosocial characteristics of the student during the assessment phase of instruction. The mobility specialist has to develop and use effective listening skills to be able to hear all that is said and understand all that is implied by each student. The more a student feels trust in the instructor, the more likely she is to share actual feelings about travel and emotional responses to various situations.

Ivey, Gluckstern, and Ivey (2006) have outlined the basic communication skills that can be used by a counselor, teacher, or any type of helper to convey a genuine interest in the student and to demonstrate effective attending and listening. Having good intentions is not enough. There are skills that must be learned or enhanced. When they are present and used properly, they help to communicate to the student that the helper is interested in understanding the student's viewpoint. These skills include attending, questioning, observing, encouraging, paraphrasing, summarizing, challenging, and fostering change (Ivey et al., 2006). Some O&M specialists as well as teachers, nurses, counselors, and other helpers bring a natural facility for these skills to their work and training. Others, however, could benefit from specific training in these skills. This training frequently uses videotaping of the interaction between the professional in training and real or simulated students and then critiquing that interaction by a more experienced professional. Feedback given to the professional in training regarding the effectiveness of his listening, paraphrasing, summarizing, and other skills can help the emerging professional improve on his ability to establish effective helping relationships with students.

Benjamin (2001) explained that there are three ways of understanding someone who has appeared to help. You can understand what others think or know about the person. You can understand what you come to understand about the person through your own interactions with him. The third and most helpful approach is to understand what the person thinks and feels about himself and his own situation. This third type of understanding is called *empathy*. The effort to understand the *student's own point of view* and the teacher's success in actually doing so has a powerful impact on the student and leads to further openness in the sharing and communication process (Carkhuff, 2000; Rogers, 1951). In order to genuinely understand some of the psychosocial reactions of a student to independent travel, a mobility specialist has to establish an empathic helping relationship. Such a relationship can improve the extent and the reliability of what is learned during the assessment process regarding the psychosocial factors related to orientation and mobility. Research reported by Ivey et al. (2006) has demonstrated that training in listening skills can improve an instructor's ability to communicate with empathy.

ASSESSMENT OF THE STUDENT'S PSYCHOSOCIAL FUNCTIONING

As discussed by Bina, Naimy, Fazzi, and Crouse (Volume 1, Chapter 12), the mobility specialist, before beginning her work with a student, has to conduct or review a thorough assessment of a student's abilities, limitations, and past experiences that relate to independent travel. Such a review is done for administrative reasons, for safety reasons, and as a part of an effective teaching process. As a part of this assessment, the mobility specialist must gather as much information as possible about the potential impact of various psychosocial factors on the student's mobility training.

Standardized Instruments and Psychiatric Diagnoses

There are very few standardized measuring instruments that are routinely available to help in the mobility specialist's effort to understand the psychosocial functioning of students that might relate directly to orientation and mobility. Efforts to assess various personality factors among people who are visually impaired through standardized instruments have encountered problems with reliability and validity, as discussed by Welsh (Volume 1, Chapter 6). Even if the results of such instruments were available and were considered valid, they would show only the performance of an individual student in relation to the reference group on which the instrument was normed. This may or may not be useful information related to the instruction or performance of a specific student with a visual impairment in an O&M situation.

Occasionally, there may be information in a case record that relates to a medically diagnosed psychiatric condition. When this is the case, the mobility specialist should be aware of the availability of the *Diagnostic and Statistical Manual of Mental Disorders (DSM-IV-TR)*, which is published and periodically updated by the American Psychiatric Association (2000). This publication reviews the entire range of psychiatric diagnoses that are used, the behaviors that typically accompany each diagnosis, and the medications prescribed for each. When a mobility specialist does not have access to a consulting psychiatrist or social worker, the *DSM-IV-TR* can help to provide basic information about a diagnosis found in a report and perhaps help inform the specialist's approach to teaching. It can also be helpful in preparing the O&M specialist for a consultation with the psychiatrist or social worker in an effort to anticipate how a diagnosed condition and prescribed medication might impact the O&M training.

Record Reviews

Lacking standardized sources of information about psychosocial factors and dynamics, the mobility specialist has to rely on personal and subjective information such as can be obtained from various records, interviews, and discussions with the student and others. From the various records and reports that may be available, it will be important to note the nature of the person's vision loss and the amount of remaining vision, if any. It will be helpful to note whether the loss of vision was sudden and complete or gradual and partial, or some variation of these two factors. Knowing when a person's vision loss occurred will indicate how long the person has been living with limited vision. These factors provide a general background against which a person's current adjustment, skill levels, and attitudes can be evaluated.

According to Erikson's Stages of Psychosocial Development (Erikson, 1982), the age at which a person lost vision may indicate the disruption of developmental goals and tasks. If vision was lost during adolescence, the mobility specialist may expect a disruption in a student's process of developing her identity as an adult. If the vision loss came later, during adulthood, the loss of vision may have disrupted that part of the person's life when personal productivity was the most important focus. These and other hypotheses drawn from Erikson's theory of psychosocial development may be helpful in suggesting motivational attitudes and goals that may help a student plan her mobility program.

Reports in the file may also refer to the nature of the student's home neighborhood as well as the structure and supportiveness of the student's family and her place and role in it. It may be helpful to understand the nature of the student's family when her visual impairment was first discovered or at the time a child was born with a congenital vision problem. It may be especially useful to understand how the student's family changed since the diagnosis was made and whether or not any changes precipitated or delayed the student's referral for O&M services. In looking for tips regarding a student's interests and motivation, reports that refer to past employment, hobbies, and community activities may suggest topics that can be used to stimulate a student's interest and motivation and to suggest goals that may be helpful in planning mobility training.

In reviewing the student's history of mobility instruction, if any, the mobility specialist should pay close attention to what was accomplished and what, if anything, is said about the student's motivation for instruction and emotional reactions to the learning process and outcomes. Is the student currently using any of the training provided? If not, why not? Were there psychosocial factors that may have intervened to make previous training unsuccessful?

Assessment Interviews

The best source for information about many of the psychosocial factors that may affect mobility training will usually be the student. This is true in spite of the fact that many of these factors may be subconscious or otherwise unknown to the student at the time. Because of the value of the interview in the assessment process, it is important that the mobility specialist develop as much skill as an interviewer as possible.

As discussed in the previous section of this chapter, the interviewing skills of the O&M specialist can be learned or improved. This begins with a focus on attending behaviors, which are those observable actions on the part of the interviewer, such as eye contact and body posture,

that indicate that the interviewer is paying attention (Kadushin & Kadushin, 1997). For students who are blind or visually impaired, the verbal component of attending behavior may be more important. This component, which is called *verbal following behavior*, includes comments by the interviewer that follow along on the comments of the student, encouraging and reinforcing the desire to continue talking. Such comments can be short utterances that do not have to contain a lot of meaning but demonstrate attentiveness to the student (Kadushin & Kadushin, 1997). If the student has vision, he may be able to tell by some of the mobility specialist's nonverbal behavior whether or not the specialist is interested. If the mobility specialist is distracted and looking everywhere but at the student, this behavior may communicate a lack of interest. But even without vision, a student generally can tell the difference between someone who is interested and paying attention and someone who is not.

As the student comes to understand that the mobility specialist is genuinely interested in what he has to say and seems to understand what he is feeling, he is encouraged to trust more and to share more. This, of course, is contrasted to an interviewing style in which the student gets the impression that the mobility specialist is not personally interested but is following a preestablished checklist. The inattentive mobility specialist may come across as already knowing what she is going to hear and may cut short the discussion before the student is finished with what he intends to say. For this reason, some interviewers choose to interview the student before reviewing reports in the file. Usually, however, the review of old reports provides the mobility specialist with a list of questions or topics on which to focus if they do not come up naturally in the conversation.

During the assessment interview, the mobility specialist can explicitly use some of the concepts discussed in Chapter 6 of Volume 1 to guide the questioning. In an effort to establish some understanding about where the student may be in the process of adjusting to vision loss, the mobility specialist may inquire about how the person is feeling about the vision loss. The O&M specialist should try to establish whether or not the person is expecting to receive a return of vision or whether the person has accepted the permanence of his loss. The mobility specialist should try to understand whether the student is angry and focused on blaming someone for his blindness or whether the student is depressed and discouraged about ever being able to get his life back on track.

If the relationship established by the interview seems solid enough, the mobility specialist may want to delve more deeply into how the student feels about himself. Some of these questions, however, may not seem appropriate until more time has passed and better rapport is established. When the relationship seems comfortable enough, the interviewer should not hesitate to ask the student questions about how he feels about himself. How has the loss of vision changed that? If the student has a vision loss as a result of a congenital impairment, how has this affected his sense of similarity or difference to peers with whom he grew up and who were not visually impaired? What does the student find really satisfying about himself? What would the student like to change?

The mobility specialist may eventually ask about the student's past accomplishments. Does he like to do things for himself, or does he not mind having other people do these things for him? In the past, has the student been inclined to take on really difficult tasks that require a lot of work, or does he usually pursue a path that is more likely to lead to an easy success? Does he feel that success depends on his own efforts, or do good or bad things happen regardless of how hard he tries?

It is also important to get a sense of the reactions of the student's family to his loss of vision. Have they been quick to provide everything the

student needed, or was that their original response until they seemed to tire of having to do things for him? Have there been other people with disabilities in the student's family? How have they succeeded?

When talking with the parents of children who are visually impaired, it is important to ask about how they feel about their child learning to become more independent. Are they afraid? Do they think it is possible? Do they think it is worth the risk? Are they worried about their child getting his hopes up and then being disappointed? Do they feel differently about their child traveling independently at school versus in their own neighborhoods? Will the neighbors be surprised to see the child traveling with a long cane?

How does the student feel about being out in public? How does he react when people ask about his vision loss or offer help? If the student has low vision, does he try to keep people from knowing about his vision loss, or would he just as soon carry a cane so that people will know he has a problem and not be surprised later?

With a student who is an older adult, the mobility specialist may inquire about how the student sees her vision loss in relation to other health problems and other losses. Is losing vision an inevitable part of growing older, or is it a problem to be addressed? What other losses has the person experienced lately? Has she lost a spouse, siblings, good friends, a career, her home? How has she coped with those losses? What has helped? What has not?

Of course, there are no right answers to questions like these. Nor is there any pattern of answers that would suggest that a person would not benefit from mobility training, either at the time of the interview or sometime down the road. It is important for the mobility specialist to not form hard-and-fast opinions about the student. The answers to these questions primarily have a heuristic value. That is, they suggest hypotheses or theories about a specific student that have to be tested through the interaction that will come with instruction. They may suggest ways to approach motivational issues, goals, or dependency issues with this student. When various methods are tried based on preliminary hypotheses, however, they may not be as successful as the mobility specialist had hoped. If not, it is important to abandon that approach and try another.

Overall, the mobility specialist is attempting to understand the student who is in front of her at that time. Experiences with other students may be helpful in suggesting possibilities, but they may not be of any help at all in relation to this particular student. The mobility specialist can think of the five superfactors that have emerged from research about personality traits (McCrae & Costa, 1990) and about what she has heard from the student and project where a particular student may fall along any or all of the continua that McCrae and Costa have presented as components of the five factors. These factors, discussed in Volume 1, Chapter 6, include (1) neuroticism/stability, (2) extroversion/introversion, (3) openness, (4) agreeableness/aggressiveness, and (5) conscientiousness/undirectedness. Thinking of the student in relation to these factors or their component continua may not give the mobility specialist an accurate or a complete understanding of the student, but it provides a place to start. It offers some basic concepts or handles to use in trying to develop a picture of a person. In all of these cases, such concepts are tentative and subject to change, but they represent a beginning in understanding motivation, attitudes, goals, and expectancies.

The purpose of these suggestions is not to turn the mobility specialist into a counselor or therapist. This is not her professional background or certification, nor does she have the time to devote to helping the student work out problems in these areas and still have time for mobility instruction. If the results of an assessment interview suggest that a person may have serious issues in any of these psychosocial areas, the mobility specialist has a responsibility to make an appropriate referral to someone who is qualified to handle such matters.

However, it is important to understand that the mobility specialist does have a responsibility to find out as much as possible about the psychosocial functioning of a student in relation to helping the student succeed as a more independent traveler than he was prior to instruction. Unfortunately, the state of most service-delivery programs is that they do not have sufficient related services and personnel to identify the kind of information that the mobility specialist needs.

The interview process, in which the mobility specialist makes a genuine effort to learn as much about the student as possible and to understand the student's situation from the student's point of view, can serve its own important purpose. It can go a long way toward establishing the kind of empathic helping relationship between the student and specialist that will prove to be of value throughout the mobility training experience.

A PSYCHOSOCIAL APPROACH TO PLANNING

Throughout this text, there are frequent references to the importance of having mobility students involved, appropriately and to the best of their ability, in planning their instruction and in choosing their goals. This is the situation for students at the preschool level and during school years, for adults, for seniors, and for students whose vision loss is combined with hearing loss, motor limitations, or any other combination of impairments, including cognitive impairments. Why is this so important?

First, student participation in planning is required by state and federal regulations that apply to most special education and rehabilitation services (see Volume 1, Chapter 12). Second, it reflects effective teaching. Providing students with an opportunity to participate in planning their own lessons communicates respect for students and for their input (see Chapter 8). This reinforces the basic attitude of respect that should be the primary purpose of the communication and listening style of the mobility specialist, as discussed earlier. Participation in selecting goals and planning the instruction encourages "ownership" on the part of the student in the plans that emerge.

Many of the theorists reviewed by Welsh (Volume 1, Chapter 6) hypothesized a connection between goals and motivation. In order to tap into the motivating force of goal setting, theorists suggested that such goals should not be vague and general. They need to be specific, challenging, and measurable in order to keep the person's attention focused on the activity, to mobilize effort, to encourage perseverance, and to generate new strategies for improving performance (Bandura, 1997).

It is especially important that the student participate in this aspect of the planning to make certain that the goals are meaningful and motivating. If the person has clearly bought into the overall purpose of the mobility training and is focused on the eventual outcome of independence, short-term goals may not be as necessary and may be perceived as intrusive. However, if the person cannot quite see the endpoint of the training, more short-term goals may be useful in helping to move the student along the process from step to step. The accomplishment of each step will provide the opportunity to add to the goals, to adjust the student's level of aspiration, and to add to the person's sense of self-efficacy. The mobility specialist's ability to understand which is the correct goal level can come only from interaction with the student during the goal-setting process. If the goals of the instruction are presented to the student as fixed and routine and the same as they are for every student, they will have a less motivating influence.

The selection of explicit and concrete goals for the instruction may be difficult. Some students see the possibility of only limited outcomes for themselves. This may be a result of having had no previous experience with successful blind people, or it may result from a particularly negative attitude toward what is possible without vision. Selecting limited goals may also be a defense mechanism for students who do not want to disappoint themselves or others. Once the mobility specialist understands the influences that result in the student's limited goals, she may see an opportunity to persuade the student to shoot higher. However, as a result of an effective assessment interview, the mobility specialist may realize that more limited goals are an appropriate starting point for this student. Once these first goals are achieved, there may be an opportunity to revisit the plan for instruction and move on to the next level.

THE PSYCHOSOCIAL VALUE OF LESSON SEQUENCING

The traditional approach to the teaching of orientation and mobility has featured the use of a client-sensitive learning sequence that emphasizes a pattern of success experiences and increased responsibility, self-efficacy, and problem solving by the student. This element traces its origins to the earliest days of mobility training at Valley Forge and Hines (Apple, 1962; Williams, 1965). In reflecting on the principles needed to run a center for the rehabilitation of people who are blind, Williams (1965) said they should include the following elements:

- the real meaning of a success pattern in activities that are tried;
- the kind of observations which tell when success is really being achieved;
- the subordination of certain basic needs on the part of the staff in favor of the satisfaction

of needs on the part of a client who, after all, is the one struggling for growth;

- the real principles behind sensitive observation or evaluation of a person;
- the gradation of activity so that there is enough to be challenging and satisfying when achieved but not so much as to bring about the negative effects resulting from failure (p. 33).

These basic principles have also been incorporated in university programs that educate O&M specialists. In learning to travel while blindfolded, the O&M student does not put on the blindfold and immediately travel in a business area, use a bus, and cross streets effectively. In the beginning, most students doubt their ability to develop these skills. However, they learn these skills through the use of teaching progressions that gradually expect better cane skills, better use of hearing, more demanding orientation challenges, more complex problem solving, more interaction with other people on the street, and, increasing confidence in their own ability to use the cane and their other senses to travel effectively.

O&M specialists since the early days of the Hines program (Malamazian, 1970; Welsh, 1972) relied on the use of well-designed learning sequences to develop what they called "self-confidence." This was before Bandura (1977) empirically verified the importance of the closely related concept of "self-efficacy." While the accomplishment of these skills and learning goals can have a positive impact on a blind student's self-concept and self-esteem, they serve an even more important purpose in the development of an individual's personal sense of self-efficacy.

The use of an effective learning sequence should not be confused with the location of the instruction or the order in which certain environments are taught. LaGrow and Weessies (1994) pointed out that the ideal sequence envisioned by the written curriculum is usually modified by the demands of each situation. For example, in

an itinerant program, the ideal learning environments may not be available, or the particular goal of a student may be to learn his way around the residential center where the program is being offered or around his apartment building. Other necessary modifications result from characteristics of the learner, including other disabilities, such as developmental delays or severe neuropathy of the feet, or limited interests that result in very narrow learning goals, such as the need only to get to a neighbor's house or a neighborhood store (Long, Boyette, & Griffin-Shirley, 1996).

Regardless of what skills are being taught and regardless of the environment in which the instruction is taking place, an appropriate learning sequence is necessary to effectively address a number of psychosocial factors. Consideration has to be given to where a student seems to be functioning and how best to help him develop the required sense of self-efficacy that leads to the level of skill that is needed to accomplish his goals.

Skill Development

Each student's learning sequence typically reflects a certain logical order of skill development, even though that order and the considerations that shape it may vary from student to student. To some extent, the sequence is affected by a natural hierarchy in which later skills presuppose the presence of more basic skills. For example, the ability to cross a street effectively requires prior skill in judging traffic, straight-line walking, and detecting veering. However, even the progression of skill development may be influenced by underlying psychosocial factors.

The learning of cane skills, sensory skills, orientation skills, and problem-solving skills frequently require the building of self-confidence. A feeling of success and an improved sense of personal self-efficacy can be important factors in learning all of the kinds of skills listed previously.

Success in learning to identify obvious sounds improves a student's chances of learning to differentiate more subtle sounds. Success in solving a simple orientation problem helps one develop a greater sense of self-efficacy, which is important when it comes to solving more complex problems. The learning sequence is more effective, however, when even the most basic learning tasks represent a challenge. If the task is too easy and the answer too obvious, and the instructor's praise too effusive for the accomplishment, the student's sense of self-efficacy is not improved, especially for adult students.

Self-Efficacy

A person's sense of self-efficacy consists of a belief on the person's part that she is up to the task at hand. This belief can have a powerful effect on behavior and motivation (Bandura, 1997). Regardless of the task or skill addressed by a lesson, the mobility specialist has to encourage a belief in the student that she can accomplish it. While the coaching by the instructor and the experience of seeing other visually impaired people accomplish the task can help, the most powerful impact on a person's sense of self-efficacy is the experience of actually doing it herself. If the task is too difficult and the student fails, it can have a negative impact on the student's sense of self-efficacy. For this reason, it is necessary to structure a lesson so that the result is success and an enhancement to the person's self-confidence. Such an outcome requires that the mobility specialist work with one student at a time. The extent to which a student changes her perceived self-efficacy through performance will be influenced by the difficulty of the task, the amount of effort expended, the amount of external aid received, the circumstances under which the student performed, and the temporal pattern of her successes and failures (Bandura, 1986).

Motivation

For a student who lacks sufficient motivation for mobility training, it is important to have the student participate in selecting the goals of the instruction and the levels of accomplishments that will signal success. It is important that these goals make sense in the plan of instruction and lead to the next set of goals. It is also important that there be agreement in advance on the measures of success. How will the student know when they have been reached? Reaching these milestones and knowing how they move a student toward certain other goals has an important impact on motivation. The sequence may include a progression of increasing success in performing travel skills or in achieving specific outcomes. This direct experience of success is the primary way in which an individual's perception of self-efficacy can be developed, leading to increased motivation to continue the training.

Independence

For some students there may be a need for a sequence of lessened dependency on the instructor. Frequently the student may depend quite a lot on the instructor, even to the point of using the instructor as a human guide in the beginning lessons. However, it is important for the typical student who eventually will be capable of independent travel that the transition to depending on oneself start during the very first lesson. For this reason the instructor talks to the student in terms of learning to *use a guide* instead of *being guided*, and the student is expected to start using his own hearing and other senses to stay oriented, even while using a guide during the early lessons (see Chapter 1).

Practically every skill can be developed and practiced in levels of increasing independent functioning. Whether it be practicing cane skills or solving orientation problems, the one-to-one instructional methodology allows the mobility specialist to structure the level of independence to match where the individual student is at any given point in the training. This is true even if the goal is limited, such as it may be with an elderly person who has the simple goal of going independently to the mailbox on the corner. The mobility specialist can structure a sequence of lessons in which more and more independent functioning is expected and required of the student. This helps the student develop sufficient confidence in his own capability so that he can accomplish even this limited goal.

Chapman (1978) described the acquisition of independence as a gradual process. The child who is blind cannot make the transition from childhood to adolescence in one step, and needs the chance to increasingly make his own decisions, decide what to eat, what to wear, what to do, what new pursuits to follow, and what new responsibilities to undertake. O&M lessons of graduated independence and responsibility should coincide with a student's perceived level of independence and lead the student toward ever-increasing levels of independent functioning.

Problem Solving

The ability to effectively solve many travel problems combines skills of orientation with the use of logic, the ability to make accurate turns and movements in the environment, and the personal sense of self-efficacy in reestablishing one's orientation when lost. When a sense of self-efficacy in regard to this skill is lacking, an appropriate sequence of problem-solving activities may be structured to reflect increasing skills in this area.

The instructor builds in graduated levels of expectations in problem solving, beginning with the student's planning of routes, alternate routes, and return routes to and from the travel objectives. For a student who is likely to experi-

ence a complete course of instruction, this will start during indoor travel and will be addressed in each new area of training. For the student who has limited opportunities and will work primarily in areas of immediate need, this progression and the building of a sense of self-efficacy in solving problems that arise still must be a part of the lesson planning.

At each level of instruction, this sequence includes learning how to recognize when orientation mistakes have been made and then deciding how to get back on track. In the traditional use of a problem-solving sequence, the student is exposed to problems of orientation from the earliest lessons in the sequence and is asked to solve these problems. Initially, these are simple and basic problems related to remaining oriented while traveling with a human guide. As the training progresses, the problems become more complex. As the student begins to travel independently, she is required to make more decisions on her own and to cope with the consequences of those decisions, including the new problems that incorrect decisions bring.

The O&M specialist typically tries to control the complexity of the problems that the student must confront through the structuring of lessons and through the specialist's own decisions about when to step into a situation and provide additional assistance to keep the problem from becoming too complex. Because the instruction is individualized, the mobility specialist can decide when to terminate a lesson or when to let it continue based on the needs of that one student. Through an effective relationship with the student, the instructor learns to evaluate how much frustration a student can tolerate and how to keep the focus on success experiences. It is unlikely that a student will develop more confidence in her ability to solve problems if the problems presented do not represent a reasonable challenge, but the problem also has to be solvable by the student at her current level of skill.

In the traditional approach to instruction, the problem-solving sequence may lead to the use of drop-off lessons (see Chapter 2). In a drop-off lesson, the student is taken to an area in which she has been training in such a way that when the lesson begins, the student is uncertain of her actual starting point but has been given a specific objective as her goal. Her challenge is to travel safely through the area until she recognizes a landmark or a series of information points that suggests where she is in the area and which way she is facing. This awareness leads to a hypothesis. For example, the student may decide that if she is on Maple Street facing east, she can walk toward the east and within a block or two come to a very busy north-south street. If she does, she can be reasonably certain that this is Main Street and that she is at the corner of Maple and Main. She then forms a hypothesis that if she turns and walks south along Main Street, she will eventually hear an opening to an arcade that has a distinctive echo, which is her objective.

This problem-solving sequence can be used during indoor travel, residential travel, or business travel as long as there are sufficient clues to allow the problem to be solved. It can even begin while the student is learning human guide techniques and focusing on orientation skills at the same time. The instructor, serving as the guide, can ask the student to identify certain environmental clues and to begin making hypotheses that she uses to direct the guide's turns in order to get to a selected objective. At each level, the problems selected have to be solvable but not so easy that they are not a reasonable challenge to the student.

It has been common practice for the O&M specialist to review each lesson with the student at its conclusion. It is especially helpful to review with the student the problem-solving and decision-making processes that the student used and to reinforce the methods that proved to be successful. This is consistent with the findings of Bandura et al. (1982) and the suggestions of Dodds et al. (1994) that it is not merely the experience of success that has an impact on a person's perception of her own self-efficacy, but it is also the personal realization that the person consciously understands and emotionally appreciates that success was due to her own efforts.

Managing Anxiety

Students who have a particularly strong anxiety response to certain situations will need to be sensitively and gradually exposed to these situations in a way that helps them develop their sense of efficacy in managing such anxiety. These situations may include increased physical danger, such as descending stairs or crossing streets, travel in busier areas, or greater interaction with the public.

Typically, an instructor will expose students to anxiety-provoking situations with a high level of support. For example, teaching techniques for crossing streets may first be done using a human guide. The student can make decisions about when it is safe to cross, and the instructor, serving as the guide, and the student can cross together. The process could then move to the instructor standing right beside the student and being clearly available to intervene if the student steps off the curb at the wrong time. Ultimately, as the student's sense of self-efficacy and skill levels progress, the mobility specialist may take a position across the street as an indication of his judgment that the student's sense of self-efficacy has progressed to the point where the student can handle street crossings independently.

INVOLVING FAMILIES

Many of the psychosocial dynamics that affect the student learning mobility without vision may also affect the student's family (Travis, Boerner, Reinhardt, & Horowitz, 2004). For this reason, it is important during the assessment process for the mobility specialist to learn as much as possible about the family's attitude and expectations regarding the student's visual impairment. The family's attitudes, feelings, and beliefs will almost certainly affect the student as well. Does the family think that the vision loss is permanent, or are they expecting a recovery? What expectations do they have of the student, whether a child or an adult, when it comes to independent functioning? What do they expect the student to do on his own at home? What does a student actually do independently at home or in his neighborhood? Of course, where multiple family members are involved, there may be multiple answers to these questions, and the mixed messages the student receives may be a problem in their own right.

While some of these questions may be answered through a review of records, the direct interview with key family members, when possible, is most useful when it comes to understanding their point of view as it relates to O&M instruction and the possibility of greater independence for their family member. Once again, the kind of helpful relationship that the mobility specialist brings to these interviews can be helpful in learning what family members *really* feel about these matters.

Tuttle and Tuttle (2004) have reviewed information that emphasizes the role of the family in developing the student's feelings and attitudes about himself. They discussed how the blind person's internal process of establishing self-esteem interacts continuously with the judgments of significant others. The emergence of the blind person's goals and aspirations has an influence on the tasks and activities he chooses to accomplish. The student's success in accomplishing these tasks is evaluated against a standard of his own choosing, and many times this standard is the judgment of significant others, especially family members. If, based on these judgments, the student concludes that he has been successful, the student may then modify future goals

and aspirations. This cyclical process continuously has an impact on a visually impaired student's feeling of competence and adequacy.

For these reasons, it is especially important that family members have a clear understanding of the goals of the mobility instruction. They should know what to expect at each level of the training and what represents a positive accomplishment that should be praised and encouraged. Occasionally, family members have expectations that are too low, and they marvel at "accomplishments" that are not truly accomplishments. This can have the effect of minimizing the value of their praise and encouragement. In contrast, family members may have fears and reservations that they communicate either directly or indirectly to the student. This can add to the student's anxiety or undermine his growing sense of self-efficacy (Cimarolli, Reinhardt, & Horowitz, 2006).

Generally speaking, it is important for a student's family to be aware of every stage of the training and to actively participate through periodic observations of the student and discussions with the student and instructor. However, there are some cases in which the family's level of anxiety and doubt may require that the student participate in training away from the family until he has had the opportunity to develop sufficient skill to convince family members that safe travel is indeed a realistic possibility.

When the student is learning to travel while attending a rehabilitation center or a residential school at some distance from his home, the family may be quite supportive of the process. However, when the student is ready to use these skills in his home community, either independently or as the training is brought to the home neighborhood, the family's support may be replaced by active resistance. When this occurs, it is sometimes caused by the embarrassment that family members anticipate as the family member who is blind is seen traveling with a cane in the neighborhood (Sebald, 1983). The family may not have been entirely open when talking to neighbors about the seriousness of the blind family member's disability, and they may have minimized the problem in an effort to protect their own self-esteem. The possibility of the family member advertising his disability by traveling through the neighborhood with a long cane may set off a credibility crisis with the neighbors. Such possibilities suggest that contact between the mobility specialist and the family should precede mobility training in the student's neighborhood in an effort to determine whether such issues exist and to plan a strategy for coping with them.

Some family members may also experience fear or anxiety as they think about the person who is blind traveling with a cane through the community. As discussed above, when such an anxiety reaction is noted in a student, a great deal of care is taken to provide an appropriate sequence of lessons in a supportive atmosphere in order to help the student learn to overcome the fear or cope with the anxiety. A similar, carefully planned sequence of exposures may need to be provided for family members, too. They may need opportunities to see the blind student travel safely first in less-threatening areas before they are ready to think of him traveling independently in his own neighborhood, with its particular level of difficulty.

Observing mobility lessons provides family members with good opportunities to ask the O&M specialist about concerns that they may have. Sometimes these concerns are a generalized anxiety that is not well formulated in their minds. The opportunity to observe lessons in real travel environments may make the threats, as well as the solutions, more concrete. Also, the opportunity to observe other students who are similar to their own family member and who are successful travelers or at similar levels in the training can help family members improve their understanding in a manner that is less threatening for them personally. When this happens, it is important for the mobility specialist to empha-

size that no two travelers are alike so that the family does not expect that their student will be able to accomplish all that they observed in another student or that their student will face the same limitations that may have been evident in the observed student.

In many respects, family members of students receiving O&M training are like most people, who have had very little exposure to blind people. As Sussman-Skalka observed, the Lighthouse National Survey on Vision Loss revealed that 23 percent of respondents who are not visually impaired feel "awkward or embarrassed" because they do not know how to behave with people who have impaired vision. This feeling is even more common (32 percent) among people who report that they have a close family member who is visually impaired (Sussman-Skalka, 2002; Cimarolli, Sussman-Skalka, & Goodman, 2004).

An important role for mobility specialists is to provide information to family members about vision loss and orientation and mobility. There are many misconceptions that serve as the basis for what may appear to be a lack of support and encouragement from the family of the student who is learning to travel. Sometimes, factual information about what to expect and what is possible can be very significant in helping family members overcome what at first appeared to be deep-seated fears and anxieties.

INTERACTING WITH THE PUBLIC

As a person with a visual disability moves through the environment, there are multiple effects on the person as well as on the environment, especially the social environment. These effects can be positive or negative and can have an impact on the person's willingness or ability to travel in that environment. According to Stotland and Canon (1972), a person's sense of competence or self-esteem can be affected by (1) her perception of the effectiveness of her own actions, (2) her perceived freedom to select from a number of possible actions, (3) her sense of similarity with others, and (4) the communications she receives about her competence from others. When the person with a visual disability has the option of traveling independently to accomplish her goals, this can contribute to her sense of competence and self-esteem, as can the positive feedback the person receives from members of the community.

L. D. Baker (1973) extended this effect to the attitudes and behaviors of other people. Using the image of a circular process (Figure 6.2), Baker proposed that the behavior of the person who is blind, who in this case is moving independently and successfully through the environment, has an impact on the attitudes of others who observe this person's behavior. This impact is usually a positive one of increased respect for the blind person and a greater likelihood of the observer seeing the blind person as being more like herself. This may lead to a change in attitude that may also lead to a change in behavior to-

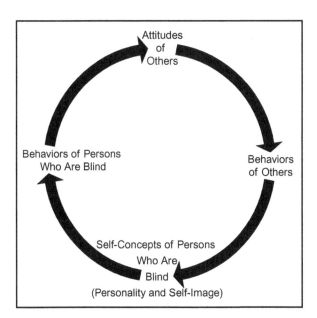

Figure 6.2. The Socialization Process for Persons Who Are Blind

ward the blind person. When the sighted observer reacts to the blind person with more respect and treats her more like a peer, this has a positive impact on the self-esteem and sense of self-efficacy of the blind person.

However, as discussed in the following sections, not all interactions with the public are the same, and some can become problems in their own right unless properly managed by the traveler who is blind.

Offers of Help

Some interactions with the public come in the form of offers of help. There are three types of offers: (1) those that are unsolicited and unnecessary, (2) those that are unsolicited and necessary, and (3) those that are solicited. Each of these types may have a different effect on the student, depending on how he is coping with his identity as a person with a disability.

The person who is feeling the conflict of *excluding overlapping roles*, as discussed by Welsh (Volume 1, Chapter 6), is torn between the role of a person with a disability who may need help in a particular circumstance and the role of a nondisabled person who can function without assistance. To the extent that the person is offered help, this excludes him from the possibility of being perceived as a person who does not have a disability. Such a person is likely to be very frustrated by offers of help, whether needed or not, and whether accepted or not. Such a person is also less likely to solicit assistance when it is needed, which may further aggravate a frustrating situation. The person who reacts to *new psychological situations* with a great amount of anxiety or emotion may be upset by offers of help and less likely to solicit assistance when necessary because of the uncertainty of how people are going to respond.

Both of these types of persons may be helped through role-playing a variety of situations that occur during travel and rehearsing different responses to each. Being prepared and having confidence in the effectiveness of certain responses will help reduce the newness of new psychological situations and the anxiety associated with them. For the person struggling with excluding overlapping roles, having effective responses to use in interactions with the public may help the person maintain his self-esteem as a person with a disability and reduce the conflicts associated with his struggle to function as a nondisabled person in situations where the disability excludes normal functioning.

Certain responses to unnecessary and unwanted offers of help are more effective than others. An effective response for one student may be ineffective for another. The role of the O&M specialist is to discuss with the student the variety of responses that are possible and help him select those that he would prefer to use in future situations.

Extracting necessary assistance from sighted pedestrians once a contact has been made is a skill that many students need to develop. Since this is usually a new situation for the sighted person, she may not know what information is useful, or because of her own anxiety, the sighted person may make rather basic errors. The person who is visually impaired must learn how to take charge of these interactions to ensure that he gets the needed information. The visually impaired person must learn how to ask specific, open-ended questions that will elicit responses other than yes or no from the helper. He must be able to break down requests for information into manageable units that the helper can provide in a way that will result in the visually impaired person getting thorough and accurate information. This structuring of the interaction by the visually impaired person will take some of the newness and uncertainty out of it for both persons, which will result in less anxiety and frustration for both and better communication between them.

Expressions of Sympathy or Curiosity

Other types of interactions may also cause problems. People may approach the person who is visually impaired with expressions of sympathy or inappropriate curiosity. This can produce anxiety and frustration if the visually impaired person is unprepared. The O&M specialist should help the student cope with the emotions that such remarks may generate and assist the student through anticipatory discussion and perhaps role-play. If a student can understand these remarks in the context of how disabilities are perceived and misunderstood by the general public, she can better prevent the negative impact of these experiences on her self-esteem and on her attitude toward and willingness to travel through the community. It may be helpful for the student to regard these interactions as opportunities to educate the public about the truth about disabilities and their effects.

While interactions with the public can be negative and can present challenges to the visually impaired traveler, the student can do a lot to structure and better manage them. In addition, the successful handling of these interactions can go a long way toward reinforcing the sense of self-efficacy that comes with success in meeting mobility goals and in maintaining high motivation for further independent travel.

Coping with Attitudes, Stigma, and Passing

If persons with low vision choose to conceal the disability components of their identities, they are spared some of the difficulties in those situations in which their vision loss does not matter. However, when they encounter situations where they cannot function visually, their inability to function or their need for assistance may stigmatize them and cause interaction problems.

For persons who choose to identify themselves as being visually impaired in mobility situations, it is frequently recommended that this can be most effectively accomplished through the use of, or merely carrying, a long cane, usually of the collapsible variety. This may result in such persons being identified as visually impaired more than is necessary, but when they do need assistance, their reasons for asking are obvious to others and the situation becomes more comfortable for them. For those who choose to remain unidentified, they frequently can learn to develop effective ways to approach others in situations where help is needed. These strategies, such as preceding a request for information with acknowledgment of the vision loss, usually require some revelation that a disability is present, but this can be done in a more focused and less public way than by carrying a cane. Persons choosing either alternative might benefit from the opportunity to role-play and rehearse responses for those situations when the alternative aspect of their identity is discovered in a social situation. They might also practice these responses with helpers who are in the know, such as coworkers or family members, before trying them out in public.

It is not the role of the O&M specialist to decide for the person who has low vision how he wants to present himself. This can be decided only by the student. The O&M specialist has the responsibility to help the person consider all of the factors associated with one approach or the other in travel situations; these may include both psychosocial and safety factors. Once the person has made a decision or is in the process of making a decision, the O&M specialist should systematically expose the student to the full range of possible situations he will encounter. The instructor should structure practice opportunities during which the student can try out a variety of solutions to the safety, psychosocial, and orientation problems that might arise in these interactions with the public. Occasionally, a person may choose to take an approach that the O&M specialist may feel is dangerous or particularly unwise for some other reason. In these rare situations, the O&M specialist should express her opinion to the student and indicate that if the student chooses to take that approach, such as refusing to use a long cane when traveling without a cane is particularly dangerous, the O&M specialist will be unable to continue to work with the student.

For many people with visual disabilities, mobility training situations might provide the first situations that bring to light the problems associated with interacting with other people. A child who is congenitally blind may have been protected from these encounters by parents and family members. The child's social experiences may have been entirely with close friends and neighbors who are in the know about the disability. The adventitiously blind person may also have had family members running interference in social situations since the disability occurred, preventing others from approaching to offer assistance or express curiosity. However, mobility training will require that the visually impaired person move through environments on his own and experience the unpredictability of these interactions with the public. The O&M specialist has to be sensitive to how the student is handling the anxieties and frustrations that often accompany these encounters, especially in the beginning. If necessary, the sequence of lessons may have to be modified to provide a gradient of more frequent and more demanding involvement with other people for students who need time to develop these skills.

Most mobility specialists plan specific lessons to work on contacting people on the street for necessary orientation information. In the beginning, the lesson may require the student to contact another pedestrian merely to confirm the identity of the street along which he is walking.

This is a significantly less demanding task than asking a person for directions to a distant objective. A beginning task may be to solicit assistance from a pedestrian in getting safely across a street. This can be much easier and much less awkward socially than getting rid of unwanted assistance. Once again, the mobility specialist, with the student's understanding beforehand, can use other staff people who can play the role of the regular pedestrian before the student actually tries out these behaviors on the street with members of the general public.

Some students may demonstrate significant anxiety when approaching lessons that will require increased interaction with the general public. This may reflect issues related to their struggle with dependency, or it may indicate only that this is another new psychological situation for which effective solutions have to be learned. An open and trusting relationship between the mobility specialist and the student can help to determine which factors are at work and how to approach effective solutions.

GROUP LESSONS

Apart from the misperceived administrative and financial advantages of mobility specialists working with more than one student at a time, there are some opportunities for group instruction that facilitate the management of some of the psychosocial factors identified and discussed in this text. As Bandura (1986) pointed out, the vicarious experiences of observing people similar to oneself performing a particular skill can contribute to a person's development of her own sense of self-efficacy related to that skill. For this reason, students who receive mobility instruction in rehabilitation centers or in residential schools have a ready-made opportunity to observe other students going through similar learning experiences. They have an opportunity to notice and hear about the small but important day-to-day accomplishments of

other students learning to cross streets successfully or solving orientation problems. These comparisons made between two students who perceive themselves as similar to each other, or one of whom is slightly behind the other in mobility progress, can have a motivating value. However, the mobility accomplishments of experienced staff members, while providing a long-range goal for the students, may not help much in the day-to-day development of a sense of self-efficacy.

Students who receive their instruction in their home neighborhoods or in school settings where they are the only student who is blind do not have natural opportunities to compare their own performance with that of their peers. In spite of feedback from their instructors, such students may develop a sense that no one has had the kinds of problems and troubles that they have, and they magnify their perceived shortcomings. On the other hand, they may have an unrealistic sense of the significance of what they have accomplished without similar students to whom they can compare themselves.

For these reasons, many mobility specialists systematically bring students together so that they can learn from one another. Sometimes this is done as a mobility group discussion in which all topics are welcomed. Sometimes, the mobility specialist sits in and participates in such groups and sometimes not. More often, group sessions are structured as seminars in which information that is needed by everyone can be shared and discussed. Such information may focus on transportation systems and how they operate, or on new automated pedestrian signals and the various ways in which they are constructed. Occasionally seminars of mobility students can take place at the bus garage, where the students are provided with opportunities to explore the buses and to practice entry and exit procedures without the anxiety of holding up other people. Frequently, such discussions may focus on the use of dog guides and how they provide an advantage or a preferred mode of travel for some blind travelers.

The interactions among mobility students that are facilitated by these group discussions and seminars can have positive impacts on the various psychosocial factors discussed in this chapter and in Chapter 6 of Volume 1 and can stimulate the vicarious comparisons mentioned by Bandura (1986). A position paper developed by the Orientation and Mobility Division of the Association for Education and Rehabilitation of the Blind and Visually Impaired lists a number of situations in which group lessons are appropriate and advantageous for students. This position paper also suggests various types of group lessons, including groups that focus on concept development, route planning, role-playing, sensory training, visual training, use of optical aids, and competitions (Orientation and Mobility Division of AER, 2006).

What is counterproductive in dealing with these psychosocial issues is for one mobility specialist to be working with two or more students in real environments at the same time. Not only does this approach create the possibility of unsafe circumstances, but it also does not allow the instructor to focus on the psychosocial experiences of each student and to structure the lesson sequence to reflect where that student is at each point in time. One student in a group may veer into a gas station and become very anxious and confused, creating an important opportunity to observe the student's reaction and to structure the problem-solving circumstance by providing enough feedback and information to make the problem manageable but still challenging for that particular student. In the meantime, what is happening to the other student or students in the group? Perhaps they, too, have encountered a significant teachable moment that is missed in the specialist's inability to focus in a detailed manner on more than one student at a time. As the O&M Division's position paper concludes,

Group lessons may be an option only as long as:

- Adequate and appropriate monitoring is provided for each student in the group.
- Students receive instruction that has been individually designed to meet their unique needs.
- Discovery learning is facilitated by providing each student with sufficient opportunities and time to analyze the features of the environment and problem-solve solutions with no more assistance than is appropriate and necessary.
- The student becomes self-reliant and confident of his ability to travel independently without peer assistance.
- the decision to provide group lessons is made by the instructor with concurrence of the consumer and, where appropriate, his family (Orientation and Mobility Division of AER, 2006, p. 1).

RISK MANAGEMENT

The quality of the relationship between the mobility instructor and his student is especially important when considered in light of the need to determine and disclose risks for a person that might result from services rendered. Debate about the intersection of patient autonomy and professional responsibility has increased during the past 20 years in the field of health care. Some of these concepts have been related to the field of orientation and mobility by Banja (1994) following the development by Blasch and De l'Aune (1992) of a computerized model for evaluating the effectiveness of cane technique coverage.

The Blasch and De l'Aune Mobility Coverage Profile and Safety Index modeling process, referred to as RoboCane, challenged some of the generally held understandings of the effectiveness of some aspects of the standard long-cane techniques. The possibility that the standard touch technique may result in less effective coverage than previously assumed by O&M specialists focused attention on the instructor's responsibility for adequately informing the student of the risks associated with mobility training and independent travel. Similar concerns have been raised more recently by Sauerburger's work on methods used to teach students how to evaluate the safety of crossing at certain intersections (Sauerburger, 2005), and in regard to travel through complex environments as discussed by Barlow et al. in Chapter 12 of this volume.

The information obtained through the use of the RoboCane with an individual student relates to one specific component of the process of independent travel. As Blasch and De l'Aune (1992) pointed out, the process of predicting risk for any aspect of independent travel, even a component as specific as the adequacy of cane coverage, is very complex. The RoboCane does not take into consideration the impact of factors such as residual vision, auditory perception, reaction time, orientation, level of attention, and motivation in determining the actual risk associated with a specific level of cane coverage given the complexity and hazards of a particular environment. However, RoboCane does represent a first step toward developing a more objective process of describing behaviors more precisely and making an objective presentation to a student about the level of risks that she might encounter in traveling independently. Similarly, Sauerburger's timing methods for determination of safe crossing can result in different determinations about the safety of the same intersection at different times of the day or on different days. While it may establish a conservative baseline for the most likely time to cross an intersection safely, it cannot determine or control the individual choices that students make in each circumstance.

The O&M specialist has to decide how to approach the discussion of the potential risks of mobility training with his students. The need for an honest and trusting relationship between the O&M specialist and the student requires that the specialist fully discuss the risks associated with independent travel. The possibility that such a discussion may dissuade a student from participating in training is not a sufficient reason to avoid it. However, it is most helpful for the process of encouraging clients whose motivation is marginal at the beginning to pace the discussion of the level of risk. Rather than laying out all the possible risks of travel that may conceivably lie ahead for a particular student, the O&M specialist should consider, in the timing of such a discussion, the individual student's skill and the environment that she will encounter in each successive phase of training. Naturally, the potential for risk typically increases as the student moves into more complex and challenging areas of travel. However, if an appropriate learning sequence has been followed, the student should not move into more complex areas until she has demonstrated the skills to handle the next level of difficulty. This changes the nature of the discussion that must take place, and the new skill levels may have enhanced the person's sense of self-efficacy to the point where she feels confident that he can manage the next level of risk successfully.

SUMMARY

From the outside, the profession of orientation and mobility is frequently seen as a specialty that primarily involves teaching a person the technical skills of using a cane and his other sensory systems as he moves safely through the environment. From the inside, mobility students and mobility specialists understand that the subplots that relate to independence, motivation, self-efficacy, family support, and interactions with the public play a much more dominant role than the aspects of the profession that are most visible. This chapter attempts to reflect how the theoretical issues related to the psychosocial aspects of orientation and mobility can be considered and applied in the day-to-day teaching of the skills of independent travel.

The history of the success of this profession provides many practical reasons to believe that these approaches are successful. However, orientation and mobility, like many practice professions, faces the challenge of documenting its successes and promoting a better understanding of how the various approaches to mobility training can have varying impact on students with different patterns of psychosocial variables.

IMPLICATIONS FOR O&M PRACTICE

1. Student or client involvement in selecting and approving individualized education or rehabilitation plans not only meets legal and bureaucratic requirements, but also can have an impact on a person's motivation for the mobility instruction that follows.

2. The person who is visually impaired or blind who travels through the environment with a cane is a significant social stimulus that can create positive, negative, or ambiguous situations. The mobility specialist has to be aware of how the blind traveler handles these different circumstances and structure learning experiences to improve these skills if necessary.

3. The person with low vision frequently has the option of making her visual disability more or less apparent when traveling. The O&M specialist tries to structure a thorough range of travel experiences that enable the person with low vision to evaluate the effectiveness of the travel method chosen.

4. Handling offers of help requires special skills by the person who is blind. The O&M specialist has to understand the full range of help interactions that might occur and the impact of each type on students with different personality characteristics.

5. The sequence of learning experiences traditionally used by O&M specialists is instrumental in addressing many psychosocial factors. It can contribute to improved motivation, a greater sense of self-efficacy, lessened dependence, and more effective problem solving.

6. The professional helping relationship that typically develops between the O&M specialist and students can itself be a tool that the instructor uses to address some of the psychosocial issues a mobility student faces. The O&M specialist has to understand how to develop and maintain an appropriate and effective helping relationship and how to use the power of this relationship to enable students to accomplish their goals.

LEARNING ACTIVITIES

1. Relate Baker's (1973) image of the circular effect of independent travel on a person's self-concept to Bandura's concept of self-efficacy.

2. Interview travelers who have low vision and identify some of the situations in which they have the most difficulty from a psychosocial perspective.

3. Role-play the range of "help" interactions that a traveler who is blind or has low vision is likely to encounter, and develop possible strategies for handling each.

4. Discuss with travelers who are blind the impact of their mobility instruction on the development of their self-confidence as travelers.

5. With other professionals in training, videotape the role-playing of typical interactions between O&M specialists and clients and identify behaviors that reflect genuine caring and honest feedback.

PART TWO

Age-Related Instruction

CHAPTER 7

Teaching Orientation and Mobility for the Early Childhood Years

Annette C. Skellenger and
Wendy K. Sapp

LEARNING QUESTIONS

- Why is the provision of orientation and mobility (O&M) during the first few years of life critical for children with visual impairments?

- What are the learning characteristics of young children that impact O&M development and instruction and what intervention strategies enhance O&M development in early childhood learners?

- How and why must O&M instructors work with families and teams to provide meaningful O&M services to early childhood learners?

- What are the components of an O&M curriculum during the early childhood years and how do these components differ based on the child's developmental level?

- What special considerations arise with O&M instruction when a child has a visual impairment and additional disabilities?

Amazing and complex changes occur within the first 5–6 years of an individual's life. Much of what the individual will become is rooted in the experiences and learning that occur in the early childhood years (Meisels & Shonkoff, 2000). It is believed that the opportunity for learning is greater in the first six years of life than in any other period (Shonkoff & Marshall, 2000). Physical, emotional, and cognitive development in this phase are rapid and interconnected, with each learned item not only affecting the next step within a particular domain but also affecting learning in many other domains (Allen & Marotz, 1994). For the most part, the wealth of information attained in the first six years is learned through activities that bear little resemblance to traditional instruction. This chapter discusses the developmental nature of the early childhood learner with a visual impairment and focuses on the necessity of facilitating the informal, incidental nature of learning when providing orientation and mobility (O&M) intervention to learners of this age.

THE IMPORTANCE OF EARLY ORIENTATION AND MOBILITY

Because of the complexity of early development, the O&M process during early childhood is very different from that faced by O&M specialists who work with the elderly, adventitiously impaired adults, or even school-age children (Anthony, Lowry, Brown, & Hatton, 2004; Knott, 2002) . For the former, orientation and mobility is primarily a process of starting with the O&M-related strengths and needs already demonstrated by the individual. During early childhood, the process must begin at a more basic step. With very young children, the process involves the initial *development* of skills both directly and indirectly related to orientation and mobility and the interweaving of these skills into the overall latticework of development. For example, an 8-year-old girl knows how to move her body in a variety of ways. The O&M process will consist of teaching her a specific way to move her hand so that she gets adequate coverage with the long-cane touch technique. In contrast, the O&M process with an infant will consist of being sure that the child includes the practice of lateral wrist movement among her earliest hand movements so that it is an internal component of her movement repertoire once she is ready to begin specific cane skills instruction. The educational process is different in these two instances, and it is important that orientation and mobility during early childhood not become a "downsizing" of processes that have been employed with adult learners. As shown in this chapter, much of the *content* of O&M instruction will remain the same, but it is imperative that processes for instilling that content be formfitted to the all-encompassing developmental nature of learners from birth to 5 years of age.

Orientation and Mobility in Early Childhood

The process of orientation and mobility during early childhood is very different because little of it consists of the types of O&M instruction provided to older learners. Because the child is "under construction" in this phase, much of orientation and mobility consists of making sure the child is aware of and can use the building blocks of later skills (Allen & Marotz, 1994). Much of the learning in orientation and mobility will occur through the practice of activities that bear little resemblance to traditionally structured O&M lessons. For example, the O&M specialist may take advantage of a "teachable moment" to explore the concept of *shoreline* when the child begins making a long path with large plastic waffle blocks during playtime. Much that may be learned to facilitate orientation and mobility will also include activities to facilitate skills such as reading (for example, concept development) or face washing (for example, body concepts). In addition to emphasizing functional use of skills, orientation and mobility with early childhood learners will focus on the developmental practice of subskills so that the child later will be ready to integrate their use in more formal O&M instructional activities. Though the definition of orientation and mobility includes instruction to facilitate travel in any environment, the process of orientation and mobility with early childhood learners may be thought of as arranging for the facilitation of travel both in current and in *next* environments. The term *O&M development* is used here to describe the process of facilitating skills and concepts with early childhood learners and *O&M instruction* refers to more systematic teaching of O&M skills and concepts.

Legislative Support

Due to the significant learning that occurs before a child enters kindergarten, federal legislation guarantees that children with disabilities have access to appropriate educational supports and services beginning at birth. Reauthorized in 2004, the Individuals with Disabilities Education Improvement Act (IDEA), Part B, Section 619, mandates a free and appropriate education for all children with disabilities from 3 to 21 years of age. Services for children age 3 to 5 are typically provided under the state department of education, are outlined in each child's Individualized Education Program (IEP), and are delivered in the least-restrictive environment. The IDEA, Part C, guarantees developmentally appropriate services and supports for children up to 3 years of age who have disabilities. Services for children up to age 3 are delivered through a state-identified lead agency, which could be the Department of Education, Department of Health and Human Services, or some other appropriate agency. Under Part C, Individualized Family Service Plans (IFSP) are written for each child who qualifies, and services are provided in the child's natural environment (for example, in the home, at day care, or in the community). O&M instructors who are not familiar with the legal requirements of the IDEA (including IEP and IFSP development) should familiarize themselves with these laws and their local interpretations. (Further details on this aspect of the legislation can be found in Bina Naimy, Fazzi, & Crouse, Volume 1, Chapter 12.)

Importance of Early Intervention

Because learning in the early childhood years normally occurs in a manner different from that commonly used with older learners, it is important that O&M specialists, as well as other professionals working with children in the early years, become familiar with the developmental stages of young children. Early learning is essential for children who are at risk for delays in development, such as children with visual impairments. Research shows that at-risk infants and

toddlers who receive early intervention services from birth to 3 years of age and preschool services from ages 3 to 5 have improved skills during elementary school compared to at-risk children who did not receive services (Berlin, Brooks-Gunn, McCarton, & McCormick, 1998). Initial studies on the long-term implications of early intervention indicate that, for many children who are at risk for delays and who received early services, the advantages of early intervention and preschool services continue to 18 years of age, as indicated by improved academic test scores compared to similar children who did not receive intervention prior to beginning school (McCormick et al., 2006). To date, no studies have looked at the long-term impact of early intervention O&M services, but the benefits of early intervention in other developmental areas underscore the importance of beginning needed interventions as early as possible to have the best long-term outcomes for children.

PREMISES RELATED TO LEARNING THAT IMPACT INTERVENTION IN EARLY CHILDHOOD

Early Learning Is Dependent on Developmental Factors

Learning and development during the early childhood years are extremely complex (see Table 7.1 for a description of theories of development). The term *development* is most often used when describing any area of learning in the preschool years. Although there is no single definition of development, there is generally agreement that development is a particular form of learning and that this type of learning has a close interaction with physical growth or aging across time. The components related to development that are most relevant to the information in this chapter are discussed below. Although learning at other stages of life can take other

TABLE 7.1

Summary of Theories and Perspectives That Influence Approaches to Teaching Young Children

Theory/Perspective	Description
Cognitive Developmental Theory (Piaget)	Learning is an active process and is related to the child's interaction with the environment.
	Children are active participants in the learning process and their interactions with the environment are how learning and development occur (for example, new structures are made).
	The environment should consist of materials and information that are not too far beyond children's current level and should include a variety of concrete experiences.
	Teachers need to understand that cognitive development is a prerequisite for learning and that it is critical to know each child and engage him or her in developmentally appropriate activities.
Ecological Systems Theory (Bronfenbrenner)	Children develop at the center of interconnected relationships and environments that all influence their development.
	Children learn and behave as a result of the interactions and influences within multiple systems.
	The many environments the child is involved in influence development.
	Teachers need to be aware of how the environment influences children's learning, and they should involve the community within the classroom and children within the community.
Learning Theory (Dewey)	Learning is a social process that occurs through daily interactions with the environment and through natural experiences.
	Children learn best by doing and by acting upon the world around them.
	The various environments in which children live should be connected and interrelated.
	Teachers need to guide children's learning by providing opportunities for experience and experimentation.
Psychosocial Theory (Erikson)	Development occurs in stages that occur throughout life and stresses the relationship between the stages and social experiences.
	Children are passive learners, developing individual personality traits and obtaining skills needed to become dynamic members of their society.
	The environment assists the child in obtaining characteristics needed to adapt to, and be a successful member of, his or her society.
	Teachers need to understand the various stages of social-emotional development and ensure that expectation and learning opportunities facilitate a child's transition from one state to the next.

(continued on next page)

Theory/Perspective	Description
Social Learning Theory (Bandura)	Learning occurs through a series of antecedent-response-consequence contingencies—in which events (antecedents) that happen before and after a behavior (response) serve to set the occasion for the behavior and the feedback (consequence) that results—which increase or decrease the likelihood that the behavior will occur again.
	Children gain knowledge from how the environment reinforces, supports, or punishes a particular behavior.
	The environment reinforces or punishes learning, causing learning to be more or less likely to occur again.
Sociocultural/ Sociohistorical Theory (Vygotsky)	Teachers need to model target behaviors and understand the importance of observation to young children's development.
	Learning occurs through interactions between a child and an individual who has more knowledge.
	A child initially learns to think and acquire knowledge through interactions with other members of society who are more knowledgeable, but the child will eventually learn to have internal dialogues that instruct and assist cognitive development.
	During the initial learning process for children, interactions with the environment facilitate learning by directly teaching the child to think and behave.
	Teachers need to incorporate social interaction and play across daily activities to promote cognitive and language development.

TABLE 7.1 (*Continued*)

forms (that is, circular, multifaceted), developmental learning is primarily linear, often referred to as a cumulative or building-block process. Most often, a skill only can be learned if the supporting skills are in place. In addition, learning in these early childhood years requires a balance of growth across multiple domains in both physiological and cognitive areas (Allen & Marotz, 1994). This requires that the progress along multiple linear paths must arrive at any one necessary point at the same time in order for learning to be most effective. For example, crawling typically occurs in sighted children when: (1) the musculoskeletal system has developed enough strength to hold the body off the floor, (2) the visual system has developed sufficiently to perceive the depth changes that occur as the

child's hand moves from the floor, upward and forward, (3) muscular patterns of leg and arm movements have been practiced sufficiently independently, and (4) the cognitive system has developed an understanding of goal-directed movement and some level of cause and effect so that the child wants to move toward and obtain some object or person. Finally, learning during the early childhood years appears to be a "continuous process of give and take between the child and the environment" (Allen & Marotz, 1994), often referred to as *transactional learning*. Learning in this phase appears to be extremely dependent on the provision of an appropriate environment that will support and respond properly to the multiple transactions occurring within the child.

In practical terms, this means that in order to increase the probability that learning will occur in the early childhood years, development needs to be facilitated by:

- Become familiar with both the typical developmental sequence (see Allen & Marotz, 1994) and the possible impact of visual impairment on the sequence.

- Provide a nurturing, responsive environment.

- Include strategies that facilitate learning in multiple domains at one time (see sensory development subsections under the section Curriculum and Instructional Strategies for Different Developmental Levels for suggestions of sensory information through infused intervention and suggestions for working with families and other team members).

- Provide intervention that is *carefully sequenced* based on the typical developmental progression but is adapted for the individual child's needs. Although careful sequencing and adaptation of intervention based on individual needs are important at all ages, these factors are critical for early learners due to the nature of development as discussed earlier (see sections on Curriculum Content and Curriculum and Instructional Strategies, which include specific instructional activities).

Young Children Are in the Sensory Motor Phase of Development

During the first five years of life, it is the child's job to experience through his senses as much as possible in the world around him. This is a time when the child learns as many new things as possible rather than delving into analyses of complex relationships. Most often, the exploration is random, unpredictable, and internally motivated. This is a period that includes much

exploration and experimentation, based on creativity and imagination. A vast majority of information is learned during play. Through play and other self-propelled exploration, the child is, in effect, creating knowledge. Although children with visual impairments have been found to play in ways different from sighted children, such as demonstrating less pretend play and engaging with adults at higher levels (Bishop, Hobson, & Lee, 2005; Lewis, Norgate, Collis, & Reynolds, 2000; Skellenger, Rosenblum, & Jager, 1997), a major overriding role of O&M specialists working with learners in the early childhood years will be the facilitation of the child's typically innate enjoyment of exploration, which is so often thwarted by absent or impaired vision. Through creative adaptations, the child should be motivated and assisted to explore his total environment. With an attitude of discovering enjoyment through exploration in the early childhood years, individuals will be more likely to reach toward independence and find a similar joy in its attainment.

Limited or Absent Vision Impacts the Ability to Integrate Information

It is presumed that the absence of vision impacts learning in multiple ways. Two factors that appear to impact learning in the early childhood years include part-to-whole learning and vision as the major integrating sense, as described below.

Whole-to-Part versus Part-to-Whole Learning

It is assumed that vision facilitates a learning process that first gives very general information about the "whole" and then allows the child to focus on the details of the "part" (Anthony, Bleier, Fazzi, Kish, & Pogrund, 2002; Fazzi & Klein, 2002; Fazzi & Petersmeyer, 2001; Ferrell, 1985). For example, when a child walks into a preschool classroom, he first gets a very general idea of the size of the room, senses bright colors and many objects, knows whether people are in the room, and so forth. The child then focuses on more specific details, such as the fact that there are children and an adult in the room, that the colors are toys and papers hanging on the bulletin board, and that there are round tables and chairs. Later, the individual can use the initial "whole" information to pull the "parts" together in a way that allows him to function in the setting, such as realizing that the papers hanging on the bulletin board are the children's artwork and that the toys are near his seat. The individual who is totally blind or severely visually impaired, in contrast, usually must rely on a part-to-whole process of obtaining information about the room. The majority of information that is provided for the student who is blind is received primarily through examination by his hands. This information is very specific, limited in size, and gives virtually no information about relative locations. The child may first feel the doorjamb, then the wall, and then walk a considerable distance trailing to find the bulletin board. Without a considerable amount of cognitive effort, each of the parts of the room may remain separate parts. Often, the result may be that the individual knows a great deal about many items but does not know their relationship or other factors that allows one to make functional use of the information from the combination of parts, and the child may never even realize that his artwork is hanging by the teacher's desk in a spot of honor.

Vision as the Main Integrating Sense

Vision is the modality that allows children with typical sight to realize that all of the sensory information received about an object, for example the sound, touch, smell, and taste of an apple, all belong to the same object (Fazzi & Klein, 2002; Fazzi & Petersmeyer, 2001). Without vision or with limited vision, a child may pet a dog, smell its breath, hear it bark, and not realize that all of

those sensations belong to the same entity. Further, if a clock were sitting on a table near the dog, it is possible that a child without vision might hear the ticking coming from a location that he or she identifies as the dog and may assume that dogs tick. In addition, the chance to experience sensory information does not necessarily provide meaning to a congenitally blind child who has not had meaningful experiences with the sound and feel of the object together. For example, a child might hear a refrigerator while eating breakfast and be told that the humming noise is the refrigerator, but the child does not necessarily understand that the item making the sound is a cold box that stores food without having direct sensory exploration of the object.

Intervention in the early childhood years needs to include both systematic practice in helping the child understand information from the senses and activities to support the child's understanding of how the sensory information is integrated to form a cohesive, total entity. Strategies for facilitating integration of information include, but are not limited to:

- As much as possible, complete daily activities and instruction using routines (Anthony, Bleier, Fazzi, Kish, & Pogrund, 2002) that incorporate all the steps or components into as cohesive a time frame as possible with an identifiable beginning and ending (see the section Create Routines to Increase Participation and Understanding).

- Include O&M skills, concepts, and intervention into daily activities. When skills such as trailing with a cane to find the swing set at the end of the garage are incorporated into a child's day-to-day life, it is more likely that the skills will be understood in their entirety and maintained across time. In addition, O&M intervention at this stage will also need to include intervention in many daily living skills such as dressing, self-help, and organizational skills in order to allow learning in each of the domains to support each other. While these are important strategies at all ages, they are critical in the initial learning period.

- Facilitate learning by providing intervention in naturally occurring environments and utilizing strategies to insure that all members of the team working with the child support and include O&M intervention. Much of O&M intervention in the early childhood years will occur in the child's home or in a day-care setting and will be infused into daily activities. Daily intervention will be provided by the O&M specialist and the other members of the team, as described later in the section on Inclusion of Significant Others on O&M Development and Intervention. Allowing the child to experience O&M skills and techniques in the same way, across the multiple people in his life and on a regular, systematic basis, will make it easier for him to understand how the parts of his life fit into the whole.

- The absolute importance of working closely with the child's family at this stage cannot be overemphasized. While working with families is always an effective and important strategy, it is of particular importance in early childhood for multiple reasons, only one of which is the need for the family to help support the child's understanding of how the parts fit into a whole. Other aspects regarding working with families are discussed later. In addition, it is strongly recommended that O&M specialists who work with young children actively seek more in-depth information about working with families (see Fazzi, Klein, Pogrund, & Salcedo, 2002; Ferrell, 1985).

- Balance the use of strategies to follow the child's lead (as discussed later) with carefully planned, sequenced intervention to assure that it is provided in a way to ensure that the child can understand the relationships between the multiple parts of whatever the total

entity is that is being taught and practiced. Random, isolated practice will have limited effectiveness.

INCLUSION OF SIGNIFICANT OTHERS IN O&M DEVELOPMENT AND INTERVENTION

Working with Families

The Family and Its Impact on Orientation and Mobility

Family is a difficult term to define in today's diverse society. We use the commonly accepted definition of family as any group of people related biologically, emotionally, or legally—that is, any group that defines itself as a family (McDaniel, Campbell, Hepworth, & Lorenz, 2005). As professionals, we may be working with the child's parent or parents (biological, adoptive, or foster), the child's extended family (for example, siblings, grandparents, aunts, or uncles), or the child's nontraditional family members (for example, unmarried homosexual or heterosexual couples raising a child of whom only one parent has legal custody).

Each individual is tied explicitly and enduringly to the family. The human infant requires a relatively long period after birth to achieve the physical stability for independence; therefore, the tie between the individual and family is particularly strong in the early childhood years to allow the child protection while learning the skills necessary for self-sufficiency. As the child matures and moves into greater contact with others outside the family system, the direct effect of the family often lessens, but emotional and indirect effects remain strong throughout the life span.

Families whose members include a child with impaired vision share the same characteristics of all families. The impact of the family on an infant or preschooler who has a visual impairment is as strong as that of other families. It is critical that O&M specialists who work with early childhood learners understand the integral relationship that exists between the learner and the family and include components in the intervention package that acknowledge this critical relationship. There are legal, theoretical, and practical reasons for O&M instructors to collaborate closely with families in providing intervention to young children.

Why We Work with Families

For children from birth to 3 years of age, the IDEA, Part C (2004), requires that all services be "family-centered," including the assessment and the components of the child's service plan. Family-centered support recognizes the complexity within families and develops supports and services that will meet the child's needs within the family structure. For preschool children, whose services are mandated under the IDEA, Part B (2004), legislative support for family involvement is not as strong, focusing primarily on the inclusion of the parent in the development of the child's educational plan and providing the parent with periodic progress reports. Despite the shift in legislative emphasis that occurs on the child's third birthday, children's families should continue to be involved in their O&M intervention, though their involvement will most likely decrease as the child matures toward school age.

Family-systems theories and an understanding of child development provide the theoretical rationale for including families in early childhood O&M intervention. According to family systems theory (Minuchin, 1974), the actions of each individual within the family system affect the actions of each of the other members, and both individual members and the system itself constantly strive to achieve balance within the system. If one member acts out or has special needs, the family system must react in a way that balances the action or need. Each family functions with particular and complex interactions that exist within the family's larger social and cultural environment. When professionals understand and work within the family's framework, families are more receptive to the services and support, and the child has a greater chance of achieving the intended outcomes (Fazzi & Petersmeyer, 2001; Turnbull, Turbiville, & Turnbull, 2000). The four basic tenets of family-centered support are: (1) an emphasis on child and family strengths rather than deficits, (2) the promotion of family choice in accessing resources, (3) a mutually respectful collaboration between professionals and parents, and (4) a holistic view of the family and the child's relationship to the family (Hatton, McWilliam, & Winton, 2003b).

From a practical standpoint, including the family as a partner in the child's O&M development is a logical way to provide the child with more learning opportunities. As a professional, the time an O&M instructor spends with a child is minimal, even if providing daily intervention, when compared to the learning opportunities that the child experiences with his or her family. Young children also learn best through daily interactions in their natural environments, meaning that practicing trailing a wall from their bedroom to the bathroom three times a day every day to wash hands or use the toilet will be much more beneficial than a 20-minute lesson once a week in which the child practices trailing a wall without a functional reason. Since we, as professionals, cannot be with children for all the "teachable moments" that arise, we must collaborate with families to ensure that children have the opportunities to meaningfully practice skills and develop concepts throughout their day. Many advantages exist when parents act as teachers, including: (1) direct and constant access to behavior as it occurs naturally, (2) an increase in the likelihood that behaviors will generalize and be maintained, (3) parents can act as natural reinforcers for the child, (4) intervention can be most effectively individualized to their child's needs, and (5) all family members can assist with learning, thereby increasing the amount of intervention that can be provided (Shearer & Shearer, 1976).

Support Provided to Families

As mentioned earlier, family systems are constantly acting to achieve balance, as members act outside normal limits or have specialized needs. Especially when the child who has a visual impairment is very young, the family may spend a great deal of energy attempting to cope with the additional stresses of having a child with specialized needs. Such stresses include the difficulty of coping with other family members' reactions to living with someone who is visually impaired, possible feelings of guilt, stress of long periods of hospitalization, and stress of additional financial considerations that may be required of some of these families. It is important to point out that not all families experience levels of stress beyond the normal; however, those who do often are especially vulnerable during the period when they are trying to find ways to balance the needs of the early childhood learner with the needs of the other family members. It is imperative that all professionals who have contact with the family during this time understand the stresses being faced and provide whatever support possible.

When working with the families of children who are 5 years of age and younger, O&M instructors and other professionals will provide three types of support: emotional, informational, and material (McWilliam & Scott, 2001). Emotional support refers to the development of a collaborative relationship in which the family members feel safe in sharing their joys and frustrations related to the child's disabilities, successes, and setbacks. Informational support is the provision of O&M- and visual impairment (VI)-specific in-

formation to the families and children. Material support is the sharing of resources such as parents' guides and adaptive mobility devices (AMDs).

Emotional Support

Though O&M instructors will never, and should never, take the place of families' informal support networks, they often provide critical emotional support related to the child's visual impairment. McWilliam, Tocci, and Harbin (1998) found that families value professionals who demonstrate positive attitudes toward the child and family, are responsive in taking action, are oriented toward the whole family, are friendly and sensitive, and who are competent with and about children and their communities. O&M instructors can provide critical support to families as they deal with the first few years of life with a child who is visually impaired, which can be overwhelming as families are inundated with new and unexpected medical and educational information. One very critical support the professional can give is to help the family realize and strengthen the social supports that are available. These systems can take the form of extended families, religious groups, or neighborhood communities. When family members are ready, their network can begin to include other families who have children with a visual impairment as well as successful adults who are visually impaired. O&M instructors can provide families with hope for their children's future by sharing success stories and connecting families to others who have had similar experiences.

Informational Support

As important as emotional support can be, most family members and professionals agree that concrete, action-oriented information is the most valuable resource professionals can provide. The act of parenting is typically learned incidentally through watching one's own parents and the parents of others. Typical experience, however, does not include information on ways to assist the child to initiate and maintain movement through the environment without sight or with limited vision. The O&M specialist working with early childhood learners will need to provide informational support to: (1) help family members acquaint themselves with the O&M process and the all-encompassing impact it can have on the development of the child, and (2) help family members learn ways to support and facilitate skills that will eventually allow the child with a visual impairment to safely negotiate the environment. Through the provision of direct service to children, O&M instructors have the chance to provide informational support to families. O&M instructors should explain what they are doing and why they are doing it. They need to brainstorm with the family about times that family members can encourage the same skill throughout the day. For example, an O&M instructor working with a young child who is not yet moving out of a sitting position may place a sound-making toy a few inches from the child's hand to encourage the child to reach out and shift his or her body weight. The O&M instructor needs to explain to the family that this activity is helping the child develop spatial awareness essential for later orientation and is providing an opportunity for the child to practice the motor skill of shifting body weight, which is a first step toward crawling. As a result of this explanation, parents will better understand the critical elements they should repeat with the child and they will be more likely to be motivated to provide the child with similar opportunities. Informational support also can include more direct parental intervention, such as the review of informational booklets or videos on orientation and mobility and motor development in children with visual impairments. Some resources to share with parents with information specific to young children who have visual impairments are: *An Orientation and Mobility Primer for Families* (Dodson-Burk &

Hill, 1989), *Pathways to Independence* (O'Mara, 1989), *Move with Me* (Blind Childrens Center, 1986), *Finding a New Path* (Gold, 2002), and *Reach Out and Teach* (Ferrell, 1985).

Material Support

Material support means ensuring that families have the resources necessary to meet their child's educational needs. Most often, children with visual impairments find common household items much more meaningful and motivational than fancy toys, but O&M instructors sometimes may need to bring toys or objects into the home or preschool for the child. These toys could be on loan while the child is learning a skill or could be used on a trial basis to help the family decide what toys or types of toys are most appropriate to help their child learn O&M skills and concepts. The provision of specialized O&M equipment such as adaptive mobility devices (AMDs) and long canes are also part of material support. On occasion, a family may lack basic material needs such as food and shelter that in turn prevent them from being able to meet their child's O&M needs. When this occurs, if the child is under 3 years old, the O&M instructor should refer the family to the child's service coordinator, or if the child is of preschool age, to the appropriate provider within the school system (for example, the school social worker).

Empowering Families

Through the provision of family-centered O&M intervention, children not only develop O&M-related skills and concepts but also their families become empowered to meet their children's needs and advocate for appropriate services and supports. Two overriding considerations should guide all interactions with families. One consideration is that all support—whether emotional, informational, or material—should be provided in such a way that the family will eventually require little or no assistance from formal support structures but will have the means to deal with future events (Turnbull & Turnbull, 2001). It is easy to fall into the trap of providing too much support for families and children rather than providing them with the skills necessary to be independent and self-sufficient. The other consideration is that the family has the right, and indeed the necessity, to chart its own course and make its own decisions. The Division for Early Childhood of the Council for Exceptional Children has time and again—in its mission statement, statement of best practices (Horn, Ostrosky, & Jones, 2004; Sandall, Hemmeter, Smith, & McLean, 2005), and organizational strategic planning—emphasized the overriding right of families to decide what assistance they wish to receive and how they wish to receive it. Professionals can and should make suggestions, provide rationale, and explain processes, but families will ultimately make the decisions.

Working with Teams

In addition to working closely with families, O&M instructors providing service to early childhood learners must collaborate with other professional team members (Anthony, Lowry, Brown, & Hatton, 2004; Blind Childrens Center, 1995; Fazzi & Petersmeyer, 2001; Pogrund & Fazzi, 2002). These teams will always include the families and the O&M instructors. Depending on the child's needs, the team may also include a teacher of students with visual impairments, an early childhood interventionist or preschool special-education teacher, an occupational therapist, a physical therapist, a service coordinator, a preschool teacher, and possibly others. Such a large and diverse team must work closely together in order to not overwhelm the child and family with service and information, as well as to insure that intervention is consistent across all factors to increase the probability that the child will be successful. The O&M specialist

can "role-release" many components (Hatton, McWilliam & Winton, 2003b; McEwen, 2000), such as teaching others how to facilitate items that will add to later O&M instruction (for example, provide opportunities to experience a variety of travel environments, even if they are not needed for current travel); develop strategies for adults to incorporate consistent terminology and routines; and monitor and provide feedback for the other adults as they provide intervention. The O&M specialist, however, needs to provide intervention directly with the child on a regular basis to insure that strategies being followed by the team incorporate ongoing evaluation of the child's progress. Four teaming roles have been identified as effective for professionals working with children with visual impairments: supportive, facilitative, informative, and prescriptive (Topor, Holbrook, & Koenig, 2000):

- O&M instructors should be *supportive* of all team members. They need to maintain contact with the family and professionals, follow up on suggestions and feedback that is given and received, provide specific examples rather than just theory, and keep notes on team suggestions. Consider an O&M instructor who is working with a child on using an AMD. Following a team-teaching lesson that included the physical therapist and the preschool special-education teacher, the O&M instructor contacts her colleagues in their preferred methods, with a phone call to the special-education teacher and an e-mail to the physical therapist. She asks specific, open-ended questions about the use of the device, concerns that may have arisen, and benefits they were seeing. On her next visit to the family, the O&M instructor also asks the family for feedback on the use of the device and shares what the other professionals were observing. In this case, the O&M instructor is providing an appropriate level of support to all team members related to an O&M-specific skill that the child is practicing throughout the day.

- The O&M instructor should also *facilitate* fellow team members in developing problem-solving skills and abilities in relation to O&M situations. To facilitate team problem solving, the O&M instructor must first be familiar with the family's and the professionals' concerns and priorities for the child as a whole and as they relate to orientation and mobility. The O&M instructor then must be willing to share expertise and knowledge with the team and be willing to learn from other disciplines while brainstorming solutions to problems. For example, a day-care provider is resistant to allowing a 4-year-old child with severely low vision to use a cane at the day care. The O&M instructor schedules a visit during nap time to talk with the teacher and discovers that the concern is *not* related to the child's use of the cane, but that the other children will get the cane and use it as a weapon in the classroom. The O&M instructor shares successful experiences of children in other preschools. The O&M instructor and the classroom teacher decide on a location to store the cane that is accessible to the child but not readily visible to all the children. They also plan to make a joint presentation on the cane to the class so that the children understand its purpose and that it is not a toy.

- O&M instructors should also *provide information* and support to the team to increase their skills and knowledge. O&M instructors can introduce the team members, including families, to adults with visual impairments. They should provide detailed information about early O&M development, maintain a library of resources to share with families and professionals, and invite team members to attend appropriate conferences and workshops. For example, an O&M instructor receives information about increasing physical activity and enhancing motor development in toddlers with visual impairments, and shares the conference flyer with colleagues. The early interventionist, the teacher of students with visual impairments, and the O&M instructor attend the conference as a team and return with numerous ideas on how they can jointly work on these skills.

- The *prescriptive* role of the O&M instructor is the most direct role through the prescription of specific actions that should be taken in response to a request for assistance. To be effective in the prescriptive role, the O&M instructor needs to make suggestions clear and succinct, follow up on progress, suggest changes as needed, and link suggested strategies to the child's overall educational plan. For example, a preschool special-education teacher reports that a child who is blind is unable to find the way to the water fountain, which is located 5 feet from the classroom door. The O&M instructor teaches this miniroute to the child, and the child is successful in walking the route with the O&M instructor. The O&M instructor invites the teacher to watch as the child walks the route during an O&M lesson. The O&M instructor writes down detailed information on the cues used so that the teacher can use the appropriate terminology (for example, "trail the wall") to prompt the child. The teacher and O&M instructor agree that the route will be practiced daily, and they will discuss the child's progress at the O&M lesson next week.

It is assumed that the strategies and activities suggested in this chapter can and will be incorporated by all members of the team, as applicable. However, the following sections are directed toward the O&M specialist, who will have primary responsibility for delivering O&M

intervention and making sure that all components of the intervention and members of the team are progressing appropriately.

INTERVENTIONAL STRATEGIES TO SUPPORT EARLY LEARNING

Assessment as a Critical but Specialized Process

As it is with learners of all ages, assessment is a critical and pivotal component of providing adequate O&M services. Assessment is equally and perhaps even more important in the early childhood years due to the absolute necessity of identifying where the child is in the developmental process to insure that instructional strategies assist global, integrative learning processes. However, the specialized characteristics of learners in the early childhood years will impact the form of assessment used with these children. The assessment process will be less structured and require much more subjective decisions than more typical assessment procedures with older learners. The actual format of the assessment will vary depending on the age of the child, but whatever the age, a major portion of assessment information will be obtained through unstructured, incidental observation of the child during naturally occurring activities. Young children do not understand the testing process, are not used to complying on command, are not capable of consistent response, or may comply on command even though it may not be indicative of their actual functioning. In addition, for most of the early childhood years, especially before the child has mastered verbal language, the child's responses are very individualized and therefore difficult to read, especially by individuals unfamiliar with the child. For these reasons and others, assessment procedures with early childhood learners will be handled differently than with older children and adults. See Table 7.2 for a

comparison of assessment procedures of adults and older children, infants and toddlers, and preschool children.

Flexible, Proactive Lesson Planning

Lesson plans with young learners need to be both proactive enough to assure that goals are being systematically addressed and flexible enough to allow for the child's inherent creativity and need to explore. Lesson planning will be a delicate balance between multiple factors, including: (1) addressing parent concerns or needs while also assuring that goals specific to typical O&M instruction are met, (2) preplanning specific objectives as well as having many activities in reserve that can be called upon when the child indicates an interest (or disinterest) in something, and (3) preplanning carefully sequenced teaching behaviors within each goal to assure that part-to-whole, integrated learning is occurring while also capitalizing on the motivation that comes from responding to unplanned child interest in other topics. Although it is important to be responsive to individual interests of young children, it is not sufficient to arrive at learning sessions and just "go with the flow." Objectives for the session, teaching strategies, and activities and materials should all be thought out in advance and specific teaching strategies described. However, planning and evaluation formats should also include a system for planning and recording activities that may have occurred by following the child's indication of interest. As the child gets older, sessions should be based increasingly on identified goals and objectives that support the typical O&M sequence.

Scheduling of Sessions

As dictated by "best practices," decisions regarding the amount, type, and duration of service should be made on an individual basis by team decision, and should be reflected in each learner's

TABLE 7.2

Comparison of Assessment of Different Age Groups

Assessment Component	Adults and Older Children	Preschoolers	Infants and Toddlers
Rapport building	Can often be accomplished by a short interview with the learner before the dynamic assessment begins.	Needs to be established in other contexts during multiple sessions before the dynamic assessment begins, one of the best being interacting with the child during play. The child is more likely to demonstrate typical functioning if the O&M specialist is familiar to the child and is familiar with the child's idiosyncratic behaviors since the child likely has not yet learned common acceptable ways of responding to requests.	Rapport is built with family members through structured and unstructured means. Family members may actually request skills from the child since the child is more likely to cooperate with someone familiar and may not develop rapport with a stranger in a reasonable amount of time
Includes information obtained from others	To direct or support more structured testing.	Parents and teachers can provide information about problem areas that can later be directly observed by the O&M specialist. Planned inclusion of the parent or teacher may be part of the assessment process. This may consist of asking the teacher to look for specific behaviors related to O&M on a daily basis or giving the teacher a list of behaviors one would like to see and asking her to include them in some way during playtime that is being observed by the O&M specialist.	As a primary source of information.
Observation of day-to-day functioning	To direct or support more structured testing, such as asking the learner to complete particular routes	Balance between observation of day-to-day functioning and more static, structured testing. Static testing might include testing of body	Reliance primarily on information obtained through observation of the child during day-to-day

(continued on next page)

TABLE 7.2 (Continued)

Assessment Component	Adults and Older Children	Preschoolers	Infants and Toddlers
	chosen to demonstrate specific skills.	image, motor skills, and concepts; however, the use of these skills should be verified through observation of day-to-day functioning.	activities. Inference may need to be made regarding O&M-related skills from observation of different yet related skill areas. For example: picking up a block using a pincer grasp during playtime may indicate the child's probable ability to isolate the index finger to place it along the cane in the normal grip.
Length of testing sessions	Typically an hour or more.	The probable necessity for multiple observations and assessment sessions to ensure the accuracy of the information obtained. Direct assessment sessions should be of short duration, sometimes no more than 5 to 10 minutes at a time.	Will be dictated by the family and the infant's daily routines.
Method for requesting information regarding skills	Verbal request to answer a question or demonstrate a behavior.	Child can be verbally requested to complete tasks, but the manner for doing this will include both playful methods and more directive methods.	Requests for behavior structured through playful activities rather than through direct request or observed "on the fly" during unstructured activities.
Content	Typical O&M sequence from indoor to downtown travel.	A similar range of behaviors may be observed at each of the sublevels within the preschool years, with more "typical" O&M behaviors included with children of increasing ages. See Appendix 7A for suggestions of skills to be included.	The majority of content will center around needs expressed by the family and may include items not typically related to O&M, such as the support system available to the

		family, or the need to identify sources of appropriate toys to facilitate sensory awareness. Observational assessment of infants may include behaviors such as object permanence, cause and effect, bringing hands to midline, strength of attachment to caregivers, and clarity of nonverbal communications.
Tools and checklists	Mostly instructor-made.	Hill Performance Test of Selected Concepts,[a] Cratty Body Image of Blind Children,[b] Teaching Age-Appropriate Purposeful Skills[c]	(1) Routine-based assessment, where the O&M specialist asks parents to describe a day's activities and information is gathered about O&M-related skills and need areas.[d] (2) Environmental assessment to gather information on factors about the environment that enhance or limit safety and facilitation of O&M development.[d]

[a] Cratty, B. J., & Sams, T. A. (1968). *The body image of blind children*. New York: American Foundation for the Blind.

[b] Hill, E. W. (Ed.). (1981). The Hill performance test of selected positional concepts. Chicago: Stoetling Co.

[c] Pogrund, R., Healy, G., Jones, K., Levack, N., Martin-Curry, F., Martinez, C., et al. (1993). *TAPS—Teaching age-appropriate purposeful skills: An orientation and mobility curriculum for students with visual impairments*. Austin: Texas School for the Blind and Visually Impaired.

[d] Anthony, T., Lowry, S., Brown, C., & Hatton, D. (Eds.). (2004). *Developmentally appropriate orientation and mobility*. Chapel Hill: FPG Child Development Institute, University of North Carolina at Chapel Hill.

IFSP or IEP. There is great variation in the way services to young learners are delivered throughout the United States, and often the amount of interventional time provided to these children and families is not based on child need but rather on local regulations. O&M specialists need to become proactive to assure that adequate time is available for O&M intervention, *by an O&M specialist*, as needed to assure that the child progresses adequately during this very important, pivotal stage of life. The more consistent the scheduling and model of intervention, the more likely the child will internalize the skills being practiced, and the more likely he or she will progress normally with independent, "typical" O&M instruction. Though skills can be facilitated and practiced through effective collaboration of instructional assistants, teachers, mobility assistants, and family members (see the section on Inclusion of Significant Others in O&M Development and Intervention), O&M specialists need to see the young child at least as regularly as they would an older learner. Ideally, intervention should be even more frequent (especially after infancy) given the critical role that developmental learning plays in later success. It is important that the O&M specialist sees the child frequently enough to observe and impact the rapid progress that can occur in the developmental stage. Hour-long sessions every other week with parents when the child is an infant might transition to 20- to 30-minute sessions three to four times a week after the child demonstrates independent mobility.

Support Learning through Playful Activities

Sessions with young learners will often look more like play than work. Play is the typical learning medium for learners in the early childhood years and therefore should be encouraged (Blind Childrens Center, 1995; Pogrund & Fazzi, 2002). Many early childhood educators have discussed ways to assess and allow learning to occur through actual self-initiated play (Linder, 1990, 1993; Musslewhite, 1986; Parsons, 1986; Tait, 1972), and this is one medium that should be explored by classroom teachers and O&M specialists. In addition, learning can be structured through *playful* activities such as games and songs. With creativity, virtually all O&M concepts can be packaged into playful form. Examples of games that have been devised to facilitate orientation and mobility can be found in *Simon Says Is Not the Only Game* (Leary & von Schneden, 1982), *Imagining the Possibilities* (Fazzi & Petersmeyer, 2001), and *TAPS—Teaching Age-Appropriate Purposeful Skills: An Orientation and Mobility Curriculum for Students with Visual Impairments* (Pogrund et al., 2003). For young children, positive reinforcement can often be provided through the natural reinforcement of an activity that is fun or playful. Therefore, playful activities increase the probability that learning will occur while also decreasing negative or inappropriate behaviors. As with other instructional strategies, the use of playful activities will need to be phased into more typical instructional routines as the child ages. If the child has received regular intervention, by 4 to 5 years of age, playful activities can be used only as reinforcement for completion of more systematic, didactic instruction.

Following the Child's Lead

All components of intervention need to be flexible to take advantage of "teachable moments" and to follow the child's lead (MacDonald & Gillette, 1984; Monighan-Nourot, Scales, VanHoorn, & Almay, 1987). While an overall plan of intervention is needed, typical learning in the early childhood years occurs incidentally and the real value of learning at this stage seems to come from the opportunity for the child to discover and "create" knowledge independently. To simulate these types of situations as closely as possi-

TABLE 7.3

Possible Items to Include in the O&M "Bag of Tricks"

Item	Potential Use
Index card sets with one goal, game, or activity per card	• Rotating "lesson planning" and data-collection system, that is, each day's lessons can be planned by selecting those objectives included in the day's lesson and notes taken on the child's success
Kitchen timer with winding knob	• Sound source to find or follow
	• Reinforcer for child to make the timer "ding" when he or she reaches the objective
Large, uncluttered pictures of animals	• Stimuli for various visual training activities
	• Prompts for stimulating gross motor movements, for example, "Hop to the picture of the bunny"
Brightly colored stuffed animal	• Stimulus for various visual training activities
	• Reinforcer—waiting at the objective to receive a hug

ble for early childhood learners with visual impairments, it is important to allow them to direct their own learning as much as possible. However, because vision often limits the ability of children with visual impairments to learn incidentally, the role of the O&M specialist will be to watch very carefully for signs that the child is interested (or not) in a topic and be ready to supply just enough support, modeling, and content information to facilitate learning. The proverbial "bag of tricks," including teaching ideas and materials to facilitate learning, is needed when teaching orientation and mobility to early childhood learners (Table 7.3).

This is not to say, however, that O&M development will be unplanned or random, or that the O&M specialist will never take total control of the learning situation. Especially as the child gets older and reaches the age to enter more typical learning situations, the O&M specialist will need to carefully balance following the child's lead with the attainment of developmentally selected objectives. With practice and genuine rapport between the teacher and learner, the two methods usually can fit together seamlessly.

Provide Opportunities for Choice

Providing the child with as many opportunities for choice as possible is one very important strategy that can be used to maintain learning that is based on the child's need to create his or her own learning process, as well as to address the need for more systematic, planned intervention to help alleviate the impact of visual impairment (Blind Childrens Center, 1995; Chen, 1999; Smith & Levack, 1996). With creativity by the O&M specialist and other adults, choices can be built into most components of a lesson that will allow the child to feel in control of the learning process, allow for learning sessions to be based on the child's interests, and meet the child's learning objectives through preplanning by the adult. Opportunities for choice should not be randomly offered but should be part of the overall sequenced instructional package. For most children, this process should also include sequenced

SIDEBAR 7.1

Incorporating Choice into Learning Sessions

The following are some examples of ways that choice can be incorporated into learning sessions:

- Plan four activities for the session, but allow the child to choose the order in which they are completed.

- Reduce potential behavior problems by giving the child a choice between the behavior or activity favored by the teacher and a choice that the teacher knows the child will not want to engage in.

- Allow the child to choose the song he wants to sing while he is practicing motor activities.

- Initially allow the child to choose the route he wants to practice. Then, after instruction in making choices, ask the child to choose between two routes—one that is efficient and will get him to the objective easily and one that may be more familiar but is complicated and contains more obstacles.

- Ask the child which toy he wants to put in his pocket while practicing a route (to be taken out only upon successful completion).

- Do not ask a child if he "wants" to do something unless the child truly has the choice to say "no." Once a choice is given, always comply with the choice made.

opportunities regarding how to make choices, eventually based not only on wants and desires but also on other factors, such as the consequences of each choice. Providing opportunities for choice also reinforces the child's movement toward more independent functioning, which is one of the goals of O&M instruction. See Sidebar 7.1 for examples of ways that choice can be incorporated into learning sessions.

Create Routines to Increase Participation and Understanding

Incorporating activities that occur as a routine will allow the child to understand how the parts of an activity fit into the whole process and increase the probability that the child will engage in appropriate behavior (Blind Childrens Center, 1995; Chen, 1999; Fazzi & Petersmeyer, 2001; Smith & Levak, 1996). A routine is an activity that is carried out in the same way during each instance of its occurrence and has a clear beginning, middle, and end. For example, an

instructor and other adults may implement a "cruising" routine with a young child (practicing early walking behaviors by providing a secure, static object to move along). The O&M specialist needs to say the same phrase whenever the child is asked to cruise; provide some object, physical gesture, or sound clue to help the child understand that the cruising routine is beginning; facilitate the child through the motions in the same way each time and use the same general wording; and then indicate that the cruising routine is finished by using a consistent phrase and object, gesture, or sound clue. As with most learning objectives, playful components can be added, for example, using the child's favorite squeaky toy ("Hector") and calling the routine the "Get Hector Game." Hector could squeak just before the routine begins, be moved just outside the child's reach to motivate each step, and then be held and squeaked repeatedly by the child once the cruising has been completed. If all adults complete the routine in the same way each time cruising is the objective, the child will learn to anticipate what is being asked and be more likely to engage in cruising behavior. In addition, the child will learn that the cruising movement is a behavior that allows him to get from a place without a toy to a place with a toy.

Inclusion of Teaching Components

Because the experience children have during O&M lessons is often the very first time they have come into contact with a particular idea or concept, it is crucial that lessons include a teaching component. The teaching component will introduce the child to the concept and allow him to completely explore it before asking him to do anything. This will require breaking all skills down to their most basic level and providing teaching at this level. For example, before being taught how to open or close doors or trail across openings, it is necessary for the child to have many experiences with doors, the components of a door, different types of doors and their movements, and so forth. In addition, the concept of "doors" needs to be broken down to the point where the door and the way it feels is

separated from the door*way* and the way it feels (that is, the way the "door" will feel when it is open when the child is trailing). The two entities will need to be learned separately and their relationship examined.

Use of Adult Attention and Behavior Strategies to Assist Motivation

Because learning and motivation often do not come from the completion of a route or objective as they do for older learners, motivation will often need to come from the attention and interaction with the adult, and from behavioral strategies used to facilitate learning. O&M specialists working with young children need to be accomplished at incorporating strategies such as prompting, reinforcement, fading, and chaining into learning sessions with young children, especially those of an age to benefit from structured intervention. See Volume 1, Chapter 7, by Jacobson and Bradley for information on these techniques. Sidebar 7.2 provides an example of the use of prompting to facilitate the initial learning of independent walking behavior.

SIDEBAR 7.2

Using Prompting and Fading to Facilitate Independent Walking

The following procedures show the use of prompting to facilitate the initial learning of independent walking behavior:

- Pattern the child through full physical assistance by holding both of the child's hands and walking quickly.

- Have the child trail the wall with one hand while the other is held by an adult.

- Have the child trail the wall and an adult occasionally touch the child's free

hand to give a feeling of pulling away (forward).

- Have the child occasionally touch the wall.

- Have the child walk down the middle of the hall with an adult who gives an occasional physical touch.

- Have the child walk down the hall with an adult providing continual verbal reminders to walk quickly.

- Have the child walk along the hall with an adult giving an occasional verbal reminder.

Use Motivating Materials

The number and variety of materials used to facilitate O&M development in the early childhood years are limited only by the creativity of the instructor and the budget available. The wide range of materials and equipment used to support intervention can be broken down into two main categories: materials that enhance learning activities and devices that enhance sensory awareness and movement (see the sections on Devices That Enhance Sensory Awareness and Movement, and Instruction in Device Use).

It is very important that materials used with young children should be motivating to the child and not be chosen solely by the teaching characteristics they offer. Especially during infancy and toddlerhood, materials that the child is familiar with and has already shown a preference for should be incorporated into learning sessions as much as possible. Sometimes even being allowed to carry a favorite toy or other material without it being the focus of the lesson can increase the comfort level of the child, as well as the probability that he or she will engage in the target activity. Familiar materials also can be paired with unfamiliar items to help the child transition to use of the new item. Another way to make materials motivating to children is to choose items with visual, auditory, or tactual enhancements that the child has shown a preference for. Care should be given, however, to insure that the enhancements do not become the child's sole focus and limit his ability to concentrate on the objectives for using the material. As with all learning components, use of preferred

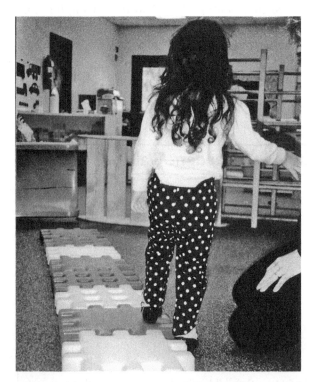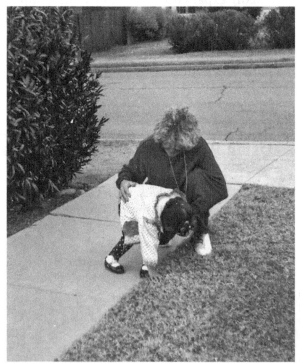

Annette C. Skellenger

Playing on these waffle blocks (left) can help a young child learn such O&M concepts as "along," "across," "side," and "shoreline." These concepts can then be transferred to learning about environments such as the sidewalk (right).

and enhanced materials should be systematically faded so the child learns to accept materials that are not of his own choice.

Materials That Enhance Learning Activities

Virtually every activity can be made more motivating and enjoyable through the use of interesting, playful materials. There are nearly endless numbers of toys and songs that can be adapted or used directly to teach O&M development.

A large set of 1-foot-square waffle blocks can be fit together to make a long "track." The child can practice balance while walking "along" the track, and then pretend to be a car and go "across" the tracks by walking from one "side" to the other. This same set can be used to explore and learn the meaning of "shoreline," and all of these concepts can later be transferred to learning about hallways, sidewalks, and streets.

A ticking kitchen timer can act both as a sound stimulus to be followed and a self-reinforcer as the child practices wrist movements to turn the knob to make the timer ring after reaching the end of the route. A feather duster can be used to practice flexion and extension of the wrist—that will be used for later cane use—as the child pretends to "dust off" the instructor or himself.

Even early mapping skills can be practiced through the use of motivating map boards made of magnets or Velcro and felt. In addition to practicing concepts such as "across" and "parallel," the use of these boards also can assist with other development skills. For example, O&M instructors can use the board to facilitate the tracking skills needed for mapping and braille reading, as well as to require the use of a fine pincer grasp (and isolation of the index finger) to remove the magnet or Velcro piece from the board. Introduced correctly, mapping boards can allow the child to learn to read maps and also make his own map of a route or simple area.

The variety of materials for use in orientation and mobility is nearly endless. Virtually any

activity can be made more fun—and therefore increase possible learning—through the imaginative selection of materials.

Devices That Enhance Sensory Awareness and Movement

Much of the early discussion related to O&M instruction with very young children focused on questions regarding whether long-cane instruction should be started in the early years. Strong arguments have been made both against (Ferrell, 1979) and for (Dykes, 1992; Pogrund, Fazzi, & Schreier, 1993; Pogrund & Rosen, 1989) long-cane instruction with young children. Current literature and practical suggestion seem to focus more on the identification of the range of devices that might benefit children's early exploration and movement. Questions regarding the benefits and limitations of specific devices and the timing of introducing a device have replaced the debate on whether or not devices should be used. A nearly endless variety of devices have the potential to enhance sensory awareness and movement. O&M specialists should seek out potential devices to facilitate intervention and carefully consider both the positive and negative impact on the child's overall development from use of the device (Anthony, Lowry, Brown, & Hatton, 2004; Clarke, 1988; Pogrund & Rosen, 1989). The range of potential devices includes, but is not limited to:

- low vision devices to allow the child to become familiar with the devices and their capabilities and to prepare for later systematic instruction in their use (Corn et al., 2003)

- long-handled wooden spoons to allow infants to extend their reach

- items such as toy shopping carts and hula hoops for use as "bumpers" (Clarke, 1988)

- swimming pool "noodles" to reach out from static or dynamic positions to locate objects

- devices constructed from PVC in a variety of forms (Foy, Kirchner, & Waple, 1991; Foy, Von Scheden, & Waiculonis, 1992; LaPrelle, 2002)

- long canes, including those with adaptations (Dykes, 1992; Kronick, 1987; Skellenger & Hill, 1991; see also Smith and Penrod, Volume 1, Chapter 8, and Rosen, Chapter 5 in this volume)

Clarke (1988) has offered many suggestions regarding the dimensions to be considered regarding the selection of devices, and other authors have discussed both the advantages and disadvantages of miscellaneous devices (Anthony, 1993; Anthony, Bleier, Fazzi, Kish, & Pogrund, 2002; Clarke, Sainato, & Ward, 1994).

Use Consistent, Specific Terminology

Because children with visual impairments will have very limited information available to them to sort out how the world is organized, it is critical, especially in the early childhood years, to be very consistent in applying labels to actions and items. When the term *door* is used, vision allows us to understand the difference between the door, the doorjamb, and the open doorway, even though each of these varies widely with respect to the sensory characteristics that a child with visual impairments will experience when trying to locate them or deal with them in a functional manner. For example if a child is asked to find the third door, yet two of the doors are open (and hence feel very different from the hard plane he usually associates with a door), he may travel past the openings and continue to try to find what he has been taught is a door. The child's behavior may be mistaken for misunderstanding or noncompliance, when it is actually a result of the instructor not using consistent, specific terminology.

CURRICULUM CONTENT

Content Areas to Address in Early Childhood

The majority of learning that occurs in the first five to six years of life focuses on experimentation in the use of the senses and the motoric system. The child learns about the information that he receives through the sensory systems and learns motoric patterns to act on this information. The child then begins to learn to organize information into categories. For this reason, much of the content of O&M learning sessions with very young children involves the areas of sensory awareness, body image, gross and fine motor activities, and conceptual awareness (Anthony, Lowry, Brown, & Hatton, 2004; Pogrund & Fazzi, 2002). In addition, however, the child in this phase is also laying the groundwork for eventual learning in all areas of orientation and mobility. While the majority of the content provided in this chapter focuses on the skill areas listed previously, the content of O&M development should include in some manner activities that focus on all areas of typical O&M instruction (See Appendix 7A).

Sensory Awareness

Before a child can make use of sensory information to assist travel, he needs to (1) become aware that the sensory information exists, (2) tolerate it, (3) discriminate it from other sensory information, (4) label it, and (5) understand its relationship to the object it is associated with. The child should be provided systematic experiences with visual, tactile, auditory, kinesthetic, and olfactory information that will later be utilized during independent travel. See Sidebar 7.3 for an example of a possible instructional sequence using auditory skills.

SIDEBAR 7.3

Hierarchy of Auditory Skills

Following is a possible instructional sequence using auditory skills:

- *Stimulate*—Demonstrates awareness by reacting to a wide variety of sounds

- *Tolerate*—Builds tolerance to variety and extremes of sounds

- *Discriminate*—Learns to distinguish one sound from another

- *Label/Identify*—Learns what name is given to a sound

- *Understand*—Learns about the object that is associated with the sound and understands that the sound represents the object

- *Reach for Sound*—Learns to reach for sound in all directions, a critical skill to motivate independent movement

- *Localize Sound*—Moves to position self in a variety of relationships to sound, moves to a static and then dynamic sound source

- *Follow Moving Sound Source*—Moves with whole body first and later by pointing

- *Identify Pattern of Moving Sound*

- *Advanced Auditory Skills to Assist Travel*—Associates sound with landmarks, identifies openings in parallel surfaces, detects objects and sound shadows, lines parallel or perpendicular to traffic, identifies safe crossing time, responds to danger signals

Body Image

It is critical that an early childhood learner develop a clear understanding of his or her body and its movements, on which to base future learning. With absent or limited vision, the child learns a body image or concept primarily through the kinesthetic (movement) sense. Cratty's phases of the development of body image can be used as an example on which body image instruction may be based (Cratty & Sams, 1968):

- *Phase 1*: body planes, parts, and movements (developed at the mental age [MA] of 2 to 5 years in children without disabilities)

- *Phase 2*: right–left discrimination (MA 5 to 7 years); this includes planes, or sides of objects in same plane as the child

- *Phase 3*: complex judgments of the body and body–object relationships (MA 6 to 8 years)

- *Phase 4*: identification of parts and relationships through another person's reference system (MA 8 to 9 years)

Motor Development, Gait, and Posture (Kinesthetic Development)

In addition to the usual benefits of health and independence of movement, for children with visual impairments, movement provides much of the information about the characteristics of the environment that is usually provided through vision. For the child with impaired vision, movement gives meaning to words and provides information regarding size, location, texture, and other qualities of objects.

Early childhood learners will benefit from engagement in virtually any and all functional motor activities. Among the types of skills to be included are those focusing on

1. movement across the midline (reaching with the right hand for an object on the left);

2. trunk rotation and segmentation ("log rolling" so that the hips roll before the shoulders);

3. isolated movement of small body parts (picking up objects with the forefinger and thumb rather than the whole palm);

4. upper body strength (pushing or pulling heavy objects);

5. full extension of joints (holding arms out to the side with elbows straight rather than bent slightly);

6. increasing stamina.

In addition to the selection of activities from the wide variety of resources pertaining to physical education and adapted physical education, Brown and Bour (1986) and Pogrund, Fazzi, and Schreier (1993) suggest activities specifically selected for children with visual impairments.

Concept Development

Concepts are mental representations, images, or ideas of what something should be (Hill & Blasch, 1980), a synthesis of sense impressions and the integration of the diverse data on a phenomenon in an orderly way. Concepts are formed by classifying or grouping objects or events with similar properties. The ability to perceive and discriminate similarities, therefore, is fundamental for concept development.

Because vision, a major source of sensory information, is limited or absent for children with visual impairments, concept formation must often be taught more directly than through the more incidental means available to children without disabilities. For the individual with a visual impairment, concept development is a continual, conscious process that requires the individual to learn to relate to objects on many different levels. For example, it is not enough for the child with

visual impairments to learn to identify the parts of a car by touch. She also must come to understand the sound a car makes as it passes on her parallel side, the way it feels when she rides inside it, and the multitude of paths a car can take in relation to the path of a pedestrian (Baird & Goldie, 1979). The individual with limitations in concept development also is likely to experience limitations in the ability to function in relation to that concept.

Because the development of adequate concepts is so fundamental to all aspects of later learning, this topic is explored in depth in the following sections.

Visual Functioning

Because vision is a learned activity (Erin, Fazzi, Gordon, Isenberg, & Paysse, 2002), it is possible that early childhood learners will benefit from intervention to help them learn to use their remaining vision more efficiently (Anthony, Lowry, Brown, & Hatton, 2004; Dote-Kwan, 1995; Harrell & Akeson, 1987. In addition to the usual strategies to facilitate vision use, such as environmental adaptations to increase contrast and providing adequate lighting, intervention with early childhood learners may include activities that have practicing vision use as their major goal. Games can be played, such as seeing who can collect the most apple shapes that have been placed along a route, or visually following lines along a chalkboard to find a treat that has been placed at the end.

Formalized Mobility Techniques

O&M development with preschool learners should include experience and practice in formal mobility techniques, such as human guide and self-protective techniques (Anthony, Bleier, Fazzi, Kish, & Pogrund, 2002; Anthony, Lowry, Brown, & Hatton, 2004; Fazzi, 1998; Hill, Rosen, Correa, & Langley, 1984). Because many very young children do not demonstrate the motor

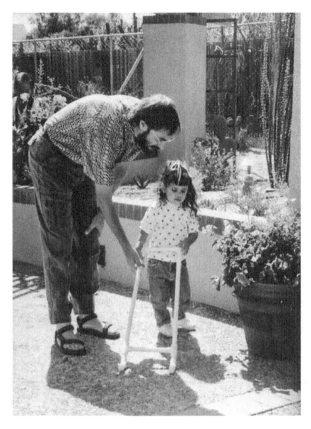 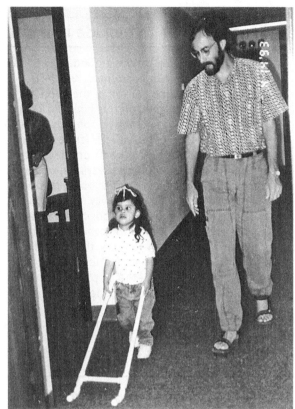

Annette C. Skellenger

Preschool learners can use adaptive mobility devices to facilitate day-to-day, functional movement in a variety of travel environments and situations, including the home.

control necessary to replicate exact technique, activities in this area may fit into "readiness" activities, or may involve adaptation of the techniques. Readiness activities might include playing statues, which will help the child learn muscle control to later hold her arm in a protective position. Adaptations may include teaching the child to grasp the guide's index and forefinger rather than the wrist or elbow (Anthony, 1993).

Instruction in Device Use

Early childhood learners often do not have the gross motor control to adequately demonstrate and maintain the protective techniques (lower hand and forearm, upper hand and forearm) that are typically taught to older learners. These children, however, can greatly benefit from feelings of protection, which will most likely increase their willingness to move about. Devices that facilitate independent mobility will fill a number of roles with preschool learners. For some children, primarily those with severe, multiple impairments, the AMD will be the sole mobility tool when they appear unable to learn the skills for long-cane use. For other children, the device will help increase the confidence to facilitate movement—possibly providing the safety and motivation to initiate independent movement—until they demonstrate higher developmental skills that indicate readiness to

---

TABLE 7.4

Possible Skills to Include in Instruction with Adaptive Canes

- Maintain cane tip on the ground.
- Maintain both hands on the cane.
- Maintain the cane in front of the body.
- When the cane goes off the sidewalk, return cane to sidewalk before foot goes off the sidewalk.
- When contacting persons or objects: (a) stop and pull the cane toward the body, (b) locate a clear area to the right or left, (c) go around object.
- Trail wall or edge of sidewalk on the right with the tip of the cane.
- When going through doorways: (a) make contact with the door, (b) walk up to the door while maintaining cane in front of body, (c) open door, (d) put cane through the doorway, and then (e) walk through the doorway, closing the door behind.
- When traveling up stairs, position the cane parallel to the body and lift it up about 1 inch from the ground. The tip of the cane should touch each step as the student moves forward.
- When traveling down stairs, the cane should be held at a 45-degree angle from the body with the tip on the lower stair. The motion of the student's body should keep the cane moving.
- When the bottom of the steps is reached, the cane tip will contact the floor first.
- When reaching the destination, park cane in designated area.
- When using a sighted guide, the child should carry the cane, resting the top parallel bar on his or her shoulder with the cane (from top to bottom) parallel with the body. One hand should hold onto the cane.

Source: Eileen Sifferman

---

begin long-cane instruction. For the majority of preschool learners, however, instruction may best include simultaneous instruction and the use of *both* an AMD and the long cane. Because the child is at such a young age, it may be difficult to determine whether he or she will have the ability to eventually use a long cane. For this reason, it may be best to include opportunities to use both types of devices. The child may use an AMD to facilitate day-to-day, functional movement, such as movement with his class between the classroom and the lunchroom, or in the backyard at home. At the same time, more formal O&M lessons may focus on beginning instruction in long-cane use and occur under close supervision (see Table 7.4).

Suggestions regarding the construction of and instruction in the use of AMDs can be found in Clarke (1988), Foy, Kirchener, and Waple (1991), Foy, Von Scheden, and Waiculonis (1992),

LaPrelle (1996), and Pogrund, Fazzi, & Schreier (1993). However, research is needed regarding the process of instruction to be followed once a device has been selected, and all learning sessions that incorporate the use of a device need to be carefully monitored and evaluated to assure that positive benefit is occurring.

Concept Development

Assessment

One of the first steps in assisting children who are visually impaired with concept development is to assess the concepts they possess. A number of assessment tools are available, including: *The Body Image of Blind Children* (Cratty & Sams, 1968); *Stanford Multi-Modality Imagery Test* (Dauterman, 1972); the Kephart Scale, in *A Journey into the World of the Blind Child* (Kephart, Kephart, & Schwarz, 1974); and *The Hill Performance Test of*

Selected Positional Concepts (Hill, 1981). It is important during any assessment of concept understanding that differentiation be made between the ability to verbally describe the concept and a concrete, functional understanding of the concept. Children with visual impairments often demonstrate inadequate understanding of the world around them and use verbalisms (when the child uses the word but does not understand the concept) rather than actual understanding. Verbalisms may be the result of inaccurate or vague concepts resulting from insufficient sensory experience (Harley, 1963). It is important, therefore, to assess not only verbal understanding of a concept but also to require a physical demonstration of functional understanding of the concept.

Sensory Information

The development of understanding a concept begins with the reception of sensory information about the entity. Instruction to facilitate concept development will begin with a multitude of sensory experiences. The type and amount of sensory experience appears to be crucial to the adequacy and variety of concepts formed by an individual, especially for children with visual impairments. Even before the child is capable of cognitively synthesizing information into an organized concept, he should be exposed to as large a variety of sensory experiences as possible. This may include taking the infant to the grocery store, helping him hold and haptically explore a wide variety of items, riding on a city bus, crawling outside on a variety of surfaces with the smell of flowers around him, and accompanying the family to a symphonic concert.

Exploration of an Entity

A further step in the development of concepts is the systematic exploration of an entity. Three premises appear to be imperative for adequate concept development at this level. The first is

that concrete *experience* with the concept appears crucial (Baird & Goldie, 1979; Fazzi & Klein, 2002; Fazzi & Petersmeyer, 2001; Hatton, Anthony, Lowry, & Brown, 2004). Rather than only reading about bus travel or even passively riding a bus with an adult, the preschool learner should be allowed to tactilely and physically explore the layout of the bus, carry the money for the fare, and be assisted in depositing the fare in the box. The second premise for complete concept development is that the breadth of experience appears to be more important than quantity (Baird & Goldie, 1979). For example, in addition to experiencing bus travel, the process should be verbally described to the child while doing it, bus riding should be compared (physically experienced) with riding in a car, and the sound of buses should be compared to other sounds while standing at an intersection. The third premise involves the necessity for the individual to internalize the concept by being able to apply a label to it. This will be necessary to facilitate generalization. In addition to these premises, it is important that the length of exposure to the concept is long enough to allow the child to fully differentiate it from other concepts.

Concepts for Travel

The list of concepts that a child will need to assist travel is nearly endless (see Hill & Blasch, 1980, for one listing). They can be roughly grouped, however, into a number of subgroups that include the following:

- *spatial and positional concepts*, such as "in front," "along," "next," and "end"
- *environmental concepts*, such as "block," "corner," "camber," and "shoreline"
- *concepts relating to the nature of objects*, such as "objects remain in the same place unless moved by someone" and "objects that move (such as cars) will change their relative location to you even if you are standing still"

- *concepts that facilitate orientation*, such as numbering systems and cardinal directions

- *concepts that facilitate mobility*, such as time and distance

The development of functional concepts to assist travel is a crucial component of instruction with preschool learners. The attainment of concrete, functional concepts will require nearly endless hours of systematic involvement. The responsibility for this involvement needs to be shared by all the significant individuals in a preschool learner's life. Concept development will be most complete if adults team together to provide as wide a variety of experiences in as systematic a process as possible.

CURRICULUM AND INSTRUCTIONAL STRATEGIES FOR DIFFERENT DEVELOPMENTAL LEVELS

The curriculum and instructional strategies used with children in the early childhood years will vary considerably between birth and 8 years of age. When working with very young children with visual impairments, it is important to plan interventions based on the child's development rather than age. Given the range of typical development and the possibility of additional disabilities, children of the same age and with the same visual condition often function at very different levels. Specific suggestions regarding intervention can be broken into three subgroups of this population: (1) children not yet walking, for whom sensory stimulation and awareness are an overriding goal, (2) children who are crawling and emerging walking, whose goals center around exploring the environment, and (3) children who are walking, who are practicing "O&M readiness," and transitioning to beginning refinement of skills. Given the introductory nature of this chapter, it is impossible to discuss the

needs of children at each level in depth. To provide a basic picture of specific strategies, we have provided a sampling of activities for sensory development, motor development, body image, device use, and concept development for each development level. Vignettes illustrating each level are provided in Sidebars 7.4, 7.5, and 7.6. As with all suggestions regarding children, these subgroups and the assignment of strategies are subjective, and decisions about using any of the suggestions with a particular child need to be based on the overall developmental picture of the child, not on any single factor. The overall format of O&M development will be jointly decided by the family and significant professionals working with each child and may vary greatly between children. The O&M specialist and the parents will be involved in these activities or in providing the required environments, as listed in the following sections.

Children Who Are Nonambulatory

Sensory Development

The awareness of sensory information does not always develop incidentally. The following activities can help the child focus on the information available to them in addition to or in place of vision.

- Items with various sensory qualities should be included in locations where the child typically spends time. For example, the child may be placed on a quilt made of squares of fabrics that have different textures, are filled with pleasant scents, or have squeaky toys in them. A bulletin board can be placed by the child's crib, where increasingly complex line drawings are posted to capture the child's residual vision (Harrell & Akeson, 1987).

- The child should be provided opportunities to meaningfully play with toys and objects that have various textures in addition to the typical infant toys, which tend to be primarily of plastic.

- Plan weekly outings that will increase the child's exposure to a variety of sensory experiences, such as taking the child to a shoe repair shop to experience the leather smell, to the transportation center to hear the buses and trains arrive, or to the downtown square to hear the sounds and to crawl or lay in the grass, cement, or mulch areas.

Motor Development

Giving young children opportunities such as the following to explore and control their motor abilities will provide an important building block to support efficient locomotion later for skills such as limiting veers while crossing streets.

- Play "horsey" games to give the child an opportunity to practice trunk control.
- Facilitate reaching for sound by using a partial physical prompt at the child's elbow.
- Encourage the child to rotate his trunk and hips separately when rolling over.
- Place the child over a bolster in a crawling position to promote weight-bearing on his hands and knees.
- Offer toys and other materials in a position that requires the child to cross a midline to retrieve the toy.

Body Image

Young children can be assisted to learn about their body parts and functions through activities such as the following.

- Name body parts and provide a consistent tactual prompt (such as tapping the part three times) when doing daily activities (for example, during bath and dressing). Play games and sing songs about body parts.

- Provide stimulation for various body parts through tickling, touching, and massaging.
- Play games taking turns, where the adult models describe movements that various body parts can do and the child is assisted to mimic the movement. Once the child has been introduced to a variety of movements, this can be accompanied with a song of "this is the way we move our (name of body part)."

Device Use

Long before the child is given a long cane or other mobility device, activities such as the following should be provided.

- Help the child to try to locate items outside her reach, then give her a long-handled spoon and show her how she can find the item using the spoon. Avoid hand-over-hand manipulation, which can discourage active learning, and facilitate by supporting the movement from the elbow or some other less-intrusive point.
- Use a stick to hit items of different materials and talk about the different sounds; then have the child look at the material with her hands.

Concepts and Orientation

Activities such as the following will provide young children with basic understanding of concepts on which more advanced concepts will be built.

- Help the child understand the "whole" concept of items by taking him to items that make sounds and allowing him to feel, smell, and hear the item while he is being told what the item is. Help the child understand *all* of the characteristics that make up the item.
- Choose three or four points in the house that can be labeled in reference to the child's compass orientation (that is, the front door is the north door, the basement steps are the west

steps) and use compass terms as much as reasonable when talking about where the child is going.

- Provide the child with opportunities to learn about his body and the environment through trial and error (for example, finding a dropped toy that is close to his body).

Children Who Are Crawling and Beginning to Walk

Sensory Development

As children begin moving on their own, activities to develop their sensory abilities will begin to incorporate the use of other domain areas such as purposeful motor use and categorization skills as shown below.

- Provide sensory-stimulating toys located in consistent places that the child can independently reach.

- Help the child learn about the variety of sensory qualities of objects and help him associate the names of these qualities (hard, bumpy, loud, and so forth). Once these are established, help the child learn how to choose objects of the same quality out of a variety of objects. Focus on providing experiences with items that might later facilitate travel, such as comparing the qualities of grass and cement areas.

Motor Development

Since vision is not available to motivate independent movement, the child should be assisted to engage in a wide variety of activities to show her ways to move through space.

- Encourage natural movements (for example, twisting to the side to move into crawling and pulling up to stand from a kneeling position) through modeling and physical assistance.

SIDEBAR 7.4

Awareness

In December, an orientation and mobility (O&M) instructor made an initial visit to a 2-month-old boy who was born without eyes and who had failed his infant hearing screening in one ear. When the instructor arrived, she noticed that the child was dressed warmly from his neck to his feet and was wearing thin mittens on his hands. After establishing a rapport with the family, the O&M instructor complimented the mother on dressing her child warmly in the cold weather and asked why the baby was also wearing mittens inside. The mother explained that his fingernails were long and he had scratched his face. When the mother cut his nails, she had cut too closely, causing her son to bleed a little and cry. She

was too distraught to try to finish cutting his nails and asked if the O&M instructor could assist her. Together, they removed the mittens and the O&M instructor cut two of the baby's nails; the mother then felt confident enough to finish.

The O&M instructor explained that since the baby was not receiving any information from his eyes and had limited hearing, his hands were going to be very important in learning about the world. The mother and instructor discussed how the child needed to explore with his hands to become aware that a world existed outside his own body. Following the discussion, the mittens were never seen again unless the child was outside on a cold day.

Help the child become aware of a variety of ways to move from place to place (for instance, "commando" crawling, scooting on bottom, and pulling self forward while prone with arms only).

- Encourage cruising (walking along furniture and walls while using them for support) as a typical initial stage of walking and as a precursor for trailing. Provide motivation by playing a game of catch by moving a favorite toy just outside the child's reach (assuming object permanence has been established).

- Play games that challenge the child's balance with her established trunk control, such as putting the child on an adult's shoulders and having her remain upright while the adult moves in a variety of patterns and speeds, or putting the child on a therapy/exercise ball and rotate the ball in a variety of planes while the child attempts to remain upright.

Body Image

As the child initiates independent movement activities, focusing on identifying and labeling body parts and functions will help him learn how his body facilitates movement.

- Play games where the child touches a named body part (Simon Says) or touches the body part when a function is named (that is, touches his leg when asked, "What do we kick with?").

- Label actions and locations as right or left (for example, "I'm putting your left arm in your jacket" or "the refrigerator is to the right of the sink), even though the child does not yet understand these terms.

- Play games that show the child the similarities and differences between his body parts and those of others (for example, the child has two eyes and his mom has two eyes that are similar; they both have two legs, but his mom's are longer; and the child has two legs

and the cat has four legs that are very different from the child's). The focus at this level is to help the child more firmly establish what his body is like rather than remembering what he learned about the other individual.

Device Use

As the child becomes aware of her ability to move, activities such as the following should be included to help her feel safe with her new ambulation skills.

- Give the child many opportunities to become familiar with the long cane while the child is stationary and before actual use. Teach the child the names of the parts of the cane and begin substituting the cane for the wooden spoon or device used previously for experiences to extend reach.

- Provide opportunities for the child to use a device to extend her reach, and play a game where the child finds two of three items that are of the same sound and material. Compare the sound made between the wooden spoon and the long cane.

- Encourage the child to use a device to reach out while she is being carried to find items around her while you are moving together. Show her how she can use the device to find a wall in front of her and show her what happens as she touches the wall with her device. Then move together toward the wall with the device on the wall and her other hand extended out to touch the wall.

- Provide alternative items to encourage waking if a child is hesitant to walk; consider the use of an item such as a toy shopping cart that is weighted to provide stability and safety when the child takes initial steps. Once the child has developed some confidence, be sure to also encourage the child to move without the device for part of the time.

Concepts/Orientation

Learning to label and note similarities and differences about the environment that the child is beginning to move through can be facilitated through activities such as the following.

- Help the child learn basic spatial concepts such as in and out and over and under by first showing the child examples of the concept and allowing him the opportunity to physically explore it, then making comparisons to situations that are not examples of the concept [for example, "I am putting the cane over the table" (and multiple other examples), then "this cane is over the table, but this cane is not" (when it is beside the table)].

- Take the child to a room in the house and look at the items in the room. Then take the child to another room and look at what it contains. Talk about why the different rooms have different kinds of things in them.

- Give the child basic experiences to begin to understand the concepts of same and different. After the child understands the sensory qualities of items (even on a very basic or limited level), provide a number of items and show the child how you can sort them based on similarity. The focus at this level is the adult's demonstration of the concept and not for the child to be able to do this himself.

- Play a game of "let's see what we can find" to encourage curiosity. Reward and praise the child for movement that results in him finding an object that he was not previously in contact with. Eventually, "plant" new or exciting items in a place where the child is sure to find them.

Children Who Are Walking

Sensory Development

Sensory development at this stage should be related to movement through activities such as the following.

Self-Initiated Movement and Exploration

Anna is a 15-month-old infant with severe low vision and mild cerebral palsy. She currently exhibits some slight delays in her overall development, but is progressing in all areas. Through the work of her early interventionist, orientation and mobility (O&M) instructor, and physical therapist, Anna has learned the motor skills necessary for crawling, but she does not move unless physically prompted by an adult.

The O&M instructor explains to the family and the rest of the team that Anna cannot clearly see things at a distance to motivate her to move and that she may be insecure about moving into a space she cannot see. Using information from the physical therapist on Anna's motor abilities, the O&M instructor and Anna's mother create a defined play space for Anna in the corner of the living room. A 3-foot square blanket is used to mark the floor. Two walls and the sofa define three of the sides. A variety of Anna's favorite toys are given "assigned" locations in the play space. The O&M instructor plays with Anna in the play space to show her where her toys are located and helps her transition from sitting to crawling to reach them. Each day, Anna's mother briefly shows Anna where the toys are and then allows Anna time to play independently in the play space while the mother works in the same room. The predictability and safety of the defined play space has encouraged Anna to begin crawling on her own to locate her toys.

- Encourage the child to use these labels himself and demonstrate understanding of these concepts in other ways, such as playing a game of "move until you find the bumpy surface, then jump up and down when you get there." Combine this with long-cane use by having the child reach or move to find specified textures with an AMD or long cane.

- Play games where the child moves in order to place himself in a specified location to a sound maker (for example, "turn so the clock is beside you"). Play games of catch while following a moving sound source.

- Take the child to streets that have a variety of traffic sounds and identify the sounds he is hearing (for example, "that is a car coming toward you," "that is a big truck," "that is a car on the street in front of you (perpendicular) and you can hear the sound of the car in your left ear, then your right ear as it moves along the street"). The focus is primarily for the child to learn that there are different types of traffic sounds and begin to have words to describe the sounds. This will also need to be paired with concept/orientation lessons to understand traffic patterns and the like.

Motor Development

Providing as wide a variety of movement opportunities is the focus of activities for children at this developmental level:

- Systematically introduce the child to as wide a variety of movements as possible: "animal walks," such as walking like an elephant and hopping like a bunny (be sure the child has had the opportunity to learn about the animals first); ways to move from place to place; ways to move other items, such as throwing and pushing; and ways to express yourself through movement.

- Provide playful practice in developing balance and coordination (for example, walking along railroad ties that line a playground area).

- Provide systematic instruction in correctly making 45-, 90-, and 180-degree turns (this will be supported by instruction in understanding the impact of these movements on the child's orientation).

- Provide experiences to practice wrist movements in playful ways that will be required for long-cane use.

Body Image

The following activities should be provided to expand and refine the child's control of his body.

- Systematically teach the child about complex body parts such as upper arm, thigh, wrist, and so forth.

- Systematically teach the child to identify the right and left sides of his body and body parts. If necessary, provide a physical prompt, such as having the child wear a bracelet on his right hand. Once he consistently identifies his right hand correctly, have the child put the bracelet on other right-sided body parts to show how they are all aligned.

- Play games where the child reaches out to touch specified body parts on another person or animal when the individual is in a variety of positions (for example, facing the child, in front of the child facing the same way, and so forth).

Device Use

Activities that focus on learning techniques for using devices for information and protection can include the following:

- Provide the child with instruction in interpreting information that is being provided by an AMD or device other than a cane. For example, walk the child through contacting an object and explain cause and effect (in appropriate terms for the child's development) or take the child to stairs and walk through an understanding of how the feel of the AMD's movement relates to the object it is touching (that is, the feeling of the AMD dropping away means you are at a down step and you need to move cautiously forward). Later, perform similar activities with the long cane.

• Teach beginning long-cane skills (for example, how to grip the cane, keeping the tip on the ground and cane in front of the body, or deciding whether to move around or up to an object that is contacted).

• Provide opportunities for the child to meet and talk with older cane users. When possible, arrange for the child and the cane user to walk together in settings such as stores and residential areas to allow the child the chance to observe how a cane facilitates day-to-day travel.

• Include parents and child-care workers in lessons on devices to increase the chances that the device will be used outside of O&M lessons.

• Give the child opportunities to explore low vision devices in controlled settings and begin to understand their capabilities.

Concepts/Orientation

Examples of concept/orientation activities that integrate sensory, motor, body image, device use skills include the following.

SIDEBAR 7.6

Readiness and Refinement of Basic Skills

Maurice is a 4-year-old boy with severely restricted visual fields in his right eye and no vision in his left eye. He attends a local preschool where he receives itinerant support from a teacher of students with visual impairments and an orientation and mobility (O&M) instructor. Maurice began using an adaptive mobility device (AMD) when he was 18 months old and received his first long cane when he was 3. Maurice is very safe in using his cane to avoid obstacles and to detect surface changes, but he does not know how to use the cane to safely go up and down stairs or curbs.

His O&M instructor arrives at the preschool 15 minutes before his class goes to the playground, which requires climbing a flight of stairs. She explains to Maurice that today he will start learning to use his cane on the stairs. They walk to the bottom of the stairs and she verbally and physically explains how to find the bottom step, align himself, find the handrail, and position the cane to go up the stairs. Providing partial

physical assistance from behind Maurice, they walk to the top of the stairs. As they climb, the O&M instructor sings a silly song to the tune of "Row, Row, Row Your Boat": "Up, up, up the stairs, up the stairs we go," she sings, raising the pitch of the song higher and higher as they move up the stairs.

At the top of the stairs, the O&M instructor applauds Maurice for climbing the stairs with his cane. They walk to the playground, arriving a few minutes before the rest of his class. The O&M instructor will continue to work with Maurice on the stairs for several weeks or months until he is safe when walking up and down stairs with the cane. She will also invite his preschool teacher and parents to observe his cane technique on the stairs. Once Maurice consistently demonstrates safe cane techniques and the adults in his life are educated about using the cane on stairs and curbs, Maurice will use the cane on stairs when walking with his parents and his class.

- Provide multiple opportunities for the child to practice skills requiring discrimination of similarities and differences, especially as this relates to concepts that facilitate travel. Give child tasks to do that require sorting objects by characteristics.

- Once examples of spatial concepts have been demonstrated and labeled, give the child simple tasks to do that incorporate both travel and understanding of a concept (for example, once the child consistently identifies the right and left sides of her body, have her find objects that are located on the right or left).

- Systematically introduce the child to objects in her environment that will be needed to facilitate travel. For example, take the child to an intersection of hallways and provide systematic instruction on the parts of an intersection, what the parts do, what the purpose of an intersection is, what the sensory characteristics of the hallway include, and so forth. As much as possible, also provide experiences with concepts of the next environments that the child will encounter, such as objects in residential areas before the child needs to travel in a residential area.

SPECIAL CONSIDERATIONS FOR CHILDREN WITH MULTIPLE IMPAIRMENTS

Data collected on very young children with visual impairments indicate that a large percentage have additional disabilities (Ferrell, 1998). These disabilities can range from very mild (for example, a slight developmental delay or mild cerebral palsy) to extremely severe (for example, multiple health, motor, cognitive, and sensory impairments). All children with visual impairments, regardless of the presence or absence of additional disabilities, have a need and the right to receive O&M services.

When working with children who have multiple disabilities, the O&M instructor needs to keep the whole child in mind rather than focusing solely on the implications of the visual impairment. The impact of multiple impairments is additive (Hatton, Bailey, Burchinal, & Ferrell, 1997), and one disability cannot be singled out for intervention without taking all aspects of the child into account. For example, a child with physical impairments may require adaptive devices or special positioning to enhance motor control and strength. These devices and positions may or may not merge effectively with the O&M activities the child needs to experience. By working closely with the other professionals (for example, physical therapist and occupational therapist) and the parents, the team can come up with creative solutions that meet the child's physical needs while allowing the opportunity to develop O&M concepts and skills.

An issue related to the concept of the "whole child" is the parental reaction to a child with multiple impairments. When a child is born with more than one impairment or health issue, parents must come to terms with each impairment and learn to meet all of their child's medical and daily needs. Each family is unique in how it deals with these issues, but most frequently, addressing the child's medical and physical needs take precedence. When this is the case, parents may choose to address medical care, physical therapy, and feeding before they are ready to discuss issues related to their child's visual impairment. Other parents will want to have information and services related to all aspects of their child's development from the beginning. O&M instructors need to be sensitive to the needs of families and provide an appropriate level of support (information, intervention, and the like) to meet the child's needs, while respecting the family's priorities.

Though no professional can be an expert on all disabilities, O&M instructors have an obligation to develop an understanding and knowledge of the disabilities of the children they serve (see Chapter 18). They need to understand the implications of all the child's disabilities and their possible interactions. They also need to know basic skills, such as how to properly position the child, how to use adaptive equipment (for example, ankle-foot orthotics (AFOs or splints), how to meet the child's physical needs (for example, suctioning), and how to identify and respond to medical emergencies (for example, seizures). Often, children's needs are unique and the O&M instructor should request that the parents and/or other professionals demonstrate techniques to be certain the child is not harmed. O&M instructors who have limited experience in working with children who have multiple impairments should pursue additional learning opportunities (for example, college courses or continuing education classes) that focus on the needs of children with multiple impairments.

All of these issues lead to the need for an O&M instructor to work closely with team members to meet the needs of the child. If a child has multiple issues, the team may include parents, an early interventionist or preschool teacher, a physical therapist, an occupational therapist, a speech therapist, a teacher of the deaf or hard of hearing, a teacher of children with visual impairments, an audiologist, an O&M specialist, and others. Such a large and diverse team provides the child and family with a wealth of resources, but also can overwhelm the family with too much information at one time. Teams must coordinate efforts to help the family and child maximize the potential benefits of intervention. In addition to the benefits of working as a team that apply to all children, children with multiple impairments need team members to work closely together to address the needs of the whole child and to meet the needs of the family. By collaborating on interventions, teams can see that the child has meaningful opportunities to learn that take into account all of the child's unique needs.

ADVOCATING FOR EARLY CHILDHOOD ORIENTATION AND MOBILITY

Despite the legal and ethical obligations to provide O&M services to infants, toddlers, and preschoolers with visual impairments, many children in this country continue to be denied this much-needed service. Parents and other service providers often do not know to request O&M services for such young children. Frequently, agencies that provide services do not have sufficient staff to serve all children. At times, O&M instructors are available, but they lack an understanding of early childhood learning, which makes them uncomfortable with providing services to very young children. It is essential that everyone concerned about the education of young children with visual impairments advocate for the provision of developmentally appropriate O&M services on a regular basis.

Several avenues exist for advocacy depending on your professional position and the specific situation. O&M instructors who may be called upon to serve very young children need to educate themselves on working with this population through readings, courses, and continuing education opportunities on typical early childhood development as well as on early childhood orientation and mobility. O&M instructors should become proactive to provide in-service workshops and other outreach methods to educate their colleagues from other areas of education about the needs of children with visual impairments and the services provided by O&M instructors. O&M instructors can meet with family support groups to provide families with information about O&M services for young children as a means for enlisting parent support and advocacy. O&M instructors can work within their agencies to advocate for service delivery policies and hiring policies that will ensure that all children with visual impairments have access to qualified O&M instructors. O&M instructors need to stay involved in the development and monitoring of state and federal legislation related to the education of young children and the provision of O&M services so that revisions of current laws strengthen the legislative support for orientation and mobility in early childhood.

CONCLUSION

The first years of life provide young learners with exciting opportunities for self-directed learning. O&M services in these years attend to the developmental nature of the child and should be based on the child's interests. It is the role of the O&M specialist to assist learners of this age, and their family members, to develop positive attitudes toward exploration and independence, and to begin to explore the myriad of skills and activities upon which more typical O&M instruction will later be based. Through the creative use of materials, including AMDs and long canes, playful activities can be incorporated into both the day-to-day activities of the child and more structured O&M lessons. The multiple "significant others" in the child's world can work together to provide a wide variety of experiences that will allow the child to begin learning in all of the multiple skills that will later constitute more formal O&M instruction. Through the creativity of O&M specialists and others, the child can begin to experience the independence provided by learning.

IMPLICATIONS FOR O&M PRACTICE

1. O&M services for young children include both typical "formalized" learning activities and learning that occurs on a more incidental basis.

2. Children of this age are in the sensorimotor phase of development, which includes much

exploration and experimentation, often in the form of play.

3. Close collaboration with the young child's family and educational team is especially important during this age. The O&M specialist should fill two major roles in this relationship: providing emotional support to families and providing O&M-specific information.

4. O&M assessments of young children primarily include observations of the child in day-to-day activities and active involvement of significant others to encourage both formalized O&M skills and skills not directly associated with orientation and mobility.

5. To allow the repeated practice that is necessary at this age, O&M services should be provided as often as possible and should be reinforced on a daily basis by the "significant others" in the child's environment.

6. O&M specialists serving young children need to become proficient at following the child's lead to take advantage of teachable moments in addition to following more formalized lesson planning.

7. For many young children, O&M services include practice in the use of both an AMD and a long cane. AMDs may be used primarily for day-to-day travel, with more advanced long-cane skills being practiced during O&M lessons.

8. The focus of much of the instruction with early childhood learners should be in the following important areas: sensory awareness, body concept, motor development, auditory development, and concept development.

9. Curricula for young children also needs to focus on developing emerging skills for all of the more advanced travel skills, even though the activities will not look the same as when practiced with older children and adults.

LEARNING ACTIVITIES

1. Give an example of a teaching component to implement for a preschool learner with visual impairments (not given in this chapter) and a playful means to provide practice.

2. Choose a toy or play material typically found in a preschool classroom and describe its use in teaching O&M-related concepts.

3. Describe at least two ways long canes can be incorporated into the O&M process with preschool learners.

4. Observe an O&M specialist working with a very young child and interview the professional about the techniques you observed.

5. Review at least three of the resources recommended in this chapter and create an annotated bibliography for your files.

O&M Content for Young Learners
Suggestions for Including Advanced O&M Skills into Preschool Lessons

O&M Skill	Age of Learner		
	Infant[a]	Toddler[b]	Preschooler[c]
Concept of turns/ accurate turns	Make distinct turns (not curves) when carrying or walking with infant.	Continue making distinct turns when walking together. When walking together, have a word or signal that you say or do whenever you make a turn to help the child clue into the fact that a difference in the movement is occurring. Show child the difference between "turn" (90°), "turn around" (180°), and "turn all the way around" (360°). Try to be consistent in your use of these terms. Play (modified) "Mother May I" by asking the child to make one of the above turns (gross approximations), and if done correctly he will "find" you in front of him— reward with hugs, tickles, and the like. Continue with previous activities.	Continue with previous activities. Play a game where the child is the "driver" and you are the "car," and you turn whenever the child tells you to (or makes motion as if turning the steering wheel). Talk about how turning changes the direction you are traveling. Put items in front of the child and to the side she will be turning, and show how the relative location changes.

[a] In the range of approximately 6–18 months old.

[b] In the range of approximately 12–36 months old.

[c] In the range of approximately 3–6 years old.

(continued on next page)

	Age of Learner		
O&M Skill	Infant[a]	Toddler[b]	Preschooler[c]
Analyzing traffic sounds and patterns	Take infant to a variety of areas with different levels of traffic. Be sure to include areas with high levels of traffic. Provide time to listen to the traffic and become used to it.		On a quiet street, talk about how the sound of the car is quiet, then gets louder as it approaches, then gets quiet again.
	Help child to localize and reach for sounds—start with hand-over-hand, then physical assistance from elbow, physical assistance from shoulder, and so forth.	Help child to learn to turn to face sounds.	As child demonstrates ability to localize sound, help him to point to and follow movement of car along the street. Do this first on a quiet street, then on busier streets.
	Use a sound maker that can be activated by hitting it and encourage child to make it sound each time he or she is correct.	While standing next to the street, talk about "loud" - and "quiet"-sounding cars.	As child demonstrates understanding of spatial concepts, show child how traffic moves from in front to behind you when you are standing with the street beside you, and how traffic moves from side to side when you are facing the street.
		While standing next to different types of streets, ask the child to tell when there are cars on the street and when there are no cars.	

(continued on next page)

	Age of Learner		
O&M Skill	Infant[a]	Toddler[b]	Preschooler[c]
		Talk about the different sounds made by "fast" cars and "slow" cars. Play games with cars and act out going fast and slow; read stories about vehicles that go fast or slow.	
Compass orientation	Begin to incorporate compass terms into your daily vocabulary. If possible, use them when giving directions to others or to describe locations of items in the house and elsewhere.	Identify three or four key locations in the house (or school) and refer to them with labels in compass terms—that is, call the front door the "east door" (or whichever direction it faces), talk about the clothes rack being on the north wall.	Continue with previous activities.
			Play a game of "detective." Take the child to locations in the house that you have been identifying with compass labels and see if he or she can tell what it is (what direction it is associated with).
			When walking between labeled compass locations, talk about how you need to turn to get from one to the other.

(continued on next page)

	Age of Learner		
O&M Skill	**Infant**[a]	**Toddler**[b]	**Preschooler**[c]
		Play games to teach and practice basic spatial concepts, specifically "in front" and "behind."	As child demonstrates understanding of spatial concepts of "in front" and "behind," talk about north being in front of you when you are walking toward the north clothes rack.
		Teach child about opposites. Use physical movements as much as possible, that is, the opposite of "stop" is "go," the opposite of "up" is "down," and so forth.	As child demonstrates understanding of opposites, talk about north and south being opposites and "when north is in front of you, south is behind you."
Public transportation	Plan periodic family "field trips." Instead of driving downtown to go to the library, park at the outskirts and take a city bus, or take a cab to the grocery store occasionally.	Continue family "field trips." Talk with student about what transportation you will take, read a story about the type of transportation, play games with toy models of the type of transportation.	Continue family "field trips." Give the child responsibility for portions of the trip, that is, have him or her hold the money and hand it to the bus driver as you get on, have the child ask the bus driver to say when you are at your stop.
Mapping skills	Accustom child to wide variety of tactual materials. Help him or her to explore/scan the entire item.	Provide child with a magnetic or Velcro map board. Encourage him or her to make designs with the pieces.	Play a game with the child where you place a magnet on the board and he or she tactually searches for it using appropriate search patterns.
			As child is able, play the above game and have the child tell where he or she found the magnet on the board (that is, "near the top and near the right side").

(continued on next page)

	Age of Learner		
O&M Skill	**Infant**[a]	**Toddler**[b]	**Preschooler**[c]
			Help child learn to make magnet lines that go all the way "across" the board or "from top to bottom."
		Walk in a hallway carrying map board and as you walk from one end of the hall to the other, place magnets in a longer and longer line going away from child's body.	
			As child is able, continue as above, but also examine an intersecting hallway and place magnets to show the intersection.

CHAPTER 8

Teaching Orientation and Mobility to School-Age Children

Diane L. Fazzi and Brenda J. Naimy

LEARNING QUESTIONS

- In addition to mastery of orientation and mobility (O&M) skills and techniques, what are qualities of the O&M specialist that contribute to success in teaching orientation and mobility to school-age students?

- What are the advantages and disadvantages of using age-level curricular guidelines in planning O&M goals for school-age students?

- How might knowledge of your students' preferred learning styles be incorporated into individualized O&M lesson planning?

- What kind of assessment activities can be used to effectively assess student skills and knowledge in each of the O&M domains?

- How does the use of instructional units improve O&M lesson planning and student outcomes?

- What are strategies for establishing rapport with students, families, and colleagues within a school system?

This chapter focuses on orientation and mobility (O&M) instruction for school-age children from kindergarten through high school. It addresses qualities of excellence in O&M services for school-age students; age-appropriate curricular guidelines; instructional planning and accountability; tools, tips, and teaching strategies; strong school and family partnerships; and ongoing professional growth. Information regarding the provision of O&M services for preschool children can be found in Chapter 7. Chapters 17 through 20 contain further information on orientation and mobility for learners who have additional disabilities.

QUALITIES OF EXCELLENCE IN ORIENTATION AND MOBILITY

Teaching orientation and mobility to school-age children and youth requires more than a working knowledge of the skills and techniques for independent travel. Successful teaching is based on a combination of depth of knowledge of orientation and mobility, varied and effective teaching skills, and interpersonal qualities for working as part of an educational team. In fact, qualities of excellence in teaching orientation and mobility include:

- high expectations for student success
- understanding the "whole" picture
- active involvement of students in the learning process
- creativity in instructional design
- good interpersonal communications
- commitment to ongoing professional development

With each of these components in place, O&M specialists will experience success in teaching and insure that school-age students develop the necessary skills for increasing levels of independence, exploration, and conceptual development.

High Expectations for Student Success

Given appropriate supports and good-quality instruction, all students can learn and all students with visual impairments can increase their levels of independence. Some students may achieve independence rapidly, such as a student of high school age who quickly masters bus travel, including complex transfer routes in the span of one semester. For other students, gains may take place over longer periods of time, such as a student who learns to do the final segment of a route semi-independently over the course of one year. Some students with additional severe disabilities may make progress that is less noticeable to the casual observer, such as a student who increases the amount of time maintaining the tip of the cane on the ground during campus travel.

High expectations for success and for increasing levels of independence drive O&M professionals to motivate and challenge students to realize their fullest potential for independence. It has been noted that lowered expectations for individuals with visual impairments are prevalent in society and often result in lessened inclusion and competition in age-appropriate activities (Tuttle & Tuttle, 2000; Wolffe, 1999). Wolffe (1999) stresses the importance of students with visual impairments having people in their lives that convey high expectations: "When people without disabilities see that young people with disabilities can do things for themselves and others, their expectations for those young people rise. Enhanced performance often follows enhanced expectations" (p. 4).

Similarly, success in orientation and mobility is positively impacted by high expectations of others. Fundamental to O&M instruction is the specialist's underlying belief that individuals with visual impairments can be independent travelers and can lead fulfilling lives.

Understanding the Whole Picture

O&M specialists must have a strong command of the content that they will teach to their students. A full review of the skills and techniques that are taught for independent travel is provided in other resources, such as Hill & Ponder, 1976; Jacobson, 1993; LaGrow & Weessies, 1994. When working with school-age students, O&M specialists must apply those skills and techniques within a developmental framework. In other words, skills cannot be taught successfully until learners have reached the appropriate level of developmental readiness to learn them. For example, cardinal directions cannot be fully learned prior to an understanding of left and right. However, that does not mean that the concepts of north and south cannot be introduced, just as young children are introduced to many concepts before they are ready to fully understand them.

Specialists should be aware that there may be individual differences in learning and development among children who are blind, and group differences for various skills and aspects of development between children who are blind and children who are sighted. An example of individual differences in mobility skill development may be one child who is visually impaired and is able to focus a monocular with ease at age five, while another child of the same age requires assistance. Much has been published about the group differences between children who are congenitally blind and children who are sighted. As a group, young children who are congenitally blind have been found to develop dynamic motor milestones (such as crawling or walking) months after children who are sighted. Ferrell (1998) has suggested that children with visual impairments may learn in a sequence that is different from what is typically expected rather than in a delayed manner. For example, in Project PRISM, a federally funded longitudinal study of child development in infants and toddlers with visual impairments, Ferrell (1998) found that children who were blind with no additional disabilities were delayed in searching for dropped objects, transfer of objects from one hand to the other, and intentional movement. In contrast, they achieved other milestones ahead of what would be expected for children who are sighted, such as playing interactive games, removing simple garments without assistance, following simple directions related to daily routines, and repeating two-digit sequences of information.

O&M specialists may look to state educational standards to understand the knowledge and skills that children of various grade levels are expected to achieve in the general-education curriculum. These general guidelines can then be applied to similar O&M skills and concepts, as discussed later in this chapter. O&M specialists can also observe the activities of students'

peers to gain perspectives on expectations for age-appropriate travel experiences.

Another important aspect of understanding the whole picture is to make the direct linkage between assessment and instructional planning:

> The O&M specialist who knows the curriculum, is familiar with the training environments, and thoroughly assesses the abilities and interests of the student is well prepared to provide high-quality instruction. Maintaining a strong connection between assessment and instruction helps ensure the relevance of the instructional program. (Fazzi & Petersmeyer, 2001, p. 32)

When the two processes are completed separately from one another, the assessment loses its purpose and the teaching and learning may fail to be meaningful or effective.

Finally, when the goals of O&M instruction are considered as a link to other aspects of student life and learning, the picture comes full circle. The ultimate purpose of independent travel for students with visual impairments is not simply to meet goals established by an Individualized Education Program (IEP) team (for more information on the IEP, see the Instructional Planning section in this chapter and also Volume 1, Chapter 12); it is to provide students with the skills that they need to participate in life to the fullest extent possible. Travel skills support enjoyment of recreational activities, success in vocational choices, and opportunities for higher education and independent living. O&M specialists who view their students in a larger life context can plan lessons, units, and goals that will reach far beyond specific skills, concepts, and route completion.

Active Involvement of Students in the Learning Process

O&M specialists can use assessment results within a developmental framework to plan goals and lessons that will be relevant, challenging, and effective for their students, but taking the extra step to involve students in instructional planning can turn a very good lesson into an excellent one. Students can be involved in helping O&M specialists to plan goals, whether there are skills that they would like to learn, areas they would like to travel more frequently, or destinations that they are interested in reaching. This process can be as complex as involving a student of high school age in self-assessment of strengths and projecting future needs or as simple as asking an elementary school student to choose between two predesigned goals. Collaborative goal setting with students helps to increase motivation for learning and provides students with opportunities for practicing self-determination. In her work on student learning motivation, Boekaerts (2002) asserts, "Recent findings indicate that learning goals that are agreed upon jointly by the students and the teacher have a better chance of being accomplished" (pp. 20–21). Students who both understand the lesson or unit goal and have a variety of strategies to use can effectively work on problem-solving skills and achieving established goals during O&M lessons.

Similarly, following a student's interest can make the planning of individual lessons fun for both teacher and pupil. For example, while on a lesson, a student of middle school age is curious about the electronics involved in controlling traffic lights and pedestrian walk signals. The O&M specialist can work together with the science teacher to modify an electric circuit lesson and follow up with a field trip to the traffic engineering headquarters for a demonstration of city traffic flow monitoring. While these few lessons may not seem to be directly related to the goals of the current sequence of instruction, as a result of being allowed to pursue a curiosity, the student may express increased interest in traveling to a variety of traffic-controlled intersections to examine how they have been designed. O&M

instruction can focus for a time on intersection analysis and safe street crossings for such a highly motivated student.

Students also enjoy participating in creating instructional materials for lessons for themselves and others. Bentzen and Marston (Volume 1, Chapter 10) and Fazzi and Petersmeyer (2001) have noted several advantages of involving students in creating maps for travel areas—school campuses, residential areas, and route planning. When students create maps and other instructional materials, O&M specialists gain an additional opportunity to assess conceptual understanding as students work to create representational layouts. While working with a student of elementary school age on a grid pattern of a residential area, the instructor may note that the student places pretend cars on the wrong sides of the street. This realization provides another chance to teach the student about lanes of traffic. Self-constructed maps are also a source of pride for many students and can serve as concrete demonstrations of growth and development in much the same way as thematic projects that students complete in general-education classes. Student work samples can be proudly displayed in classrooms or as appropriate at school open houses.

Creativity in Instructional Design

Can O&M specialists teach lessons without attempting to add some creativity? Certainly it can be done, but without creativity, the instruction may not be effective with all students and the motivation of students may be hard to maintain. Creativity is the process by which O&M specialists tailor lessons to meet the individual abilities, learning styles, and interests of students. With an ounce of creativity, a lesson on cane skills, for example, can become a fun music lesson by incorporating rhythm with interesting percussion instruments.

Appropriately used instructional materials support learning of O&M skills and concepts in just the same way that manipulatives, visuals, and workbooks are used in the classroom to support learning of math and reading. Fazzi and Petersmeyer (2001) suggest experimenting with a variety of exciting instructional materials that can lead to innovative lessons. For example, transparent sheets of differently colored plastic have been overlaid on visual graphics to highlight scanning patterns or other points of emphasis for students with low vision. Less-expensive substitutes can also be used, such as a variety of plastics found in common office supply stores. Regardless of what is used, the point is to create teaching materials to help students learn advanced concepts for independent travel.

Packaging creative lessons and materials into an instructional unit that maintains a theme of interest to the student helps to build a logical sequence within which a student can learn, practice, and master important concepts and skills. Highly motivating culminating activities at the end of instructional units build anticipation for future lessons and provide an interesting approach to applying skills in an integrated fashion. For example, a monocular training unit could culminate in solving a secret code based on signs read throughout the unit. The secret code could be a message to locate a coupon to use in purchasing a specialty item. Culminating activities also provide the instructor and student with an opportunity to assess concepts and skills learned during the unit and give direction to future areas of learning.

Good Interpersonal Communications

The best O&M school programs enjoy the support of families, school personnel, and community partners. The level of support obtained for educational programs is partly based on the rapport, trust, and open communications established. Many schools have family communication systems already in place with which O&M

specialists can work. For example, weekly folders that go home and must be signed by parents can contain notes and reminders from O&M specialists. O&M specialists can work with their students to keep an O&M journal that goes home on a monthly basis for family review. They also can invite families to observe O&M lessons. Informed families have served as strong advocates within school districts to ensure that adequate numbers of teachers are hired to maintain reasonable caseloads and adequate service hours for students, and they have even sponsored fundraising activities for field trips and independent living activities.

It is also important that school personnel understand what O&M instruction is all about. Educating school and community personnel about orientation and mobility for students with visual impairments can be done in many ways, including:

- describing the purpose of various lessons to colleagues

- volunteering to prepare one of the school bulletin boards that is rotated throughout the year

- inviting a colleague or administrator to observe a lesson in the community

- providing opportunities for families, colleagues, and administrators to participate in various activities of daily living wearing a sleep shade or low vision simulator

- assisting a student in preparing a presentation to his or her own classroom about O&M accomplishments

- contacting the local police department to notify them about O&M lessons that will be taking place in their community

- supporting local merchants and explaining why there will be students with visual impairments having lessons in their stores or places of business

- volunteering to conduct an in-service training to the local transportation company

Commitment to Ongoing Professional Development

In order to maintain excellence in teaching, O&M specialists must be engaged in a process of reflection, improved teaching, and ongoing professional development. O&M specialists benefit from learning new strategies, revisiting proven methods, and expanding teaching repertoires. In the 2004 reauthorization of the Individuals with Disabilities Education Improvement Act (IDEA), there is an emphasis on the need for special educators to document the use of research-based practices in educational programming. School professionals must stay current in order to ensure that they are using educational practices that are grounded in accepted research (see Wiener & Siffermann, Volume 1, Chapter 14).

As part of the expanded core curriculum (Huebner, Merk-Adam, Stryker, & Wolffe, 2004), professionals need to be familiar with relevant student and family resources that support independent living, recreation, social, transportation, and vocational development. For example, O&M specialists need to be familiar with city or county guidelines for eligibility for paratransit for school-age students with visual impairments. Students with visual impairments may be interested in recreational activities available after school or on weekends—either in the local community or at an agency that supports activities designed for youth who are blind or visually impaired. Families of students with visual impairments and additional disabilities may need contact information for agencies and/or developmental centers to obtain services such as assistance for respite care. Similarly, families may need information on negotiating rehabilitation services as their children approach transition age. O&M specialists who maintain access to current support services provide students and families with a valuable resource.

KNOW THE GRADE: AGE-APPROPRIATE CURRICULAR GUIDELINES

Unlike academic subjects that have state-published grade-level guidelines for core content, O&M curricula have traditionally been tailored for individual students as deemed appropriate by the O&M specialist in collaboration with the educational team. There are many clear advantages to this approach. School-age students with visual impairments represent a heterogeneous group of learners who absorb information at vastly different rates. For example, despite the fact that many students may not have the physical coordination to use well-refined two-point touch technique until the age of 5 or 6, it does not mean that a child with strong motor coordination could not develop such skills at age 3 or 4. Furthermore, it is estimated that more than 50 percent of school-age children with visual impairments have additional disabilities (Erin & Spungin 2004; Silberman, 2000), many of which may directly impact a student's physical, sensory, or cognitive ability to learn or apply various O&M skills (see Chapters 17–20).

Students with visual impairments also live and travel in a wide variety of environments (for example, rural, suburban, or urban areas, which may or may not have sidewalks) and these areas often dictate the need to prioritize O&M skills that are critical to developing levels of independence (LaGrow & Weessies, 1994; Welsh, 1997). For example, while rural travel experiences are typically reserved for older students after residential and light business travel skills are mastered, it is obvious that a student living in a rural or other area without sidewalks must learn these skills at an earlier age. Clifton (2003) examined the travel behaviors of teenagers and found that independent travel varied by age, gender, household income, and geographic location. Teenagers living in urban areas were clearly more likely to walk or use public transportation than those living in suburban and rural areas. However, teens in suburban and rural areas had greater distances to travel and often had greater access to rides. McDonald (2008) found significant differences in rates of students who walked or rode bikes to school that were related to racial group and family-income level, with white children having the lowest walking rates, but also living greater distances from schools and similarly having greater vehicle access.

Additional travel behavior research has examined factors related to parental perspectives and permissiveness toward allowing children to travel without supervision. McMillan (2007) reported that the percentage of children walking/biking to school decreased from 87 percent in 1969 to 55 percent in 2001. Neighborhood and traffic safety concerns, household transportation options, cultural norms, and caregiver attitudes were all cited as contributing factors. These same factors may be considered when developing individualized O&M programs for school-age students. O&M specialists need to listen closely to their students and their students' families to determine what levels of independence might be deemed appropriate in a given year for a specified goal. Cultural expectations, student age level, cognitive and physical capabilities, family resources and safety concerns, community norms, and environmental access play an important part in determining how independence and interdependence might be achieved for a given student.

While individualization of O&M curricula remains essential (Orientation and Mobility Division of AER, 2006), many O&M specialists can still benefit from general age-appropriate O&M curricular guidelines during educational planning. O&M specialists serving school-age students working in public and private sectors may collaborate with colleagues to establish such guidelines at a district, residential school, agency or other education consortia level. Such guidelines may be based on consensus of practice (Azusa Unified School District, 1984; Ministry of Education, British Columbia, 2000), extensions of previously established state academic standards (Lohmeier, 2003, 2009; Wisconsin Department of Public Instruction, 2005), or both.

Such age- or grade-level guidelines can assist educational team planning of individual student goals within the context of a larger picture of assessed needs and provide a framework for team discussions. Similarly, they can serve as a tool for O&M specialists who are educating students, families, colleagues, and administrators as to the scope of concepts and skills that are important to be addressed across each learner's school career. Connecting O&M practices with academic standards may help both to strengthen program justification and to ensure that students with visual impairments are fully engaged in learning activities similar to same-age peers by providing supplemental, hands-on learning opportunities within the context of O&M learning. For example, as fourth-grade students are working on computing perimeters of various rectangles and squares from a workbook, students receiving O&M instruction might apply this skill and practice computing the perimeter of their home residential block by using a measuring stick with wheels while traveling around the block.

Upon a review of the current literature, a limited number of resources on grade-level O&M curricula were located—possibly because relatively few O&M specialists have yet to publish the guidelines from which they work. Pogrund et al. (1995) published a useful O&M curriculum for school-age children and youth that is both comprehensive and sequential, and the corresponding curriculum-based assessment helps the O&M specialist with instructional planning. The advantage of the curriculum is its emphasis on individually tailored behavioral objectives for students. It does not, however, provide guidance as to what might be considered age-appropriate O&M concepts and travel-related experiences. Lohmeier (2003) identified state standards in Arizona (Arizona Department of Education, 1997) that were parallel to skills and concepts incorporated within the expanded core curriculum for blind and visually impaired students (Huebner, Merk-Adam, Stryker, & Wolffe, 2004). Ambrose (2000) looked at the knowledge and ability of children with sight to solve spatial orientation tasks at age 10 and 6, and considered implications of age differences for teaching orientation and mobility to children of elementary school age with low vision. These studies and others help to create a body of work that can further support grade-level O&M guidelines.

The information presented in Tables 8.1A–D (age-appropriate curricular guidelines) represents an attempt to connect general development in O&M practices in mobility, orientation, concept, and sensory skills to state published academic standard areas, including math, science, English language arts, and visual and performing arts. Levels were grouped as follows: Kindergarten to third grade, fourth to sixth grade, seventh to ninth grade, and tenth to twelfth grade, respectively. The list of O&M skills and concepts is not intended to be exhaustive. More items were found in the primary grade standards because of the greater focus on hands-on learning and building foundational concepts (for example, creating a map of the school in kindergarten or learning concepts of parallel and perpendicular in the third and fourth grades. Concept areas (for example, money skills or cardinal directions) were easier to align with standards of specific O&M techniques and skills (for example, stair travel with a long cane). In some instances, no skills or concepts specific to orientation and mobility were identified and grade-level "products" (for example, creating a multimedia presentation or finding a variety of research sources) were included as a means for expanding upon, deepen-

ing understanding, or demonstrating competence in a given domain area.

Initially, O&M skills were identified and delineated in the charts that follow. Then, the state academic standards were used to assist in refining selections and were later cross-referenced within the charts. Finally, additional resources (Ministry of Education, British Columbia, 2000; Wisconsin Department of Public Instruction, 2005) were consulted to determine if certain skills and/or concepts were appropriately placed according to age level. Each source is identified with a code within each chart. Groups of practicing O&M specialists may wish to expand on these charts, consult with each of the individual resources listed, and reference their own state standards to create a document that is meaningful and useful for them. Additional sources of information that can be reviewed include adaptive skill inventories (for example, *Vineland Adaptive Behavior Scales* or *Wisconsin Adaptive Skills Resource Guide*); general pedestrian safety guidelines; current reports from local, state, or federal transportation agencies; and research on pedestrian behavior, such as those previously noted (Clifton, 2003; McDonald, 2008; McMillan, 2007).

Certain assumptions should be adhered to when consulting the charts:

- Individualized assessments and team input must drive educational decisions and goal setting.

- These guidelines are intended to be general in nature and students will perform according to their individual abilities.

- A myriad of factors may impact the applicability of grade-level curricular guidelines for a given student, including:
  - the presence of additional disabilities,
  - family priorities,
  - student goals,
  - influence of the nature of the environment where the student lives on independent

TABLE 8.1A

Age-Appropriate Curricular Guidelines—Mobility

Mobility	Kindergarten–3rd grade	4th–6th grade	7th–9th grade	10th–12th grade
Basic skills	• Use human guide skills (A3) • Demonstrate protective techniques (A3) • Demonstrate trailing techniques (A3) • Align and square off in indoor environments (A3)	• Correct improper human guide techniques (A8) • Anticipate the need for and use protective techniques and trailing skills in familiar environments • Demonstrate alignment and squaring-off techniques in residential environments (for example, curb or grass line)	• Teach human guide skills to others • Anticipate the need for and use protective techniques and trailing skills in unfamiliar environments • Demonstrate alignment and squaring-off techniques in light business environments (for example, storefront) (A8)	• Create pamphlet to describe the "Do's and Don'ts of Human Guide Technique" (ELA11/12)
Long cane	• Demonstrate diagonal cane techniques (A3) • Demonstrate two-point touch technique and constant-contact technique (A3) • Demonstrate touch-and-drag technique (A3) • Demonstrate cane skills to negotiate doors and stairs (A3) • Fold, unfold, store cane and identify parts (A3)	• Demonstrate three-point touch technique (A6) • Use various cane techniques in familiar indoor/outdoor environments • Bring cane to and from school • Demonstrate cane skills to negotiate escalators and elevators (WM C4,3)	• Anticipate the need for and use various cane techniques in unfamiliar indoor/outdoor environments	• Order appropriate cane • Demonstrate awareness of use of various electronic travel devices
Street crossings	• Cross streets with guide • Identify timing of crossings at residential streets (WSS E.4.6) • Identify basic residential intersection shapes and traffic controls	• Complete semi-independent residential street crossings (A6) • Demonstrate basic elements of intersection analysis (A6)	• Complete independent residential street crossings • Complete supervised light business crossings (A8) • Analyze residential and simple light business intersections (WSS E.4.6)	• Complete independent light business crossings • Analyze complex intersections (A8)

	• Cross residential streets with supervision (WSS E.4.6) (A3)		• Complete crossing at railroad crossing (A8)	• Complete supervised crossings at complex intersections • Complete crossing in metro/urban area (A12)
Mall, stores, etc.	• Use human guide travel in markets and local stores	• Travel with supervision in markets and local stores • Make simple purchases (WM B.4.7)(M4) (A6)	• Travel with supervision in malls and department stores • Travel independently in small stores (A8) • Make complex purchases (WM B.4.7)	• Travel independently in markets, malls and stores (A12)
Use of transportation	• Use seatbelt independently	• Locate bus stop • Ride bus with others	• Use public bus with supervision (WM C.4.4) • Obtain public transportation schedule from a variety of sources (ELA7)	• Research independent transportation options, for example, ride share, private driver, taxi, etc. (WM C.4.3) (ELA9/10) • Apply for paratransit services (ELA8) • Complete transit transfers independently

A = Azusa Unified School District Priority Goals Checklist (Kindergarten –12th grade)

FIT = Framework for Independent Travel
- Level 1 (L1) = coincides with Kindergarten –3rd grade
- Level 2 (L2) = coincides with grades 4–7
- Level 3 (L3) = coincides with grades 8–12

H = California Health Standards

M = California Math Standards

S = California Science Standards

ELA = California English-Language Arts Standards

VPA = California Visual and Performing Arts Standards

WM = Wisconsin Model Academic Math Standards

WSS = Wisconsin Model Academic Social Studies Standards

Sources: Azusa Unified School District. (1984). *Priority goals checklist for orientation and mobility.* Azusa, CA: Author; California State Board of Education. (1997). *Mathematics content standards for California public schools: Kindergarten through grade twelve.* Sacramento: Author; California State Board of Education. (1997). *Physical education guidelines for kindergarten through grade twelve.* Sacramento: Author; California State Board of Education. (1998). *Science content standards for California public schools: Kindergarten through grade twelve.* Sacramento: Author; California State Board of Education. (2005). *Visual and performing arts: Dance content standards for California public schools: Kindergarten through grade twelve.* Sacramento: Author; Ministry of Education, British Columbia (2000). *Framework for independent travel: A resource for orientation and mobility (RB0094).* Province of British Columbia: Ministry of Education. Available from www.bced.gov.bc.ca/specialed/docs/fit.pdf; and Wisconsin Department of Public Instruction. (2005). *Wisconsin adaptive skills resource guide.* Available from http://dpi.wi.gov/sped/adaptskills.html.

TABLE 8.1B

Age-Appropriate Curricular Guidelines—Orientation

Orientation	Kindergarten–3rd grade	4th–6th grade	7th–9th grade	10th–12th grade
Landmarking	• Describe characteristics of landmarks, cues, and clues (FITL1, SK, A3) (ELA1) • ID appropriate home, school, and residential block landmarks (FITL1)	• ID residential landmarks in residential blocks and routes (FITL2) • Anticipate sequential landmarks during route travel in familiar areas (FITL2, WM F.4.4)	• Use effective questioning strategies to elicit landmark or destination information from others (ELA7)	• Create multimedia presentation of familiar city and key landmarks that can be used for orientation (ELA11/12)
Route travel	• Maintain orientation for simple route shapes (for example, "I", "L", etc.) in home and school environment (M2) • Follow and give simple route directions (for example, left/right) (M1, FITL1) • Maintain orientation for simple route reversals (FITL1)	• Use street names, directions, route shape, and landmarks to maintain orientation (WM F.4.1) • Maintain orientation during complex routes (e.g. "U", "Z", etc.) in home, school, and residential block environments (FITL2, A6) • Maintain orientation for more complex route shape reversals (for example, within a residential grid) (FITL2) • Plan routes and route alternatives to destinations within familiar residential environments (WM C.4.3, A2, A6)	• Plan alternative routes/detours within familiar light business environments	• Plan routes using public transit to unfamiliar destinations
Orientation strategies	• Use sun to aid direction of travel (S3) • Describe spatial layout (that is, survey-level cognitive map) of familiar school, home, and neighborhood locales (FITL1)	• Use sun and time of day to ID cardinal direction (S3, M8) • Use self-orientation strategy for room orientation (FITL1)	• Apply use of sun, compass, and landmarks to orient self when dropped off in familiar residential area (A6, M6, M8, FITL2, FITL3)	• Orient self when dropped off in familiar business area (M6, M8, FITL3)

Orientation aids (maps, GPS technology, etc.)	• Use problem solving strategies when disoriented in familiar environments (FITL1, M1) • Use and construct simple tactile, visual, auditory maps (M1, VPA1, WM C.4.4, FITL1)	• Use spatial updating and time distance estimation during route travel in familiar areas (VPA2, MK) • Employ effective recovery strategies after veering into driveways, streets, etc. (M5, A6) • Problem solve using task analysis and hypothesis testing (M3, M7) • Use compass to establish direction (S4, FITL2) • Use and construct detailed tactile, visual, or auditory maps to assist orientation in semifamiliar areas (A5, M4, S7, FITL2)	• Use effective questioning (in person and via telephone) to elicit route and destination information from others (WM C.4.3, FIP – L2, L3) (ELA7) • Locate destinations using indoor numbering and outdoor address systems (M2, FIP-L2) • Use detailed tactile, visual, or audio to orient self to shopping malls and outdoor areas (FITL3) • Use available/ accessible business directories (for example, mall) (FITL3) • Use commercially available or Internet map tools (ELA7) • Use GPS technology to establish orientation, plan routes, find outdoor destinations (FITL3) • Familiar with remote infrared audible signage (for example, Talking Signs) (FITL3)

A = Azusa Unified School District Priority Goals Checklist (K–12)

FIT = Framework for Independent Travel

- Level 1 (L1) = coincides with Kindergarten –3rd grade
- Level 2 (L2) = coincides with grades 4–7
- Level 3 (L3) = coincides with grades 8–12

H = California Health Standards

M = California Math Standards

S = California Science Standards

ELA = California English-Language Arts Standards

VPA = California Visual and Performing Arts Standards

WM = Wisconsin Model Academic Math Standards

WSS = Wisconsin Model Academic Social Studies Standards

Sources: See Table 8.1A.

Age-Appropriate Curricular Guidelines—Concepts

Concepts	Kindergarten–3rd grade	4th–6th grade	7th–9th grade	10th–12th grade
Environmental	• Identify/describe common textures and terrain features (FITL1) (SK) (A3) (ELAK) • Identify/describe basic indoor features (for example, doors, stairs, windows) (FITL1) (A1) (ELAK) • Identify/describe basic outdoor features (for example, grass, asphalt, cement, trees, fences, mailboxes) (FITL1) (S1) (MK) (A3) (ELAK) • Identify/describe basic residential block concepts (M4) (WM D.4.5) (A3)	• Identify/describe advanced and atypical residential block and grid features (for example, parkway, gutter, hedges, alley) (WM D.4.5) (A3) • Identify/describe complex indoor features (for example, escalators and elevators) (WM C.4.3)	• Identify/describe light business features (for example, street hardware, bus benches, sandwich boards, manhole covers) (FITL1) • Identify/describe features of grocery, department, and convenience stores and malls) (WSS A.4.5) • Identify/describe features of rural and other areas without sidewalks.	• Identify/describe atypical features in light business areas (for example, construction areas and scaffolding, outdoor cafes) • Identify/describe atypical travel features (for example, railroad track features, roundabouts, pedestrian bridges) • Identify/describe features of urban travel environments (for example, high-rise building, multilane and/or one-way major traffic thoroughfares, subway transit)
Spatial (directional / positional, etc.)	• Identify self-object relationships (VPA2) • Identify left/right sidedness—self/others (FITL2)/objects and turns (A3) (WSS A.4.1) • Identify basic positional concepts (S1) (FITL1) (A3) • dentify clock face points (M1) • Identify object-object relationships (S1) • Identify basic compass points (WSS A.4.1) (FITL2) (A3)	• Reverse right/left turns on return route • Identify parallel and perpendicular (M3) (A6) • Apply compass points in route travel (FITL2) • Make 90-, 180-, 360-degree turns (FITL2) (A3) • Identify clockwise and counterclockwise directions (FITL2)	• Identify midcompass points (FITL2) (A6) • Apply midcompass points in identifying corners for intersection analysis	

	Level 1	Level 2	Level 3
Numbering systems	• Count to 100 and above (M1) • Identify odd and even numbers (M1) • Determine greater and less than up to 100 (M2)	• Identify characteristics of indoor numbering systems (A6) • Identify characteristics of outdoor numbering systems (A6) • Use indoor numbering system to determine side of hallway of a destination • Use outdoor numbering system to determine proximity to a destination	• Determine relative location of destination based on numbering system and street name (WM F.4.1) • Determine direction of travel based on numbering system • Plan simple route using indoor/outdoor numbering system	• Independently plan complex routes using indoor/outdoor numbering systems • Apply numbering system in use of commercially available maps
Traffic concepts	• Describe basic pedestrian safety rules • Identify basic traffic controls (A3) • Identify intersection shapes • Identify parts/functions of cars, buses and other vehicles (ELAK)	• Describe relevant road markings and elements (for example, limit line, islands, medians) (FITL2) (A6) • Identify parallel and perpendicular traffic flows (FITL2) • Identify near/far lanes of traffic (A6) • Describe basic traffic patterns (FITL2) • Describe pedestrian/traffic timing at basic traffic light controls • Describe basic driver rules (for example, right turn on red, left-turn arrow) Estimate volume, speed, acceleration of traffic (S2) (S8)	• Describe complex road elements (for example, yield access lanes, double yellow lines, slip lanes) (FITL3) • Describe complex traffic controls/phasing • Compare timed versus actuated control traffic patterns • Describe traffic flow at one-way and atypical intersections	• Identify complex intersection configurations (for example, roundabout) • Describe freeway/interstate systems • Describe rail systems • Describe role of traffic engineer • Describe approaches to consumer advocacy in intersection accessibility

A = Azusa Unified School District Priority Goals Checklist (K–12)

FIT = Framework for Independent Travel
- Level 1 (L1) = coincides with Kindergarten–3rd grade
- Level 2 (L2) = coincides with grades 4–7
- Level 3 (L3) = coincides with grades 8–12

H = California Health Standards

M = California Math Standards

S = California Science Standards

ELA = California English-Language Arts Standards

VPA = California Visual and Performing Arts Standards

WM = Wisconsin Model Academic Math Standards from *Wisconsin adaptive skills: Resource guide.*

WSS = Wisconsin Model Academic Social Studies Standards from *Wisconsin adaptive skills: Resource guide.*

Sources: See Table 8.1A.

TABLE 8.1D

Age-Appropriate Curricular Guidelines—Sensory Skills

Sensory Skills	Kindergarten–3rd grade	4th–6th grade	7th–9th grade	10th–12th grade
Visual skills	• Process/analyze sensory information (AK) • Trace a stationary line • Use appropriate scanning patterns to locate people/objects while stationary • View objects eccentrically (as appropriate)	• Systematically scan the environment while moving • Track familiar moving objects	• Interpret visual cues to anticipate mobility challenges (for example, parked car with wheel half covered=curb) • Track unfamiliar moving objects	• Independently use visual cues • Integrate selective use of visual skills
Auditory skills	• Localize sound source • Identify/discriminate sound sources • Use basic reflected sounds for travel (for example, identify presence of object in travel path) • Create a sound source for echolocation	• Align/square off to sound sources • Use reflected sound to identify interior/exterior corners and recesses • Track a moving sound source	• Use reflected sounds to describe characteristics of objects (for example, height, density) • Explain the Doppler Effect (S9)	• Integrate selective use of all auditory skills
Optical and nonoptical device use	• Use low-power optical devices in familiar areas	• Use optical devices independently for O&M activities	• Use optical devices in daily routines	• Describe needs for optical devices to optometrist or others

Understanding pathology	• Offer simple explanation of how eyes do/don't work • Identify eye pathology	• Identify/describe eye pathology in simple terms • Identify/describe visual functioning	• Wear protective eye wear (for example, filters) • Label the parts of a monocular or other optical device	• Describe eye pathology and visual functioning in detail (S7) • Use model of the eye to describe the anatomy and physiology (S7)	• Select/order appropriate optical and nonoptical devices • Research eye pathology and synthesize information (ELA9/10)

A = Azusa Unified School District Priority Goals Checklist (K–12)

FIT = Framework for Independent Travel

- Level 1 (L1) = coincides with Kindergarten–3rd grade
- Level 2 (L2) = coincides with grades 4–7
- Level 3 (L3) = coincides with grades 8–12

H = California Health Standards

M = California Math Standards

S = California Science Standards

ELA = California English-Language Arts Standards

VPA = California Visual and Performing Arts Standards

WM = Wisconsin Model Academic Math Standards from *Wisconsin adaptive skills: Resource guide.*

WSS = Wisconsin Model Academic Social Studies Standards from *Wisconsin adaptive skills: Resource guide.*

Sources: See Table 8.1A.

travel expectations (for example, urban versus residential),

- parental perceptions of neighborhood, personal, and traffic safety, and
- parental comfort and typical family practice related to allowing children to travel with differing levels of supervision.

The development of age-appropriate O&M-related concepts and skills for school-age students can be very helpful in assisting O&M specialists in designing instructional programs. However, caution should be taken to ensure that age-based parameters such as those presented here are never used in place of O&M goals based on assessment of student needs, strengths, family priorities, and input from the educational team. To serve a heterogeneous population of school-age pupils with visual impairments, including students with additional disabilities, quality O&M instruction will always be individually designed (Orientation and Mobility Division of AER, 2006).

WHERE TO START: INDIVIDUALIZED ASSESSMENT AND INSTRUCTIONAL PLANNING FOR SCHOOL-AGE STUDENTS

Comprehensive O&M assessments involve students, families, and a host of teachers and related service professionals. These assessments are used for educational decision making, including eligibility for services and instructional planning. Decisions made based on a collection of assessment data can be high stakes for some students and families, making the difference as to whether or not a student receives appropriate services and determining the frequency and duration of those services. Considering the high-stakes nature of assessments, it seems that all children with visual impairments should receive O&M assessments from a qualified O&M specialist when the visual impairment is first identified. In fact, Goal No. 1

of the *National Agenda for the Education of Children and Youths with Visual Impairments, Including Those with Multiple Disabilities* (rev. ed.) (Huebner, Merk-Adam, Stryker, & Wolffe, 2004), states: "Students and their families will be referred to an appropriate education program within 30 days of identification of a suspected visual impairment. Teachers of students with visual impairments and orientation and mobility (O&M) instructors will provide appropriate quality services."

Goal No. 6 further supports the importance of O&M assessments for all students with diagnosed or suspected visual impairments. However, actual assessment practices may vary. In conducting a Delphi study with O&M specialists, Wall Emerson and Corn (2006) found most panelists agreed that the time of identification of visual impairment was the appropriate time to initiate the O&M assessment. There was lesser consensus about the impact of a child's visual status on the need for assessment. While some specialists felt that students with a visual acuity of 20/70 (6/21)–20/199 (6/60) should receive an O&M assessment, all agreed that students with a visual acuity of 20/200 (6/61)(or worse) or those who had a peripheral or central field loss should receive an O&M assessment. Recognizing the importance of O&M assessments for school-age students with visual impairments, it is essential that O&M specialists develop sound skills for conducting quality assessments.

Individualized Assessment

The ability to conduct quality O&M assessments with school-age students is a multifaceted skill set. O&M specialists need to

- understand the purpose for the given assessment (for example, IEP goal setting, monitoring of instructional effectiveness);
- identify domain areas to be assessed (for example, mobility skills, concepts, functional vision, and so on);

- select and/or adapt assessment instruments;
- plan ahead for age-appropriate assessment activities and materials;
- adapt assessment approaches for a wide range of student developmental and chronological abilities (K–12).

For a thorough review of the purposes, domains, and methods for O&M assessments, see Volume 1, Chapter 12. The following ideas build upon the foundational materials contained in that chapter, with additional considerations for conducting O&M assessments with school-age students that may assist O&M specialists to be increasingly successful in planning and conducting assessments with the K–12 population.

Developmental and Chronological Considerations

A unique aspect of conducting O&M assessments with school-age students is the need to plan for a very wide range of developmental abilities occurring in a mere span of 12 years. Just within the typical six years of elementary school, students go through dramatic changes in physical coordination, cognitive abilities, conceptual understanding, social maturity, and independent living skills that directly impact O&M skill development. Age differences often dictate the environments (for example, school campus, home neighborhood, local community, and businesses) in which children are expected to apply various skills and whether or not they do so independently or with supervision. O&M specialists need to be sensitive to age and developmental differences when selecting

- *which* domain items to assess
- *where* assessments should be conducted
- *what* assessment materials and activities to use accordingly

See Know the Grade: Age-Appropriate Curricular Guidelines in the previous section for a gen-eral guide or starting point for selecting items to assess within specific domain areas (individual differences will apply) and which environments may be appropriate.

Assessment Activities

Creativity in the selection of assessment activities can render great dividends in terms of student motivation (Boekaerts, 2002). Fun activities need not be reserved for instruction alone. Incorporating O&M assessment activities can enhance student participation and decrease student performance anxiety that is associated with the assessment process. For example, a kindergarten-age student might become withdrawn when told she will be asked to identify a list of body parts for an assessment. However, when incorporated within a fun and familiar game of Simon Says, the student may relax and perform to ability level. Table 8.2 provides an assortment of additional assessment activities that can be used with school-age students from kindergarten through high school.

Some professionals may assume that older students are not interested in games and activities and rely solely on O&M self-reports and skill demonstrations; however, individuals of all ages may enjoy participating in motivating activities for assessment, as evidenced by the popularity of game shows and "reality television." For example, students of high school age may be interested in demonstrating orientation skills in a challenge that is modeled on a popular reality television program, such as one fashioned after traditional orienteering challenges that incorporates competitions. Television game shows provide other possibilities for game themes that can be incorporated in assessments. For example, driving time can be optimized en route to the assessment by playing an O&M version of a trivia-type game show, full of address system questions or cardinal direction challenges. Common sense should be used when selecting the environment within

Ideas for Use of Demonstration, Games, and Activities in O&M Assessment

O&M Domain	Ideas for Conducting Demonstrations, Games, and Other Assessment Activities
Mobility skills • Protective techniques • Trailing • Human guide • Use of various cane techniques or other mobility devices in various environments	• Prepare a human guide obstacle course • Use role-playing, such as having young students pretend to be robots and they must follow every command • Create fun challenges for students to demonstrate skills • Reverse roles and ask the student to teach a technique via demonstration • Incorporate demonstrations in age-appropriate games or activities • Quiz students on when a given technique should be used
Orientation skills • Ability to detect and use landmarks • Ability to follow directions • Spatial updating • Plan and execute routes	• Incorporate landmarks within a treasure or scavenger hunt that is age-appropriate for the student • Ask student to serve as a "tour guide" to demonstrate orientation skills on a school campus or in a community area • Have student tape record each change of direction made along a travel route like a narrator or tour guide • Give student pushpin, Velcro, or magnet markers to place along a tactile map to designate a planned travel route
Concepts • Body concepts and body awareness • Spatial and positional concepts • Environmental concepts	• Do the Hokey Pokey with the youngest students to assess body part concepts and left and right. • Use a compartment hardware organizer and place nuts, bolts, screws, etc. using spatial terms to assist the adult in locating them in different spots • Prepare an incomplete map of a familiar area and have the student add labels or environmental features • Analyze games and activities for relevant concepts that may be assessed • Role-play money-use scenarios, such as banking, bus fare, etc. • Create a matching game using photos or drawings of environmental features and definition cards for students with low vision • Use toy cars on an intersection model to have students demonstrate understanding of traffic patterns
Visual functioning • Functional fields • Functional acuity • Visual skills such as tracing, scanning, and tracking • Use of optical devices	• Use age-appropriate targets (for example, toys for young children, CD jacket covers for teenagers, and playing cards for older students) to assess functional fields and acuity • Ask students with low vision to label monocular parts on a worksheet • Attach inflated balloons to a wall for students to locate via visual scanning—O&M coupons are contained inside balloons • Arrange a guessing game of "which street has more?" and have the student visually count moving traffic volume on two different streets • Play "The Price Is Right" at a fast food restaurant, having the student use a monocular to identify three food items that total less than $5.00

(continued on next page)

TABLE 8.2 (Continued)	
O&M Domain	Ideas for Conducting Demonstrations, Games, and Other Assessment Activities
Auditory functioning • Ability to identify, localize, and track sounds • Ability to adjust body position in relation to sounds	• Ask young children to track a moving toy with an auditory sound source • Practice locating dropped objects • Arrange a guessing game of "which street has more?" and have the student count moving traffic volume using hearing on two different streets • Identify prerecorded sound sources on an audiotape • Challenge student to align and square off to recorded age-appropriate music

which an assessment activity is conducted. For example, while high school students may enjoy an obstacle-course activity in an individual or small group setting, they might be embarrassed to engage in the activity on the high school campus, where the possibility exists of peers passing by. The O&M specialist must also effectively set the tone for the activity with a positive demeanor and in an age-appropriate manner.

Instructional Planning

A fundamental aspect of instructional planning is the development of the IEP. The purposes of the IEP are to create a blueprint of the student's educational program, set priority goals and benchmarks for the year, and set the stage for a team approach to education. In addition to the development of appropriate goals and benchmarks based on comprehensive O&M assessment, O&M specialists are advised to consult with students, families, and other educators regarding their priorities, which can be considered, as appropriate, for goal setting. At the start of the written document, the O&M specialist will prepare a written narrative description of the student's present level of O&M skills that is based on assessment. The description should be clear, concise, and specific and avoid professional jargon. It also should have

a positive tone and include student strengths and areas of improvement, addressing goals that were met and those not met from the previous year. This section of the IEP should be a logical link to future goals.

Clearly defined behavioral measures, either quantitative or qualitative, noted at the beginning of the IEP year, enable O&M specialists to document student outcomes. For example, an assessment may yield quantitative data such as the percent of time that a specific cane technique is executed properly or the distance at which a student can accurately recognize a visual target. The same items would then be assessed during and at the end of the year so that growth can be demonstrated. Similarly, qualitative assessment results, such as stated attitudes toward cane use or teacher-reported satisfaction with level of independent campus travel, can be compared with results obtained following instruction. A high mark of professionalism is maintaining concrete and accurate records of student achievement that demonstrate accountability.

O&M goals should be directly related to assessed student needs and family priorities and be clearly described in the description of present levels of performance. Goals are intended to be broad in scope. Two to three annual O&M goals in an annual IEP are typical; however, the

---

SIDEBAR 8.1

Sample O&M Goal and Benchmarks

GOAL

Casey will safely cross at four-way residential intersections that are controlled by stop signs.

Benchmarks

1. Casey will identify "all quiet" traffic patterns at four-way residential intersections that are controlled by stop signs with 100 percent accuracy, as observed by the O&M specialist by December 2006.

2. Casey will demonstrate appropriate cane techniques for completing street crossings at four-way residential intersections that are controlled by stop signs with a maximum of one instructor prompt, as recorded by the O&M specialist by April 2007.

3. Casey will complete crossings at four-way residential intersections that are controlled by stop signs with minimal veering, 9 out of 10 attempts, as recorded by the O&M specialist by June 2007.

---

exact number is determined by the needs of the individual student and with input from the educational team. While benchmarks are no longer required for students who are assessed according to general-education standards, it still may be appropriate to develop O&M benchmarks since there are not standardized assessments available to use. Benchmarks are required for IEP goals for students who are being assessed according to alternative standards. They are logical steps to be accomplished in efforts to achieve the identified goal and to monitor progress along the way. Benchmarks should include:

- *Who*—target student

- *What is expected*—behavior or skill

- *Conditions*—for example, student is given a tactile map

- *Criterion for measuring goal attainment*—level of accuracy, percent, or number of trials

- *How it will be measured*—for example, by observation of O&M specialist

- *By when*—date leading up to the goal

- *Who is responsible*—O&M specialists and possibly others

Benchmarks are described in behavioral terms (for example, cross, identify, complete, demonstrate, use, and so on). They are measurable steps that are required to reach the goal(s) recommended by the O&M specialist and agreed upon by the educational team. For a sample O&M goal and benchmarks, see Sidebar 8.1

At the IEP meeting, the O&M specialist should be prepared with a written statement of present level of functioning and a written draft of O&M goals and benchmarks. Input from team members should be solicited at the meeting and O&M specialists need to be prepared to edit goals accordingly. Once the blueprint is established, O&M specialists can focus on instructional planning and teaching strategies.

O&M TEACHING APPROACHES, TOOLS, AND TIPS

Good teaching in orientation and mobility requires selecting an appropriate instructional approach and skillfully applying it with an individual student. Regardless of the approach selected, the O&M specialist will need a toolbox full of creative teaching strategies, relevant instructional units, well-thought-out lesson plans, and meaningful learning activities. When exploring creative ideas, O&M specialists may consider individual learning styles and the use of interesting teaching materials, activities, games, role-playing, and group lessons.

Instructional Approaches

With careful thought, O&M specialists can select from general teaching approaches, including teacher-directed and student-initiated approaches and discovery learning. The use of individual learning styles, such as those proposed by Gardner's *Multiple Intelligences* (1993), can be used to enhance any of these approaches (see Volume 1, Chapter 7 for additional information on learning theories). Considering student strengths in various areas of intelligences and incorporating student learning styles in O&M teaching can enhance teacher-directed, student-initiated, and discovery-learning approaches.

Teacher-Directed Learning

The teacher-directed approach to designing lessons is familiar to most instructors, as it is commonly used in K–12 and higher-education classrooms. Teacher-directed experiences, also referred to as guided learning (Jacobson & Bradley, Volume 1, Chapter 7), consist primarily of verbal explanations, behavioral modeling, and guided and independent practice. For example, O&M specialists may choose to describe with words the centered hand position to use with two-point touch cane technique, while the student uses listening skills to process the information and perform the technique. Alternatively, O&M specialists may elect to actually demonstrate the hand position to a student who has low vision (with or without the accompanying verbal description) or use hand-under-hand modeling for a student who is visually impaired (when the instructor's hand is under the student's hand, allowing the student greater control of the situation). (For more

information on the use of the long cane, see Chapter 1.) In each instance, the student is directly told or shown how to perform a skill and is then provided with opportunities for guided practice, with feedback from the teacher, so that the skill or concept is refined. Independent practice can be encouraged in the form of classroom assignments or homework.

When used with creative teaching strategies, directed learning can be very effective and efficient with school-age students in:

- providing an introduction to new content
- teaching a physical skill with specific steps
- helping a student to memorize important facts
- presenting a sequence of skills in a preferred order

The success of this method relies heavily on the skills with which the instructor presents new information through verbalizations or demonstrations and the quality of practice opportunities provided. The instructor must be clear, accurate, and skilled at keeping the student's attention and give feedback that is specific and encouraging. Broad guidelines suggest that primary-grade students are able to best maintain attention during lesson chunks of approximately 15–20 minutes, upper elementary school students in chunks of 20–30 minutes, and secondary school students up to 45 minutes.

In order to maximize this teaching approach with school-age students, O&M specialists may want to consider creating

- interesting lesson introductions;
- varied methods of presenting information or modeling techniques;
- fun approaches to rehearsing verbal information or practicing physical skills;
- Ample success-oriented, guided practice opportunities.

As an introduction, an O&M specialist may choose to start the lesson by piquing the student's curiosity with a story that encourages the child to wonder about the best or safest manner to approach the given O&M task. For example, the O&M specialist may relay a short story to a very young student about the "three little pigs and the big bad wolf" in which the mother sent the little pigs off to cross a very big street, asking them to be very careful. As the story unfolds, there will obviously be two bad examples of street crossings and one positive example that keeps the third pig safe from cars and the big bad wolf. Following the story, the student is interested and engaged in thinking about street crossings and the specialist then proceeds to instruct the student in a sequence of steps that can be used for safe street crossings with supervision at the given intersection—just like the third pig, who saved his brothers from the big bad wolf.

While the teacher-directed approach relies heavily on instructor presentation of information, there is nothing that precludes the information from being presented in an interesting fashion. For example, a student of middle school age might like an audiotape presentation of the steps to a new skill in a "Mission Impossible" theme. Other students might benefit from route directions that are accompanied by tactile flip cards that are helpful for remembering the route segments. Teacher-directed learning experiences also can be followed up with interesting opportunities for practicing newly learned skills, such as reversing roles in which the student then teaches the skill to the teacher or completing a mobility obstacle course to refine the newly learned cane skills. The obstacle course can be designed to accommodate a variety of age and ability levels. For more examples of teacher-directed instructional activities for students of elementary and secondary school ages, see Table 8.3.

Planned opportunities for guided and independent practice are essential if students are to fully learn physical skills or to apply concepts in natural settings. While repetition is necessary for learning many skills and concepts, it does not have to take the form of drill practice. Taking a simple-to-complex approach to practicing newly learned skills may mean that the practice of a physical skill (such as touch-and-drag technique) initially may be isolated in drill fashion (simple), but as the motor skill becomes more automatic, cane skill practice can be integrated into functional routines (complex), such as delivering notes to the office or orientation tasks, such as challenging scavenger or treasure hunts on campus. Independent practice occurs during the natural routine at school or home, and teachers and families need to be well informed as to expectations for skill use in various environments and the frequency of practice needed.

While the advantages of teacher-directed learning approaches are clear, an overreliance on this approach can result in students becoming passive recipients of information rather than actively engaged learners. As O&M specialists work to promote independence, they need to encourage critical thinking (such as choosing between two orientation strategies), risk taking, and problem solving in their students. Doing so may require the use of additional and complimentary learning approaches.

Student-Initiated Learning

For school-age students, the IEP drives the instructional process and sets the stage for the teaching and learning that is to happen during the year. Unless the student is invited to participate in designing goals (which is highly recommended, but not always a practical reality), the instructional sequence is typically teacher-directed. However, students can initiate learning by sharing with the O&M specialist a specific need for a skill, orientation challenges for a particular route, or general areas of interest. These occasions can be used to motivate students and to increase their under-

TABLE 8.3

Instructional Approaches for Students of Elementary and Secondary School Age

Instructional Approaches	Elementary School-Age Students	Secondary School-Age Students
Teacher initiated	• Using a Dora the Explorer theme, take student for an adventure walk on the school campus. Afterward, have student note key locations, landmarks, buildings, etc. on a skeleton map (orientation skills) • Plan for student to make three consecutive street crossings en route to a local park for playtime (mobility skills)	• Assign student with low vision to use MapQuest to obtain directions from his home to a local mall (orientation skills) • Create a student street-veering challenge that requires the student to make five crossings, measure the inches of veer for each, and compute an average veer in inches (mobility skills)
Student initiated	• Ask student to identify a favorite place on campus and assist in building a map of the area (orientation skills) • After student expresses interest in being able to walk to neighbor's house, street-crossing lessons are focused within that route (mobility skills)	• Student identifies interest in summer jobs and after generating a list of possibilities together, calls for directions to pick up job applications (orientation skills) • Along an O&M route, student expresses curiosity when hearing an audible pedestrian signal (APS), and a mini-unit on street crossings at APS-controlled intersections is conducted (mobility skills)
Discovery learning	• There is construction on the school campus that interferes with usual route to playground; give student the opportunity to plan and try out an alternative route (orientation skills) • A student explores tactile models of different intersection shapes and discovers different characteristics between plus-shape and T-shape intersections (street crossing)	• Student is given an address to locate that does not follow the typical local address system and must problem solve how to locate the destination (orientation skills) • Student encounters an anomaly (for example, a crowd or construction) at an intersection that prevents him from independently crossing the street; after student brainstorms possible alternative methods to cross, he selects one to try (with instructor approval) and evaluates effectiveness afterward (street crossing)

standing of the purpose and perceived relevance of O&M training.

In order to successfully incorporate student initiatives within the O&M instructional process, the O&M specialist should be able to

- encourage student curiosity as part of orientation and mobility;
- plan lessons around student interests;
- make good use of spontaneous learning moments;
- allow students to share in aspects of instructional planning.

Student curiosity can be encouraged in many ways (Fazzi & Petersmeyer, 2001). O&M specialists can prepare students to ask questions on each O&M lesson or take time to answer student questions. *Where's Waldo?* is a familiar book and associated game for school-age children. A similar theme can be developed for O&M lessons to help students of elementary school age wonder where Waldo may be hiding on the school campus today. A similar elementary-level theme is based on the book series *Flat Stanley* in which a flat paper doll is made and sent to friends and family members around the country and the world and returned with photos from the many interesting destinations. Such activities can be adapted for students with visual impairments in the local or global community and help build strong interest in unfamiliar areas and a general interest in travel.

Once a student's area of interest is known, lessons can be planned in advance to incorporate motivating features. For example, if a student of high school age has a strong interest in architecture, the O&M specialist can arrange for a variety of interesting travel destinations that involve residences or buildings with interesting architectural styles. In fact, the student may use the Internet to locate particular buildings of interest and plan routes as homework.

Following student initiatives can sometimes be planned in advance, but other opportunities may arise when least expected—sometimes in the middle of O&M lessons. For example, while working on cane skills on campus, a student of elementary school age encounters a ladder being used by the custodian. While the ladder is not related to the lesson objective, the O&M specialist must quickly decide whether or not it is meaningful to sidetrack to explore the ladder and the many related concepts that can be experienced firsthand. There will be many instances during orientation and mobility in which the student's interest in an object or event will be worthwhile to pursue and there will be times when it is prudent to stick to the lesson plan (see Bozeman & McCulley, Chapter 2).

Student initiatives also can be encouraged when students are actively involved in the construction of tactile maps, models, and other instructional materials. For example, when a middle school student is asked to construct an ideal residential or light business neighborhood on a given map or diagram, the perceptive O&M specialist may begin to notice areas of student interest or curiosity. Those areas can be incorporated in actual travel lessons later.

Making good use of student initiatives means that O&M specialists allow students to be either directly or indirectly involved in some aspects of instructional planning. This does not mean that the start of each lesson begins with the question: "Where would you like to go today?" Rather, it means that school-age students can be involved in short- and long-term planning for O&M goals. (See Table 8.3 for additional examples of student-initiated approaches to instruction).

Discovery Learning

Different from the teacher-directed approach, "in discovery learning the material to be learned is not taught by the instructor, but it is discovered by the learner while working through a problem"

(Jacobson & Bradley, 1997, p. 378). Discovery learning works particularly well with some orientation and problem-solving tasks; however, it would be less effective and efficient in teaching specific skills that have step-by-step procedures (for example, two-point touch technique). Montessori schools are well known for their emphasis on creating child-centered learning environments in which the focus is on discovery—"children learning, not on teachers teaching" (Montessori method, 2009). The design of Montessori learning is based on the premise that children have an intrinsic desire to learn about the world, master skills, and become independent beings. The use of external motivators (for example, stickers, praise, and other rewards) is discouraged, as they are believed to create passivity and dependence in otherwise self-motivated learners. Montessori classrooms are designed and modified to meet the abilities and interests of the children as they move about freely to engage in hands-on activities with real items of their own choosing. O&M instruction for school-age children can readily incorporate many aspects promoted in Montessori's teachings. O&M learning already takes place in natural settings and presents many real-life challenges from which children may engage in problem solving under the supervision of the O&M specialist. Discovery learning challenges students to construct their understanding of the world through manipulation of objects and application of problem-solving strategies at the developmental level of the child (Piaget, 1963). Hands-on activities clearly have been shown to be an effective method of teaching concepts to students who are blind and visually impaired (Fazzi & Petersmeyer, 2001; Recchia, 1997; Skellenger and Sapp, Chapter 7).

In order for the discovery-learning approach to be successful with school-age students, these students must have the developmental readiness (cognitive and physical ability) to learn from the level of orientation challenge or mobility skill application required on a given lesson. In addition, the student must have the motivation and confidence to attempt to solve the problem presented. Motivation may be intrinsic (within the child) or extrinsic (reinforced by the environment or directly by people). Confidence can be developed or maintained over time, when success is experienced in foundational lessons (see Welsh, Volume 1, Chapter 6).

There are a variety of purposes for which O&M specialists may elect to employ discovery approaches to learning within the sequence of instruction. Discovery-learning approaches can be helpful in moving students from passive recipients of knowledge given from teachers to an active role of seeking answers from trial and error. This active role can ultimately support a higher level of independence for students. Discovery learning also can be an effective tool in helping students to understand the importance of using appropriate cane or related travel skills when O&M specialists are not present to serve as a safety net. Students can learn from mistakes that might result in light encounters with obstacles caused by using the long cane inappropriately, or in occasional periods of disorientation when they fail to establish landmarks along a route. However, it is ultimately the responsibility of all credentialed or certified teachers in public schools to take the necessary procedures to ensure student safety at school and during school activities.

For school-age students, discovery learning is not simply something that should always happen by chance; rather, it is a well-planned emphasis of the training process. In other words, lesson plans can include discovery learning as part of the planned methodology to achieve established goals. Learning through student discovery can be optimized when:

- Students are ready to learn from the selected travel environment.

- Previously learned concepts or skills are reviewed to help focus students on the task.

• Learning environments are well chosen so that students experience an exciting challenge without high levels of frustration.

At the elementary school age, students are most ready to benefit from the orientation challenges of discovery learning after they have the prerequisite concepts and skills. For example, students need to use landmarks and have successful experiences in designing independent routes and route reversals before route detours can be discovered independently. O&M specialists might review the importance of appropriate cane skills to use before asking a student of middle school age to explore one block of a light business area in order to discover the different environmental features from those previously experienced in residential travel environments. A high school student may discover the exceptions to the address system layout in an area with many open businesses from which information can be readily obtained. For additional ideas on instructional approaches that incorporate aspects of discovery learning, see Table 8.3, in which the teacher-directed, student-initiated, and discovery-learning approaches were compared, incorporating appropriate activities for both elementary school and secondary school. Similar curricular areas were used to highlight the differences between the instructional approaches. O&M specialists easily can expand the activities presented and incorporate different learning approaches that will most effectively meet the needs of their students.

The ability to distinguish among the different teaching approaches leads to the instructor's ability to purposely select a given approach that will best suit the curriculum covered, the environment taught in, and the student's individual abilities. In a simplified manner, teacher-directed approaches are effectively employed when specific skills are introduced, and discovery learning works well when students are equipped to handle problem-solving situations. Incorporating student initiatives creates greater interest and potential for increased investment in learning. There are instances when elements of all three instructional approaches can be combined to create very effective lessons and learning outcomes.

Use of Learning Styles

Not all students learn best in the same manner and not all teachers have the same instructional strengths. With this fact in mind, O&M specialists can assess student learning styles and adjust instructional approaches accordingly to optimize success in the achievement of independent travel skills and knowledge. Gardner (in Guignon, 1998, p. 3) states: "It's very important that a teacher take individual differences among kids very seriously. . . . The bottom line is a deep interest in children and how their minds are different from one another, and in helping them use their minds well." Researchers with Project SUMIT (school using multiple intelligences theory) reviewed the performance of a number of schools using multiple intelligences theory and reported significant improvements in the areas of Scholastic Aptitude Test (SAT) scores, parental participation, and discipline (Kornhaber et al., 2000).

Fazzi and Petersmeyer (2001) have applied the multiple intelligences theory (Gardner, 1993) to teaching and learning styles in orientation and mobility. While many different learning style theories have been postulated, the multiple intelligences theory allows for individualization of teaching so that O&M specialists can plan to vary their own teaching styles to match those of their students. Eight distinct intelligences identified by Gardner (1993) are:

• linguistic (language, both written and spoken)

• musical (auditory, linked to pitch, rhythm, and timbre)

• logical-mathematical (numbers, symbols, physical, and abstract reasoning)

• spatial (shapes, forms, and design)

- bodily-kinesthetic (movement with coordination and perception)
- interpersonal (awareness of others' needs and intentions)
- intrapersonal (sense of self)
- naturalist (observe, understand, and organize patterns in nature)

Each of these areas of intelligence can be incorporated easily through various instructional strategies. O&M specialists can optimize success in orientation and mobility when teaching approaches match their students' strongest learning styles, such as teaching a student with high linguistic intelligence by using verbal explanations, word challenges, and puzzles. A student's learning style can then be paired with the skill that is challenging to acquire, such as using a metronome to teach the rhythm of the cane movement to a student who is strong in musical but weak in the bodily-kinesthetic intelligence.

Assessing intelligence strengths is not an exact science, but rather a reflective process that may combine a variety of approaches, including review of student records, student-family interviews, observation of lessons, and completing a brief inventory. Fazzi and Petersmeyer (2001) provide information on assessing student learning styles and adapting O&M instructional methods accordingly. Table 8.4 provides sample instructional strategies that are categorized according to five of the eight intelligences.

Instructional approaches provide the blueprint for designing customized lessons, but are of limited use without the specific tools necessary to implement an effective lesson. Teaching strategies are the tools with which O&M specialists implement lesson plans.

Teaching Strategies and Tools

Regardless of the learning approach being utilized, O&M specialists need to be prepared to incorporate a variety of specific teaching strategies to organize and sequence lessons in order to optimize student learning.

Lesson Format and Strategies

Madeline Hunter (1979) is well known in educational fields for her expertise in educational planning. She emphasized the importance of planning meaningful objectives, creating student anticipation for learning, and using guided and independent practice. Hunter suggested a variety of strategies for introducing key lesson content, modeling, and checking for understanding. Sidebar 8.2 provides a sample O&M lesson plan that incorporates several of these elements.

Lesson objectives paint a clear picture of what the student is expected to learn by lesson completion. The lesson objective should be measurable and indicate the level or degree of proficiency the student is expected to achieve so that lesson success can be clearly measured, for example: "The student will spot a traffic light and identify the changing colors four of five times using a monocular telescope."

O&M specialists can help students prepare for what will occur during the upcoming lesson by creating an anticipatory set. Lesson introductions can be used to:

- focus the student's attention
- engage the student's interest
- provide an organized preview of the lesson
- relate new information to previously learned skills or concepts

A creative anticipatory set can pique student interest and engage participation in learning. In the example provided earlier for monocular use at a traffic light, the student might be hooked by reminding him that a destination of interest can only be reached by crossing a particularly complex intersection. The monocular skills previously learned and practiced will need to be

TABLE 8.4

Orientation and Mobility and Five of the Eight Intelligences

Type of Intelligence	Cane Skills	Intersection Analysis	Visual Efficiency Skills	Maps and Mapmaking	Auditory Training
Linguistic	Recite rhymes or poems while practicing the two-point touch cane technique	Select the correct order of cards that describe individual procedures for crossing light–controlled traffic intersections	Spot-on letter targets of different sizes, colors, or fonts	Give an oral report to the class about a map you have made of a certain travel area	Listen to environmental sounds; write what each sound is on a card; use the cards to make sentences
Musical	Practice wrist movements with the "grip cane" (grip with marshmallow tip on end) on a table to music or metronome	Identify by sound: trucks, cars, buses, and motorcycles	Use a monocular to view an orchestra, choir, or band	Write lyrics to recall a route; sing them while traveling	Use a tape recorder to identify, compare, and contrast sounds heard during a lesson
Logical-mathematical	Keep chart for the number of times specific cane skills were used correctly	Use a stopwatch to compare the timing of traffic light–controlled intersections	Assemble a large visual puzzle (of the world, states, continents, and so on)	Use a ruler to make a grid pattern for a map	Count the number of cars passing through streets at a stop sign–controlled intersection
Spatial	Use arc to compare the width of objects or distance between objects	Photograph/ draw shapes of different types of traffic light housings and their signals (housings with 3, 4, 5, or 6 lights in them)	Visually trace or scan lines or shapes on a target with a monocular	Assemble LEGO pieces to make a map of a real or imaginary place	Identify pictures/ shapes of different utility vehicles heard (garbage truck, street cleaner, and so forth)
Bodily-kinesthetic	Perform feet and leg warm-ups before stair travel with the use of the long cane	Play "Red Light, Green Light" with a group on parallel and perpendicular hallways/ pathways	Learn correct hand/eye/ head coordination to use a monocular effectively	Act out a neighborhood block on a rug with props (interactive model)	Practice keeping the feet still while turning the head to hear a traffic surge

Source: Adapted with permission from "Integrating Individual Teaching and Learning Styles: Motivating O&M Instruction," in Diane L. Fazzi and Barbara A. Petersmeyer, *Imagining the Possibilities: Creative Approaches to Orientation and Mobility Instruction for Persons Who Are Visually Impaired* (New York: AFB Press, 2001), p. 164.

SIDEBAR 8.2

Sample Lesson Plan

Student: Mackenzie

Instructor: Earl

Date: 01–14

Time: 10:15–11:45 a.m.

Lesson Location: Doverwood Drive and Bristol Parkway

Lesson Objective: Mackenzie will spot a traffic light and the changing colors four of five times using a monocular telescope.

Lesson Materials: monocular telescope, long cane, visor

Lesson Introduction (anticipatory set): Ask student to recall her favorite bakeshop, the Robinson Bakery, located on Bristol Parkway. Note the complex phasing of the intersection needed to be crossed in order to get there. Give student challenge to identify light change four of five times and be given opportunity to travel to Robinson Bakery and purchase a treat.

Instructional Steps:

1. Begin lesson at simple traffic light–controlled intersection south of Doverwood Drive and Bristol Parkway.

2. Ask student to demonstrate skills by instructing me on how to use the monocular at this intersection.

3. Verbalize any missing information to student. Use effective questioning to check for student understanding.

4. Provide student with opportunity for guided practice in use of a monocular at a simple intersection. Provide verbal prompts as needed.

5. When student demonstrates proficiency, move to complex intersection and provide opportunity for independent practice.

Evaluation: Ask student to identify when she is ready for a challenge, and evaluate to see if the student meets lesson criteria (four of five trials). If student does not meet competency, provide additional guided practice.

Lesson Culmination: End lesson with trip to Robinson Bakery.

---

used skillfully at this new intersection in order to get to the destination. Other "hooks" might incorporate a lesson challenge (for example, a taste-testing challenge at three different bakeries), the start of a collaborative project (for example, building a map of a local community together), or reviewing the student's O&M travel portfolio to determine areas that need additional practice.

The lesson content (for example, diagonal cane technique method or compass directions) is commonly presented through verbalization of information and modeling of techniques.

Verbalization may include specific step-by-step instructions, labeling of environmental features, comparing similarities and differences of skills or concepts, categorizing techniques and information, using analogies, and discussing new material. Recorded or written information can also be used to teach O&M content. Modeling may include physical demonstration, presentation of examples and products, observation of others, and role-play scenarios. It is important to plan to check for understanding throughout the presentation of new learning material. Students also can be asked to demonstrate techniques, repeat route directions back to the instructor, or reverse roles by teaching the instructor the concept or skill. Use of questions can be an effective means to gauge the student's level of comprehension and recall of information. Bloom's taxonomy (Bloom, Englehart, Furst, Hill, & Krathwohl, 1956) identifies specific levels of learning and cognitive complexity in a hierarchy that has been translated to levels of O&M questions in Table 8.5. Fazzi and Petersmeyer (2001) discuss effective questioning techniques and how to avoid common questioning mistakes in orientation and mobility.

Practice is an essential element of learning. O&M specialists provide feedback, assistance, and supervision during guided practice. This opportunity is important for refining techniques and conceptual understanding. Instructor assistance and feedback gradually will be reduced as students gain in competence. Once students have mastered the content, they need to be provided with opportunities for independent practice. Independent practice is important so that students maintain skills and concepts and are able to apply them with ease. In O&M lessons, independent practice presents an interesting conundrum because of the safety considerations for school-age children; therefore, independent practice during the school day should include planned safety monitoring when it is expected that all students will be under the direct supervision of a certificated/credentialed teacher/specialist during school hours. Families may provide additional opportunities for independent practice as appropriate during home hours. See Creative Ideas later in

---

TABLE 8.5

Levels of Questions

Level of Learning	Cognitive Activity	Sample Question
Knowledge	Recall	*"What bus number are you supposed to take?"*
Comprehension	Interpret, translate, summarize	*"How do you know this intersection has a four-way stop?"*
Application	Use information in a new situation	*"Which lining-up technique would you use at this crossing?"*
Analysis	Separate the whole into parts until the relationship between them is clear	*"What category of intersections does this one belong to?"*
Synthesis	Combine elements to form a new entity	*"What is an alternate route to locate your classroom from the bus stop?"*
Evaluation	Act of decision making, judging	"What is the most appropriate technique to use at this crossing, and why would you use that one?"

Source: Reprinted with permission from "Preparing for Teaching: Comprehensive Assessment," in Diane L. Fazzi and Barbara A. Petersmeyer, *Imagining the Possibilities: Creative Approaches to Orientation and Mobility Instruction for Persons Who Are Visually Impaired* (New York: AFB Press, 2001), p. 18. Based on Bloom's Taxonomy of Learning; see B. Bloom, M. Englehart, E. Furst, W. Hill, & D. Krathwohl, *Taxonomy of Educational Objectives.* Handbook 1: *Cognitive Domain* (New York: David McKay, 1956).

this chapter for ways to enhance guided and independent practice.

Fundamental Teaching Tools

In addition to the effective verbalization, modeling, questioning, and guided and independent practice strategies described previously, there are other basic teaching tools that will help O&M specialists teach school-age children in an effective manner. Teaching tools addressed in this section include: instructional prompting, task analysis, behavioral chaining, scaffolding, and positive behavior supports. O&M specialists may find individual techniques or a combination of these techniques to be particularly useful with given students and lesson content (see Jacobson & Bradley, Volume 1, Chapter 7).

Instructional Prompting

Natural cues can be found in the environment that will prompt students to initiate or complete given tasks. For example, the sound of the bell ringing at the end of recess prompts most children to get in line to return to class. For those children who do not line up, there are typically consequences, such as being sent to the principal's office, which help them learn to complete the task in the future. Teachers and school staff need to make sure that students with visual impairments also experience these natural consequences so that they have equal opportunities to learn from them. Still, there may be some children for whom natural cues and consequences are insufficient, and they require instructional prompting to learn the task at hand.

Instructional prompts are additional cues designed to encourage students to perform specific behaviors or tasks. For students who need instructional prompting, a hierarchy of prompting techniques that go from least to most intrusive can be used (for sample hierarchies, see Dote-

Kwan, 1995). A simple hierarchy of prompts, ranging from least to most assistance, may include:

- natural cue (no instructor prompt)
- indirect verbal prompt
- direct verbal prompt
- modeling
- light physical prompt
- physical guidance

For example, while traveling a campus route to the music room, a student consistently does not make the appropriate turn onto the intersecting walkway. The natural consequence of reaching the end of the path does not seem sufficient to trigger the response to turn. The O&M specialist may next try an *indirect verbal prompt*, such as: "I think I hear someone playing the piano." If this level of prompt is not successful, then the next level would be to provide a *direct verbal prompt*, such as: "Turn right now." Increasingly more intrusive prompts might include modeling, a light physical prompt, such as tapping the right elbow, coactively moving with the student to make the turn, or by physically guiding the student to make the turn. Once the student is able to successfully complete the task with instructional prompts, the teacher will want to make sure to gradually *fade* the use of prompts through either progressively moving to a less-intrusive form of prompting or by decreasing the number of prompts provided so that the student can complete the task with less assistance.

Some students may benefit from other visual and tactile/object cues that can be used as instructional prompts and routine markers throughout the student's day, as needed. An example of a visual cue for a student with low vision would be a picture (or series of pictures) of the next landmark(s) to be sought along a route. Calendar boxes can incorporate a variety of object cues (for example, a washcloth, milk carton, cane tip, and so on) to prompt a student as to the order of events on a given school day. (See Chapter 20 for additional information on instructional prompting and the use of object cues and calendar boxes.)

Task Analysis

A task analysis is the key ability to break down a lesson, task, or skill into smaller, sequential, and manageable parts. The purposes of the process are to ensure that:

- The task or lesson does not overwhelm the student or teacher.
- Key elements of the task are not skipped over.
- The task is taught in a sequential manner.

The task analysis may clearly provide a step-by-step lesson plan or may result in a series of nicely sequenced lesson plans. A lesson on street-crossing skills easily can be broken into a sequence of steps to be followed at an intersection for a student able to learn at a rapid pace or into a series of sequenced lesson plans in which each step is further broken down to be learned. For example, one lesson for a particular student could contain the following seven steps to be learned:

1. alignment
2. intersection analysis
3. determine safe timing
4. initiate crossing
5. maintain straight crossing
6. negotiate up curb
7. recovery from veer

In contrast, for a student with a slower learning pace, each of the steps above could be broken down into much smaller segments and be taught over a series of lessons. In both cases, completing the task analysis has been worthwhile because it has provided a sequential approach and it will help to ensure that students are only taught as much as they can handle in a given lesson. The task analysis also will help the O&M specialist better analyze student strengths and weaknesses related to the given task. For example, in the seven-step lesson outlined earlier, the O&M specialist could readily note which skill is presenting a student with difficulty rather than simply noting that the lesson objective was not achieved.

For students who require the use of a frequent or complex combination of instructional prompts, it may be useful for the O&M specialist to create a task analysis and instructional prompting chart, as shown in Figure 8.1. The use of a chart assists the instructor in establishing a systematic approach and provides a means for documenting progress. The results of such charting can be shared with the educational team as appropriate.

This chart uses a scoring system in which the highest score is given for steps completed without instructional prompts; therefore, the higher the total score, the higher the overall level of student independence. The percentages are helpful in representing the student's degree of growth.

Forward and Backward Chaining

Chaining (also referred to as *behavioral chaining*) is a process closely related to task analysis by which an instructor can string together the sequential behaviors required of a given task. In forward chaining, the first step of the sequence is mastered before the second step is introduced to the child. In an example of forward chaining used in teaching residential street crossings, the student is introduced to a given alignment procedure and helped to learn the technique until it is mastered. The second step is then addressed similarly. Mastery may occur in one lesson or over a series of lessons, depending on the child and the lesson time frame.

In contrast, backward chaining requires that the teacher perform all of the steps in the sequence (through modeling, physical guidance,

Objective: Counterclockwise Street Crossings (Low Vision Traveler)								
Date Collection: *At end of O&M Instructional Session* (final trial)								
Instructional Prompts:								
3 = No Prompt (natural cue/independent)								
2 = Indirect Verbal Prompt								
1 = Direct Verbal Prompt								
0 = Did Not Demonstrate								
Date:	4/01	4/03	4/05					
Instructional Prompt Used:								
1. Identifies type of traffic light *control*	2	2	2					
2. Identifies *shape* of intersection	1	2	2					
3. Identifies *traffic patterns*	1	1	2					
4. Actuates pedestrian button (if present)	2	3	3					
5. Positions self appropriately on corner for crossing (has cane "on display")	1	3	3					
6. Identifies safe time to cross (near-side/surge or sees pedestrian light)	1	3	3					
7. Looks over the shoulder to left (for potential right-hand turners) *prior to* stepping off curb	1	1	2					
8. Looks to direct left *prior to* stepping off curb	0	0	0					
9. Signals long arc *prior to initiating crossing*	0	0	3					
10. Looks to left and ahead during first half of crossing (lane by lane)	2	2	1					
11. Looks to right *prior to* entering second half of crossing	2	2	1					
12. Looks to right and ahead during second half of crossing (lane by lane)	2	2	1					
13. Looks for up curb	3	3	3					
14. Clears up curb with cane and steps up	0	2	1					
TOTAL SCORE (INSTRUCTIONAL PROMPTS)	18	26	27					
TOTAL POSSIBLE SCORE	42	42	42					
PERCENTAGE: (Level of Independence)	43%	62%	64%					

Figure 8.1. Sample O&M Task Analysis

or coactive movements) except for the last step, which the child is taught to complete. In learning a school campus route, the O&M specialist may incorporate backward chaining by walking the student through the first five segments of a six-segment route and having the student complete the final segment. Once the final segment is mastered, the student will be expected to complete the last two and so on. This teaching strategy can be very effective when traveling routes, because the student is successful in completing the route more frequently and experiences the satisfaction of reaching the desired destination.

Some students will do well when introduced to the entire task in sequence (whole-task chaining) and then practice each of the steps during every lesson or attempt. When addressing the total task in this manner, the student is afforded more opportunities for practicing each step.

Scaffolding

The instructional strategy known as *scaffolding* is an important feature of Vygotsky's (1978) theory of social cognition. (For more information on social cognitive learning theories, see Volume 1, Chapters 6 and 7.) Social cognitive theory emphasizes that children (novices) learn from problem-solving experiences mediated by teachers (experts). O&M lessons can clearly provide children who are visually impaired with a vast array of problem-solving opportunities to support cognitive development and learning. In scaffolding, the teacher initially guides much of the problem solving and then lessens the amount of help given as the child gains in skill and confidence (Doolittle, 1997). The term *zone of proximal development* (ZPD) has been coined to describe the difference between what children can do independently and what they can do with help (Vygotsky, 1978). When discovered through assessment, this area of learning potential is the perfect developmental level to target O&M instruction. For example, if an elementary school student is able

to independently plan travel routes in a familiar residential area and with guidance is able to solve problems through a drop-off lesson in the same area, the child's zone of proximal development and target for instruction may be the planning of alternate and detour routes.

Closely related to scaffolding is the teaching strategy of *shaping*. When teachers or parents attempt to shape a student's behavior, they reinforce successive approximations of the desired behavior. For example, prior to a kindergarten student being able to properly use an arc for two-point touch technique, the O&M specialist would initially praise the child for any attempt to move the cane with the cane tip on the ground. Gradually, the child would only be praised when the cane movement more closely approximated the appropriate arc for the technique. Shaping allows teachers to start with what children are able to do and encourage them to move forward to build up to their potential.

Supporting Positive Behaviors

O&M specialists need to design lessons that will support learning and manage dynamic learning environments to ensure that students are encouraged to demonstrate positive behaviors that will help them learn and to succeed in life. Lessons designed to support positive behaviors will provide students with opportunities for:

- making positive choices (for example, a choice between two reasonable travel destinations provides positive options versus giving a choice between having an O&M lesson or not)
- experiencing success in skills and concepts learned
- learning from mistakes in an honest yet compassionate manner from a respected teacher

O&M specialists, because of the necessity to teach outside of classrooms, have the added responsibility to manage dynamic learning environments in a way that also supports positive behaviors from their students. For example, if a young student expresses self-abusive behaviors when anxiety levels are elevated and if the student is very fearful of dogs, the O&M specialist must initially attempt to plan lessons in areas where dogs are not expected. In the event that a stray dog approaches, the O&M specialist must be ready to respond appropriately to lessen the student's anxiety.

When O&M lessons are meaningful, creative, and involve active participation, many students will find learning new concepts or techniques to be highly rewarding and they will strive to do their best because they *enjoy* the process of O&M instruction! As young students mature, it is hoped that they will view the ability to travel independently to desired destinations as intrinsically rewarding and serve as motivation to learn new O&M concepts and techniques. For highly motivated students, specific recognition and sincere praise of the student's efforts and achievements may provide sufficient reinforcement to support ongoing positive behaviors during O&M instruction. However, some school-age students may require additional tangible activity or edible reinforcers or rewards to increase their motivation for mastering the skills necessary for independent travel (see Jacobson & Bradley, Volume 1, Chapter 7, for additional information on reinforcement procedures).

One method of reinforcing positive behaviors that easily can be applied in orientation and mobility for school-age students is the use of a token economy system. Basic elements of a token economy system include small tangible items that serve as tokens (for example, stickers, tickets, magnets, or coins) that students can earn after demonstrating specific identified behaviors (for example, student maintains appropriate arc coverage for five consecutive minutes). After a predetermined number of these tokens have been earned over a period of lessons, students may "exchange" the tokens for desired rewards (for example, a music CD or time spent at a preferred activity). When carefully selected, the tokens themselves can serve as immediate reinforcement for specified behaviors during individual O&M lessons, and students learn that continuing the specified behavior can result in a desired reward.

Table 8.6 provides examples of different types of reinforcement strategies that may be used with elementary and secondary school students.

While it is common practice in O&M lessons, the use of candy, soft drinks, or other edible items to reinforce desired behaviors best occurs after careful consideration and only with parental permission. When linked with a specific O&M task, such as independently locating a fast food restaurant and ordering a soft drink, students may find the reward of the soft drink or meal motivating for future independent travel to other restaurants. However, when edible treats are not linked directly to the achievement of a desired skill or concept, they may not promote a student's intrinsic value of the O&M skill or his increased desire for independent travel. Furthermore, parents may object to the use of food as a reinforcer, especially if a child has dietary restrictions, specific food allergies, or the family is encouraging a healthy diet.

Some children may exhibit behaviors that interfere with their ability to stay on task during O&M lessons. Repetitive behaviors such as eye poking or rocking may compete with the child's ability to use the cane for extended periods of time. In some instances, the O&M specialist may see an improvement in behaviors when lessons are carefully designed to match the child's attention span, stamina, and ability level. This can increase success and enjoyment and limit stress and frustration. In other cases, O&M specialists need to work together with the educational team in efforts to determine the function of such disruptive behaviors and design interventions that can be used consistently on lessons, at school, and at home to reduce the negative behaviors and replace them with positive ones. It is important for

TABLE 8.6

Sample Variations of Token Economy Systems

	Tokens and Display Boards/Collection Containers	Possible Behaviors Resulting in Earned Tokens	Possible Rewards That Can Be Earned with Tokens
Elementary school students	• Stickers on a poster board chart • Small polished rocks or marbles collected in a drawstring pouch • Various shapes attached with Velcro to a mat or foam board • Pieces of a puzzle (can be made from cutting up laminated photo of desired item or activity) assembled and taped on poster board	• Absence of undesired behavior (for example, crying, rocking, eye poking) for set periods of time during a lesson • Presence of desired behaviors (for example, set time "on-task," use of proper grasp for human guide, cane moving in appropriate arc, locating landmarks, finding specific destinations)	• Healthy snack • Time on swings, playground equipment at end of lesson • Pencils, pens, crayons • Small toy cars • Small action figures • Lunch at a fast food restaurant • Outing to a local petting zoo, • Visit to a pet store • Student lesson choice
Secondary school students	• Raffle tickets kept in a wallet or waist pack pocket • Magnets on a magnetic board	• Absence of undesired behaviors (for example, excessive talking, complaints) • Presence of desired behaviors (for example, does bus route planning for homework)	• Consider allowing choices for exchange of tokens, for example: • 5 tokens = healthy snack • 10 tokens = fast food restaurant coupon • 25 tokens = lunch at a fast food restaurant • 50 tokens = baseball cap with favorite team logo, video, music CD, or DVD • 100 tokens = day activity outing

professionals and families to learn the function of such a behavior (for example, avoiding a task, expressing anxiety or boredom, or seeking attention). Once the function of the behavior is accurately identified, a more acceptable substitute behavior can be introduced to replace the target behavior. For example, if a student exhibits hand-flapping behavior, presumably to express boredom during cane skill practice, the O&M specialist can then design a more motivating cane skill lesson in which the student's free hand is kept busy carrying an attendance report to the office. (See Chapters 17–20 for more information on working with students who have multiple disabilities.)

Creative Ideas

All of the previously described basic teaching tools can be further maximized by using creativity to plan for O&M lessons that are engaging for students with visual impairments. Interesting instructional materials (commercially purchased or handmade), age-appropriate games and activities, creative use of role-playing, and small group instruction can be used to motivate students during O&M lessons.

Instructional Materials

In addition to standard vendors that carry long canes, adaptive mobility devices, and low vision aids, there are some sources of O&M-related instructional materials that can be bought through various companies, such as Independent Living Aids, American Printing House for the Blind, Exceptional Teaching and MaxiAids (see the Resources section for more information).

Mapmaking materials, adapted board games, cards and dice, beeper balls, braille compasses, measuring tapes, survival signs, flash cards, Wikki Stix, puffy paint, and other assorted educational games and materials can be purchased from such companies. O&M specialists also will find a plethora of materials at educational, craft, hobby, hardware, and discount stores from which simple or complex maps, games, and other teaching aids can be constructed prior to or during O&M lessons with students.

Activities

When teaching school-age students the vast array of concepts and skills they need to travel independently, O&M specialists certainly need

strategies that extend beyond verbal explanations, skill drills, and route practice. "Activities that are most meaningful are those that provide concrete, hands-on experiences and promote positive interactions with the physical and social travel environment" (Fazzi & Petersmeyer, 2001, p. 113).

To capture a student's interest and participation, the instructor should plan to incorporate engaging activities in lessons and along routes by using interesting or relevant destinations. For example, elementary school students might quickly lose interest if simply asked to walk from point A to point B on a school campus—however, the incorporation of a scavenger hunt with interesting items to be found at each destination may hold their attention. When planning residential route travel for a high school student, a functional task may be incorporated. For example, the instructor might choose a mailbox within the neighborhood as the route destination and plan to bring a braille or large-print greeting card for the student to sign and mail to a family member or friend. Teaching mobility skills in business areas can be designed easily to incorporate a student's interest by choosing destinations of interest, such as a music store or an ice cream shop.

Field trips, whether a whole class school trip or an individually planned O&M outing, can be excellent opportunities for concept development when students are given hands-on opportunities to learn about new things. Other activities and instructional units can center around a large or small O&M project. For example, together with the O&M specialist, a student could create an O&M scrapbook with photos, business cards, brochures, maps, bus schedules, and other items from O&M travels. Other students may enjoy constructing a small-scale model of a residential area that corresponds with a series of exploratory lessons. After-school activities, such as scouting, may provide additional opportunities for projects like environmental-awareness efforts that could be incorporated into O&M lessons. High school students may like to create their own college catalog or portfolio. The catalog may contain information obtained via the Internet and from campus visits. For example, the student may like to organize information on admissions, student disability resources, financial aid, and transportation options from various community colleges visited during O&M lessons in the area.

The practice of physical skills required for mobility can be enhanced through the incorporation of imagination and age-appropriate pretend scenarios for younger children, such as a princess preparing for the royal ball for girls or robot command station routes for boys. Challenge scenarios like those found on some reality television programs could provide opportunities for cane skill refinement for older students. For example, a simple L-shaped relay could be set up and the student travels back and forth gathering puzzles pieces that will need to be placed together at the culmination. Relays can be timed or scored according to quality of cane skills used. Alternatively, practicing mobility skills during real-life functional tasks can make lessons more meaningful and provide students with additional opportunities for social interactions. O&M specialists will need to collaborate with teachers and school personnel on occasion to plan regular on-campus tasks that can be completed, such as delivering attendance reports or lunch counts, placing items in teacher mailboxes, and similar activities for students who are working on campus routes.

Games

A wide variety of games can be incorporated into O&M learning. Games can be competitive, cooperative, or a combination in nature, and the right type of game depends on which one the student may respond to most positively. Board games can be adapted, such as "O&M Monopoly," in which students are given a set amount of money at the beginning of an instructional unit.

Houses or other destinations within a specific training area are assigned values and at each lesson the student is given the opportunity to reach a new destination of his choice. Easiest destinations are of lesser value and more complicated destinations are of greater value. If the student is successful in reaching the destination, he is given the opportunity to use his money to "purchase" it. If he is not successful, then the O&M specialist gets to buy the property. At the end of each lesson, the student marks the chosen property (perhaps on an instructor-created game board) as belonging to either the student or the instructor. At the end of the unit, the property value is added up to see who won the game. A variation of this approach would be to include additional students who are traveling in the same training area and play the game with three or more players or to create game boards for separate training areas and students, but everyone's progress should be charted on one master board.

Any O&M activity can be turned into a game simply by adding a twist like keeping score, adding an element of time, or incorporating any sort of challenge. Similarly, two students (even those not attending the same school) can play an O&M game and compete with one another or work together to locate the pieces of a puzzle that will be completed together. Travel time can also be used to play games that serve as a review of concepts, such as "O&M Jeopardy" or "20 Questions."

Role-playing

Role-playing is frequently used as a teaching strategy in orientation and mobility. It is commonly used to practice the interpersonal skills required to be successful in soliciting assistance, making purchases, declining unwanted assistance, and interacting with bus drivers. Role-playing can readily be used in the car en route to the O&M lesson as a review of interpersonal skills to use in the community. Role-playing has the advantage of providing ample practice opportunities in a safe environment with a known person. As the student gains in skill level and confidence, the instructor can be less predictable and more challenging to interact with in order to prepare the student for more dynamic travel environments.

Small Group Lessons

O&M instruction, as both a tradition and as a necessity, has been provided primarily to one student at a time. However, there are instances in which group instruction, when planned appropriately, can be highly motivating and productive (see Orientation and Mobility Division of AER, 2006, for guidelines on creative uses of group lessons). It can be fun for an experienced bus traveler to pair up with a peer who is a novice and complete a basic bus route together with instructor supervision. Treasure hunts can be completed in small groups or two teams so that peers have an opportunity to problem-solve clues together and experience how different individual strengths can contribute to a successful team. Orienteering activities in local parks or hiking areas have been adapted for students with visual impairments (Blasch & Penrod, 2006, AER O&M Division Day presentation) and provide great opportunities for students to work in tandem to solve orientation challenges, increase confidence, and develop a healthy sense of the interdependence of teaming. Reality television programming may provide themes that easily can be incorporated, such as the "Great O&M Race"—which is simply a popular variation of orienteering. Road car rallies, complete with braille maps, have been sponsored by various organizations as a weekend youth outing.

Whether O&M instruction is provided in groups or in its primary format with individual students, creative lesson planning is sure to make the time spent more fun and will hopefully lead to positive learning outcomes for students. Lesson ideas can be found easily and the challenge is simply to match the lesson to the correct student and implement it in a manner that will be both fun and educational.

Developing Instructional Units

Quality instruction in orientation and mobility is not only tailored to meet the individual needs of students with visual impairments but also is designed in a sequential manner that affords learners the best opportunity to learn, practice, and apply new skills and concepts. Instructional units serve as an organizer for planning, instruction, and assessment, in much the same way that K–12 school curricula are presented in integrated thematic or content units.

Classroom teachers commonly rely on commercially available curricula that include well-developed instructional units in academic areas. In contrast, O&M curricula are comprised of a set of techniques, skills, and concepts necessary for independent travel. Since instruction must be so highly individualized for a wide range of students, there is no commercially available curriculum full of lesson plan ideas for the O&M specialist to follow. The traditional O&M curriculum has frequently been divided into units according to travel areas (such as residential or light business travel) or skill areas (such as basic skills, cane skills, or street-crossing skills) (Hill & Ponder, 1976; Jacobson, 1993; LaGrow & Weessies, 1994; Pogrund et al., 1995). Such organizers are especially useful for university teacher preparation and for working with adults who receive intensive services in rehabilitation settings because they may be able to cover a great deal of content rather quickly. These large topical units are often less useful for school-age students, who may receive shorter lessons of less frequency throughout the school year, and whose developmental level and need for foundational concepts for younger students may preclude rapid acquisition of the same skills. Instructional units should be designed to have a clear beginning and ending and involve a series of graduated experiences in which the student learns and utilizes new skills and information. Culminating activities designed at the end of the unit can help the instructor assess learning objectives and provide the student with a strong sense of accomplishment. Units can also incorporate age-appropriate themes that are motivating for students and create a sense of anticipation for future lessons as the lessons progress toward a highly rewarding end.

Thematic units can be developed for O&M curricula to create an engaging series of learning activities for school-age students in which concepts and skills are integrated. For example, "All about Transportation" could be a thematic unit for a first-grade student who is visually impaired. The unit may be designed to address a limited number of objectives that will be introduced, reviewed, applied and assessed over a four-week period across 12 individual lessons—each with a nicely linked transportation focus.

Games, such as "On the Move" bingo, might be used to teach transportation-related concepts or "Red Light, Green Light" might be used to practice visual scanning or specific cane skills. Throughout the unit, the student might earn points to use toward a bus or light rail token for a culminating lesson in which the instructor and student ride together.

In the design of O&M instructional units, Fazzi and Petersmeyer (2001) focus on:

• a traditional sequence of skill development from simple to complex

• a critical skills approach to meet immediate travel needs

• a segue to a short-term unit to more fully address a tangential skill or concept of interest

• an in-depth extended unit featuring instruction in an area of assessed need

O&M instructional units can be developed around age-appropriate activities that similar-age peers enjoy. For example, preschool students may like units designed around themes related to adventures of popular cartoon characters. Elementary school students may be highly motivated with an instructional theme that incorporates collecting a trendy toy or playing card. Older students are commonly engaged in social activities that easily can be adapted into an O&M unit, such as cruising the mall or exploring transportation options. Academic curricula are another source of instructional unit ideas for orientation and mobility. For example, mapmaking units can be linked to geography units and sight word vocabulary can be incorporated into a monocular training unit (Fazzi & Petersmeyer, 2001).

GETTING ORGANIZED

O&M specialists need to be organized in order to successfully implement instructional units and creative lessons. Whether working at one school or traveling to multiple schools, setting a logical O&M teaching schedule, planning itinerant services, managing paperwork demands, selecting training environments, organizing teaching supplies, and planning for emergencies will all support effective instruction.

Setting the Instructional Schedule

An essential step for managing time and getting organized is establishing a weekly teaching schedule. While it is important that instructors aim for consistency, they need to be flexible and keep in mind that schedules will need to be adjusted frequently to reflect school holidays, teacher training days, minimum days, assemblies, and testing dates. Thus, one of the first steps for setting a schedule should include getting a copy of each school calendar. Most school offices post (either in print or online) monthly or annual calendars that indicate the typical daily schedule (for example, class periods) and reflect anticipated special events in student schedules. This information is typically available for educators and families.

Developing a weekly schedule can be a complicated task that requires both an agile mind and expert diplomacy. O&M specialists must plan their schedule to avoid interfering with other teachers and service providers and minimize pulling students out of academic subjects to the extent possible. Dunham-Sims (2005) suggests the following tips to help O&M specialists with caseload scheduling:

- Gather student IEP goals to determine the lesson locations, frequency, and length of each instructional period.

- Set priorities for which students should be scheduled first (for example, first schedule high school students, who have more academic subjects and thus fewer flexible opportunities to be pulled out, and then schedule elementary school students, who tend to have more-adaptable schedules during the day).

- Contact teachers to determine possible days and times for your lessons for students who receive direct service. Olmstead (2005) recommends starting with itinerant teachers of students with visual impairments (TVIs), resource room teachers, and special day class teachers first—as they may be waiting for schedule feedback from all the educational team members before making their classroom schedules. Because of the many complications present at the start of each new school year, contact with general education teachers may need to wait until the end of the first week of school.

- Ask about specific restrictions on when students can be taken from class to receive O&M instruction. For instance, high school students nearing graduation may not be able to miss any academic subjects.

- Start organizing your schedule with self-stick notes that have the student's name, school site, and service time printed on them. These can be shuffled around on your schedule form like pieces of a puzzle.

- Be sure to incorporate adequate travel time to commute from site to site and, to the extent possible, organize schedules so that students at the same or nearby schools can be scheduled back-to-back.

O&M specialists should keep in mind that they very possibly will compete with other service providers (for example, speech therapist, adaptive physical education teacher, and teacher of students with visual impairments) for a time slot with a particular student. In order to find time to serve each of their students appropriately, instructors need to be prepared to negotiate time slots, take their lunch period at odd hours, and consider seeing some students before or after school. Dunham-Sims (2005) has a sample weekly O&M schedule that can be seen in Figure 8.2.

Planning Itinerant Services

While a small number of O&M specialists, such as those working at residential schools for the blind, teach at one school—the vast majority who serve school-age students work on an itinerant basis. With a philosophical trend toward inclusive education in the United States, an increasing number of students with disabilities are receiving education in the general education classroom. As of 2002, 85 percent of students with visual impairments spent at least part of their day in the general education classroom (U.S. Department of Education, 2002). With less than 1 percent of the total school population identified as having visual impairments (U.S. Department of Education, 2006), it is not unusual for a child to be the only student with a visual impairment at his school. This means that most O&M

	Monday		Tuesday		Wednesday		Thursday		Friday		
8:45–9:30	SEAVIEW Juan Diaz Campus routes & consult	8:30–9:10	DE ANZA Sam Barnaby Campus routes & consult Monitors: Joanna Simpson Lisa Wagoner	8:30–9:20	CANTERBURY Mahmood Abdul Canterbury routes & consult	8:30–9:30	Prep 3	8:45–9:30	SEAVIEW Juan Diaz Campus routes & consult	_Canterbury_ M. Abdul _Transition_ T. Wilson
	Travel		Travel		Travel					_De Anza_ S. Barnaby J. Simpson
10:00–11:00	TARA HILLS Alan Edwards 1 & 3 IH. routes 2 Appian 80 4 Hilltop Mall 5 Pinole Vista	9:30–10:10	TARA HILLS Susan Abbot Concepts & consult Monitor: Lenny Cravets	9:30–10:40	TARA HILLS Kathy Kellog 1 & 3 IH. routes 2 Appian 80 4 Hilltop 5 Pinole Vista & consult	9:30–10:30	Prep 4	9:30–10:30	SEAVIEW Julia Thomas 1 & 3 IH. routes 2 Appian 80 4 Hilltop 5 Pinole Vista & consult	L. Wagoner I. Williams _Ellerhorst_ Y. Morgan I. Viceroy M. Gonzales
					Travel	10:30–11:30	Prep 5		Travel	_Seaview_ J. Diaz J. Thomas
11:00–12:00	TARA HILLS Carmen Jiminez 1 & 3 IH. routes 2 Appian 80 4 Pinole crossings 4 Hilltop Mall 5 Pinole Vista	10:10–12:00	TARA HILLS All consults	11:00–12:00	ELLERHORST Yolanda Morgan 1 & 3 IH. routes 2 Hilltop Mall 5 Advanced & consult Monitor: Ishmael Viceroy	11:45–1:30	1st Thursday Visually Impaired Program Staff Meeting PERES Maria G.	11:00–11:30	CCC TRANSITION Toby Wilson Campus routes	_Tara Hills_ S. Abbot L. Cravets A. Edwards M. Finkle

	Lunch		Lunch		Lunch		Travel		Lunch		J. Hinman C. Jiminez K. Kellog
1:00–2:00	TARA HILLS Marianna Finkle 1 & 3 IH. routes 2 Hilltop Mall 4 Appian 80 5 Pinole Vista	**1:00–2:00**	TARA HILLS Josh Hinman 1 & 3 IH. routes 2 Hilltop mall 4 Appian 80 5 Pinole Vista	**1:30–3:00**	CCC TRANSITION Toby Wilson Bus travel		Lunch		**11:30–3:00**	Special Consult	
2:15–3:00	Prep 1	**2:15–3:00**	Prep 2				Travel	**2:00–3:00**	TARA HILLS Josh Hinman Bus travel		Assessments	

Figure 8.2. Sample O&M Schedule

Source: Reprinted with permission from Faith Dunham-Sims, "Orientation and Mobility and the Itinerant Teacher," in Jean Olmstead, *Itinerant Teaching: Tricks of the Trade for Teachers of Students with Visual Impairments*, 2nd ed. (New York: AFB Press, 2005), p. 134.

specialists serving school-age students are traveling teachers, going from school to school and visiting multiple classrooms over the course of a day.

Itinerant teaching presents distinct challenges that must be addressed so that burnout can be avoided and career satisfaction preserved. Some challenges, common to many itinerant teachers, include:

- finding enough time to provide quality instruction to students

- adjusting to unanticipated changes in student schedules

- establishing positive relations with multiple administrators and teachers from different schools

In order to optimize itinerant teaching, O&M specialists need to be flexible, have strong time-management abilities, and use effective communication skills (see Volume 1, Chapter 12 for more information on service delivery options).

Finding enough time in the day is a quest for all educators, particularly for those who are itinerant. The demands of consulting with teachers and families, planning lessons, completing paperwork, driving to and from schools, attending meetings, and developing or adapting materials are all crucial but take time away from providing direct instruction to students. To address the need for increased time with students, O&M specialists must use every minute of their time effectively. To the extent possible, the instructor's schedule should be organized to minimize driving. Students who are at the same school or at nearby schools should be scheduled back-to-back on the same days. Consultations with teachers and families can be scheduled into regularly established lunch meetings, allowing the opportunity to build professional connections in a social manner.

O&M specialists who work as itinerant teachers need to be flexible and willing to respond to changes in school schedules with little or no notice. Unannounced assemblies, field trips, medical appointments, or exams can result in a student being unavailable for a scheduled lesson. Although these disruptions can be frustrating, particularly when one has just spent time traveling to see the student, the trip need not be wasted. Specialists may consider making a few quick telephone calls to check on the availability of seeing another student in that time slot. Free time also can be used for catching up on lesson planning or daily notes, reviewing training sites for future lessons, or consulting with general education teachers.

Strong communication skills will aid in establishing positive relationships with the various people that the itinerant O&M specialist interacts with on a daily basis. Perhaps one of the most fundamental steps toward initiating these connections is to ensure that one is well known to the office staff, school administrators, and teachers at each of the schools visited. Instructors should be prepared to introduce themselves to significant personnel the first several times they visit a school campus, and to always wear appropriate photo identification when arriving to check in at school offices. Of course, the process of developing positive interactions assumes that O&M specialists reciprocate by making every effort to learn the names, titles, and responsibilities of those they encounter at the various schools. When educators become a "familiar face" at each school, they begin the steps toward establishing long-lasting collaborative relationships with students, teachers, administrators, and families.

Managing Paperwork Demands

Paperwork seems to be an unavoidable obligation of all educators and requires good organization and time-management skills to stay ahead of the pile. O&M specialists write lesson plans, document daily progress in notes, develop annual IEPs and Individualized Transition Plans (ITPs), compose periodic progress reports, complete attendance records and mileage forms, make records for parent conferences, and fill out emergency and other miscellaneous forms, as required.

A good system for managing forms may first involve the identification of all ongoing documentation requirements, mandated timelines, and the procedures for submitting the documentation to school personnel. A helpful program assistant, administrator, or experienced O&M specialist may be of assistance with this task, as there may be different expectations, forms, and timelines required by different employers. Next, the instructor may develop a tickler file, which is a calendar-dated file system that can be in either paper or electronic format, containing daily, weekly, monthly, and annual reminders of documents to be completed. For itinerant O&M specialists, portability of the file system will be imperative so that it is easy to carry in their vehicles. It is important to establish easy access to the forms needed to complete documentation—in either electronic or paper format. A tickler system also can be useful to remember important meeting dates. For example, it is not unusual for O&M specialists to be surprised with last-minute notification of an impending IEP meeting. Knowing that IEPs typically are conducted on an annual basis, the O&M specialist can enter reminders one month in advance to contact the student's teacher or case manager to check the date and time of an upcoming meeting.

Use of electronic technology is essential to complete paperwork in a time-efficient manner. In many cases, it may be a worthwhile investment of time to convert existing forms or other paperwork into electronic format on a computer and save them as electronic files for easy future access. Saved lesson plans written in an electronic for-

mat for a specific student may be reworded or modified easily for another student. If the school or agency does not already have an existing database of previously written O&M IEP goals, the O&M specialist may want to keep a personal electronic database for future reference. A portable laptop computer or handheld personal digital assistant (PDA) will allow itinerant O&M specialists to use free moments effectively to document daily progress notes or write up future lesson plans. Where Internet access is available, O&M specialists on the go can communicate important messages with the educational team via use of e-mail.

Selecting Training Environments

Ideally, the selection of training environments will consider each student's age, abilities, home and school areas, cultural background, and favorite activities and interests so that they may be incorporated into motivational lessons. A thorough discussion of desirable environmental features for indoor, residential, and light business training areas as well as strategies for locating these environments, and multiple teaching tips for creative teaching, organizing environmental information, and addressing imperfect environments can be found in Fazzi and Petersmeyer (2001).

Although it is desirable to find training sites near students' schools or homes, instructors may have to search outside the neighborhood to locate desirable training areas. There are several strategies that may be used to begin a search for desirable training sites. First, if there are other O&M specialists working in the same school or district, it will be beneficial to tap their knowledge of the training areas they have used. Instructors also may use printed maps or Internet mapping programs to find possible instructional locations. Several online map programs have satellite imagery that may be viewed to gain basic topographical information of the area, including information about curbs, sidewalks, houses, and other details relevant to travel. Students and instructors should keep in mind that not all map sources are up-to-date. When a general area has been selected, the instructor should plan to walk each section of it, drawing a map (by hand or electronically) and noting significant features for training, such as the type of traffic controls at each intersection, addresses of homes, points of interests (like parks or schools), and names of businesses and shops. Much of this information also may be available for certain locations through a Geographic Information System (GIS) (see Bentzen & Marston, Volume 1, Chapter 10). Additionally, areas of potential hazard—for example, broken sidewalks or obstructed visibility—should be recorded on the handwritten map. A sample instructor-made map of a training area can be seen in Figure 8.3.

Organizing Teaching Supplies, Office Space, and the Car Trunk

Well-prepared O&M specialists have carefully chosen teaching supplies for a variety of school-age children yet rarely find enough room to store them! Office space for many O&M specialists is nonexistent, shared with other professionals, or only accessed on an infrequent basis. Regardless of whether the instructor works from an office or the trunk of a car (or both, in many cases), it is important that appropriate instructional materials are selected, well organized for effortless accessibility, and easily portable for transport between office, car, and multiple lesson sites.

Teaching supplies for the O&M specialist may range from instructional materials (such as high-contrast toys, stickers, interesting sound sources, and mapmaking supplies) to appropriate items for emergencies and inclement weather (such as a first aid kit or rain ponchos in various sizes). Careful thought must be given to ensure that the instructor has necessary items,

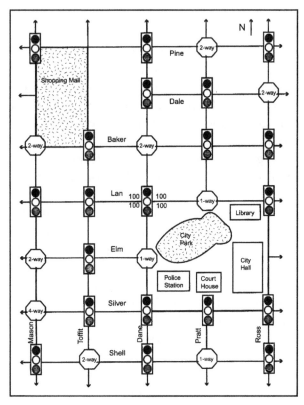

Figure 8.3. Sample Training Map

Source: Reprinted with permission from "Selecting Training Environments: Sites for Different Students," in Diane L. Fazzi and Barbara A. Petersmeyer, *Imagining the Possibilities: Creative Approaches to Orientation and Mobility Instruction for Persons Who Are Visually Impaired* (New York: AFB Press, 2001), p. 244.

as needed. In addition to motivating toys and manipulatives, Knott (2002) has an extensive checklist of materials that are appropriate for the O&M specialist's mobile office, otherwise known as one's car. An adapted version of this checklist can be seen in Sidebar 8.3.

Fazzi and Petersmeyer (2001) provide several tips for storing and organizing instructional materials in the trunk or backseat of a car. Specialists may choose to organize materials, for example, by size and shape (small cane tips together), function (assessment materials together), need (most frequently used near the front of the trunk), and age group (concept toys for young

SIDEBAR 8.3

Adapted Checklist for the Mobile Office

- Critical information for each student—*vital contacts, addresses, phone numbers, and release forms for medical treatment*
- Teacher identification—*ID badge, business cards*
- File for record-keeping forms
- Cell phones—*one for you and your student*
- Walkie-talkies—a fun way to keep in verbal contact with students
- Change for pay telephone and parking
- Maps—*of areas where you are traveling and schools you frequent*
- Current transit schedules and transit company phone numbers
- First aid kit
- Moist towelettes
- Facial tissues
- Sunscreen
- Visors, caps, and hats—*that can be thoroughly cleaned after each use*
- Monoculars, magnifiers, and various tinted sunglasses with broad-spectrum protection—*for trial comparison and assessment purposes*
- Lens cleaner and lens tissues
- Spare canes in several sizes

- Cane tips—*consider a variety for comparison*
- Measuring tape and measuring wheel
- Steel wool, wax, or bar soap—*for cleaning joints of folding canes*
- Red and white reflective tape—*for replacing worn tape on canes*
- Heavy-duty fabric tape—*for multiple uses, including reinforcing cane tips and curb detectors*
- Waist pouch and backpack—*for use by you or student*
- Tape recorder and blank tapes
- Rain gear (for example, a poncho, waterproof headgear that doesn't cover the ears, umbrellas, rubber shoes or boots, gloves without fingers)
- A tactile diagram kit or self-constructed tactile maps and models
- Felt-tip pens, heavy-duty drawing paper, or raised-line drawing paper
- Dry-erase board and markers
- Compasses (braille, large-print, and auditory)
- Tote bags, plastic bags, heavy-duty shopping bags with handles, wheeled luggage, or collapsible carts—*for storing and moving items*

Source: Adapted with permission from "Professional and Strategic Issues," in Natalie Isaac Knott, *Teaching Orientation and Mobility in the Schools: An Instructor's Companion* (New York: AFB Press, 2002), p. 211.

children in one area). A box with hanging files is recommended for organizing student lesson plans and other paperwork. Storage boxes of various sizes, with and without handles, are suggested for holding and organizing instructional materials. Clear plastic sandwich bags can be used to easily store and identify small items such as compasses, bus tokens, or pens. The authors also suggest carrying cloth tote bags for storing and transporting a variety of small items to and from the office, car, classroom, and training sites.

Preparing for Emergencies

Over the course of an O&M specialist's career, situations are likely to occur that will call for emergency action. To lessen the impact of emergency situations, instructors need to be prepared. By obtaining, organizing, and carrying critical student information and appropriate materials for off-campus instruction, the O&M specialist will be ready to act quickly in the event of an emergency.

O&M specialists also need to be knowledgeable about individual school procedures for evacuation drills (for example, fire, tornado, or earthquake drills) and instances in which the school may be on "lockdown" because of a potential threat or criminal activity in progress. These two types of emergency preparedness at schools also reinforces the importance of itinerant professionals adhering to school sign-in and sign-out procedures so that administrators can conduct an accurate head count and be aware of all individuals who are permitted to be on campus.

O&M specialists need to ensure that they are easily accessible to others, as well as have immediate access to essential student information. They should carry a reliable cell phone and ensure that families and school administrators have the number.

As noted in Knott's checklist for the mobile office (see Sidebar 8.3), when off-campus with students, O&M specialists should carry critical contact information for:

- families (addresses and phone numbers for work and home, cell phone numbers, and so forth)
- schools (administrators' names and phone numbers)
- emergency treatments (911, the school nurse, or student's personal physician)

Phone contact information may be organized in print format or programmed into a cell phone for quick access.

In addition to contact information, important student documentation must be gathered and organized prior to off-campus instruction. O&M specialists carry data relating to each student's health conditions, medications, and known allergic reactions. Additionally, signed release forms for medical treatment need to be prepared and updated periodically, and carried on all off-campus lessons. Some itinerant O&M specialists organize this information at the beginning of each school year and store it in a portable box with hanging file folders to be held in their vehicle.

ESTABLISHING STRONG SCHOOL AND FAMILY PARTNERSHIPS

It is well known that at the center of every successful O&M teaching program is the positive rapport between instructor and student (see Welsh, Chapter 6, and Volume 1, Chapter 6). However, educating children with visual impairments presents multifaceted challenges that cannot be met by any one individual. As a result, it is important that good working relationships extend to other teachers, specialists, administrators, and families. Parental involvement, in particular, has been shown to be a predictive factor for a student's success in school (for example, higher grades, better attendance, more follow through with homework, increased graduation rates, and more enrollments in college) (Dettmer, Dyck, & Thurston, 2002; Thomas, Correa, & Morsink, 2001).

Student Rapport Building

The earliest O&M professionals clearly understood the importance of the student-instructor relationship in ensuring a successful O&M training experience (Bledsoe, 1980; Williams, 1965). Collaboration, trust, genuine caring, sensitive and honest observations and evaluations of performance, and challenging yet success-oriented lessons have all been identified as key factors in establishing positive student-teacher relationships. These important elements are fundamental to high-quality O&M instruction regardless of the age group served. The following list includes general strategies that may assist O&M specialists in achieving rapport with school-age students (many of these strategies also may be useful when working with adults):

- Research age-appropriate trendy games and toys to incorporate in lessons (Fazzi & Petersmeyer, 2001).

- Watch some youth-oriented television and listen to popular radio programs to have items of interest to chat about with students.

- Carefully listen to students' concerns and, whenever possible, plan O&M goals in collaboration with students (at a minimum, seek age-appropriate input for goal setting).

- Take time to learn about students' interests and strengths so that they may be fully incorporated into O&M lessons and goals.

- Carefully plan O&M lessons to ensure that they are challenging but success-oriented.

Projecting a Positive Image with Colleagues in the School System

Whether O&M specialists are based in residential or itinerant programs, they are an important part of the educational team. Professionals who have earned the respect of their colleagues are most able to contribute to the team as everyone works toward a common goal. O&M specialists have a somewhat unique working environment since they serve students on a one-on-one basis and are frequently working off school grounds. It is not uncommon to hear work descriptions from school personnel such as "they are out on their walk." Educating peers as to the scope and complexity of assessment and instruction in orientation and mobility is sometimes a challenge,

but a worthwhile endeavor. The following strategies may help O&M specialists to establish positive working relationships, respect, and collegiality in the school workplace.

To increase visibility:

- Take time to get to know school personnel, including administrators, teachers, and custodial, secretarial, and security staff.

- Follow sign-in and sign-out procedures according to individual school policies.

- Dress professionally and wear or carry appropriate school identification.

To establish reliability:

- Provide teachers and school supervisors with a written work schedule and contact information.

- Maintain a consistent schedule that others can rely on.

- When changes to schedules are necessary, make sure to contact involved individuals as soon as possible.

- Be on time for starting and ending lessons and administrative meetings.

- Complete reports and other documentation in a professional and timely manner.

To educate others:

- Conduct in-service training with educators and administrators—including simulated and sleep shade experiences, as appropriate.

- Carry professional literature (brochures, business cards, and so forth) that can be readily handed to individuals who may make inquiries.

- Provide opportunities for colleagues and administrators to observe lessons when feasible.

- Have a ready-made list of professional and consumer resources to share with others (for example, web sites, contact numbers, and videos).
- Volunteer to create an O&M bulletin board display in a school classroom or hallway (Fazzi & Petersmeyer, 2001).

Communication with Families

Ongoing communication with families is an important aspect of serving school-age students with visual impairments. In much the same way that parents can monitor their child's academic achievement by helping with homework, reviewing graded assignments, reading notes from teachers, attending parent-teacher conferences, and receiving report cards throughout the year, parents can also be involved in and informed about progress in orientation and mobility. Such standard forms of communication may not be established for related service personnel, but O&M specialists can take the time to prepare meaningful homework to support family follow-through on O&M goals, send monthly notes home to families for review, and maintain e-mail or phone communication with parents throughout the year. While IEPs typically occur once per year, communication patterns established throughout the year are particularly helpful when designing student goals. The IEP process can be enhanced when families are given an opportunity to provide informal input for preplanning goals. The more families understand about orientation and mobility and their child's individual gifts and talents, the better prepared they are to participate in educational planning in a meaningful way. In addition, unpleasant surprises and the potential for animosity at IEP meetings can be greatly diminished when there is communication between families and professionals prior to the annual meeting. It will benefit the O&M specialist to make inquiries of families regarding preferred methods of communication. While some professionals and family members are comfortable with impromptu phone calls, others may prefer e-mail or scheduled face-to-face meetings. O&M specialists may select from a variety of strategies for communication that fit within the school system or service delivery model and seem appropriate to the age of the student and family interest level, as follows:

- Prepare monthly newsletters (for example, individualized letters, O&M news in general, or checklists that can be quickly individualized for a variety of students) to be sent home to families.
- Create a Listserv, which is a form of e-mail where one communicates with a group of individuals simultaneously, for either family or student use. When an e-mail is sent to the list server, it is automatically sent to everyone on the list. A Listserv provides a wonderful opportunity to communicate with an entire group. Students and family members on the mailing list may begin to interact with each other, sharing resources and providing support and direction. As a cautionary note, school districts frequently have student e-mail and confidentiality policies that should be adhered to.
- Use video teleconferencing or Internet video phone service as available and when appropriate. With increased public access to advances in technology, it can be expected that in years to come, more "face-to-face" discussions, observations, consultations, and IEPs will take place over the computer or via videoconferencing.
- Work with students to create an O&M journal of travel experiences from O&M lessons that goes home weekly or monthly and requires a parent's signature.
- Establish a school web site (with possible family log-in password protection if using photographs or identifying student information) with O&M updates and other interesting facts about travel, public transportation updates,

environmental accessibility issues, and so on. Students may contribute to the web site with information that they have obtained in their travels. Again, school districts frequently have confidentiality policies regarding school web sites and use of student photographs or personal information.

- Provide families with e-mail and cell phone contact information and guidelines for when calls or contacts can be made or returned.

- Attend back-to-school nights and open houses when possible to showcase student work, set student expectations, and provide opportunities to talk with families in an informal setting.

- Meet, e-mail, or call families prior to scheduled IEP meetings in order to find out about their priorities and concerns for orientation and mobility for the upcoming year and to obtain their input prior to designing annual student goals.

- Design meaningful O&M homework assignments to support follow-through on O&M skills (for example, similar to reading clubs in which children and families are expected to read a required number of minutes per month, establish a travel club in which children and families are required to log in travel destinations and note cane usage).

School organizational climates and the dynamics of student-teacher and professional-parent relationships vary greatly and the most effective rapport-building and communication strategies change similarly. Resourceful O&M specialists will make use of a variety of team-building tools to fit the situation.

MAINTAINING HIGH-QUALITY PROFESSIONAL PRACTICE

Once a level of effective professional practice in orientation and mobility with school-age students is established, a concerted effort to maintain and improve upon that practice is essential. Maintaining high-quality professional practice often involves self-reflection, consideration of personnel evaluations, student and family satisfaction with O&M programming, and peer support as part of ongoing professional development.

Importance of Self-Reflection

O&M specialists who provide quality instruction to their students on an ongoing basis are likely engaged in a process of self-reflection in which they consider:

- the strengths of their teaching strategies
- the quality of student outcomes achieved
- the need for new and creative lesson plans and materials
- the importance of dedicating time to communication with families
- the ongoing collaboration with colleagues and administrators

For some O&M specialists, this process may be formalized through a professional development plan associated with either the employer or perhaps with the renewal of a state teaching credential or national certification. For other O&M specialists the process may take a less formal shape and occur either on a regular basis due to personal choice or happen sporadically when talking with colleagues or attending interesting conferences or workshops. Regardless of the means, the end is a worthwhile endeavor for any teacher. Self-reflection can help professionals to ensure ongoing improvement in teaching practices and result in greater job satisfaction.

Personnel Evaluations

Many O&M specialists teaching school-age students will work in a system in which formal personnel evaluations are conducted. A typical form of evaluation is lesson observation by a direct supervisor. Such observations will likely occur one to three times per year and are commonly followed up with a supervisor conference or written document in which plans can be made for any needed improvements. Supervisors typically schedule such observations in advance since O&M specialists are not teaching in an easily accessible classroom. Many supervisors assigned to conduct observations may have little experience in the field of orientation and mobility. For specialists working in larger school districts, their supervisors may even know little about students with visual impairments. This observation then becomes a perfect opportunity to educate the administrator about the scope and practice of orientation and mobility. O&M specialists should welcome these observations and be prepared with written lesson plans and any appropriate literature about orientation and mobility in the event that it is requested. While supervisors may not be knowledgeable about orientation and mobility, this does not negate their input into teaching effectiveness, and O&M specialists can consider their suggestions carefully as they work to constantly improve their effectiveness.

Student and Family Satisfaction

When working with school-age students, the IEP process assures that student outcomes for learning are assessed at least annually. It is a less-frequent occurrence that students and families are provided with informal opportunities to provide feedback to O&M specialists regarding their satisfaction with the instructional program. O&M specialists who are interested in obtaining such feedback can carefully design an informal survey to give to families at the beginning and end of the year. The questions can be targeted so that O&M specialists may examine student and family understanding of O&M goals, family satisfac-

tion with services provided, or even differences that O&M instruction may have made in the family home (for example, more frequent cane usage during family outings).

Peer Support

Some O&M specialists are fortunate to work in a school setting where other O&M specialists also are employed. In such instances, peer support may be readily available. While not all instructors are open to sharing ideas and concerns related to teaching effectiveness, others use peer support to build upon their teaching repertoire and individual strengths. Informal monthly meetings can be used to share "best practices" or "teaching tips" with one another. Some O&M specialists who serve as supervisors for student teachers report feeling a sense of reinvigoration from sharing with a novice instructor and from learning about new techniques and strategies that may be taught at the university.

SUMMARY

O&M specialists who plan for and conduct appropriate and thorough assessments establish a good starting point for developing individualized instructional programs for school-age students with visual impairments. Creative lesson plans within well-sequenced instructional units provide students with an opportunity to learn the O&M skills necessary for age-appropriate travel experiences that are both fun and meaningful.

As part of the educational team working with school-age students, O&M specialists must fully consider the logistical details of providing school-based or itinerant services in school, home, and neighborhood communities. The most effective team members within the school system are O&M specialists who project a positive image with colleagues and communicate consistently with families, teachers, and administrators.

Regardless of the form that it takes, evaluations of teaching practices are a mark of excellence in orientation and mobility that propel specialists to try new strategies, maintain enthusiasm, and experience the satisfaction that comes with helping students achieve their fullest potential. High quality practice ensures that all students receiving O&M services have the opportunity to learn from age- and ability-level travel experiences as they develop increased skills and concepts necessary for progress in orientation and mobility in a range of environments.

IMPLICATIONS FOR O&M PRACTICE

1. Successful teaching is based on a combination of depth of knowledge of orientation and mobility, varied and effective teaching skills, and interpersonal qualities for working as part of an educational team.

2. Age- and grade-level guidelines can assist educational team planning of individual student goals within the context of a larger picture of assessed needs. Similarly, they can serve as a tool for O&M specialists who are educating students, families, colleagues, and administrators as to the scope of concepts and skills that are important to be addressed across each learner's school career.

3. One of the keys to good O&M instruction is to know how to choose and skillfully apply the most appropriate teaching approach with an individual student in a given learning environment.

4. Thematic units can be developed for O&M curricula to create an engaging series of learning activities for school-age students in which concepts and skills are integrated. They provide an organizer for sequential instruction, themes that are motivating for school-age stu-

dents, and incorporate culminating activities that can be used to assess instructional outcomes.

5. O&M specialists providing quality educational services make use of a full set of basic teaching tools, including: verbalization of information, modeling, guided and independent practice, effective questioning, task analysis, instructional prompting, and behavioral chaining.

6. Use of games, activities, interesting materials, role-play, incentives, and reinforcement strategies make O&M lessons fun for school-age students. Students who are actively engaged in the learning process are more likely to master the appropriate O&M skills being taught.

LEARNING ACTIVITIES

1. Create an O&M resource kit that contains assessment and instructional tools and materials specific to working with school-age students with visual impairments. For example, file a selection of assessment tools that would be age appropriate and that you would like to have quick access to. Many useful instructional materials and tactile mapmaking tools are often made on the spot, so an assortment of construction materials may be very useful (for example, Wikki Stix, scissors, felt-tip markers, foam board, Velcro with adhesive, and nonskid carpet runners). Choose to organize by grade level or by domain area.

2. For one week, make a list of the different television programs that you have watched. Examine the list and determine how you could incorporate some aspect of the programming into a motivating O&M instructional unit theme (for example, "Survivor Orientation and Mobility," which includes

weekly survivor challenges and a reward system).

3. Select a mobility skill or route that might be taught to a school-age student and develop a task analysis. If you are actually teaching this skill to a student, then determine the types of instructional prompts that will be used and develop a chart for tracking student progress (see Figure 8.1 for a sample).

4. Generate a list of games and activities that can be used to assess concepts for students in elementary school.

5. Look at the O&M Age-Appropriate Curricular Guidelines (see Tables 8.1 A-D)) and obtain a copy of your own published state academic standards. After comparing the two, add five new items to the existing chart that are supported by your research.

CHAPTER 9

Teaching Orientation and Mobility to Adults

Richard L. Welsh

LEARNING QUESTIONS

- What are the leading causes of visual impairment among adults and what are related health issues that can impact their ability to travel?

- What are various options for delivering orientation and mobility (O&M) services to adults with visual impairments?

- What are some of the common characteristics of adult learners that may impact O&M instruction and what are the teaching strategies that O&M specialists use with adult learners?

- How does an O&M specialist assess the travel skills and potential for adult learners?

- How can O&M services interact with vocational rehabilitation and employment services for adults?

Systematic instruction in orientation and mobility (O&M) first began with adventitiously blinded adults. Attempts to rehabilitate military personnel who had lost their vision in combat and in military-related activities led to the development of methods of traveling safely and independently without vision or with reduced vision. More im-

portant, these efforts resulted in the development of and the commitment to teaching methodologies to help each person attain the most independent level of travel of which that person was capable.

Initially, simulated vision loss played a central role in training people to enter this profession and to develop the skill of teaching the techniques of independent travel without vision. While wearing blindfolds, students learned to use techniques in the same way that the blinded soldiers had been taught. As adults who had grown up with vision, these professionals in training were deprived of their vision by blindfold and required to learn the techniques of independent travel. As a result of this history, the methods of teaching orientation and mobility to adventitiously blinded adults has been considered the most basic approach to O&M instruction and formed the fundamental training of each O&M specialist. As O&M services were extended to visually impaired people other than adventitiously blinded adults, the basic education of O&M specialists was expanded to include special information about how best to teach orientation and mobility to children, to adults who were congenitally blind, to older adults, to persons with multiple disabilities, and to persons with low vision. It was assumed that O&M specialists already knew how to teach adventitiously blinded adults.

This third edition of *Foundations of Orientation and Mobility* is the first to include a chapter that specifically addresses the topic of teaching orientation and mobility to adults. This chapter discusses the specific needs of adults who have to learn how to travel independently without vision or with impaired vision while in the prime of their lives. An effort is made to identify the characteristics of adults as learners that may have an impact on this process. This includes the appropriate participation of adult learners in the assessment and planning process. It also includes a discussion of how O&M instruction interacts with the central issues of vocational rehabilitation and employment of adults.

PREVALENCE AND DEMOGRAPHIC CHARACTERISTICS OF ADULTS WITH VISUAL IMPAIRMENTS

Wall Emerson and De l'Aune (Volume 1, Chapter 16) reviewed the complications associated with estimating the numbers of people who are visually impaired in any segment of the population. These complications include the various definitions of severe visual impairment used, the methods of assessing the presence of severe visual impairment in members of the population being studied (ranging from self-reports to clinical examinations), and the varying age groupings of the population used by researchers. With these complications noted, Wall Emerson and De l'Aune used data from the National Health Interview Survey (NHIS) done by the National Center for Health Statistics (1994) to estimate that the number of legally blind adults (visual acuity <20/200 [6/60]) between the ages of 20 and 60 was 450,000 in 2003. They also projected that this number would increase to 486,000 by 2010 and to 492,300 by the year 2020.

When the definition of visual impairment was expanded to include low vision (visual acuity <20/70 [6/21]), the estimated number of people between the ages of 20 and 60 was 3,044,000 in 2003. This estimate was projected to increase to 3,282,000 by 2010 and drop to 3,279,000 by 2020. In summary, it is expected that more than 3 million people in the United States between the ages of 20 and 60, who are generally in the most productive years of their lives, may need vision rehabilitation services, possibly including orientation and mobility. This, of course, does not include children, adolescents, and older adults in these projections, but as the population ages, the numbers of people overall who may need O&M services are likely to increase dramatically (see Griffin-Shirley & Welsh, Chapter 10).

CAUSES AND CHARACTERISTICS OF SEVERE VISUAL IMPAIRMENT AMONG ADULTS

The leading causes of blindness and severe visual impairment among adults in the United States are glaucoma, cataracts, diabetes, and macular degeneration (Prevent Blindness America, 2008; Ferris and Tielsch, 2004) Among older adults, the four leading causes are the same, but macular degeneration moves ahead of all the others in the ranking of prevalence. Other frequent causes of vision loss among adults are retinitis pigmentosa, retinal detachment, optic atrophy, trauma to the eye or to the brain, vitamin deficiencies, drug side effects, and other systemic diseases such as multiple sclerosis. In some cases, the cause of visual impairment may not be known (Ward & Johnson, 1997).

It is important for the O&M specialist to know the cause of vision loss for the person who has been referred for training. In some cases, this information may suggest that the vision loss is likely to worsen. In other cases, the disease that causes the vision loss may have other implications for the health and functioning of the student. This is especially true when the cause of the vision loss is diabetes. As Rosen and Crawford (Chapter 18) discuss, there are a number of health and functional complications from diabetes, such as neuropathy, pressure sores, and hyperglycemic and hypoglycemic reactions that have a direct impact on a student's ability to travel independently. An adult's other health complications may not be responsible for vision loss, but may have a direct impact on O&M training and outcomes. Rosen and Crawford discuss the mobility implications of a wide range of conditions that might be seen among adult students, such as neurological impairments, seizure disorders, multiple sclerosis, hemophilia, cardiac and blood pressure disorders, asthma, the human immunodeficiency virus (HIV), acquired immunodeficiency syndrome (AIDS), and orthopedic impairments.

The eye conditions and visual disorders that result from this wide range of etiologies found among adult students can themselves span a wide distribution. Typically, there is no way to determine from the cause of the visual impairment whether the person who has been referred for instruction is totally blind or has low vision. If the person has low vision, the range of acuities and the remaining fields of vision can be quite wide. Whether the eye condition is stable or fluctuating will vary. The length of time that a person may have had a visual impairment depends on many factors. One person may see more poorly as the amount of light decreases, another may have more problems as the amount of light or glare increases, and a third student may have the most difficulty when transitioning from one level of light to another.

Just as the actual amount of vision will vary among adult students, so too will the ability of each student to cope with his own vision loss. Some students may be coping quite well with a severe loss of vision, while others may be having serious difficulty adjusting to relatively minor losses. In some cases, these differences may re-

flect variations in students' cognitive and physical abilities; in other cases, they may be caused by variations among students in their psychosocial reactions to loss. *There is no shortcut to the process of thorough and individualized assessments in determining the abilities and disabilities of each person who appears for services.* The essential concept of individualized assessment is discussed later in this chapter.

ADJUSTMENT TO LOSS OF VISION

A large majority of the students encountered by O&M specialists in rehabilitation training programs will be persons who grew up with vision and who have lost all or part of their vision either suddenly or gradually. As a result, understanding a person's adjustment to that loss is central to the provision of appropriate and effective O&M instruction. Occasionally, however, O&M specialists in rehabilitation settings also will encounter adults who have congenital visual impairments. Thoughts about the special needs and abilities of that group of students are discussed in Sidebar 9.1.

Impact of Vision Loss on the Individual

Losing vision as an adult frequently has a strong impact on a person's psychological well-being and on his social interactions with others. Welsh (Volume 1, Chapter 6) reviews literature that is relevant to the history of the various theories regarding a person's adjustment to the loss of vision. Welsh focuses on the value of Tuttle and Tuttle's (2004) eclectic theory of adjustment with vision loss that draws from both psychoanalytic and cognitive personality theories. Tuttle and Tuttle posit a sequence of psychosocial responses to vision loss that are frequently observed in adults who are faced with this challenge. While some observers note that not every adult who experiences vision loss necessarily experiences

Adults with Congenital Visual Impairment

There may be a tendency on the part of orientation and mobility (O&M) professionals to believe that adults who grew up with visual impairments already will have received all of the O&M instruction they need during their school programs. This has become increasingly true as school-based programs have grown and expanded. However, for a number of reasons, adults with congenital impairments may show up in adult agency programs as well.

Occasionally, a child grows up with a visual impairment that is short of total blindness and may have learned to travel by using her residual vision and supplementing it with other senses and mobility tools as needed. As a young adult, this student may have experienced a change in vision and further deterioration causing a need for additional training and a greater reliance on other senses.

Other students may not have been ready to benefit from O&M training when it was offered to them as adolescents. For one reason or another—perhaps because of new education or employment opportunities—they recently have come to appreciate the importance of mobility training, and may turn to the adult agency for assistance. Still other students may have attended a school program that was not extensive enough or effective enough to help them achieve full confidence in their ability to travel independently. In other situations, students' families or living circumstances may not have permitted them to practice the learned skills to the point where they felt able to use these skills independently when their circumstances changed.

Whenever an adult with congenital visual impairment and a history of previous instruction comes to an adult program for additional training, services must begin as it does for every other adult student, with a thorough assessment of her current skills. The O&M specialist cannot assume that a person should be able to travel effectively because of previous instruction, or that she will have difficulty with independent travel because of congenital blindness.

When assessing the skills of an adult with congenital impairment and when planning instruction with such a student, the O&M specialist needs to be aware of some of the factors that *may* be likely to have an impact on instruction. Such factors may include restricted concept development, limited life experiences, an overprotective family environment, and unusual gait and posture (See Bina, Naimy, Fazzi, & Crouse, Volume 1, Chapter 12). Welsh and Tuttle (1997) have reviewed research literature relating to adults with congenital impairment. While there are few if any characteristics that are consistent for all adults in this category, there are tendencies for some of these students to have gaps in their conceptual development, especially in the areas of spatial, directional, and environmental concepts. There is no research to support the misconception that students who grew up without vision necessarily have better than average abilities in other sensory areas. While there is some evidence that such students may learn to use their other senses more effectively, these skills result from practice and not from some type of automatic compensation (see Lawson & Wiener, Volume 1, Chapter 4, and Rosen Volume 1, Chapter 5).

In recent years, great strides have been made in helping students with low vision learn to use their vision more effectively and to take advantage of low vision aids and devices. It should not be assumed, however, that all students

(continued on next page)

SIDEBAR 9.1 *(Continued)*

who have come through special programs for children with visual impairment have had appropriate assessments and services. In a similar way, it is generally understood that students who lose their vision as adults will frequently have serious adjustment issues as they cope with this loss. However, it should not be assumed that an adult with a congenital impairment does not have similar concerns. Life circumstances change for adolescents and

young adults, and a student's lack of vision suddenly can become an emotional issue when it had not been previously. While certain tendencies for students who are congenitally impaired versus those who are adventitiously impaired may be valuable in suggesting certain skills or concerns during assessments, there is no substitute for a thorough and individual evaluation of each student who appears for O&M services.

a sequence of emotional reactions that must be addressed before rehabilitation training can take place (Bledsoe, 1980 and Volume 1, Chapter 13; Dodds, 1989; Dodds et al., 1994), the sequence described by Tuttle and Tuttle is helpful in guiding how O&M specialists initially approach their adult students.

Usually, a mobility specialist will not encounter students who are in the early phases of adjustment to vision loss that are described by Tuttle and Tuttle (2004). Persons who are still experiencing the trauma of vision loss or who are still in the shock, denial, mourning, withdrawal, and depression phases typically will not present themselves for rehabilitation training. It is not until such individuals have begun to move on toward the reassessment, reaffirmation, coping, and mobilization phases described by the Tuttles that they agree to take advantage of orientation and mobility and other rehabilitation training services (Welsh, Volume 1, Chapter 6). At this point, they have begun to come to grips with the loss of vision and have begun to focus on the other skills that are available to them as alternatives to vision. However, the proposed phases of adjustment do not always flow in a clear and distinct manner. They tend to overlap, and people who seem to have reached one phase, may regress to

an earlier phase of adjustment (Tuttle & Tuttle, 2004). Sometimes these regressions are occasioned by a specific event, perhaps a situation on the street in which the person becomes especially frustrated by his inability to handle a task without vision. They may be occasioned by an encounter with an acquaintance who was not previously aware of the person's vision loss, or with a would-be helper who is especially condescending. For these reasons, the O&M specialist needs to be aware of all the phases of adjustment to vision loss and to respond to whatever emotions—whether denial, mourning, or depression—the student is expressing at that particular time.

Frequently, an opportunity to discuss these feelings with the O&M specialist or with other adult students who are going through the training at the same time will be all that is needed to help the student get back on track and continue to focus on learning new skills. If, however, these regressions occur frequently or they do not resolve easily, the O&M specialist may need to refer the student to a counselor or social worker who is better able to help the student focus on the emotional issues that may be getting in the way of O&M training.

For many adults who lose vision, this loss has a serious impact on challenges and issues that are central to being an adult. Many adult students feel very negative about the loss of independence that accompanies their inability to drive. Being able to come and go on their own helped to establish them as adults in their own minds. Learning to drive and owning their own automobiles defined for them their status as adults. When vision loss occurs, they not only face the practical problems of getting to where they want to go but also begin to feel less capable than they did before (Corn & Sacks, 1994).

Adults who experience vision loss may also face difficulty in continuing with their responsibility for their families. This is another of the major challenges of adulthood, and the fear that they may not be able to care for and provide for their families weighs heavily on the minds of many adults who lose their vision (Carroll, 1961). Related to this psychosocial challenge is concern about employment. Succeeding in the right job and establishing oneself in an appropriate profession are highly valued accomplishments for adults. The loss of vision frequently disrupts these goals or accomplishments and contributes to the psychosocial adjustment difficulties that many adults experience.

In a parallel manner, these major challenges for adults provide opportunities for motivation that O&M specialists can harness as they work with students in learning how to travel independently. The ability of an individual to care for himself and his family and to succeed in his occupation or profession are immediate and practical goals for adults. The O&M specialist should identify practical steps toward meeting these goals and relate the learning of O&M skills to those steps. Learning to cross streets independently or to travel on a bus are concrete goals that are easily shown to be directly connected to regaining independence as a family provider. While these activities may not be as directly related to the motivation of children or older adults, it is easy for the O&M specialist to connect them

directly to the training for adults in their productive years.

Impact on Families

The importance of families in the O&M instruction of children who are visually impaired is well understood, and the involvement of families is necessitated by law and regulations. This importance is also apparent when services are provided to older adults, especially those who are dependent on their families (Bambara et al., 2009). However, the importance of family involvement and participation in the provision of O&M services to adults is less well understood and frequently not addressed. However, as Tuttle and Tuttle (2004) point out, the support of the family plays a significant role in helping the adult student begin to reassess his loss, to consider the need for rehabilitation, and to follow through with rehabilitation training successfully.

The involvement of family members in an adult student's rehabilitation training must begin with the adult himself. The rehabilitation agency and the O&M instructor cannot assume to engage family members in the process without first obtaining the permission of the adult student. For a variety of reasons, an adult student may prefer not to have his family involved. The rehabilitation counselor, the social worker, or the O&M specialist may have to discuss the importance of family involvement with the student before the student agrees to his family's participation.

Once the student has given permission to contact his family, the attitudes and dynamics of family members will have to be evaluated as part of the assessment process. Some family members may have a positive and encouraging attitude toward a person's ability to cope with vision loss, but others may have a negative or patronizing point of view. Some may have a disbelieving attitude toward the student's ability to achieve increased independence because of his lack of vision. Others may feel as if their responsibility is to protect their family member from injury, exploitation, and the disappointment that may result from false expectation of success. Negative attitudes that are encountered may reflect the family member's negative attitude toward the disability itself or they may reflect interpersonal dynamics between family members that go beyond the disability and its impact.

As Sussman-Skalka (2002) discovered, the family members of the person who is visually impaired will most likely have the same level of misinformation about blindness and visual impairment that is characteristic of the population in general. As family attitudes and dynamics are evaluated, the O&M specialist or other team members should provide basic information about vision loss and the possibilities of rehabilitation. Anxieties that are expressed about the dangers of O&M training may reflect a lack of information about what is possible and how a blind person is able to travel. Observation of effective blind travelers or of other students in training may begin to provide family members with realistic information about what their spouse or sibling will be doing in O&M training. Better information may begin to break down some of the concerns and resistance that the student is feeling from his family. Another method of approaching the information needs of family members of adults with visual impairment was researched by Cimarolli, Sussman-Skalka, and Goodman (2004).

If family members tend to be overprotective toward the student, it may be important to begin the instruction in areas away from the student's home or neighborhood in order to avoid interference from the family. This is one of the advantages of a rehabilitation center program that brings the student to a center away from his home community or neighborhood. As Williams (1965) pointed out in his discussion of the dynamics related to the running of a rehabilitation center for people who are blind:

Family involvement can be a problem in a center, but it is many times more difficult in the client's home and neighborhood. The classic by-stander, moreover, who always thinks the instructor is "mean" when he offers a challenge to the pupil is next to murderous when a member of his own family is the victim, or, once he gets a little sophistication, more demanding than any instructor would ever dream of being. The emotional load is greatly reduced away from all of this. (p. 36)

The reactions of family members tend to be exaggerated much more than those of unconnected observers on the street. Whether they believe that the O&M specialist is being too easy on the student or too demanding, the responses of the family member may be especially upsetting to the student. In some cases, it is important for the student to have developed beginning skills and, most important, confidence in his own abilities, before facing the challenges and anxieties of travel in front of family members. As is true of every other aspect of O&M instruction, the best approach for each individual student will depend on the specific analysis of that student's abilities and family dynamics.

As Sussman-Skalka (2002) discussed, spouses or close family members are frequently in a position to encourage independent functioning in keeping with the goals of O&M instruction or to subvert the training that has been provided. Encouraging and allowing the spouse or the visually impaired family member to use his new skills and to figure out how to reorient following a wrong turn requires that the family member have the time and patience to support the learning process and know when to step in or not to step in. While the family member cannot be expected to be as skilled as the O&M specialist in making such judgments, time spent in helping family members to learn how best to support the learning process can pay important dividends.

ISSUES IN ADULT LEARNING

Cognitive Theory and Andragogy

Jacobson and Bradley (Volume 1, Chapter 7) have reviewed the primary theories of learning and how they relate to teaching methodologies used in O&M instruction. While most approaches to teaching and learning initially were grounded in behavioral theory, Jacobson and Bradley have demonstrated how teaching has been influenced in more recent decades by cognitive learning theory and especially social cognitive theory, which is a combination of behavioral theory and cognitive theory.

Cognitive theory emphasizes the learner's active involvement in the learning process. It holds that learning is most successful when the learner is aware of the purpose of the instruction, the plan for instruction, and the cognitive scheme in which the new learning fits. According to Zimmerman (1989), social cognitive theory supports the value of self-regulated learning, which involves the learner in goal setting, self-motivation, self-instruction, and self-evaluation.

Cognitive theory also supports a growing interest in recent years in the concept of "andragogy." While people are generally aware of the term "pedagogy," which is defined as the art and science of teaching, the term is considered to apply primarily to the art and science of teaching children. Andragogy has received greater attention in the field of adult education as a result of the work of Knowles (1980). According to Knowles (1980, pp. 44–45), andragogy focuses on four basic assumptions about adult learners that reflect adults' abilities, needs, and desires to take responsibility for their own learning:

1. Adults' self-concepts move from dependency to independency or self-directedness.

2. They accumulate a reservoir of experiences that can be used as a basis on which to build learning.

3. Their readiness to learn becomes increasingly associated with the developmental tasks of social roles.

4. Their time and curricular perspectives change from postponed to immediacy of application and from subject-centeredness to performance centeredness.

Unlike a child in a school setting who may be preparing for some future need or responsibility, the adult learner typically is focusing on an immediate objective. This is especially true for adults in rehabilitation settings. Their lives have been disrupted by disabilities, and they are eager to have their lives and their independence restored. As a result, whatever is being taught should clearly relate to the adult's immediate and practical needs.

In discussing the differences between pedagogy and andragogy, Hiemstra and Sisco (1990) focused on the role of the teacher versus the role of the student. Traditionally, pedagogy is teacher-directed instruction that places the student in a submissive role dependent on the instructor. Andragogy, however, acknowledges that as adults mature, they need to become more responsible for their own actions. They need to learn what is immediately required to solve present problems, but they need to learn *how to learn* so that they can adapt to a constantly changing world. A similar distinction is that between guided learning and discovery learning, discussed in Sidebar 9.2.

The principles of andragogy are relevant to all kinds of instruction and for learners of all ages. However, these principles seem to be especially helpful for adult learners who are facing life situations, as in O&M instruction, in which they are required to learn a new set of necessary skills and to develop a method of solving similar problems in the future. According to Knowles (1984), these principles can be summarized as follows:

SIDEBAR 9.2

Guided Learning versus Discovery Learning

Jacobson and Bradley (Volume 1, Chapter 7) have discussed the concepts of guided learning and discovery learning, and compared the two. The primary differences between these approaches seem to be in the amount of didactic teaching or guiding that is provided by the instructor when compared to the amount of experiential learning that results from the learner's active involvement. This distinction is similar to the point made by Knowles (1980), when he clarified that pedagogy and andragogy are not dichotomous but rather are most useful when they are seen as two ends of a continuum. Learners in a given situation fall somewhere in between the two extremes of needing to be taught everything by the teacher in a didactic manner and needing to be totally responsible for their own learning.

The teaching of orientation and mobility (O&M) has always promoted the active participation of the student in actual travel situations in natural environments. While instruction begins with the presentation of mobility techniques and the skills of orientation by the mobility specialist, it also includes opportunities for the student to demonstrate the use of these techniques and orientation problem solving in practically every lesson. LaGrow

(Chapter 1) demonstrates how the development of perceptual skills is integrated into every lesson, while Bozeman and McCulley (Chapter 2) do the same in demonstrating how orientation skills are taught. Mettler (1995) and Altman and Cutter (2004) have suggested a dichotomy in two different approaches to teaching orientation and mobility. They believe that the traditional approach has relied solely on guided instruction, in which the instructor presents techniques to the student and expects no demonstration of effective use of the skills. They also suggest that the alternative approach they favor uses a structured discovery approach that requires participation from the learner. However, Malamazian (1970), Welsh (1972), and Williams (in Welsh, 2005) have noted that the teaching of orientation and mobility from its earliest days required an active participation on the part of the student, with many opportunities at every level of instruction to use the skills that were being developed, including the problem-solving skills of orientation. This level of participation effectively communicated to the student that he was responsible for his own orientation and that he had to learn how to orient himself to new locations and to solve orientation problems as they arose in the future.

1. Adults need to know why they are learning particular skills or information.

2. Adults learn through experiences as opposed to just being told what to do.

3. Adults learn most effectively when they approach learning as problem solving.

4. Adults learn best when they understand the immediate value of the topic they are studying or the skill they are developing.

A Problem-Solving Approach to Teaching

Perla and O'Donnell (2004) have explicitly addressed the manner in which O&M specialists can teach problem solving. While all mobility students will benefit from a teaching method that helps them learn to solve problems, as Knowles (1984) points out, adults learn most effectively when they approach learning as problem solving.

Perla and O'Donnell point out that problem solving will not occur if lessons are structured in such a way that problems do not occur. Students are unable to learn from their mistakes if mistakes are never allowed to happen. Similarly, students never have an opportunity to develop confidence in their problem-solving ability if lessons are not structured to allow time for the students to actually solve the problems that occur. Perla and O'Donnell (2004, p. 49) have suggested a number of steps that O&M specialists can take to create an atmosphere in which problem-solving skills can be developed, as follows:

1. Discuss with students the value of making mistakes.

2. Praise students for their willingness to try, whether or not they are successful.

3. Encourage students to take risks.

4. Praise students for considering other options, not just the "first impulse."

5. Work from students' strengths to improve their weaker skill areas.

6. Plan problem-solving learning experiences in a sequenced manner so that tasks are both attainable and challenging.

ASSESSMENT AND PROGRAM PLANNING

Bina, Naimy, Fazzi, and Crouse (Volume 1, Chapter 12) present a thorough review of the need for and importance of assessment as an essential component of O&M instruction. While this applies to all students, it is *especially* important for adults. Most of the time, services provided to adults are not mandated, unlike those available to children. As a result, the assessment may play an important role in helping to determine the adult's eligibility for services and the extent of the services offered and provided. The O&M services provided to adults are usually part of a vocational

rehabilitation plan, and eligibility for such services is based on the likelihood that they will result in employment. Services are usually not provided through the state-federal vocational rehabilitation program if the goal is merely to enable the adult to learn to cope more effectively with vision loss. The limited availability of funding through the vocational rehabilitation program also may result in a limited amount of services. For this reason, it is important that the assessment done with adults be as accurate as possible. There are no resources to spare, and the pressure is on the adult student and the O&M specialist to use these limited resources as efficiently as possible. An effective assessment may help the student and instructor avoid spending time focusing on the use of remaining vision only to find that vision is insufficient to assure the student's safety in travel. Or, a good assessment may show that time spent trying to develop O&M skills in the student's home environment under the interfering eye of protective family members may be time wasted. In this case, the student may need to attend a rehabilitation center away from home to develop confidence in travel skills before convincing his family that he can be a safe traveler.

An effective O&M assessment also can have an impact on the nature of the vocational rehabilitation plan being developed. If the student and rehabilitation counselor are focusing on an employment goal that will require extensive travel either for training or for the work itself, it may be important to the consideration of that goal for the results of the O&M assessment to be available as soon as possible. Significant challenges to independent travel need to be identified, if present, and their impact on the rehabilitation plan assessed by the student and the rehabilitation counselor. Adult students, in representing themselves to their counselors, may under- or overestimate their present level of skills. Because the counselor may not be able to evaluate these representations himself, it is important to have the O&M

specialist, as a member of a comprehensive rehabilitation team, carry out a functional evaluation with the student.

Performance Domains and Functional Measures

Bina, Naimy, Fazzi, and Crouse (Volume 1, Chapter 12) present a comprehensive list of the various performance domains that need to be included in an O&M assessment. These include: (1) background information, (2) mobility skills, (3) orientation skills, (4) conceptual understanding, (5) vision functioning, and (6) auditory functioning. They also discuss a number of methods of assessing these various areas of functioning. Some of these domains, such as vision and auditory function, are evaluated through standard clinical assessment procedures. Others, such as orientation skills and environmental concepts, are reviewed in an interview format with the student. An assumption is made that if the adult student grew up with vision, many of these basic concepts are present. However, experienced O&M specialists have come to appreciate the need for functional evaluations in real settings. It is not unusual to find students who are unable to interpret what they hear or see when their clinical measurements suggest that they should be able to see or hear certain environmental stimuli. Others may be able to describe a car or a bus, but they are unable to translate those concepts into functional skills without vision. For these reasons, the O&M specialist tries to base assessments on observations of the student's actual performance at whatever level of skill he can demonstrate at that point in learning to cope with his vision loss.

For the adult student who has lost vision relatively recently and who has only begun to pursue O&M training, it is difficult to truly assess his ability to learn certain advanced skills until the learning of more basic skills has been accomplished. Acknowledging this reality, some program settings authorize and fund a beginning segment of the instruction with the expectation that the student's success or difficulty in learning these basic skills of orientation and mobility will provide the O&M specialist with an opportunity to make a more accurate assessment of the amount of time and instruction that will be needed to accomplish the ultimate goals of the rehabilitation plan.

Permission to Contact

When providing services to adults, it is especially important to obtain the student's permission before interviewing family members, employers, and others. This allows the adult student to play a role in determining how his situation is presented to these other important people his life. It is also a way in which the O&M specialist communicates respect for the student as a full participant in the learning process. As the specialist contacts these other people in the adult student's life, it provides the opportunity to communicate the basic premise that this contact is happening only with the permission of the student. This sets a tone of respect for the student and reinforces the student's role and importance in all planning related to his future.

Goal Setting

The earlier discussion regarding the principles of andragogy emphasized the importance of having adult learners involved in the setting of goals for the instruction and the selection of methods to reach those goals. As Welsh has discussed (Chapter 6 and Volume 1, Chapter 6), the selection of appropriate goals interacts closely with the student's feelings about himself and especially his feelings of self-efficacy with regard to coping with vision loss. They also may reflect more basic aspects of the student's personality, adjustment to vision loss, and expectations for the future. Selecting lesser goals may reflect a realistic assessment of the student's knowledge of himself or it may be a way in which the student is avoiding the risk of failure. For some students, however, the choice of a higher goal may be a subconscious strategy for later explaining why they did not succeed.

Ultimately, however, the adult student must feel part of the team that chooses the goals and sets the plan. He must be personally invested in the plan, and the goals have to make sense to him, regardless of the psychosocial dynamics that may underlie the selection. The adult student needs to understand why the approach suggested by the O&M specialist is important, and has to be fully committed to it. Students whose programs are funded by the state-federal vocational rehabilitation program are required to participate in a formal planning process that results in an Individualized Plan for Employment (IPE). This document must be reviewed and signed by the student, and it becomes the legal basis and the accountability document for the services that are provided for that student.

Evaluation of Progress

Involvement in the planning also means that the student plays a role in determining how the ongoing assessment of progress will take place. The benchmarks indicating that the plan is working must be determined in advance and not after the fact. This approach can help adult students and their service providers know whether or not they are making progress and, if necessary, make corrections in the approach while the instruction is taking place. This participation in the evaluation process helps students develop their own evaluation skills, which is an important component of developing problem-solving skills and is necessary as students leave the program and assume an independent lifestyle.

Cultural Diversity

Another category of information to be considered when doing assessments and planning the delivery of services to adult students relates to cultural diversity and its impact on assessment and teaching situations. Most of our discussion in the United States about the impact of impairment and disability on people reflects the perspective of the mainstream or majority point of view in the culture. However, various ethnic groups can have very different points of view from that of the majority culture about disability and about attempts to help people with disability become more independent. O&M specialists need to consider how these differences may impact the way they assess their students' attitude toward disability and their motivation for O&M training. In some cases, these differences also may have an impact on the working relationship between the O&M specialist and the student from a different ethnic background and on the reactions of the student's family.

Rogers, Schmitt, and Scholl (1997) discuss some of the conceptual difficulties associated with a discussion of ethnic and cultural differences. They note that the concept of a "majority" culture is relative. What constitutes a majority in one community may be a minority in another. Also, differences *between members within an ethnic group* may be greater than the differences *between one ethnic group and another*. Because of these differences, O&M specialists have to be careful not to allow information about characteristic ways in which members of an ethnic group may react to disability to become stereotypes that influence their judgments and assessments about specific students. As Orlansky and Trap (1987) emphasize, it is important that students who need specialized services be treated and assessed as individuals and not be perceived as stereotypes.

O&M specialists and other professionals working with people should become as knowledgeable as possible about other cultures and ethnic differences. They should bring this information to bear when their observations about students from such groups do not fit the expected pattern in a particular community. Some of these observations may be explained or better understood by considering the impact of the student's unique culture or ethnic background. Ponchillia (1993) discusses a number of Native American cultural beliefs that may have implications for those providing rehabilitation services to people with diabetes-related blindness or other visual impairments. Also, Rogers, Schmitt, and Scholl (1997) review a number of rehabilitation-relevant attitudes, values, behaviors, and communication styles for which the Eurocentric perspective may differ from the perspectives of other cultures.

In addition to increasing their awareness of the impact of various ethnic perspectives on the attitudes, behaviors, and communication styles of students from cultural backgrounds different than their own, O&M specialists need to become sensitive to the way their own attitudes or biases may influence their communications with and decisions about such students. In any profession that requires close and personal interactions between the student and the professional, university educators and agency supervisors need to help beginning professionals identify, understand, and move beyond their own cultural biases and perspectives to the point where they can serve all students objectively.

Multiple Impairments

The traditional understanding of the demographics of adults who are visually impaired seems to be that such adults are more likely to have only a visual impairment to contend with, but children and seniors more frequently have multiple impairments. While prevalence statistics may show this perception to be statistically accurate, there is no lack of visually impaired adults in rehabilitation settings who have other disabilities as well. Chapters 17 through 20 of this volume contain information that can be helpful in knowing how best to assess and address these other impairments, whether they are found in children, adults, or seniors. These other impairments in-

clude hearing loss, motor and neurological problems, serious health concerns such as diabetes with all of its related issues, emotional and cognitive impairments, and an increasing frequency of brain trauma and related impairment. The presence of any of these additional impairments will have consequences on both the assessment of the adult student's needs and abilities, on the development and structure of lesson plans, and on the implementation of the agreed-upon program of training.

IMPLEMENTING O&M TRAINING FOR ADULTS

Structuring Lessons

The original curriculum for O&M instruction was developed with the needs of adventitiously blinded adults in mind. The lesson plan sequence that most O&M specialists encountered when learning to travel under blindfold during their university training can trace its origin to the Blind Rehabilitation Center at the Hines VA Hospital in the 1950s (Bledsoe, Volume 1, Chapter 13). The initial publications that addressed curriculum and lesson planning for orientation and mobility (Hill & Ponder, 1976; Jacobson, 1993; LaGrow & Weessies, 1994) reflect this same general pattern, although each with certain modifications to reflect the special insights of the authors. The appropriateness of this original curriculum or the ability to follow it closely for each adult student must be evaluated in light of the many factors discussed earlier. These factors relate to the individual student, the setting in which the instruction is being provided (discussed later in this chapter), and the amount of funding and time available to support the instruction.

Instruction that is provided in established centers, whether residential or day centers, offer the advantage of clearly identified internal and external areas that offer the opportunity to teach most of the lessons and skills covered in the typical O&M curriculum. Even when the standard curriculum has to be modified in view of the special needs or interests of a particular student, an inventory of alternative locations usually exists, for example, where the lighting may be different, where accessible environments allow the use of a wheelchair, or where routes do not require the same level of stamina. Planning and keeping records of lessons in such well-established settings are more easily accomplished, and preprinted goals, objectives, and evaluation forms may be available.

When instruction is provided in a community-based service delivery setting, more time is required on the part of the O&M specialist to identify and analyze nearby and accessible locations that offer the opportunity to expose the student to the range of skills and experiences required by that student's plan of instruction. Additional effort is required on the part of the O&M specialist to note the location of these areas for future reference and for use in evaluating and reporting on the student's experience and progress. Many areas may not offer the appropriate and necessary range of travel situations that will permit the instructor to cover all of the skills and experiences that are needed by a given student. This may require greater time and travel on the part of the instructor and student to more distant areas to fully implement the plan that was written. Or the plan may have to be modified to eliminate some of the skills that may not be able to be taught in that community, such as the use of some types of public transportation, larger intersections, or rural travel. One advantage of community-based settings may be the opportunity to help the student learn the required skills in the exact areas where they will be used. This can eliminate the loss of skill and confidence that sometimes accompanies the transfer of skills learned in established training areas to the student's home or employment community. This

may be especially helpful when teaching students who have limited understanding or memory issues that make the transfer to new areas very difficult.

Motivating and Rewarding Adults

Having engaged the adult student in a thorough assessment and planning process, the O&M specialist should have a good understanding of what is most likely to motivate the student for the instruction to come. Theories of andragogy suggest that the adult learner should have a good understanding of and agreement with the reason the instruction is taking place and what goals will be accomplished as a result of the student's success. It is not enough for O&M specialists to approach adult students with the vague explanation that they should learn to travel independently because it is the thing to do or merely because it can be done. There needs to be an understanding between the instructor and the adult student that the purpose of the instruction relates to goals and outcomes that are meaningful to the student.

Usually, adult students will have immediate goals that motivate them, for example, traveling independently to a place of employment. Adult students typically will be motivated by any activity that they view as related directly to that goal. Such a goal, however, based as it may be on rather complex and sophisticated skills, may require that the student develop more basic skills first. Before crossing a street successfully, the student first needs to be able to walk in a straight line and hold that line for the width of the street. When working with an adult student, the O&M specialist has to take the time to explain how certain skills must come first and how these more basic skills relate to later skills. This cognitive understanding will help the student see the importance of the sequence in which these skills have to be learned.

As Williams (1965) points out, there is nothing more important or more motivating for adult students than successful experiences. For each learning experience to represent a successful experience for students, the task must be achievable, but also of sufficient difficulty that its accomplishment feels like a significant success. While adult students may want to start directly with learning to use the bus that goes to the neighborhood where they hope to be employed, if they are not successful in the lessons leading up to bus travel, they will probably not succeed in bus travel either. As a result, the goal that is so relevant to them will not prove to be motivating if they cannot accomplish it. Welsh (Chapter 6 and Volume 1, Chapter 6) cites the research of Bandura (1986), which provides the theoretical and research-based support for the observations of Williams that the experience of success in the accomplishment of more basic skills can improve the student's sense of self-efficacy as it relates to the motivation to try more advanced skills.

As LaGrow illustrates in Chapter 1, lessons that are important for learning human guide skills or cane skills will be most helpful if they also contain the seeds for learning or reinforcing basic environmental concepts or problem-solving skills. Similarly in Chapter 2, Bozeman and McCulley show how the process of learning to use basic orientation skills will be most effective if the student can see how these basic skills relate to more complicated orientation skills down the road. Even when learning to use human guide techniques, the adult student can be practicing more sophisticated orientation problem-solving skills that will be needed when traveling independently in more complex environments.

As the necessary sequence of learning emerges for an individual student, it is important for the O&M specialist working with an adult student to keep that student involved in the planning and decision making regarding how the learning sequence will proceed. This will require frequent discussions about the next steps and how they relate to the specific goals of the student. In the situation where a student wishes to proceed more rapidly than the O&M specialist thinks is manageable, the O&M specialist should try to work out a compromise that may require trying the student's preferred approach first, with an understanding that if certain problems are encountered, a different approach will be tried that addresses skill development in the sequence more likely to lead to success.

ORIENTATION AND MOBILITY AND EMPLOYMENT

The Vocational Rehabilitation Process

Most adults are referred for O&M training through the vocational rehabilitation system. While some adults are referred for personal adjustment training by medical or social service personnel or by family or friends, most adults enter the rehabilitation system as a result of their loss of employment following their loss of vision, or because of their difficulty in entering the employment market as a person with a visual impairment. In the United States, the state vocational rehabilitation agencies, funded largely with federal dollars, are the most common sources of funding for rehabilitation training, including O&M training.

In some instances, rehabilitation counselors who manage the vocational rehabilitation system recognize that a newly referred person who is visually impaired will require personal adjustment training to learn to cope with the basic problems of vision loss before considering employment opportunities. On such occasions, the rehabilitation counselor first will refer the student for personal adjustment training, including O&M training. For other students, either because of previous personal adjustment training or because of less-severe vision loss, the rehabilitation counselor may not be sure whether or not personal adjustment training is needed before considering employment possibilities. These students may be referred for an assessment of their independent travel abilities before a decision is made regarding the need for training.

The Role of the O&M Specialist in Vocational Rehabilitation

In providing an employment-related O&M assessment, the O&M specialist needs to work closely with the rehabilitation counselor and the student to understand the type of employment that is being considered and the type of travel that might be required for the student to be able to access employment opportunities. For example, will the use of public transportation be required, or will employment require travel through a complex and changing factory environment? Once the agreed-upon goal is known and considered, the O&M specialist's assessment may suggest that more comprehensive O&M training will be required than was anticipated by the counselor or by the student. This may have the impact of delaying the start of job training or the process of employment placement.

It is important that the O&M specialist be an active member of a student's rehabilitation team. Luxton, Bradfield, Maxson, and Starkson (1997) review the roles of various team members and discuss the particular role that the O&M specialist plays in the vocational rehabilitation process. In addition to providing basic O&M training, the O&M specialist can play a role in evaluating the travel aspects of specific employment options and can provide placement counselors and employers with feedback on how the work environment or its neighborhood complies with the accessibility guidelines discussed by Barlow, Bentzen, and Franck (Volume 1, Chapter 11). Some job sites will require travel skills that are beyond the ability of the student who is being considered for placement. In some cases, getting to the site

will present a challenge for any blind employee or at least for this particular employee. In other situations, getting to the site will not be as difficult as the travel will be at the site itself.

Orientation and Mobility and the Placement Process

In some instances, the O&M specialist will be the best person to accompany the student to the location for a specific assessment of the student's ability to access this location or for focused training at the location itself. Mobility training at the site can be an important part of the placement process. Such training can provide the employee who is visually impaired an opportunity for an informal introduction to the site and to other employees prior to the pressure of job responsibilities. The O&M specialist can also play a helpful role in answering the questions of other employees who may have concerns about having a coworker who is blind. Like most people, if coworkers have not had interaction experiences with people who are visually impaired, they may require some guidance and training in what to expect and in human guide skills. The O&M specialist, with the approval of the employer, can arrange time for guide training, for training in basic interaction skills with a person who is blind, and to answer questions that other employees may have.

When such training occurs, it may be helpful to have the new employee who is visually impaired present and participating, or it may be best for some employees to have this training take place before the student's arrival. In the latter instance, it is important that the O&M specialist or whoever is conducting the training provide the employee who is visually impaired with a summary of what took place and what other employees have been told with regard to having a coworker who is visually impaired.

As Harkins and Moyer (1997) explain, the process of job development and job modification can require an ongoing process of interactions between the rehabilitation staff and the employer to assure the success of employees who are visually impaired. O&M specialists can play an ongoing role in this communication and education process as new mobility challenges arise for employees who are visually impaired. These challenges may arise as a result of changes in the impairments of the employees or in the employment environment, or because of the emergence of new technology that can be of use to employees who are visually impaired. Some employees with multiple impairments may require the ongoing support of job coaches who work closely with the employee on-site. Because job coaches work so closely with employees, they may require extra training from the mobility specialist because they are in a good position to support and reinforce the everyday travel skills of the employee. They also need assistance in recognizing when they are doing too much for the employee who is visually impaired, and that additional instruction by the O&M specialist may be needed from time to time. The job coach may be in the best position to recognize that need and to communicate it to the rehabilitation counselor or the O&M specialist.

OPTIONS FOR THE DELIVERY OF O&M SERVICES TO ADULTS

O&M services for adults in their working years can be provided through either center-based or community-based programs. Center-based programs may operate as a part of a residential program or can be a day program without a residential component.

Center-Based Programs

Historical Background

The first rehabilitation center for adults who lost their vision was established at St. Dunstan's in England in 1915 to serve veterans blinded dur-

ing World War I. "The main idea . . . in establishing this Hostel for the blinded soldiers was that the sightless men, after being discharged from the hospital, might come into a little world where the things which blind men cannot do were forgotten and where everyone was concerned with what blind men can do" (Pearson, 1919, p. 14). The first rehabilitation center for blind adults in the United States was begun at a special U.S. Army General Hospital in Baltimore in 1918, on an estate called Evergreen that had been taken over by the government. Those who developed the center at Evergreen emphasized that its purpose was to equip the blinded soldier to take his place in society as a self-supporting and self-respecting individual (Fitzgerald & Asenjo, 1965). As responsibility for Evergreen was transferred to the American Red Cross and then to the Veterans Bureau, its focus was further sharpened to target the educational needs of the blinded soldiers. However, a concentration on the systematic teaching of orientation and mobility was not a part of this post–World War I program.

A similar time-limited focus was included in the designation of two military general hospitals, Valley Forge and Letterman, which were selected for the "special treatment of blinded casualties" during World War II (Greear, 1946). Letterman was later replaced by Dibble. In addition to these specially designated hospitals, a social rehabilitation center was established in June 1944 at Avon Old Farms in Connecticut (Fitzgerald & Asenjo, 1965). Through the work of Avon Old Farms and Valley Forge Army Hospital, formal instruction in orientation and mobility became a central part of the rehabilitation program for blinded veterans, which was passed on to the Veterans Administration (VA) and further developed at Hines VA Hospital in Hines, Illinois.

Leaders of civilian programs that served adults who were visually impaired visited the Avon Old Farms, Valley Forge, and Hines programs, leading to the establishment of numerous rehabilitation centers around the country. Between 1945 and

1950, approximately 30 agencies—both government and private—claimed to have rehabilitation centers that offered comprehensive personal adjustment to blindness centers (Fitzgerald & Asenjo, 1965).

Purpose of Rehabilitation Centers

The purpose of rehabilitation centers is to provide personal adjustment to blindness programs addressing the needs of recently blinded adults as comprehensively as possible. O&M training is usually most efficiently and thoroughly provided through such center-based programs. Center-based O&M programs play a central role in the Blind Rehabilitation Centers of the U.S. Department of Veterans Affairs. It was in the first of these programs at Hines Hospital that the most widely replicated model for center-based O&M training was developed.

Center-based O&M training programs are characterized by well-established assessment and training areas that offer comprehensive opportunities for evaluating and teaching the entire range of O&M skills. The staffing of such centers also provides the opportunity for comprehensive interdisciplinary inputs that address low vision needs, health needs, communication skills, other personal adjustment skills, and psychological, social, and employment needs.

Center-based programs provide opportunities for intense programming that might include as many as two O&M lessons per day or a minimum of three lessons per week. Such intense instruction can more readily identify needs and weaknesses and reinforce emerging skills. Reinforcement also can be provided by center staff in addition to the O&M staff because they are typically aware of what is expected of students in the center when it comes to independent travel.

Center-based programs allow for the natural interaction of O&M students with other students, which can be important in addressing a number of psychosocial issues (Welsh, Chapter 6). In some settings, meetings among students are arranged for the purpose of discussing various aspects of O&M training, including social and emotional reactions to the process. However, even when formal meetings are not part of the schedule, interactions between students take place during meals, in lounges, or during recreation times that result in helpful discussions of O&M training and comparison of successes and challenges.

Nonresidential Programs

Not all center-based programs are residential in nature. In some large cities and well-populated suburban areas, some center-based programs operate on a day basis. Students are transported to a center every day or several days per week where they participate in programs that vary in intensity. Depending on transportation options, funding, and demand for the services, some students may attend the program every day until they have reached predetermined goals. Others, especially older adults, may attend less frequently and extend their rehabilitation training over a longer period.

Most centers that provide O&M services are primarily focused on serving people who are blind or visually impaired. Some may offer a special unit for people with visual impairments within a more broad-based agency that serves people with a wide range of disabilities. Some center-based programs may be located in a community college setting or in some other type of vocational education or adult education facility. To the extent that an O&M program is housed within an agency that serves only people with visual impairments, it is more likely that the O&M services will be supported by other services related to coping with vision loss. In more broad-based rehabilitation centers or adult education centers, students who have other disabilities in addition to their vision loss may be more likely to receive needed services such as physical therapy, occupational therapy, speech services, or basic education and vocational training.

Funding for Center-Based Programs

Rehabilitation centers that serve visually impaired students may be state agencies funded as a line item in the budget of a larger state agency or department. Typically, some of the funding for such centers comes from the cooperative state-federal vocational rehabilitation program. State residents are usually referred to such centers by state-employed rehabilitation counselors. Other centers are private not-for-profit entities that operate on grants obtained from state rehabilitation departments or on fee-for-service arrangements that cover the costs of students referred by state-employed rehabilitation counselors. Such arrangements may arbitrarily limit the amount of time a student is able to attend the center and therefore limit the extent and the thoroughness of the O&M training provided.

Most private, not-for-profit rehabilitation centers also pursue other sources of funding as they become available (Welsh, 2001). This includes local, state, and national government program funding and a wide variety of private fund-raising activities. Students also are able to pay out of pocket for their own services at some private agencies.

Community-Based Services

Increasingly, O&M services are provided through community-based programs. In some communities or states, a comprehensive rehabilitation center is not available for students who are blind or visually impaired. In other situations, state funding through the state-federal vocational rehabilitation program is insufficient to cover the cost of referring students to comprehensive center-based programs, especially when residential support is required.

Among the advantages of community-based programs is the opportunity for the student to stay home and continue to function as a member of the family and community, while still receiving O&M training. In these settings, the rehabilitation training does not have to disrupt other aspects of the student's life, even though separation from the home setting may be very helpful for some students (Welsh, Chapter 6).

Community-based programs also allow the student to receive training in the areas where the skills will be used. This can be helpful for some students and can eliminate the problem of the student having to transfer skills learned in the training area to the home or employment area, which may or may not be similar to the training area. Community-based training is more likely to engage family members in the observation and support of the training. While this is typically a helpful process, if it is not, community-based training will provide more opportunities for intervention with family members who may be purposefully or inadvertently sabotaging the instruction.

On the negative side, instructors who provide services through community-based programs spend more time locating and evaluating assessment and training areas near each student's residence or place of employment. This can translate into more of the mobility specialist's time being spent traveling between students and setting up assessment and training areas and less time spent teaching. In community-based programs, there are usually fewer team interactions to discuss students and less time spent in consultation with members of other disciplines who may also know the student.

Students who receive their training in community-based programs are less likely to know and interact with other students who are experiencing visual impairment and participating in rehabilitation training. As a result, it is sometimes difficult for them to set appropriate goals for themselves, to evaluate their own performances effectively, and to sort out which of their problems are characteristic of the condition and which are the result of personal decisions and efforts that can be remedied through additional training or greater effort on their part. Students in such programs are also less likely to receive a comprehensive array of services designed to address many different aspects of their adjustment to vision loss.

FUTURE DEVELOPMENTS

Less-Comprehensive Services and Fewer Instructors

Formal instruction in orientation and mobility began with adults, specifically adults who had lost their vision during World War II. Civilian agencies that provided rehabilitation services to adults were among the first to send staff members to Valley Forge Hospital, Avon Old Farms, and the Hines Blind Rehabilitation Center to learn what they could about teaching independent travel in their own agencies (Blasch & Kaarlela, 1971). Shortly after university training programs began to turn out formally trained O&M specialists, research and demonstration programs were funded to show how these new professionals could be of service to children who are blind or visually impaired in local and residential schools (Blasch & Kaarlela, 1971).

As university-based training programs began to expand, more of them came to be associated with education-based teacher training programs. In part, this was responding to the needs of children with visual impairments for formal training in orientation and mobility. However, as an increasing number of job openings appeared for O&M specialists in residential schools and public school systems, more and more O&M specialists turned to schools for employment. While some O&M specialists preferred to work with adults rather than children, many school positions were more attractive. In general, school salaries were more than competitive with the salaries offered in adult agencies, but when the 9-month school year was compared to a 12-month position in an adult agency, the school position fre-

quently turned out to be more attractive. This was also true when other employee benefits and retirement plans were considered. This advantage for school-based employers was further strengthened when federal special-education legislation mandated fair and appropriate education for children with disabilities in all school systems.

This trend toward the employment of increasing numbers of O&M specialists in school-based programs has been aggravated by level funding of federal programs that support university training in orientation and mobility focusing on rehabilitation services. When compared to programs that focus on children and the dual preparation of teachers of the visually impaired and O&M specialists, the university programs for training O&M specialists to work with adults have not been able to compete.

When this pattern of greater employment in school systems is considered alongside the growing focus on the development of funding opportunities for O&M services for Medicare-eligible older adults (Griffin-Shirley and Welsh, Chapter 10), a concern arises regarding the ability of service programs for adults to compete for O&M specialists with schools and services for older adults. Not only is the funding for comprehensive O&M services for adults less available, but agencies serving adults are having increasing difficulty in attracting and retaining O&M specialists. As members of the baby boom generation reach their senior years, it is expected that the demand for services for older adults will increase. While this is not expected to minimize the demand for mandated services for children, it may very likely impact the available funding for services for adults in their working years, which are not mandated.

Greater Reliance on Technology

Barlow, Bentzen, Franck, and Sauerburger (Chapter 12) discuss the changes in the travel environments that are making travel for people without vision more complex. Also, Bentzen and Marston (Chapter 11) and Penrod, Smith Haneline, and Corbett (Chapter 14) review the emergence of new technology, especially for orientation, and how that may affect independent travel in the future. These changes and the growing complexity that they are likely to add to travel, especially for adults, imply the need for more thoroughly trained O&M specialists and for increased training time and funding for adult students. These needs contrast starkly with the insufficient funding and the reduced number of O&M specialists discussed in the previous section.

Independent Living Services for Adults with Multiple Impairments

In Chapters 17 through 20 of this volume, information is presented about the growing numbers of students who are blind or visually impaired with additional disabilities and health impairments. This is a reflection of improvements in health care that are resulting in the survival of increasing numbers of people with multiple impairments. As more and more of these adults with multiple disabilities take advantage of increasing opportunities for them to live independently or with support in the community, those with blindness or visual impairments will most likely need additional O&M training in order to succeed. Once again, it appears that the delivery systems that provide O&M services to adults with visual impairments will need substantially more funding and service providers in order to deliver the increased skill training that is implied by the expansion of community-based independent living services that have been promised to these adults. This, too, represents a major strain on services to adults with visual impairments as services to adults with multiple disabilities expand in order to provide the increased level of services required by the commitment to providing independent living services in the community to all adults with disabilities.

Health Care–Based Services

In recent years, O&M services have begun to be associated with the health care system in an attempt to identify and take advantage of potential sources of payment for these services and other rehabilitation services for people with visual impairments. In response to many other types of disabilities, the health care system has accepted the responsibility for helping people who are functionally impaired return to full functioning through the services of physical therapists, occupational therapists, and speech therapists, among others. For a variety of historical and social reasons, the health care system had not embraced responsibility for addressing the independent living needs of people who lose their vision (Lidoff, 2001; Wainapel, 1995). Such services had developed as educational and vocational rehabilitation services rather than medical services, and some blind consumer advocates, rejecting the medical model as applied to blindness, made every effort to reinforce that separation.

Massof and Lidoff (2001) reviewed efforts that are under way to integrate O&M instruction and other vision rehabilitation services into the health care system. As low vision services have expanded within the health care system, the inclusion of rehabilitation services, especially orientation and mobility, has begun to be offered in health settings. In some settings, vision rehabilitation services have been provided by occupational therapists, but low vision programs in some other health care settings have begun to employ certified O&M specialists. While these services are primarily focused on providing O&M training to older persons who are visually impaired and eligible for Medicare (Griffin-Shirley & Welsh, Chapter 10; Wiener & Siffermann, Volume 1, Chapter 14), it is possible that the success of this expansion for that segment of the adult population will represent a preview of the eventual expansion of such services for all adults through the health care system.

Expanding Needs of Blinded Veterans

Recent military conflicts in Iraq and Afghanistan have seen an increase in the number and variety of multiple injuries caused by powerful explosives detonated in the immediate vicinity of military personnel. This change in the nature of combat-related injuries has corresponded with advances in the medical interventions used in the field of combat to result in more military personnel surviving serious multiple wounds. As a result, the number of disabled veterans surviving with combinations of vision loss, brain injury, hearing loss, and loss of limbs has increased dramatically. The rehabilitation of these veterans with severe multiple disabilities will increase the number of hours of mobility instruction needed by such veterans and will challenge the O&M specialists who serve such veterans to find additional ways to help them cope with these multiple losses.

CONCLUSION

Formal instruction in independent travel first began with attempts to meet the needs of adults who were blind or visually impaired, specifically veterans who lost vision during World War II. As the outcomes achieved by this new service came to be appreciated by consumers and other service providers throughout the system, the skills and services of O&M specialists became increasingly sought after. This has created an expanding demand for O&M specialists that is expected to continue. The providers of services for adults who are blind or visually impaired will vie with other providers throughout the field for the services of O&M specialists.

As adults who have lost their vision in the prime of their lives are able to receive and benefit from mobility instruction, one of the most important benefits of this service will be clearly evident. Effective O&M instruction plays a sig-

nificant role in helping adults who have experienced a vision loss regain their independence as full-functioning and employed individuals. This is an important role for the profession of orientation and mobility and it should not get lost in the equally important expansion of O&M services to all other people who experience visual impairment.

IMPLICATIONS FOR O&M PRACTICE

1. Estimates suggest that 3 million adults between the ages of 20 and 60 are considered to be severely visually impaired to the extent of having low vision or less. Of these, nearly 500,000 meet the definition for legal blindness.

2. Generally speaking, the cause of an adult's visual impairment does not indicate whether the person is totally blind or has low vision, his visual acuity or visual field, whether the eye condition is stable or fluctuating, or how this person will relate to varying amounts of light.

3. Students who have lost their vision as adults frequently pass through stages of adjustment, as identified by Tuttle and Tuttle (2004). It is not until the later stages of this sequence that many students are ready to consider the need for and actually begin to receive O&M training.

4. Family members may have a positive or negative attitude toward a person's ability to cope with vision loss. Some may feel that it is their responsibility to protect their family member from the disappointment that may result from false expectation of success. Negative attitudes may reflect the family member's attitude toward the disability or interpersonal dynamics between family members that extend beyond the disability.

5. Receiving O&M training at a center away from the student's home may allow students to develop sufficient confidence in their skills before having to demonstrate to their famillies that they can travel safely on their own.

6. The principles of andragogy emphasize the need for adult learners to be able to focus on concrete matters that enable them to achieve the practical demands of everyday living and, in doing so, improve or affirm their concept of themselves as independent adults.

7. According to the principles of andragogy, adult learners should be involved in the setting of goals for instruction and selection of methods to reach those goals. Adult learners have to be invested in the plan and the goals have to make sense to them.

8. Students funded by the state-federal vocational rehabilitation program are required to participate in the planning and review and must sign the resulting Individualized Plan for Employment (IPE).

9. Center-based programs encourage the interaction of O&M students with other students, facilitating the discussion of psychosocial issues and the comparison of successes and challenges.

10. O&M services play an important role in the development and implementation of vocational rehabilitation services by helping the counselor assess a student's ability to handle the travel demands of various employment situations, by providing the instruction that is necessary, and, in some cases, assisting with placement and orientation at the work setting.

LEARNING ACTIVITIES

1. Interview adult clients who are congenitally visually impaired and receiving O&M services through an adult program to determine how their experiences as children or adolescents with visual impairment contributed, if at all, to their need for O&M services as adults.

2. Discuss with practicing O&M specialists the phases of adjustment to blindness identified by Tuttle and Tuttle (2004), and discuss the frequency with which they see evidence of these stages in the students they serve.

3. Discuss with adults who have adventitious visual impairment their particular reactions to the loss of their ability to drive, and identify interventions by family and professionals that they feel helped them cope with this loss.

4. Interview family members of adult students to discover their attitudes toward O&M training, as well as whether or not their attitudes changed during the period of O&M training and what was responsible for those changes.

5. Through discussions and interviews with O&M specialists in both center-based and community-based programs for adults, compare the typical amount of services provided to students in each program.

6. Discuss with vocational rehabilitation counselors their perceptions of the role and importance of O&M training in the development and implementation of successful vocational rehabilitation plans.

CHAPTER 10

Teaching Orientation and Mobility to Older Adults

Nora Griffin-Shirley and
Richard L. Welsh

LEARNING QUESTIONS

- What are the leading causes of severe vision loss among older adults?

- In general, how do older adults adjust to visual impairment?

- What percentage of older adults who are visually impaired experience depression, and how can it be managed?

- How can orientation and mobility (O&M) training help reduce the incidence of falls among older adults who are visually impaired?

- How can teaching strategies be modified for older adults to improve the effectiveness of O&M training?

Formal instruction in orientation and mobility (O&M) for persons who are visually impaired began in rehabilitation programs for military personnel. It then spread to vocational rehabilitation programs for civilians and was later adopted by educational programs for school-age children. In part, this pattern reflected the availability of funding for such services and society's perspec-

tive on who could benefit from the rigorous training that this new service entailed. Missing in the early decades of the development of O&M instruction was the systematic offering of such training to older adults who had experienced vision loss. This pattern also reflected a bias in society regarding the perceived interest among older people in this type of training to help them cope with vision loss, a condition that many regard as an inevitable part of growing older.

Writing in 1972 about social services and blindness, Douglas MacFarland, director of the Office for the Blind and Visually Handicapped in the Rehabilitation Services Administration of the U.S. Department of Health, Education and Welfare, reflected the rather limited but prevailing view of what was needed by older adults who are blind:

The greatest problem we face today is that of providing social services for the older blind person. We have only begun to demonstrate in a few areas of the country how the social needs of this large group can be met. The services are relatively simple: regular social visiting for the person living alone; reading mail and writing essential correspondence when necessary; accompanying the blind person on special shopping tours; orienting the blind person to immediate surroundings so that he can find restaurants, laundry, and other essential facilities; making certain that the person receives special training in home management if desired; and obtaining assistance to help the blind person make full use of recreational facilities that may be available to him. In order to implement these services to any great degree and have an appreciable impact on the total population that can profit from them, state and private agencies must recruit, train, and supervise vast numbers of volunteers. (Mac-Farland, 1972)

As the average life expectancy lengthened and the general health of older adults continued to improve, this expanding population became more vocal in expressing their right to continue to enjoy their lives and to participate in all aspects of living. This trend was reflected in the growing number of older people who were surviving injury and disease and who were challenged to live their lives with impairments and disabilities. As a result, O&M specialists who work in systems that serve adults have increasingly found that significant portions of their caseloads are comprised of older adults. While many such adults participate fully and successfully in such services as routinely provided, some older people require adjustments and alterations in O&M services that are tailored to their particular needs.

GENERAL CONDITIONS RELATED TO AGING

Myths and Stereotypes about Aging and Older People

There are a number of myths and stereotypes that many people in Western cultures have about aging and older adults. Older people themselves, as members of their culture, can hold these same stereotypes, as can people who serve them. Butler and Lewis (1973) identified certain myths that may have an impact on decisions made by service providers or by older adults themselves about the suitability of rehabilitation services:

- The myth of chronologic age, which mistakenly relates advances in chronological age with the effects of aging

- The myth of unproductivity, which suggests that because a person is old he cannot contribute to society

- The myth of disengagement, which implies that older people prefer being alone or associating only with their peers

- The myth of inflexibility, which suggests that older persons are resistant to change

- The myth of senility, which attributes normal emotional reactions of grief, anxiety, and depression to irreversible senility

- The myth of serenity, which implies that old age is a period of tranquility and few concerns

Individual Differences

Similar to these common myths and stereotypes is the more basic notion that all older adults are alike. This is even more fallacious than the stereotypes listed above. Birren (1959) made the observation that older adults are *more unlike* each other than they are *similar* to each other. Birren also pointed out that: "The student of aging must continually be aware of the uniqueness of individuals and that man and other organisms possess a genetical system which keeps that diversity permanently in being" (p. 36). Both Schonfield (1974) and Tobin (1977) have demonstrated that on virtually any psychological test and on many physiological measures, there is greater variance among older persons than among younger persons.

Emerging Patterns

In an effort to dispel some of the stereotypes that an O&M specialist may bring to working with people in this age category, it is helpful to consider some of the patterns that emerge from a review of statistics gathered about older adults by various government agencies in the United States. Many of these findings are available for review on the web sites of the National Center for Health Statistics (NCHS) (2006) of the Center for Disease Control of the U.S. Department of Health and Human Services (www.cdc.gov/nchs/agingact.htm). Another source that overlaps somewhat with the NCHS site is the Federal Interagency Forum on Aging-Related Statistics (2006) (http://agingstats.gov/agingstatsdotnet/Main_Site/Data/Data_2006.aspy).

Average life expectancy continues to expand. The life expectancy for people born in 1900 was 47.3 years, and people who were 65 years old could look forward to an average of 11.9 more years of life. In 2003, life expectancy for newborns had increased to 77.5 years (National Center for Health Statistics, 2006). Those who were age 65 in 2003 could anticipate an average of 18.4 more years, and those who were age 85 could anticipate another 6.8 years. One effect of these projections is that people who lose their vision later in life will most likely have a good number of years to live with that condition. Efforts to help them live more effectively and independently will pay significant dividends.

In 2006, while 54.5 percent of people over the age of 65 lived with a spouse and 12.5 percent lived with other family members, more than 30 percent lived alone. This indicates the importance of rehabilitation services to reinforce a person's ability to live independently. Also, dependence on family members for day-to-day support becomes less burdensome for every task and activity that the person with a visual impairment can do independently.

Many surveys quantify the functional status and the level of disabilities among older adults, evaluating limitations in *activities of daily living* (ADLs), *instrumental activities of daily living* (IADLs), and *physical tasks*. For this discussion, the following definitions apply:

- ADLs—personal care needs, such as bathing, showering, dressing, eating, getting in and out of bed or a chair, using a toilet, and walking

- IADLs—using a telephone, doing light or heavy housework, preparing meals, shopping, and managing money

- Physical tasks—stooping, lifting, reaching, grasping, and walking

Among all Medicare beneficiaries 65 and older living in community dwellings in 2004, 57 percent had no functional limitations or physical task limitations only; 13.4 percent had limitations in IADLs but not in ADLs; 18.9 percent had limitations in one or two ADLs; and 10.4 percent had limitations in three to six ADLs. These numbers suggest a minimal level of functional limitations among adults age 65 and older in the community (National Center for Health Statistics, *2006).* The picture changes somewhat when those who live in more supportive environments are also considered. In community housing where services are provided, 31 percent had no limitations or physical task limitations only; 22 percent had IADL limitations only; 28.4 percent had limitations in one or two ADLs; and 18.7 percent had limitations in three to six ADLs. In long-term-care facilities, only 3.8 percent had no limitations or only physical task limitations; 13.8 percent had IADL limitations only; 16.3 percent had one or two limitations in ADLs; and 66 percent had three to six limitations in ADLs (Federal Interagency Forum on Aging-Related Statistics, 2006).

Travis, Boerner, Reinhardt, and Horowitz (2004) interviewed 155 older adults who were predominately Caucasian (80 percent), female (53.5 percent), lived with others (55 percent), and who reported having three other health problems in addition to their vision loss. This study's purpose was to explore the degree to which subjects had problems with ADLs and IADLs due to their vision problems and to determine "if there are distinct or shared predictors of functional disability that are due to visual problems and functional disability that are due to other problems" (p. 535). Subjects had more problems with IADLs due to visual loss; however, difficulty performing ADLs was due to other health conditions. When other conditions are present in older adults, O&M specialists should inquire about the cause of their difficulties. Not all problems are due to vision loss and amenable to the interventions of vision rehabilitation specialists.

General Health Status

As the population of older adults lives longer, they are more likely to be diagnosed with chronic conditions. The most commonly occurring conditions for people age 65 and older and the percentages of people who have been diagnosed are:

- hypertension—51.9 percent.
- arthritis—49.9 percent.
- heart disease—31.7 percent.
- cancer—20.6 percent.
- diabetes—17 percent.
- stroke—9.2 percent.
- asthma—8.9 percent.
- emphysema—5.2 percent.

In addition to these specific conditions, 47.7 percent of men and 33.9 percent of women report trouble with hearing, and 14.4 percent of men and 18.7 percent of women report trouble with seeing. Despite the prevalence of these conditions, when people age 65 and older respond to

general questions about their health status in various surveys, 76.2 percent of those who are white report that their health is good to excellent. Of those who are black, 57.9 percent report that their health is good or excellent and 61.6 percent of Hispanics do as well (Federal Interagency Forum on Aging-Related Statistics, 2006).

Older adults are also thought to have serious problems with memory loss and depression. Based on various health surveys as of 2002, moderate or severe memory loss was diagnosed in 12.7 percent of adults age 65 and older. This was more characteristic of men (14.9 percent) than of women (11.2 percent) (Federal Interagency Forum on Aging-Related Statistics, 2006). In addition to the numbers of people with moderate or severe memory loss, the O&M specialist should be aware of the fact that *normal* aging affects the memory of individuals in the following ways (Johnson, Bergtson, Coleman, & Kirkwood, 2005):

1. A deficit occurs in *working memory*, which refers to the storage and processing of information. A reduced processing speed is evident.

2. *Episodic memory* is also affected, as people have problems with the temporary retrieval of information and are susceptible to false memories and inaccurate rote memories.

3. *Explicit memory* declines.

4. *Prospective memory*, or remembering things to accomplish in the future, may be compromised.

It is important to keep in mind that even with these normal age-related changes, the consequences of these typical decreases may be rather trivial for daily life performance (Verhaeghen, Marcoen, & Goossens, 1993), but are usually frustrating to older people.

Of all people age 65 and older, 15 percent have been diagnosed with some level of depression (Federal Interagency Forum on Aging-Related Statistics, 2006). For men and women, the pattern for depression is opposite the pattern for moderate or severe memory loss. Depression is more prevalent among older women (17.8 percent) than among older men (10.9 percent) (Federal Interagency Forum on Aging-Related Statistics, 2006). In spite of the frequency of the diagnosis of depression, only 2.5 percent of persons age 65 and older report that they have talked to a mental health professional (National Center for Health Statistics, 2006). It may be that older people are more likely to have these issues handled by their general practitioners than by mental health professionals.

One other general condition for older adults that has been documented by various federal surveys is the high frequency and danger associated with falls. The National Center for Health Statistics (2006) reported that falls are the most frequent type of injury that can result in death for adults age 65 and older. The rate of deaths from injuries associated with falls is 37.6 per 100,000. This is almost double the rate of deaths associated with motor vehicle accidents, which is 20.2 per 100,000. This is a problem that occurs too frequently for older adults in general and it becomes even more of a problem for older adults with vision loss.

The previous paragraphs attempt to provide O&M specialists with an understanding of the general health status of adults who are age 65 and older. As life expectancy increases and greater numbers of people survive into their 80s and 90s, there will be a higher frequency of chronic health conditions and the functional limitations related to these conditions. However, the average condition of people over the age of 65 is remarkably good and getting better. While the needs and circumstances of each older adult who appears for services as a result of vision loss must be carefully assessed, there is every reason to expect that older adults can benefit from rehabilitation services and can continue to enjoy a high quality of life in spite of vision loss.

DEMOGRAPHICS OF AGING AND VISION LOSS

Consistency in the Estimates

Wall Emerson and De l'Aune (Volume 1, Chapter 16) and Horowitz (2004) discuss the difficulty of obtaining exact numbers of the population of people with blindness or low vision in the United States. Because researchers in various studies use different definitions of visual impairment, different methods of sampling the population, different assessment methods, and different age groupings when they project population numbers, obtaining exact numbers of older adults with vision loss is difficult. The findings of such research studies have to be considered *estimates* of the prevalence rates of visual impairments. However, across many different studies, one estimate continues to be made consistently: the majority of all people who are considered to be blind or visually impaired are older than age 65, and in some studies, this is a large majority (Crews, 1991; Friedman, Congdon, Kempen, & Tielsch, 2002; Lighthouse International, 1995; National Center for Health Statistics, 1994 and 2004; Nelson, 1987; Nelson & Dimitrova, 1993; Tielsch, 2001; Tielsch, Sommer, Witt, Katz, and Royall, 1990).

Wall Emerson and De l'Aune (Volume 1, Chapter 16) estimate that in 2003, the number of people over 60 years of age who were legally blind (visual acuity of $< 20/200$ [6/60]) was 734,900 and that this number would grow to 1,081,900 in 2020. The estimated number of people with low vision or blindness (visual acuity of $< 20/70$ [6/21]) in 2003 was 1,192,300 and is expected to grow to 1,620,500 in 2020. Orr (1992) helped to clarify the estimated rapid growth of people with visual impairments by explaining that gerontologists categorize older adults as being in one of three cohorts: (1) age 65 to 74, the *young* old; (2) age 75 to 84, the *middle* old; and (3) over age 85, the *old* old. The group of adults age 85 and older is the most rapidly growing cohort (American Association of Retired Persons, 1990). Because the leading causes of visual impairment among older adults are age-related, the rapid growth of the oldest cohort is primarily responsible for the rapidly rising estimates of older adults who are visually impaired over the next 20 years.

Currently, the highest prevalence rate of people with visual impairment is in the group of those older than 75 years of age (Friedman, Congdon, Kempen, & Tielsch, 2002). According to Rovner, Zisselman, and Shmuely-Dulitzki (1996), age-related eye diseases affect 25 percent of people 75 years and older.

Leading Causes of Visual Impairment

The leading causes of visual impairment among older adults are cataracts, diabetic retinopathy, glaucoma, and macular degeneration (Rosenbloom, 1992). These eye conditions typically occur gradually and usually do not result in total blindness. They can cause functional problems such as glare, reduced contrast sensitivity, poor depth perception, impaired distance vision, reduced light adaptation, and field restrictions (Crone & McKinney, 2004). Other problems may include blurred vision, nausea, headache, seeing halos around bright lights, and blind spots (Orr & Rogers, 2006). Tielsch, Sommer, Witt, Katz, and Royall (1990) performed clinical examinations of 80 percent of the population over the age of 40 in three residential areas in Baltimore. They found that two-thirds to three-fourths of the visual impairment observed through these clinical examinations was able to be improved through better refraction. Even after these improvements were made, however, the rate of severe visual impairment and legal blindness among these groups was consistent with many other studies.

One other eye condition that may affect from 10 to 40 percent of older adults with macular degeneration is Charles Bonnet syndrome (CBS).

This condition can cause visual hallucinations lasting for a few minutes or longer and usually occurring at night or when the person with visual impairment is alone. CBS first appears after the person's sight has worsened and it can last from 12 to 18 months. O&M specialists need to be aware of this condition because it can sometimes be mistaken as the onset of dementia or mental illness. While there is no cure at the present time, a good knowledge of one's surroundings can help a person cope with CBS (Orr & Rogers, 2006).

ISSUES AND STRATEGIES FOR TEACHING ORIENTATION AND MOBILITY TO OLDER ADULTS

Many of the issues discussed by Welsh (Chapter 9) that are related to teaching orientation and mobility to adults apply equally well to the circumstances of older adults. The authors recommend a review of the sections of Chapter 9 that discuss adjustment to loss of vision and to theories of adult learning.

Assessment

As discussed by Welsh (Chapter 9) and Bina, Naimy, Fazzi, and Crouse (Volume 1, Chapter 12), an assessment of a person's need and readiness for O&M instruction should include a review of the individual's (1) background information, (2) mobility skills, (3) orientation skills, (4) conceptual understanding, (5) vision functioning, and (6) auditory functioning. In addition to reviewing information obtained through an interview, through records that may have accompanied a referral, and through clinically based vision and hearing tests, it is important to assess how the student actually functions in real environments. As compared to services provided to children and adults who are referred through the vocational rehabilitation process, older adults frequently come with fewer records and prior evaluations to consider. The service delivery systems for older adults are, generally speaking, less comprehensive and less formal. As a result, O&M specialists have to depend on their own observations and information gathering to a greater degree. As with all adults who are adventitiously blinded, an assumption is made that if older adults lived many years with vision, they understand the basic concepts of the travel environment and have had many travel experiences from which to draw when learning to move through the environment without vision or with reduced vision.

As discussed in the chapter on teaching orientation and mobility to adults (Chapter 9), it is important to establish an effective partnership with the older student. During the assessment process, this is done in part by requesting the student's permission before contacting family members or medical personnel when seeking additional information about the student's health, adjustment, or daily functioning. Typically, an older adult is accompanied to the rehabilitation program by a family member. Frequently, the family member is in the room during the assessment interview and supplements or contradicts what the older student reports regarding her functioning or problems. Usually, the student is aware of these comments, but occasionally, the family member is sitting out of view from the student and commenting nonverbally on what the student is saying. This creates a fair amount of uncertainty for the O&M specialist regarding who has the correct story. It also runs the risk of undermining the specialist's goal of establishing a trusting relationship with the student. In an effort to avoid this situation, the O&M specialist may want to interview the student alone and then ask permission to also interview her family member about that person's view of the student's functioning and coping challenges. This additional interview can be done without the student present as long as the student knows that it is taking place and has given permission.

Program Planning

Also, as discussed by Welsh (Chapter 9), the principles of andragogy, the science of teaching adults, stress the importance of having the adult student participate in the selection of goals for the instruction and be fully supportive of the plan. It is typical for the older student to choose less-extensive goals for the training than may be realistically accomplished. This may reflect self-esteem issues for the older student (see Welsh, Chapter 6, and Volume 1, Chapter 6) or, more likely, lessened feelings of self-efficacy related to the task of moving safely and successfully without vision. This may also reflect a realistic view of the student's own travel needs and opportunities, or concerns about her ability to afford more extensive instruction. This is especially true because of the lack of third-party funding for rehabilitation training for older adults who do not have employment goals. This can create a critical juncture in the older student's training program. The O&M specialist who pushes for or insists on a more thorough and complete program for which the older student is not motivated or not prepared to embrace may lose the opportunity to engage the student in any instruction at all.

The selection of more limited goals as a starting point for the instruction can be an important strategy for older students—whether the issue is gaining sufficient value for the investment that will be made for the service, or whether the student does not feel up to the task. As the person begins to experience success and see the value of additional training, the goals can be expanded from the use of a sighted guide in familiar areas to more independent travel in familiar areas to travel in new and less familiar areas. Whatever the starting point and the progression, not much progress will be made unless the older student is supportive of the plan.

Adjustment to the Loss of Vision

Stages of Adjustment

The readiness of an older student for O&M instruction will depend to a large degree on her adjustment to the vision loss. Tuttle and Tuttle (2004) present a model of adjustment to blindness that includes seven phases that people may experience. These phases are sequential and overlapping. People who have lost their vision may not experience all of the phases or they may become stuck in one phase or another. Coping with a vision loss is individually determined. Adjustment is influenced by the coping mechanisms that an older person has developed when dealing with other traumas in her life and by her own personality and personal attributes. The phases that a person may experience in adjusting to vision loss as identified by Tuttle and Tuttle are:

1. *Trauma, physical or social*: The actual diagnosis of an eye condition or the sudden onset of blindness.

2. *Shock and initial denial*: This phase is characterized by people experiencing the shock that occurs after the onset of blindness, where they may deny the situation is occurring or refuse to deal with it.

3. *Mourning and withdrawal*: Individuals may grieve the loss of their vision and the way their life circumstances were prior to the blindness and engage in self-pity.

4. *Succumbing and depression*: People think of the repercussions of being blind. They may become depressed, negative, pessimistic, lethargic, withdrawn, isolated, angry, and frustrated.

5. *Reassessment and reaffirmation*: During this phase, people reassess the meaning of their lives while possibly participating in rehabilitation programs.

6. *Coping and mobilization*: People learn new skills and apply them to accomplishing the tasks in their everyday lives.

7. *Self-acceptance and self-esteem*: During this phase, a person accepts her blindness as a part of her being.

A more-detailed discussion of each of these phases as they relate to orientation and mobility is provided by Welsh (Volume 1, Chapter 6).

The extent to which an older adult experiences any of the phases identified by Tuttle and Tuttle will vary according to that individual's personality characteristics and life circumstances. It also will depend on whether her vision loss is sudden or gradual and whether it is total or partial. During the assessment process, it is important that the O&M specialist try to determine where the older adult is in her own individualized process of adjusting to the loss of vision. Tuttle and Tuttle (2004) have pointed out that a person who is in any of the first four phases of their model of adjustment is not likely to be interested in rehabilitation training. However, once the person has moved forward to Phase 5 (the reassessment and reaffirmation stage), she is more likely to be open to instruction and intervention.

Most older adults who experience severe visual impairment do not lose all of their vision, but function as persons with low vision. Welsh (Volume 1, Chapter 6) reviews many of the special adjustment and identity issues that confront people with low vision. Older adults may not want to use a long cane because it identifies them as being blind, a label that they are desperately trying to avoid. Kleinschmidt (1999) found three categories of resources that older adults felt helped them adjust positively to loss of vision: (1) prior life experiences, taking strength from past accomplishments and from dealing with adversity; (2) internal resources, such as positive attitudes, a sense of humor, problem-solving ability, deciding to remain active and productive, and religious beliefs; and (3) external resources, such as support from family, neighbors, and friends, professional support from medical personnel and rehabilitation personnel, the good example of other successful blind people and comparisons with less-fortunate people.

Giving Up Driving

A very important step in the process of adjusting to vision loss for older adults occurs in relation to the ability to drive a car. For many people in Western cultures, owning a driver's license and a car are signs of independence and control over one's life. When a license is given up as a result of vision loss, older adults have to learn to cope with being nondrivers. This may trigger a loss of independence, termination of employment, and relocating to a new residence. According to the Tuttle and Tuttle phases, this can push the person deeper into Phase 4 (succumbing and depression).

Corn and Sacks (1994) surveyed 110 adults with visual impairments to explore the issues facing nondrivers, including the impact on their lifestyle, the frustrations of being a nondriver, and how their transportation needs were met. The frustration of being a nondriver was higher for individuals with low vision than for those who were totally blind. The two most frustrating experiences were waiting for rides that were late and being unable to find a ride for an important occasion. Other disadvantages of not driving included lack of spontaneity in their lives and not being able to go places that mass transit did not serve. While there were some advantages to not driving, such as reduced stress and money saved by not owning an automobile, the number one negative effect of being a nondriver was the limited choice of residence for those who depend on public transportation.

Rosenblum and Corn's (2002) survey of 162 older adults with vision loss who had stopped driving found that 18 percent of the participants did not travel in unfamiliar areas, and only 66.7 percent used public transportation, paratransit, or taxis, even though more than 75 percent resided in areas that had these services. About one-third of the participants used public transportation, one-third used paratransit, and one-third used taxis. About 19 percent of those interviewed hired drivers.

The majority of the participants in this study had low vision, and half had received O&M services. When participants were asked about their worries as nondrivers, they identified the top three concerns as not getting to their destinations, loss of independence, and being a burden to others. Those who used public transportation were less apt to be worried about being isolated than those who did not. Men seemed to worry more than women about being isolated, not having as much fun, and being a burden to others after becoming a nondriver. In addition to the reduction in travel, participants also reported changes in their lifestyles, such as moving to a new home and no longer working or volunteering. While 61 percent reported a decrease in travel at night and to friends' homes, participants reported an increase in attending senior centers and other groups.

The research studies by Corn, Rosenbloom, and Sacks cited above document the important lifestyle changes that occur when an individual has to give up his driver's license. This leads to adjustment difficulties and sometimes provides the initial motivation for the older adult to seek rehabilitation services and especially O&M instruction.

Stuck in Depression

Some older adults experience serious difficulty in moving beyond Phase 4 of the model by Tuttle and Tuttle (2004). The negative emotions associated with the loss of vision overwhelm them and they cannot escape the depression that settles in and keeps them from moving forward. The degree of depression experienced by any one individual may be related to the psychodynamics of past experiences or it may reflect serious concerns about the impact of vision loss on future plans. It is also possible that the level of depression results from the interaction between the person who is visually impaired and those upon whom she depends for day-to-day support. The person who has experienced a vision loss necessarily goes through a time of increased dependency on others for everyday functioning and safety. Ponchillia (1984) points out that family members' lack of accurate knowledge about the impact of visual impairments on their ability to function can result in their offering assistance that is perceived by the person who is visually impaired as unnecessary or insufficient. Cimarolli, Reinhardt, and Horowitz (2006) have demonstrated that a person with low vision may sense that family members are offering unnecessary assistance, which can be perceived as overprotection. This perception can result in poorer adjustment and in an increase of depressive symptoms. Additional studies have documented other relationships between depression and vision loss (Casten, Rovner, & Edmonds, 2002; Horowitz, 2004; Horowitz, Reinhardt, & Boerner, 2005; Travis et al., 2003).

Reinhardt (2001) studied 570 older adults who were visually impaired and whose average age was 80 years. Participants "who received affective support from friends had fewer depressive symptoms, greater life satisfaction and better adaptation to vision loss" (p. 76). Those who received instrumental family support had greater life satisfaction. Participants who themselves "provided greater affective support to their families had higher life satisfaction" (p. 76). More depressive symptoms occurred for those who engaged in negative interactions among their family and friends. Realizing that these interactions and depressive symptoms can negatively affect students' adaptation to their vision loss, Reinhardt encouraged professionals to identify and involve the supportive family and friends of their students as well

as those whom the students support. He also encouraged professional personnel, family members, and students to deal with issues of overprotectiveness and dependence in an open and candid manner.

Some older students will require treatment with physician-prescribed medication to enable them to move beyond the depressive symptoms and to reengage in everyday living, especially in rehabilitation activities. Others will respond to empathic conversation with family, friends, or professionals to help them move to the phase of adjustment where they will learn to cope with vision loss. For those who do engage in rehabilitation activities, the success that comes with this new learning can have a positive effect on their depression. A study of 95 older adults with vision loss who received low vision clinical services, counseling, and optical devices found that their level of depression improved after receiving these services (Horowitz, Reinhardt & Boerner, 2005).

Horowitz, Reinhardt, and Kennedy (2005) found that 7 percent of the applicants for vision rehabilitation services who were over the age of 65 met the diagnostic criteria for a major depressive disorder and 27 percent showed subthreshold depression. Casten and Rovner (2008) have indicated that for persons with age-related macular degeneration, both major and subthreshold depressions are a problem because they seriously compound the disability caused by vision loss. Horowitz, Reinhardt, and Kennedy (2005) demonstrated that persons with subthreshold depression who applied for low vision services had levels of disability that were comparable to a person with major depression and both had significantly greater disability than did those with no depression.

Horowitz and Reinhardt (2006) have pointed out that older visually impaired adults with depressive symptoms frequently fall between the cracks of the vision rehabilitation system and the mental health systems. Mental health practitioners may feel that they are incapable of addressing mental health issues that are complicated by vision loss. In the vision rehabilitation systems, there is insufficient funding to provide mental health services directly, and some professionals may feel that depression may be alleviated by services that reduce the impact of the disability by helping students learn how to cope. While some students with depressive disorders may be helped by rehabilitation training, there are others who need pharmacological and psychotherapeutic interventions.

O&M Strategies for Older Adults

When teaching older adults with vision loss, O&M specialists use most of the same teaching strategies and equipment they use with adults of all ages. However, the assessment process will sometimes indicate the need for a modification to the typical approaches to teaching orientation and mobility based upon the presence of other disabilities, chronic illnesses, limited goals, or limited financial resources. The following list offers suggestions for modifications to teaching strategies and equipment that an O&M specialist may find helpful with some older adults:

- *Use an andragogical approach to teaching* (see Welsh, Chapter 9):
  - This is a *learner-centered approach* in which the O&M specialist works with the student to identify what she wants to learn; the benefits of learning O&M skills can be used immediately.
  - Choose the locations and content of lessons that will contribute to *meeting the most immediate O&M goals* of a student. Initial lessons need to incorporate in some way the most immediate goals identified by the student. For example, if a student's goal is to learn how to use public transportation, initial lessons can teach the use of a human guide while getting on and off a bus.

- Provide initial objectives that are meaningful, readily attainable, and lead to successful experiences. Success during the initial O&M lessons is essential for developing and sustaining motivation (see Welsh, Chapter 6). Use a task-analysis approach to carefully plan each lesson to allow for successful experiences while learning meaningful skills at every level in the O&M process.
- Discuss the objectives for each lesson with the student and obtain her opinion of the value of these objectives. Assure the student of the connection between each lesson and her O&M goals.
- Choose routes for instruction that are highly motivating to the student. Ask the student to prioritize the routes she wants to learn and discuss what O&M skills are needed to travel these routes. Working as a team, re-prioritize the routes, if necessary, to reflect the sequence of skills that are needed to be successful on each route. With this information in hand, reach a mutual agreement on the most important route to teach next.
- Teach to the level of independence the student chooses. This could include a simple route from the ranch house to the barn or travel in a complex urban environment. A student may be content learning only human guide technique, even though she might have the ability to learn to travel independently in a shopping area. The O&M specialist must respect the student's choices and be ready to offer more instruction at a later time.
- Assign homework. Students can be encouraged to keep an O&M journal—on a computer, on a tape recorder, or written in a notebook—that describes their thoughts and feelings, actual task analysis of important O&M skills, and tips they want to remember about traveling in certain areas.
- Share observations of performance and evaluation reports with the student. Students

should be encouraged to evaluate their own progress on a regular basis and share their evaluations with the O&M specialist. O&M specialists should share their reports with their students. This develops a positive rapport and trust. Continuous feedback between the student and the O&M specialist ensures that the O&M program is on target with the original O&M goals.

- *Schedule the time and duration of lessons to reflect any limitations in the student's abilities:*

  - Some older adults and especially those with diabetes may function better at certain times of the day than others. For example, a lesson right before lunch, when a diabetic's blood sugar may be going down, may not be a good idea. Asking older students what times are best is highly recommended.
  - Other older adults have multiple health conditions like orthopedic and cardiovascular problems. They may be able to walk only one or two blocks on a day when they feel well. A 20- to 30-minute lesson may be all they can tolerate. When it is extremely hot or cold outside, they may not be able to travel outdoors at all. Indoor lessons, therefore, may be indicated on such days.

- *Implement special communication considerations for older adults with a hearing loss or comprehension difficulties:*

  - Bagley (1994) suggests that the O&M specialist: (1) before speaking, make sure that the older adult acknowledges his presence; (2) find a quiet place to explain directions for a lesson; (3) reconfirm that the student has understood the information; (4) rephrase a message if the older adult does not understand his instructions; (5) ask the student what he (the O&M specialist) can do to improve communications between the two of them; and (6) be patient and positive. Law-

son and Wiener (Chapter 4 and Volume 1, Chapter 4) provide thorough information for assessing and improving the student's hearing, if necessary.

  - Information presented to an older adult during O&M lessons needs to be delivered in such a way that the student can easily comprehend and apply the information. To determine if a student understands a lesson's content, the O&M specialist can ask a student to identify the two most important points learned during the lesson and to record the points in an O&M journal.

- *With the student's permission, involve the student's family members:*

  - Discuss O&M goals with the student and her family members together and discuss their feelings about the student's independent travel and how it fits into their lifestyles.
  - Ask family members what their hopes and expectations are for the student. Do they have fears and concerns about the student traveling independently? If so, what are they? Their fears could be unfounded or based on their lack of experience with vision loss and insufficient knowledge about the positive outcomes of O&M training.
  - Empower the student to tell family and friends what she expects from them when they are traveling together, whether the student is using a human guide or a long cane. Role-playing how a student would approach her family about using a cane rather than using the human guide technique (which the family member might prefer) can be an effective teaching tool. Discussing possible family reactions and possible responses to each reaction can empower the student to be assertive.
  - When appropriate, include caregivers in your lessons, teaching them ways to support the student's independence and safety. For some students who require personal assistance due

to physical or mental health problems or a combination of problems, it may be necessary to teach the human guide technique to family members, hospice workers, or personal care attendants. Film your lesson using a DVD recorder to archive it.

- *Be aware of and provide the special psychosocial support that an older adult student might need:*

  - Make sure the older adult does not think you are being overprotective because of her age. The student's perception of overprotectiveness could interfere with her desire to become an independent traveler (Cimarolli, Reinhardt, & Horowitz, 2006). The student has agreed to participate in an O&M program after understanding the potential risks involved. The design of challenging lessons that can be successfully completed will demonstrate to the student that the O&M specialist is not being overprotective.

  - Have high expectations for the student and articulate these to her. Clearly defining what an O&M program entails and believing that students can succeed in the goals they set will assist older students in believing they can attain these goals. Having other students who have completed their O&M programs meet with current students who are beginning their training can also be helpful.

  - Respond promptly to students who are crying or extremely emotional during O&M lessons. The O&M specialist should acknowledge the emotional responses of students and, if possible, redirect them for the duration of the O&M lesson. Students can sometimes be redirected by asking them to focus on something else for a few minutes. For example, a chance to examine a new orientation tool or a talking compass may take their mind off what is bothering them and allow the lesson to go forward. However, if students are distraught for the majority of the

lesson time, a referral to the rehabilitation agency's social worker or rehabilitation counselor may be indicated. It is important to inform the student of your concern and to request permission to make the referral in order to maintain an open and trusting relationship.

- *Use the teaching materials and special equipment that will improve a student's chances for success in orientation and mobility:*

  - Create teaching materials that enhance a student's comprehension of lesson content, involve a multisensory approach, and tap into the student's needs or interests. Using a tactile-graphic and low vision map to teach the layout of the cardiac rehabilitation center where the student will go three times a week to improve her cardiovascular functioning is a great way to encourage the use of the student's kinesthetic senses and remaining vision to learn the new area.

  - Recognize that older adult students may benefit from a variety of mobility tools and orientation aids, such as global positioning systems (GPS), hearing aids, walkers, support canes, wheelchairs, scooters, and long canes. O&M specialists need to be well versed in their use and maintenance and in how to train the students to use them.

  - Due to the number of problems some older adults with vision loss may have, a team approach may be needed. Some students may require many different types of mobility or orientation tools to travel safely. A person who is totally blind with a cardiovascular problem and emphysema may need to use a support cane in and around her home, but may require a scooter when traveling to the grocery store or longer distances. The O&M specialist needs to be able to teach the student how to use a long cane with each of these other mobility tools if possible and when required. It may be necessary to consult with a physical therapist in the evaluation of a support cane and scooter for the student. Effective communication between all members of the team will help to meet the student's requirements (see Rosen & Crawford, Chapter 18).

- *Help the student evaluate and select environmental modifications when appropriate:*

  ■ Assist the student in considering and selecting environmental modifications when needed for her home and workplace to maximize safety and travel efficiency. One of the roles of an O&M specialist is to help older adults with vision loss to review their homes and workplaces to see what modifications can be made to improve accessibility and safety and to reduce the possibility of falls. Lighting, color contrast, rearranging furniture, changing architectural features, and constructing landmarks to easily distinguish the student's residence from others on the street are some of the modifications to investigate.

  ■ The "Home Survey Checklist" developed by Orr and Rogers (2006, pp. 138–144) is an easy tool to use. "A Checklist for Safety and Access" in *Prescriptions of Independence* (Griffin-Shirley & Groff, 1993, p. 47) is useful when evaluating a community center, residential facility, or nursing home (see also Barlow, Bentzen, and Franck, Volume 1, Chapter 11, and Rosen & Crawford, Chapter 18).

- *Use memory techniques and devices if a student has memory problems:*

  ■ The areas of mental functioning that typically decline with age relate to secondary memory that stores information such as abstract symbols and the relations between them, execution of tasks that are fast paced,

tasks that require constant switching of attention between them, and tasks requiring free recall. Some older adults may have problems with absentmindedness, not recalling what they said 15 minutes ago or what they planned to do in 15 minutes (Schulz & Salthouse, 1999). The rate of learning also can decrease with age, but given enough time and practice, older adults with vision loss usually are able to learn O&M skills unless certain types of brain deterioration are present.

  ■ The O&M specialist should tailor the use of memory assist techniques to the student's cognitive abilities and life experiences. O&M specialists should ask students what helps them remember things and how they recall important information, and then incorporate these ideas into the O&M lessons.

  ■ Other memory strategies that may be helpful are: rehearsal, association, categorizing, mnemonics and visualization (Hardman, Drew, & Egan, 2005). *Rehearsal* involves repetition of items an older adult wants to recall. *Association* is relating new information to something the older adult already knows. *Categorizing* is grouping words into category labels. *Mnemonics* is using acronyms, poems, rhymes, or nonsense phrases so that the first letter of each word represents the information to be remembered. With *visualization*, older adults organize the new information into a clear mental picture.

- *Teach safety and self-defense techniques:*

  ■ Include in the training personal safety techniques, self-defense techniques, and guidance on when and how to ask for assistance.

  ■ Some rehabilitation centers for adults with visual impairments offer self-defense courses for their students. In some of these courses, law enforcement professionals offer a presentation on safety techniques. Others consist of a self-defense class at the agency or at a local community senior center.

As with all students, specific teaching techniques may include modeling, task analysis, role-playing, chaining, positive reinforcement, and effective communication techniques, especially for students with hearing impairments or those who do not speak English. Whatever works for a student should be used if it enables the student to successfully learn O&M skills. Sometimes the O&M specialist may have to problem-solve with the student and with other O&M specialists and develop or incorporate an unfamiliar or innovative approach. If it works for a student, use it; or if it appears that it may work, try it (see also Fazzi & Naimy, Chapter 8; Jacobson & Bradley, Volume 1, Chapter 7; and Welsh, Chapter 9).

Orientation and Mobility and Concern for Falling

As the average age of the population increases, so does the incidence of falls among older adults. The injuries that frequently accompany such falls can have devastating and sometimes fatal results. In addition, the costs of caring for older persons injured in falls can have a serious impact on the health care system. Falls can lead to reduced functioning, nursing home placement, morbidity, and mortality (Kenny, 2005).

Woollacott, Shumway-Cook, and Nashner (1986) discuss how the loss of bone mass among older adults, especially women, can limit intense physical exertion, but that it alone should not affect walking. However, this loss can combine with losses in sensory and cognitive abilities to create significant loss of functional capabilities, including mobility. The authors describe the cyclical aspect of exercise in which the stress on bones and muscles builds strength. However, lack of exercise allows physical loss to escalate and increases the likelihood of falling and, therefore, the hesitancy to travel.

The benefits of exercise for older adults with visual impairments are discussed by Ross (1984):

Physical exercise can help develop and maintain flexibility for daily activities, whether in the home, in stores, or in the streets. Both strength and coordination are needed for everyday tasks such as opening doors or windows, pushing shopping carts, carrying packages . . . A reserve in strength is helpful in order to meet unforeseen emergencies or simply to reinforce independence in daily living skills. (p. 3)

Additionally, exercise can reduce falls; assist with controlling weight and chronic health conditions (that is, coronary artery disease, diabetes, osteoarthritis); and improve mental health, functional capacity, and certain brain activity (that is, performance to attention-taxing tasks) (Colcombe et al., 2004; Ettinger, 1997; Johnson, Bengston, Coleman, & Kirkwood, 2005; Ponchillia, Powell, Felski, & Nicklawski, 1992; Walling, 2003). Strength training, walking, and Tai Chi (Li, Harmer, Fisher, & McAuley, 2004) are some of the exercises recommended for older adults to be physically active and engage in regular exercise.

O&M instruction for older adults with visual impairments can play an important role in breaking into the cycle of losing vision, which leads to lack of exercise, which causes additional physical losses and weakness, which causes hesitancy to walk and get exercise. In Appendix 10A, Couturier demonstrates that falls among older adults have become an international concern. She presents a comprehensive view of how O&M specialists can play a role in disrupting the downward spiral that can result from loss of vision.

Disorientation and Cognitive Impairment

A very important part of the process of orientation and mobility with impaired vision is to establish and maintain one's location while moving through the environment. When older adults with vision loss experience cognitive problems, difficulty with independent travel may occur. While technology of the future may offer solutions for older adults with vision loss who are having problems with their memory (Baldwin, 2003), current interventions are much less dramatic.

The effects of various comorbid conditions on the physical functioning, social participation, and health functioning of older adults with visual impairments were reviewed by Crews, Jones, and Kim (2006). They were surprised to note the high correlation of vision loss with many conditions, especially depression, and the impact of these multiple impairments on older adults. Warren (2008) discusses the implication of memory loss, dementia, and stroke for rehabilitation activities for older adults with age-related macular degeneration. The cognitive impairments related to these conditions can have an impact on the orientation aspects of travel without vision. An earlier section of this chapter offers suggestions for how to help older adults who are having memory problems related to orientation and mobility.

LaGrow and Blasch (1992) discuss the difficulty and the lack of research in determining whether a resident in an extended care facility who is disoriented because of her visual impairment is a wanderer or has dementia and may require a medical intervention other than rehabilitation training. Wanderers in nursing homes tend to be individuals with severe cognitive impairment who exhibit socially inappropriate behavior and refuse medical treatment, take antipsychotic drugs, and are able to ambulate but need assistance with ADLs (Schonfeld et al., 2007). When teaching these individuals, LaGrow and Blasch recommend breaking a complex route into small, logically contained sections that are taught successively. The individual can remember them, they can be written in braille, or recorded on audiotape. Practice with a smaller section of the route should be provided until it is successfully

learned before moving on to the next section. Other suggestions included the use of simple routes and teaching students how to solicit aid and to know when they need to travel with a guide who has vision.

THE STUDY OF O&M OUTCOMES FOR OLDER ADULTS

Over the years, research studies have demonstrated the positive effects of O&M services for older adults with vision loss. For example, after interviewing 70 adults with vision loss who were 60 years of age and older and had received rehabilitation training, including orientation and mobility, Engel, Welsh, and Lewis (2000) found that participants experienced a decline in falls, less difficulty with using public transportation, more confidence while using transportation, and an increase in their sense of control over their environment.

Kuyk et al. (2004) interviewed 128 mostly older veterans using a mobility questionnaire that consisted of 34 mobility situations and questions pertaining to falls, use of mobility devices, including anti-glare devices and their levels of satisfaction with their travel abilities. Significant differences were found in 76 percent of the situations when scores from before the training were compared to scores afterward. This was especially evident in relation to using "public transportation, avoiding tripping over uneven surfaces, seeing cars at intersections, and detecting descending and ascending stairwells." After veterans completed rehabilitation training, their confidence level "increased for travel in unfamiliar areas, in stores, and outdoors" (p. 340). Veterans reported that the number of falls they experienced decreased by 50 percent after training. Post-training, the usage of long canes and human guides by veterans increased, satisfaction with their travel abilities increased, and they tended to limit their travel less often.

Long, Boyette, and Griffin-Shirley (1996) interviewed 32 older adults with visual impairments and 28 older people who were sighted about their travel habits and perceptions. One-third of the older adults with visual impairments reported having other disabilities that affected their mobility. More than half of the older adults with visual impairments had mobility training. More than one-third of the participants with visual impairments reported being dissatisfied with their travel independence, while one quarter of these individuals were satisfied with their travel opportunities. One quarter reported they had traveled independently outside their homes in the past week to an average of 2.2 destinations. Forty-five percent of the travelers with visual impairments reported never traveling independently outside their homes. Sidewalks proved to be an environmental factor that enabled participants with visual impairments to travel independently outdoors. Implications for O&M training for older adults with visual impairments gleaned from this research include:

- O&M specialists need to accept the specific goals of older adults with visual impairments and help them achieve these goals.

- A client-centered approach to training should be used.

- Training needs to be easily accessible, short training periods should be offered to deal with specific problems, and training should be offered when the life circumstances of older adults with visual impairments change (for example, relocation or the death of a spouse).

- A caregivers' training program may include human guide training, "environmental modifications to improve O&M, the psychosocial implications of visual impairment, the functional implications of various types and degrees of visual impairments, and how to access related services" (p. 311).

De l'Aune, Welsh and Williams (2000) developed a functional outcomes measurement instrument for veterans with visual impairment. It was called the Blind Rehabilitation Services Functional Outcomes Survey (BRSFOS). It was also modified for use with a sample of nonveteran adults with visual impairments who were served by private rehabilitation agencies or state vocational rehabilitation agencies. Data was collected on 3,403 veterans and 389 nonveterans. Of the 389 nonveterans interviewed, the majority were females (66 percent), Caucasian (90 percent), living alone (51 percent) in private residences (81 percent), with an average age of 70.1 years (SD = 18.1). The veterans were mostly Caucasian (72 percent) males (96 percent) who lived with their wives (42 percent) in private residences (92 percent). The mean age was 67.2 years (SD = 12.6).

Overall, 93.7 percent of the veterans self-reported that they were either "satisfied" or "completely satisfied" with the VA's blind rehabilitation program. For the non-VA participants, 99 percent indicated that they were satisfied or completely satisfied. The results of data from a retrospective pretest on 759 veterans and 175 nonveterans and 6-month follow-up data on 248 veterans and 47 nonveterans have indicated that virtually all average changes associated with the rehabilitation experience were in a positive direction. And, even though the most objective item of the responses (the frequency of accomplishing a specific task) does not always show a major positive change, two other items (self-perceived level of independence and satisfaction with performance of the task) generally show larger positive changes.

In relation to a sample O&M task, when asked, "Since your discharge from the blind rehabilitation program, have you crossed a street with a traffic light?" veterans reported changes in the performance of this task on a daily or weekly basis from 37 percent pre-rehabilitation to 87 percent post-rehabilitation. For perceived independence,

45 percent stated they could do the task independently before rehabilitation versus 84 percent afterward. Before rehabilitation, 56 percent were satisfied with their ability to perform the task versus 97 percent who were satisfied after rehabilitation. Data from the nonveterans on a similar task showed a slight decrease in their performance of street crossings from before rehabilitation (32 percent) to after rehabilitation (25 percent). Their perceived independence before rehabilitation was 55 percent and 65 percent afterward. Their satisfaction with completion of this task before rehabilitation was 71 percent, but 86 percent after rehabilitation.

The documented positive-outcome studies reviewed previously offer clear evidence of the value of providing O&M instruction to older adults with vision loss. This information will be helpful to the ongoing advocacy efforts to develop third-party reimbursement for orientation and mobility and other rehabilitation activities for older adults who are visually impaired.

PROGRAM STRUCTURES FOR PROVIDING O&M SERVICES TO OLDER ADULTS

The Blindness System

Older adults with visual impairments have been served for many years by various organizations that operate within the "blindness system." The latter is a loosely organized, informal network of public and private organizations that share the common purpose of providing services to people with visual impairments.

In the late 1800s, home teachers emerged to teach older adults who were blind. This approach first was used in the United States when William Moon trained volunteers in Philadelphia to teach blind adults in their homes to read Scripture (Hanson, 1976). This group of volunteers grew

to form the basis of the profession of rehabilitation teaching (now known as vision rehabilitation therapy), which continues to provide a wider array of services in the homes of older adults with visual impairments.

As private agencies for the blind began to form in the early 1900s, they provided a diverse range of services. While many were focused on vocational training and employment, some also provided social services for older adults, including casework, recreational, and transportation services (Lowenfeld, 1975).

In some states, private and state rehabilitation agencies had already begun to tap into vocational rehabilitation funding and private funding to cover the cost of rehabilitation services for older adults. These adults were not likely to be employable, but it was expected that rehabilitation training would make a qualitative difference in their lives or would free another family member for employment (Orr, 1992). The practice of providing rehabilitation services for independent living came to be reflected in the congressional debates in the 1970s on the Rehabilitation Act. Finally, in 1978, the amendments to the Rehabilitation Act included for the first time the concept of independent living services. Part C of Title VII of the amended Rehabilitation Act called for the provision of training in independent living skills for older persons who were blind or visually impaired. While these services were not funded until 1986, and then only minimally, this legislation marked a major breakthrough for the concept of providing older adults with rehabilitation training to help them learn to cope with vision loss and to support maintaining their independence (Orr, 1992).

Low Vision Services

Most older adults who receive formal instruction in orientation and mobility will have entered the blindness system through their use of low vision services (Massoff et al., 1995). "Low vision services" refer to any of a diverse array of services designed to help people with low vision use their vision more effectively and improve their efforts to cope with their visual disability (see Geruschat & Smith, Volume 1, Chapter 3). While some low vision services have developed in ophthalmology and optometry practices or in hospital settings, others have emerged in rehabilitation agencies and schools, frequently with the collaboration of medical personnel. While some low vision services provide only medical diagnoses, interventions, and the prescription of and training with low vision devices, others provide additional social and rehabilitation services, such as O&M instruction, to help people with low vision cope with visual disabilities that cannot be corrected through medical interventions (Massoff et al., 1995). For many older adults, the services of the low vision provider may be their only contact with the blindness system. In other cases, a low vision service may not provide the additional services themselves, but may refer patients to social and rehabilitation programs or to independent O&M practitioners.

Older adults are more likely to begin with a low vision service provider for several reasons:

1. Their eye diseases typically do not result in total blindness. It is natural that they would pursue their vision problems with an eye care provider who may then make a referral to a medically based low vision service.

2. Older adults with low vision are hesitant to think of themselves as "blind" and therefore are not quick to identify themselves as needing the services of a specialized agency that primarily serves people who are "blind" (Zarit, 1992).

3. The traditional jurisdictional boundaries between education, vocational rehabilitation,

and health care have left older adults who are visually impaired "unclaimed" (Wainapel, 1994). Unfortunately, however, the health care funding that usually covers most of the cost of services provided through health care providers does not yet routinely cover the cost of vision rehabilitation services such as orientation and mobility.

The availability of funding for services through health care can make a significant difference in the likelihood that older adults will avail themselves of these services. As Mogk and Goodrich (2004) have discussed, the regionalization of certain Medicare funding decisions had temporarily permitted some service providers to have vision rehabilitation services funded by Medicare as long as they were provided incident to and under the general supervision of an ophthalmologist or optometrist. Welsh (2001) has reported that the availability of Medicare funding for orientation and mobility and vision rehabilitation services made a significant difference in older adults opting for the service. When the sole option for payment for the services was self-pay, only 1 out of 10 clients accepted vision rehabilitation training. When Medicare funding was available for the vision rehabilitation training, 9 out of 10 clients accepted it (Welsh, 2001).

Advocacy efforts have been pursued in recent years to obtain routine funding from Medicare for O&M training for a larger percentage of older adults. An update on these efforts is provided by Bina, Naimy, Fazzi, and Crouse (Volume 1, Chapter 12).

Community-Based Services

Some O&M services are provided to older adults through community-based itinerant services. Such services may be provided by a state-funded agency, using funds from Title VII, Part C of the Rehabilitation Act or state general funds. Others may be provided by a private rehabilitation agency under contract to the state or using privately generated funds.

Some older adults contact rehabilitation service providers on their own or through their families and others are referred by a low vision service provider. For community-based training, a social worker or counselor typically will visit the person in her home, explain the availability of services, and attempt to deal with issues of depression and family support, which may be primary at that time. If the older adult has not already been seen by a low vision service provider, a referral may be made to determine if there are any medical interventions that may help improve her vision. In some settings, the visit of the social worker is followed by visits from a rehabilitation teacher who will help the older adult develop daily living skills for coping with vision loss and perhaps provide basic indoor O&M training. If the older adult shows an interest in additional O&M training, an O&M specialist may visit her home to provide services.

Center-Based Services

Older adults may also receive O&M training in a center attended by other visually impaired adults who attend on a residential basis or on a day basis. In these settings, O&M training is usually only one of several rehabilitation and social experiences offered. In addition to having the opportunity to address O&M skills along with other skills needed for coping with vision loss, an opportunity is provided to interact with other people who are also learning to cope. Interactions with others who are experiencing the same thing can help a person identify issues that are common to the condition for many people versus those that are particular to an individual (see Welsh, Chapter 6).

Providing services through a center-based program is usually a more expensive option. Typically, the student is involved in a whole day or at least a partial day of training. As other services are provided, the cost naturally escalates. When a residential program is a part of the experience, dormitory and food services costs are added. While the additional experiences and learning opportunities are generally worth the expense, when this fact is combined with the lack of a reliable source of funding for such comprehensive programs for older adults, the problem is apparent.

Teamwork

Because older adults may have multiple health problems and resulting functional limitations, the interaction of professionals from different disciplines can be particularly important. In low vision settings, O&M specialists can draw directly from the input of optometry and ophthalmology professionals, social workers, low vision specialists, and occasionally from occupational therapists. When low vision services are in hospital settings, the input from physical therapists, nurses, and nutritionists also may add to the resources from which the older student and the O&M specialist can draw.

In comprehensive rehabilitation centers, the disciplines specializing in blindness—such as rehabilitation teachers, low vision specialists, and access technology specialists—are available, along with the frequent participation of rehabilitation counselors, social workers, optometrists, nurses, recreational and vocational specialists, as well as physical and occupational therapists on occasion.

When providing services on an itinerant basis, consultation from other professions is less readily available. While the social worker and the rehabilitation teacher may have visited the older adult in the home, and there may have been a report from a low vision clinic, the day-to-day consulting that is available in other settings is less likely.

The Aging System

Area Agencies on Aging (AAA)

The aging system provides an integrated service delivery system to older adults living in the community. These services may include transportation, senior centers, congregate dining, and Meals on Wheels programs. Many of these services are funded by the Older Americans Act, which was passed in 1965 and requires every state to develop and file a comprehensive outreach and service plan to reach older adults, identify their needs, and provide services that are needed to help older adults continue to live independently in their homes and communities. Comprehensive plans can include assistance with obtaining housing, repair and maintenance of homes, long-term care, home health care, advocacy, health screenings, legal services, social and recreational programs, and employment and training programs. Most state plans identify local Area Agencies on Aging (AAA) that fund and coordinate these services and provide information and referral to people in these areas (Orr, 1992).

In some areas, agencies that serve older adults with visual impairment have been able to build collaborative relationships with AAAs, as these two groups have many clients in common and have similar purposes. Both organizations are focused on helping older adults remain independent in their communities. In some instances, funding for specialized services such as orientation and mobility for older adults who are blind has come from local AAAs (Welsh, 2001; Orr, 1992). In addition, agencies for people who are blind or visually impaired can provide educational and screening programs in senior centers, as well as needed staff training opportunities. Similarly, agencies that focus on aging can provide training and staff support to blindness agencies.

Assisted Living and Nursing Facilities

There is a range of congregate living facilities for older adults that reflect a corresponding range of health and daily living needs among this population. Typically, the prevalence of visual impairment among the residents in such facilities is much higher than for adults of similar age in the community (Tielsch, 2001). This statistic indicates the need for close collaboration between agencies and professionals who serve people with visual impairments and such facilities.

Relocation to a nursing home for older adults can be stressful for them and for their families. Preparing older adults for the move ahead of time can alleviate some of the stress (Washburn, 2005). By providing a higher quality of care for older adults, nursing homes improve residents' well-being (Capezuti, Boltz, Renz, Hoffman, & Norman, 2006). To help with this transition to a nursing home, O&M specialists can familiarize the older adult with the facility. They can also share information with family members and facility staff about techniques to help the older adult with daily living skills, how to organize her living area for safer and more independent living, and how to adapt the environment to assist with orientation and mobility.

As with all services for older adults, funding is limited. The funds that have been identified for older adults through the Independent Living Title of the Rehabilitation Act and through the Older Americans Act are designated to help keep people in the community. Once they are placed in a nursing facility or in an assisted-living facility, they are frequently considered ineligible for funding designed to keep them in the community. In some states, initiatives have been organized to extend state Medicaid funds that are used to fund placement in nursing facilities by using some of them to provide alternative services ahead of such placement to help keep older adults in their community homes or in assisted-living facilities rather than in nursing facilities.

Cross-System Collaboration

One of the challenges in service delivery for older adults with vision loss is information and referral. Awareness of vision rehabilitation services by the general public, seniors and their families, and professionals working with the elderly is limited. Over time, awareness has improved somewhat, as people are living longer, experiencing vision loss more frequently, and accessing services. Organizations such as the American Foundation for the Blind, the American Association of Retired Persons (AARP), and the National Eye Institute have made information available on vision problems affecting older adults and available vision rehabilitation services through a variety of media, including print publications, television, the Internet, and radio (Mogk & Goodrich, 2004).

Funding for services provided to elderly people with vision loss comes from two systems: the vision-related system and the aging service delivery network. Many barriers to collaborative efforts between the two systems currently exist (Orr, 1992). Service providers in the aging network assume that vision-related service providers take care of the elderly who experience vision loss and they have the notion that vision loss is a natural consequence of aging; therefore, acceptance of this loss is not difficult (Branch, Horowitz & Carr, 1989). These barriers have been addressed in a positive manner through national and state memoranda of understanding to advocate for and provide increased services to improve the quality of life for older adults with visual impairments.

Orr (1992) states: "In light of the current and projected number of older persons living longer and experiencing multiple problems, it is becoming increasingly difficult to serve these clients without cross-disciplinary efforts across many systems" (p. 357). Unfortunately, neither system has sufficient funding to meet the needs of this population; however, some progress is being made (see Bina, Naimy, Fazzi, & Crouse, Volume 1, Chapter 12).

SUMMARY

As the population ages and more people live into their 80s and 90s, the number of people with visual impairments will continue to grow in absolute numbers and as a percentage of the population. In spite of stereotypes to the contrary, many older adults who experience vision loss are capable of and interested in learning how to cope with these losses so that they can continue an independent lifestyle as long as possible. These trends will continue to increase the need for and the opportunity to provide O&M training for older adults with visual impairments.

In spite of research indicating the success and cost-effectiveness of O&M services for older adults, there continues to be insufficient funding to provide these needed services. Growing collaboration between the blindness, health, and aging networks will continue to bring older adults with visual impairments into contact with services that can help them function independently. While, in the short term, this may aggravate the lack of sufficient funding to meet the identified needs, it may also produce new ways that these systems can solve this emerging problem.

As O&M specialists have more opportunities to serve older adults with vision loss, they should rely on individualized assessments that are not influenced by stereotypes and generalizations about the needs and abilities of older adults. However, they should also consider some of the special strategies that may be needed to help older adults overcome the limitations of additional health conditions that are seen among this population with greater frequency.

As increasing numbers of older adults come to need O&M services and to benefit from them, one impact may be a rise in the need for O&M specialists who are trained for and interested in serving this emerging population of people with visual impairments.

IMPLICATIONS FOR O&M PRACTICE

1. Even though the growing number of older adults with vision loss is creating a public health concern, rehabilitation services, including O&M services, are not readily available to help these individuals remain independent.

2. Older adults with vision loss may have additional disabilities and health problems that will need to be assessed and addressed when planning an instructional program.

3. Older adults with vision loss who received low vision clinical services, counseling, and use of optical devices found that their level of depression declined after receiving these services.

4. O&M training has many benefits for older adults with vision loss. These may include: a reduction in the number of falls, an increase in the use of human guides and long canes, an increase in their satisfaction with travel, fewer limitations of travel after training, and an increase in their confidence level for travel in unfamiliar areas, outdoors and in stores.

5. Older adults with vision loss experience certain health and functional problems more frequently than older people with unimpaired vision. These problems include strokes, falls and subsequent hip fractures, hypertension, diabetes, heart disease, and arthritis, as well as more difficulty with walking, getting in and out of a chair or bed, getting outside, and shopping for groceries.

6. When planning and implementing O&M programs for older adults with vision loss, using an interdisciplinary team model, effective communication, and collaboration techniques will assist them in attaining their goals.

7. O&M specialists can help older adults who become nondrivers cope by finding travel alternatives.

LEARNING ACTIVITIES

1. Interview three older adults with vision loss and their families to see what their concerns are with regard to O&M services. Write a report highlighting your findings.

2. Interview older adults who have lost vision with regard to the special impact of their losing the ability to drive.

3. Interview two O&M specialists who provide services to older adults with vision loss concerning effective teaching techniques, lessons learned, and what changes they would like to see in the rehabilitation system to provide better O&M services to these students. Write a report summarizing your findings to be shared with your classmates.

4. Develop a case study of an older adult with vision loss to be used by other classmates in developing an O&M program for this sample student. Develop a form for your classmates to complete that highlights their assessment findings and the important aspects of an effective O&M program.

Falling: Prevalence, Risk Factors, and Interventions
Julie Anne Couturier

According to the World Health Organization (WHO) (2007) and the American Geriatrics Society (AGS), the British Geriatrics Society (BGS) and the American Academy of Orthopedic Surgeons Panel on Falls Prevention (2001), approximately 35 to 40 percent of generally healthy, community-dwelling people older than age 65 fall each year; the rates are higher after the age of 75. They also report that falls are three times more frequent among people living in residential homes or long-term care institutions and that fractures or hospitalization occur in 5 percent of falls. Risks of falls are higher and more serious for women (for example, hip fracture), although men suffer from more comorbid conditions than women of the same age.

The risk of falling increases dramatically as the number of risk factors increases. The rates of falling increase from 27 percent for people with no or one risk factor to 78 percent for persons with four or more risk factors. Falls are associated with mortality, morbidity, reduced functioning, and premature nursing home admissions. Falls and resulting injuries have become major public health problems worldwide. The World Health Organization (WHO, 2007b) pinpoints that if preventive measures are not taken in the immediate future, the number of fall-related injuries would be 100 percent higher in 2030. However, there is evidence that most falls are predictable and preventable (WHO, 2007b). Special consideration will need to be given to the oldest segment of the population, age 80 and older, who are more prone to falls, as this special group is expected to be the fastest growing subgroup within the older population in the next decades.

RISK FACTORS FOR FALLS

Factors that contribute to falling have been classified within four dimensions: biological, behavioral, environmental, and socioeconomic (WHO, 2007b). *Biological* risk factors relate to age, gender, race, chronic illness, and to a decline in physical, cognitive, or affective capacities. Visual impairment is among these factors, in addition to balance, muscular strength, and gait impairments. *Behavioral* factors may include multiple or psychotropic medication use, excessive alcohol intake, lack of exercise or inactivity, poor nutrition, fear of falling, and inadequate footwear. *Environmental* factors relate to home hazards, such as slippery floors and stairs, loose rugs, insufficient lighting, and absence of handrails; they also include uneven and cracked sidewalks. Environmental factors are not by themselves causes of falls, but they interact with other factors. Finally, *socioeconomic* factors include low income and educational levels, isolation, limited access to health and social services, or lack of community resources. A history of falls is also a risk factor for recurrent falls (WHO, 2007b).

Many studies have been done on the causes and treatments that could prevent or reduce falls. In the review of this research, experts have applied scientific standards and criteria to evaluate the quality of such studies and to grade the level of scientific evidence supporting the association of a risk factor with fall occurrence (that is, high, moderate, or poor). At this point, some risk factors (for example, balance and gait impairment, medication uses, and history of falling), have shown a *high* level of evidence; that is, their relationship with falls have been *continuously* confirmed in studies that respect quality criteria

(continued on next page)

recognized by the scientific community (Francophone Network for Injury Prevention and Safety Promotion #IPSP], 2004, [English version] 2008).

Other risk factors, like chronic illness and fear of falling, have been evaluated to produce a *moderate* level of evidence, while other factors, such as inappropriate footwear, risk-taking behaviors, and environmental hazards, show *poor* levels of evidence. This grading system is a tool that helps professionals in defining priorities for fall prevention; for example, a person presenting a risk of falling, that is, with a history of falls and/or gait or balance impairments, should receive priority attention for fall prevention intervention (FNIPSP, 2008).

FALL PREVENTION AND INTERVENTION

Various preventive measures have been developed and tested and are presented according to a grading system (that is, highly recommended, recommended, or promising). Overall, meta-analyses have concluded that multifactoral interventions are more effective than interventions targeted on single factors (American Geriatrics Society [AGS] & British Geriatrics Society [BGS], 2006).

Assessing the Risk of Falling

Screening and assessing the risk of falling should be the first step of an intervention program (AGS & BGS, 2006; FNIPSP, 2008). The O&M specialist needs to be alert to the need for screening for falls and may play an important role in detecting a history of falls and making appropriate referrals to medical professionals when necessary. A history of a person's falls should be done once a year. Looking at a history of falls should include two main questions: Have you fallen during the last year? How many times?

A screening test serves in identifying those people who are at high risk of falling and those who are at a moderate or low risk of falling. An example of a screening test for balance and gait impairments is the "Timed Up & Go" (TUG) test (FNIPSP, 2008). The TUG test takes ten minutes, is simple to use, and provides satisfactory sensitivity. It can be administered by health, rehabilitation, and social service professionals. Once a person's level of risk has been assessed, specific intervention recommendations may be used according to the level of risk. The FNIPSP's (2008) practice guide presents types of prevention and intervention measures recommended for each risk level.

Medication and Exercise Programs

Clinical trials have demonstrated that reducing the number and dosage of medication decreases the risk of falling (AGS & BGS, 2006). Particular attention needs to be given to people taking four or more medications, as well as those taking psychotropic medication. The O&M specialist may want to review information on drug effects associated with risks of falling and the prevalence of depression among people with age-related macular degeneration (AMD) (Casten & Rovner, 2008). Secondary effects of antidepressants—such as drowsiness, dizziness, orthostatic hypotension, and blurred vision—may cause falls (FNIPSP, 2008).

Findings from several high-quality meta-analyses and randomized controlled trials have shown the benefits of exercise programs on the reduction of falls (AGS and BGS, 2006; WHO, 2007b). An interna-

(continued on next page)

tional consensus has emerged on the health benefits of regular exercise (that is, approximately 30 minutes per day) for cardiovascular problems, diabetes, hypertension, depression, and the like (FNIPSP, 2008). In this respect, an exercise and physical activity guide has been developed by the National Institute on Aging (NIA, 2004)). Exercises focus on endurance, strength, balance, and flexibility, all of which enhance gait, balance, and coordination while walking. Some exercises also slow the loss of bone mineral density in the older person (FNIPSP, 2008) (for more information on this topic, see Couturier and Ratelle, Chapter 15).

Many community exercise programs have been developed and implemented for the older population (FNIPSP, 2008). O&M specialists may want to consult with their local public health services to identify such programs and to assist on a consultation basis for persons with visual impairments who wish to participate in such programs.

Visual Impairments and Fall Prevention

Older people with visual impairments have an increased risk of falling (Campbell et al., 2005), but despite a significant relationship between falls, fractures, and visual acuity, there are very few studies on specific vision-related interventions to reduce falls. Studies have demonstrated, however, that cataract surgery performed early on decreased fall rates by 34 percent (AGS & BGS, 2006).

Campbell et al. (2005) conducted a study with 391 participants who are visually impaired, age 75 years or older, and showed the effectiveness of a home safety and modification program on reduction of falls, especially for persons with a history of falls. The environmental modification components included: avoid loose floor mats, paint the edge of steps with a contrasting color, reduce glare, install grab bars and stair rails, remove clutter, improve lighting, and provide advice on how to negotiate environmental hazards more safely. The researchers also included a one-year exercise program on muscle strength and balance, and a walking plan that had to be practiced three times a week. However, compliance with the program is a major concern. The data showed that a higher level of adherence to the prescribed program resulted in lower fall rates (that is, a lower fall rate for persons walking three times per week than for those walking one time per week).

The O&M specialist may be involved in assessing parts of a home environment and providing advice and instruction on the safe negotiation of environmental hazards in and around the home. For pedestrian traffic areas, it may be worthwhile to consult the *Guide on Global Age-Friendly Cities*, developed by the World Health Organization (2007a). Some guidelines are offered regarding environmental modifications for safer walking on sidewalks, in parks, and in public buildings.

PART THREE

Adapted Tools and Complex Environments

CHAPTER 11

Teaching the Use of Orientation Aids for Orientation and Mobility

Billie Louise Bentzen and James Robert Marston

LEARNING QUESTIONS

- In what ways does the age of the user, the cognitive level of the user, the tactile sensitivity of the user, and the reason for developing or using a map influence design decisions about information content, size, scale, information density, and symbols used on tactile maps?

- Why may single-copy maps made using household and craft materials be more interesting and easier to read than maps reproduced using heat-sensitive material such as microcapsule paper, Flexi-Paper, or vacuum-formed plastic?

- What kits or materials can visually impaired students easily use to make maps?

- What is the role of a geographic information system (GIS) in making tactile and large-print maps? How are GIS and the global positioning system (GPS) combined to provide information for route planning and ongoing guidance for travelers with vision impairments?

- What concepts and skills are needed by proficient map users?

This chapter begins by presenting principles for designing maps; subsequent sections describe some common materials for producing maps, and provide strategies for teaching map-reading concepts and skills. The chapter concludes by describing the use of geographic information system (GIS) devices and GIS–GPS (global positioning system) devices for wayfinding. This chapter is not a "cookbook" for making orientation aids using any one system; rather, it includes principles for designing and using orientation aids that cut across production techniques. (An excellent reference that provides detailed instructions for mapmaking using one or more techniques is *Tactile Graphics* [Edman, 1992].)

The chapter also describes a number of orientation aids that were available in the United States at the time of publication. Since the first publication of *Foundations of Orientation and Mobility* (1980), there has been an explosion in the

315

number of products available. By the time you read this chapter, additional products will doubtless be available, some products may no longer be available, and some will have changed. This is particularly true of electronic wayfinding technologies. There has been no attempt to include the many excellent products for making orientation aids that are available outside the United States.

In Volume 1, Chapter 10, spatial concepts and cognitive maps (that is, a person's knowledge of the layout of a specific place) were discussed as central to independent travel of people with visual impairments at any level of independence. Orientation aids including route descriptions, models, and tactile, large-print, and tactile and large-print maps were defined and described in terms of their usefulness for promoting spatial concepts and cognitive maps, and supporting research was presented. GIS databases were also described as a way to have a potentially infinite amount of information available on one digital map that could be accessed by people with visual impairments using tactile and audio interfaces. The use of GIS coupled with GPS technology for guidance of active travel was also introduced. This chapter builds on that knowledge and its application to everyday use.

DESIGN PRINCIPLES FOR MAPS FOR PEOPLE WHO HAVE VISUAL IMPAIRMENTS

Maps are appropriate for many students or clients, and many learning situations. However, whether or not a student or client benefits by using a map in a particular situation often depends on the creativity and skill of the specialist in designing, making, and using a map appropriate to the skill level of the user. The materials and design of any map must be able to convey the information needed, and be used in such a manner that users will understand the map itself, and, most importantly, be able to understand the relationship between the map and the environment.

There are a number of issues in the design of tactile, large-print, or tactile and large-print maps. The visual acuity and visual efficiency of intended users will determine whether a given map will be most useful if it is tactile, large print, or both tactile and large print. Other issues include information content, size, scale, choice of symbols, information density, labeling, and provision of supplementary verbal information. Design decisions about each issue impact all the others, so mapmakers need to be aware of the implications of decisions with regard to all these issues. While simply enlarging print maps sometimes makes them usable by persons who have low vision, it is rare that simply raising all information on a print map to make it tactile will result in a map that is very useful to persons who rely on touch for reading; it is likely to have too much information too close together.

In this section of the chapter, map design is discussed and guidelines for making map design decisions are provided. Where guidelines are based on research, a reference will be given. Other guidelines reflect the authors' judgments, based on experience. A comprehensive review of research prior to 1980 can be found in Bentzen (1980).

Information Content

The content of the information that needs to be included in a map depends on both what one wants to communicate and to whom. There are two basic rules concerning information content for maps for persons who are visually impaired, regardless of map type (tactile, large print, or tactile and large print).

- Include only information that is absolutely necessary.

- Err on the side of providing too little information.

The amount of usable information on a tactile map is less than the total amount that can be recognized (Angwin, 1968a, 1968b). The user may be able to identify all of the symbols on a map, but if much more information is presented than is needed for the user to perform the necessary tasks with the map, relevant information and important relationships may be obscured (Berlá & Murr, 1975). Information to be included should be selected by personal inspection of the area by someone experienced in selecting those elements of the environment that are of greatest significance for travelers who are visually impaired (Wiedel & Groves, 1969a, 1969b).

Map designers need to bear in mind that there are a number of environmental features that are not commonly represented on print maps, which are either so salient to travelers who are visually impaired that they are excellent nonvisual landmarks, or so important to the safety of travelers who are visually impaired that they are beneficial when included on tactile, large-print, or tactile and large-print maps (or in verbal information accompanying these maps). Examples of such features are slope, changes in walking surface, obstacles, unenclosed stairs, the nature of traffic controls at intersections, and the presence of an accessible pedestrian signal. Inclusion of pushbutton information is particularly important if it is necessary to push a button to get the pedestrian phase of a traffic signal. (See Volume 1, Chapter 11.)

The amount of information to be included is greatly influenced by the cognitive level of the user, the tactile skill of the user, and the purpose of the map. Maps for people who are just beginning instruction in orientation and mobility (hereafter, O&M) may need to be very simple, contain very few symbols, and represent relatively small spaces or short routes. Maps for people who are elderly, who may have reduced tactile sensitivity or who may be easily confused, may also need to be very simple. Maps intended to enable users who are proficient and generally well-oriented travelers to plan and travel new routes in unfamiliar environments may require a lot of information.

Size

The overall size of a tactile map is probably best if it is no larger than the span of two hands placed together with the fingers outstretched, about 16–18 inches (400–450 mm). Smaller maps are often better, provided that they are low in information density and the user understands the scale. Perception of both distance and direction on maps is complex. Both the person who reads a map using touch and the person with low vision who reads a map (particularly persons with a reduced visual field or who read using a magnifier) are able to perceive only very limited portions of a map at one time. They must, therefore, integrate over time the spatial relationships that a person with unimpaired vision can see in one glance. Therefore, maps to be used by persons with impaired vision need to be as small as possible. Decisions about map size cannot, however, be made independently of decisions about information content and scale; these decisions are always compromises.

Scale

Absolute Scale

Absolute scale on a map expresses the relationship between the size of the area mapped and size of the map. It may be expressed as a simple fraction or ratio, called the *representative fraction* (RF). For example, the ratio 1:1 means that the map is the same size as the area mapped; an example of this would be a map of a child's desk that is the same size as the desk. The ratio 1:100 means that one unit on the map corresponds to 100 units in the physical area being mapped. Scale may also be written as a statement of map distance to earth distance, for example 1 inch = 10 feet. A third way in which scale is commonly indicated on maps is a line with a label indicating that, for example, one segment equals 100 feet or 30 meters. Any of these ways of indicating scale can be used on either large-print maps or tactile maps.

Depending on the purposes for which a map is to be used, it may be unnecessary to indicate scale at all. Nonetheless, the map designer has to decide at what scale a map will be made. Decisions about scale will be influenced most by how much information the map is to contain, and how the map is to be used. Secondary considerations will be the actual map space needed for legibility of symbols and labels. For example, a map intended for planning and traveling the long bus route to work may be most useful at a relatively small scale, but maps for walking the short distances to and from the bus stops on both ends may be most useful at a relatively large scale.

One important determination of scale is the level of graphic abstraction that is meaningful to the map user. Users who are still learning basic environmental concepts may best understand large-scale maps that have rather literal representations of features of the environment. For example, a student who is beginning to learn the predictable, useful relationships between streets, curbs, sidewalks, and inside shorelines may benefit greatly by having a large-scale map of an intersection, including sidewalks, curbs, inside shorelines, streets, and crosswalks.

There is, however, a good reason for keeping scale as small as possible to show the needed information and perform the necessary tasks. One of the most difficult map-reading tasks for persons who are visually impaired is shape recognition. This is true regardless of whether readers use low vision or touch. Most persons who are visually impaired find shapes easier to recognize in relatively small scale than in relatively large scale. Therefore, if the primary purpose of

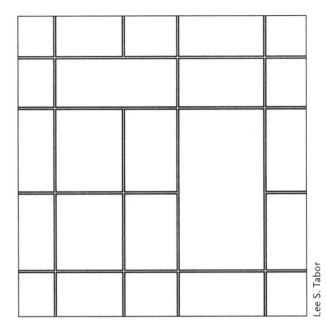

Lee S. Tabor

Figure 11.1. Example of a Small-Scale Map
If this small-scale map were raised, it would be easy for most users to identify the *plus* and *T* intersections.

an aid is to demonstrate a shape, it needs to be no larger than necessary for good discrimination. It is easy to identify *plus* ("+") and *T* intersections in the small-scale map in Figure 11.1. It is much more difficult to understand that the Velcro map shown in Figure 11.2 shows a *plus* ("+") intersection.

Consistency of Scale

Although persons who are visually impaired can probably acquire the most accurate cognitive maps by use of maps in which every feature is shown at the same scale, it is fortunately not essential for scale to be *absolutely* consistent in all parts of a map for the map to be useful (Armstrong, 1973; Bentzen, 1972; James, 1972; Kidwell & Greer, 1973; Wiedel & Groves, 1969b). There are limitations of the haptic perceptual system, which also apply to perception with impaired

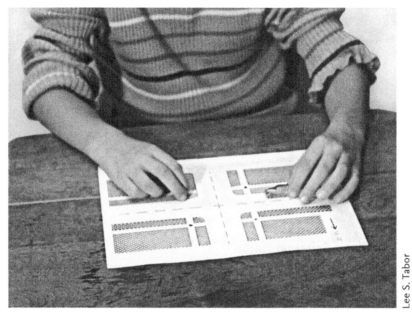

Lee S. Tabor

Figure 11.2.

This tactile and large-print map of an intersection can be used to teach the concepts of inside and outside shorelines (grasslines) and their relationship to streets, the travel paths of vehicles, and recognizing and recovering from veers while crossing at intersections.

vision, which make consistency in scale throughout a map very difficult.

- Symbols that are closer together than 1/8 inch (3 mm) tend to be perceived as a single symbol. Braille and large print should be a minimum of 1/8 inch (3 mm) from the nearest symbol.

- Symbols of the same type, for example, filled circles, must vary from one another in size by at least 25 to 30 percent to be perceived as different in size by most users (Pick, 1980). Larger differences may be better. Inconsistencies in scale may therefore be necessary in order to make differences in the sizes of symbols perceptible.

- Braille and large print have fixed dimensions that have been determined to result in the best legibility. A feature to be labeled may be too

small to contain a legible label, and may need to be larger in order to accommodate the label.

Schematization

A tactile map or tactile and large-print map that is in a simplified form, or is schematized, may be easier for users to read than a map that shows forms in all their complexity. It is easier to perceive a shape that is simplified than one that is complex (see Figure 11.3). It is easier to trace lines that are relatively straight than lines that show every slight bend in a road. It is easier to find landmarks on a map that omits elements that are not needed for understanding key spatial relationships.

It may also be easier to form a cognitive map from a tactile or tactile and large-print map that is schematized (Kidwell & Greer, 1973; Wiedel & Groves, 1969b). It is common for regular print

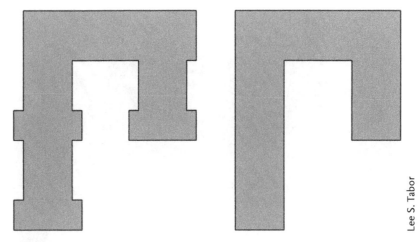

Lee S. Tabor

Figure 11.3. An Example of Schematization
The drawing on the left shows the actual footprint of a building. The drawing on the right shows a schematized footprint.

maps to be schematized; for example, maps of transit systems are typically schematized.

Symbols

Kinds of Symbols

There are three basic kinds of symbols: point, line, and areal. *Point symbols* show the location of a landmark, clue, or particular travel situation, but say nothing about its shape or dimension. A point symbol may show the location of a certain landmark, such as a specific pedestrian pushbutton, or it may indicate only that a particular intersection is signalized.

Line symbols convey information that is linear in nature. They indicate both location and direction. A line symbol may represent the location and direction of a specific linear feature such as the Long Island Railroad track, or a particular line symbol may be used generically—the same type of line used, for example, to represent the location and direction of all streets in the area shown. Line symbols do not typically convey information about the width or height of what they represent (although they may be modified in width and height to do so, especially in

situations where a student's conceptual level requires a somewhat literal representation).

Areal symbols convey information about the location of a feature and its shape and size as seen from above. A particular texture or color may be used to show the location, shape, and size of one particular building on a campus; alternatively, the same texture or color may be used in different locations, and in varying shapes and sizes, for all buildings on a campus.

Choice of Symbols

While it seems like a desirable goal to standardize symbols for tactile maps, as consistency is generally of great benefit to people with visual impairments, standardization of symbols may not be advantageous for some purposes, and may be difficult to achieve across different mapping techniques and materials (Edman, 1992; Tatham, 1991). Nonetheless, a considerable amount of effort and research has been conducted with the goal of standardizing symbols for tactile maps (First European Symposium on Tactual Town Maps for the Blind, 1984; Jehoel, Ungar, & Rowell, 2005; Rowell & Ungar, 2003). Because of the characteristics of different materials used for reproduction of multicopy maps, symbols that appear the same in print may feel quite different in different materials; thus, symbols that are very discriminable in one material may be difficult to discriminate in another material (Edman, 1992). For example, symbols reproduced using vacuum-formed plastic can vary noticeably in height and roughness. Similar symbols reproduced using microcapsule paper do not differ as noticeably in height and roughness. Therefore, choice of symbols for maps is somewhat dependent on the materials in which they are to be produced or reproduced.

The symbols for a particular map need to be ones that are not easily confused with each other, and that are easily perceived and recognized as representing the information they are intended to show. Symbols that are to be used together on a map should differ from each other in as many ways as possible to be most discriminable (Leonard, 1966; Nolan & Morris, 1971; Schiff & Isikow, 1966; Wiedel & Groves, 1969b). Edman (1992) contains illustrations of the large number of symbols that were in use on multicopy tactile maps in 1992. Use of some of these symbols in combina-

tion is supported by research, and some of these symbols are included in standardized sets (both noted in Edman). People who are engaged in designing multicopy maps of areas, buildings, and facilities are encouraged to base symbol choices on the examples and guidelines available in Edman.

Point symbols. Point symbols can be varied by altering their shape, size, elevation from the background (for tactile maps made using some materials and techniques), and color (for print maps), as well as the nature of their outline (smooth, broken, filled in). Four tactilely different circles are visually represented in Figure 11.4. If two circles are to be used as point symbols on the same map, they need to differ from one another in two or three characteristics. For example, a 1/8-inch (0.3 cm) diameter solid raised circle could represent the location of bus stops indicated only by a sign on a pole, and a 1/4-inch (0.6 cm) diameter open circle could represent bus shelters. Other point symbols on the map can also differ in shape. Point symbols need to fit under the reader's fingertip, but be large enough to be

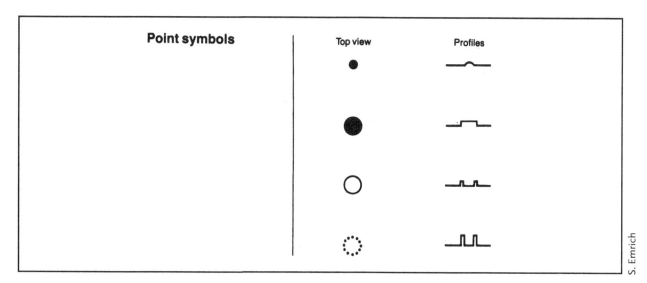

S. Emrich

Figure 11.4. Point Symbols
Point symbols with the same shape can be varied to make them discriminable.

haptically discriminable. If symbols are to be discriminated as different solely on the basis of size or elevation, then the difference in size or elevation should be a minimum of 25 percent (Pick, 1980). Point symbols that are outlined and have straight lines and sharp corners are generally the most legible (Austin & Sleight, 1952; Gill & James, 1973; Lambert & Lederman, 1989).

Symbols that are meaningful, such as a raised shape of a telephone receiver; a sharp, pointed symbol meaning stop or danger; or a miniature staircase, are quickly recognized and accurately identified (James & Gill, 1974; Lambert & Lederman, 1989). Use of such meaningful symbols reduces the need to refer to a key. On highly schematic maps, two-letter (or two-braille-cell) mnemonic codes may function better than abstract point symbols, whose meaning must be ascertained and remembered (Preiser, 1985).

Line symbols.   Line symbols can be varied by making lines continuous or interrupted, thick or thin, smooth or rough edged, and single or double (multiple) (see Figure 11.5). Height and profile of lines can also be varied for tactile maps, as can color for visual maps. As with point symbols, line symbols that differ from each other only in width or in height need to differ by a minimum of 25 percent in width or height (Pick, 1980).

In choosing line symbols, it is important to consider the tasks for which they will primarily be used, as well as their discriminability. For example, the line symbol that will be used for the greatest number of tracing tasks on a map should be the one with the best traceability; for example, the major streets shown on a neighborhood map. Narrow, single lines are the easiest to trace by touch, particularly when they are to be traced

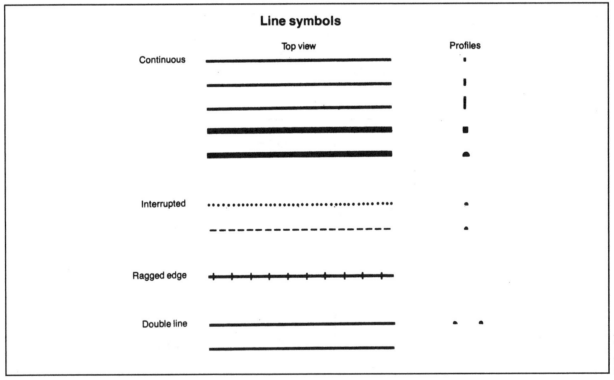

Figure 11.5. Line Symbols
Line symbols can be varied to make them discriminable.

across intersecting lines (Bentzen, 1983, 1989; Bentzen & Peck, 1979; Easton & Bentzen, 1980). Double raised lines that are more than 1/8 inch (0.3 cm) apart are difficult to trace, as both sides of the line are unlikely to be encountered by the fingertip at the same time, and the touch reader must go back and forth, or use more than one finger simultaneously, to locate both sides. There are, nonetheless, times when it may be desirable to use wider lines—for example, maps of intersections used for teaching recovery from veers at intersections. Double lines also enable the depiction of more detailed information, such as the shapes of curbs or islands. It needs to be kept in mind, however, that where the width between double lines representing roads is varied, the traceability of the line symbol will vary, and a change in width between the two lines may cause the line to be perceived and interpreted as an entirely different symbol. For example, a street divided by a wide median may be represented by a double line; but if the lines are too far apart, the single street may be understood to be two different streets. Incised lines are very difficult to trace and should not be used on tactile maps (Nolan, 1971). Channels 1/4 inch (0.6 cm) wide are, however, acceptable. Jehoel, McCallum, Rowell, and Ungar (2006) found that wide single raised lines were sometimes perceived as double lines, and that double lines were more accurately perceived as double lines when the individual lines comprising the double-line symbol were thin rather than thick.

Areal symbols.   Areal symbols should be used to differentiate adjacent areas on a map so that users do not have to trace an outline to determine whether they are "in" or "out of" a particular area. Areal symbols may differ from one another in density of texture elements (spacing between elements), regularity of element spacing, size of elements, shape of elements, and direction of elements (see Figure 11.6). On tactile

maps made by some production techniques, areal symbols may also differ in intensity or sharpness (rough versus smooth) of the haptic sensation produced, and height in relation to surrounding areas. On print maps they commonly differ in color or gray value. Differences in intensity and height make it possible to include more information on a tactile map of a given size. For example, a smooth solidly raised areal surface may represent a pond, an area surface that is raised and rough may indicate main buildings on a campus, and an area that is designated by a low, slightly rough surface may represent service buildings.

On tactile maps, differences in intensity or perceived "sharpness" make symbols highly discriminable (Levi & Schiff, 1966), and are easily achieved in some techniques. Four different grades of standard sandpaper reproduced in vacuum-formed plastic can be readily discriminated in areas as small as 3/4 square inches.

Variations in density of texture elements are more distinguishable to touch readers than differences in the shape or orientation of the elements (Levi & Schiff, 1966). So a texture composed of parallel lines spaced very close together is readily distinguished from parallel lines at the same angle but spaced farther apart. Parallel lines oriented having the same spacing, but oriented in different directions, are more likely to be confused with one another. A texture composed of circles is not easy to distinguish from a texture composed of squares.

Differences in the size of elements can also be a distinguishing characteristic (Nolan & Morris, 1971). However, when an areal symbol is to be used in a small area, it must be a symbol with small elements close together (Levi & Schiff, 1966; Morris & Nolan, 1963).

Areal symbols may obscure line and point symbols on a tactile map (Berlá & Murr, 1975), especially where line or point symbols are within the field of an areal symbol. Areal symbols should therefore be avoided on areas where line

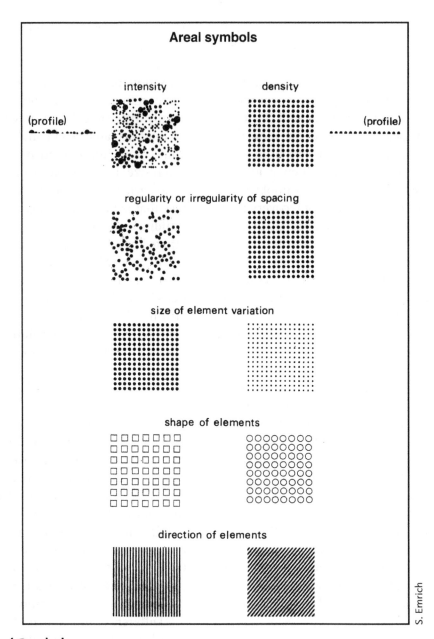

Figure 11.6. Areal Symbols
Areal symbols can be varied to make them discriminable.

or point symbols are needed to represent significant information or on maps where line tracing is a major component of the tasks to be performed with the map. Examples of maps requiring accurate line tracing are maps of cities and maps of transit routes.

Information Density

Information density for a particular map should be determined by consideration of the user's tactile or visual acuity and tactile or visual perceptual ability. For example, a person whose tactile acuity is reduced by environmental conditions such as cold, or physical conditions such as peripheral neuropathy or calluses, will best be able to use an aid that has maximum spacing between all symbols. A person who has difficulty isolating figures from ground, for example, a person who concentrates on the spaces between lines instead of the shape defined by the lines, needs maps with minimal information density.

Information density is influenced by other design factors such as information content, scale, size, symbols, and construction materials. There are a number of techniques for reducing information density:

- Use the smallest discriminable symbols.
- Use single-line symbols rather than double lines or a channel.
- Increase the scale.
- Delete unnecessary information, such as borders around maps.
- Place keys on a separate page.
- Place some information on an overlay or underlay.
- Use two-letter or two-cell mnemonic labels.

Overlays and Underlays

A map with an overlay consists of pages that are hinged together and carefully aligned so that the information on the overlay is directly over related information on the map itself. The reader places one hand on the overlay and the other hand on the page below to read related information. An underlay is made with related information shown on the underside of the same sheet. Underlays are also read with two hands, one on the top and one on the underside.

The photos in Figure 11.7A–D show a portion of a primarily tactile map of Boston and Cambridge, Massachusetts. This map is composed of four registered layers (see Figure 11.7A). The top layer is a transparent print map with labels of major areas and neighborhoods; this layer enables a person with vision to assist a map reader who is blind. Beneath this transparent layer, and visible through it, is a second layer having a high-contrast tactile map using different line symbols to differentiate between highways, minor roads, major roads, and shopping streets; different point symbols to indicate universities, squares, and points of interest; and different area symbols to indicate water, parks, and industrial areas. A third layer is on the reverse side of the second layer. It contains braille labels for major streets and neighborhoods. The braille is intended to be read with one hand palm-side up, while the hand reading the map is above it, palm-side down; thus opposing fingers can follow a street on top and read the name of the street on the bottom (see Figure 11.7B). The fourth layer is a tactile map, with braille labels, depicting rail transit lines and stations (with variations of point symbols showing whether a station is above or below ground, and whether it is a transfer point between two or more lines), and major bus lines. With both hands palm-side down, fingers of the hand on the second layer can, for example, find the location of Copley Square, while the other hand, on the fourth layer, locates the two rail transit lines that converge at Copley Station (see Figure 11.7C). The upper hand can then be turned palm-side up, to read the names of the two streets under which the two transit lines run (see Figure 11.7D). The original tactile map measured 16 by 23 inches (41 by 58 cm). Proficient travelers who were visually impaired were able to use this map set to plan and travel unfamiliar routes (Bentzen, 1977).

Labels

Adding labels to tactile maps often increases the problems of information density, scale, and symbol size. Braille labels are most legible if they are

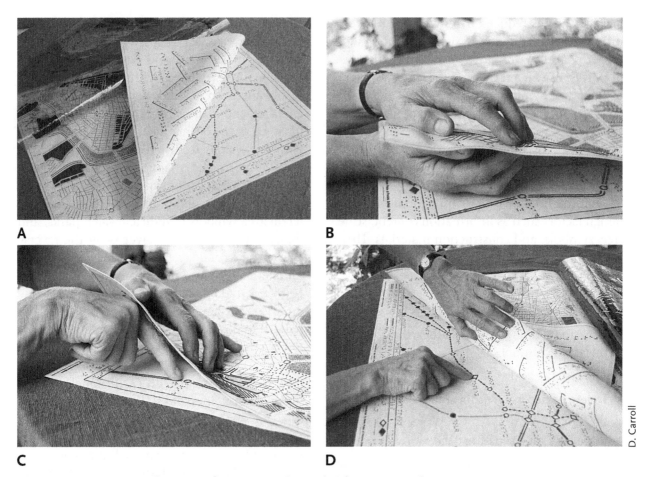

D. Carroll

Figure 11.7A–D. Tactile Map of Boston and Cambridge, Massachusetts

The four layers of this map include a transparent print map with labels of major areas and neighborhoods on top (A); a high-contrast tactile map using different line, point, and area symbols (A); a third layer containing braille labels on the reverse side of the second layer (A and B); and a tactile map, with braille labels, depicting rail transit lines and stations and major bus routes on the bottom (C and D).

horizontal, particularly for nonexpert braille readers. However, many users can readily read labels placed in other directions (Ungar, Blades, & Spencer, 1998). Where labels are to be abbreviated, abbreviations need to consist of a minimum of two braille cells, and they need to be mnemonic, for example *BC* for Boston College, or *Pk* for Park Station. Mnemonic labels reduce the need for reference to an index. On any one map, labels need to be placed in consistent positions relative to their referents. In the map in Figure 11.8, each street is labeled where it intersects the

edge of the map. Interior streets are not labeled. In the map in Figure 11.7, streets are labeled (on an underlay) above the street and parallel to it.

A solution to clutter or density added by the use of braille labels is to put them on an overlay or underlay. Overlays and underlays are also suitable for showing multilevel environments such as levels of malls or transit stations.

Preiser (1985) found that symbols for landmarks could simply be replaced by two-letter abbreviations, for example *ph* for telephone, reducing clutter on the map.

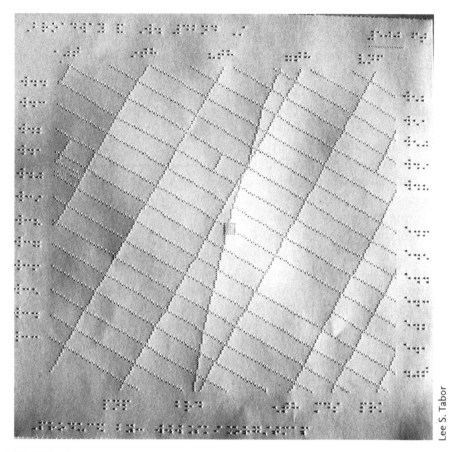

Figure 11.8. A TMAP Map

Tactile Map Automated Production (TMAP) maps, generated by software developed at Smith-Kettlewell Eye Research Institute from a commercial GIS, label streets with three–braille-cell mnemonic abbreviations where they intersect the edges of the page. A key relates abbreviations to the full names of streets, and also provides information about the orientation of streets.

Grids

On a map of an extended area, it is often desirable to have a *grid* to facilitate locating specific points given in a verbal index. This system is commonly used on print maps with indexes and can also be used on tactile maps (Bentzen, 1972; Edman, 1992). Tactile scanning, or scanning with low vision, is much more time-consuming than scanning with unimpaired vision. A grid system narrows the field that needs to be searched to find a destination on a map. A tactile or large-print grid can be provided along the margins of a map, or a complete raised or large-print grid can be provided on an overlay or underlay (Armstrong, 1973; Edman, 1992). A marginal grid can be seen along the left side of the Boston and Cambridge map shown in Figure 11.7A.

MATERIALS FOR TEACHING O&M CONCEPTS

As described in Volume 1, Chapter 10, different materials and models can be used to teach spatial and map concepts. In addition to materials that can be created by an O&M specialist, two kits available from the American Printing House for the Blind (APH) are useful for this purpose.

The O&M Tactile Graphics kit (available from the APH) provides ready-made tactile and large-print graphics for teaching concepts such as position, direction, hallways and rooms (with landmarks and objects), parallel and perpendicular streets, compass directions, city blocks, types of intersections, movement of vehicles at intersections, street crossing (including recognizing and recovering from veers), shapes of routes, and reversal of routes. See Figure 11.2 for a sample graphic.

Picture Maker: Wheatley Tactile Diagramming Kit (available through the APH) consists of a folding Velcro board with a great many pieces in a variety of shapes, sizes, textures, and colors (see Figure 11.9). The pieces can be used by O&M specialists and students or clients to teach, or

demonstrate mastery of, spatial concepts. The varied textures and colors make maps using Picture Maker interesting to students or clients who are totally blind as well as to those who have low vision (see Sidebar 11.1). Additional symbols can be made by gluing "hook" Velcro onto other types of pieces.

MATERIALS AND TECHNIQUES FOR MAKING TACTILE MAPS

A variety of easily purchased materials as well as ready-made kits can be utilized in making different kinds of tactile maps for teaching students map skills and concepts. The examples of commercial products mentioned here were available at the time of publication, but availability and contents of such products can change over time.

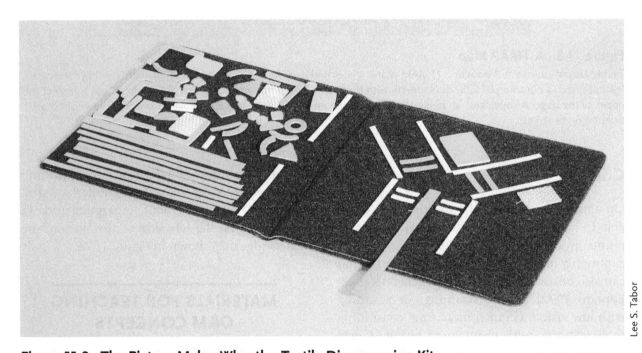

Lee S. Tabor

Figure 11.9. The Picture Maker Wheatley Tactile Diagramming Kit
On the left half of the folding Velcro board are samples of the symbols in the kit. On the right half, some of the symbols are used to show the geometry of a *Y* intersection.

SIDEBAR 11.1

Using Picture Maker to Share the World

As the inventor of Picture Maker, I created it to meet my own needs as an orientation and mobility specialist for flexible mapping materials (see Figure 11.10). It worked so well that I use it on a daily basis with all of my students, from preschool age to the elderly. The board has proven to be a versatile tool for instruction. It is lightweight, portable, and convenient to use on street corners, in the car, at home, or in the classroom. It is very handy for instruction and assessment of positional concepts, single-block orientation, grid-pattern development, and building and room familiarization, and to illustrate intersection design. I also create quick diagrams with the Picture Maker to answer tough spatial questions like "What does a Ferris wheel look like?"

The Picture Maker allows me to present the world as I see it, but more importantly, my students with visual impairments and blindness can share their perceptions of the world with me. I use the Picture Maker to teach concepts and routes; my students use the Picture Maker to

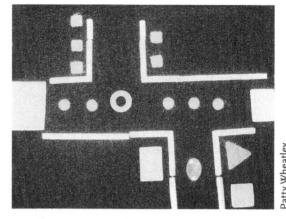

Patty Wheatley

Figure 11.10.
A map constructed using Picture Maker of the central part of a shopping mall, including the food court, anchor stores, and kiosks.

demonstrate what they understand. In this way, the Picture Maker enables me to assess the thoroughness of my own instruction.

PATTY WHEATLEY

Making Single-Copy Maps from Readily Available Materials

Excellent single-copy maps for individual students can be made by gluing commonly available materials onto a base of braille paper or cardboard. Various kinds of string, wire, and even pasta can be glued on for line symbols, or lines can be stitched into the base. Buttons, paper fasteners, and staples all make satisfactory point symbols, and various papers, fabrics, and sandpaper make good areal symbols. Maps made of such varied and readily available materials may be more interesting to touch than maps reproduced on a single substrate such as plastic or paper. These maps may also have superior discriminability, because of differences in texture, softness, resilience, slipperiness, and thermal conductivity of the varied materials (see Sidebar 11.2 and Figures 11.11A&B).

Small "minute maps" can be created by O&M specialists during lessons by using either a tracing wheel or chart tape on file cards. Tracing wheels with differently spaced teeth can be used to make lines that are discriminable from one another, such as different transit lines. Tracing wheels that are small in diameter and have closely spaced teeth are particularly easy to use. Various tracing wheels can be obtained from the APH, Howe Press, and leather working and

Preschool Tactile Map Concepts

I teach my preschool students, whose classmates are learning colors and shapes, to recognize colors (if applicable), shapes, and textures that I then use for orientation to their school. I cut 3-inch squares out of white foam board and put a symbol on each square, and use games to teach the children to say the shape, texture, and color (again, if applicable) of each symbol. I also put tactile arrows on two cards to show left and right turns.

I then place the same symbols around the school to mark important rooms. For example, I place a small orange foam square on the wall beside a child's classroom door, a "carpet" circle on the wall beside the music room door, and a red felt circle beside the resource room. I encourage the child to find *and name* the tactile markers every time she comes to a room with a symbol. In this way, she learns that the symbols represent real places. She can then put the square cards in order, including the arrow cards to show the action at each landmark. (See Figure 11.11A.)

Next, I introduce a basic tactile map of the school. I make both the map base and rooms of the school out of foam board, and glue on small symbols corresponding to the symbols they already associate with key landmarks. A child can literally run her finger down the hallways just like she is trailing the wall. More symbols are added when the child is ready. (See Figure 11.11B.)

DIANE BRAUNER

A

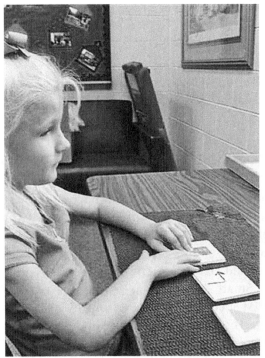

B

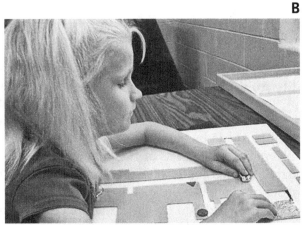

Diane Brauner

Figure 11.11.
(A) This 4-year-old girl places tactile cards in sequence to form her route: "From the cafeteria (pink square) make a left hand turn (left arrow) to go the bathroom (felt triangle)." (B) Then she moves a little car (in her left hand) along the route from her classroom to the cafeteria (under her right hand).

sewing stores. To produce a map using a tracing wheel, you must work in reverse, on the back side of the paper, so that when it is embossed and the map is turned over, it will read correctly. The paper must rest on a somewhat resilient surface to make good raised lines. Chart tape comes in different widths, textures, and colors, and is available at some graphics supply stores. It is also available through the APH (called Graphic Art Tape). It is excellent for quick production of simple tactile-visual maps. A great advantage of these two systems is that supplies for both can be in a shirt pocket, enabling maps to be made and modified quickly and easily on-site. These materials can be combined on the same map to create more discriminable symbols (see Figure 11.12). The materials are not easy for students to use to create their own maps, however.

Wikki Stix, a product consisting of sticky waxed cords, can be used both by teachers and students to make simple tactile-visual maps. An advantage of Wikki Stix is that they can be

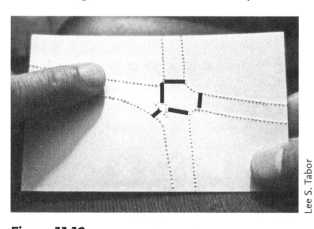

Lee S. Tabor

Figure 11.12.
This 3″×5″ "minute map" was created during a lesson to help a client understand the geometry of a complex intersection, including the relationships between crosswalks, corners, and parallel traffic. The map took no more than two minutes to make, using a tracing wheel for lines representing curb lines, and chart tape to represent crosswalks. To provide the resilient surface that is necessary for making good raised lines using a tracing wheel, the O&M specialist held the card against her leg as she drew with the tracing wheel.

repositioned to correct a mistaken perception, or additional information can be added (see Figure 11.13).

Making Tactile Maps Using a Braille Writer or Braille Embosser

Maps consisting primarily of labels and straight lines that intersect at right angles can be produced by teachers or students on a standard braille writer. Smoothly curved lines cannot be produced on a brailler, but they can be added using a freehand drawing stylus or tracing wheel. For individuals who are blind and highly familiar with a brailler, the brailler can be an excellent means for creating simple tactile maps.

Most embossers for producing braille from digitized input can now produce tactile maps based on GIS databases, and can produce curved lines. Embossers vary considerably in the quality of the raised image, however. Most embossers are not capable of making symbols that vary in height, and all are limited in the number or types of symbols they can produce. The best embossers for producing tactile graphics are designed with this function in mind.

Typical data in a GIS is far too detailed to be represented in an easy-to-understand tactile format. In order to make tactile maps from a GIS, the amount of tactile information needs to typically be reduced to simpler lines and labels limited to the information that is absolutely necessary for a particular student or purpose. Care also needs to be taken so that street name labels are not confused with and do not overwrite raised lines representing streets.

Kits and Materials for Producing Single-Copy Maps by Hand

There are a number of kits and materials for producing single-copy maps, some of which can be used by persons who are blind, as well as by O&M specialists.

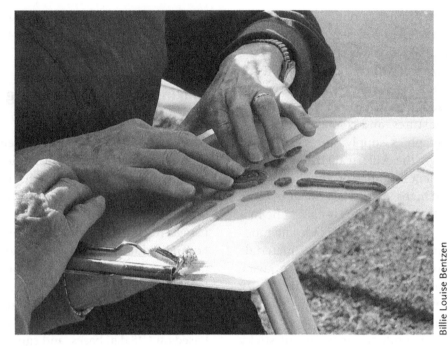

Billie Louise Bentzen

Figure 11.13.
A map made from Wikki Stix to familiarize a client with a particular roundabout.

Chang Tactual Diagram Kit

The Chang Tactual Diagram Kit (available from the APH) consists of a Velcro loop board, geometric shapes of graduated sizes backed with hook Velcro, and plastic stick figures. The Chang Kit is particularly easy for young children to manipulate, and is pleasing to touch. It is good for showing room arrangements or street layouts. Its large rectangles can be used to represent blocks, and the spaces between them can represent streets; alternatively, long narrow rectangles can represent streets, and the spaces between them can represent blocks (see Figure 11.14).

The kit does not contain small point symbols, but these can be glued onto the smaller plastic shapes, or they can be made by gluing Velcro directly onto items selected for symbols. Braille labels can be glued onto the plastic shapes.

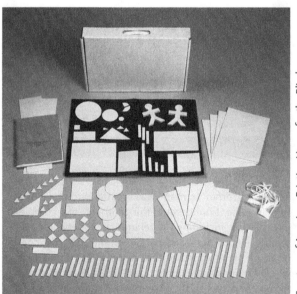

Courtesy of American Printing House for the Blind

Figure 11.14. Contents of the Chang Tactual Diagram Kit

Teachers can also make inexpensive Velcro kits that are particularly suited to the needs of their students. Velcro can be purchased by the yard or in small shapes, with or without self-adhesive backing.

Tactile Drawing Equipment

Stiff rubber boards to which transparent or translucent sheets of textured plastic or Mylar are clamped can be used to make tactile maps. Raised graphics are produced by drawing on the sheets with a ballpoint pen, a braille stylus, or specialized drawing tools provided with the drawing board. The pen, stylus, or drawing tool produces lines that are raised on the same side of the plastic or Mylar as they are drawn. Blind children or adults can draw on the sheets, and receive instant feedback regarding what they have drawn. They do not need to reverse the image or draw on the reverse side of the plastic or Mylar. The system enables students or clients who are visually impaired to communicate their understanding of spatial arrays such as simple room arrangements or complex intersections. Teachers can then correct misunderstandings either on the drawing system or in the environment. Two examples of such items are the Draftsman Tactile Drawing Board (see Figure 11.15, available from the APH) and the Raised Line Drawing Kit (available from Howe Press).

It is difficult using just a pen, stylus, or drawing tool to produce line, point, or areal symbols that are highly discriminable from one another, and there is no visual contrast. However, braille can be added using a braillewriter or slate and stylus, and point symbols such as those contained in Feel 'n Peel point symbols and adhesive braille (available from the APH) can be added. Additional discriminable lines may be added by drawing on the reverse side of the plastic or Mylar using a tracing wheel. Some people find the smooth plastic irritating to read by touch, and young children may lack the control needed to produce legible symbols.

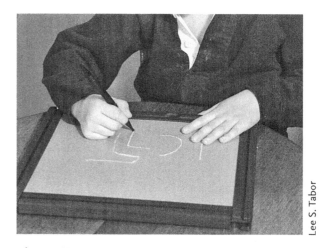

Lee S. Tabor

Figure 11.15.
This kindergarten student is using the Draftsman Tactile Drawing Board to demonstrate his understanding of routes that go straight, curve, or have a turn (corner).

Another system for drawing images that are raised on the side of the material on which they are drawn is somewhat thick, textured paper that swells when drawn on using a water-based pen. This material is easier for many young children to handle, and it has the additional advantage of producing print images, including color, at the same time as raised images, thus being more suitable for people with low vision than maps drawn on translucent or transparent plastic or Mylar (see Figure 11.16). One product using this system is Quick Draw Paper (available from the APH). Additional symbols and braille can be added to these maps in the same ways they can be added to maps produced using raised-line drawing boards.

One-of-a-kind maps can also be made using paper point symbols, puffy craft ink, and fabrics. These materials are combined into the Tactile Graphics Starter Kit (available from the APH).

Stencils and Special Tools for Making Tactile Maps by Hand Using Web-Based Maps

Web-based maps such as those available on Mapquest, AAA, or Google Maps can be used for

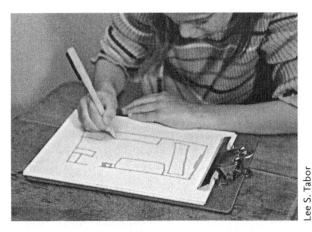

Lee S. Tabor

Figure 11.16.

This second-grade student is using Quick-Draw Paper to represent the layout of objects in her bedroom. As she draws, she tells her teacher what each outline represents. Through both her drawing and her verbal description, the teacher learns that while the child's drawing is not very accurate in scale (that is, the large bed and small table are shown the same size), the student has a good idea of relative sizes of objects in her room and their spatial relationships.

manual production of tactile maps or tactile and large-print maps. Figure 11.17A–C shows one method for making a tactile map of a neighborhood using a map printed from the Internet. First, streets and landmarks selected by the mapmaker are transferred onto the reverse side of a sheet of braille paper by laying the printed map on top of a sheet of braille paper, and these two on top of a sheet of carbon paper, then drawing the streets and landmarks on the printed map. Next, a tracing wheel is used to emboss the streets into the reverse side of the braille paper, following the carbon paper lines. Finally, point symbols for landmarks are embossed onto the reverse side of the map using a stencil and a stylus. The map is placed reverse-side up, on a light-box or window, with the stencil between the map and the glass. This makes it possible to position the stencil accurately for embossing the point symbols.

A variety of stencils and tools are included in the Crafty Graphics: Stencil Embossing Kit and the Crafty Graphics Kit II (both available from the APH), including stencils for braille and a variety of serrated tracing wheels and other embossing tools.

Making Multicopy Tactile Maps

There are three primary methods for making multicopy tactile maps: vacuum forming in plastic, copying on microcapsule paper, and ink-jet printing with thick ink. Vacuum-formed plastic maps are capable of greater symbol definition, and consequently a larger number of discriminable symbols than microcapsule maps. The maps are not damaged by moisture. However, they cannot be folded without wrinkling, making them hard to read.

A disadvantage of the microcapsule technique is that very little variation in symbol height is possible, and symbols, including braille, are less sharply defined than they can be in vacuum-formed plastic. However, a great advantage is the ease of making the original drawing and the fact that when produced on Flexi-Paper (an alternative to microcapsule paper), they can be folded or crumpled without affecting the map. Flexi-Paper maps are also weatherproof.

Research has been conducted to determine the relative suitability of different materials for making multicopy maps. It is difficult to compare the legibility of tactile maps made with different substrates because although the same symbols on maps produced using materials such as microcapsule paper (which is heated to raise images) or Brailon (which is vacuum-formed to raise images) look the same, they feel very different. In general, results of research examining speed of extracting information from maps using different substrates, as well as preference for substrate, suggest that tactile map readers perform faster with and prefer maps made on rougher substrates such as rough plastic, rough paper, or microcapsule

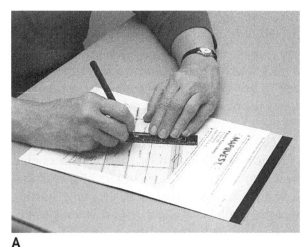

A

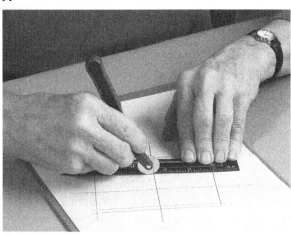

B

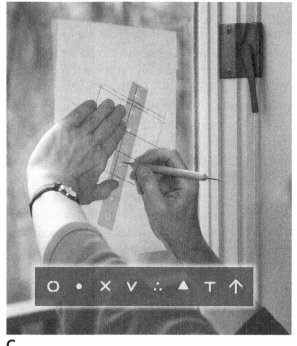

C

Lee S. Tabor

Figure 11.17. Making a Tactile Map from a Web-Based Map

(A) Transferring selected streets and landmarks from the map to the reverse side of braille paper by tracing them using carbon paper. (B) Creating raised lines for the streets using a tracing wheel. The paper is placed on a rubber mat to provide the resilient surface necessary to achieve good tactile lines. (C) Embossing point symbols on the map using a stencil and stylus. Placing the paper on a window or light box helps to position the symbols accurately.

paper than those on smoother surfaces such as Brailon, smooth plastic, or aluminum (Dacen-Nagel & Coulson, 1990; Horsfall, 1997; Jehoel, Ungar, McCallum, & Rowell, 2005; Pike, Blades, & Spencer, 1992).

Jehoel et al. (2005) produced identical sets of symbols on seven substrates using ink-jet technology. Thick ink that dries when exposed to ultraviolet light can be used to print onto many different sorts of media, including paper, card, plastic, clay

tile, and metal. The height of tactile symbols can be controlled (Ahmed, McCallum, & Sheldon, 2005; Pike et al., 1992; Shoufeng & Evans, 2005).

Map masters for vacuum forming by equipment such as that available from American Thermoform Corp. can be made of craft materials glued onto cardstock, or embossed into heavy, soft, aluminum foil. With craft materials, care must be taken in choosing and gluing them so that it is not possible for the plastic to be pulled under the materials in the process of vacuum forming; if this happens, it is likely that both the master and the copy will be unusable.

The Tactile Graphics Kit (available from the APH), developed on the basis of research on a discriminable symbol set for reproduction in vacuum-formed plastic (Barth, 1982), contains equipment and supplies for the creation of aluminum master copies of maps to be duplicated in plastic by vacuum forming. Tools are included to produce eight point symbols, seven line symbols, and four areal symbols, all of which have been demonstrated to be highly discriminable from one another (see Figure 11.18). The aluminum is heavyweight aluminum that is very malleable (dead-soft), available in the kit or in bulk from APH. In addition to the tools provided in the kit, a variety of tools available for leather or woodworking, as well as tracing wheels for sewing, and various styluses can be used to make symbols. Textured materials, point symbols, and braille labels can also be glued onto the aluminum.

Microcapsule paper is coated with plastic microcapsules that expand when they are exposed to heat. When a graphic is drawn, photocopied, or printed onto this paper and then exposed to a heat source, the microcapsules expand the most where the paper is darkest (that is, gets the hottest), which results in a raised image (Andrews,

1985). Any information drawn, printed, or photocopied onto microcapsule paper is raised when the paper is heated. Darker lines result in slightly higher raised images, and broader print lines result in broader raised lines. Heat sources (sometimes referred to as *fusers*) may be infrared heaters, heat lamps, or stereocopiers.

Flexi-Paper is another product on which a graphic image is raised by passing it through a heat source. An advantage of Flexi-Paper is that it can be folded without creasing or distorting images. Available at the date of this book's publication through Repro-Tronics, Inc., and other sources, Flexi-Paper is specifically recommended for use with the Tactile Image Enhancer (TIE) fuser. In addition to producing tactile maps on Flexi-Paper using the TIE, a heat pen (Thermo-Pen) is available for producing freehand raised images directly, without need for an additional heat source (see Figure 11.19).

Geographic information system databases make it possible to print maps of a desired location in a scale that is appropriate for touch reading. If these maps are printed on microcapsule paper or Flexi-Paper, they can then be readily turned into tactile maps. However, extensive editing is usually required to delete unnecessary or confusing information, to add landmarks of particular interest, and to add braille labels.

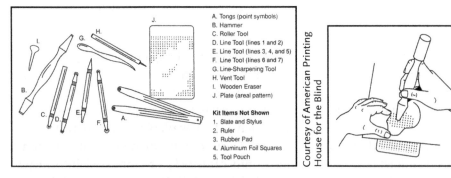

A. Tongs (point symbols)
B. Hammer
C. Roller Tool
D. Line Tool (lines 1 and 2)
E. Line Tool (lines 3, 4, and 5)
F. Line Tool (lines 6 and 7)
G. Line-Sharpening Tool
H. Vent Tool
I. Wooden Eraser
J. Plate (areal pattern)

Kit Items Not Shown
1. Slate and Stylus
2. Ruler
3. Rubber Pad
4. Aluminum Foil Squares
5. Tool Pouch

Courtesy of American Printing House for the Blind

Figure 11.18. The Tactile Graphics Kit

(A) Tools for producing line, point, and areal symbols on aluminum master copies of maps to be reproduced using vacuum-formed plastic. (B) The hammer being used to create a texture, and the tracing wheel being used to create a line.

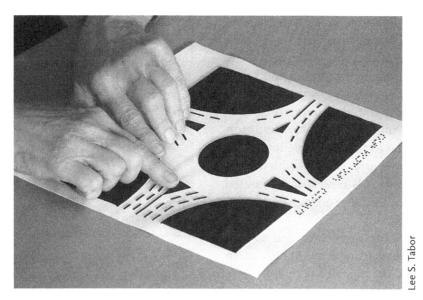

Figure 11.19.
A schematic map of a roundabout is reproduced in Flexi-Paper.

Computer-Aided Design (CAD) and Production of Tactile Maps

CAD design and production of tactile (or tactile-visual) vacuum-formed maps, pioneered by Gill (1973a, 1973b), has been further developed at the Computer Center for the Visually Impaired, Baruch College, City University of New York and by Touch Graphics, Inc. Graphics are designed using CAD software, and are then translated into negative relief by a computer-guided milling machine. A positive master is created by coating the negative created by the milling machine with silicon. Vacuum-formed copies are then produced from the positive master. Maps produced using this process can contain a number of levels of relief as well as braille. The precision in this production process makes symbols particularly discriminable.

CAD systems are also being adapted to produce raised graphics using other technologies, including braille printers, silk screening, and ink-jet printing (McCallum, Rowell, & Ungar, 2003; McCallum & Ungar, 2003).

Automated Production of Tactile Maps with the Possibility of Additional Information

Tactile maps may be quite labor intensive to make, and they vary greatly in quality. However, there is increasing interest in automating the design and manufacture of tactile maps. The Tactile Map Automated Production (TMAP) project was initiated by Miele at the Smith-Kettlewell Eye Research Institute, Rehabilitation Engineering Research Center in 2003 with the goal of developing a web-based software tool for rapid production of high-quality, standardized, tactile street maps of any location in the United States (Miele, 2005; Miele & Marston, 2005a, 2005b). Readers can find out more about the TMAP project at www.ski.org/tmap. The TMAP web site allows users to select various scales for a desired area, and instantly produce tactile maps that have standardized information, legends, and feel, using any tactile-graphics-capable embosser. Maps may be customized to be labeled in contracted or uncontracted braille, and specific landmarks can be indicated. If users do not have a braille embosser, the data can be e-mailed to a braille production facility for embossing. The data used for this automatic production come from a GIS database, and are customized using software developed by Miele. Users are able to produce and keep multiple maps having information almost equal to that available to readers of print maps (see Figure 11.8). Production of tactile maps in Slovenia is now also automated as well as standardized by processes developed by Rener (2005a, 2005b).

Verbal information can be provided when a tactile map is created using the TMAP system and used in combination with a touch tablet to which verbal information supplementing the map has been added. Touch Graphics, Inc., whose Talking Tactile Tablet (TTT) is a simple device that connects to a USB port on a user's computer, has teamed with TMAP developers to add auditory information to the TMAP. This system, called TMAP Reader, is a program that runs on the computer to which a TTT is connected (Miele & Gilden, 2004; Miele, Landau, & Gilden, 2006; Miele & Marston, 2005a, 2005b). A TMAP map is placed on the TTT, and a user can press on a location and hear synthetic speech giving names, or other information, about that location. In this way, street names, block addresses, and other information can be heard. Users can also receive this information from a refreshable braille display. A user can scan an alphabetical list of street names, select one, and let the TTT give audio cues that allow the user to touch the map and be guided to that particular street by a series of audio instructions (see Figure 11.20).

Spatial information such as maps of a transit station or campus can now be provided on interactive kiosks. The names of buildings are provided when users touch their location on maps displayed on the kiosk screen. Accessible, interactive kiosks provide information that is especially useful for visually impaired travelers negotiating complicated multimodal transit hubs.

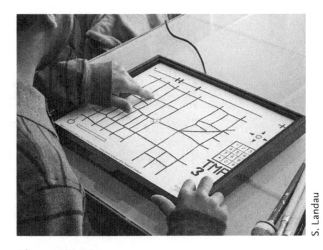

Figure 11.20.
This student is using a Tactile Map Automated Production (TMAP) map on a Talking Tactile Tablet. Touching the street might cause the tablet to speak not only the name of the street, but also the destinations of buses traveling on that street.

Examples at the Staten Island Ferry Terminals and Penn Station in New York City (see Figure 11.21) include touchable three-dimensional maps produced in a translucent material and illuminated from below to make them especially useful for travelers with low vision. As various features are touched, they are described verbally, and also visually highlighted for greater comprehension by a variety of user populations. The kiosks emit a bird chirp sound to help users who are visually impaired locate them.

Another kind of interactive kiosk uses three-dimensional scale models of outdoor environments that can be explored manually; as features are touched, they are described. This approach takes advantage of rapid prototyping technology that allows producers to make low-cost models in very low quantities.

NARRATIVE MAPS

Narrative maps provide verbal wayfinding instructions for following routes and for maintaining

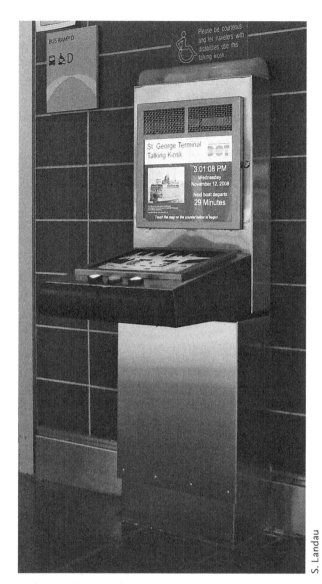

Figure 11.21.
This interactive kiosk provides traveler information in the St. George Terminal of the Staten Island Ferry in New York City.

orientation along those routes. They may be made by O&M specialists to enable clients to travel routes with which they have been familiarized, but which they may not remember well. Even better is teaching students to make narrative maps for themselves, using whatever technology is best for themselves, such as making a digital recording

describing a route as they travel, making hand-written notes, or using a portable braille computer. Travelers who are blind who have become adept at making narrative maps for themselves are well equipped to map routes they travel with a friend, or for which they get directions from other people.

InTouch Graphics provides ClickAndGo Way-finding Maps modeled after the "get directions" features of such digital wayfinding programs as Yahoo Maps, Google Maps, and MapQuest. ClickAndGo Wayfinding Maps provide walking directions for blind and deaf-blind travelers; these maps include landmarks and routes that are especially relevant for travelers with little or no vision. These text-based maps designed for auditory and braille output are also available as MP3 downloads, podcasts, and RSS audio text feeds, and using an interactive voice response service accessed via telephone.

A feature called Find a Point of Interest (POI) allows a user to select a "point of interest" from a drop-down list of choices. In response, a text-based visual description of that POI is provided via speech or braille. The level of detail for each POI can range from basic address and location to a full 360-degree text-based tour of the surrounding area. This is essentially the blind user's equivalent to a pinpoint viewing of POIs with a satellite image, including a street view "pan." The POI details are compiled individually for each property that has included this service in its ClickAndGo map database.

ClickAndGo maps are developed by O&M specialists who have completed training in standard narrative mapping conventions. The map service is marketed to such properties as transit systems, airports, campuses, schools and agencies for the blind, public parks, libraries, museums, hotels, and convention centers. Once an area is mapped, the route information is available at no cost to travelers. Neither the property nor the ClickAndGo map users need to purchase and maintain any specialized equipment.

TEACHING MAP-READING CONCEPTS

Teaching map-reading concepts and skills to visually impaired persons differs little from teaching the same concepts and skills to persons without visual impairment. In the following section are some general suggestions for teaching these concepts and skills: linear continuity and directionality, symbolic representation, size and scale, shape, and advanced concepts. Materials for each concept should be selected or designed according to the visual, haptic, and cognitive abilities of the students. Some specific impairment-related suggestions are made below. Otherwise, it needs to be assumed that these suggestions apply equally to teaching students who are blind to use tactile maps; teaching students with low vision to use specially prepared large-print or tactile and large-print maps; or teaching students with low vision, who read regular print, to use regular-print maps. In all of these suggested activities, the student is asked to draw inferences from a map, travel in the environment to demonstrate the transfer of each concept from a map to the environment, and, finally, become a mapmaker.

Linear Continuity and Directionality

A line conveys linear continuity. To isolate this concept for evaluation or teaching, begin with a map consisting of one straight line. Place the map in front of a student with the line running toward and away from him. Tell the student that the line shows something about where he will be going, and ask the student what he thinks it shows. Many students will be able to generalize that the line means they will go straight ahead, in the direction they are then facing. Another straight line can be connected to the far end of the first line, forming an angle to the left. Students who have good concepts of laterality typically understand that the line means that they

will then turn left and walk straight ahead in the new direction. Walk this route in an open space, keeping the map aligned with the environment at all times. When you are at the end of the route, have the student add a line showing a right turn. Then turn right and walk that segment. Continue the lesson by taking turns drawing and walking routes consisting of straight lines and turns of varying angles (see Figure 11.15).

Transfer this concept to a short *L*-shaped route in a bounded space in intersecting hallways, or along two sides of a rectangular room. Have the student place on the map an appropriate symbol, such as an acute triangle, to indicate his location and heading at the beginning of the route, and then move the symbol along as he travels the route. The sharp point of the triangle may be thought of as representing the student's nose, so the symbol can indicate both location and heading. Take care to keep the map correctly oriented as the student turns the corner. Later this understanding of the directional quality of linear information will be related to other environmental features, such as streets and sidewalks.

Size and Scale

Size at which information is portrayed on the map is related to the relative sizes of objects displayed and to their relative distances from one another. Many students use maps very well without ever learning to convert scale to actual distance, but relative distance is a necessary concept for the understanding of nearly all maps—for example, "I am going from my house, which is a small building, to my school, which is a large building. First I travel a long block, and next, a short block." To relate the concept of scale to mobility in a practical way, the specialist might begin with two lines that point toward and away from students, a short line and a long line. Students may be asked which line is longer, and which line would mean a long walk. Then students might walk different distances in a straight line, and show these distances by making a map. The concept can be extended by straight lines of different lengths, combined with turns in different directions.

Ungar, Blades, and Spencer (1997) observed children who were blind who used a particularly effective strategy for judging distances on a tactile map, and subsequently taught the strategy to others. The strategy involved using the number of fingers that could be placed between symbols to estimate distances in terms of fractional relationships with a known distance (that is, a distance of "two fingers" was half as long as a known distance of "four fingers").

The mathematical concept of scale such as 1 inch = 100 feet (or 1:100) is taught only after the student has some familiarity with estimating actual distances of travel and has the arithmetical skill necessary to relate the numerical value of scale to the actual distance to be traveled. One way that may be used to estimate actual travel distance is for a person to count steps, and multiply by the length of her stride.

Symbolic Representation

Symbols represent real objects. Models are a good way to help students who are blind begin to learn this concept, although simple, high-contrast photographs may work better for children with low vision. (Fully sighted children understand photographs before they understand models [DeLoache, 1991].) Students can progress to drawings of objects and to more abstract symbols through repeated association of the symbol (for example, a red dot for the classroom that has a red door or a square for a square table) with travel to the destination (see Sidebar 11.2).

Most students can begin by choosing, from preselected materials such as those contained in the Chang Tactual Diagram Kit, symbols to represent objects such as tables that are square, round, or rectangular, and then placing these on a map. They should talk about why, for example, a circle is a good symbol for a round table. Stu-

dents should also be taught, in an appropriate context, that a graphic symbol may also occasionally be used to represent other kinds of information, such as a place to observe caution, a fixed sound source, or a point at which to solicit aid.

Shape

Shapes on maps are related in an understandable way to shapes in the environment that is mapped. In teaching this concept, it can be helpful to begin by having young children who are visually impaired match drawings of shapes with corresponding plane shapes. The task is easiest if the drawings and plane shapes are at a scale of 1:1, the shapes fit easily into one hand, and the shapes are presented in the same orientation as the corresponding drawing. Students may then match small drawings with larger plane shapes in different orientations, and next match drawings with objects that have a dominant (top) plane surface in a simple shape, such as jar lids and box tops. Later they can match drawings with larger objects such as tables, which they must walk around in order to understand their shapes.

Now students are ready to make very simple maps of objects on a rectangular table. Lines of different lengths will be used as well as symbols having a shape related to the shape of the object. A Velcro board such as the Chang Tactual Diagram Kit or the Wheatley Tactile Diagramming Kit can be used for this activity.

The next activity could entail mapping a small, simply furnished room. In mapping a room, the following sequence of activities is recommended. The room should first be explored; have students note its shape and the furnishings that will be represented on the map. This exploration needs to be done from a home base along one wall. When finished, students need to sit at home base, facing the opposite wall, and hold a map base (such as a Velcro board or tray) to correspond to the orientation of the room. A symbol should then be placed along the edge of the map closest to the student's body to represent home base. Students need to then make tentative selections, from available materials, of symbols to represent furnishings. If necessary, guidance needs to be given in choosing symbols appropriate in size and shape to what they represent. This is very reinforcing to the learning of the concepts of symbolic representation, size and scale, and shape. Students need to arrange the symbols along the opposite wall on their maps, in positions corresponding to their memories of the relative positions of the furnishings. Accuracy can be confirmed by another trip to explore the opposite wall, paying more attention, if necessary, to relative distances between furnishings. The walls to the right and left can be mapped in the same way. Pointing to actual objects as their symbols are placed on the map helps to further connect map location with actual location.

It can be helpful to have students change perspective before they map the wall against which they were originally seated. They need to sit against the wall that they were previously facing, so that they now face the original home base. The maps need to remain oriented correctly in relation to the room, so that the side of the map that was closest to the student's body is now farthest away. Students need to again point to symbols on the map and the furnishings each represents. They need to notice that they point generally to the left for things that are shown on the left side of the map and that previously they pointed generally to the right to point toward these same objects before they changed position. It is important at this point to help students understand that the map did not turn, nor did the room turn; *they* turned. When students have mapped furnishings along the walls, they may add central furnishings.

Concluding tasks can involve pointing to objects in the room from different vantage points, planning routes on the map, verbalizing routes, and traveling routes from various starting points. Each trip will further confirm the relationship between the location of symbols on the map and landmarks in reality. Even in early stages of mobility, maps can be used for drop-off lessons in a room in which students, who have been disoriented, first find their location on the map, and then travel to a destination. They can be challenged to find the shortest route, a new route, or a "funny" route.

Advanced Concepts

Actual location on earth of things portrayed on a map can be understood by relating their location on the map to compass directions, and by converting distance on the map to actual distance. The student who has fully grasped the concepts involved in the preceding tasks is ready to learn to use compass directions as they are shown on a map. This should be taught in conjunction with actual travel in which compass directions are being learned, and it can complement such lessons.

In using the map during actual travel, it is helpful to keep the map oriented so that the northern edge is always toward the north (Rossano & Warren, 1989). In this way, whatever is farthest from the student on the map corresponds to the environment in front of him. For example, if the student is facing south, the southern edge of the map will be toward the south, that is, on the side furthest away from the student. Objects ahead of the student's location on the map will be ahead of the student in travel space, objects on the left side of the map will be to the student's left, and so on. Having the student frequently touch symbols on the map and then point to the objects they represent will reinforce this concept as well as the ability to relate the items shown on a map to one's actual body position within the area mapped. Having students tell the direction in which they need to travel to reach a landmark shown on a map reinforces the use of compass directions. A tactile or talking compass can provide feedback to students. It is helpful to use a map that has a number of distinctive landmarks. Choose some kind of a moveable symbol with a "nose" to represent a student. Have the student stop frequently to place herself on the map, being careful to point the "nose" in the correct direction. When students no longer need to have a symbol for themselves, have them place a finger on each landmark as they come to it.

Many students experience difficulty in transferring what they observe on a map to travel in the environment. The best way to help students transfer map observations to travel is to have them regularly travel with a map, and often a compass, in hand, repeatedly showing their location on the map and pointing toward other locations as well as compass directions. This activity will quickly reveal to a specialist the gaps in the students' knowledge of spatial concepts and the areas mapped; it is a key activity in teaching and diagnosing difficulties in spatial updating.

Orienteering is an excellent, fun way to promote map use, in combination with other O&M skills and concepts and the use of a compass (Blasch & Brouwer, 1983). Traditionally, orienteering is a timed cross-country race in which the participants use a map and compass to plan the most efficient route between controls (checkpoints) on an unfamiliar course set in a large undeveloped area or any environment appropriate for the skill level of the participants. For O&M, orienteering courses might also be in a building, campus, or city (Langbain, Blasch, & Chalmers, 1981).

TEACHING MAP-READING SKILLS

Identifying Symbols

When teaching students to identify symbols, the specialist needs to begin with maps that have just a few, highly discriminable symbols. Students need to readily be able to identify each symbol used before they are given tasks requiring the combination of symbol identification with other information-gathering techniques. There is some evidence that touch readers perform best on discrimination tasks when only the index fingers are used (Berlá & Butterfield, 1977; Lappin & Foulke, 1973).

Scanning Systematically

Scanning in a systematic pattern to locate graphic symbols is essentially the application of organized search procedures to the map. In teaching this skill, maps with few and highly discriminable symbols should be used. First, the student needs to be shown an isolated sample of a symbol. Then the map needs to be systematically searched for examples of the symbol, using both hands beside each other in a top-to-bottom pattern, and working from left to right (Berlá, 1972, 1973). This systematic scanning of an entire tactile map should give the reader some idea of the size of the map, information density, concentrations of information (if any), and the symbols used. Subsequent tactile or visual scanning for specific symbols may start and go outward from an easily recognized feature on the map. Use of two hands should always be encouraged (Russier, 1999).

Ungar, Blades, and Spencer (1995) demonstrated the importance of having effective strategies for learning spatial layouts portrayed by maps. Children whose learning was most accurate frequently related map features to the frame of the map, and also mentioned relationships between features.

Tracing Line Symbols

Visual or tactile tracing of line symbols may be facilitated by keeping one index finger at a starting point. This will make correction easier if one "gets off the track." The direction of motion of the hand as it explores a tactile line appears to influence the perception of the direction of that line in space (Pick, 1980). Thus, it is important to encourage students to hold maps squarely in front of their bodies, and aligned with the environment, for the most accurate perception of the directions of lines.

There is some evidence that guiding the finger of a tactile reader along lines results in a more accurate mental image of the shape described by that line than free haptic exploration (Kennedy, 1995). The probable reason for this is that haptic line tracing is not a particularly easy task, and is often accompanied by a good deal of offline searching, especially if the shape is complex. Touch seems to be poorly suited for the acquisition of two-dimensional spatial information, even when it is raised. Inexperienced students have difficulty independently examining unfamiliar two-dimensional shapes using exploration that is continuous and fluid enough to result in accurate cognitive maps. Thus the preferred strategy for introducing a map to students may be to first guide a preferred finger along the most important lines and then encourage students to retrace the lines until they can do this smoothly without hesitation. When they have done this, they are ready to talk about what those lines mean.

Recognizing Shapes

The ability to recognize a shape requires the skills of tactilely or visually tracing the outline of a shape, recognizing distinctive features of that shape, and comparing the distinctive features with the remembered features. Both touch readers and persons with reduced visual fields may need practice in combining these skills into shape recognition.

It is of critical importance that such readers have a *system* for shape recognition tasks, as the relationship of distinctive features (hence shape) may appear different if each feature is not perceived, and these features are not perceived in the same order each time the reader looks at the same shape (Gibson, 1966). For example, students may be trained to trace a shape with the index finger of their preferred hand, while using the index finger of their other hand as a reference. Tracing needs to begin and end at the reference finger. Students need to be trained to recognize distinctive features such as "parts that stick out, parts that are pointed, parts that go in, and parts that are curved" (Berlá & Butterfield, 1977). Remember that it is the *outline* of the shape that conveys shape, not any texture that may fill an enclosed shape.

Special Considerations for Map Readers with Low Vision

Whenever a map is to be read by a person with low vision, lighting should be glare-free. Each kind of map-reading task should be tried with and without any optical aid normally used for near work. The specialist should remember that tasks especially requiring acuity, such as the identification of small symbols, may be easier with an optical aid. Tasks facilitated by a full field—for example, gaining a general idea of the utilization of space or relating widely separated areas of the map to each other—may be easier without an optical aid that magnifies, but also reduces the user's visual field.

Well-designed maps are particularly useful when orienting persons with peripheral field loss, as they are less likely to accurately perceive spatial relationships in large-scale environments than persons with acuity loss (Rieser, Hill, Taylor, Bradfield, & Rosen, 1992).

EXPLORATION AND ROUTE PLANNING USING DIGITAL MAPS WITH AN ACCESSIBLE INTERFACE

As of the date of publication, there are three accessible interface systems providing access to

Teaching the Use of Orientation Aids for Orientation and Mobility   345

GIS. The features of these systems will doubtless continue to change rapidly. Some GIS interface products that are accessible to people with visual impairments include BrailleNote GPS (with a refreshable braille keyboard) or VoiceNote (with speech output and a QWERTY keyboard) from Sendero Group, LLC; Trekker from HumanWare; and StreetTalk from Freedom Scientific (see evaluations by Denham, Leventhal, & McComas, 2004; National Federation of the Blind Access Technology Staff, 2006). Each uses different means to access the stored data. Instead of explaining specific commands valid for only one system, we offer examples that are somewhat generic so that the reader can understand the underlying uses of these powerful devices. These three systems all access a GIS database; they differ in how the user interacts with the system (see Figures 11.22, 11.23, and 11.24). Additional information about GPS devices may be found in Chapter 14.

In addition to these three self-contained units, Wayfinder Access, powered by Nuance TALKS,

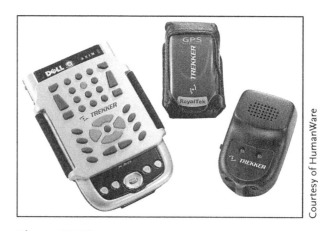

Figure 11.23.
Close-up of the Trekker system.

Courtesy of HumanWare

offers a cell phone interface that communicates to a user's GPS receiver to provide navigation information. Unlike the other systems, it also offers visual information in addition to voice output.

In Volume 1, Chapter 10, the authors told the story of Bob, a blind traveler going to a new city for the first time. He was able to use his digital map to query the system for locations and directions to various places, including searching for a hotel near the convention center, and for various attractions. Bob was able to find specific types of restaurants, and other places of interest that were nearby. He was able to ask for route directions to and from any two locations. These queries could be used without using a GPS signal, so Bob could pre-plan routes and destinations from any location. Depending on the system, he might use a braille or typical (QWERTY) computer keyboard, and the requested information might be delivered through synthetic speech, or from a refreshable braille display. For example, Bob might input "Chicago, IL" into the device and then search for or "find" the convention center. He could search by street intersection, by address, or in a point of interest (POI) file. He could then do another "find," this time searching for names of hotels. He could input a minimum and maximum

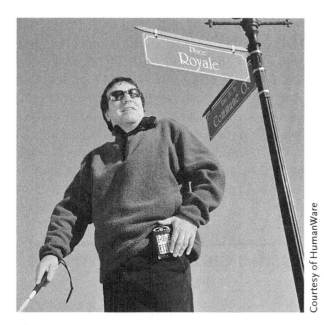

Figure 11.22.
The Trekker system used during travel.

Courtesy of HumanWare

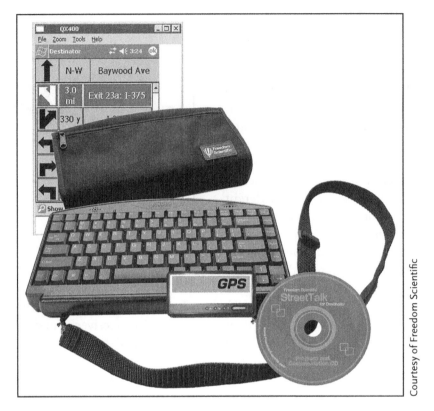

Figure 11.24.
The user interface for StreetTalk-accessible GPS system.

distance from the convention center, or just receive the hotel names in order of their proximity to the convention center. When Bob found one he was interested in, he could further query it, and get the address and phone number. He could set the convention center and the hotel as the origin and destination of his trip, and be able to get step-by-step route descriptions in either direction. He could also explore the virtual city in a "look-around" mode, listening to various attractions and landmarks as he mentally traveled the route he chose. The database has millions of places identified and sorted by categories, so Bob could look for specific types of places. Bob could choose to look for a nearby ATM machine, a dentist, a police station, a library, or anything else in that area. Once he

had located and stored all the points of interest and routes, he would be ready to make the physical trip; using this "virtual" mode could allow him to safely and easily "explore" the new city before leaving home, assured that he has a good idea of the layout and routes he will face. He could "practice" routes between various POIs, or explore the surrounding area to learn the spatial arrangements of this part of town.

USING GIS COUPLED WITH GPS FOR TRAVEL

The great advantage of coupling GPS with a GIS when compared to a print map is that when a print map is used to plan travel, the user needs to first determine where he is on the map. In an unfamiliar area, this means looking for nearby locations, landmarks, or streets that may be difficult to find on the map, especially if the user is confused and not looking in the right area on the map. The GPS component of a navigation system *always* knows where the user is; the user only needs to enter the standard command, and he instantly gets the information identifying the street, the block number, and the names of nearby intersecting streets. See Figures 11.22, 11.23, and 11.24 for illustrations of accessible GPS.

"Where Am I?" Plus Highway and Pedestrian Route Guidance Modes

When the digital map is used with the GPS signal, much more can be done to make travel easier and more independent for the user. In Volume 1, Chapter 10, Bob used the GPS to plan a trip to a conference in Chicago and to plan and guide his travel while there. Anytime Bob needed to know where he was, he just entered a command and the system located his position through the GPS signal, and told him what street he was on, and the name of the nearest intersection. When he arrived at the airport, he input the hotel name and put the device in "highway mode," and tracked the cab driver and the route to the hotel. In highway mode, limited-access highways with no pedestrian facilities are included, but one-way streets are not included if the car is going in the other direction. For walking, Bob uses a "pedestrian" mode, where he couldn't be routed along a limited access road, but could be routed to walk the wrong way on a one-way street. When he left the hotel, he could input the restaurant that he wanted to visit, or, if he had saved that as one of his POIs he could find the restaurant in the file; then the device would tell him, using either

speech or refreshable braille, a route to the restaurant.

Look-Around Mode

While Bob traveled, he could also go to "look-around" mode and find out what was in the vicinity. By changing the size of the "bubble" that surrounded him, he could hear about locations as far away or as close as he desired. He could learn what kinds of locations and businesses were nearby, and learn about ATMs, restaurants, medical services, or whatever was in his database. Note that the number of locations in different GIS is different, but by using "Where am I?" and then using "look-around" to find the closest POI, Bob could find the address nearest to where he was very handy thing to know when calling for a cab or waiting to be picked up by a friend.

Leaving "Breadcrumbs" and Other Personal Information

In addition to being able to find millions of locations and POIs, and to find routes to destinations, Bob can also personalize his database. If he would like to remember where he has traveled for future reference, he can press another command to tell the device to leave data points (referred to as *breadcrumbs*) whenever he wants to mark a route or special POI. He can name these personal POIs in any way he likes. While doing his free exploration after finding the convention center, he could mark the sculpture gallery he found, so he could bring a friend there the next day. He might also find a park that does not have any GIS database information, and wander around and find some interesting spots he would like to revisit. He could leave "breadcrumbs" to record his path through the park and mark those places of interest with his personal POI names. Additional information can be found in Volume 1, Chapter 14.

Sharing Files

Bob could use his personal navigation device to go back and forth from the hotel to the conference, find interesting places for lunch, and locate some excellent ethnic places for dinner. He would be able to take new friends to places he had visited and could enjoy being able to show sighted people how to get around.

After the convention, Bob might plan to visit a new friend in a nearby town. Perhaps his friend's child is sick and the friend cannot leave his home to meet Bob at the train station. It might be a very complicated route from the train station to the friend's home, including walking through a very large park, with many winding trails. However Bob's friend, who is also blind, has probably walked that route many times. He may have recorded it, and can simply e-mail that route file to Bob as an attachment. Bob can then take the train, listening to geographic information along the way; get off in the right town; and simply follow the route his friend has already recorded. Bob may notice that his friend also has a favorite restaurant listed along the route, and stop to pick up a surprise take-out meal for his host's family.

Learning to Use a GPS

O&M teachers and GPS users need to be aware that these are very powerful systems unlike anything else they might have learned. In stand-alone devices, the user needs to usually learn many commands and finger positions. Other GPS devices are attached to existing accessible personal digital assistants (PDAs). Users of different kinds of accessible PDAs might already know how to input queries or information and maneuver through that interface. It is understandable that in order to access the many features, it will take time for students to learn to use the system efficiently. Beginning users in most cases can easily find out how to locate their position, "look around," and input destinations to have a route produced. More advanced features will require more practice. Computer savvy and expertise are valuable whenever learning new electronic devices, but using an accessible PDA is not like using a regular PC. For example, BrailleNote GPS uses Windows CE, so prior knowledge of other Windows products is not an asset. It is important for teachers to have a basic understanding of braille, and it is very helpful for them to be able to understand rapid synthetic speech, although the rate of speech is likely to be adjustable.

GOALS IN ACCESSIBLE WAYFINDING TECHNOLOGY DEVELOPMENT

As development of accessible wayfinding technologies continues, we are likely to see increases in the amount of information stored in digital maps. This information will then be readily available to mapmakers as well as to blind travelers who use GPS. Simpler user interfaces will be available so a wide variety of people will be able to use their features, including people who have limited knowledge of or experience with electronic technology, people who are unable to remember or follow multistep procedures, and people whose manual dexterity is compromised. Miniaturization is likely to continue. Finally, a variety of accessible wayfinding technologies will be integrated into a common device such as a cell phone.

SUMMARY

Many travel concepts and skills can best be taught using orientation devices; therefore, each O&M specialist should be thoroughly familiar with orientation devices, design principles, materials available for production, and techniques for aid use. O&M specialists should have materials appropriate for their students readily available for use on many lessons.

O&M specialists need to also be involved in the design of special-purpose orientation devices for schools, agencies, metropolitan areas, or transit systems that wish to provide mobility maps, including narrative maps, to visually impaired persons who use their facilities. An informed O&M specialist is the professional most capable of judging which information is most appropriate to promote independent travel in any situation, along with its purpose and the way it is displayed. Any O&M specialist participating in the design of such a device should be certain that it will be made available in ways that facilitate its optimum use and the best understanding.

O&M specialists need to be alert to the development of new technologies that may speed up familiarization with new areas, or enable travelers who are blind to obtain real-time information about their locations and routes to destinations. They need to be prepared to suggest new wayfinding technologies to their students, provide information about obtaining wayfinding technologies, and help students learn to use new technologies to maximum advantage.

IMPLICATIONS FOR O&M PRACTICE

1. Whether or not a student or client benefits from a tactile map depends on the skill of the designer as well as the skill of the teacher.

2. Rules of thumb for making design decisions:

   a. Information content: Include only essential information; err on the side of providing too little information.

   b. Size: When possible, keep map size less than the span of two hands touching.

   c. Scale: Keep scale as small as possible to show the necessary information.

   d. Schematization: Schematized maps are often easier to read than more literal maps for people who are blind or who have low vision, and they may also lead to easier formation of cognitive maps.

   e. Symbols: Choose all tactile symbols on the basis of what they feel like, not what they look like.

   f. Information density: Minimize information density as much as possible, especially for map users who have reduced tactile sensitivity or haptic perceptual ability.

   g. Labels: Keep labels to a minimum; where they are needed, use two braille-cell mnemonic abbreviations.

3. Maps made from craft and household materials may be superior for use with individual clients to maps made using standard materials.

4. Tactile or large-print maps made by students or clients from materials that are easy for them to use can tell the O&M specialist much about the spatial understanding of these students or clients.

5. Tactile or large-print maps that provide verbal information are preferable to ones that provide only tactile or visual information.

6. Geographic information systems can be used by O&M specialists to make single-copy maps by hand; they can also be used with special software, to automatically produce tactile maps having the area, at the scale, and including the features desired by the user.

7. Concepts that are necessary for students to make maximal use of maps include linear continuity and directionality, symbolic representation, scale, and shape. Having students

or clients make maps helps them master these concepts.

8. Skills necessary for students or clients to make maximal use of maps include scanning systematically, identifying symbols, tracing line symbols, and recognizing shapes.

9. Geographic information systems with accessible user interfaces can be used for complex route planning and for exploration of unfamiliar areas.

10. Geographic information systems coupled with accessible global positioning system technology can provide continuous verbal guidance toward a destination, revising the guidance if the traveler misses a landmark or turn.

LEARNING ACTIVITIES

1. Practice designing tactile and large-print maps for different students or clients and different purposes by answering the following questions for each of the scenarios below.

Questions

a. What information will be shown on the map, and where will you get the information?

b. How large will the map be?

c. What scale will the map have?

d. To what extent will inconsistency in scale be needed and acceptable?

e. What symbols will you use, and how will you create them?

f. Will the map require labels? If so, how will you provide them?

g. What materials or techniques will you use to make the map?

Scenarios

i. You have been asked to design a map of a college campus for use by students with vision impairments.

ii. You are teaching a 4-year-old student to travel independently between the door of her school and her own classroom. You want a map that both of you can use to show your understanding of spatial relationships.

iii. You are teaching a student to make crossings at a complex intersection, and the student is having difficulty understanding the patterns of vehicular movement.

iv. Your student, who has a very constricted visual field, needs to remember the routes to many specific destinations in her city.

2. You find that you often have trouble helping your adult, adventitiously blinded students understand complex spatial relationships such as complex intersections or transit stations, and you want to be prepared to create tactile, large-print, or tactile and large-print maps on the spur of the moment when you are in a perplexing environment.

3. Describe the mapmaking materials and techniques you would like to have available to use in the following jobs. Briefly tell how you would use each material or technique in each job.

- Orientation and mobility specialist in an early intervention program
- Itinerant O&M specialist serving K through 12
- Orientation and mobility specialist in an agency-based program serving primarily elderly students

- Orientation and mobility specialist orienting college students to new campuses

4. How do decisions regarding the following aspects of tactile map design influence one another?

- Information content
- Size
- Scale
- Symbols

- Information density
- Labels

5. Why is it important to teach young children who are visually impaired to be mapmakers?

6. If you had a student who was a well-oriented and active traveler, how would you prepare her to learn about new areas and travel unfamiliar routes?

CHAPTER 12

Teaching Travel at Complex Intersections

Janet M. Barlow,
Billie Louise Bentzen,
Dona Sauerburger,
and Lukas Franck

LEARNING QUESTIONS

- What are some of the changes in intersection design that affect the techniques and skills we teach for street crossing?

- What problems do curb ramps introduce for pedestrians who are visually impaired, and what are some techniques and strategies that can be taught to ameliorate these problems?

- What are some techniques and strategies for alignment for street crossings?

- Why is it unwise to assume that because no vehicle can be heard approaching, the pedestrian has sufficient time to cross the street safely?

- How can you teach your students to judge whether a location is a place where they can hear well enough to cross?

- What are some of the various signal phasing plans, and how do they affect pedestrian crossings? What are some of variations on pedestrian signal operation that affect pedestrians who are blind or visually impaired?

- What effect do pedestrian pushbuttons have on intersection timing?

- What are the advantages and disadvantages of clockwise and counterclockwise crossings?

- What cue should pedestrians who are blind use to determine the appropriate crossing time at signalized intersections?

- Describe the approach to an intersection and appropriate use of accessible pedestrian signals by a pedestrian who is blind or visually impaired.

This chapter discusses street crossings, and how intersections and traffic controls vary and affect the ability of blind or visually impaired people to cross safely. It will present research that documents the problems that these changes in infrastructure have generated for people who are blind or visually impaired. It will then explain how street infrastructure is designed, including both the complexities of intersection geometries and traffic control, and the intended interactions between pedestrians and vehicles. Strategies, skills, and concepts that may enable people who are blind or visually impaired to navigate our streets and intersections safely and efficiently, as well as suggestions for teaching them and discussion of the issues of risk taking, alternatives to crossing, and decision making, will all be integrated into the chapter.

In the 1940s, when the profession of orientation and mobility (O&M) was founded, intersections and traffic controls were simple and predictable and the information needed to cross streets safely without vision existed readily in the environment. The founders of O&M developed and codified street-crossing concepts and techniques that exploited the infrastructure created by the civil engineers of that era, so people who were blind or visually impaired were able to evaluate intersections and cross independently. Traditional strategies for street crossing included using a curb to recognize the end of the sidewalk and the edge of the street, using traffic sounds or the edge of the sidewalk or curb to align to cross, and using the surge of traffic on the parallel street to determine when to cross at signalized intersections, and using quiet as a cue to assure a sufficient gap to cross streets with no traffic control (Allen, Courtney-Barbier, Griffith, Kern, & Shaw, 1997; Jacobson, 1993; LaGrow & Weessies, 1994; Pogrund et al., 1993). However, for reasons that are discussed in this chapter, these strategies can no longer be used reliably, either because they depend on features or sounds that do not always exist (such as a curb, or traffic sounds) or because they can mislead the traveler who is not aware of the traffic patterns and features of modern intersections. The world has changed tremendously—in ways that drastically affect street crossings of people who are blind or visually impaired.

CHANGES IN INFRASTRUCTURE

Although the skills, concepts and techniques that the founders of the O&M developed after World War II continue to be the foundation of independent travel, they are insufficient on their own at some intersections. Modern traffic engineers (a specialty which began to develop at precisely the same time as O&M) have been modifying intersection designs and increasingly incorporating computer technology to cope with the increase in the driving population, the move of large segments of the population to the suburbs, and the changing demands on the roadways that have resulted.

Many of these changes wrought by traffic engineers are highly visible. Travelers of 50 or 60 years ago would not recognize some of the intersection designs of today. For example, arterial highways, often seven or eight lanes wide, cut through residential communities and intersect streets that have little or no traffic most of the day. Corners are rounded so squaring off with a curb can lead a pedestrian who is blind or visually impaired to cross diagonally into the intersection, and traffic in some cases barely needs to slow down to make a turn. Islands separate right turning lanes so drivers can bypass the traffic signal and turn into the intersecting street, sometimes in an acceleration lane that makes it unnecessary to yield to perpendicular traffic. Curbs have been replaced by curb ramps that round the corner and blend into the street. Roundabouts exist as intersections with no traffic control and no corners (see the section on Intersection Geometry).

Other changes are subtle and could be detected by visitors from the past only after careful observation. For example, laws in the United States and parts of Canada now allow drivers to turn right when facing a red signal, after stopping briefly. Actuated signals make the timing and pattern of traffic movement unpredictable, even to the engineers who designed them, and require that pedestrians push a button in order to get enough time to walk across the street. Regulations and environmental policies make cars generate less than half the sound they did before 1972 (Wiener, 1997). There is an increasing presence of hybrid and electric vehicles that are not audible while waiting at traffic signals and whose surge may be difficult to hear. The mindset of traffic engineers and designers as well as drivers reflects a change from the culture of the 1940s, when cities and towns were designed around pedestrians and transit systems, to an autocentric culture that minimally accommodates pedestrians and discourages the use of public transportation.

For people who are blind or visually impaired, these changes, both obvious and subtle, render many traditional street-crossing strategies unreliable or useless in some situations, and dangerous and potentially fatal in others. Experienced blind travelers have reported having their confidence shaken because of traffic patterns that they had not been taught to recognize and deal with (Terlau, 1997). Research documented that pedestrians who are blind are often not completing their crossings before the perpendicular traffic gets a green signal, even when they started to cross with a "fresh green" signal (Bentzen, Barlow, & Bond, 2004a).

Changes in the design of streets and intersections require changes in some of our teaching strategies, and require that O&M specialists and the people they teach clearly understand how the street infrastructure is designed, know about strategies for negotiating these intersections and, just as importantly, understand when these strategies can or cannot be reliably used. The Association for Education and Rehabilitation of the Blind and Visually Impaired, Orientation and Mobility Division (AER O&M Division) has adopted position papers which specify information and changes in strategies required for crossing at traffic signals and at crossings where there is no traffic control (AER O&M Division, 2006, 2008). The new strategies and information that should be taught to O&M students are covered in this chapter, including the ability to recognize situations where these concepts,

skills, and strategies for dealing with modern street crossings are not sufficient, where the available information is inadequate to enable pedestrians who are blind or visually impaired to determine some of the intersection features or to determine the appropriate time to cross safely. Students should be prepared with alternatives for crossing as well as information about environmental modifications that can help provide information (see Volume 1, Chapter 11, on environmental accessibility).

The authors' choices of terminology in this chapter generally reflect the U.S transportation industry standard terminology, as used in the *Manual on Uniform Traffic Control Devices* (FHWA, 2009), *A Policy on Geometric Design of Highways and Streets* (AASHTO, 2004a), *The Traffic Control Devices Handbook* (Pline, 2001), *Roundabouts: An Informational Guide* (FHWA, 2000), *Signalized Intersections Informational Guide* (FHWA, 2004) and *The Guide for the Planning, Design, and Operation of Pedestrian Facilities* (AASHTO, 2004b). Throughout the chapter, where transportation engineers and orientation and mobility specialists use different terms, terminology differences are clarified where authors are aware of them. There are regional differences and international differences in some of the terms used to describe intersections, signalization, sidewalks, curb ramps, and crosswalks. Some engineers and transportation professionals can be very precise in discussing traffic signals and signal phases, intervals, and cycles, or curb ramp design features and O&M specialists using the wrong term may find that they have been completely misunderstood.

STREET-CROSSING TASKS

Street crossing involves the following tasks:

- Detect the street.
- Locate the crosswalk and crossing location.

- Determine traffic control.
- Locate and use pushbuttons (at signalized intersections with pedestrian pushbuttons).
- Align to cross.
- Determine time to begin crossing.
- Initiate crossing.
- Maintain alignment while crossing.

In general, the tasks of detecting the street, locating the crossing location, aligning to cross, and maintaining alignment while crossing are affected by intersection geometry. Tasks of using pedestrian pushbuttons and determining when to begin crossing are affected by traffic control. There is some overlap.

Throughout each of these tasks is embedded the need for the traveler to analyze the intersection using all clues available to determine traffic patterns, geometry, and other information needed to travel safely in that environment. Although students will be performing all tasks in conjunction with street crossings, for purpose of discussion here, tasks are discussed separately. Instructors may find it useful to focus on some aspects of the crossing on some lessons and others on different lessons. In some cases, being guided in some portion of the crossing may allow the student to focus on certain aspects of the crossing. In the end, for proficiency, instructor and students need to put all tasks together. None of these tasks are taught completely in isolation, but they may be sequenced differently in different situations and teaching areas, and with different students.

RESEARCH EVIDENCE OF THE PROBLEM

Research has verified some of the problems that present themselves when traditional street-crossing techniques are used in today's world. Guth, Reiser, and Ashmead (in Chapter 1, Volume 1) note that the perceptual demands of street crossing have increased and discuss how this has affected several of the street-crossing prerequisite tasks: detecting the street, aligning the body toward the street-crossing destination, initiating the crossing, and walking a straight path across the street. In 1998, the American Council of the Blind (ACB) and the Association for Education and Rehabilitation of the Blind and Visually Impaired (AER) conducted parallel surveys to determine problems experienced by pedestrians with visual impairments while crossing streets. The ACB surveyed pedestrians with visual impairments (Carroll & Bentzen, 2000), and AER surveyed orientation and mobility specialists (Bentzen, Barlow, & Franck, 2000). Respondents to both surveys reported difficulty with several tasks when crossing at signals: knowing when to begin crossing; determining whether there was a pushbutton to activate a pedestrian signal; and finding and using the pushbutton. Of the 163 respondents in the ACB survey, 13 reported that they had been hit by a vehicle and 47 reported that their canes had been run over. Although the survey questions mainly focused on signal issues, 97 percent of the AER respondents indicated that their students sometimes had difficulty aligning to cross the street. Sixty-six percent (229 of 347) of respondents indicated that their students sometimes had difficulty knowing where the destination curb was and 64 percent (223 of 347) of respondents indicated that their students were sometimes confused by unexpected features such as medians or islands.

Traffic Signals

For crossing at traffic signals, a number of research projects have studied blind or visually impaired travelers crossing with and without accessible pedestrian signals (APS). The results of the installation and use of APS are discussed in Volume 1, Chapter 11, on environmental accessibility, but the data collected without APS provide valuable information about the safety, orientation, and independence of pedestrians who are blind or visually impaired when using traditional strategies to cross modern signalized intersections.

In one study, field testing was conducted at six complex, signalized intersections (two each in Portland, OR; Charlotte, NC; and Cambridge, MA) with and without APS. In each city, data were collected with 16 pedestrians who are accustomed to crossing streets independently. The results formed the first large data set (over 400 crossings by 48 unique individuals) available to researchers on measures of safety, orientation, and independence of pedestrians who are blind when crossing at unfamiliar, complex, signalized intersections without APS (Barlow, Bentzen, & Bond, 2005; Bentzen et al., 2004a). Among these findings were that participants (1) started crossing during the walk interval less than 50 percent of the time, (2) were still in the street after the perpendicular traffic had a green signal 27 percent of the time, (3) started from outside the crosswalk 28 percent of the time and were misaligned 27 percent of the time, and (4) traveled or ended outside the crosswalk 42 percent of the time (Bentzen et al., 2004a).

Other research has looked at crossings at signalized intersections. Marston and Golledge (2000) compared crossings by blind or visually impaired participants with and without APS. Without APS, almost half (48 percent) of the participants attempted to cross during the steady Don't Walk interval, a time recorded as unsafe by the researcher. In similar research, 20 experienced pedestrians who were blind crossed at four intersections (80 crossings) in downtown San Francisco, both without and with APS. Intersection signal phases were pre-timed (the same every cycle) and pushbutton use was not required. At crossings without APS, participants requested assistance to determine the onset of the walk interval on 24 percent of crossings, and

for crossings on which they independently initiated the crossing, participants began crossing during Walk on only 66 percent of crossings (Crandall, Bentzen, & Myers, 1998). Williams, Van Houten, Ferraro, and Blasch (2005) assessed participants on the total number of signal cycles missed before crossing. Without APS, mean wait time was almost two full cycles (1.91), while with either of two types of APS, the mean wait time was just over a half a cycle (0.51).

Latency to begin crossing, the time between onset of the Walk signal, or near-lane parallel traffic green, and the participant beginning to cross, can be an important factor in crossing safely at traffic signals. Typical latency for sighted pedestrians is assumed to be less than two seconds (Stollof, McGee, & Eccles, 2007). Mean latency to begin crossing for pedestrians who are blind, combining data from Portland, OR; Charlotte, NC; and Cambridge, MA, was 6.41 seconds (Barlow et al., 2005). Williams et al. (2005) found latency of more than 5 seconds.

Judging Traffic Gaps

Research has also studied and documented problems for people who are blind or visually impaired when crossing where there is no traffic signal or stop sign, such as at roundabouts, channelized turn lanes (that is, those separated from the main traffic flow by an island), or at streets and intersections with two-way stop control when crossing the street that has no stop sign. In these situations, pedestrians are expected to cross during a gap in traffic or when drivers have yielded.

Several research projects studied the ability of blind travelers to determine when there is a gap in traffic at roundabout crossings. Adults who were totally blind and adults who were sighted made judgments at three roundabouts about whether gaps in vehicular traffic were "crossable," that is, long enough to permit crossing to the splitter island before the arrival of the next vehicle (Ashmead, Guth, Wall, Long, & Ponchillia, 2005; Guth, Ashmead, Long, Wall, & Ponchillia, 2005). Trials were conducted at both exit-lane and entry-lane crosswalks. Overall, blind participants were about 2.5 times less likely to make correct judgments than sighted participants, took significantly longer to detect crossable gaps, and were more likely to miss crossable gaps altogether. The errors of blind participants were much more likely to be "high risk" than the errors of sighted participants at the two roundabouts that carried moderate and high volumes of traffic. In a follow-up study, the same procedures were used at roundabouts where there were large and predictable variations in traffic volume over the course of the day (Long, Guth, Ashmead, Wall, & Ponchillia, 2005). Relative to the sighted participants, blind participants made more "high-risk" judgments during rush hours than during off-peak hours.

These studies involved participants making judgments about crossing without actually crossing, possibly using different judgment criteria than would have been the case had they actually crossed. To address this possibility, as well as to follow up several differences found in the earlier studies, research was conducted at a high-volume, two-lane roundabout (Ashmead et al., 2005). Participants who were blind and participants who were sighted made judgments without actually crossing on half of their trials and crossed on the other half. Those findings demonstrated the validity of the judgment-only measure, and confirmed the serious safety problems associated with unassisted crossings at that roundabout, with nearly one in six crossings by a blind pedestrian requiring the intervention of an O&M specialist to avoid an unsafe situation. Interventions occurred on only a small percentage of trials; however, a 99 percent probability of a serious pedestrian-vehicle conflict at this intersection was calculated if a person who was blind crossed it daily for three months. (A *conflict* is a

situation in which a crash is likely unless the driver or pedestrian takes immediate evasive action.) Most participants who were blind told researchers that they would not cross at the intersection if they had any other option.

At a study of pedestrians crossing at channelized right turn lanes, it was found that crossings were significantly more difficult for pedestrians who were blind than for sighted pedestrians. Pedestrians who were blind faced a greater risk and a greater amount of delay (Schroeder, Rouphail, & Wall-Emerson, 2006). Another study conducted at three streets where the crossing had no traffic control found that in some situations, people who are blind and have normal hearing cannot hear all the vehicles well enough to know there is a gap long enough to cross, even when it is quiet (Wall-Emerson & Sauerburger, 2008).

If it is not feasible to determine when there is a gap in traffic, one might consider crossing when drivers in all approaching lanes have yielded or are expected to yield. However Guth et al. (2005) observed that blind pedestrians often fail to realize when drivers yield to them at roundabout crossings. This appears to result from the sounds of nearby yielding vehicles being masked by the sounds of other vehicles traveling in or near the roundabout and by vehicles yielding several car lengths away from the crosswalk. In another study at a two-lane roundabout crossing (Inman, Davis, & Sauerburger, 2005), five participants who were blind detected only one out of every five two-lane yields, and were incorrect 14 percent of the times that they thought drivers had yielded in both lanes (there was not a yielding driver in both lanes). Drivers who yielded stopped an average of 7 feet (2 m) away from the crosswalk. In an informal survey of 15 blind or visually impaired travelers (Sauerburger, 2003), only three travelers were confident that they could always detect the yielding cars (at least two of these three had functional vision).

Curbs and Curb Ramps

Another change that has affected the crossing of blind or visually impaired pedestrians is the removal of curbs and their replacement with curb ramps or blended transitions to the street. This has negatively affected the street detection and alignment techniques and strategies used by pedestrians who are blind or visually impaired. As described in Volume 1, Chapter 11, two research projects (Bentzen & Barlow, 1995; Hauger, Rigby, Safewright, & McAuley, 1996) confirmed that the removal of the curb resulted in the inability of even skilled, frequent travelers who were blind to detect some streets. Bentzen and Barlow (1995) found that on 35 percent of approaches to unfamiliar streets where curb ramps were encountered, blind travelers who used a long cane failed to detect the presence of an intersecting street before stepping into it; this was true even when there was traffic on the intersecting street. Some of the curb ramps used in the study had steeper slopes than allowed by the Americans with Disability Act Accessibility Guidelines (ADAAG) (U.S. Department of Justice, 1991). On curb ramps with slopes of 1:12 or less, as required by ADAAG, travelers who were blind stepped into the street on 48 percent of approaches.

Alignment Issues

With the increasingly complicated geometry of modern intersections, the tasks of finding the crosswalk, aligning to cross (establishing a heading toward the opposite side of the street), and maintaining crossing direction while crossing have also become increasingly difficult (Barlow, 2004; Bentzen et al., 2000, 2004a; Guth & LaDuke, 1994, 1995). Finding the crosswalk can be difficult when the crosswalk does not begin from a corner, such as at the channelized right turn lanes of signalized intersections, at roundabouts, and at mid-block crosswalks. Figure 12.1

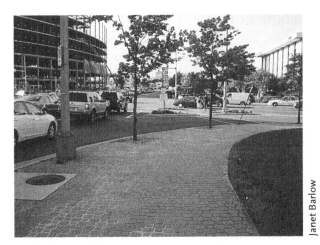

Janet Barlow

Figure 12.1.
The crosswalk location at this channelized right turn lane is not obvious to pedestrians who are blind or visually impaired.

shows a signalized intersection with a channelized right turn lane. Because the crosswalk is located off to the left of the traveler's path as the sidewalk gently curves around the corner, it is difficult for blind or visually impaired pedestrians to locate.

Traditionally, the principal alignment cue has been sounds of traffic moving parallel or perpendicular to the crosswalk (Chew, 1986; Guth, Hill, & Rieser, 1989; LaGrow & Weessies, 1994; Willoughby & Monthei, 1998). This pattern of traffic movement almost never exists at roundabouts and channelized right turn lanes, and may not exist at some signalized intersections. Similarly, the traditional cue for maintaining one's intended heading while crossing has been the sounds of parallel traffic, which also may not be present because of intersection geometry, intermittent traffic and/or inaudible vehicles. At the intersection in Figure 12.1, blind or visually impaired pedestrians may have difficulty aligning to cross after locating the crosswalk because there is no traffic moving parallel to the crosswalk. The orientation task is further complicated because after arrival at the island, the pedestrian needs to identify the direction to walk in order to find the second crosswalk and then needs to re-align to cross the signalized portion of the intersection. Subjective data from the ACB and AER surveys of street-crossing problems both confirmed that pedestrians who were blind or visually impaired had problems aligning to cross streets (Bentzen et al., 2000; Carroll & Bentzen, 2000). Objective data in San Francisco demonstrated that, in the absence of accessible signals, participants who were blind were misaligned on 52 percent of trials (Crandall et al., 1998).

All these studies indicate that pedestrians who are blind or visually impaired are having difficulty at signalized and unsignalized intersections, including roundabouts, with tasks of detecting the street, locating the crosswalk, aligning to cross and maintaining alignment while crossing, as well as determining the appropriate time to cross. At all kinds of locations, it is necessary for blind or visually impaired pedestrians to be able to adequately assess the risk of crossing, identify options and alternatives and make decisions about where and when to cross. The O&M specialist of today should be prepared with information and strategies to enable people who are blind or visually impaired to deal with modern intersections. The rest of this chapter will address these issues.

Intersections Today

Before teaching street crossings, O&M specialists need to understand the environment and functioning of intersections. Two aspects of an intersection, geometry and traffic control must be thoroughly evaluated before the functioning of an intersection can be understood and an appropriate judgment about a street crossing can be made. Each person, before crossing a street, needs to determine the geometry of the intersection and the type of traffic control provided at

the intersection (see Figure 12.2). Sighted pedestrians make these determinations and evaluations quickly at new intersections, usually without thinking much about them. Pedestrian signals are often provided where crossing timing is difficult for sighted pedestrians to determine based on the vehicular traffic signal. Some aspects of intersections are hard to determine nonvisually, and this is much more complex than it used to be.

INTERSECTION GEOMETRY

O&M specialists may not know that intersections have geometry but they do. This is an example of traffic engineering jargon. It can be important to learn to speak this language to communicate effectively with traffic engineers. Understanding the language of traffic engineers is as important to the field of O&M as understanding the language of ophthalmologists and the optometrists.

Intersection geometry generally refers to the shape of the intersection, as well as slopes and curves or angles of the sidewalk and roadway surface. The intersection shape or geometric dimensions include the angle of the intersection of the streets; the width and placement of sidewalks; the width and number of travel lanes, islands, and medians; the shape of islands and medians; the turning radii of each corner; the curb ramp location and slope; and other intersection details and dimensions. These features can affect location of pedestrian crossings or crosswalks, width of the crossing, whether traffic is traveling parallel to the crosswalk, whether traffic provides a good cue to alignment and travel directions across the street, the speed of traffic crossing the crosswalk, and other aspects important to crossing. In general, geometry affects the street-crossing tasks of detecting the street, locating the crosswalk, aligning to cross, and maintaining alignment while crossing.

The intersection geometry of unsignalized and signalized intersections can be quite similar.

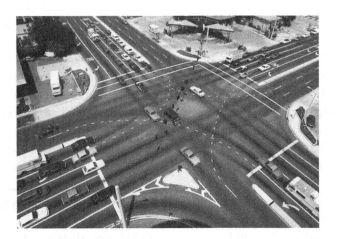

Figure 12.2.

Intersections today may be quite large, with complex lane configuration and geometry. Only two pedestrian crosswalks are provided at this intersection.

Source: Federal Highway Administration, *Signalized Intersections: Informational Guide* (Washington, DC: U.S. Department of Transportation, August 2004), Figure 11. http://www.tfhrc.gov/safety/pubs/04091/04091.pdf.

Traditionally in the United States, intersections with high volumes of traffic are signalized.

Intersection Categories

Each roadway radiating from an intersection is called a *leg*. There are three basic categories of at-grade intersections (intersections where the two streets meet at the same grade, without overpasses or underpasses), determined by the number of intersecting legs. They are the T intersection (three approach legs), four-leg intersection, and multileg intersection (five or more approach legs). Most intersections have four legs, which is generally accepted as the maximum recommended number; however, there are many existing intersections with more than four legs.

Intersection Shapes

Square or Right-Angle Intersections

In addition, the intersection can be considered *square*, or *right angle*, where each street intersects at approximately a 90-degree angle. Orientation and mobility specialists often refer to these as *plus* intersections; however, traffic engineers do not typically use that term and may not understand it without explanation. Traffic engineers will usually call a *plus* intersection a four-leg right-angle intersection, or a right-angle intersection with four legs.

Skewed Intersections

At skewed intersections, streets, or legs, intersect at an angle less than 75 degrees and may be described by traffic engineers in terms of the degree of skew (for example, Portland crosses Grand at 60 degrees; see Figure 12.3).

In general, at skewed intersections, blind or visually impaired pedestrians can use parallel traffic for alignment information, but cannot use a curb, or traffic traveling on the street they are crossing because the vehicles are not traveling perpendicular to their path. Some crossings at the intersection may be more difficult, because the wider angle on some corners will usually allow cars to turn faster. The location of

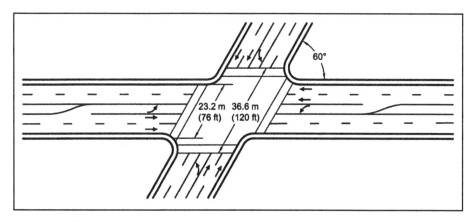

Figure 12.3. A Skewed Intersection Showing Crosswalks Parallel to Traffic Movement

Source: Federal Highway Administration, *Signalized Intersections: Informational Guide* (Washington, DC: U.S. Department of Transportation, August 2004), Figure 15c. http://www.tfhrc.gov/safety/pubs/04091/04091.pdf.

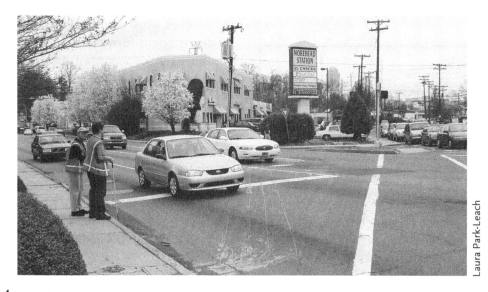

Figure 12.4.

At skewed intersections the location at which vehicles stop can provide misleading cues to visually impaired pedestrians.

perpendicular cars, which is sometimes used by pedestrians who are blind or visually impaired in judging their crossing location and alignment, may not provide a good indication at a skewed intersection. For example, at the location pictured in Figure 12.4, perpendicular traffic is stopped considerably back from the crosswalk, so using the angle of the curb and waiting traffic is misleading. Pedestrians who began crossing near the waiting traffic, as shown in the figure, were outside of the crosswalk area when starting and were aligned toward the center of the intersection.

Offset Intersections

At an offset intersection, the legs of one street do not continue straight across the intersection, but instead are offset from each other to the right or left. The amount of the offset is often given as a distance such as "Haywood Street is offset to the right by 30 feet." This means that the center of Haywood Street on one side of the intersection is 30 feet (9 m) to the right of the center of Haywood Street on the other side of the intersection. This type of intersection may be informally referred to as a "dog-leg" intersection. Unmarked crosswalks exist, under many state laws, between each corner, as shown in Figure 12.5, in gray.

Crosswalks may be marked only for the four crossings on the outside of the intersection as shown in Figure 12.6, or only where one leg intersects the through street. For blind pedestrians who are unfamiliar with the intersection, this

configuration can lead to crossing the major street at locations outside the crosswalk area, and was a major problem noted at offset intersections by Bentzen et al. (2004a). In addition, an offset intersection can cause orientation problems and confusion if pedestrians who are blind or visually impaired cross without being aware of the offset. After crossing, they may find that the parallel street is on their right instead of their left (Willoughby & Monthei, 1998).

Channelized Turn Lanes

Where there is a lot of traffic turning from one street to another, an intersection may be designed with a channelized turn lane (CTL) from one leg to another. Most commonly, CTLs in the United States are right turn lanes. The turning traffic is channelized (or separated) from the main traffic flow, by a triangular, or "pork chop" island, which may be raised or just painted (see Figure 12.7).

The island provides a refuge, or stopping point for pedestrians between the turning traffic and the main intersection crossing. However, islands that are delineated by painted lines are not detectable by most pedestrians who are blind or visually impaired. At intersections with CTLs, pedestrians are expected to cross to the island, turn and locate the main crossing, wait for the

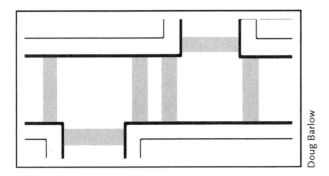

Figure 12.5. Offset Intersection Showing All Possible Crosswalk Locations

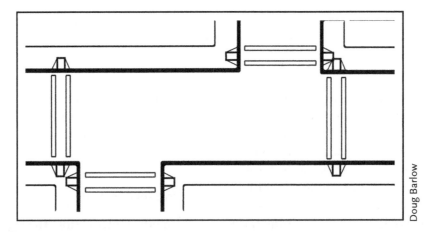

Figure 12.6. Offset Intersection with Two Marked Crosswalks Outside the Intersection

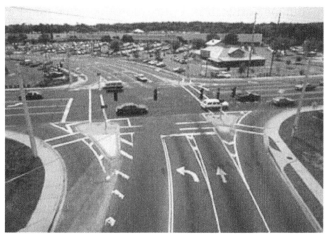

Dan Burden

Figure 12.7.
The behavior of vehicles at channelized turn lanes may vary. At this intersection, there are four channelized turn lanes, each designed slightly differently. The one in the left foreground is an acceleration lane, so vehicles are not likely to slow at the crosswalk. The one in the right foreground is a deceleration lane approaching the crossing and has a sharper merge angle, so cars may tend to yield more to pedestrians.

appropriate time to cross, then cross the main intersection lanes. The main intersection crossing and the CTL crossing may be unsignalized or signalized, or a combination of signalized and unsignalized. Intersections may have CTLs on one or all corners. Some pedestrian advocates consider channelized right turn lanes to be an advantage for pedestrians because right turning traffic is separated from the main traffic flow; however, pedestrians who are blind or visually impaired often find it difficult to determine when to cross the turn lane (see the section on Unsignalized Intersections), and may have difficulties with orientation as well.

CTL designs can vary and the design may make a difference in drivers' willingness to yield to pedestrians. As shown in Figure 12.7, vehicles exiting the CTL on the right side of the photo have to yield to traffic on the main street, usually requiring drivers to stop when traffic is heavy on the cross street. At the CTL shown on the lower-left side of the photo, there is an acceleration or merging lane, so vehicles seldom have to stop, and yielding to pedestrians may be less likely (see

the section on Drivers' Yielding Behavior, and see Volume 1, Chapter 11, for discussion of modifications). The crosswalk may be marked at different locations along the turning lane. Current design guidance favors marking the crosswalk in the center of the curve, as shown in the photo. Locating crosswalks, both for right turn lanes and for the main crossing, may be problematic for pedestrians who are blind or visually impaired because of continuous movement of traffic, and confusion with the sound of traffic stopping or moving within the main part of the intersection (Barlow, Bentzen, Bond, & Gubbe, 2006).

Medians

Medians, or *center islands*, are provided on some roadways to separate the lanes of traffic, to prevent cars from turning in the middle of a block, and to give pedestrians a place to wait for their opportunity to cross another section of the roadway. At intersections, medians should be cut-through level with the street, or have ramps on each side to allow crossing by people who cannot manage a step up or down, but medians can still be found that are not cut through or ramped. However, cut-through islands may be undetectable to blind or visually impaired pedestrians, particularly dog guide handlers. Detectable warnings are now required in the United States to indicate the island location, but detectable warnings at cut-throughs are not universal at this time. Figure 12.8 shows a cut-through island at an unsignalized crossing.

A median or island may also be designated simply by markings on the street, but a painted median or island is undetectable to a pedestrian who is blind, although a person with low vision may be able to recognize it. Medians may also be located completely outside the pedestrian crosswalk area. But even when they are outside the crosswalk area, pedestrians who are blind may contact and be confused by medians if they veer slightly away from the parallel street while crossing (Barlow et al., 2005; Bentzen et al., 2000).

Medians are often installed at unsignalized crossings to separate the crossing task into two stages, allowing pedestrians to focus on one direction of traffic at a time. At signalized intersec-tions, the signal may be timed for pedestrians to cross the entire street at once, or may be timed for a two-stage crossing, stopping in the median. It may be very difficult to reliably determine the signal timing plan because the timing may be different at different times of the day or days of the week, and may also change moment to moment, depending on the presence of vehicles and pedestrians.

Roundabouts

Roundabouts are circular intersections with specific design and traffic control features, including yield control of all entering vehicles. The approaching roadways are channelized with markings or islands to direct vehicles around the central island, and to slow traffic, but vehicles do not have to stop, except to yield to vehicles in the circulating roadway before entering the roundabout, or possibly to yield to pedestrians crossing at crosswalks. Small roundabouts have single lane entries and exits and a single lane circulating roadway (see Figure 12.9), and most in the United States currently are of this type.

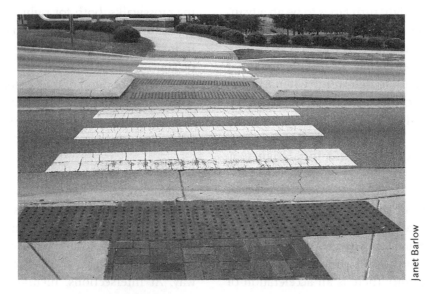

Janet Barlow

Figure 12.8.
A midblock crosswalk with a cut-through island with detectable warnings.

Large multilane roundabouts do exist, however, and more roundabouts are being planned and built with three- and four-lane entries and exits, as shown in Figure 12.10.

At roundabouts, the pedestrian crosswalks are along the roadways entering or exiting the roundabout, set back from the circulating lanes, usually with a raised island (referred to as a *splitter island*) in the middle of the crossing (see Figures 12.9 and 12.10). Pedestrians are expected to cross in two stages, stopping on the splitter island and waiting for a gap in traffic or a yielding vehicle before crossing the second half of the street. Sidebar 12.1 presents an example of typical instructions for pedestrians at roundabouts.

The configuration of roundabouts means that sidewalks at roundabouts often curve in large arcs and, unlike traditional intersections, rarely lead directly to crosswalks. Instead, crosswalks are typically positioned to the side of the pedestrian

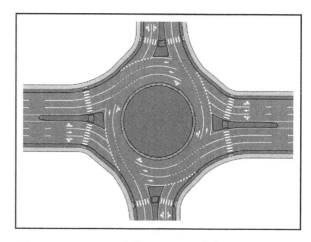

Figure 12.10. Multilane Roundabout
A three-lane roundabout with marked unsignalized pedestrian crosswalks, all on outside legs.
Source: Federal Highway Administration, *Manual on Uniform Traffic Control Devices for Streets and Highways* (Washington, DC: Department of Transportation, 2009).

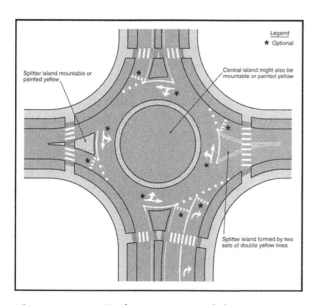

Figure 12.9. Single-Lane Roundabout
Pedestrians cross one lane at a time on the outside legs and are not supposed to go to the center island.
Source: Federal Highway Administration, *Manual on Uniform Traffic Control Devices for Streets and Highways* (Washington, DC: Department of Transportation, 2009).

and need to be located using different strategies and sources of information than those used at traditional intersections (Access Board, n.d.; see Figure 12.11). Even though guidance from the U.S. Access Board (Access Board, 2005) suggests landscaping or fences to provide a cue to crosswalk location, sidewalks are often paved right up to the curb all the way around the circulatory roadway. Failure to cross from the correct location may result in completing crossing where there is landscaping or a barrier that prevents pedestrians from stepping out of the street.

Traffic sounds at roundabouts provide ambiguous cues. Vehicles circulating in the roundabout often mask the sounds of vehicles approaching the crosswalk, making it difficult to hear approaching vehicles from an adequate distance and identify an appropriate time to cross. At exit legs, auditory information may not be adequate to reliably convey whether circulating vehicles will exit or continue around the roadway (Guth et al., 2005; Access Board, n.d.). In addition, pedestrians who are blind have difficulty recognizing when a vehicle has yielded (Guth et al., 2005; Long et al., 2005).

SIDEBAR 12.1

Typical Instructions for Pedestrians at Roundabouts

- Walk on the sidewalk at all times.

- Cross only at the designated crosswalks.

- Never cross the circular roadway to the central island.

- Look in the direction of the oncoming traffic and wait for a safe gap before entering the crosswalk.

- Proceed to the splitter island.

- Look in the direction of oncoming traffic and wait for a safe gap before proceeding to cross.

Source: Town of Ajax, *Information on Roundabouts* (n.d.), retrieved February 12, 2010, from www.townofajax.com/ Page1724.aspx.

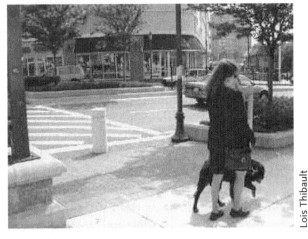

Lois Thibault

Figure 12.11.
This guide dog user has no cue to help her detect the crosswalk at a roundabout.

Volume 1, Chapter 1, provides some information about perceptual information at roundabouts.

Curb Radius

Another aspect of intersection geometry that affects crosswalks and sidewalk design is the *curb radius*. The curb radius varies from intersection to intersection and is related to the traffic expected and to the design speed of the intersection. Large radius corners allow vehicles to turn faster, and make it easier for large vehicles such as buses or trucks to make turns.

Figure 12.12 shows corners with three different curb radii, 15 feet, 25 feet, and 50 feet. The small radius, 15 feet, results in relatively square corners, and is used in some residential areas and older business districts. In suburban areas, curb radii of 40 to 50 feet are quite common now. The rounded curbs at large radius corners can make aligning to cross difficult, since the sidewalk curves around the corner. Large radius corners also result in longer crosswalks and longer time needed for pedestrians to cross the street. As shown in Figure 12.12, a curb radius increase from 15 feet to 50 feet increases the pedestrian crossing distance from 62 feet to 100 feet, when all other aspects of the intersection remain equal (Federal Highway Administration, 2004).

In addition to the longer crossings, the large radius corners along with the required curb ramps can have a significant effect on the alignment skills and techniques of pedestrians who are blind or visually impaired. The next section discusses the construction of curb ramps on corners with larger radii and the resulting intersection geometry.

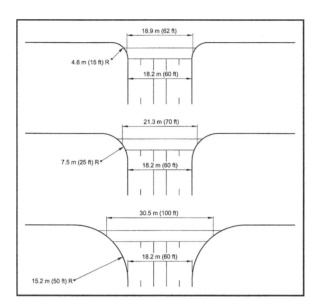

Figure 12.12. Increases in Crosswalk Distance Resulting from Larger Curb Radii

An increase in the radius of a curb from 15 feet (4.6 m) to 50 feet (15.2 m) increases the pedestrian crossing distance from 62 feet (18.9 m) to 100 feet (30.5 m), all else being equal.

Source: http://www.tfhrc.gov/safety/pubs/04091/04091.pdf

Curb Ramps

Requirements for Curb Ramps

The installation of curb ramps, required for access to sidewalks and street crossings for people who are unable to negotiate a step, has been a change that has complicated the travel of pedestrians who are blind or visually impaired. Two issues have been noted: difficulty detecting the street when approached on a curb ramp (Barlow & Bentzen, 1994; Bentzen & Barlow, 1995; Hauger et al., 1996), and the negative effect on alignment of various sloping surfaces at the corner (Whipple, 2004). Since the early 1970s, curb ramps have been required at intersections to provide access to street crossing for pedestrians who cannot step up or down curbs. Curb ramps are also useful to pedestrians pushing strollers,

or those with carts or luggage. Minimum standards for curb ramps are provided in ADAAG (U.S. Department of Justice, 1991) and in *Draft Public Rights-of-Way Accessibility Guidelines* (Draft PROWAG; Access Board, 2005), requiring that curb ramps cannot be steeper than 1:12 (8.33 percent slope), and should be built with the least slope possible. Curb ramps also cannot have more than 2 percent cross slope (the slope perpendicular to the travel direction).

Since 2001, in order to provide a tactile cue to the edge of the street for pedestrians who are blind or visually impaired, truncated dome detectable warning surfaces have been required on new curb ramps in the United States. For a review of the research on detectable warnings, see the section on detectable warnings in Volume 1, Chapter 11. The detectable warning surfaces should be the full width of the ramp or level transition area, and 2 feet (0.5 m) deep in the direction of travel, at the base of the ramp/edge of the street. However, it will be many years before detectable warnings are in place at all curb ramps in the United States.

At this time, there is no requirement for the slope of the ramp to be aligned with the direction of travel on the crosswalk. ADA standards and guidelines (Access Board, 2004, 2005; U.S. Department of Justice, 1991) do not require two ramps at each corner (one for each crosswalk), or standardized placement or configuration of the ramp, except that the ramp must be within the crosswalk lines. Detectable warning surfaces must be aligned so the domes are in line with the slope of the ramp in order to make it easier for wheelchairs users to traverse the dome surface, and this means that usually the domes and detectable warning surface cannot be aligned in the direction of travel on the crosswalk.

The Institute of Transportation Engineers and the Access Board have been working on developing guidance on curb ramps designs that would be more helpful to orientation of pedestrians who are blind. Some suggested designs were developed, but have not been widely implemented (Stollof, 2005a, 2005b).

Types of Curb Ramps

The following examples show some of the more common types of curb ramps and blended transitions. Curb ramp construction is affected by topography, weather conditions requiring the need for drainage or snow storage, curb radius, sidewalk location and width, location of existing buildings and facilities, and other factors, including scope of work in constructing the curb ramp. A sidewalk may be located at *back of curb*, which means right next to the curb line and street, or separated from the curb by an area that may be called the *landscape strip, furniture zone, boulevard, tree lawn, snow zone*, or some other name. The different sidewalk configurations can affect the design of the ramp and the information that is available to pedestrians who are blind or visually impaired. The following section describes the various types of ramps, mostly as described in Draft PROWAG (Access Board, 2005).

Ramp terminology. An understanding of the engineering terminology for different types of ramps and blended transitions will be helpful in the descriptions that follow. *Running slope* refers to the slope of the ramp in the direction of travel. *Cross slope* is the slope perpendicular to the direction of travel. Each ramp has a *landing*, or level area, with no more than 2 percent cross slope in any direction, which is a turning space, located either at the top or bottom of the ramp. The *grade break* is the line where there is a change in slope. For example, it is where the slope of the ramp down changes to go up at the gutter. Various curb ramp alignments are required in order to design for the front wheels of wheelchairs to contact the grade break squarely, because hitting it at an angle can cause tipping and loss of control. Usually the grade break is at the gutter but

that may not be true in some curb ramp designs, which could cause confusion for pedestrians who are blind or visually impaired. The ramp *flares* are sloped sides on the ramp, required where pedestrians may walk across the ramp. Flares are not required where there is a landscape strip or other feature, such as a pole, blocking pedestrians from walking across the ramp (see Figure 12.13).

Perpendicular curb ramps. *Perpendicular ramps* are ramps that are perpendicular to the curb line. As shown in the graphic, in a wide sidewalk, flares are provided on each side of the ramp and the detectable warning surface is at the bottom of the ramp by the curb. Figure 12.14 shows two typical perpendicular ramps installed on a small radius corner.

The landing is at the top of the ramp. Where curb radii are small, curb ramps are often perpendicular to the street and aligned with the direction of travel on the sidewalk and the crosswalk. The amount of slope of the ramp depends on the topography and design. At a small radius corner, blind or visually impaired pedestrians will usually contact a curb that is relatively perpendicular to the street, as shown in Figure 12.14. If there is no landscape strip, the

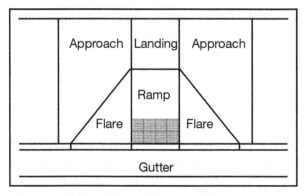

Figure 12.13. Parts of a Curb Ramp

Source: J. B. Kirschbaum, et al., *Designing Sidewalks and Trails for Access*, Part II of II: Best Practices Design Guide (Washington, DC: Federal Highway Administration, 2001).

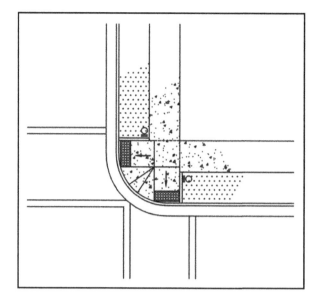

Figure 12.14. Perpendicular Curb Ramps

Perpendicular curb ramps at a location with landscape strips are aligned with the sidewalk and crosswalk.

Source: Access Board, *Special Report: Accessible Public Rights-of-Way Planning and Design for Alterations* (Washington, DC: U.S. Architectural and Transportation Barriers Compliance Board, 2007), Chapter 6, Perpendicular Curb Ramps, Example 6.

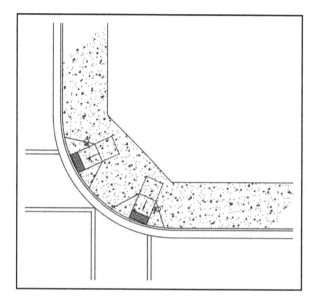

Figure 12.15. Perpendicular Curb Ramps at a Corner with a Large Radius

These ramps point toward the center of the intersection.

Source: Access Board, *Special Report: Accessible Public Rights-of-Way Planning and Design for Alterations* (Washington, DC: U.S. Architectural and Transportation Barriers Compliance Board, 2007), Chapter 6, Example 14.

curb ramp and crosswalk may not be directly in the line of travel.

The above example of perpendicular curb ramps is probably not the most common. Draft PROWAG requires that "perpendicular curb ramps shall have a running slope that cuts through or is built up to the curb at right angles or meets the gutter grade break at right angles." At large radius corners with wide sidewalks, this requirement often results in ramps that slope toward the center of the intersection, as shown in Figure 12.15. The ramps point toward the center of the intersection because the grade break is in line with the street gutter. If pedestrians who are blind or visually impaired think that the curb ramps are sloping in the direction of travel on the crosswalk, or that the edge of the detectable warnings can be used as an alignment cue, they may align facing toward the center of the

intersection, rather than in line with the crossing. The curving approach sidewalk and curb line shown in this drawing also provide confusing information.

Parallel curb ramps. *Parallel ramps* lower the sidewalk to a level landing at the street level. Parallel ramps are often used on narrow sidewalks that are at back of curbs (sidewalks installed right next to the curb), where there is not room to install a perpendicular ramp. The ramp slope parallels the direction of travel on the sidewalk. As shown in Figure 12.16, at a small radius corner, the arrows indicate the downslope of the sidewalk; the level landing is at the bottom of each pair of parallel ramps, centered on the crosswalk. The detectable warning surface is installed along the street edge on the landing, which should be level with the street.

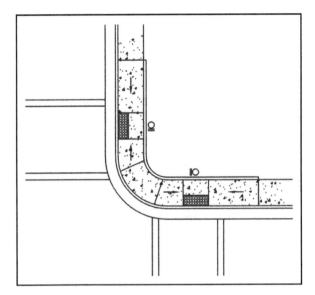

Figure 12.16. Parallel Curb Ramps in a Narrow Sidewalk

Source: Access Board, *Special Report: Accessible Public Rights-of-Way Planning and Design for Alteration* (Washington, DC: U.S. Architectural and Transportation Barriers Compliance Board, 2007), Chapter 6, Example 1.

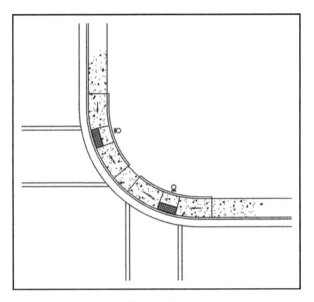

Figure 12.17. Parallel Curb Ramps at a Large-Radius Corner

Source: Access Board, *Special Report: Accessible Public Rights-of-Way Planning and Design for Alterations* (Washington, DC: U.S. Architectural and Transportation Barriers Compliance Board, 2007), Chapter 6, Example 10.

At a large radius corner with two sets of parallel curb ramps installed in a narrow sidewalk (see Figure 12.17), the slope of the ramps, the location of the crosswalks and the curvature of the corner can be particularly confusing for pedestrians who are blind or visually impaired. The ramps slope down to a level landing, which should have detectable warnings at the crosswalk, but the sidewalk/corner curve makes it necessary to for pedestrians to turn to align for crossing. At this large radius corner, the pedestrian who begins crossing from the location where a curb is first contacted would be crossing close to the parallel traffic, possibly too close, and would not be within the crosswalk area when crossing.

Blended transitions. At *blended transitions*, which include blended curbs, depressed corners, raised crosswalks or tabled intersections, the en-

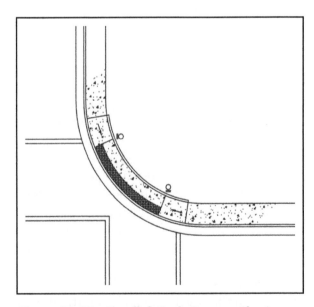

Figure 12.18. Parallel Curb Ramps Sloping Down to a Blended Transition Area

Source: Access Board, *Special Report: Accessible Public Rights-of-Way Planning and Design for Alterations* (Washington, DC: U.S. Architectural and Transportation Barriers Compliance Board, 2007), Chapter 6, Example 11.

tire sidewalk area blends with the street. The entire corner area may be flat with the street or may slope gently toward the street as shown in Figure 12.18. Detectable warnings may be the only indication of the edge of the street for pedestrians who are blind or visually impaired; they need to be installed behind the curb line for the entire distance that the corner is level with the street.

Diagonal or apex ramp.   A *diagonal* or *apex ramp* is when one perpendicular ramp is provided for both crossings of an intersection. The ramp often points directly toward the center of the intersection, as shown in Figure 12.19. Diagonal or apex ramps are not desirable for wheelchair or walking device users since the user needs to turn immediately upon reaching the street and is required to travel a further distance in the street.

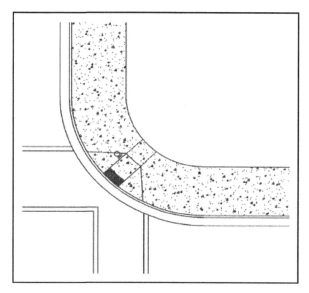

Figure 12.19. Diagonal or Apex Curb Ramp

Source: Access Board, *Special Report: Accessible Public Rights-of-Way Planning and Design for Alterations* (Washington, DC: U.S. Architectural and Transportation Barriers Compliance Board, 2007), Chapter 6, Example 16.

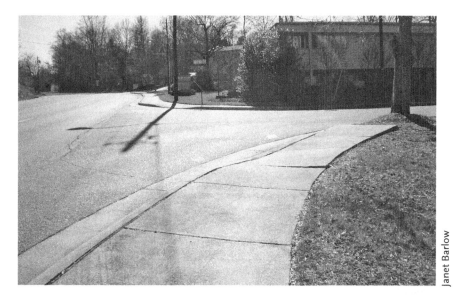

Janet Barlow

Figure 12.20.
At this location the entire sidewalk slopes sideways, a situation not allowed by ADA.

Although the above descriptions cover the types of curb ramps that are currently allowed under ADA, there are many ramps on the street that do not meet those requirements. In some areas, curb ramps are still being built that do not conform to the above descriptions. A common mistake is a ramp built so the entire corner area has a significant cross slope, as shown in Figure 12.20.

EFFECT OF DIFFERENT RAMP AND CORNER CONFIGURATIONS

Detecting the Street

Curb ramps that are in line with the sidewalk, particularly if other cues are not available such as detectable warnings, traffic, building lines, or steep slope, can lead to difficulty detecting the street (Barlow & Bentzen, 1994; Hauger et al., 1996). Hauger et al. (1996) found that apex ramps were more easily detected, but led to a

higher number of unsuccessful street crossings for pedestrians who were blind.

Parallel curb ramps vary in width and location in relation to the street; the slope does not usually aim directly into the street, because the ramped portion is parallel to the direction of the sidewalk. Pedestrians turn on the level landing at the bottom of the ramp in order to step into the street. However, if there are no detectable warnings installed, it can be very difficult to discern the street from the landing. Checking for curbs on the sides of the landing may be helpful. The other confusing part of a parallel ramp is that there is often a curb on the back edge of the landing (the side away from the street) that can be confused with the street curb (see Figure 12.21).

Locating the Crossing Location or Crosswalk

Blind or visually impaired pedestrians and O&M textbook authors have typically assumed that

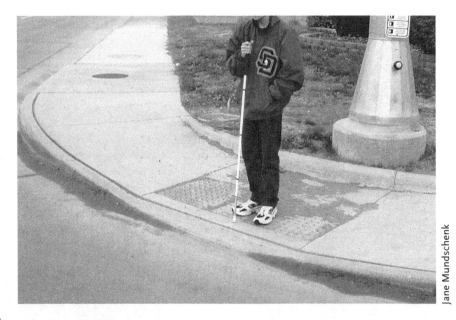

Jane Mundschenk

Figure 12.21.
Parallel ramps to a shared landing may cause confusion. This student first felt the major slope leading down the parallel ramp to the landing with truncated domes; he then felt the curb on his left and detectable warnings on his right. Aligning with the detectable warnings would have sent him out into parallel traffic.

the crosswalk or appropriate crossing location is at the corner where the curb is first contacted on approach to the street/intersection. Most describe approaching the intersection, contacting the curb, and anchoring the cane on the curb while maintaining approach alignment for crossing. As described in the discussion of intersection geometry above, at some types of intersections, including one with offsets or large radius corners, the crosswalk will not be located where pedestrians first contact the curb or curb ramp. Multileg intersections often have crosswalks at unusual locations, depending on the street angles. The sidewalk may lead directly toward the center of the intersection, as shown in the photo (see Figure 12.22). And, as discussed earlier, crosswalks at roundabouts and channelized turn lanes are deliberately set back from the intersection, intending that pedestrians will cross behind the point where drivers are required to yield for vehicles. All these issues are common situations

that blind or visually impaired pedestrians need to be prepared to recognize in the current intersection environment.

Establishing and Maintaining Crossing Alignment

Various ramp configurations affect techniques for establishing alignment. Traditionally, three basic alignment strategies have been taught and used: (1) maintaining approach line of travel, (2) parallel alignment with the grassline or perpendicular alignment with the curb, and (3) auditory alignment with parallel and perpendicular traffic (Hill & Ponder, 1976; LaGrow & Weessies, 1994; Willoughby & Monthei, 1998).

While many residential intersections are relatively square and seem simple to cross, the lack of traffic sound cues may make alignment difficult there, particularly with curb ramps sloping in different directions toward the intersection.

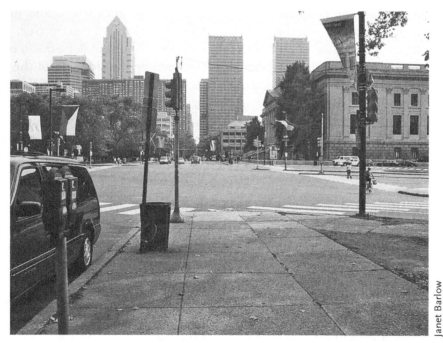

Figure 12.22.
At this multileg intersection, typical strategies for determining where to begin crossing will not work.

Maintaining the approach line of travel or parallel alignment with grassline still works quite well in residential neighborhoods if there are small radius corners and the sidewalk edges align in the direction of the crosswalk. However, it is common for suburban neighborhoods to have large radius corners and sidewalks that are back of curb, or sidewalks that widen as they approach the intersecting street, where the techniques above do not work well.

As shown in Figure 12.21, where the sidewalk is narrow and at back of curb and the curb radius is large, it is common to find two parallel curb ramps that slope down and curve to a shared level landing right at the corner for crossing both streets. This is a situation that pedestrians who are blind or visually impaired need to be prepared to detect and recognize.

In addition, at signalized crossings, using a pedestrian pushbutton is often required in order to call the pedestrian timing. After using a pushbutton, the pedestrian must realign quickly and be prepared to cross with the next parallel surge of traffic, or go back and push the pushbutton again. Going to find and use the pushbutton and having to cross when the parallel traffic begins moving prevents using traditional techniques. It is no longer possible to listen through the cycle and check alignment after arriving at the curb. The section on pedestrian pushbuttons later in this chapter discusses this issue further.

Detection, Location, and Alignment Techniques

Techniques to Detect the Street

In discussing street-crossing techniques, orientation and mobility programs and textbooks typically have described detecting the street when the cane tip drops off the curb (Hill & Ponder, 1976; Jacobson, 1993; LaGrow & Weesies, 1994;

Willoughby & Monthei, 1998). Since curbs have been replaced with curb ramps, these techniques need to be adapted to detecting curb ramps, detectable warnings, and the street gutter. Using touch and slide technique or constant contact technique is suggested to detect drop-offs, changes in texture, or slopes (Allen et al., 1997; Jacobson, 1993; LaGrow & Weessies, 1994). Being alert to the variety of clues that could indicate the approach to a perpendicular street, and understanding and using a combination of clues, was found by Barlow and Bentzen (1994) to result in more accurate street detection.

The "best" travelers in that study demonstrated a combination of various strategies for detecting the street or avoiding the curb ramp area. Some of the clues that were noted include awareness of slight changes in slope, both up and down, with the cane as well as underfoot, changes in building lines and shorelines, parallel and perpendicular traffic, the open sound of an intersection, pedestrians or other sounds on the perpendicular street, poles on the side away from the parallel street, and judgment of distance traveled. A primary clue, when available, was the curb or the slope down of the curb ramp followed by the slope up of the street. Changes in building lines and "shorelines" were also recognized as indicators of the presence of a street. The end of a building line, which might be detected by changes in reflected sound or sound shadow, or by haptic information provided by trailing, led to behaviors by participants that indicated anticipation of a street. Such behaviors commonly included a decrease in rate of travel, a switch from touch technique to constant contact technique, and/or an increase in other exploratory activity with the cane, checking for a sidewalk edge or building line. All these are strategies and techniques that are useful to include in training, and to practice in approaching unfamiliar streets with a variety of sidewalk and curb ramp configurations.

Teaching Techniques for Street Detection

Information about curb ramp requirements and characteristics of various ramps is primary knowledge needed for blind or visually impaired pedestrians to understand what they might find on approaching the street. Students need experience recognizing and negotiating a great variety of curb ramp slopes and configurations, with variations in the approach sidewalks. Teaching areas can include urban and suburban environments with some large radius, rounded corners, and wider streets so students learn to recognize and handle those features.

Use of a particular cane technique (such as use of constant contact or touch and slide technique; see Chapter 1) does not guarantee detection of the street, nor does addition of modifications such as truncated dome detectable warnings. Awareness of all the clues, as discussed above, and using a combination of information is needed for successful travel.

At some locations, traditional techniques work well. When individuals think that they have reached the street, it may be confirmed by exploring with the cane in a wide arc to either side of the body to locate a portion of a curb or the flare of the curb ramp, or stopping and drawing the cane back to check for a texture change or gutter (Hill & Ponder, 1976). When using this technique, pedestrians who are blind or visually impaired need to first plant their feet and hold their position and line of approach while checking. However, on a very wide curb ramp or blended transition, the street may not be detected with this technique.

When familiarizing themselves to a new area, pedestrians who are blind or visually impaired may find that shorelining is helpful for detecting each street and determining the sidewalk and curb ramp location. After locating the street and curb ramp, and developing an understanding of the configuration and layout, they may walk back up the block and approach the intersection again, checking their cues to help detect the street and to use for alignment.

Students need to be taught to use efficient and effective techniques when they recognize that they are close to a street, changing their technique from the one used while traveling mid-block. They need to be taught to avoid searching around with ineffective and unsafe techniques, and need to learn to look for cues to the street, such as the presence of vehicular traffic in front of them, detectable warnings, slopes, slight texture changes, and poles, fire hydrants, or mailboxes located near the corner. Students with low vision may be able to detect visual contrast of curb, sidewalk and street, and possibly of detectable warnings, crosswalk lines, groups of pedestrians, and vehicles on the perpendicular or parallel street. Smith and O'Donnell (2001) provide detailed suggestions for teaching students to use visual cues to recognize the street, slopes, and curb ramps, and to estimate curb height.

Instruction needs to include practice recognizing changes in running slope and cross slope, both underfoot and with a cane. Instructors can point out the downslope of a curb ramp, followed by a characteristic upslope toward the crown of a street. However, the wide variety of curb ramp designs and the increased use of parallel ramps can make it more difficult to determine where the street edge is located (see Figure 12.22). Cross slope is more easily recognized underfoot than running slope (Barlow & Bentzen, 1994; Cratty, 1965; Cratty & Williams, 1966), so ramps at the apex of the corner that slope toward the middle of the intersection, or the flare of a perpendicular ramp may be more easily detected than perpendicular ramps. As noted above, Hauger et al. (1996) found that apex ramps were more easily detected, but led to more unsuccessful crossings.

However, all the techniques listed may not be enough to enable consistent detection of low slope ramps or locations where the street and sidewalk are on the same level. Detectable warnings are now required in the United States at curb ramps (see Volume 1, Chapter 11), but it will be many years before all curb ramps have such detectable warnings installed. Meanwhile, it is important to include curb ramps and level crossings with and without detectable warnings in the O&M curriculum, and to teach students where the detectable warnings need to be installed, and how to recognize the detectable warning surface underfoot and under cane. Information on installation and advocating for environmental modifications can be found in Volume 1, Chapter 11.

Techniques for Locating Crossings (Crosswalks)

Barlow, Bentzen, and Bond (2005) observed that participants were most successful at starting within the crosswalk when they used the location of curb ramps to indicate the location of the crosswalk. Curb ramps are required by the Americans with Disabilities Act at all marked and unmarked crosswalks, and are required to be within the width of the crosswalk, unless crossing is prohibited at that location (marked with a sign or barrier). Curb ramps are almost always indicators of the location of the crosswalk, although they are not reliable clues to the alignment of the crosswalk and direction of the destination curb. Even when there is one apex ramp, it is generally within the marked crosswalk, so the crosswalk is very close to the parallel traffic. Appropriate techniques are needed to explore safely and to maintain alignment and orientation while locating the curb ramp, and for aligning while on or beside curb ramps that may not slope in the direction of travel on the crosswalk.

Students need to understand that the mere presence of a curb ramp does not indicate that the crossing is marked or that the location is a safe place to cross. They still need to use other information, and assess traffic and other features at the location to decide if it's a reasonable place for them to cross.

Markings for crosswalks may be in several different styles, ranging from a white line on each side of the crosswalk, to wide lines across the crosswalk (Continental), or a combination of the two (ladder). Students with low vision may be able to locate the contrasting crosswalk lines, depending on the width and contrast at each location. Some individuals who are totally blind are able to find some types of markings made of thermoplastic, which results in slightly raised lines. While not always reliable, since markings fade and wear over time, instruction can develop awareness of all possible clues and techniques for students to choose from.

Traffic can also be used to confirm the crosswalk location by listening to patterns on approach to intersections and after arriving at intersections. Sounds of traffic stopping and starting can be used to verify the appropriate location to cross, although right turning cars now commonly pull into the crosswalk area before stopping. It is generally easiest to use the vehicular traffic in this manner when making a clockwise crossing because the lanes of stopped perpendicular traffic are close to the student preparing to cross. In some locations, the perpendicular cars lined up waiting can be heard well even when preparing for a counterclockwise crossing. However, at skewed intersections, the location of waiting cars can be misleading, as shown in Figure 12.4.

If grass, bushes, or poles are located where the curb or curb ramp is expected, they may indicate that crossing is prohibited or that the crosswalk is not located in line with the approach sidewalk.

Teaching Students to Locate Crosswalks

Students may practice finding the curb ramp, then listening through a cycle or two of traffic movement to determine intersection layout, and confirm that they are at the correct location for crossing. Informing students with low vision about different crosswalk marking styles, and going to intersections marked with the different markings can be helpful.

Students may be taught that, when they recognize that they are approaching or have come to a curb ramp, they may be able to locate a straighter portion of curb by moving to the side away from the parallel street. However, when making such a maneuver, the student also needs to maintain her orientation and recognition of location of parallel and perpendicular traffic while changing her position. On rounded corners this tends to position the traveler within the crosswalk, and on the side farthest from parallel traffic, and may help pedestrians avoid aiming toward the center of the intersection at diagonal ramps.

At channelized turn lanes and roundabouts, Draft PROWAG (Access Board, 2005) requires landscaping or "barriers" to prevent crossing at incorrect locations and to guide blind or visually impaired pedestrians to crosswalk locations. While such landscape features may not be consistent design features, students should have practice trailing around corners to the crossing at a roundabout or channelized turn lane looking for a break in the landscaping, an intersecting sidewalk, or the slope of a curb ramp on the street side, then assessing the crossing location. Practice is needed to recognize the curving sidewalk path and changes in sound of intersecting traffic. Once students have practiced this skill when they are informed that they are approaching a roundabout or channelized turn lane, lessons should include some approaches in which they need to recognize the traffic patterns and locate the crossing location without prior familiarization.

Bar tiles across the sidewalk are used in Australia and a number of other countries to indicate the crosswalk location (see information in Volume 1, Chapter 11). There is potential for similar installations in the United States at roundabout locations, since the Roundabout Bulletin published by the Access Board (n.d.)

suggests that as one option. If bar tiles or similar materials are not installed in teaching areas, instructors can get samples of various materials from manufacturers and introduce students to the materials and their potential use to indicate a crosswalk or similar feature.

Techniques for Alignment

At many locations, useful alignment cues are traffic sounds and maintaining the approach direction at signalized and unsignalized intersections. Crossings of a major street may have very little traffic parallel to the crossing to use as an alignment cue, while crossings of streets alongside a major street will have plenty of useful parallel traffic.

At locations with rounded curb lines and adequate parallel traffic traveling straight through the intersection, students can explore the corner, and then align using the sound of traffic on the parallel street. Using the sounds of parallel traffic can be difficult at noisy or congested intersections or at intersections with heavy turning movements. However, research indicates that individuals are able to use traffic for alignment even after hearing only a small part of the vehicle path (Guth, Hill, & Rieser, 1989). If pedestrians know that the streets at the intersection cross at approximately 90-degree angles, both the traffic on the street being crossed, and the line of cars at the stop line, can be used for alignment. However, without knowledge that streets are at a 90-degree angle, perpendicular traffic cannot be relied on as an alignment clue.

Another strategy for aligning is to move away from the parallel street far enough that the curb is straight, and square off on the curb or edge. However, when using this strategy, especially if the radius is large, the traveler may not be in the crosswalk where drivers expect pedestrians, and may be at a distance from the corner at the completion of the crossing. The distance that it is necessary to walk from the corner in order for the curb edge to be straight varies. This technique should not be used where the traveler might have to walk through a line of waiting perpendicular traffic or where vehicles turning from the parallel street could be traveling at higher speeds.

Sometimes it is not possible to use any of the above strategies, such as at intersections where the crosswalk is not parallel to the traffic, or when it's necessary to move out of alignment to push a pedestrian button just before crossing. It is often possible to align in these situations by locating a physical feature that can be used as an alignment aid. To do this, pedestrians who are blind or visually impaired find a physical feature near the crosswalk that is unique, easy to find, and has (or is close to) a tactually detectable line such as a curb, grass line, a square pole or wall. Then, they establish alignment to cross (with assistance if needed), and determine the angle of the physical feature in relation to their body when aligned. On later approaches, they again find the physical feature and use it to align. People can usually learn how to align with tactually detectable lines at various angles if they have practice with feedback. Where there is adequate traffic, a person might get the alignment feedback without assistance. Where traffic is sporadic, or not parallel to the crosswalk, pedestrians may need to ask another pedestrian or a friend for assistance and feedback in aligning to cross. Knowing good questions to ask others can be important in this task. For example, pedestrians who are blind or visually impaired might stand at the location and ask another person to tell them if they are in line with the crosswalk lines or if they need to angle to the right or left. It can also be important to find out whether the crosswalk continues straight all the way across the street, since there are some locations that have "bend" or "jog" in the marked crosswalk.

When using pushbuttons at intersections, a strategy suggested by some experienced O&M specialists is to first travel to the edge of the street, maintaining approach alignment, and then assess the street crossing, including locating a tactile clue to use in realigning. After determining a clue for realignment, pedestrians can use systematic search patterns to determine if there is a pushbutton for the crossing, and then return to the predetermined location and tactile cue. Even at locations where an accessible pedestrian signal with a pushbutton locator tone is installed, travelers need to locate the street, analyze the intersection, and determine appropriate crossing alignment before pushing the pushbutton, because it will not be possible to use the sound of parallel traffic to align after pushing the pushbutton since it will be necessary to cross during the next parallel traffic surge (see the subsection on Strategies for finding and using pushbuttons under the section on Signalized Intersections).

In the United States, tactile arrows are often mounted on the face of APS (see Volume 1, Chapter 11) and the arrow is supposed to be aligned with the direction of travel on the crosswalk that the pushbutton controls. Research (Harkey et al., 2007) found that some blind pedestrians did not understand tactile arrows and could not identify the direction to which the arrow was pointing, nor could they align well to travel in the direction indicated by the arrow. However, this may be a skill that can be improved through training and experience.

As discussed earlier, truncated dome detectable warnings are required in new construction and alterations in the United States. However, the domes are intended in the United States to be an indication of the location of the edge of the street at the base of a curb ramp, not an alignment cue. O&M specialists and pedestrians who are blind or visually impaired need to understand that detectable warnings cannot be used for alignment, at least not as currently specified in ADA guidelines. In other countries, such as Australia, the tactile bar tiles and truncated domes are often aligned with the direction of travel on the crosswalk, rather than with the slope of the ramp, so they may be useful for alignment in those countries. See Volume 1, Chapter 11, on environmental accessibility for information on alignment surfaces used in other countries.

Teaching Strategies for Alignment and Maintaining Alignment while Crossing

Maintaining the line of travel direction when approaching the crosswalk usually requires training and practice to ignore the angle of the curb and the curb ramp. The novice will often turn unaware to face perpendicular to the edge of the curb or parallel to the slope of the curb ramp. This tendency can usually be overcome by practice with feedback, such as walking across a diagonal ramp while following a sound source that is straight ahead and then trying it without the sound source, checking for accuracy each time. It can be helpful to practice on several different types of ramp alignment, slope, and configuration, and to focus on maintaining a straight travel direction despite changes in running slope and cross slope.

Individuals can learn to align with traffic by standing beside a straight street, midblock, where there are no clues about their position except for the sound of the traffic (for example, no sun, or cracks or slopes or edges underfoot, or steady sound sources). Have students begin in a position of alignment and listen to how the traffic sounds when aligned, and then listen to the traffic when standing slightly misaligned. If the difference in the sounds isn't apparent, have students turn until the difference can be detected, and/or listen to the vehicles as they recede into the distance as well as when they are close. Once students are able to correctly identify when the traffic sounds seem parallel and when sounds seem angled, the next step is to disorient them and then have them reposition themselves to stand so that the traffic again sounds aligned and parallel (also see Chapter 4). Lessons can begin midblock beside a one-way street, with only two lanes, but fairly regular traffic. It is best if platoons (groups of cars) can be heard from signals several blocks behind and in front of the student. Practice with cars coming from behind the student, then turn around and practice with cars coming toward the student. It can be useful to also practice while facing the street, listening to the vehicles traveling across in front of the student, from both directions. After the student has developed the ability to align with traffic on the street at a midblock location, similar activities and exercises can be done at intersections. It may work best to begin at an intersection with a steady stream of traffic parallel to the direction of the crosswalk, and then move to locations with more intermittent traffic. Intersections of two one-way streets can be a good starting place. After developing proficiency at aligning while standing on a level sidewalk with good traffic sounds, practice can take place while standing on various angled curb ramps or sloping areas to help students develop the ability to align with traffic sounds while standing on various slopes. Throughout a training program, it can be useful to occasionally practice just one skill in isolation, such as alignment with traffic at complex locations.

Reviewing various possible sidewalk and ramp design configurations on tactile maps can help students understand the alignment of ramps and landings in relation to pushbuttons, crosswalks, sidewalks, and intersections. Models of ramps, constructed from layered foamcore or other materials that show the various slopes, work well for this purpose, combined with actual experience with similar ramp configurations in the community.

Where APS with tactile arrows are installed, individuals who attempt to put their palm or fingers on the arrow tend to turn away from the travel direction, due to the awkward position of their hand (Bentzen et al., 2006). Some O&M instructors teach students to use the APS arrow by lining up with the outside of their forearm along the face of the device and the arrow, so their hands and arms are pointing in the direction of the arrow, and aligned with the crosswalk travel direction. While tactile arrows did not help participants align to cross in the research cited above, all participants attempted to align with their palms or fingers on the arrow, rather than with the above technique. This technique needs to be used with caution, however, as installation of APS is still quite inconsistent, with installers not understanding the critical nature of orientation of APSs on poles.

Students need to understand the construction of streets and typical street camber (varies somewhat in different areas of the country) in order to recognize street slopes and effectively correct their travel path. Practice might take place first walking with a human guide to allow students to focus on street contours and traffic sounds, on different paths on both residential and wider streets, understanding and estimating distances. It is best to practice alongside steady parallel traffic on streets of varying widths and slopes.

TRAFFIC CONTROL

Traffic control takes a number of forms, and pedestrians, especially blind or visually impaired pedestrians, need to recognize and understand the variations, because traffic control affects the movement of both vehicles and pedestrians.

At intersections, the streams of traffic may be controlled by signals, stop signs, or yield signs or they may be uncontrolled. Various types of unsignalized controls (stop signs, yield signs, and crosswalk markings) can be combined with signal control. For example, an intersection may have yield signs controlling traffic in the channelized turn lane, but signals for crossing the straight-through lanes of the roadways.

Although the operation of streets and sidewalks is predicated on an assumption of relatively orderly response to controls provided, drivers of vehicles still sometimes ignore the traffic control, or make errors in responding to signals or signs (Stollof et al., 2007). Therefore, pedestrians should never assume, for example, that approaching vehicles whose drivers have a yield sign preceding a crosswalk will yield for them to cross, or that all drivers of vehicles on the perpendicular street will stop before the onset of the Walk signal to begin crossing that street.

Pedestrian Right-of-Way Laws

Crosswalks

In addition to signals and signs, pavement markings are considered to be traffic control devices. According to the definition in the *Manual on Uniform Traffic Control Devices* (MUTCD; Federal Highway Administration, 2009), crosswalks exist at almost every intersection, regardless of whether they are marked by lines on the road surface or unmarked. Crosswalks exist at other locations, such as midblock locations, if the crosswalk is indicated by markings, as indicated in (b) of the MUTCD definition of a crosswalk:

> MUTCD, Part 1A.13. **44.** Crosswalk—(a) that part of a roadway at an intersection included within the connections of the lateral lines of the sidewalks on opposite sides of the highway measured from the curbs or in the absence of curbs, from the edges of the traversable roadway, and in the absence of a sidewalk on one side of the roadway, the part of a roadway included within the extension of the lateral lines of the sidewalk at right angles to the centerline; (b) any portion of a roadway at an intersection or elsewhere distinctly indicated as a pedestrian crossing by lines on the surface, which may be supplemented by contrasting pavement

texture, style, or color. (Federal Highway Association, 2009)

The legal requirement for vehicles at crosswalks is stated in the Uniform Vehicle Code (UVC):

11-502(a) Pedestrians' right of way in crosswalks [Yield to pedestrian in crosswalk] When traffic-control signals are not in place or not in operation, the driver of a vehicle shall yield the right of way, slowing down or stopping if need be to so yield, to a pedestrian crossing the roadway within a crosswalk when the pedestrian is upon the half of the roadway upon which the vehicle is traveling, or when the pedestrian is approaching so closely from the opposite half of the roadway as to be in danger. (National Highway Traffic Safety Administration, 2002)

Note that this requirement for vehicles to yield to pedestrians applies only at crosswalks, marked or unmarked, where traffic signals are not operating. Different states have enacted variations of this law, so it is important for O&M specialists and pedestrians who are blind or visually impaired to know the laws of the state or area in which they reside or teach. For example, in some states the pedestrians need to be in the roadway before the driver is required to stop, and in others, the person needs to just be approaching the street crossing (National Highway Traffic Safety Administration, 2002). In most jurisdictions, pedestrians who are crossing outside a crosswalk are required to yield to vehicles. Where there are signals, pedestrians are required to obey the signal (see the section on Vehicle Signalization and Phasing Plans).

The law, the level of enforcement of the law, and the level of driver compliance with the law vary from jurisdiction to jurisdiction, and from street to street. At times yellow flashing beacons, or pedestrian flashers, are installed on poles at unsignalized marked crosswalks to call attention to the crosswalk. These flashers may be pedestrian activated, requiring pedestrians to push a button to activate them, and then flashing for a specified amount of time after activation. These are considered warning beacons and must be used as supplementary to warning signs and crosswalk markings. Pedestrian-actuated in-roadway warning lights may also be installed at crosswalks, along with warning signs. However, the legal requirement to stop is based on the crosswalk laws of the state.

Practical and Legal Implications of Using Crosswalks

While it can be difficult or impossible for a pedestrian who is blind or visually impaired to know for sure where the crosswalk is located, drivers may be expecting pedestrians to cross within the crosswalk. As noted above, pedestrians crossing outside of crosswalks are legally required to yield to vehicles in most states.

White Cane Laws

While some individuals believe that white cane laws allow pedestrians who are blind or visually impaired to cross at any location and require vehicles to yield, that is not true in every state and location. The model white cane law in the U.S. Uniform Vehicle Code (UVC) states, "The driver of a vehicle shall yield the right of way to any blind pedestrian carrying a visible white cane or accompanied by a guide dog" (National Highway Traffic Safety Administration, 2002). However, the white cane laws of various states have different wording, such as the Colorado law § 42-4-808, which "requires any pedestrian (other than a person in a wheelchair)" and any driver of a vehicle to "immediately come to a full stop and take such precautions before proceeding as are necessary to avoid an accident or injury" to a person who has an obvious apparent "disability of blindness, deafness, or mobility impairment." In some states, the law has specific wording about the pedestrian's location and may only require the driver to yield to a pedestrian who is "crossing the street at an intersection and carrying a white cane" (National Highway Traffic Safety Administration, 2002).

However, the UVC also includes a statute requiring all pedestrians to obey the traffic control signals (UVC11-50) and another statute that prohibits walking into the path of a vehicle unexpectedly: "No pedestrian shall suddenly leave a curb or other place of safety and walk or run into the path of a vehicle which is so close as to constitute an immediate hazard" (11-502 UVC). These laws basically leave an area of confusion for drivers, pedestrians, and enforcement personnel. (See the section on Pedestrian Signals and Timing.) In a recent situation, a person who was blind was hit by a car and injured, but was ticketed for crossing outside a crosswalk (Margaret Stroud, personal communication, August 31, 2007). A few states use variations on the white cane law that clarify the intent. For example, the Wisconsin White Cane Law includes the following statement: "The fact that the pedestrian may be violating any of the laws applicable to pedestrians does not relieve the operator of a vehicle from the duties imposed by this subsection." That law clearly addresses the conflict between typical pedestrian laws and white cane laws. However, most states' laws do not address the legal conflict.

In any case, education about white cane laws is poor and enforcement is nonexistent in most areas. Students need to be informed of the risk of relying on drivers to stop, based on their use of a white cane. It may be appropriate to also discuss and consider the potential for negative perceptions that could come from emphasis on the responsibility of drivers to stop and from improved enforcement of the white cane law. It

might have the unintended effect of reinforcing the image of pedestrians who are blind or visually impaired as unable to determine appropriate times to cross and being unable to travel independently. O&M specialists and pedestrians who are blind or visually impaired may want to consider whether it is better to encourage enforcement of general pedestrian right-of-way laws, rather than the white cane law.

Drivers' Yielding Behavior

Despite laws that give all pedestrians right of way when crossing in a crosswalk, marked or unmarked, and white cane laws that give right-of-way to pedestrians who are blind or visually impaired, yielding behavior of motorists at uncontrolled locations or yield controlled locations has been found to vary, with from 17 to 97 percent of motorists yielding to pedestrians waiting to cross (Fitzpatrick et al., 2006; Geruschat & Hassan, 2005). While Geruschat & Hassan (2005) found significantly more drivers yielded to pedestrians using a long white cane than to those without a cane, the percentages of drivers yielding varied from below 40 to over 80 percent, depending on other factors at the crossing. For example, at one location, 63 percent of the drivers yielded to pedestrians with a long cane while 52 percent yielded to pedestrians without a long cane. Individuals who are blind or visually impaired should not expect that the presence of a long white cane will consistently result in drivers yielding.

There are a number of factors that affect the likelihood that drivers will yield. These factors include the following:

- The laws regarding pedestrian right of way in the situation and, more importantly, how well the drivers understand and obey those laws
- The drivers' expectation of pedestrians to cross at the particular location, which is af-

fected by the number of pedestrians normally crossing there, as well as features such as the presence of a marked crosswalk or signage

- The location of the crosswalk in relation to other traffic control or vehicle conflict, for example, the entrance vs. exit lanes crossing of a roundabout
- The visibility of the pedestrian to drivers
- Whether the pedestrian is using a white cane or dog guide
- The speed of the vehicle
- Road conditions

Multiple Threats

Even if the legal issues with pedestrian laws and white cane laws are clarified, there are situations where drivers are unable to see pedestrians adequately or in time to avoid conflict. For example, well known in the literature about pedestrian safety at multilane streets is what is called the *multiple-threat situation* (Zegeer et al., 2002). As shown in Figure 12.23, the view of an approaching driver in the second lane of a street may be blocked by another vehicle, parked or yielding in

the first lane, until it is too late for the driver to stop for pedestrians in the crosswalk. Even drivers who are willing to stop for pedestrians may not be able to see crossing pedestrians in time to stop for them.

Vehicle Stopping Distance

Other impediments to pedestrian visibility, such as hills or curves, may also make it impossible for a driver to see pedestrians far enough away to yield the legal right-of-way to them. Many people underestimate the distance drivers need to stop. Traffic-engineering design guidelines estimate braking distance of 155 feet (47 m) for a vehicle traveling at 25 mph, and more than 360 feet (110 m) for a vehicle traveling at 45 mph (American Association of State Highway and Transportation Officials [AASHTO], 2004a). O&M specialists might benefit from measuring stopping distances on several streets with different speed limits to prepare to evaluate the visibility of crossings and ability of drivers to stop for a pedestrian crossing the street. Bear in mind that on most streets, more than 15 percent of drivers will exceed posted speed limits (AASHTO, 2004a).

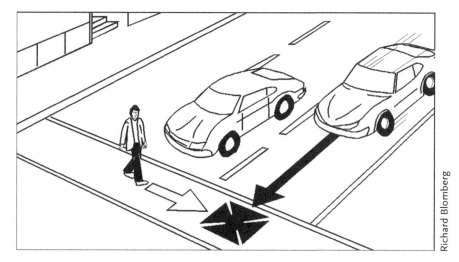

Richard Blomberg

Figure 12.23. Example of a Multiple-Threat Collision

Detecting Yielding Vehicles

When vehicles do yield, pedestrians who are blind often are unable to detect that they have yielded (Guth et al., 2005; Inman et al., 2005). When this happens, drivers will sometimes move on, or attempt to assist pedestrians who are visually impaired by honking, calling out, or getting out of their vehicles to guide them. However, at locations with two lanes, other vehicles may come around stopped vehicles, or otherwise endanger pedestrians, as noted in the discussion above of "multiple threats" (Inman et al., 2005). When pedestrians wait to be sure a vehicle has yielded, they also may begin to cross at the same moment that the driver has decided that the pedestrian does not intend to cross, and begins to accelerate.

UNSIGNALIZED INTERSECTIONS

Unsignalized intersections include locations without any traffic control and locations where traffic is controlled by stop signs or yield signs. In many residential areas, there are no signs or official traffic control indications posted. Even then, all traffic is assumed to be governed by the following right-of-way rule: "When two vehicles approach or enter an intersection from different roadways at approximately the same time, the driver of the vehicle on the left shall yield the right of way to the vehicle on the right." If stop or yield signs are installed to designate the right-of-way, the road or street is "controlled." As discussed above, marked and unmarked crosswalks are considered another aspect of traffic control, although this is poorly understood by pedestrians and drivers.

Among the skills that students should have for crossings with no traffic control (AER O&M Division, 2008) are strategies to maximize their detection of approaching vehicles by audition and/or vision, and be able to recognize situations where they cannot hear or see well enough to reliably predict gaps in traffic (situations of uncertainty for gap judgments), as well as determine the risk of crossing there. Students should also be able to implement any alternatives that may exist for crossing streets independently, and advocate for features of accessibility and pedestrian safety as needed. O&M specialists need a clear understanding of traffic control at unsignalized crossings, yielding behavior of drivers, and issues related to gap judgment.

Stop Signs

Stop signs can be installed to require traffic on all streets at an intersection to stop, called a four-way stop or all-way stop, or for only certain streets to stop, three-way stop, or two-way stop. Vehicles approaching a stop sign are required by law to come to a full stop before entering an intersection.

Four-Way Stop

At a *four-way stop* or *all-way stop intersection*, stop signs are provided for all intersecting legs. This is usually used when the roads have approximately equal amounts of traffic. Each vehicle approaching the intersection is supposed to stop. The usual rule for such intersections requires that vehicles entering the intersection yield the right of way to pedestrians who are in a crosswalk, and yield to vehicles that entered the intersection, or stopped at the stop sign before them. If two vehicles arrive at the same time, the vehicle on the right has the right-of-way. The sound signature of a four-way or all-way stop intersection is of traffic pulling up to the intersection, stopping, then moving through the intersection, generally in a fairly random pattern and sequence.

Two-Way Stop

At a *two-way stop intersection*, traffic on one of the intersecting streets has to stop and wait for a gap in traffic on the intersecting street to cross or turn onto it. Two-way stops are usually installed when one road at an intersection has more traffic than the other.

There are two types of crossing situations for blind or visually impaired pedestrians at a two-way stop-controlled intersection. At an intersection with four legs, two crossings will be across the streets controlled by the stop signs, and two crossings will be across the uncontrolled street of the intersection, typically the one having greater traffic volume moving at higher speeds.

For drivers, the advantage of a two-way stop is that the major traffic does not have to stop and they incur almost no delay at the intersection. This can be a disadvantage for pedestrians, particularly pedestrians who are blind or visually impaired, because they need to cross the uncontrolled roadway in a gap in the traffic, and traffic may be moving at a high speed. Paradoxically, these may be crossings at which there are normally few pedestrians, so drivers are not prepared to see and yield to them.

Yield Sign

Where yield signs are installed, traffic from one leg of the intersection must yield upon entering another. Vehicles are not required to come to a full stop and can continue to move into a gap in traffic. Drivers are required by law to slow down and prepare to stop (usually while merging into traffic on another road), but do not need to stop if there is no reason to stop. Yield signs are typically used at channelized right turn lanes and at roundabout intersections, where traffic is merging at an angle into another roadway or the circulatory roadway of the roundabout. In both situations, the driver is likely to look left (in the United States and Canada) for approaching vehicles while continuing to move forward, and then possibly look to the right.

At roundabout intersections, if there are crosswalks, the crosswalks are supposed to be one or two vehicle lengths away from the circulatory roadway, before the yield sign where vehicles merge into other vehicular traffic at the roundabout entry. At channelized turn lanes, the crosswalk and yield sign relationship is much more variable, but drivers often encounter the yield sign after they have passed the crosswalk to the island. This means that while drivers may be legally required to yield, or stop, for pedestrians in crosswalks at channelized turn lanes and roundabouts, drivers may not see a yield sign until after they have crossed the crosswalk! That legal requirement to yield to pedestrians is supposed to be communicated to drivers by the crosswalk markings.

Issues of Gap Judgment

Crossable Gaps

A gap in traffic that is long enough to allow a pedestrian to complete the crossing has no vehicles approaching so close or fast that they can reach the pedestrian before the crossing is completed. That is, the time in which approaching vehicles will reach the pedestrian is as long as or longer than the time the pedestrian needs to cross. This gap in traffic will be called a *crossable gap*. Its length varies according to the time needed to cross, which depends on the width of the street and the speed of the pedestrian's movement.

Acceptable Gaps

An *acceptable gap* is one that pedestrians think is as long as or longer than they need to allow them to cross. People vary in what they consider to be an acceptable gap. Some people cross only when they feel that there is not only enough time to finish their crossing before a vehicle arrives, but there is additional time (a *safety margin*) that is long enough for them to feel confident and secure about crossing. The length of the safety margin can vary, depending on the frequency of crossable gaps (Guth et al., 2005), as well as the person's motivation to cross and level of risk acceptance. Other people cross during gaps that are shorter than their crossing time—that is, when there is a negative safety margin (Guth et al., 2005). This may be because either they are unaware that the gap in not long enough to cross because they misjudged the speed and distance of the vehicles or how much time they need to cross, or they are relying on the drivers to slow down or stop for them.

Detectable Gaps

In addition to the gap being long enough to be crossable or acceptable, the gap needs to be detectable—that is, the pedestrian needs to have some way of knowing that there is time enough to cross before the next vehicle arrives. In order for gaps to be detectable, and accurately judged as crossable, the approaching vehicles need to all be detectable from a sufficient distance. For example, if the crossing time for a given person at a particular crosswalk is 8 seconds, all the approaching vehicles need to be detectable (visible or audible) to that person at least 8 seconds before the vehicles reach the crosswalk, or the safety margin for detection of those vehicles will be negative.

There are many instances where it is not possible to hear and/or see all the approaching traffic far enough to know whether the gap is long enough to cross. Factors that affect the ability to hear approaching vehicles were studied by Wall-Emerson and Sauerburger (2008) using 22 blind or visually impaired subjects listening to vehicles at three different sites. The subjects all had normal hearing and were experienced with using sound to cross streets independently. All sites were quiet, residential two-lane streets—at one site the street was straight and unobstructed for about 1,000 feet (305 m) in both directions, and the other two sites had obstructions or hills or bends in the road. The subjects were positioned facing the streets and asked to indicate when they heard a vehicle approaching. The de-

tection of 805 approaching vehicles was analyzed; of these, 360 approached during quiet. The time from when the subjects first heard a vehicle until the moment that the vehicle arrived was measured and compared to the crossing time to determine the safety margin (positive or negative) for the detection of that vehicle.

As expected, the factor that most affected the ability of the subjects to detect the approaching vehicles was the level of ambient sound that existed at the time when the vehicle was detected. That is, when it was quiet and there were no other sounds present when the approaching vehicle was first heard, it was easier to hear it than when the ambient sound was higher. When the ambient masking sound was loud enough, none of the approaching vehicles was heard well enough to have any positive safety margin. This result validates the rationale for the traditional strategy that streets with no traffic control should be crossed when it is quiet. At the site where the street was straight, whenever it was quiet (no more than 40 dB(A)), all vehicles were heard well enough that there were no negative safety margins.

At the time that the O&M profession and street-crossing strategies were developed, whenever it was quiet, it was possible to hear the traffic well enough to be assured that there was a gap long enough to cross (Sauerburger, 1999). However, today there are situations where the traffic cannot be heard well enough, even when it is quiet (Sauerburger, 1989, 1995). In the study by Wall-Emerson and Sauerburger (2008), at the sites where there was a hill or a severe bend in the road, the vehicles could not all be heard as well, even when the ambient sound was lower than the average level of "quiet" measured at these residential intersections (38 dB(A)). At the site with the severe bend, three vehicles that approached during quiet could not be heard until they were only 4 seconds away from the crosswalk, making a negative safety margin of about 3 seconds.

Situations of Uncertainty

Although there are situations (such as at the straight residential street in the study described above) where the traditional strategy of crossing when quiet is effective for determining that there is a gap long enough to cross, there are situations where the strategy is not reliable. When that is the case, such as at the narrow residential street with a bend in this study, even when it is quiet and no vehicles are detected, there is a "situation of uncertainty for gap judgments" because undetected vehicles may be just a few seconds away.

The profession has asserted (AER O&M Division, 2008) that pedestrians who are blind or visually impaired need to be able to recognize these "situations of uncertainty for gap judgments" where they cannot hear or see the approaching traffic well enough to know if there is a gap long enough to cross. In these situations, even when it is quiet and they hear or see nothing coming, they do not know whether there is enough time to cross before another vehicle reaches them, and if they start to cross, there may be a driver who will have to take evasive action to avoid hitting them if they do not turn back. Pedestrians, even those with normal hearing, should realize that in these situations, even when it is quiet, it is uncertain that there is a gap long enough to cross.

In addition to being able to recognize situations of uncertainty for gap judgments, pedestrians should know how to ascertain the level of risk involved when crossing during gaps in traffic. The risk that a vehicle, which was undetected when the crossing was started, will reach the crosswalk before the crossing is completed and will not yield varies with different traffic levels and speeds, and different detection distances of the approaching vehicles. For example, the risk of being hit by a vehicle that was undetected at the beginning of the crossing is higher where the traffic volume and speed are high or where many vehicles are undetected until they

are very close, or where drivers are unable to anticipate the need to stop far in advance (for example, when their view of the pedestrian is blocked), than it is where there are few approaching vehicles or where the vehicles are detected further away, or the drivers have longer sight distances and good road conditions.

The Issue of Judgment

The previous sections discussed the ability to see or hear the vehicles far enough away to know that, when no vehicles are detected, it is clear to cross. This section addresses the situation where pedestrians are able to see or hear the approaching traffic from a distance and they need to determine whether the gap before the next vehicle arrives is long enough to cross. Being able to judge the length of gaps in moving traffic requires the ability to judge one's own crossing time, and judge the time of arrival for approaching vehicles—that is, being able to determine that none of the approaching vehicles will arrive before the crossing is complete.

Pedestrians vary in their judgment of the approaching time of vehicles. Research on visual determinations of *time-to-contact* (TTC, a term used in psychophysical research that combines speed and distance of both vehicle and perceiver) of sighted individuals has found that there are consistent errors in judgment of TTC (Schiff & Detwiler, 1979). Observers made underestimation errors of between 34 and 40 percent, so they thought the time to contact was shorter than it actually was. Gray and Thorton (2001) note that "although underestimation errors err on the side of caution, they could be dangerous, since if a TTC estimation is made too early, the observer is vulnerable to other approaching objects and any change in velocity of the initial object." Note that this research was all done using objects approaching from distances closer than those typical for street-crossing decisions. Seward, Ashmead, and Bodenheimer (2007) found that performance worsens at longer time ranges, those that pedestrians typically use in street-crossing decisions.

In research with individuals with low vision (RP), participants overestimated but were basically able to make TTC estimations that were comparable to sighted observers (Jones, 2006). But Guth et al. (2005) found that blind pedestrians are much more likely to accept gaps that are too short (risky decisions) than sighted pedestrians. Collapsing across three roundabout sites in their studies, sighted pedestrians accepted risky gaps on only 13.4 percent of their decisions, compared to 28.9 percent of the decisions for blind pedestrians. This direction of results was confirmed by the research of Bond (2006) with sighted participants who used their vision or were blindfolded. Participants who had access to visual information made fewer risky decisions.

Strategies for Crossing at Unsignalized Locations

Unsignalized crossing locations may include crossing where the vehicles have stop or yield signs and situations where there is no sign or marking requiring the drivers to stop or yield—that is, no traffic control. The following sections will outline strategies for crossing at stop or yield signs and at locations where there is no traffic control, and the risks involved in each of those strategies.

Strategies for Crossing at Stop or Yield Signs

One strategy is to cross when no traffic is present that is close enough to reach the crosswalk before the crossing is complete. Using that strategy, there are no risks from vehicles if there are no vehicles approaching that are close or fast enough that they can reach the pedestrian before the crossing is finished, but the challenge is to determine with certainty that no traffic is present or approaching too close or too fast.

There are many situations, including multiple-threat situations, where it is not possible to see or hear all approaching traffic far enough away (see the previous section, Issues of Gap Judgment). Idling cars waiting at the stop or yield sign, even those with gasoline engines, can be difficult to hear above ambient sound; electric or hybrid cars are often not audible when idling.

Another strategy is to cross when a vehicle in the nearest lane on the parallel street is just entering the intersection, while going fast enough that it cannot turn, thus assuring that no perpendicular traffic can enter the street, and traffic from the parallel street cannot turn left into the crosswalk. However, with multiple lanes and quiet cars, it is becoming increasingly difficult to distinguish in which lane the vehicles in the parallel street are traveling. If a vehicle approaching in a far lane is mistaken for one in the nearest lane, the crossing may be initiated when that car enters the intersection while a car in the nearest lane is turning right into the crosswalk. Even when this strategy is done correctly, there is considerable risk that after the fast-moving parallel vehicle passes, drivers whose view of the pedestrian was blocked by the passing vehicle will turn left from the parallel street into the crosswalk.

Others cross with the expectation that all approaching drivers will stop or yield to pedestrians. The problems or risks with that strategy are that drivers will fail to yield (see Drivers' Yielding Behavior earlier in this chapter), or will be unable to see the pedestrian in time to yield or stop. If a person is unable to hear cars adequately, or if traffic sounds are masked by other sounds, the person who is blind or visually impaired may step out when a vehicle is too close to stop. And a fourth potential strategy is to cross when drivers in all approaching lanes have stopped. In this case, one risk is that the drivers have stopped for a reason other than waiting for the pedestrian, such as to make a turn or to yield to a vehicle, and did not intend to wait for the pedestrian. Or a driver may have yielded to the pedestrian, but then decided that the pedestrian was not going to cross, and moves forward just as the pedestrian steps in front of the vehicle. Another risk at locations with more than one lane to cross is that the pedestrian thinks that drivers in all lanes have yielded when, in fact, not all lanes are blocked. In a study at the two-lane exit of a roundabout, blind subjects were asked to report when they detected that drivers in both lanes had yielded. Fourteen percent of the time that they thought both lanes were blocked with a yielding driver, there were not drivers yielding in both lanes (Inman et al., 2005)

Strategies for Crossing Where There Is No Traffic Control

When crossing at locations with no traffic control (the through street at a two-way stop, midblock, etc.), the strategies may be more limited. One, as discussed above, is to cross with the expectation that drivers will all yield. The risk there is that the drivers will not or cannot yield, as discussed above and in the section on the yielding behavior of drivers. Another is to cross when pedestrians have recognized that drivers have yielded. If the crossing is more than one lane, this strategy can be very difficult and dangerous due to the multiple threat (discussed earlier) of the second lane of traffic (Guth et al., 2005; Inman et al., 2005). However, at a one-lane crossing (channelized right turn lane, one lane roundabout), it may be a feasible strategy for some pedestrians (Ketts & Barlow, 2008).

Another is to cross when there is a gap in traffic long enough that no approaching vehicles can reach the pedestrian before the crossing is completed. If there is indeed a crossable gap in traffic the risks are minimal, but it is difficult and in many cases impossible to know for sure that there is a gap in traffic long enough to cross, even when it is quiet. The traditional strategy for

ensuring that there is a sufficient gap, which is to cross whenever it is quiet (Allen et al., 1997; Hill & Ponder, 1976; Jacobson, 1993; LaGrow & Weessies, 1994) is no longer reliable in all situations (see the section on Issues of Gap Judgment).

Assessment of Crossings and Detection of Gaps and Uncertainty

Safe, efficient street crossing at unsignalized intersections requires the ability to determine gaps that are crossable or acceptable, and to recognize situations of uncertainty for gap judgments. This section will consider the issues involved in assessing and developing these abilities.

Many people who recently lost their vision require training and experience to become proficient at using their hearing to determine crossable gaps and situations of uncertainty, because even though using hearing has some features in common with using vision, there are some features that are different. For example, like visual information, which is affected by visual conditions such as fog or glare, auditory information about the approaching vehicles can be affected by acoustic conditions (see Volume 1, Chapter 4). However, when using vision for making crossing decisions, the approaching vehicles cannot be seen beyond blockage, but they may still be audible. And, unlike visual information about the approaching vehicles, the sound of approaching vehicles can be masked and even obliterated by sounds that emanate from places that are nowhere near the approaching vehicles, such as the sound of vehicles receding in the opposite direction, airplanes, lawn equipment, or construction equipment. Students need to learn when the masking sound or acoustic conditions are such that auditory detection of approaching vehicles has been compromised enough to cause an uncertainty for gap judgments. This can be taught by providing the student with experiences such as observing how the sound of one car can make it impossible to hear another car until it is very close.

In addition, students who rely on hearing for street-crossing decisions need to be able to recognize when a situation of uncertainty for gap judgment exists even when it is quiet. Students can be taught to recognize when a situation of uncertainty for gap judgment exists by using the Procedure to Develop Judgment of the Detection of Traffic (see Sidebar 12.2) after they learn to determine the width of various streets and how much time they need to cross them (Sauerburger, 2006). The procedure to develop judgment of the detection of traffic uses the Timing Method for Assessing the Detection of Vehicles (TMAD) (see Sidebar 12.3) to provide students with objective feedback about their ability to hear approaching vehicles in various conditions.

People with both functional vision and hearing may find that in some situations, such as in noisy environments, their vision provides more reliable information for gap judgment than their hearing. In other situations, such as when the vision is limited or when vehicles can be heard but cannot be seen beyond a hill, their hearing provides more reliable information. As already explained, there are also situations where neither vision nor hearing is sufficient for gap judgment. Students need to learn when to use which sense, and when neither is reliable—feedback from the TMAD can be useful for helping them evaluate the effectiveness of their vision and hearing.

Pedestrians who use vision to detect approaching vehicles and judge if gaps are crossable may need to learn how to judge the approaching time of vehicles, how to scan or glance efficiently, and how to assess gaps in multiple lanes or from multiple directions. The ability to judge the approach time of vehicles can be assessed and developed using the Timing Method for Assessing the Speed and Distance of Vehicles (TMASD) (see Sidebar 12.4).

For streets with traffic coming from two directions, students should also develop an efficient strategy for scanning to determine when the street is clear (or the gap is crossable) in both directions. Once the road appears to be clear or crossable, the student scans toward the traffic coming in the nearest lanes, then approaches the other half of the street while attending to traffic from the other direction. People with less than 5 degrees of central vision usually need to scan more slowly than they did when they had more vision because otherwise they will miss seeing even large objects. If they glance too quickly, they often miss seeing cars that are approaching from about two car lengths to their left (where the driver would be unable to stop if the student suddenly started to cross). People with a central scotoma also have a problem glancing quickly for cars, even after they've become skillful with eccentric viewing, because they cannot see objects of low contrast at a distance unless the object moves. Thus, they cannot glance quickly toward the left or right to see if there are any cars coming—they need to learn to hold their gaze long enough to see if there are any vehicles moving. These skills can be taught using scanning practice with feedback about whether the student misses seeing any of the approaching vehicles.

SIGNALIZED INTERSECTIONS

The functioning and complexity of traffic signals have changed significantly as computer control has become more prevalent, and signal functioning can be expected to continue changing and becoming more interactive and complex. Among the skills and knowledge that students need to have for crossings at signalized intersections are accurate information about functioning of modern traffic signals, including their unpredictability, techniques for finding and using pedestrian pushbuttons to provide adequate time to cross, and how to cross with the near parallel traffic. Students need to also understand

Procedure to Develop Judgment of the Detection of Traffic

This procedure teaches people to be able to recognize situations where they cannot detect traffic well enough to know if there is a sufficient gap to cross. A prerequisite is that students must understand how much time they need to cross streets of various widths.

1. Go to an intersection that has frequent but intermittent traffic (that is, traffic with sufficient gaps).

2. Have the students determine the street's width and understand how much time they need to cross (one of the most common reasons for students being unable to recognize situations of uncertainty for gap judgment is a lack of understanding of their need for time to cross).

3. Have the students try to judge whether they can hear or see the traffic well enough to know when it is clear enough to cross or, conversely, whether the vehicles are appearing without enough warning (there is a situation of uncertainty for gap judgments). Allow them as much time as they need to observe and listen, and perhaps prompt them with questions about the traffic such as "If you had started to cross just before you heard (or saw) that car (that is, when it was still quiet or you didn't realize something was coming), would you have finished your crossing before it passed, or would it have to slow down to avoid hitting you? Listen to (or watch) the approaching traffic as long as you need, and tell me if you think you can hear (or see) all vehicles here well enough to know you have time to cross, or if you think some of them aren't audible (or visible) until they are too close."

Note: Students should be judging conditions when it is quiet (or, if they are using vision, when the visibility is good). Many students who rely on hearing to cross are unaware of the presence of noise and how much it impacts their ability to

hear approaching traffic—if they try to draw conclusions about how well they hear traffic when there is masking noise, encourage them to notice that there is a noise present (an airplane, receding car, lawnmower, etc.), and notice the effect that the noise has on their ability to hear the approaching traffic.

4. Use the timing method for assessing the detection of vehicles (TMAD) to provide them with feedback to help them improve their judgment.

Note: Many students are able to understand the effect of noise on their ability to hear approaching traffic by simply noticing how close the vehicles can get before they are heard when there is a masking sound from receding vehicles or other noise. For students who have difficulty understanding this, it can be effective to use the TMAD to compare the detection time of vehicles that approach when it is quiet to those that approach when it is noisy.

5. Repeat this procedure of providing feedback and testing their judgment under a variety of conditions, until they can accurately judge when the conditions are such that they can recognize when it is clear to cross, and when they cannot. Conditions in which their judgment is tested should include those in which they are able to hear or see the traffic well enough, and those where they cannot, to ensure they can tell the difference.

Note that the conditions (masking sounds, lighting conditions, etc.) must remain relatively steady long enough to test whether the student judged the situation accurately.

To test a variety of conditions, you can go to various intersections, or vary the conditions at one intersection (for example, with various masking sounds, or objects to block the sound or the view).

SIDEBAR 12.3

Timing Method for Assessing Detection of Vehicles (TMAD)

This procedure answers the question: "Can I see/hear vehicles far enough away to be certain that when it is quiet, it is clear to cross?"

PROCEDURE

1. Determine the time needed for the crossing, either by an estimation based on walking speed and the width of the street, or by timing several crossings and using the longest time (do not use the average time, since you are looking for the worst-case scenario).

2. While standing at the curb, wait until no approaching vehicles are detected (a perceived lull in traffic). If you depend on hearing, this should be at a time when you think it is quiet enough to hear approaching traffic sufficiently.

3. Start a stopwatch when something is seen or heard that might be an approaching vehicle.

4. Stop the watch when the approaching vehicle passes in front of you. If the time recorded is less time than you need to cross (the time determined in step 1), then you know that if you had started to cross just before it was detected, the vehicle would have reached you before you finished your crossing. If the recorded time is longer than your crossing time, you would have completed the crossing before the vehicle arrived, even if you had started just before it was detected.

5. Continue timing the detection of approaching vehicles until sufficient samples have been taken to conclude whether you can detect vehicles well enough to know when there is no vehicle approaching close or fast enough to reach you before you finish your crossing.

   a. If you started the timer the instant you first detected anything that might possibly be a vehicle, yet a vehicle reached you in less time than you need to cross, there is no need to continue. You now know you cannot detect all the vehicles sufficiently under the condition that it was detected, and you should consider alternatives, or be aware that if you cross there, you are depending on drivers to see and avoid you.

   b. If you detected all the vehicles, including one of the "worst cars"[1] with enough warning to allow you time to cross, then you can conclude that you can cross there with confidence under those conditions.

---

[1] The "worst cars" are those vehicles that reach you in the shortest time once you detect them. We want to know whether even the "worst cars" can be detected with enough warning. Thus, we continue to time our detection of approaching vehicles until we are satisfied that we have timed the approach of at least one of the "worst cars." That is, we continue until we are confident that if we timed the approach of any more cars, we would be very unlikely to find one that reaches us in less time than the cars we have already observed.

---

that even when using best practice techniques there may not be adequate time or information available to cross at some intersections and learn methods for determining where and when that is the case, and be prepared with alterna- tives. They also need information about accessible pedestrian signals, regulations regarding accessibility, and strategies for advocating for accessibility features when needed (AER O&M Division, 2006).

Timing Method for Assessing Speed and Distance of Vehicles (TMASD)

This procedure answers the question "Can I determine the speed and distance of approaching vehicles well enough to know when they are sufficiently far or slow that it is clear enough to cross?"

PROCEDURE

1. Define an arbitrary length of time, which we will call X seconds. If the purpose of this procedure is for you to learn to judge when you have a gap long enough to cross, X seconds should be the time needed to cross, including some clearance time (see note below). If you simply want to improve your judgment of the speed and distance of traffic, X seconds can be any randomly selected time.

2. Stand at the curb and, as a vehicle or vehicles approach, try to judge (based on their speed and distance) when you feel that you could still start crossing and reach the other side with sufficient clearance time before the first vehicle reaches you (or try to judge when a given vehicle is X seconds away). Start a stopwatch when you think it is the last possible moment that you could safely start a crossing (or when you think that a given vehicle will reach you in exactly X seconds).

3. Stop the watch when the vehicle reaches you. If the lapsed time is significantly longer or shorter than X seconds, you did not accurately perceive or judge the vehicle's speed, distance, or both (or you do not have a good understanding of your crossing time).

   Use this feedback to modify when you start the timer the next time.

   Note: If a vehicle changes speed while being timed, disregard that trial, since in that situation it is not possible to know whether you judged its initial speed and distance accurately.

4. Continue to judge the vehicles as in steps 2–3, with the goal of improving your judgment until you can discern when the vehicles, regardless of their speed, are approximately X seconds away from you (that is, you will start the stopwatch for faster vehicles when they are further from you than you will for slower vehicles). (Accuracy can be expected to be within one second of the arbitrary time X—see note below.)

Many people will simply start the timer every time the nearest vehicle passes a certain landmark. Although this is an effective alternative strategy that can be used by people who cannot develop the ability to judge the speed and distance of vehicles, doing it during this training will not enable the development of an accurate judgment of the speed and distance of vehicles because it does not provide any feedback about that judgment.

If your judgment does not improve, perhaps you are unable to perceive the speed and distance of vehicles accurately because of impaired depth perception or acuity or you are unable to cognitively process the speed and distance; in such cases, you should consider alternatives to determine when there is enough of a gap in approaching traffic to start crossing. One such alternative is to choose a landmark (such as a driveway, pole, or tree) at a distance such that even the fastest vehicles take more time to reach you from that spot than you need to cross.

HOW TO DETERMINE HOW MANY SECONDS IS X SECONDS

When developing judgment of gaps for crossing, X seconds is typically the time needed to cross either the whole street (for analyzing traffic from the right) or half the street (for analyzing traffic

(continued on next page)

from the left), plus a safety margin (*clearance time*), plus an extra second to allow for error.

The one-second error margin is needed because most people can learn to make this judgment accurately within 1 second or less. That is, they can determine when the vehicle is *X* seconds away, give or take 1 second or less.

The safety margin and clearance time is the time from when you complete the crossing until the first vehicle passes your crosswalk. The preferred clearance time will vary, depending on the situation and the person. People may want more clearance time for fast-moving traffic than

they do for slow traffic, and cautious people may want a longer clearance time than do high risk takers.

The crossing time, preferred clearance time, and error margin should all be considered when determining how many seconds *X* will be. For example, if you need 6 seconds to cross and want a safety margin and clearance time of 3 seconds, you want to be sure the traffic is at least 9 seconds away when you start to cross. Thus, your *X* should be 10 seconds, so that if you misjudge a car by 1 second, you'd still have the full 9 seconds of clearance that you want.

How Traffic Signals Have Changed

The traffic signal controller at each intersection is a computer with complex programming, often interlinked with other controllers along a traffic corridor. Many intersections today are part of an Intelligent Transportation System (ITS) controlled from a Transportation or Traffic Management Center (TMC). TMCs were first installed to provide freeway monitoring and incident clearance, and in some locales that is still the focus of the TMC; however, many TMCs also can adjust signals and signal timing along surface streets (not freeways) to improve traffic flow, or to provide faster travel for an emergency vehicle. In other words, it is possible for signal timing to be quickly changed from a center located miles from the intersection, at any time of the day or night (Hicks, 1999).

Traffic Signal Functioning

In order to discuss the functioning of traffic signals, it is necessary to use accurate terms for the various sections of the traffic signal sequence. A signal "cycle" encompasses the entire set of potential traffic movements at an intersection. A typi-

cal simple cycle, for example, could include green, then yellow, and red for one street, followed by green, then yellow, and red for the other street. Each set of traffic movements in that cycle is called a *phase*. The cycle that was just described has two phases—one for each street. The phases may then be broken down into segments called "intervals," which are the parts of the cycle during which the signal indications do not change, such as the green or "right-of-way" interval, yellow or "vehicular change" interval, and the red or "clearance" interval. Another example might be the intervals of the pedestrian phase, such as the Walk interval, the pedestrian change interval (flashing Don't Walk), and the Don't Walk interval.

Traffic signal control logic fits into two general categories: *pre-timed signals*, which are also sometimes called *fixed-time signals*, and *actuated signals*.

Pre-Timed Signals

Pre-timed signals have a consistent and regularly repeated sequence of signal indications and are common in central business districts of major cities. This type of control, and its predictability, had a strong impact on the development of the field of orientation and mobility.

Actuated Signals

At *actuated signals*, the duration of some or all of the signal intervals varies from cycle to cycle, or some phases may be omitted during a cycle, depending on the vehicular and pedestrian traffic detected at the intersection. Traffic-actuated control of intersections is now common, with some engineers estimating that 95 percent of all signals are traffic actuated (D. Fullerton, personal communication, March 9, 2005; J. Hereford, personal communication, March 8, 2005). Where signals are actuated, there are detectors for some or all of the traffic. It is also possible for a street or intersection to operate on a pre-timed basis at some times, and on fully actuated or semiactuated control at other times.

Actuation is based on the detection of traffic. There are a number of different types of traffic detectors. At this time, vehicle detectors are usually magnetic loops buried in the roadway or video detectors mounted overhead. For pedestrians, the most common type of pedestrian detector is a *pedestrian pushbutton*.

At locations where pedestrian pushbuttons are installed, the pedestrian needs to interact with the signal by pushing the button in order to get a pedestrian phase. Pedestrians need to push the pedestrian button to get the Walk signal and enough time to cross the street. The green phase programmed for a single car may be as short as 5 seconds, which is just enough time for one car to move through the intersection, and not long enough for pedestrians to safely cross more than a lane or two. If pedestrians push the pushbutton, rather than 5 to 7 seconds for a single car, they will get a longer calculated time based on typical pedestrian walking speed to cross the street, but not unless the intersection "knows" the pedestrian is there.

If the intersection was designed for pedestrian use, there will usually be a pedestrian signal. Pedestrian signals are installed where pedestrians may not be able to see the vehicular signals or where the vehicle signal may provide incorrect or misleading information to pedestrians. However, some jurisdictions do not design all or even a majority of their intersections for pedestrians, and do not provide pedestrian signals or pushbuttons, even though the signal is actuated. Pedestrians at these intersections are not assured of having enough time to cross because the green signal for the vehicular traffic may not be long enough for them to cross the street.

Semi-actuated intersections.   At *semi-actuated intersections*, the major street has a green signal unless there is traffic on the side street. An intersection is called semi-actuated because only the minor street has sensors or detectors in it. A car on the side street triggers a detector, traffic on the major street is then given a red signal and the side street is given a green signal to allow the vehicle on the side street to pull out. The signal on the main street doesn't turn red unless traffic is detected on the side street. This is very common on arterial roadways, where there may be long periods of time where no traffic pulls out of a side street. Enough time for pedestrians to cross the major street is provided only in response to a pedestrian pushing the pushbutton.

Fully actuated intersections.   At *fully actuated intersections*, detectors are installed for each lane of traffic, and usually for pedestrians. Signal phases and cycles are highly variable with the sequence and timing changing constantly, depending on the traffic detected in each lane moment by moment. The signal phase for each lane or movement, including the pedestrian phase, may be omitted if there are no vehicles or pedestrians detected. Some signal controllers even extend the vehicular green signal if a car is approaching and is moving too fast to stop safely.

Coordinated Systems

A coordinated system comprises a number of consecutive signalized intersections along an arterial street where the signals are timed together, possibly through a TMC. Signals can be coordinated for several miles to keep the traffic moving, "to maintain the progression between signals" (Federal Highway Administration, 2004). This is quite common, particularly at rush hours. In a coordinated system of traffic signals, the controller may give a short green phase to vehicles on the side street and hold the pedestrian phase until the next cycle, if the pedestrian phase would interfere with the coordination and traffic progression. Pedestrians who are blind or visually impaired may be unaware that the pedestrian phase has been omitted.

For example, a blind or visually impaired pedestrian wants to cross the arterial street after getting off the bus at a crossing with a traffic signal that has a pedestrian pushbutton but no accessible pedestrian signals (APS). He uses his knowledge of signal and traffic patterns to determine the time to cross. He pushes the pedestrian pushbutton and gets ready to cross and hears a car waiting on the side street beside him. However, the system controller determines that it is possible to provide 8 seconds for a vehicle to pull out without interfering with the coordination with other signals on the arterial, but the pedestrian phase, at 22 seconds long, would interfere with the traffic flow, so the pedestrian phase is held until the next cycle.

The pedestrian who is blind or visually impaired may hear the vehicle beside him pull out, assume he has a Walk signal and enough time to reach the other side, and start to cross. BUT he may not have a Walk, and the perpendicular traffic on the arterial receives a green in less than 10 seconds, before he can complete crossing three of the five lanes. The pedestrian was supposed to wait for the next cycle, when the visual Walk was displayed, and pedestrian time is allowed in the cycle. If pedestrians cannot see the visual signal, and no accessible (audible and/or vibrotactile) signal is provided, those pedestrians have no

way to know that the pedestrian phase has been skipped. The typical technique of using the vehicle movement as a cue to start crossing does not work at those locations. The pedestrian who is blind or visually impaired may be caught in the middle of the street when a "platoon" of vehicles approaching a green signal reaches the intersection traveling at or above the speed limit. There is no way for pedestrians who are blind or visually impaired to know when the controller has held the pedestrian phase, unless an APS is installed. On O&M specialist or pedestrian who is blind or visually impaired evaluating an intersection may not see this situation occur in several hours of observation; the only way to know about the potential is to discuss the intersection timing and phasing with traffic engineers responsible for the programming and timing. Sidebar 12.5 provides another example of an intersection timing situation that could be dangerous to pedestrians who are blind or visually impaired.

Preemption

When *emergency vehicle preemption or transit vehicle priority preemption* is installed, an emergency vehicle or transit vehicle approaching the intersection can change the signal cycle to allow continued movement of that vehicle. Emergency preemption is even allowed to shorten the length of the flashing Don't Walk, assuming that pedestrians will move quickly out of the roadway if an emergency vehicle is approaching. The problem is that the preemption changes the signal, so in addition to the emergency vehicle seeing a green signal, all the cars on that street also have a green signal. There is normally no way for a pedestrian or a driver to know when preemption is in effect, thus pedestrians do not know that they have to hurry, and drivers are not expecting to see pedestrians in the crosswalk. Transit preemption is allowed to shorten the Walk indication, but is not allowed to shorten the flashing Don't

SIDEBAR 12.5

When Observing an Intersection Is Not Enough

The following situation is an example of how observation of an intersection alone may not be sufficient to judge the timing and phasing of traffic and signal cycles. An orientation and mobility (O&M) specialist was evaluating routes to teach clients to get to their jobs at a large hospital and went to an intersection that had pedestrian pushbuttons and obvious loops in the roadway. However, after timing the crossings for a number of phases at different times of the day, whether the pedestrian pushbutton was pressed or not pressed made no difference. There was adequate time for a pedestrian to cross on every phase without using the pushbuttons. He decided to ignore the pushbuttons because using them would require his clients to deviate from their approach path along the sidewalk.

However, as a precaution, he called the local traffic engineer to confirm the timing of the intersection. The engineer explained that the intersection operated as pretimed during the week, but was actuated on the weekends. On the weekends, the signal for crossing the major street had a minimum green time of 5 seconds, which was not enough time for pedestrians to complete the crossing. It was essential for pedestrians to use the pushbuttons on the weekends. Since the students were going to be working some weekend shifts at the hospital, simply observing the intersection at various weekday times could have led the O&M specialist to teach dangerous crossing techniques. Calling the local traffic engineer can be essential to understanding intersection timing.

Walk indication, so pedestrians should have time to complete their crossing in a transit preemption situation.

Vehicle Signalization and Phasing Plans

In teaching and making street crossings, some understanding of typical signalization plans and traffic signal terminology, in addition to the above, is helpful. Signal controllers and controller programs are sophisticated. Two to eight phases are commonly used, depending on the complexity of the intersection, although some controllers can provide up to 40 phases to serve complex intersections or sets of intersections.

In particular, it is important to understand the differences in what are called permissive and protected turn indications for vehicles, the effect of vehicular phasing plans on pedestrian phas-

ing, and how that affects pedestrian crossing. Since signal phasing plans affect the timing and legality of pedestrian crossings; an understanding of the signal-phasing possibilities is essential in order for O&M specialists and pedestrians who are blind or visually impaired to correctly analyze and interpret intersections.

Each signalized intersection is governed by both a signal-phasing plan and timing plan. The phasing plan shows the sequence of various traffic movements and which traffic moves concurrently. The timing plan shows the minimum and maximum length of time programmed for each phase. Some of the most common terminology and phasing plans are described in this section based on descriptions in the *Traffic Control Devices Handbook* (Pline, 2001) and the *Signalized Intersections: Informational Guide* (FHWA, 2004). A sample phasing and timing plan is also provided at the end of this section.

Two-Phase (Permissive-Only Left Turn Phasing)

Two-phase signals are the most basic, in which no vehicular turn arrows are provided. For example, all traffic on the north-south street has a phase, including pedestrian traffic and vehicles turning right and left, then all traffic on the east-west street has its phase. Left turns are made, when gaps in opposing traffic permit, which is called permissive phasing. There may be a separate left turn lane, but there will not be a separate time in the signal phase for turns from that lane. As noted above, the timing plan will be a portion on the phasing plan, but can vary. Two-phase intersections can be pre-timed or traffic-actuated.

With permissive phasing, turning vehicles are legally required to yield to pedestrians in the crosswalk, however, many do not. This is probably because drivers are focusing on the oncoming traffic and judging the gap in traffic and don't check the crosswalk for pedestrians before they begin turning (Stapin, Lococo, Byington, & Harkey, 2001). This may be a problem for pedestrians who are blind or visually impaired, particularly when making clockwise crossings, because they will be crossing the lanes that the left turning driver will be turning into later in the light cycle, when there are typically more gaps in a parallel stream of traffic. The benefit of two phase signals for pedestrians who are blind or visually impaired is that all of the traffic (in both directions) on a street begins moving at the same time, except for the possibility of vehicles turning right on red, so it may be easier to detect the surge of traffic on the parallel street.

Protected-Only Left Turn Phasing

Protected-only left turn phasing provides a separate phase for left turning traffic and allows left turns only when green left turn arrows are displayed. There is no pedestrian movement or vehicular traffic movement that conflicts with left turning cars during the left turn arrows. A separate left turn lane and a separate signal indication for that lane is usually provided. For example, traffic turning from northbound to westbound may have a left turn arrow and can turn at the same time as traffic turning from southbound to eastbound. All other vehicular traffic, and pedestrians, have a red or Don't Walk signal during this turning movement. Then the turning traffic is stopped with a red signal, often a red arrow, and all straight-through and right turning north-south traffic moves, including pedestrians. During the next phase, either all east-west traffic begins moving or, if there are protected turns for that road also, the protected left turn traffic may move before the straight-through east-west traffic.

Protected-only left turn phasing is considered safer for pedestrians in general (Zegeer et al., 2002), because no cars are allowed to turn left across the crosswalk during the pedestrian phase. The above paragraph described *leading protected* left turns. The left turn phase can also be provided at the end of the straight-through traffic movement; those are called *lagging protected* left turns. Lagging turn phases, rather than leading turn phases, are somewhat better for pedestrians who are blind or visually impaired; the surge of straight-through and right turning traffic first, just after the traffic has stopped on the perpendicular street, can be easier to detect. Lagging turns are less commonly used because of vehicular safety issues related to driver confusion at the end of the left turning movement and the need for some more complicated signal phasing.

At intersections with protected left turn intervals, pedestrians who are blind or visually impaired may mistakenly begin crossing with the sound of the left turning cars moving parallel to their path. Drivers turning across the crosswalk are not required to, nor expecting to, have to yield to pedestrians when turning with a green arrow signal. However, in protected-only phasing, all left turning traffic will be held during the pedestrian phase, minimizing concerns about turning traffic that were discussed in the earlier section on permissive-only phasing.

Protected-Permissive Left Turn Phasing

Protected-permissive left turn phasing are commonly combined at fully actuated intersections (and called PPLT by traffic engineers), to allow for the most efficient movement of traffic. The phasing for PPLT is most complicated, and intersections using PPLT can be extremely difficult to decipher by listening. This type of phasing can be implemented in many different ways, and the timing and sequencing often change with every cycle. For example, when vehicles are waiting in the left turn lane on the south approach (facing north), they may receive a left turn arrow at the same time the straight-through traffic on that approach receives a green signal. All traffic on the north leg (traffic facing south) will still have a red signal for 5 to 30 seconds or longer, depending on the amount of traffic in the left turn lane from the south leg (traffic turning from northbound to westbound). After a programmed time (set through the timing plan), or after all left turning vehicles have cleared, through movement in both directions will begin, but left turn lanes may still have a green ball signal (rather than an arrow), so vehicles can turn from those lanes when there is a gap in oncoming traffic.

Protected-permissive phasing can be sequenced in various ways and the variations have implications for blind or visually impaired travelers because the pedestrian phase is provided at different times, depending on the sequence of the left turn phases. In general, the pedestrian phase is provided when the traffic in the near parallel lane begins moving (see the description in the section on Using Near-Lane Parallel Traf-

fic). However, the two parallel pedestrian phases (the ones crossing the same street) may be provided at different times. Pedestrians need to be aware that vehicles may be legally turning right or left across the crosswalk during the pedestrian phase, but are legally required to yield to pedestrians. However, vehicles commonly do not yield to pedestrians.

Split Phasing

In split phasing, the two opposing approaches of vehicular traffic on one roadway are timed consecutively rather than concurrently, so all traffic movements from the north are at a different time than all movements from the south. This means that all the southbound traffic, including right and left turning traffic, will move together. A protected left turn arrow is usually displayed for the left turning traffic, so drivers do not expect pedestrians at that time. Generally, at locations with split phasing, pedestrians on the parallel crosswalks are given a Walk at different times. For example, pedestrians on the west side of the intersection receive a Walk when the traffic from the north (southbound, straight-through, and turning right and left) is moving; pedestrians on the east side of the intersection receive a Walk when the traffic from the south (straight-through, right turning, and left turning, generally northbound) traffic begins moving.

Where there is split phase timing, if the pedestrians who are visually impaired or blind are not cognizant of only using the "near-lane parallel" traffic, the surge of parallel vehicles could be mistaken as indicating the onset of the Walk interval, and pedestrians could cross into the path of left turning vehicles. In addition, the heavy flow of turning traffic, often dual lanes, can be mistaken for the surge of traffic on the street beside the blind pedestrian, when the traffic is actually on the street the pedestrian is crossing.

Right Turn Overlap Phasing

To add to the difficulty of interpreting traffic at busy intersections, a right turn overlap may be provided at any time when other traffic moving at the intersection does not conflict with the right turn movement. A right turn overlap is an additional opportunity for traffic to turn right and is provided by displaying a right turn arrow for traffic during another traffic movement, The most common use of right turn overlap is when right turning traffic receives a green arrow during the left turn arrow for traffic on the cross street. There is no conflict between these vehicles; pedestrians are not legally allowed to cross either street during those protected phases and drivers will not be prepared to stop for them.

Blind or visually impaired pedestrians waiting to cross with the parallel street on their right side could step into fast moving right turn traffic that has a green arrow indication, if they mistakenly begin crossing with the left turning vehicles. Or pedestrians waiting to cross with the parallel street on their left may hear the right turning cars moving and incorrectly believe that there is also a green signal for the straight-through traffic; if so, they may begin crossing lanes that are about to receive a green signal.

Pedestrian Signals and Timing

Pedestrian signals are installed to provide information to pedestrians about when they are supposed to begin crossing an intersection and when enough time has been provided in the signal cycle for the "typical pedestrian" to cross at that crossing. Pedestrian signals display the underlying pedestrian timing. See Sidebar 12.6 for an explanation of timing calculations. Often pedestrian signals are installed where left or right turn arrows are used, since, as discussed above, pedestrians are not supposed to be in the crosswalk when a vehicle has a green arrow to turn

across the crosswalk. In most states, if pedestrian signals are installed for a crosswalk, it is legal to begin crossing only during a Walk indication (National Committee on Uniform Traffic Laws and Ordinances [NCUTLO], 2000).

Typical Pedestrian Signal Operation

Pedestrian signals in the United States are often misunderstood, and signs are usually posted to explain the signal, as shown in Figure 12.24. With that sign, pedestrians are instructed to push the button for a Walk signal and to begin crossing during the walk interval, which is symbolized by the white "walking man" symbol. During the flashing Don't Walk, shown by an orange flashing hand, the instruction on the sign is "Don't start, finish crossing if started." Many newer signals have a pedestrian countdown signal feature which provides a numerical countdown of the time left during the flashing Don't Walk signal. At the end of the flashing Don't Walk, a solid or "steady" orange hand symbol is displayed. Pedestrians are supposed to have completely finished crossing the roadway. In many other countries a "green man/red man" pedestrian signal is used, with somewhat similar timing.

As mentioned earlier, the Uniform Vehicle Code (UVC) in the United States provides standard laws that form the basis for traffic laws in the

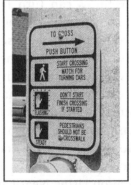

Figure 12.24. A Standard Pedestrian Sign

How Pedestrian Crossing Times Are Calculated

The Walk sign comes on and the pedestrian starts to cross the major street, all eight lanes of it, at an intersection with a minor street. She has pushed the pedestrian pushbutton, so is sure it is safe. Suddenly, long before she is halfway across, the light starts flashing an orange hand—a warning, but of what? Suddenly the pedestrian realizes she is in . . . the Twilight Zone!

A bit dramatic but oddly true. How are these times calculated, and what do those flashing lights—or *signal indications*—actually mean?

REGULATION
Traffic signal pedestrian indications are governed by standards and guidance set forth in a guidebook issued by the Federal Highway Administration (FHWA) called the *Manual on Uniform Traffic Control Devices* (MUTCD). Should they be sued, states, counties, and municipalities leave themselves open to lawsuits if they are out of compliance with the standards laid out in the MUTCD.

The Walk indication used to be the word "walk" in white. Several years ago FHWA decided to get away from words in signal indications and to use symbols. Hence the current and ubiquitous walking person symbol in white has replaced Walk, and an orange hand is the symbol for the old Don't Walk.

The MUTCD also spells out standards and guidance for pedestrian timing.

THE TIMING OF THE WALK INTERVAL
The walk interval is intended for pedestrians to start their crossing. The pedestrian clearance time is intended to allow pedestrians who started crossing during the walk interval to complete their crossing. (MUTCD, 2009, Section 4E.06, paragraph 13)

In addition, the MUTCD provides the following guidance regarding the length of the walk interval in Section 4E.06, paragraphs 11 & 12:

Guidance:
Except as provided in Paragraph 12, the walk interval should be at least 7 seconds in length so that pedestrians will have adequate opportunity to leave the curb or shoulder before the pedestrian clearance time begins.

Option:
12 If pedestrian volumes and characteristics do not require a 7-second walk interval, walk intervals as short as 4 seconds may be used.

When crossing an "arterial roadway," the short Walk indication is followed by a longer Flashing Don't Walk (FDW or orange hand) indication. This indicates the pedestrian clearance interval.

THE PEDESTRIAN CLEARANCE INTERVAL
Guidance:
07 . . . the pedestrian clearance time should be sufficient to allow a pedestrian crossing in the crosswalk who left the curb or shoulder at the end of the Walking Person (symbolizing Walk) signal indication to travel at a walking speed of 3.5 feet per second to at least the far side of the traveled way or to a median of sufficient width for pedestrians to wait. (MUTCD, 2009, Section 4E.06, paragraph 7)

10 Where pedestrians who walk slower than 3.5 feet per second, or pedestrians who use wheelchairs, routinely use the crosswalk, a walking speed of less than 3.5 feet per second should be considered in determining the pedestrian clearance time. (MUTCD, 2009, Section 4E.06, paragraph 10)

So, that time is calculated by the width of the street, divided by a walking speed of *3.5 feet per second* (an "average" speed).

(continued on next page)

SIDEBAR 12.6 *(Continued)*

So if we have 10-foot-wide lanes (many are 11 or 12 feet wide), our eight-lane street would be *80 feet wide.*

80 feet/3.5 feet per second = 23 seconds

That means that in this instance we would have 23 seconds of FDW or pedestrian clearance time.

THE CLEARANCE INTERVAL

This is what traffic engineers call the period when the vehicular indication (the traffic signal) is yellow. It is timed to allow cars that have entered the intersection late in the green to *clear* the intersection before a red signal indication is shown. Of course, it also is intended to warn oncoming drivers to slow and prepare to stop.

During this period, which may last 3 or 4 seconds, the pedestrian indication is typically a *solid orange hand,* or *steady Don't Walk.*

The opposing traffic flow has not yet begun. The solid orange hand is also shown during the opposing traffic flow. Pedestrians need to be out of the street during the (vehicular) clearance interval.

IMPLICATIONS

It is important that travelers who are blind be aware of the visual signal indications. Many sighted people are not clear about them and, meaning well, will sometimes shout something like "Watch out—it is flashing red!" Only with knowledge can the traveler maintain composure and confidence.

Also, this information is fundamental to understanding the variability of the timing of actuated signals, and what pedestrian pushbuttons actually do, both for O&M specialists and for the pedestrians who are blind or visually impaired that they are teaching.

---

individual states. The UVC specifically limits pedestrian right-of-way where pedestrian signals are installed (NCUTLO, 2000). UVC § 11-501(a) requires pedestrians to "obey the instructions of any official traffic control device specifically applicable to such pedestrian" and UVC 11-203, Pedestrian-control Signals, explains the meaning of the pedestrian control signals. As shown on the sign described earlier, at locations with pedestrian signals, the pedestrians are legally crossing only if they begin their crossing during the Walk signal. It is legal to complete their crossing during the flashing Don't Walk, if they began crossing during Walk, but it is not legal to begin their crossing during the flashing or steady Don't Walk signals. Since pedestrians who are blind or visually impaired are often delayed in starting their crossing because they need to wait to be sure vehicles are

moving through the intersection, or that no vehicle is about to turn across their path of travel, they may often begin crossings late and "illegally," during the flashing Don't Walk signal (see Sidebar 12.7).

As discussed above in the section on vehicular phasing, when vehicles have a green arrow signal, they are allowed to turn in the direction indicated by the arrow and they have the legal right-of-way across the crosswalk at that time, and do not expect to yield to pedestrians. During the pedestrian Walk and flashing Don't Walk intervals, vehicles usually have a "green ball" or "circular green" signal, which usually means that vehicles that are turning are supposed to yield to pedestrians in the crosswalk. However, drivers commonly do not do so. The Walk signal should not be taken as an indication that it is safe to cross without checking vehicle movement either visually or auditorally, and pedestrians should remain alert to turning vehicles during their crossing.

Usually, the pedestrian crossing time begins with the movement of straight-through parallel traffic in the near travel lane. However, there are some types of pedestrian timing that provide for pedestrian movement at different times, generally intended to improve pedestrian access and safety.

Atypical Pedestrian Signal Operation

Leading pedestrian intervals.   Where there is a *leading pedestrian interval* (LPI), the Walk begins 3 to 6 seconds before the vehicular green so pedestrians can establish their presence in the

crosswalk before turning vehicles receive a green. Several studies have documented improved safety for pedestrians and a reduction in conflicts with turning vehicles (FHWA, 2004). However, blind or visually impaired pedestrians who wait for the parallel traffic to begin moving will be crossing behind most other pedestrians, just as vehicles begin to turn across the crosswalk, and when drivers have no reason to expect pedestrians who have been waiting at the curb to begin crossing. In addition, the timing may not be adequate for pedestrians to cross if they wait and begin crossing after vehicles begin moving.

Lagging pedestrian intervals.   With a *lagging pedestrian interval*, the pedestrian Walk begins a

---

SIDEBAR 12.7

What the Pedestrian Pushbutton Does

Traffic engineers sometimes refer to pedestrian pushbuttons as pedestrian "detectors." This phrase accurately describes the function of the pedestrian pushbutton, which alerts the "controller" (the computer that controls the intersection) to the fact that a pedestrian is present.

When a pedestrian pushbutton is installed and when it applies to a major street or "arterial roadway," it does more than "give the pedestrian the Walk signal." In fact, pushing the button can change the timing of the intersection very significantly. Orientation and mobility (O&M) specialists should understand the function of these pedestrian detectors.

- If there is a pedestrian pushbutton:

  - Walk may not be displayed unless the button is pressed.

  - *Pedestrian timing* will *not* be provided unless the pushbutton is pressed.

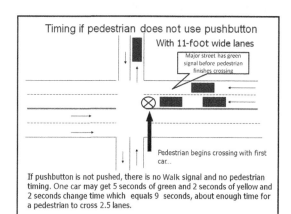

Timing if pedestrian does not use pushbutton
With 11-foot wide lanes

Major street has green signal before pedestrian finishes crossing

Pedestrian begins crossing with first car...

If pushbutton is not pushed, there is no Walk signal and no pedestrian timing. One car may get 5 seconds of green and 2 seconds of yellow and 2 seconds change time which equals 9 seconds, about enough time for a pedestrian to cross 2.5 lanes.

In the above illustration, pedestrians attempting to cross the major roadway have not pushed the pushbutton, so the signal controller, unaware of the pedestrians, applies a vehicular timing. That is, the single car on the parallel (N/S) street will get 5 seconds of green time, followed by 2 seconds of yellow time, followed by 2 seconds of time for the light to change back to green on the arterial. Pedestrians will be in the

(continued on next page)

SIDEBAR 12.7 *(Continued)*

middle of crossing when the light changes against them.

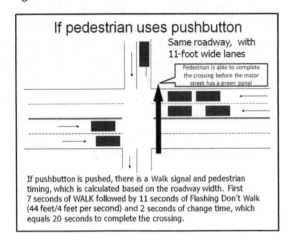

If pedestrian uses pushbutton

Same roadway, with 11-foot wide lanes

Pedestrian is able to complete the crossing before the major street has a green signal

If pushbutton is pushed, there is a Walk signal and pedestrian timing, which is calculated based on the roadway width. First 7 seconds of WALK followed by 11 seconds of Flashing Don't Walk (44 feet/4 feet per second) and 2 seconds of change time, which equals 20 seconds to complete the crossing.

In this illustration, the pedestrians have pushed the button and, when they begin crossing with the surge of the single parallel car next to them, an entirely different timing applies to the same intersection. The Walk indication will last at least 4 seconds, and likely 7 seconds. When the Flashing Don't Walk (FDW) begins, it will last for about 11 seconds. These 11 seconds are based upon the 44-foot width of the street, divided by the 4-foot per second (FPS) rate of the "average walking speed" used by engineers to calculate pedestrian timing. Just as in the prior example, another 2 seconds will be tacked on the end to allow the light to change back to the main street. The total: about 20 seconds!

So pushing the button in this instance gives pedestrians an additional 11 seconds of crossing time, which is a possibly a critical and essential safety margin.

OTHER FACTORS TO CONSIDER

If there were other cars on the side (N/S) street, each car passing over the diamond-shaped sensors would have added about 2 seconds to the timing allocated to that side street. In our first example, the single car got 5 seconds to green time. Two cars would have gotten 7 seconds total, and 3 cars would have gotten 9 seconds (5+2+2) of green time, followed by the yellow clearance and change interval. This variability may mislead pedestrians (with or without visual impairment!) into believing they always have sufficient time to cross the street without using the pushbutton, until they get caught—or worse.

At some intersections, the controller may disable the pedestrian pushbuttons at certain times of the day or week, and bring up Walk indications, with attendant pedestrian-friendly timings, on every cycle. This may be temporary, however, and the intersection may change back to an "actuated mode" at other times when fewer pedestrians are expected.

The moral of the story:

O&M specialists must be careful about what they teach, and not trust casual observations. Talk to the engineer who controls the intersection.

few seconds after the vehicular green. This can be an advantage to vehicles when there are lots of pedestrians or one-way turning movement. It is not considered advantageous to pedestrians.

Exclusive pedestrian phase. An *exclusive pedestrian phase*, also *called Barnes Dance, scatter light,*

or *pedestrian scramble timing*, provides a completely separate phase for pedestrians. When the pedestrian Walk signal is displayed, all vehicles have a red signal and the pedestrians may cross in all directions, including diagonally. If this type of signalization is provided, No Right Turn on Red (NRTOR) should also be posted, but may not be, and may not be enforced even if posted. If NRTOR is not posted and enforced, there will still be right turning vehicles during the exclusive pedestrian phase. Exclusive phases can be a disadvantage for all pedestrians, if they only wish to cross one of the streets, because they have to wait through both vehicular phases for their turn. For blind or visually impaired pedestrians, exclusive phases can be difficult to recognize and there is no parallel traffic moving to use for alignment during the crossing. However, there is also, if NRTOR is enforced, no turning traffic during the crossing. Pedestrians are typically permitted to travel between diagonal corners if they choose to do so.

Concurrent and Nonconcurrent Phasing

Other terms that are helpful to know and understand are *concurrent* and *nonconcurrent* phases. Phases most commonly run concurrently; for example, a Walk displayed while parallel traffic is moving. When there is nonconcurrent Walk phasing, no other phase is active at the same time, for example, an exclusive pedestrian phase. At locations where the pedestrian Walk is not displayed at the same time that parallel traffic begins moving, the *Signalized Intersections: Informational Guide* (FHWA, 2004) recommends installation of APS to provide information to pedestrians who are blind or visually impaired about when the Walk is displayed.

Intersection Diagram and Phasing Plan

To summarize the discussion of signalization and intersection phasing and timing, let us review a typical intersection diagram and timing plan. Figure 12.25 is an intersection diagram, with the phasing diagram. Table 12.1 is an example of one page of the accompanying signal timing plan, which provides the timing of each of the phases shown on the diagram. These illustrate just two

pages of an 18-page document that is used in programming the signal. These pages show some aspects that are of most interest or concern to O&M specialists.

The intersection diagram (see Figure 12.25) shows the intersection wiring details, the location of signals, poles, sidewalks and curb ramps, detector location, and the intersection phase information. The phase diagram is shown in the upper left section, made up of arrows that describe the phasing set up in the signal controller. At this intersection, protected left turns are provided first (labeled 01 and 05), moving concurrently. The next phase (02 and 06) is north-south traffic, including pedestrians (double-headed arrows with dotted lines, shown beside the vehicular traffic arrows). This is followed by protected left turns for the east-west street (03 and 07). However, note that these left turns are also accompanied by a right turn overlap (the additional arrow in the 03 box). The next phase is for straight-through traffic on the east-west street and for pedestrians traveling east or west on either side of the intersection.

The timing plan (see Table 12.1) provides details about some of the issues described earlier in the discussion of actuated timing. The timing plan sets the times for each phase. The labels at the top of the columns are the lanes and the phases, for example west approach, left turns (moves with east left turns).

In looking at the first column of this chart, the first line is minimum green (min grn) time, which is 4 seconds. That's the minimum time that the green left turn arrow will be on, if there is a one car in the left turn lane. Remember that phase could also be skipped, if there's no car detected in that lane. "Gap, Ext" refers to the amount of gap between vehicles crossing the detectors in order to extend the green time. So if there is another car detected in that lane within 0.5 seconds of the first one, the green is extended to a longer time than the minimum 4 seconds, up to the time shown on the next line (Max 1). If

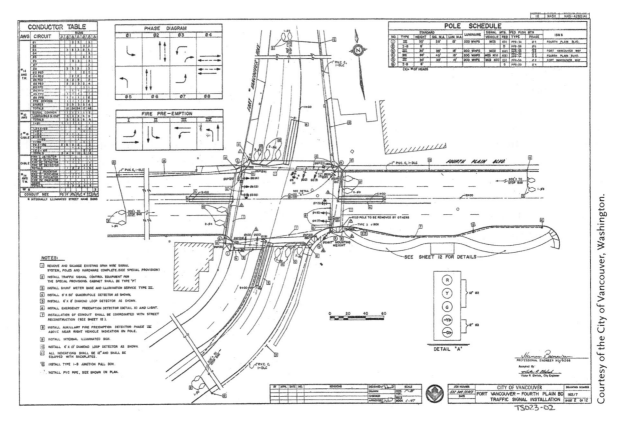

Figure 12.25. Intersection Diagram, Including Phasing Graphic

TABLE 12.1

One Section of an Actual Signal Timing Plan

	WL	E	SL	N	EL	W	NL	S
	1	2	3	4	5	6	7	8
Min Grn	4	4	4	4	4	4	4	4
Gap, Ext	0.5	0.5	0.5	0.5	0.5	0.5	0.5	0.5
Max 1	40	96	24	64	40	96	24	64.5
Max 2								
Yel Clr	4	4	4	4	4	4	4	4
Red Clr	1	1	1	1	1	1	1	1
Walk		6		6		7		7
Ped Clr		21		15		23		15
Red Revt	2	2	2	2	2	2	2	2

Source: City of Vancouver, Washington.

there are a lot of cars in that lane and they keep coming over the detector, the left turn arrow may be displayed for up to 40 seconds (the number shown in Max 1). The "yel clr" and "red clr" lines show the yellow and red clearance time, so there are actually 5 more seconds for that turn lane in the cycle, when the arrow is displayed as yellow, then red.

Then, look at the second column for the straight-through traffic from the east approach, probably moving at the same time as the straight-through traffic from the west approach. This is for a street that is seven lanes wide or about 80–85 feet. The minimum green time is still 4 seconds, and the gap extension is still a half second, but the max green is longer, up to 96 seconds. The min green, yel clr, and red clr add up to 9 seconds, which is the timing for the signal for that street if just one car is detected on that street. That's not enough time for a person to walk across those seven lanes even if they begin to cross with the first car.

The next two rows are important ones for O&M specialists and pedestrians who are blind or visually impaired, the Walk and "ped clr" or pedestrian clearance times. If the pushbutton is pushed, the walk signal is 6 seconds long and the pedestrian clearance time (flashing Don't Walk) is 21 seconds, giving a pedestrian up to 27 seconds to cross that seven-lane roadway. If the pushbutton is not pressed, the Walk is not displayed and the pedestrian timing is *not* called.

The "ped clr" time is a calculated time, based on the width of the street. Typically, that time is calculated at 4 feet per second, as shown in this plan (see Sidebar 12.6 for an explanation of pedestrian signal timing). That time will probably be calculated in the future based on 3.5 feet per second walking speed (FHWA, 2009). The other street is just 60 feet (18 m) wide, and note that the pedestrian clearance time is shorter, 15 seconds (column 4 and 8).

The timing at this intersection completely depends on the traffic. This is where O&M spe-

cialists sometimes get in trouble in analyzing intersections. At that intersection when traffic is heavy, observing the intersection, without seeing the timing plan, could lead someone to decide that there is no need to use the pushbutton because the green time for the vehicles provides plenty of time to cross. While that may be true at that time of day, or on that particular day, since the green time for vehicles could be extended to almost 100 seconds when there is a lot of traffic, the timing plan indicates that it will not be true at some times. At a time with low traffic (midmorning, or evening, or on the weekend), pedestrians may not even get across two lanes of traffic before the signal changes if they do not use the pushbutton. The 14 other pages of the signal timing plan address coordination, emergency preemption timing, times of day for different plans (if they are set up), and other issues, all of which might affect the signal timing. This discussion just looks at one small part of the timing plan.

Analyzing Signalized Intersections

Before and during crossing, pedestrians who are blind or visually impaired should analyze the intersection and features that affect the street-crossing tasks. Some aspects of the crossing task are essentially the same for signalized and unsignalized intersections. These include locating the street, aligning to cross, and maintaining alignment while crossing. The cues available vary depending on width of the street and volume of traffic, but basic techniques remain the same, whether intersections are signalized or not. However, the task of determining when to begin crossing the street is quite different at an unsignalized location from the task at a signalized location.

Signalized intersections are usually characterized by the sound of several cars stopping or starting up together, in alternating flows. However, semi-actuated intersections, when crossing the major street, might sound like an intersection that is not signalized if there is no traffic on the side street, or a pedestrian does not push the button, because the traffic on the major street will not get a red signal unless there is traffic demand on the minor street. In research by Crandall et al. (1998), blind participants crossed at fixed-timed signalized intersections, and were unable to say whether the intersection was controlled by a signal or stop sign.

Finding Landmarks or Pushbuttons

Analysis may include listening to determine features, lane widths, and traffic patterns, and physically exploring the intersection area. For those with low vision, it includes visually scanning in an organized manner to evaluate the area. A systematic method for exploring to find landmarks and pushbuttons at intersections is needed. Jacobson (1993) describes a method for people with visual impairments to familiarize themselves to corner and sidewalk features and landmarks by going to the street edge, then turning around and shorelining along both sidewalks to locate features at corners. Similar techniques may be employed to explore the corner at an intersection to find equipment such as pedestrian pushbuttons and to locate landmarks and cues for alignment.

Clockwise or Counterclockwise Crossing

Before beginning crossing, pedestrians who are visually impaired or blind need to determine whether to cross in a clockwise direction (parallel street on their right) or counterclockwise direction (parallel street on their left). The complete route may affect their decision, as well as traffic patterns at the intersection. Understanding the advantages and disadvantages of each crossing direction needs to be included in instruction.

Disadvantages of Clockwise Crossing

- Traffic clue to begin crossing is lane coming toward pedestrians from across the intersection, which may not be clearly audible until

several seconds after traffic begins moving, delaying pedestrians' start.
- Pedestrians reach the middle of street late in phase and at a time that cars turning on permissive left may be turning across crosswalk.
- RTOR on perpendicular street—drivers are looking left and may be blocking or pulling across the crosswalk at beginning of pedestrian crossing time, when pedestrians are approaching from or waiting on the drivers' right, and may accelerate without ever seeing pedestrians crossing in front of them.

Advantages of Clockwise Crossing

- Perpendicular traffic that is stopped (if several lanes) may provide beginning alignment clue.
- Parallel traffic cannot turn into lane as pedestrians are starting to cross (at a two-way street).
- Cars waiting on the perpendicular street have a clear view of crosswalk (which is across intersection from them) on last part of crossing, which may be helpful if pedestrians are late completing the crossing.
- Drivers of right turning vehicles from parallel street, near the end of the crossing, are more likely to see the cane and may yield.
- Vehicles running the red light on the perpendicular street are likely to be past pedestrians who are blind or visually impaired before the pedestrian begins crossing.

Disadvantages of Counterclockwise Crossing

- Drivers turning right on green may not see a long cane and may beat pedestrians who are blind or visually impaired into crosswalk, delaying pedestrians' start.
- Vehicles running the red light on the perpendicular street might get to crosswalk just as pedestrians begin to cross.

Advantages of Counterclockwise Crossing

- Near lane of traffic is moving in the same direction as the pedestrian, which is easier for some pedestrians to use for alignment. Also, pedestrians can often hear the traffic start up better.

- Idling perpendicular traffic near the end of crossing may help in maintaining alignment.

- RTOR drivers on perpendicular street will be looking left, toward pedestrian when pulling into the crosswalk.

- Left turning traffic (permissive) across crosswalk at the beginning of the walk interval is likely to be blocked by traffic moving in the near lane beside pedestrian.

Lane-by-Lane Analysis

While crossing, pedestrians who are blind or visually impaired need to understand the traffic movement well enough to recognize from what direction conflicting vehicles could come at different times during the crossing (Scheffers & Myers, 2006). The task of determining time to begin crossing includes the discussion of lane-by-lane analysis. Instructors need to help students recognize and think ahead to recognize potential conflicts on each part of the crossing. Before starting to cross, for example if the parallel street is on the pedestrians' left, as they begin to step off, they need to be aware of potential cars running the red light, coming fast from their left, and potential cars turning right across the crosswalk, usually just starting up on the parallel street behind them. Potentially, there could also be a left turning car crossing in front of them as they step off, particularly if there has been a leading protected left turn phase on the parallel street. Then, as they get to the middle of the street, they can use the waiting cars on the perpendicular street as an alignment confirmation. At the last lane, they need to pay attention to cars coming from the right that are potentially making a right turn on red, and may not be planning to actually stop.

Determining When to Begin Crossing

Where pedestrian signals are installed, pedestrians who are blind or visually impaired need to begin to cross during the walk interval, if at all possible. Traffic patterns at many intersections are dangerous if pedestrians are not crossing at the time designed for pedestrians. Understanding the earlier discussion of signals and how they work is essential for O&M specialists and blind or visually impaired pedestrians.

Determining when to cross is particularly difficult where there is no parallel traffic, such as when crossing the through street at three-leg intersections, crossing where there is actuation and intermittent or variable traffic, and crossing where complex vehicular or pedestrian phasing is used, such as split phasing, LPI, or exclusive pedestrian phasing.

Using Pedestrian Pushbuttons

It has become essential for blind or visually impaired pedestrians to use pedestrian pushbuttons effectively. Some common problems with pushbuttons are knowing whether there is a pushbutton, determining which street the pushbutton controls, having to use the pushbutton again if the pedestrian misses the walk interval or the surge of parallel traffic, realigning after using the pushbutton, and not having enough time to get back to the crossing location and get ready before the signal changes.

In research by Barlow et al. (2005), participants who were blind looked for, found, or used the pedestrian pushbuttons on 16.3 percent of actuated crossings in Portland, OR, and 0 percent of crossings in Charlotte, NC. This resulted in a high proportion of crossings during the Don't Walk, which were not covered by any legal provision of right-of-way. Of greater concern, on nearly half (45.4 percent) of all crossings where signals were pedestrian actuated, participants were still in the street when the perpendicular traffic began moving. Participants' responses to questions after their crossings indicated that many did not understand the function of pedestrian pushbuttons, thinking they would make the signal change faster. Many participants stated that they only used pushbuttons when they knew they were there and knew where to find them. At the time of this writing, there were no techniques described in the orientation and mobility texts (other than this volume) for searching for and using pedestrian pushbuttons. The need to use pedestrian pushbuttons can affect all aspects of the street-crossing task.

Strategies for finding and using pushbuttons. It is most effective for pedestrians who are visually impaired or blind to, as much as possible, continue facing the perpendicular street while exploring for the pole. Where new types of APS are installed, a pushbutton locator tone lets pedestrians know there is a pushbutton and the tone helps them locate the button. A tactile arrow on the pushbutton, which should be oriented parallel to the associated crosswalk, lets a user know which crossing is controlled by the pushbutton. However, research investigating the use of several types of APS at intersection in two cities (Bentzen, Scott, & Barlow, 2006) found that blind participants needed hands-on training to recognize and use pushbutton locator tones and to understand and appropriately use tactile arrows.

Strategies to Determine When to Begin Crossing

Most O&M textbooks state that pedestrians should start to cross with the surge of parallel traffic, delaying the initiation of the crossing until they are sure that the traffic is going straight and is not turning right on red (Allen et al., 1997; Hill & Ponder, 1976; Jacobson, 1993; LaGrow & Weesies, 1994; Willoughby & Monthei, 1998).

Willoughby and Monthei (1998) state that using parallel traffic moving in the same direction as the pedestrian should be the first choice. However, at complex intersections, this strategy can lead to crossing into moving traffic and when drivers have the right-of-way. Left turn arrows and/or right turn overlaps may result in blind or visually impaired pedestrians crossing at the same time that vehicles turn across the crosswalk, when drivers who are turning with an arrow signal and do not expect pedestrians to be in the crosswalk turn across those crosswalks.

Using Near-Lane Parallel Traffic

Crossing with the "near-lane parallel through traffic" has been recommended as one strategy for dealing with left turn arrows and other complex signalization and phasing schemes (Barlow, Bentzen, & Bond, 2005; Frieswyk, 2005; Scheffers and Myers, 2004). The timing of the pedestrian walk signal is usually coordinated with the movement of the traffic in the parallel through lane nearest to the pedestrian (near-lane parallel). As shown in Figure 12.26, traffic in this lane may be traveling in the same direction as the pedestrian, or it may be coming toward the pedestrian from across the intersection. Near-lane parallel through traffic begins moving after any protected left turn phase is completed; if the left turn is protected-permissive, vehicles may still be permitted to turn left, but they no longer have the right-of-way and are required to yield to oncoming traffic or to pedestrians in the crosswalk. When traffic in the near parallel lane is moving and steady, it blocks left turning traffic from crossing the crosswalk.

Crossing with near-lane parallel traffic does not mean to cross with traffic traveling in the same direction as the pedestrian; this is only accurate for counterclockwise crossings. On clockwise crossings, the near-lane traffic to use for a cue to begin crossing is the traffic coming toward the pedestrian from across the intersection. With

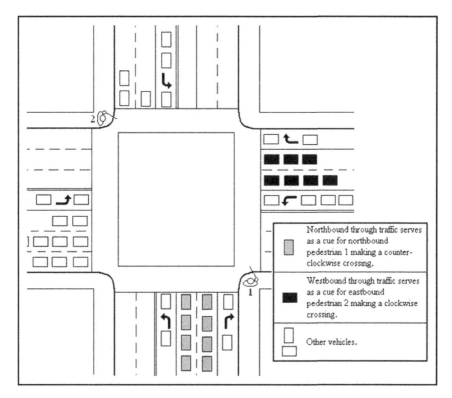

Figure 12.26. Using Near-Lane Parallel Traffic as a Cue for Crossing
Source: Reprinted from J. M. Barlow, B. L. Bentzen, and T. Bond, Blind Pedestrians and the Changing Technology and Geometry of Signalized Intersections: Safety, Orientation, and Independence, *Journal of Visual Impairment & Blindness*, 99 (October 2005): 596.

complex signalization patterns that are being implemented at most intersections, it is essential for students to understand and be able to use "near-lane parallel" traffic. This strategy is not well understood and used by blind or visually impaired pedestrians. In research on crossings at complex intersections (Barlow et al., 2005), participants were observed to start crossing with any traffic moving on the parallel street, which was often traffic beginning to move with a leading left turn phase, which was the cause of many interventions while crossing the street.

Although this technique prevents crossing while traffic has a protected left turn and the pedestrian does not have the right-of-way, it requires excellent listening skills to discern which traffic is moving. At wide streets when the pedestrian must use the traffic across the intersection as a cue, it may take several seconds for traffic to get across the intersection to the pedestrian and the pedestrian signal may actually be in flashing Don't Walk by the time the pedestrian is able to determine that the appropriate lanes are moving. In addition, there are many intersections where there is intermittent or no parallel traffic, and the signal status cannot be adequately determined by traffic sounds. At such intersections, including three-leg intersections, multileg intersections, intersections in a coordinated system that allow the pedestrian phase to be skipped after a call, or those with exclusive pedestrian phasing, or an LPI, APS may be necessary to determine the appropriate time to begin crossing. At busy intersections with lots of turning traffic, even very skilled students can sometimes have difficulty distinguishing each lane of traffic and which lanes of traffic are moving, particularly if students are slightly misaligned. Also, when no traffic is moving parallel to students' direction of travel, they may not be able to reliably discern the time to begin crossing.

Other Strategies

Some strategies may work in some situations but not in others. For example, timing the signal for the perpendicular street to determine when the signal for the parallel street will change (Stevenson, 2001) is appropriate only for crossings where signals are pre-timed. Except for central business districts, most signalized intersections are actuated. With traffic actuation and constantly changing length of signals in response to the traffic on the street, that strategy could lead to unsafe crossings at the wrong time in the cycle, when the perpendicular street has a green signal (Barlow, Franck, Bentzen, & Sauerburger, 2001; Sauerburger, 2005). The strategy for individuals with low vision to look at the traffic signal for the perpendicular street to determine the color of the signal for the parallel street (Smith & O'Donnell, 2001) is not reliable at locations where there are complicated signal phases, since different lanes and directions of traffic may be released at different times.

Use of Accessible Pedestrian Signals (APS)

Accessible pedestrian signals notify pedestrians of the onset and duration of the Walk signal, that is, the time during which pedestrians may legally enter the crosswalk. They provide other information as well, and this is covered elsewhere in Volume 1, Chapter 11. It is important to recognize that APS information is supplemental to traffic and environmental cues, and the APS Walk indication indicates only that the Walk signal is on, not that it is safe to cross. Cars can still be turning across the crosswalk or running a red light. The APS Walk sound can be compared to the *on your mark* instruction at the beginning of a race.

It means that the signal has changed, however, it is still important to *get set* (assess the traffic), then begin to cross (*go*) (Barlow & Franck, 2005).

APS that are recommended in the United States by Draft PROWAG (Access Board, 2005) include an APS speaker that is integrated with the pushbutton and located at approximately waist height, a pushbutton locator tone, automatic volume adjustment, a tactile arrow, and vibrotactile and audible Walk indications. Some of these features have been common in APS in some European countries and in Australia for many years. These APS provide information throughout the pedestrian phase. (See Volume 1, Chapter 11.) Older types of APS are still installed in the United States too. These usually provide a cuckoo or chirp walk indication from a speaker mounted on the pedestrian signal head and they provide a sound only during the walk interval, which usually ends well before pedestrians have finished crossing.

Misunderstanding of APS functioning. Research also suggested some confusion for blind or visually impaired pedestrians with new types of APS (Barlow & Franck, 2005; Bentzen et al., 2006). Some individuals thought that when the pushbutton locator tone got louder, in response to ambient noise, that the fact that the sound was louder was an indication of the correct time to cross. Individuals need to understand that both the APS locator tone or walk tone could increase in volume as louder vehicles pass, due to the automatic volume adjustment, and know the difference between the pushbutton locator tone (one repetition per second) and a Walk indication (much faster repetitions or a speech message). O&M specialists need to teach the use of APS and include experience with different APS installations in their instructional programs.

APS effect on street crossings. Several studies have found improvements in crossing timing with APS (Marston & Golledge, 2000; Scott, Barlow, Bentzen, Bond, & Gubbe, 2008; Williams et al., 2005), particularly at pedestrian actuated crossings. See Volume 1, Chapter 11 for a review of the research and detailed information about APS and regulations regarding APS in the United States.

Strategies for using APS. A systematic approach is needed when using APS. Specific techniques are suggested in a draft curriculum on APS, developed for Easter Seals Project ACTION (2003), and in an article by two of the authors of this chapter (Barlow & Franck, 2005). The following techniques provide a starting point for instruction:

- Approach the intersection and stop at the curb or curb ramp/street edge, maintaining initial alignment. Check alignment for crossing by listening to traffic. Even if a pushbutton locator tone is noticed during approach, pedestrians who are visually impaired should first continue to the curb or edge of the street.

- Determine the starting location for crossing, and identify tactile cues to use to realign after pressing the pushbutton, because after pushing the button, there may be no time to listen to parallel traffic and realign before the next Walk signal.

- Listen and evaluate the intersection. Determine traffic patterns and intersection geometry and listen for a pushbutton locator tone, or a tone or speech Walk indication.

- Leave the curb and search for a pedestrian pushbutton using a systematic pattern, starting by making a 180-degree turn and looking on the side of the sidewalk away from the intersection. Even where there is a pushbutton locator tone, a systematic search pattern is needed to maintain orientation. Because dog guides are trained to avoid obstacles, they may be reluctant to approach poles supporting pedestrian pushbuttons. It may be more

efficient for the handler to use a cane to search initially before teaching the dog to locate the pole.

- Once the pushbutton, with or without APS, is located, explore the device and its functioning, including locating the tactile arrow, if there is one, to confirm that the arrow is pointing in the direction of the street to be crossed.

- Stand at the pushbutton and while maintaining awareness of crossing location, listen to traffic and the APS for a full cycle to make sure that the audible Walk signal corresponds with traffic information.

- Press the pushbutton at the beginning of the perpendicular surge and return to the predetermined spot at the curb, realign, and prepare to cross.

- When the Walk indication is heard, confirm that traffic on the perpendicular street is stopping or stopped, and listen for the initial surge of near-lane parallel through traffic movements, when available.

- Cross the street using typical alignment techniques (traffic, straight line travel, etc.) while continuing to listen for turning cars. As discussed earlier, in many cases, cars can turn right and left across the crosswalk during the pedestrian phase. Although drivers are supposed to yield to pedestrians, they often do not. Listen for the pushbutton locator tone on the destination curb, which may provide additional wayfinding information.

In some locations, it is necessary to hold the pushbutton for more than one second to call an audible Walk indication. Holding the pushbutton for more than one second may also actuate a louder, beaconing, signal. Some APS provide additional information through a speech message, including street names and special signalization and geometry information. It may be necessary to depress the pushbutton for one or more seconds to actuate this additional information.

If a tone or speech Walk indication is audible on every cycle, the intersection signals are probably pre-timed (fixed timed) without a pedestrian pushbutton, so listen through a cycle to confirm sounds and the street they apply to, then cross, using traffic sounds to confirm the APS information.

Sequence of Instruction at Signalized Intersections

The following sequence of instruction can be used at signalized intersections:

- The first lessons may be conducted at the intersection of two one-way streets, or the intersection of a small one-way street and a major street, a crossing where no cars can turn into the lanes being crossed and preferably where there is a line of idling perpendicular traffic to use as a cue to maintaining crossing direction while crossing, along with a good stream of traffic on the parallel street.

- Cross in both directions with the major street on the right and on the left, pointing out the near-lane parallel traffic, and using that traffic as a cue to begin crossing.

- Move to two-way crossing beside a major street, at a two phase intersection. It may be better to consider an intersection with protected left turns, if available, so students do not have to deal with left turning traffic immediately, but protected signal phases can be hard to find where minor and major streets intersect. The advantage of crossing minor streets beside a major street is that the minor street is usually a smaller street with less rounded corners, and there is lots of traffic on the major traveling parallel to the pedestrian's path, to provide easily recognizable

surges of traffic. Some instructors prefer to begin all street-crossing instruction in a situation with good parallel traffic to assist in alignment and maintaining alignment while crossing.

Additional Considerations

Small business areas and downtown commercial business districts may not have the complexity of signals typically found along major commuting arterials and in suburban shopping districts. Training should cover intersections with split phasing, roundabouts, and channelized right turn lanes, as well as intersections that are fully or semi-actuated. Arterials in suburban areas (often along bus routes) are generally fully or semi-actuated. Most town and cities have most or all of these complexities for pedestrians who are blind or visually impaired to deal with. Roundabouts will become increasingly common, as they have been found to significantly decrease the severity and number of vehicular crashes (FHWA, 2000).

Some instructors choose to begin teaching street crossing in a small business area rather than a residential area. It is relatively easy to cross a small street beside a major street because of the traffic sounds to use for alignment and for a starting cue. Working in an area with traffic cues can assist in developing orientation and listening skills from the beginning. If programs spend too much time in a quiet area, students may become more focused on the cane tip and tactual information, rather than the auditory environment and may have more difficulty learning to attend to traffic cues.

RISK ASSESSMENT AND CLIENT DECISION MAKING

Decisions about Risks

Almost any activity involves some element of risk. One primary goal for crossing streets is safety (Jacobson, 1993; LaGrow and Weessies, 1994). Every crossing has associated risks that should be recognized and addressed. As indicated previously, common risks at signalized intersections include conflicts with turning vehicles and drivers running the light just as it turns red, and common risks at unsignalized crossings include conflicts with vehicles that are undetected or unexpected and do not yield to the pedestrian. With these inherent risks, what crossings could be considered "safe"? Lowrance (1976, quoted in Kraft, 1988, p. 189) concluded that "a thing is safe if its risks are judged to be acceptable."

Using this definition, decisions must be made about whether or not a given street-crossing risk is acceptable. The person who makes that decision is the student or his or her guardian. Each person's acceptance of risk is individual, and depends on such factors as the person's values, motivation, and level of risk taking. However, individuals often are not aware of the risk involved in some activities and can have an incorrect and exaggerated perception of the risk of some types of activities. One example is people who are fearful of flying but take a long trip by car instead. In actuality, the risks of death or injury from a motor vehicle crash are much higher than the risk of an airplane crash—according to the National Safety Council an individuals' lifetime probability of dying in a motor accident are about one in 83, whereas the chances of dying in an airplane crash in our lifetime is one in 5,000. Therefore, an essential aspect of O&M training in complex environments is to provide accurate information about the possible risks in various travel situations, and ways to minimize risks. As much as possible, this information should be based on reliable facts and research.

The decision of the student or his or her guardian needs to be respected by the O&M instructor. However, O&M instructors need to also respect their own feelings and concerns, and avoid participating in activities or instruction with which they are not comfortable. The role of O&M specialists is to ensure that the decision maker (student and/or guardian) is aware of and fully understands the risks. In addition, his or her role is to prepare students to make informed decisions by teaching them:

- effective street-crossing strategies and helping them become reliably skillful in those strategies;
- techniques and strategies to determine what risks and possible consequences are involved in each situation and how to reduce those risks as much as possible; and
- alternatives that can be considered when the risk of crossing independently is not acceptable.

Students may be concerned about common risks, such as the risk of cars turning into their path, or about risks that are extremely unlikely, such as the risk that an airplane will crash-land on the crosswalk. Each of their concerns needs to be respected and addressed, regardless of how likely they may be. Strategies need to be discussed and considered for reducing the level of associated risk, and the student or appropriate decision maker needs to determine if the resulting level of risk is acceptable.

Alternatives to Crossing

Alternatives to consider when the risks for crossing at a given intersection are not considered acceptable include the following:

- Getting assistance to cross
- Crossing elsewhere, such as at an intersection where there is better or different traffic control, or where the drivers expect or can see the pedestrians better, or where the traffic is moving more slowly or the street is narrower

- Avoiding the crossing (by getting a ride, taking the bus to the end of the line and back, having food or merchandise delivered)

- Requesting intersection alterations from traffic engineering or public works departments to make the crossings more accessible or pedestrian-friendly (see Volume 1, Chapter 11)

WHAT DOES THE FUTURE HOLD?

Technology Developments Related to Street Crossings

The Federal Highway Administration in the United States is funding an ongoing activity, now called Intellidrive, which is building on systems developed in the earlier Vehicle Infrastructure Integration project and Intelligent Vehicle Initiative (IVI). The goal is to deploy communication technologies in all vehicles and on all major U.S. roadways, so data transmitted from the roadside to the vehicle could warn a driver that it is not safe to enter an intersection or trigger a collision avoidance system in the vehicle. Vehicles could serve as data collectors and anonymously transmit traffic and road condition information from every major road within the transportation network. Implications for pedestrians at this point are not clear. Applications of this technology may eventually focus on providing information to drivers about pedestrian presence, or it may result in vehicles that are on "autopilot." Radio and wireless capability may open the possibilities of remote signaling devices for pedestrians who are blind or visually impaired that communicate with traffic signal controllers.

New Intersection Designs

However, designers and engineers are continuously experimenting with ways to move traffic faster, more efficiently, and more safely. New intersection designs are not always best for pedestrians, and even if they are better for pedestrians, the sound patterns can be unusual and confusing for visually impaired pedestrians. Roundabouts are an example of a new intersection design that is being used at thousands of intersections and O&M specialists can expect their use to become common.

There are many other new intersection designs being developed. For example, several locations have recently been experimenting with what is being called a continuous flow intersection. Design methodologies for providing pedestrian access were evaluated. Jagannathan and Bared (2005) suggest that such a design is better for pedestrians than a conventional intersection with similar volumes of traffic. However, the patterns of traffic and unusual locations of crosswalks may be confusing to pedestrians who are blind or visually impaired. This is just one example of newer complex intersections designed to move large volumes of traffic and pedestrians.

Quiet Cars

Another trend that is starting to affect the safe travel and wayfinding of blind pedestrians is the increasing number of electric, hybrid, and quiet cars on our streets. Starting in 1996, the O&M Division and AER passed a series of resolutions regarding this issue. The most recent resolution, in 2004, urged that research evaluate the effect of quiet vehicles on pedestrian safety, and determine techniques for providing information that is equivalent to the acoustic cues that are currently provided by vehicle engines. It also urged studies to evaluate the broader issues of the effect on the environmental access to street crossings and the wayfinding of blind pedestrians that may occur if there are large numbers of quiet vehicles on our streets, and to develop techniques and technologies to address whatever problems are found. Research is being conducted by a number of institutions (see Volume 1, Chapter 4).

Responsibilities of O&M Specialists

Instructor Awareness of Environment and Its Complexity and Changeableness

O&M specialists need to remain alert and aware of changes in the environment and in the complexity of intersections. Communicating with transportation engineering professionals can provide insight into issues that should be included in instruction. Participation in citizen advisory groups is discussed in Volume 1, Chapter 11. Preparation for lessons may require calls to traffic engineers to get accurate information about signal systems and students should learn to make such calls, as well.

Working with Traffic Engineering Professionals

Transportation engineers and transportation planners design the roadways and intersections and have developed specific terminology to describe intersection geometry and signalization. With the new developments in traffic engineering and design and changes in accessibility guidelines and regulations, there is a host of new terms to describe intersection features, signalization schemes, curb ramps designs, and traffic calming features. In this chapter, the authors have chosen to use terms common to the transportation engineering profession in describing intersections, intersection geometry, and intersection control and have attempted to explain where those terms conflict with traditional O&M terminology. O&M specialists have developed their own terms, but may find that they are talking at odds with traffic engineers in using those terms.

O&M specialists and their students need to be able to understand some of the traffic engineering jargon in order to discuss intersections and signalization in terms that make sense to transportation engineers and planners. Terminology differences can result in misunderstandings between traffic engineers and O&M specialists. O&M specialists may describe intersections

as plus, T, or Y, but traffic engineers may describe the same three intersections as a right-angle four-leg, a three-leg, or a skewed three-leg intersection. If an O&M specialist uses the term *plus intersection* with a traffic engineer, it may conjure up another idea completely. For another example, what O&M specialists and O&M texts call the inside shoreline or inside crosswalk line (the crosswalk line further from the center of the intersection) is typically called the outside crosswalk line by traffic engineers. And more than one O&M specialist has requested a signal or intersection modification and been taken aback when the engineer responded that the signal or modification was not warranted. However, engineers have specific "warrants" that must be met to install signals or stop signs, according to the *Manual on Uniform Traffic Control Devices* (FHWA, 2009) and the engineers are responding based on the terminology of their field. Another example is our title, O&M specialist; in the field of transportation, an O&M specialist is responsible for Operations and Maintenance. Transportation engineers also use the term *mobility* in discussing travel between locations, but they usually are referring to the speed of travel, with a recent emphasis on increasing mobility through roadway design, and their focus is usually on the mobility of vehicles, or the people in vehicles, not of pedestrians. These differences in training and emphasis can be challenging at times, but continuing to work with transportation engineering professionals and recognizing their effect on what we teach at street crossings can be an important part of the O&M specialist's job.

IMPLICATIONS FOR O&M PRACTICE

1. Traditional O&M techniques for street crossing are inadequate in many situations because the information provided by the environment is less consistent and less predictable, and

intersection geometry and signalization are far more complex, than when the techniques were developed in the 1940s and 1950s.

2. Research in which pedestrians who are blind, who are experienced travelers, made crossings at unfamiliar complex signalized intersections, revealed problems in locating crosswalks, aligning to cross, determining when to begin crossing, and traveling straight across the crosswalk.

3. At crossings with no traffic signal or stop sign, pedestrians who are visually impaired cannot assume that they can cross safely because it is quiet. In many situations, it is impossible to hear or see all the approaching traffic far enough away to know whether a gap in traffic is long enough for a pedestrian to cross. Students need to learn to judge traffic and assess the risks at each street crossing.

4. At roundabouts and channelized turn lanes, pedestrians with normal vision are fairly good at detecting gaps in traffic that are long enough for them to cross safely, and they can accurately judge when drivers have yielded. Pedestrians who are blind are not able to detect gaps as readily, and are more likely than fully sighted pedestrians to accept gaps that are not long enough to complete crossings, and have difficulty detecting that drivers have yielded, particularly at multi-lane crossings.

5. Curb ramps enable people who cannot negotiate a step to use public rights-of-way; however they also can result in blind pedestrians' entering streets unaware, and misaligning for crossing. A variety of cues must be used for identifying the boundary between sidewalk and street, and updated cues and techniques need to be used for alignment for street crossings.

6. Intersection design, or geometry, has become much more complex and O&M specialists and pedestrians who are blind or visually impaired need to develop an understanding of intersection design and intersection terminology to have a common language for discussing intersections among themselves and with traffic engineers.

7. A majority of signalized intersections are now actuated, that is, the presence of vehicles in each lane, as well as pedestrians pushing buttons, determine the length and presence of signal phases moment by moment. Signal timing cannot be determined by observation alone.

8. At intersections having a pedestrian pushbutton, use of the pushbutton is typically required to get a Walk signal and sufficient time to cross the street. Pedestrians who do not begin crossing during the walk interval (walking person symbol) may not have enough time to complete their crossing before the perpendicular traffic starts moving and they are illegally crossing the street, under the laws in most states.

9. At complex signalized intersections it is necessary for pedestrians who are visually impaired to begin crossing with the onset of parallel through traffic on the nearest side of the street (near-lane parallel traffic), regardless of whether that traffic is going in the same direction as or coming toward the pedestrian.

10. Accessible pedestrian signals (APS) make Walk signal timing accessible to pedestrians who are blind. Techniques for using APS need to be introduced as part of O&M instruction.

LEARNING ACTIVITIES

1. Go to five intersections with different intersection geometry and note issues for blind pedestrians at each intersection. Identify crossings where it would be relatively easy to align with traffic or other cues and ones that

would be difficult, and describe what the determining features are. Practice aligning by memorizing your position when aligned compared to using a physical line (such as the curb or grassline). Does time of day matter?

2. Go to an actuated intersection with pedestrian pushbuttons at three different times of day: at rush hour, non–rush hour, and late at night. Select one crossing of the major street to evaluate. Time the "green time" for the parallel street traffic (the time available for crossing using surge of traffic), with and without pushing the pushbutton. Time it for five cycles pushing the button, and five cycles without pushing the pushbutton. (Make sure no one else on another corner presses the button.) Record the length of the green signal for parallel traffic, and the Walk and of the flashing Don't Walk intervals. Compare times.

3. Find 10 different curb ramps and try to detect the edge of the street accurately (nonvisually) while approaching the street (noticing what cues are useful and not useful). Compare the abruptness of the changes in slope, and notice the effect on detectability. Notice what happens if you use the ramp to align to cross the street, and how the slopes feel when you stand on the ramp while aligned correctly.

4. Meet with a city traffic engineer and discuss the traffic engineer's training and priorities, and policies for adding vehicular signals, pedestrian signals, crosswalks, and accessible pedestrian signals. Educate the engineer about travel by blind pedestrians.

5. Visit two uncontrolled crossings along a street, one with a hill or curve to the right or left, and time your detection of cars approaching (using TMAD) to determine whether you can hear cars far enough away to make a good judgment about whether you have time to cross. Where you cannot make a good judgment, move up or down the street and evaluate other options nearby.

Teaching the Use of Transportation Systems for Orientation and Mobility

Bonnie Dodson-Burk, Laura Park-Leach, and Linda Myers

LEARNING QUESTIONS

- What are the various types of transportation systems, and what do O&M specialists need to know about them?

- What tools and strategies can persons with visual impairments use to gather information needed to plan and to travel on transit trips?

- What instructional strategies are recommended for teaching bus travel and rail travel to adults with visual impairments? Children? People with vision loss and cognitive or mobility challenges? People who are deaf-blind?

- How can O&M specialists advocate for accessible, user-friendly transit systems?

- How can technology such as online trip planning, cameras on transit vehicles, audible real-time information, remote infrared audible signage, and global positioning systems help with bus and rail travel tasks?

- What are the Americans with Disabilities Act regulations in regard to paratransit eligibility for persons with visual impairments?

- What are some considerations for air travel?

- What are considerations for persons who use dog guides when using transportation systems?

This chapter covers all transportation modes as well as O&M instruction in how to use various modes of public transportation. Public transportation systems transport passengers within cities and between cities on a continuing basis. Learning to use public transportation is crucial to many persons with visual disabilities. O&M specialists play a vital role in sharing information about public transportation with their students. Public transportation is also referred to as *mass transportation* and *mass transit*. Persons, referred to in the transit industry as *passengers* or *riders*, pay a fee for the service. Transportation systems along fixed routes within cities include service by buses, subways, light rail, and trolleys. Public transportation also includes federally mandated paratransit service for seniors and persons with disabilities, vanpool, limousines, and taxi services operated under contract with a public transportation agency (American Public Transportation Association [APTA], 2007). Transportation systems between cities include air travel, over-the-road buses, and long-distance rail, which are owned and operated by private entities.

OVERVIEW OF TRANSPORTATION SYSTEMS

Transportation Modes

A *transportation mode* is the system for carrying transit passengers described by specific right-of-way, technology, and operational features. Large urban areas have more transportation modes than small towns. Some rural areas have no modes of public transportation. Trips that require a passenger to transfer from one transportation mode to another are referred to as *multimodal trips*.

Types of Service

There are two basic types of service: fixed–route and demand response. Fixed-route service is provided on a repetitive, predetermined fixed schedule basis along a specific route with vehicles stopping to pick up and deliver passengers to specific locations. Each fixed-route trip serves the same origins and destinations. Intercity buses and subways are examples of fixed-route service.

Demand response service is a transit mode comprised of passenger cars, vans, or class C buses operating in response to calls from passengers to a transit operator, who then dispatches a vehicle to pick up the passengers and transport them to their destinations. Typically, the vehicle may be dispatched to pick up several passengers at different pick-up points before taking them to

their respective destinations and may even be interrupted en route to these destinations to pick up other passengers. Americans with Disabilities Act (ADA) complementary paratransit services and taxis are examples of demand responsive service.

Benefits of Public Transportation

Access to public transportation gives mobility to people from all walks of life, including those with disabilities, allowing them choice and freedom to accomplish what is important to them. Public transportation provides persons with severe visual impairments the opportunity to access employment, services, and other places which are essential for everyday living. According to data from APTA, in 2008 Americans took 10.7 billion trips using public transportation (APTA, 2009). APTA estimates that more than 34 million trips are taken each weekday in the United States. Fifty-four percent of all trips end at workplaces, 15 percent of trips go to schools, 9 percent to shop, 9 percent to social visits, and 5 percent to medical appointments. Forty percent of residents in the United States have no access to public transportation services and another 25 percent have negligible access (APTA, 2006a). This is particularly burdensome to individuals with severe visual impairments that live in rural areas.

In comparison to the general population, persons with visual impairments are overrepresented in cities and nonmetropolitan areas and underrepresented in the suburbs (Schmeidler & Halfmann, 1998). Although no data are available to explain this phenomenon, the availability of public transportation systems in cities is most likely one important factor. Some persons with visual impairments choose their place of residence based on the availability of nearby public transportation. An accessible, user-friendly public transportation system provides opportunities for them to have an independent lifestyle.

Decisions Relating to Transit Usage

According to survey data from the Transit Cooperative Research Board (TCRB), factors rated as most important to transit customers (in the following order) are on-time service, frequency of service, employee courtesy, safe facilities, safe vehicles, clean facilities, clean vehicles, and pricing (Transit Cooperative Research Board, 2002). Persons with visual impairments add the following to the list of factors:

- Accessibility of a next stop signal device
- Driver announcing the route number to those waiting at the stop
- Availability of bus stops near home and destinations
- Drivers' sensitivity to passengers with disabilities
- Availability of information in a usable format

Many persons with visual impairments use public transportation. If a destination cannot be reached by walking or if the decision is made to use public transportation for convenience, the person should determine the nearest intersection to the destination. Individuals can call the local transit office or get information online to determine if the destination can be reached by bus or train, or a combination of both (LaGrow & Weessies, 1994). Some trips require a transfer between vehicles within the same mode of transportation or a transfer to a different mode. Many transit system web sites have trip-planning features. This allows persons with accessible computers to find out independently which modes serve destinations, as well as route, scheduling, fare, and other information.

Persons with visual impairments have varying levels of independent usage of transportation systems. Some persons travel to new cities and countries independently and use various public transportation modes by applying "system" knowledge. They know how to seek fare, stop, and route information, how to plan trips, and can generalize skills to new transit systems. Other persons are limited to familiar routes. After receiving O&M instruction, they can travel on bus routes to places they go to frequently, such as work and shopping. Because they do not have a full understanding of the system, they would most likely have difficulty adapting to route changes or problem solving when unforeseen events occur. Some persons with additional disabilities are not able to use public transportation independently. These persons may use private transportation or Americans with Disabilities Act (ADA) complementary paratransit services for all of their trips. ADA paratransit service is a federally mandated service in which persons with disabilities schedule rides in advance. These persons are picked up and driven to their destinations using a shared ride system.

Components of Transit Trips

The Transit Cooperative Research Project (2001b) summarizes the elements of a typical transit trip into six basic functions:

1. *Understanding the system*: Schedules, fares, stops or stations, route planning, transfers, and special services and provisions for persons with disabilities.

2. *Accessing the correct vehicle*: Find the correct stop or station, move to and wait in the proper boarding area, identify the correct incoming vehicle, and move to the vehicle doorway. For rail, locate and access the fare system, and activate and pass through the fare gate.

3. *Entering a vehicle*: Move through the doorway, ascend the stairs or use the lift, pay the fare, identify a vacant seat or standing space, and move to it.

4. *Traveling in a vehicle*: Handle the movements of vehicle and other passengers, and comprehend and respond as needed to special announcements.

5. *Exiting a vehicle*: Identify the desired stop, station, or terminal; notify driver of desire to stop (where necessary); move to the doorway; descend the stairs or use the lift; exit the vehicle and reach the stop area or platform.

6. *Exiting the stop or station*: Determine the desired exit direction. For rail stations, activate and pass through the fare control gate, and exit the station.

O&M Specialist's Role

Direct Instruction

O&M specialists need to know about all the transportation systems within their local instructional areas. They should be prepared to provide instruction in all aspects of transit system usage to individuals of all ages with varying levels of ability and system knowledge. O&M instruction ranges from providing a system overview to a person who recently moved into the area, to strategies persons can use to obtain route, stop, and fare information from transit system personnel, web sites, and printed schedules. O&M instruction may include intensive instruction over several lessons with a particular individual along a specific route. Instruction may also incorporate technology such as online trip planning, remote infrared audible signage (RIAS), and using a global positioning system (GPS) both to locate bus stops and to stay oriented while riding in vehicles. This chapter covers O&M instructional strategies for all elements of a typical transit trip as well as recovery strategies for handling atypical events, situations, and emergencies. Specific techniques used when traveling on public transportation are covered more in depth in O&M techniques textbooks (Hill & Ponder, 1976; Jacob-son, 1993; LaGrow & Weessies 1994; Uslan, Peck, Wiener, & Stern, 1990).

Emergency Situations

All passengers must be able to comprehend and respond appropriately to an emergency situation while utilizing any type of transit system. Emergencies may include everything from unforeseen or unusual weather conditions, route deviations, and canceled routes, to more serious conditions such as accidents, evacuations, and fire. As part of a comprehensive program, O&M specialists must discuss or role-play how to deal with emergency situations. O&M specialists should also provide training to drivers so that they are knowledgeable about how to provide assistance to persons with visual impairments in emergency situations.

Rural Areas with No Public Transportation Services

Some O&M specialists teach individuals who do not live in an area that has public transportation. The nearest town that has public transportation may be an hour or more away. As part of a comprehensive program, O&M specialists should include instruction on public transportation options. Individuals can make informed choices about where to live when they understand the freedom public transit can provide. Although scheduling lengthy lessons to incorporate travel time to an area with public transportation is challenging, it is important. Thus, O&M specialists must make every effort to take these individuals to the nearest area that has bus, rail, paratransit, or taxi service to expose them to the strategies utilized for planning and taking trips.

Partnerships with Transit Systems

One method of partnering with transit systems is for O&M specialists to provide quality training to vehicle operators (drivers), customer service staff, and other transit system personnel. Inservice training may help to increase driver sensitivity and to improve the quality of the information provided to customers with visual impairments during all phases of transit usage including trip planning, boarding, riding, and disembarking. Another method of partnering is to be involved with the design of transit systems making sure accessibility is considered.

Participation on Committees or Advisory Boards

O&M specialists, along with persons with visual impairments, are encouraged to become members of transit system advisory boards and committees for accessible transportation. Individuals may contact the transit system's ADA coordinator to obtain information about participating on advisory boards and committees. Subsequent dialogue between O&M specialists, persons with visual impairments, and transit system personnel can lead to practical, up-to-date information about how to make systems more accessible and user-friendly for persons with visual impairments. Participation with these groups can help O&M specialists and consumers keep abreast of current transit-related information because vehicles, accessibility regulations, ways to access transit-related information, technology, trip planning, and other transit factors change rapidly.

Dog Guides on Public Transportation

By law, dog guides are allowed to travel with their handlers in all public transportation vehicles (see Volume 1, Chapter 9). Neither charging additional fares nor denial of service is allowed. Dog guides must ride on the floor of the vehicle, not on the seat. Handlers must ensure that their dogs are well behaved at all times. Dogs must also be well groomed so that the dog does not smell or shed an unreasonable amount of hair during trips.

School-Age Children

School-age children should be introduced to the transit systems in their local areas long before they will be expected to ride alone. Assessment, instructional strategies, and goals and objectives in the area of public transportation which may be included on the child's Individualized Education Program (IEP) can be found in the *Teaching Age-Appropriate Purposeful Skills* (TAPS) curriculum (Pogrund et al., 1993).

Familiarization to transit vehicles, role-playing, trip planning and taking trips with an O&M specialist under close supervision can allow students to develop confidence and to realize the potential benefits of public transportation in helping them to lead more independent lives. Exposure can begin as early as preschool. Older children who use computers can learn how to plan trips on fixed-route service online. Children may also role-play scheduling a trip, and then listen to their O&M specialist calling to schedule an actual trip by taxi.

The decision about when someone is mature enough to ride alone needs to be made by that child's family, after input from the O&M specialist documenting that the child has mastered all transit-related skills consistently using safe travel practices. In general, the goal might be to prepare children to be able to use mass transit for independent travel by high school (Uslan et al., 1990). O&M specialists working with children must be knowledgeable about their school district's policies and procedures in regard to transporting students to and from lesson sites and monitoring students on transit lessons. Because transit lessons may be lengthy and schoolchildren often cannot miss classes, some O&M specialists work with students after school hours.

Transportation System Accessibility

The U.S. Department of Transportation (DOT) has issued regulations mandating accessible public transit vehicles and facilities. (See Volume 1, Chapter 11 for more information on environmental access.) The regulations, which are revised periodically, include requirements that all new fixed-route, public transit buses and trains be accessible and that complementary ADA paratransit services must be provided for those individuals with disabilities who cannot use fixed-route bus and rail service. The DOT regulations for publicly operated mass transit are found online in the Code of Federal Regulations (49 CFR Parts 27, 37, 38) available from the Federal Transit Authority web site (2007).

The lack of uniformity within and between transit systems can create significant challenges for persons with visual impairments. Inconsistency is not the exception but the rule in mass transit structures (Uslan et al., 1990). The locations of bus stops vary from street to street and from municipality to municipality. It is often difficult to determine bus numbers or routes. The layout of rail stations is inconsistent. The locations of platforms, exits, stairs, turnstiles, fare machines, ticket booths, restrooms, and telephones vary from station to station (LaGrow & Weessies, 1994).

Features of an Accessible Transit System

Transportation systems vary in their degree of accessibility. Within the past decade, some transit systems have made significant improvements in accessibility. Transportation systems in cities such as Lansing, Michigan, and Colorado Springs, Colorado, use remote infrared audible signs (RIAS) that transmit the bus number and destination. When an individual wearing a pocket-size receiver enters the field of transmission, audible information on mass transit vehicles and public transit stops is transmitted through the receiver's speaker.

The bus system in Charlotte, North Carolina, is an example of a system that is user-friendly and accessible to persons with visual impair-

ments. Riders can access information on eleven bus stop amenities through customer service including the cross street, through street, street address, landmarks, sidewalk availability, whether it is a transfer point, if there is a route deviation, distance to the intersection from the stop and whether there is a shelter, lighting or an emergency phone. A portion of this information is also available using a BrailleNote GPS. The bus stop poles are standardized square poles with an

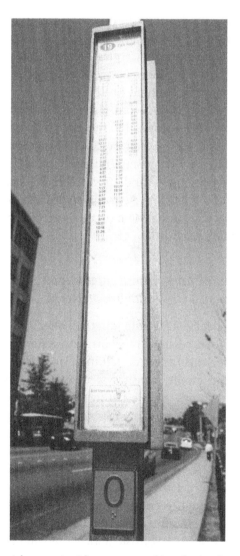

A bus stop with a square pole and raised-letter and braille route identification from Charlotte Area Transit System.

attached rectangular schedule holder placed at waist height. The Charlotte Area Transit System (CATS) has initiated a project to include bus route information in braille and raised letter signage at bus stops.

Route maps and web scheduling are accessible. Real-time bus location is available through customer service and on audio and visual signage at the transportation center. Audible bus bay information is available by depressing a button on a column near the stop at the transportation center. Each bus has an automated enunciation system for ADA stop announcements which uses GPS. On passenger request, specific stops are added to the automated enunciation system. Cameras are mounted on the interior and exterior of the bus to record visual activity. An audiotape also records interactions between the driver and the passenger. Such information is useful for customer service issues and the safety of the passengers and driver. All drivers employed by CATS have participated in sensitivity training to educate them on the needs of passengers with disabilities.

Communicating Transit Information to Persons with Visual Impairments

O&M specialists should join their clients in advocating for accessible transportation systems. Technologies such as RIAS, talking directories, auditory and tactile transit system maps, accessible fare machines, tactile pathways, and detectable warnings at platform edges can provide significant benefits to passengers with visual impairments. Online trip planning, transit schedules in accessible formats, and well-trained customer service personnel are useful for planning trips. Signage with high contrast, large-print raised letters and braille mounted at eye level in well-lit areas with predictable, consistent locations can improve accessibility at transit stations (LaGrow & Weessies, 1994). See Volume 1, Chapter 11 for more information regarding ways to make transit stations,

trip planning, fare systems, signage, and other transit-related areas more accessible for persons with visual impairments.

URBAN BUS TRAVEL

Buses are vehicles powered by diesel, gasoline, battery or alternative fuel engines contained within the vehicle. Buses travel on congested city streets, through suburban neighborhoods and on highways. The vast majority of scheduled fixed-route transit service operates in bus and trolley-bus modes on streets and highways using rubber-tired vehicles. In all but about 50 metropolitan areas and small cities in the United States, bus service is the only fixed-route transit service available (APTA, 2006a). A rider accesses most buses by waiting at a bus stop. Buses operate along fixed routes, with specified time schedules and fares.

The Department of Transportation (DOT) ADA regulations at 49 CFR sections 37.167(b) and (c) require that stop announcements must be made on fixed-route systems as follows:

1. The entity shall announce stops at least at transfer points with other fixed routes, other major intersections and destination points, and intervals along a route sufficient to permit individuals with visual impairments or other disabilities to be oriented to their location.

2. The entity shall announce any stop on request of an individual with a disability.

3. Where vehicles or other conveyances for more than one route serve the same stop, the entity shall provide a means by which an individual with a visual impairment or other disability can identify the proper vehicle to enter or be identified to the vehicle operator as a person seeking a ride on a particular route.

The DOT ADA regulations do not require the use of automated audio equipment. The requirement is for stop announcements to be made in such a manner that everyone riding the bus can hear them. If the stop announcements are not audible, regardless of whether or not audio equipment is used, the requirement is not being met.

Types of Bus Service

Local service, where vehicles may stop every block or two along a route several miles long, is by far the most common type of bus service. When limited to a small geographic area or to short-distance trips, local service is often called *circulator*, *feeder*, *neighborhood*, or *shuttle service*. Such routes, which often have a lower fare than regular local service or no fare, may operate in a loop-and-connect pattern, connecting at a bus transfer center or rail station to major routes for travel to more-far-flung destinations. Examples are office park circulators, historic district routes, transit mall shuttles, rail feeder routes, and university campus loops (APTA, 2006a). This service may be easy to access for persons with visual impairments because bus stops are numerable.

Local service is different from *express service*, which speeds up longer trips (especially in major metropolitan areas during heavily patronized peak commuting hours) by operating for long distances without stopping. Examples include park-and-ride routes between suburban parking lots and the central business district that operate on freeways, and express buses on major streets that operate as a local service on the outlying portions of a route until a certain point and then operate nonstop to the central business district.

Limited-stop service is a hybrid between local and express service, where the stops may be several blocks to a mile or more apart to speed up the trip or the bus may skip stops during non-peak hours. Thus, people may have to walk farther to access the bus stop. Persons with visual impairments that live in limited-stop or express service areas might have fewer opportunities to come and go from their homes because service

to a nearby bus stop may be restricted to just early mornings and late afternoons. This may limit trips for elderly persons who do not have the stamina to be away for most of the day.

Bus rapid transit (BRT) is a type of limited-stop service developed in the 1990s that relies on technology to help speed up the service. It can operate on exclusive transitways, high-occupancy vehicle lanes, expressways, or ordinary streets. A BRT line combines priority for transit vehicles as well as rapid and convenient fare collection to substantially upgrade bus system performance.

Route Deviations

Upon customer request, some bus systems will make route deviations to pick up or drop off a customer at an off route location. Customers must call the transit system to request route deviations. This service may be beneficial to persons with visual impairments in situations where certain bus stops are inaccessible. These persons can request that a bus make a slight route deviation to pick them up or drop them off at an accessible location. On the other hand, an unexpected route deviation may cause confusion for a passenger with a visual impairment who is familiar with the regular route.

Types of Vehicles and Route Identifiers

Bus systems may have several types of vehicles including buses with steps and lifts, low-floor buses, double-deck buses, and articulated buses. For some buses, persons enter the front door and exit via the "back" door, which is located on the side of the bus near the back. Exceptions can be made for passengers with visual impairments, if needed. Other buses allow persons to enter and exit via the front door. Some buses have raised seating in the back of the bus resulting in one or two steps in the aisle or a step up from the aisle to seats over the front wheels. Thus, O&M specialists should teach persons to visually scan or use their canes while inside vehicles to locate steps.

Bus route numbers and names are located on the mastheads, which are across the top of the front, back, or side of the vehicle as well as inside near the front of the bus. Some systems also have large high contrast route numbers in the bus window either in the front or side window near the entry doors to increase visibility. Persons who are unable to see the bus signage can either ask another pedestrian for help or rely on the bus driver or automated route announcements for stops that serve more than one bus route. Persons with low vision may use a telescope to locate route information.

To help find the correct stop, deaf-blind persons with low vision who cannot hear the enunciator may be able to use the light-emitting diode (LED) display inside the bus to read the stop announcements.

O&M specialists must inform their students about the vehicle identification number at the front of the bus that identifies that specific vehicle. Students should not confuse this number with the route number. The vehicle identification number is used by the transit systems for purposes such as fleet inventory and repair. It is also important information for a customer service complaint. If needed, passengers with visual impairments may get this information from another passenger.

Trip Planning

Routes and times of departure will vary during the course of the day (rush hour versus midday) or day of the week (weekday versus weekend). Routes, location of bus stops, timetables, fares, and accessibility information can be obtained via telephoning customer service or online. When planning a trip, the rider must know the locations of the starting point and destination as well as the time of day she plans to travel. Some individuals have found that by mentioning that they are visually impaired they get more and better information from the customer service

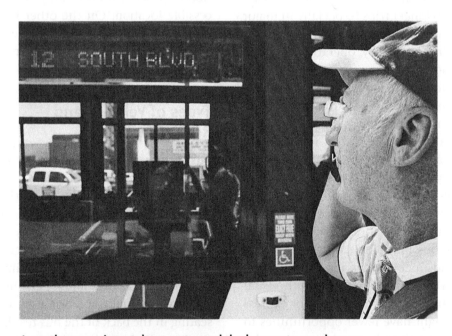

A gentleman using a telescope to read the bus route number.

Key Questions for Obtaining Bus Information

BEFORE CALLING CUSTOMER SERVICE

1. Know the address, intersection, or landmark of your starting point.

2. Know the address, intersection, or landmark of your destination.

3. Know the day and time you want to begin your trip or arrive at your destination.

4. Know if you want the fastest trip, fewest transfers, or shortest walking distance.

TRIP TO DESTINATION

1. What bus route will I take? What is the endpoint for the bus I want?

2. On what street and in what direction will the bus be traveling when I board?

3. What is the exact location of the bus stop where I'll board the bus? Which of the four corners? Is the bus stop before the intersection, just after it, or midblock?

4. Does the stop have a shelter, bench, or pole? Is there a landmark near the bus stop?

5. What time is the bus scheduled to arrive at this stop?

6. Where can I get off the bus so that I will be as close to (destination address or nearest intersection) as possible?

7. In which direction will the bus be traveling when I get off?

8. Will I have to transfer buses? If yes, where? (Then repeat questions 2–5.)

9. What is the fare?

For the return trip—repeat relevant questions from this list.

---

personnel. Refer to Sidebar 13.1 for questions to ask when soliciting bus information.

Many transit systems are moving to computer-assisted systems versus human operators. This can be confusing and frustrating for some callers. O&M specialists may suggest their students use a direct telephone number which will be answered by a human operator. Printed bus schedules need to be made available in accessible formats (braille, large print, audiotape, or CD) upon request. Schedules typically include a route map, timetables that list times the bus arrives at major stops, fare, and other general system information. O&M specialists should also teach their students how to access whatever information is available from their local bus systems.

Planning trips has become much easier for persons who use computers due to the availability of online trip-planning software.

Persons must enter the address of the origin and the destination. Most trip planners accept street addresses, names of the streets at the nearest intersection, or landmarks, such as medical centers, transit stations, schools, colleges, major commercial facilities, and government office buildings. Dates and times of travel must be entered. The software program adds walking time to the time entered for arrivals and departures. If the inbound stop is some distance from the origin, the trip planner assumes the person will leave the location at the time they enter and allows walking time to the stop. Additional information available from transit systems' trip-planning software varies and may include detailed walking directions, walking distance to the specified stop, and accessibility information. The accessibility information may include grade, whether the bus is lift equipped or low floor

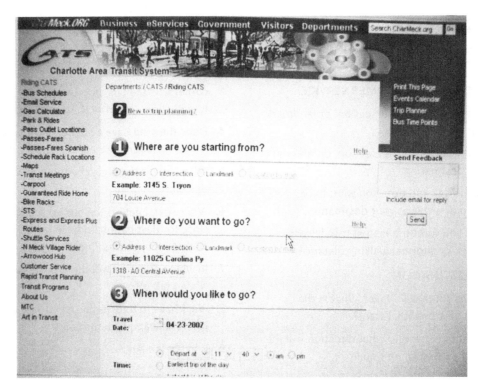

Screen from trip-planning software used by the Charlotte Area Transit System.

with a ramp, and whether stop meets the federal operational standards for lift or ramp deployment. Some systems also have a listing of bus stop amenities such as shelter, bench, public telephone, or a photo of the bus stop area. Because accessibility information is often geared toward accessibility for those who use wheelchairs, O&M specialists should encourage their local transit authorities to include environmental information that is useful to passengers with visual impairments, such as a change in the walking surface and lighting.

Bus Stops

The lack of clear landmarks and standardized locations of bus stops are often the biggest challenges to using the bus system for persons with visual impairments. Finding unfamiliar stops can be difficult or impossible without assistance.

Bus stops may be designated by signs, benches, shelters, or a combination of these. Some stops are not marked at all. The bus stop signs and types of poles used for mounting the signs used within a municipality may not be standardized. Some cities have unique bus stop poles that are tactually different from all other sign poles. Although this does not help a person who is blind find the pole, it can help the person verify that the pole they have located is the pole for a bus stop.

When traveling to an unfamiliar stop, it does help to have an understanding of the path the bus will travel along a route. Bus stops are usually located on the corner before the bus travels through the intersection. This is referred to as a *near-side stop*. For example if the bus is traveling north, the bus stop would be located on the southeast corner. If the bus is heading east, the bus stop would be on the southwest corner.

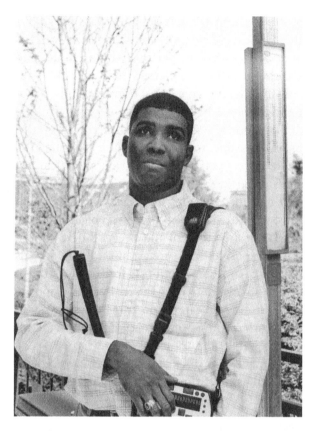

A gentleman using a global positioning system (GPS) at a bus stop.

Because transit systems have data on the latitude and longitude of the bus stop, personal data assistant devices with GPS software can be used to find stops.

As technology such as GPS information through personal devices and RIAS become more prevalent, locating bus stops will become an easier task. Using a virtual globe browser such as Google Earth or Streetview allows the O&M instructor and student with low vision to explore geographic information such as intersections, bus stops, and buildings. A combination of satellite and aerial images as well as street level photographs is possible. These tools provide a first-person perspective of the street at the bus stop location, and can provide the O&M instructor with a useful way to remotely view the potential starting point or destination of a planned transit trip.

Transfer Points

Transfer points can be crowded and noisy with multiple buses arriving at the same time. Some transfer points are outdoors in a specified block along a busy street or on a loop while others can be indoors at transit stations. Finding the correct bus at a large transit station can be challenging for persons with visual impairments. ADA requires bus drivers to open the bus door and announce the route name and number. However, when there are two or more buses pulling up simultaneously, it is often difficult to find the desired bus. Many cities have bus identification kits which consist of large high contrast numbers held up by the rider. This enables the driver as well as nearby pedestrians to know which bus the rider is seeking. Bus identification kits are especially useful in areas where different transit systems use the same stop because often buses will not stop unless flagged down. Although anyone can use these bus ID kits, they can be particularly useful for persons who are deaf-blind. Some cities provide deaf-blind riders with differently colored bus ID kits so that the driver will know the passenger is deaf-blind.

Bus Fares

Fare systems vary between transit systems. Riders may pay cash, use smart cards, or purchase daily, weekly, monthly, or yearly passes. Many systems require that riders have the exact change. In most systems, frequent riders save money by purchasing long-term passes. Passes and smart cards can be purchased at transit customer service buildings, shopping centers, and other designated places. Trips can require the rider to pay the fare on entry or when exiting. Some systems have reduced fares for riders with disabilities and give O&M specialists free passes to be utilized when providing direct instruction to students.

Bus Accessibility Issues

Boarding and riding in the vehicles generally do not pose challenges related to a person's visual impairment. ADA requires priority seating for elderly persons and persons with disabilities on all transit vehicles. Sitting in the priority seating area on the front door side may facilitate communication between the passenger and the driver. Also, it may help the driver remember to call out requested stops as the passenger remains in the driver's line of sight every time the driver opens the front door. Although ADA requires priority seating, it also has language specifically prohibiting an entity from requiring an individual with a disability to use a priority seat, if the individual does not choose to use such a seat. Any persons who cannot or does not want to use the steps can have the lift deployed for his or her use. Occasionally a driver will kneel a bus when he sees a rider with a visual impairment. O&M specialists may teach students to recognize the sound of the bus lowering.

O&M specialists should advocate for system-wide accessibility and improvements at bus stops by encouraging transit authorities to use consistent signage with large print and braille, adequate lighting, and predictable bus stop locations. One resource for universal design at bus stops is a *Toolkit for the Assessment of Bus Stop Accessibility and Safety* from Easter Seals Project ACTION (2006) available at www.projectaction.org/clearinghouse. This tool kit is designed for inventorying bus stops to determine whether they meet the ADA requirements. The tool kit includes principles of barrier-free design, two sample bus stop checklists with instructions for their use, guidelines for creating safe and accessible bus stops, considerations for rural stops, and case studies with examples of agency coordination.

There may be a number of accessibility challenges for riders with visual disabilities. Transit authorities frequently must add or delete routes, change bus numbers, move bus stops, and re-route buses. Although signs are posted at bus stops to inform riders of the changes, these signs are not accessible to persons who are unable to see them. Other challenges may include difficulty finding the right bus at transfer points, negotiating large, noisy transit stations, and walking to bus stops along paths that have no sidewalks or inaccessible intersections (see Chapter 11). There are several options for riders who cannot cross a particular street to get to a bus stop or destination. The rider might stay on the bus to the end of the line, and then loop back to get off on the desired side of the street. Riders should not be required to pay an additional fare for this method. Another solution is to ride to a transit center and change to a bus going the opposite way. Upon request, some transit systems will make minor bus route deviations to provide for an accessible stop for a passenger. Otherwise, a rider may exit the bus and solicit assistance with street crossings from the public, if necessary.

Technology

With advances in technology, access to information is slowly beginning to improve. It is possible to find bus stops and station entrances using accessible personal data assistant devices with GPS, such as the BrailleNote GPS or Trekker as well as RIAS, such as Talking Signs. RIAS also allows access to audible real-time bus information so persons with visual impairments can know when the next bus or light rail vehicle is scheduled to arrive at the stop.

Automatic Vehicle Locators and Real-Time Bus Arrival Information Systems

In the early 1990s many transit and paratransit systems began to deploy automatic vehicle location (AVL) systems to better monitor and control operations. Some vehicles are fitted with a satellite or other type of tracking system that monitors the location of the bus along its route. The initial focus of the AVL system was to increase operational efficiency, not provide customer information. As years passed and AVL systems became more sophisticated, transit agencies realized data from the AVL system could be utilized to provide customers with real-time predictions of bus arrivals (TCRP, 2003). This information can then be displayed on the World Wide Web, on screens at transfer stations, mobile phones, and on bus pole signs. From the comfort and security of a protected place, people can learn when the next bus will arrive at their stop. Having audible real-time information at bus stops can allow riders with visual impairments more independence. Real-time information can also reduce anxiety if individuals are fearful of waiting for prolonged periods at bus stops as they can get to the stop shortly before the bus arrives if they know when it is coming.

Mobile Digital Video Recorders

The use of video recorders in buses, on rail vehicles, and in transit stations is increasing. Cameras are placed onboard, outside the vehicle, or both.

Digital or analog audio and video recordings are made. Information from the recordings can be used:

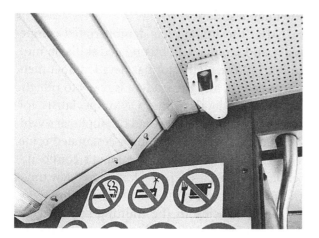

A mobile digital video recorder mounted on bus.

- To determine whether ADA stop announcements were made both inside vehicles and outside at transit stops
- As evidence in disputes
- In emergency situations such as hostage takeover or accident
- As a permanent driver training aid
- To verify whether a passenger with a disability was passed by at a stop
- To document potential troublemakers aboard the vehicle
- To document interactions between drivers and passengers

Cameras with wireless transmitting equipment will allow personnel at transit stations, police officers in squad cars, and first-responder vehicles to see what's happening "live."

Role of O&M Specialist

Transit Driver Training

According to the DOT ADA regulations at 49 CFR section 37.173, each public or private entity which operates a fixed-route or demand responsive system shall "ensure that personnel are trained to proficiency, as appropriate to their duties, so that they operate vehicles and equipment safely and properly assist and treat individuals with disabilities who use the service in a respectful and courteous way, with appropriate attention to the differences among individuals with disabilities." O&M specialists need to teach drivers how to serve the needs of passengers with visual impairments, multiple disabilities, and deaf-blind persons. One safety issue that should be addressed is the risk of falling or being thrown off balance due to the bus accelerating before the person finds a handhold or seat. Training benefits both the transit agency and the passengers with visual impairments. It helps transit agencies fulfill their legal obligations to ensure "personnel are trained to proficiency" and may improve route and stop announcements, and the quality of information and assistance passengers receive.

Sequence of Instruction

Several O&M textbooks offer instructional strategies for teaching bus usage. Detailed information for planning the bus route, locating the bus stop, locating the front door of the bus, boarding the bus, paying the fare, finding a seat, and exiting the bus can be found in several texts (Hill & Ponder, 1976; Jacobson, 1993; LaGrow & Weessies, 1994; Uslan et al., 1990). Other than increased use of technology for trip planning and access to route and time information, the techniques utilized in bus travel have not changed considerably over the years. The proposed sequence that follows is intended for students of any age who have little or no prior experience with bus travel.

Ideally, the first exposure to buses would be a hands-on experience without the time pressure of a bus en route. If possible, O&M specialists should take the student to the bus storage area (depot, garage, or yard) to familiarize the student with the various types of buses. If this is not possible then a familiarization might be done for one type of bus at the end of a line with a layover. Familiarization lessons should provide an opportunity for the student to explore the interior of the bus, including the fare box, driver's seat area, arrangement of seats, front and back door, and pull cord or push strips used to request a stop. Students need to practice boarding and exiting the bus. Role-playing various scenarios can be an effective instructional strategy for O&M specialists working with children or adults with multiple disabilities. Students need to be informed of the rules posted, such as no food or drink on the bus.

Next, O&M specialists need to teach persons about the various ways to obtain route and scheduling information and the specific locations of bus stops. During O&M lessons, students need to call customer service, use large-print, braille or audio bus route schedules and maps, and seek information online using the transit system's web site. O&M specialists can model procedures for how to obtain information by having students listen as the instructor calls customer service. Instruction in how to enter data into online trip-planning software programs should be provided, where appropriate.

Taking trips on the bus is the next step. It is best to select a trip that is relevant to the student's interest or need. Depending on the student's abilities, the instructor may want to select a simple trip initially, and then involve a transfer or other complications on subsequent trips. The student needs to complete a round trip because the return can involve different skills. On initial trips, the O&M specialist rides with the student, sitting next to him to narrate events as they unfold. As the student's skills progress, O&M specialists increase the monitoring distance by sitting in the back of the bus. When the student is ready, he can plan the route, board the bus, pay the fare, locate the destination stop, get off the bus, and travel to the destination without the instructor's assistance. The student needs to complete several trips in which the only time the O&M specialist converses with the student is at the final destination.

After the student has demonstrated competency and safety on all bus-related skills on multiple trips, the instructor has detailed documentation of this, and the student is ready to ride the bus independently, some O&M specialists follow the bus in their personal or employer's vehicle as the student rides along a designated route. This can help to build the student's confidence while providing a safety net for the first few times the student is riding the bus independently.

The final step in the training sequence for some students may be the student riding the bus alone, meeting his O&M specialist at a predetermined destination. Traveling unsupervised during training is referred to as a "solo" lesson. Solo lessons may occur at any time during an individual's O&M instructional program from indoor routes up to using public transportation. Written permission from the parent or legal guardian is recommended for solo lessons for students who are under 18 years of age. Some service providers may not allow children or adults to travel unsupervised while in training. If the school district's or agency's policy states that the student must be under direct supervision at all times, then following in another vehicle and solo lessons are not options.

Some O&M specialists do not see a need for unsupervised travel during training as they believe that the same goal can be accomplished with lessons in which the instructor observes from a long distance without any interaction with the student or the public. The student has mastered bus travel when he can complete trips without instructor intervention. In essence, students who are making decisions and traveling on the bus to the destination without help are completing a solo lesson, as per this alternative definition of "solo."

Other O&M specialists feel that the benefits of solo lessons outweigh the risks. The potential for confidence boosting, the affirmation that the instructor believes the student can complete the trip on his own, and the lessons learned from the student solving any problems that may arise, without the instructor being there, are deemed more important than the potential liability issues. Whether or not solo lessons are part of an individual's O&M training, it is important to be honest with the student about whether or not he will be observed during a lesson.

For those O&M specialists who do choose to incorporate solo lessons for some of their students, documentation and set procedures are crucial. In addition to student performance data depicting competency on bus travel–related skills, the O&M specialist needs to be assured, through sufficient observations, that the student can handle whatever arises during the bus trip (Jacobson, 1993). It is crucial to develop an agreed-upon plan for what to do during solo lessons in the event the O&M specialist or student does not arrive at the correct bus stop or other specified destination within the specified time frame (Pogrund et al., 1993). It is recommended that persons of all ages carry cell phones during solo trips as part of the backup plan.

Recovery Strategies

Students must have a planned course of action to follow in the event that they miss their bus or stop, get off at the wrong stop, cannot find a return bus, or realize that the bus they are on is taking an alternate route. Since it is unlikely that all these occurrences will happen during O&M lessons, strategies need to be role-played or discussed. Strategies to use after missing a stop include the following:

- Stay on the bus to the end of the line or a transfer station and then ride back to the desired stop (which is likely to be on the opposite side of the street).
- Get off and walk back (if it is not too far).
- Ask the driver for assistance.
- If the student is familiar with the areas along a bus route, he can get off the bus at a familiar location and call a taxi, family member, or friend for a ride.

Strategies to use after getting off at the wrong stop include the following:

- Determine one's exact location, soliciting assistance as needed.
- Use a cell phone to call a family member or friend to inform them of the situation and get advice.

- Wait for the next bus, get on it, then ride back to the desired stop, which is likely to be on the opposite side of the street, unless it is at a transit center.

Students with multiple disabilities may not be able to problem solve in these situations without assistance. These students need to be taught what to do if they miss their stop or what to do if they get off at the wrong stop. Having a written copy of a recovery plan and knowing that they need to show it to the driver for assistance can be helpful. Students need to carry self-identification and emergency contact information. It is also helpful if the student and the adults responsible for them each have a copy of the travel plans that includes locations of all bus stops as well as departure and arrival times.

Dog Guides

Individuals who use a dog guide need to work the dog onto the bus and may heel the dog up the steps to the fare box, and then to the nearest available seat. A seat running sideways is preferable as it allows more room for the dog. Dog guides often ride in a sitting position, facing the same direction as the owner. This allows the dog to brace itself and decreases the likelihood of getting its tail stepped on. Some individuals put one leg over the dog for its increased protection.

RAIL TRAVEL

Rail travel is linear by nature (LaGrow and Weessies, 1994). Trains may operate at (surface), below (subway), or above (elevated) the ground level. Trains are typically accessed from stations and boarded from platforms, although some trains operating at the surface level allow for direct boarding from the ground. In some large cities, the subway system operates 24 hours a day, seven days a week. Routes are usually identified using letters, numbers, colors, or end-of-the-line station names. Trains stop at specified stations, having fewer stops than buses. Detecting the platform edge and the space between rail cars are two safety concerns specific to rail travel.

Types of Rail Service

Light Rail

Light rail (streetcar, tramway, cable car, or trolley) is a transit mode that typically is an electric railway with light volume traffic capacity. *Light* refers to the number of riders that the train can carry, not the weight. It is characterized by passenger rail cars operating singly (or in short, usually two-car trains) on fixed rails in a right-of-way that is not separated from other traffic for much of the way. Stops typically are surface level on-street locations at the curb or in a median, sometimes with a shelter, signs, or lighting. Light rail systems can have low or high platform boarding with vehicle power drawn from an overhead electric line via a trolley (APTA, 2006b).

Commuter Rail

Commuter rail (regional rail, suburban rail) is a transit mode that is an electric or diesel propelled railway for urban passenger train service consisting of local short distance travel operating between urbanized areas and between a central city and adjacent suburbs. Such rail service operates on a regular basis and is generally characterized by multitrip tickets with specific station-to-station fares. Vehicles are either locomotive hauled or self-propelled railroad passenger cars (National Transit Database Glossary, 2001).

Rapid Rail

Rapid Rail (metro, subway, heavy rail, or rapid transit) is an electric railway with the capacity for heavy volumes of passengers. It is characterized by high-speed and rapid-acceleration passenger cars operating in multicar trains on fixed rails. Rapid rail has separate rights-of-way from which all other vehicular and pedestrian traffic is excluded. Trains have a variable number of rail cars, depending on the line, time of day, or day of week (APTA, 2006b).

Locating Rail Stations

Stairs leading down to a subway station or up to an elevated platform located on the sidewalk in the path of travel can be a safety issue if come upon unexpectedly and are not detected. Although transit systems use signs to signify a rail station entrance, recessed entrances may be difficult to find. Some visually impaired travelers may use a low vision device such as a telescope or be able to recognize the sign even if they cannot read it. Station entrances may be labeled with tactile signs but locating them can be an issue. Access to the station entrance, fare gates, platforms and other amenities can be labeled with RIAS which can provide detailed and precise directional information that allows a blind traveler with a receiver to accurately and discretely navigate through areas where the RIAS system is installed.

Rail station entrance areas generally include steps, escalators, and/or elevators to take passengers either aboveground or underground to the platform area, fare machines, fare gates, and possibly public and courtesy telephones. Stations can have one or more entrances, concourses, levels, and platforms. The complexity and irregularity of rail station design, signage with low visibility, and poor lighting can make unfamiliar rail stations difficult to negotiate for persons with visual impairments. Individuals who are unable to access information on signs can use the auditory cues from escalators, the flow of pedestrian traffic, and turnstile noises to help with orientation and travel through stations.

Platforms

There are two basic types of platforms, a side platform and a center platform. Some stations may be a combination of two side platforms with a center platform. This can be particularly confusing if the person is not familiar with it. Knowing the type of platforms within a station is important to the orientation and safety of persons with visual disabilities.

Side Platforms

A side platform (single track) has a wall on one side. Two side platforms have both sets of tracks, for trains in opposite directions, running between them. Pedestrians with visual impairments may walk along the wall to locate the stairs or escalators and to keep a large distance from the platform edge. In doing this, they will have to negotiate obstacles such as signs, system maps, and benches as these are typically located near the wall.

Center Platform

A center platform, which is also referred to as an island platform, is a platform located between two or more sets of tracks. Trains usually run in one direction on one side of the center platform and in the opposite direction on the other side. Larger stations can have two center platforms each serving different lines or local and express trains. This configuration may be used for transfer stations. Center platforms usually are not as common as side platforms so knowing that you are on a center platform with two platform edges is critical information for the visually impaired person. It is also helpful for visually impaired riders to know the track numbers to better understand the announcements of track changes and that they may have to go up or down a level to get to the track they need.

On center platforms, escalators, elevators, and stairs are positioned at intervals in the center

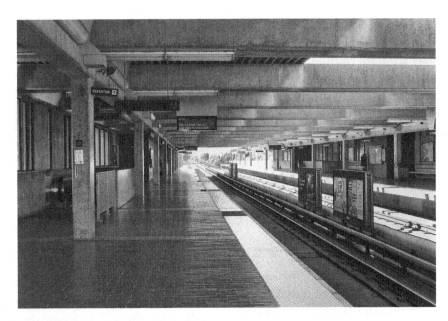

A side platform at a Bay Area Rapid Transit rail station.

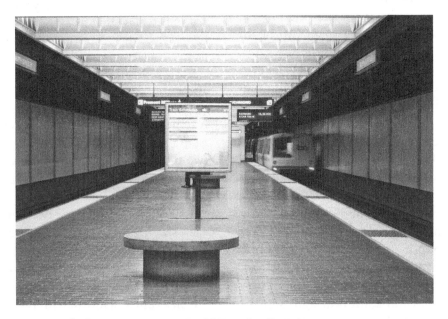

A center platform at a Bay Area Rapid Transit rail station.

of the platform width, parallel to the tracks. Typically there are obstacles such as benches, trash cans, and signs in the center of the platform. Some O&M specialists teach students to trail along the inner edge (away from the tracks) of the detectable warning strips when they walk along center platforms to reduce the possibility of veering, approaching the platform edge at an angle, and needing to frequently negotiate obstacles. This can be difficult in crowded stations.

Platform floors can be made of tile, brick, or aggregate concrete. By law, in the United States platform edges are marked with truncated dome detectable warning surfaces. See Volume 1, Chapter 11 for photos and specifications for detectable warnings.

Rapid Rail Track Area

Rail systems may use a third rail, located farthest from the platform, as a source of high voltage electricity. The other two rails also conduct electricity when the train is in proximity. The rails must never be contacted with a metal cane because the cane will act as a conductor of electricity. Carbon fiber canes do not conduct electricity. The platform may overhang the track area such that a 3- to 4-foot deep crawl space or refuge area is formed alongside the wall. In an emergency after a fall to the tracks, this refuge area is large enough to allow a person to lie safely while a train passes. The person must lie against the wall, as far away as possible from the train, to be safe in this refuge area. O&M specialists must teach their students about the refuge area. With the permission and supervision of transit system personnel and under controlled circumstances, O&M specialists have provided students an opportunity to explore the track area to familiarize them with the refuge area (Uslan et al., 1990).

Trip Planning

Planning trips using rail service is similar to planning trips using buses. Individuals can call customer service, obtain printed schedules in large print, braille, or audiotape or use the system's online trip-planning software. Rapid rail trains usually have fewer stops than buses and trains may go through some stations without stopping. Light rail trains may have frequent stops. Refer to Sidebar 13.2 for information about questions to ask when planning rail trips.

Entering Stations

Because many underground stations have very dim lighting, there is a significant change in the illumination level when a person enters the station from outdoors, especially on a sunny day. Underground stations can be very loud with echoes. Pedestrians with visual impairments can follow the general flow of other pedestrians to the fare gate, turnstile, and platform boarding area. One type of turnstile system is a series of rotating bars positioned horizontally from the floor to several feet above head level that allow one person at a time to go through (Jacobson, 1993). The horizontal bars move in only one direction as each person pushes through one at a time. The O&M specialist should demonstrate how the turnstile operates, then go through behind the student. Stairs and escalators are areas where accidents may occur due to slips, falls, or trips. Students may need instruction on escalators if they have not previously used them.

Tactile and auditory maps are installed in some rapid rail stations in Japan (Uslan et al., 1990). These maps utilize different textures for rail tracks, stairs, entrances and exits, restaurants, fare machines, newsstands, and other relevant station features. A description of the texture representation is provided on the left side of the map. Audiotape messages on maps provide verbal directions to major public facilities. These messages can be accessed through switches that are labeled in braille. Some stations have high contrast light-colored raised blocks that lead travelers from the entrance to the platforms.

Fare Machines and Fare Gates

Fare cards, tokens, or passes can be purchased a variety of ways including online, through the mail, at retail locations, at fare machines, or at ticket booths, which are usually located near the station entrance. Discount tickets for some

Key Questions for Obtaining Rail Information

BEFORE CALLING CUSTOMER SERVICE

1. Know the address, intersection, or landmark of your starting point.

2. Know the address, intersection, or landmark of your destination.

3. Know the day and time you want to begin your trip or arrive at your destination.

4. Know if you want the fastest trip, fewest transfers, or shortest walking distance.

TRIP TO DESTINATION

1. Which station is closest to my starting point?

   a. What entrance should I use, and where exactly is the entrance? (Which corner of intersection or midblock between what two cross streets?)

2. What type of station is this?

3. Will I have to go down or up to get to the platform?

4. Will I board from a center platform or a side platform?

5. Which line(s) serve my destination?

6. Will I need to transfer? If so, where? What is the stop immediately before that? How many stops before the transfer stop?

7. How often do trains run on this line, or what time is the train due at the station?

8. What exit station is closest to my destination?

9. How many total stops? What is the name of the stop immediately before my stop?

10. Does the exit station have a center platform or a side platform?

11. What station exit should I use to get to my destination?

12. In what direction and along which street should I travel to get to my destination?

13. What is the fare?

For the return trip—repeat relevant questions from this list.

---

transit systems are not available at the stations but must be purchased ahead of time and require the user to have a discount identification card. At some stations, the fare card, token, or pass is then used at a turnstile. Fare machines typically have slots for coins, bills, and credit cards. Accessible fare machines may be hard to find and difficult to use even if they have audio, raised characters, braille, and a tactile pathway. O&M specialists should familiarize students with these machines even if they typically use a discount ticket that is purchased by the month in case riders experience difficulty with their ticket.

Fares for rail travel are usually paid for in advance at a fare gate with a turnstile or at a ticket counter with payment in the form of a token, ticket, pass, or a smart card. A smart card is like a debit card. Each time an individual takes a ride, the fare is deducted from the balance. Knowing the balance may be an issue for those who are unable to see the digital display or printed receipt. Monthly passes can help avoid the issues of frequently needing to find and use the fare machine, or finding oneself with too little on a ticket and having to find an add-fare machine. Some systems sell unlimited ride cards for the day, week, or month.

Passengers with visual impairments can use auditory cues of pedestrian movements to help determine which fare gate is for entry and which is for exit. Different systems use various methods to orient the fare card or pass in the correct direction prior to placing it in the slot in the fare gate. Some tickets have holes punched in them or a cut corner to help with card orientation. Passengers can feel and hear the machine taking in the card or pass. The fare card or pass may come out in various locations depending on the fare gate. After it is removed, the person proceeds through the turnstile or gate opening.

Detecting the Platform Edge

Finding the edge of the platform is a crucial safety concern because the tracks are about five feet (1.5 m) below the platform. A fall from the platform could cause severe injury. Individuals who use long canes need to approach the edge of the platform perpendicularly walking at a slower pace using constant contact technique. Using constant contact technique instead of touch technique makes it easier to identify the detectable warnings and to find the platform edge.

When traveling along platforms, some O&M specialists teach their students to trail the edge of the platform's detectable warning surface that is farthest from the platform edge (Uslan et al., 1990). This allows the individual to constantly be aware of where she is in relation to the platform edge. Persons are taught to trail the edge of the detectable warning surface because walking directly on it puts the person too close to the platform edge. Other O&M specialists object to even trailing the detectable warning surface because it requires the individual to walk relatively close to the platform edge and increases the possibility of collisions with pedestrians, especially on crowded platforms. One problem reported by pedestrians with visual impairments is that other pedestrians often interfere with them by pulling them away from the platform edge. When sighted passengers see a pedestrian with a white cane or dog guide they may overreact and feel the need

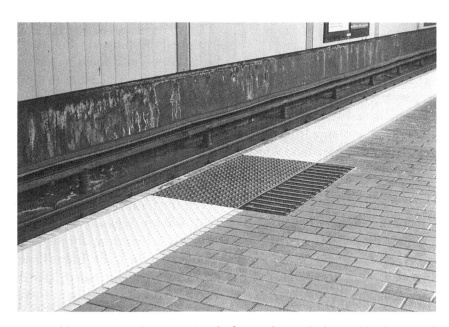

Detectable warnings along a train platform edge with detectable directional textures showing the location of doors.

to warn the visually impaired pedestrian that he or she is too close to the edge. Persons with visual impairments can either ignore others or assure them that they are confident about their own travel skills. Platform screen doors, which are full height total barriers between the station floor and the ceiling, are now being used at some stations to prevent people from falling into the rails.

Waiting at Platform

Once passengers with visual impairments find the platform edge, they need to remain well back from the edge while waiting for the train. All passengers should wait behind the detectable warnings. Some systems have high contrast tactile markings or directional strips to indicate where the door opens, depending on the length of the train. Trains have bright headlights and make a loud noise when they enter a station. Moving trains also cause the platform to vibrate. Some trains may go through the station without stopping. In some stations, trains pass along both sides of the platform, so the student must learn the directions the trains are going.

Boarding Trains

To find the correct train at platforms that serve multiple rail lines, passengers with visual impairments can listen for automated announcements, use LED signage, or ask for assistance from other passengers. It is important to understand which direction the desired train will be traveling as it enters the station.

After the train comes to a complete stop, persons with visual impairments can use the sound of the doors opening and the people entering and exiting to help locate the door. Some O&M specialists teach their students to trail a stopped train using modified three-point touch to find the door, when necessary. A safety concern is that passengers who are blind may step into the space be-

tween cars because they mistake it for the open rail car doorway. Thus, it is crucially important for passengers to check for and contact the train floor with their cane before boarding to confirm that it is the floor and not a gap or another part of the train that is at the same level as the floor. After locating the gap between the platform edge and the train floor, persons need to step over it into the car. Platform screens which close off the platform edge and open only when trains are correctly aligned with the doors are the best solution, but many systems do not use them.

Some transit systems have installed between-car barriers (BCBs) on the trains, such as chains or collapsible gates, to prevent visually impaired patrons from stepping into the space between rail cars and falling from the elevated platform to the trackway below. Other systems have installed bollards, which are flexible poles at least knee height mounted on the platform. Train operators need to berth, or stop the train such that the open space between cars is behind the bollards and the front door of the train stops in the same place each time, regardless of the number of cars in the train. Some transit agencies have received exemptions from installing required between-car barriers.

A sound indicates that the train doors will soon close. Train doors are not like elevator doors and will not reopen automatically. In addition, passengers need to make sure that pocketbooks, knapsacks, clothing, packages, umbrellas, and other personal items are clear of the closing doors. If an object or person is caught in the door a different sound signals the train operator and the train cannot move until the doors are closed. However, the train can move if an item is stuck in a closed door. Typically, each of the train doors is directly across from another door on the opposite side of the train. Trains have priority seating near the door for elderly persons and persons with disabilities. It is best if passengers with visual impairments sit or stand close to the doors to enter and exit efficiently. Many trains are packed with riders, especially during peak hours. Thus, individuals with visual impairments may need to learn to ride standing up while holding the vertical bars or hand loops. O&M specialists need to teach students how to go from car to car in the event they wish to move away from someone who is bothering them or the intercom is not working in that car. They need to familiarize students with the location of the intercom for calling the train operator and posted emergency information.

Identifying Station for Train Exit

Visually impaired riders need to be made aware that in some rail systems the doors that open will vary depending on the type of platform at the station. Is it important to note that some doors are passenger activated so the door will not open unless someone presses a button. Passengers with visual impairments may use the following strategies to identify the exit station:

- Count number of stops by door opening (not train stopping).
- Use distance between stops as a cue.
- Memorize order of the stops.
- Listen for automated announcements (sometimes difficult to hear or understand).
- Use which side of the car the door opens as a cue.
- Seek assistance from other passengers.
- Call the train operator on the intercom (if available).
- Use RIAS when available.

Exiting Station

Passengers with visual impairments can follow the sounds of pedestrians, ask for directions, or walk along the platform until they hear an escalator or stairs. Passengers can transfer to another rail line at transfer stations. To do so, they may need to locate the transfer fare machine and walk to the correct platform to continue their trip. There are many variations on what happens when transferring between trains depending on the transit system, the configuration of the station, and the fare system. Some rail stations have a bus area for multimodal trips. Passengers who are finished using the rail system must find the station exit. Stations with multiple exits typically have signage on the platform level that indicates the street name or points of interest below the exit sign.

Passengers leaving the station through an exit turnstile may or may not have their ticket or fare card returned, depending on whether it has expired, has no remaining balance, or can be used again. O&M specialists need to make students aware of the emergency bar which allows a passenger to release the lock for exiting if necessary. This typically activates an alarm and alerts the station agent. The bar can be used in an emergency or might have to be used if the person's ticket does not work and an agent is not available.

Light Rail Transit (LRT) System Safety Issues

The Transit Cooperative Research Board (TCRB) continues to conduct research regarding pedestrian safety for light rail service. Because some light rail systems operate on fixed rails in shared rights-of-way (not separated from other traffic), vehicles and pedestrians cross the tracks. To board the train in some systems, pedestrians must cross to median islands in wide streets. Some islands are not detectable as they have no tactile or level change from the street. It may be difficult for persons with visual impairments to recognize they have reached the island until their cane or foot contacts the tracks. Light rail vehicles are moving at high speeds and are relatively quiet. Sighted pedestrians have been hit by trains. Sometimes the sound from a train coming in one direction may mask the sound of a train coming from the opposite direction. Passengers may be caught off guard when they enter a train at a station from a surface-level platform, and then must exit via stairs because vehicles go from underground to aboveground during a trip. Issues related to detecting the gap between rail cars used in light rail service are similar to those in rapid rail systems.

After TCRB (2001a) addressed safety issues for pedestrians and vehicles by compiling accident data from systems throughout the United States and Canada, it began researching what types of devices might improve pedestrian safety, including pedestrians with visual impairments. The goal of TCRP Project D-10, "Audible Signals for Pedestrian Safety in Light Rail Transit Environments," is to develop a guidebook for LRT systems on the use of audible signals and related operating procedures for pedestrian crossing safety.

Monorails

A monorail is a transit mode that is an electric railway of guided transit vehicles operating in single-car or multicar trains and suspended from or straddling a guideway formed by a single beam, rail, or tube. Monorail vehicles are wider than the guideway that supports them. Because a monorail is elevated, accidents with surface traffic are impossible, thereby increasing pedestrian safety. Monorails are quiet and environmentally friendly. Monorails are used worldwide, with increasing popularity in the United States.

Role of O&M Specialist

O&M specialists need to give input to rail transit systems regarding system operation and station design. This is especially beneficial during the planning phases of new stations. Sidebar 13.3 includes suggestions from Uslan et al. (1990) to increase station accessibility for persons with visual impairments.

In addition, O&M specialists need to provide train operator training, reminding them of the importance of stopping at the same place every time such that tactile indicators line up with the doorways and the gap between rail cars lines up with the between-car barriers, when present.

Sequence of Instruction

Sometimes O&M specialists can take students to the end of the line where a train waits out of service to familiarize the student with the train. Some rail systems periodically bring a train to a platform not being used and let people get on and off and even go down in the tracks to familiarize them with the refuge area. Students need to have opportunities to practice approaching, boarding, locating a seat, and exiting a parked train. Utilizing empty parked vehicles provides an opportunity for the student to practice identifying the door opening versus the space between cars in a nonthreatening, controlled environment.

Following the general instructional sequence of simple to complex environments, initial instruction usually begins during nonpeak hours in a relatively quiet station with a simple layout, such as a station with a single-access corridor. The other possibility is to begin instruction at the station the student will use most frequently. Some students need step-by-step practice of every aspect of negotiating the station while more advanced students can be taught station self-familiarization techniques.

The O&M specialist needs to help the student become familiarized with the operation of the turnstile, fare machine, and fare gate. Next, the student needs to practice locating the platform edge until both the student and the O&M specialist have confidence that the student can consistently locate it, and then position himself safely to wait for the train. As the student gains proficiency, complex stations with multiple entrances, levels, corridors, and platforms that serve trains traveling in different directions

SIDEBAR 13.3

Accessibility Features for Rail Stations

1. Trip-planning information from customer service staff sensitive to the needs of visually impaired riders as well as an accessible web-based system

2. Accessible ticket vending machines, add-value machines, and card interface devices through speech, large-print raised letters, and braille

3. Access to signs including real-time information by complying with visual signage standards and audible signage such as remote infrared audible signage (RIAS)

4. Accessible route and station maps

5. Auditory or tactile pathways from station entrances to platforms

6. Easy-to-understand automated announcements

7. High levels of no-glare, artificial lighting in underground stations

8. High-contrast signs with raised large-print letters and braille mounted on walls at eye level in well-lit, predictable areas

9. Follows specifications for detectable warnings at platform edges

10. Between-car barriers (BCBs), such as safety gates between rail cars or on platform barriers that prevent individuals from falling into the gap between cars

11. Train operators informed of needs of visually impaired passengers who stop the train so that the doorways align with the tactile markers

12. Obstacles placed out of pedestrian travel paths with benches parallel to platform edge and no poles in doorway openings

13. Single-access corridor to the platform edge is ideal

14. Stairs and escalators (in access corridors) should be side by side

15. Elevators placed consistently in all stations within the system

16. Handholds available at both waist level and above head level

17. Seating within cars for persons with disabilities near the doors

Source: Adapted in part from M. M. Uslan, A. F. Peck, B. R. Wiener, and A. Stern, *Access to Mass Transit for Blind and Visually Impaired Travelers* (New York: American Foundation for the Blind, 1990).

---

along multiple routes should be introduced (La-Grow & Weessies, 1994).

Recovery Strategies

Students need to have a planned course of action to follow in the event that they miss their train or stop or get lost. To get reoriented, individuals need to determine their exact location. This can be done by reading either signage in the station or street signs near the station, or by asking tran-

sit system personnel or other passengers. Another basic strategy is to go to a known location and start the trip again. This strategy can be used effectively in cities that have a central station in the heart of the city (LaGrow & Weessies, 1994). Passengers who miss their stop can exit at the next stop, locate the track going in the opposite direction, and then board that train to go back to the desired stop. In underground rail stations, persons who wish to use their cell phones to call coworkers, family members, or friends to inform them that they are running late due to disorientation may need to move toward the station entrance to obtain a sufficiently strong phone signal.

Safety Concerns

In rail stations, persons with visual impairments might want to avoid using elevators that are located in remote areas and not monitored by video camera. Assistance phones, which are typically located near the fare gates, connect the passenger to transit system personnel. Some systems use closed-circuit televisions so that they can see persons at the phones. Personnel can give basic directions or send a police officer to the person in the event of an emergency. The O&M specialist may advocate for increased lighting in targeted areas within rail stations.

Falls from Platform

At most stations, a passenger who falls down to the track area needs to do the following (Uslan et al., 1990):

1. Yell for help.
2. Listen for and orient himself using sounds of pedestrians on the platform.
3. Stand and reach out to touch the platform edge. If possible, let someone pull him up immediately.
4. If the train is coming or if people are not available to help, duck under the platform edge and contact the wall of the refuge area or crawl space, if available.
5. Lie down along the wall as close as possible, making oneself as small as possible.
6. Continue to yell for help.

Emergency Evacuations

Persons should use the emergency cord only to prevent an accident or injury. If an evacuation is necessary, the most important thing is to follow the instructions of the train operator. This may mean staying on or leaving the train. According to Uslan et al. (1990), the safety evacuation procedures for passengers with visual impairments are nearly the same as those for people who are sighted. In most situations it is safer to remain inside the train to wait for rescue personnel. However, persons need to leave the stalled train if the situation is life threatening. Passengers with visual impairments need to follow a designated "lead" person by holding onto the guide's arm. All evacuees need to walk along the track bed to the nearest rail station, paying close attention to avoid the high-voltage third rail, and wet, slippery portions and switching devices located along the track bed.

Dog Guides

Dog guide users should inform the O&M specialist what procedures they would like to use for rail station familiarization. Before working the dog in the station, O&M specialists may familiarize the individual with the station using a long cane (without the dog). The next step might involve repeating the familiarization using human guide techniques with the dog at heel. Finally, the O&M specialist can observe the individual working with the dog through the station. This sequence of instruction may not be necessary for individuals who are experienced with using the rail system. The user and his dog guide should wait for the train approximately 4–6 feet (1–2 m) from the edge of the platform, facing the edge with the dog at sit and relaxed. While working the dog onto the train, the individual assumes the modified upper-hand and forearm technique (Hill & Ponder, 1976) to prevent the doors from closing on him. During the ride, the dog sits in front of the owner facing in the same direction. The owner can help support the dog, as needed, and keep it relaxed. The user exits the train, again using the modified upper-hand and forearm technique. The dog guide user walks a few feet away from the platform edge and pauses while trains leave the station, if the dog needs this for stress reduction.

PARATRANSIT SYSTEMS

The ADA clearly emphasizes nondiscriminatory access to fixed-route service, with complementary paratransit acting as a "safety net" for people who cannot use the fixed-route system (ADA Paratransit Eligibility Manual, 1993). Each public entity operating a fixed-route system is required by law to offer comparable ADA paratransit service to persons with disabilities and others not able to use fixed-route service (intercity bus, subway, light rail).

Paratransit is a type of demand response service. Persons schedule rides from a specified origin to a destination. The decision as to whether paratransit service is *door-to-door* or *curb-to-curb* is not federally mandated, but rather an operational decision made at the local level. Door-to-door means that the drivers escort the passengers along the path between the pick-up and destination doors and the paratransit vehicle. Curb-to-curb means that passengers walk between the doorway and the vehicle on their own. Generally, ADA paratransit within three-quarters of a mile of any fixed-route service needs to operate during the same hours and days of the week as the fixed-route service. Because paratransit has high per-trip costs, fares up to double the fixed-route fare are permitted under the ADA. Many paratransit agencies sell prepaid books of tickets with no expiration dates and/or monthly passes. Others accept cash. Paratransit service may be provided by the fixed-route bus agency or by a completely separate agency. Typically, the vehicles are dispatched to pick up several passengers at different pick-up points before taking them to their respective destinations.

Eligibility Standards

Only some persons with visual impairments are eligible for all trips using paratransit services.

There are three statutory eligibility categories that deal with a person's functional inability to use fixed-route transit arising from a combination of a disability and circumstances. The first eligibility category concerns individuals who cannot board, ride, or disembark from an accessible vehicle. These people cannot "navigate the system." The second eligibility category consists of people who can use an accessible vehicle but cannot use a route on the fixed-route system for lack of accessible vehicles. The third eligibility category pertains to people who have specific impairment-related conditions that prevent them from getting to or from a transit stop.

Persons with visual impairments are eligible for paratransit services under the first and third categories. These persons may not be able to "navigate the fixed-route system" due to any of these reasons:

- An environmental barrier (e.g., inaccessible intersection, no sidewalks along a busy street on the walking route to the bus stop)
- Additional disabilities
- Lack of safe, independent travel skills

Eligibility is granted only if the interaction of the environmental barrier and the visual impairment *prevents* the individual from getting to the stop. For example, consider a trip that involves crossing a four-lane highway with a lot of fast-moving vehicles in an area without a traffic signal to get to the bus stop. The necessity of crossing a busy, dangerous, uncontrolled street *prevents* some persons who are blind from using fixed-route transit for this trip. It's not just an inconvenience. Thus, eligibility would be granted for this trip.

A visual impairment does not confer eligibility if it simply makes use of fixed-route transit less comfortable, or more difficult, than use of fixed-route transit for persons who do not have the condition. For example, fear of crime when using the fixed-route system, or fixed routes with infrequent times or widely spaced bus stops do not confer eligibility.

Conditional Eligibility

Many persons with visual impairments can use the fixed-route service for some destinations but not for others. Thus, they are eligible for some, but not all, trips on paratransit. For example, someone who can navigate the fixed-route system to and from work may not be able to navigate the system to a different destination. Someone who can get to the bus stop in the summer may not be able to get there on icy or snowy winter days. This type of eligibility is known as conditional eligibility.

Unconditional Eligibility

Unconditional paratransit eligibility means that a person is eligible to use paratransit for all trips. Persons with visual impairments who also have a cognitive or physical disability or health condition that prevents them from independently using the fixed-route bus or rail systems for any trips may be granted unconditional eligibility. If requested, O&M specialists need to provide information to the paratransit agency for students with multiple disabilities who are deemed unable to travel safely and independently.

It should be noted that some paratransit agencies question eligibility for persons with visual impairments because many persons with visual impairments can and do use fixed-route services. Because these agencies believe that persons with visual impairments are not eligible for any paratransit trips, they may refuse service to all persons with visual impairments who apply. The statute makes clear, however, that persons with visual impairments are eligible if they cannot "navigate the system." A paratransit system cannot require the instruction necessary for a person to become able to "navigate the system."

In other areas, persons with visual impairments who could be using fixed-route service are using paratransit service for all of their transit trips. O&M specialists need to work with students who use ADA complementary paratransit as their only mode of public transportation to be sure they are knowledgeable about fixed-route service options.

Feeder Service

Feeder service meets the ADA requirements for people in the third eligibility category, which pertains to people who have specific impairment-related conditions that prevent them from getting to or from a stop. Feeder service refers to the paratransit agency giving persons a ride on a paratransit vehicle from their origin (often home) to the bus stop or station or from the bus stop or station to their destination. The person then uses the fixed-route service for the rest of the trip. Thus, the trip is multimodal as it combines both paratransit and fixed-route service.

Trip Planning

Individuals contact the paratransit agency to schedule trips. There are no restrictions on the number of trips any individual can schedule or on the purpose for the trips. Paratransit agencies across the United States have different procedures for scheduling trips. However, ADA does dictate some parameters for scheduling trips. Generally, to schedule a ride, a person must call the paratransit agency at least a day, but no more than 14 days in advance and provide the following information:

- Name as it appears on the paratransit application
- Complete addresses of pick-up and destination, including zip code, name of building (if applicable) entrance location, and cross street or nearest major street
- Desired arrival time at destination
- Need for special requirements, such as a vehicle with a lift and tie-downs for a wheelchair

or an oversized wheelchair, or scooter, and whether the person can transfer to a sedan

- Intention to have a personal care attendant or human guide companion accompanying person

Most systems do not provide same day trip requests except in the event of an emergency. Reservation service must be available during the normal business hours of the provider's administrative offices. Paratransit authorities can negotiate pickup times but cannot insist on pickup times (either to destination or return trip) that vary by more than an hour from the user's desired travel time. That hour must be consistent with the purpose of the trip. For example, if an individual calls to request a 7:00 A.M. pickup as he needs to be at work by 8:00 A.M., the system could offer an hour earlier (6:00 A.M.) pickup. The system could not offer an hour later (8:00 A.M.) pickup as that would not serve the purpose of the trip, causing the person to be late for work.

If an individual's transportation needs require him to be at the same place, at the same time, from the same location, on the same days of the week, he should request a "subscription trip." There is no ADA requirement that paratransit systems offer this scheduling convenience, but most do. Subscription trips are provided, except on holidays, on a "standing basis," unless a person cancels them. If a trip is not cancelled it is considered a missed ride or "no show." Persons must call in advance to cancel trips. Policies about how far one must call in advance are made at the local level. Individuals must be familiar with these policies regarding "no shows." Paratransit agencies may suspend services to otherwise ADA paratransit–eligible individuals who engage in a pattern or practice of missing scheduled trips. This involves intentional, repeated incidences of "no-shows" and is determined by a percentage computed by number of trips a person schedules in relation to the number of "no-shows." Before imposing a sanction, the entity would have to pro-

vide basic administrative due process to the individual, and this system's administrative appeal mechanism would be available in cases decided against the individual.

Service Cancellations

During severe weather, such as ice and snow, paratransit service may be delayed or cancelled. Agencies must make every attempt to operate as long as local law enforcement and traffic agencies permit vehicles to remain on the streets.

Role of O&M Specialists

Working with Students

In situations where persons with visual impairments cannot use fixed-route service, O&M specialists should facilitate the application for paratransit services. In addition to a report from an eye care practitioner, most paratransit agencies require documentation of a person's travel abilities, and conditions under which the person would be unable to use fixed-route service. With permission for release of information from the student, the O&M specialist needs to provide this documentation. After individuals are determined eligible for ADA paratransit, instruction may be necessary on how to buy tickets and how to schedule and cancel trips. For students with disabilities in addition to visual impairment, O&M specialists may need to provide direct instruction on how to count tickets and have them ready for the driver, as well as how to board and exit vehicles. If paratransit service is denied, the person with a visual impairment may need assistance or instruction on how to use the appeals process. The O&M specialist may advocate for the student in the appeals process.

Some clients may need information in order to determine if they can use fixed-route service or paratransit service for a particular trip. O&M specialists can provide information about the travel path to and from fixed-route stops or travel with a client along the walking route to a fixed-route stop to help the client determine if a particular trip is possible using fixed-route service. If the route from the person's home to the closest bus or rail stop is not accessible, the O&M specialist can discuss feeder service as an option.

Upon paratransit staff request, O&M specialists may preview a walking route to refute or confirm the presence of an environmental barrier which prevents the person from getting to a fixed-route stop or station. Some paratransit agencies will provide trips on a temporary basis during the time an individual is receiving O&M instruction. Sometimes clients are reluctant to receive O&M instruction to learn the skills required to use fixed-route service because they fear losing their rides on paratransit. If the client does not have the O&M skills to use transit, the paratransit system cannot refuse to give them continued service even if they refuse to receive O&M instruction. In this situation, the O&M specialist should discuss the potential benefits of increased flexibility, independence, and lower fares when using fixed-route service with their client.

Driver Training

O&M specialists need to provide training to both the paratransit customer service staff and drivers. Instruction for paratransit drivers might include basic information about what riders with visual disabilities need to know such as the driver's name, presence of other passengers in the vehicle, available seating, and a description of what is happening in an emergency. Inform drivers not to beep the horn when they arrive for a pickup but rather to go to the door (door-to-door service providers) or get out of the vehicle (curb-to-curb service providers) to greet the passengers. Some persons will prefer to walk to the vehicle with the driver using human guide techniques while others will follow behind the driver. The use of short videos, such as *What Do You Do When You See a Blind Person?* available through the

American Foundation for the Blind (2000), may be included in the training. Demonstration of and practice in using basic human guide techniques for negotiating stairs, doors, and finding a seat would be more relevant for drivers who work in systems with door-to-door service. Optimally, drivers should practice human guide techniques by guiding other drivers who are blindfolded and by being guided while they are under blindfold themselves. Drivers need to also learn how to give a brief orientation of the area immediately inside the destination building upon passenger request.

TAXI SERVICE

Taxis are generally the quickest and most convenient type of travel within cities. Unfortunately, they are also the most expensive. Taxis will pick up a person at his specified location and drop him off at his destination. Taxis usually operate 24 hours a day, seven days per week. They typically carry up to four passengers. Most taxis are not accessible for travelers who use wheelchairs or some other type of bulky travel aid.

Under the ADA, taxis are in the category of demand response service. Taxi companies may not refuse to provide services to individuals with disabilities. Private taxi companies are also prohibited from charging higher fares or extra fees for transporting individuals with disabilities and their service animals than they charge to other persons for the same or equivalent service. Persons can get a taxi by scheduling one, going to a taxi stand, or by hailing a taxi at curbside.

Trip Planning

Scheduling trips can be done over the telephone and with some companies over the internet. When scheduling a trip, the customer is typically expected to give the following information: location of both the pickup and drop-off, number of passengers, time the taxi is needed, and contact information. When calling, a customer can ask the dispatcher to estimate what time the taxi should arrive for pickup, the approximate trip duration, distance, and approximate fare for the scheduled trip. Some companies will not give an approximate fare, but rather will provide the flag drop and mileage fees so people can figure fares out themselves. Before they enter the taxi, customers can confirm this information with the driver (Jacobson, 1993). It would be helpful if passengers could direct taxi drivers by providing directions to their home, place of employment, doctor's office, salon, and other destinations they travel to frequently.

A person who uses taxi services regularly in his home area might find a driver he likes, call to request him or her by name or by taxi number, and tip well. This generally leads to improved service. Many companies allow regular customers to set up a call time for routine service, such as a ride on weekdays to and from work, so that a driver is dispatched to the designated place at a set time on the set days.

Taxi Stands

Another option for getting a taxi is locating a taxi stand. Visually impaired travelers may find this a useful approach if the taxi stand is within walking distance. The most common places to find taxi stands are airports, major hotels, shopping centers and transit stations. Additionally, in some cities taxi stands may be located at large office buildings and apartment buildings. Some of these buildings have a doorman, bell captain, security staff, or other employee who will assist a person with getting a taxi. These types of helpers may assist an individual with a visual impairment even when there is no taxi stand present. It is customary practice to tip such persons.

Hailing Taxis

A third option is to hail a taxi. In some cities, such as New York City, pedestrians must hail a taxi by standing along the street curb and flagging down a vacant taxi. People with visual impairments must step to the edge of the curb, put their hand up, make their cane visible, and wait for a taxi to pull to a stop. This approach is particularly challenging for persons with severe visual impairments as it is difficult to distinguish approaching taxis from other vehicles. It also may pose safety risks. Before getting into the vehicle, customers should wait for the driver to identify himself. They can also ask the driver for identification but may be unable to see well enough to read it. In a few cities, taxis have a sign on the passenger door with braille and large print stating the name of the company and the taxi ID number. Also, people can solicit aid from other persons on the street to hail a taxi.

Fares

Fares differ between geographical areas, so people need to check the fare rates with taxi companies to be sure they understand what the costs can be and what form of payment is accepted. Although the rates for taxi services are regulated and posted in all taxis, rate information is not in an accessible format for persons who read braille or large print. Most fares are paid in cash, but some companies can be paid with a voucher and some accept credit cards. Vouchers are documents that allow persons to take a taxi for free or at a reduced rate. Vouchers may be allocated to eligible persons by human service agencies or other organizations. Many passengers, whether using vouchers or paying cash, tip the driver for good service. When requested, the driver needs to give the customer a receipt.

Most companies do not allow set fees except for trips from airports to certain destinations. Taxi fares are determined by the distance of the trip and are often calculated on a meter mounted on the dashboard. Some cities are divided into zones with additional fares when traveling through various zones. Most taxi companies require their drivers to use a fare meter. There is an initial charge for engaging a taxi plus a distance charge for each fraction of a mile traveled. Taxi meters often have a small flag that operates as a switch to start and stop the meter. The meter starts when the driver "drops the flag" as he arrives at his scheduled pickup and stops when the taxi arrives at the final destination. Some companies charge extra fees for waiting time if customers are late for a pickup and for traffic delay time. The fare may also include an additional fee for extra passengers, toll roads, bridge tolls, airport surcharges, luggage, and other fees where applicable. Many taxi companies do not charge for children or for personal care attendants accompanying a person with a disability.

Driver and Passenger Responsibilities

Taxi drivers should provide professional and courteous service. They should identify themselves, provide identification when possible, and assist passengers with stowing luggage in the trunk. They must take the most direct route to the passenger's destination, charge metered rates, accept any passenger unless the taxi is engaged or off duty, and give a receipt when requested. If the passenger asks the dispatcher to tell the driver she is blind, the driver can tell the dispatcher to call the passenger when he is in the vicinity or get out of the vehicle and go to the person's door to let her know he has arrived for a pickup. It has been reported by persons with visual impairments that drivers have pulled up, waited, and then left, thinking the service was no longer needed without the passenger ever realizing the taxi had arrived.

Passengers should wait at the curb or be prepared to come out to the taxi immediately upon its arrival, pay the fare, and enter and exit the vehicle away from the traffic lane. Passengers need to cancel reservations if the taxi is not needed. It is suggested that passengers request receipts so they have a record of the trip.

In order to remain oriented during the ride, passengers may periodically question the driver regarding the direction being traveled, street name, and distance to the destination. Use of accessible GPS technology allows passengers with visual impairments to track their progress independently. This also helps to ensure that any agreed-upon route is being taken. Upon arrival at the destination, the passenger can ask the driver to identify the exact location at which he is being dropped off, where he should go to reach the destination, and nearby landmarks. After the driver tells the amount of the fare, the passenger pays his fare and exits the taxi. The driver may walk to the door with the passenger if requested to do so.

Dog Guides

Dogs should be in a sitting position on the floor, not on the seat (Greenwald, 1979). Persons who use dog guides are responsible for keeping their dogs well groomed, quiet, well behaved, and under good control at all times when riding in the taxi. Taxi drivers are required to respond to dog guide users.

Safety Considerations

Persons with visual impairments should use a taxi company or a driver that has a good reputation. When scheduling a trip, passengers may be able to get the approximate trip distance and fare amount either from the dispatcher or online. Passengers may wait for the taxi inside as the dispatcher can call when the taxi arrives. When a scheduled taxi arrives or a vehicle believed to be the taxi pulls up to the curb, the person should wait for the driver to identify himself as the taxi driver instead of asking him if he is the driver. Taxis usually operate 24 hours, seven days a week and can be a safer option than buses late at night. Persons must be wary of private cars posing as taxis.

LIMOUSINES

A *limousine* refers to a large passenger vehicle, especially a luxurious automobile, usually driven by a chauffeur and sometimes having a partition separating the passenger compartment from the driver's seat. A limousine can also be a van or small bus used to carry passengers on a regular route, as between an airport and a downtown area. Trips are scheduled by calling the limousine company.

Not much is written in the literature regarding utilization of limousines by passengers with visual impairments. O&M specialists who teach in areas with limousine service need to help their students learn about this transportation system.

AIR TRAVEL

Planes tend to be the quickest form of travel between distant cities. Airline travel can be the most expensive, serve the fewest locales, and is often the most difficult transportation mode to access (LaGrow & Weessies, 1994). Many people with visual impairments travel independently all over the world via air travel. Discrimination by air carriers (in areas other than employment) is not covered by the ADA but rather by the Air Carrier Access Act (49 U.S.C. 1374 (c)), which passed in 1986.

Trip Planning and Fares

Trip information including dates, times, flight numbers, number of stops, transfers, and fares can be obtained online from travel and airline web sites or by phone from an airline or travel agency. Tickets may be purchased online, through a travel agent, in advance from the airline by phone, or at the airport ticket counter. Different airlines have discounted ticket prices for tickets purchased a minimum number of days in advance. If several carriers service the same route, it is best to check

all of them to determine the best schedule and fare. The availability and cost of ground transportation between the airport and the destination may also be an important factor in the decision about which air carrier to utilize.

Packing

Packing as little as possible can make the trip easier. For short trips, packing everything to carry on the plane helps to avoid checking a bag. Use of a backpack or a rolling suitcase allows persons with visual impairments to use their cane or dog guide while carrying or pulling their luggage behind them. All luggage must be marked with the traveler's name, address, and telephone number. Luggage should not be locked as airport security may need to open it to inspect the contents. If checking a bag, passengers with visual impairments must make sure they can identify it to others and put something on it to make it easily identifiable, especially if they plan to ask for help with finding their luggage at the baggage claim area. Passengers need to have a doctor's note for any medical equipment (such as diabetes syringes) that they need to bring onboard. Check first with the airline to learn its policies about medical equipment.

Airlines allow only one small carry-on bag which cannot exceed maximum size requirements to fit under the seat or in the overhead compartment and one personal item, such as a purse or briefcase. As per the Air Carrier Access Act, disability-related medical supplies, equipment, mobility aids, or assistive devices do not count against any limit on the number of pieces of carry-on baggage.

Getting to the Airport

Intercity buses, express bus service either from downtown or from a regional collection point, shuttle buses from hotels, rail service, and taxis are usually available for transit to get to/from large airports. Airport shuttles will often serve a more limited number of stops than a taxi, but will often cost less.

Check-In

All adult passengers must take a valid, current photo ID for the check-in process. Check-in procedures vary and change over time. Luggage may be checked in at either the ticket counter or at curbside with a skycap. Many larger airports have self-check-in kiosks, which allow customers with e-ticketed, domestic reservations to bypass the ticket counter. Self-check-in kiosks allow passengers to check in, change a seat assignment, check baggage, and receive a boarding pass. To use the kiosk customers must enter their confirmation number or insert a major credit card (for identification only), then follow the directions on the touch screen. At this time, kiosks are not accessible to customers who cannot see the directions. Kiosk agents are usually available for assistance but not always.

Obtaining Assistance

Passengers with visual impairments who chose to travel through airports independently have reported that they are often offered assistance repeatedly from the time they enter the airport until they board the plane. This can be quite bothersome. Some individuals report that when they are simply asking for directions to a specific place such as the departure gate area, airline personnel or other persons may become insistent about taking the person to the area or trying to get them to ride in a cart or use a wheelchair to get there.

Some passengers with visual impairments do choose to obtain assistance when negotiating an airport. Airline staff will assist a passenger with a disability with check-in, security screening, boarding, deplaning, and locating connecting flights, baggage claim, and ground transport. This is called the "meet and assist" program. The law requires a

passenger to give the airline 48 hours notice if requesting this service. For many airlines, this service needs to be requested when the flight is booked. If the passenger alerts the airline of her arrival time at the airport, unnecessary delays in obtaining assistance can be avoided. Allowing additional time for delays in obtaining assistance during heavy traffic periods helps avoid a high-stress situation and the possibility of missing a flight. Airport personnel may offer human guide assistance or drive the visually impaired person in a cart for the sake of expediency between connecting flights.

Assistance varies from airline to airline and airport to airport. It is best to find out what type of assistance is offered beforehand. Some airports have Travelers' Aid services, which are available for no charge to all passengers. Services may include helping people find hotels, providing information about local community attractions, providing an escort who accompanies persons as they move from arrival to departure at the airport, or helping with emergency situations. Services may be provided by volunteers.

Airport Security

All passengers must go through a security checkpoint screening (metal detector). Regulations for security checkpoints are established by the Transportation Security Administration (TSA). Security procedures and policies are subject to change so it is important for travelers and O&M instructors to check for updated information from the TSA web site before trips. Every airport has a security checkpoint designated for people with disabilities. Travelers with visual impairments have the option of using the regular security line, the security checkpoint for persons with disabilities, or a private, pat-down screening. They can listen and look for conveyor belts or for passengers waiting in lines to help locate the security checkpoint. Long canes must be put on the conveyor belt. Folding canes need to be folded. Passengers can talk to the security person to use his voice as a sound cue, using self-protective techniques when walking through. Passengers should know that searches can now also be done with the front of the hand instead of the back to check for plastic explosives. If a passenger with a disability wishes to have a companion or an assistant to accompany him through the security checkpoint and to his gate or meet him at his gate, it is recommended that he check with the airline for procedures for getting authorization for this person.

Mobility aids and assistive devices permitted through the security checkpoints include: canes, walkers, crutches, prosthetic devices, body braces, wheelchairs, scooters, augmentation devices, braille note takers, slate and stylus, service animals, and diabetes-related equipment/supplies (TSA, 2007). Passengers need to notify the screener if X-ray inspection will harm the equipment (i.e., braille note takers). Passengers may ask for the device to be visually and physically inspected instead of X-ray inspection. Regulations regarding what items may not be carried on to the plane change frequently due to security threats.

Boarding and Riding in Airplane

Boarding may involve going outside and then negotiating stairs to reach the plane. A corridor called a *jet way*, which may have a downward slope, may lead directly from the boarding gate to the plane. Passengers must step over the lip of the airplane door to enter the plane. Taller persons may want to use upper hand and forearm technique or reach up to contact the top of the door frame and duck their heads when moving through the doorway. Once inside the plane, flight attendants will escort passengers to their seats. Although most airlines will offer assistance at boarding gates, passengers with visual impairments may choose to board the plane independently. They may preboard, but they are not required to do so.

Airplanes may have one or two aisles with varying numbers of seats in each section, depend-

ing on the size of the plane. Passengers can find out about the seating arrangements when they make reservations. At the time this chapter was written, passengers who are visually impaired are forbidden to sit in emergency exit row seats. Carry-on items may be stored in overhead compartments or under the seat in front of the passenger. For easy access, folding canes can be stored in the magazine pocket of the seat in front of the passenger. Most rigid canes will fit on the floor under a row of three consecutive seats. Passengers should become familiarized with the location of emergency exits and restrooms as well as the operation of the seat mechanism, seat belt, food tray, air vents, and overhead lights. If needed, flight attendants may familiarize passengers with the opening and closing of restroom doors as they can be tricky for people who have never flown before. Federal Aviation Regulations require flight attendants to explain evacuation procedures to travelers with disabilities. Written safety information should be made available in braille or large print, upon passenger request.

Collecting Baggage

Persons with visual impairments may follow the crowd or ask for directions to the baggage claim area, which is most likely on the ground floor of the airport. Passengers who ask for assistance in locating their luggage must be able to give a visual description of their luggage. Skycaps will bring luggage to the ground transportation or pickup spots. Tips are usually given for this service.

Leaving Airport

Passengers who need ground transportation can plan ahead with hotels or commercial transportation agencies. Ground transportation is near the baggage claim area at most airports. Ground transportation at large airports has separate places for city buses, taxis, and shuttles to hotels. Sometimes getting to the designated area may require street crossings. Many airports have free phones for ground transportation connecting passengers to hotels. These phones have signs identifying the hotels but they all look and feel alike so passengers who cannot see the signs may want to use a cell phone or pay phone. If taking a taxi, passengers can call to find out the cost. For people getting picked up by friends, family, or coworkers having a cell phone facilitates communication about when and where to meet.

Dog Guides

There is no documentation required to take a service animal through the security screening checkpoint. The dog guide and its belongings (collar, harness, and leash) may require a physical inspection, whether they walk through the metal detector together or the animal walks in front or behind the owner with the owner continually maintaining control of the animal with the leash or harness. It is possible for the handler to purchase a temporary lead without metal that is made of twine or a synthetic material. Prior to entering the security checkpoint, the handler can place the harness, collar, and regular leash into a bin before passing through the metal detector, by looping the temporary lead around the dog's neck. This negates the necessity of a physical inspection. Passengers may need to advise the screener on how to best screen their dog guide, reminding them not to take off the animal's belongings during the inspection. Dog guides should never be separated from their owners.

Passengers with dog guides do not need to notify the airline that they have a dog guide when they book a flight. Airlines have differing policies about handlers and dogs sitting in the bulkhead seat. Bulkhead seats are usually located in the first row of coach. They have a wall or curtain in front of them instead of another row of seats. Although airline personnel often believe there is more room in the bulkhead seating area, there may actually be less. The passenger should determine what type of seating is most comfortable for him and his dog. In any case, when booking a flight the person should request to not be put in an emergency exit row and to ask for a window seat. Window seating helps to ensure that the dog's paws or tail will not extend out into the aisle, and that people will not have to step over the dog when they enter or exit the row.

Many airlines will pre-board the owner and dog guide. This is a convenience but not a necessity. During takeoff and landing the dog should be in a sitting position with the harness on, in front of the owner. During flight the dog's harness may be removed and the dog may lie down. For very long flights, such as flights overseas, it might be best to feed and water the dog a little less than usual and take the dog out for a long walk beforehand, allowing the dog to relieve itself in a designated dog relief area as close as possible to boarding time.

Complaints

Each air carrier must have at least one Complaints Resolution Official (CRO) available at each airport during times of scheduled air carrier operations. The CRO can be made available by telephone. Any passenger with a complaint of alleged violations of the Air Carrier Access rules is entitled to communicate with a CRO. The CRO has authority to resolve complaints on behalf of the air carrier and will try to solve problems on the spot. Passengers who complain to the airline must be concise and give specific information regarding wrongdoing or discrimination. For additional information, travelers can also go to www.dot.gov/airconsumer/DiscrimComplaintContacts.doc.

Role of O&M Specialists

Airport travel incorporates many skills, such as negotiating escalators and elevators, and traveling in irregularly shaped areas that may be heavily congested. In large airports, persons may ride a bus or rail car to get to the gate area. Finding the airline baggage and check-in counter, negotiating the airport to locate the gate, handling carry on luggage, and locating one's seat can be accomplished independently. The O&M specialist may teach a student how to travel through the airport, seeking assistance at strategic areas as needed (Jacobson, 1993). Some agencies teach group lessons at airports, familiarizing clients with various parts of the airport and relevant airline procedures. O&M specialists need to get permission from airport personnel to provide instruction in the airport that requires familiarizing clients with the security checkpoint or traveling beyond the checkpoint.

OVER-THE-ROAD BUS SERVICE

Over-the-road buses are characterized by an elevated passenger deck located over a baggage compartment. Some buses also have luggage storage areas above the seats. Over-the-road buses provide long-distance service between municipalities, and are owned and operated by private carriers. Most buses make intermediate stops to pick up additional passengers en route to their destinations. In addition to stops en route, buses make rest stops every few hours, and meal stops are scheduled as close to normal mealtimes as possible. This information may be useful for individuals with diabetes or those who travel with dog guides.

Greyhound, a company that provides over-the-road bus service in the continental United States, Canada, and Mexico, provides assistance to customers with disabilities with boarding and exiting buses, luggage, transfers, and stowage and retrieval of mobility devices. This service is provided during transfers, meal and rest stops and other times as reasonably requested. Personal care attendants who travel with customers with disabilities pay reduced fares. Priority seat-

ing is available for the elderly and customers with disabilities. However, all customers may sit wherever their needs are best accommodated. O&M specialists should help clients seek information via telephone or online regarding services provided by their local over-the-road bus service providers.

Trip Planning

Depending on which carrier is used, reservations may not be necessary for over-the-road bus service. Passengers simply arrive at the terminal at least an hour before departure to purchase a ticket. Boarding generally begins 15 to 30 minutes before departure. Seating is on a first-come, first-served basis. Advance purchase tickets do not guarantee a seat. Tickets can be bought at the terminal, online, or over the phone.

Dog Guides

In the United States, over-the-road bus companies welcome customers with dog guides. The dog guide must ride in the bus within the customer's space, not in the aisle or on a seat. The service animal is the responsibility of its owner and must be under the control of its owner at all times. When traveling long distances, it is imperative that the handler takes the dog's needs into consideration by cutting back on food and water as needed.

LONG-DISTANCE TRAIN SERVICE

Trip Planning

Schedules and timetables can be obtained online or by calling customer service. Self-service kiosks are available at most larger train stations. Persons who booked reservations and paid for their tickets online can pick up and print out their tickets at a self-service kiosk. However, these kiosks are not accessible to persons who cannot see the printed directions on the touch screen.

Trains often have steps and side rails. Each car is a self-contained seating unit (Jacobson, 1993). At some point near the beginning of the trip, the conductor may pass through the cars to collect prepaid tickets or fares from passengers who do not have tickets. The conductor also announces the upcoming train stops.

Fares

Fares vary based on day and time of travel. Amtrak, one of the few companies in the United States that provides long-distance rail service, offers a rail fare discount to passengers with disabilities. To receive this discount passengers must book their reservations by telephone or at a ticket counter and provide written documentation of their disabilities when requested. On most Amtrak trains, seating is on a first-come, first-served basis. Once onboard, the conductor may assign seats. Carry-on baggage is typically limited to two pieces per passenger (with few exceptions). Meals and sleeping accommodations are offered for a fee on Amtrak long-distance train routes. Meals are provided as part of the cost of travel for passengers traveling in a sleeping accommodation. Countries in Europe and other parts of the world have many companies that provide long-distance train service.

Dog Guides

In the United States, trained service animals accompanying passengers with disabilities are permitted in all customer areas in stations and on trains. The laws vary in other countries. If the train schedule permits, a person may walk his or her dog guide at station stops provided the unit stays within reasonable proximity to the train and reboards promptly when the conductor informs passengers that the train is about to depart.

PERSONS WITH ADDITIONAL DISABILITIES

Many persons with visual impairments and mobility, cognitive, or health challenges and those who are deaf or hard of hearing use transportation systems independently. For these individuals, learning specific O&M techniques makes traveling unassisted to a transit stop, boarding, paying the fare, identifying the destination stop, getting off the vehicle, and traveling to the destination a reality. Even after completing O&M instruction, some individuals may need assistance with certain portions of the trip. For example, a person who has poor balance and limited stamina may not be able to walk to the bus stop if the route involves walking up a long, steep hill. This person may get a ride to the bus stop, and then ask the driver to deploy the lift when boarding and exiting the bus. A person with a medical condition such as multiple sclerosis may be able to handle the demands of light rail travel some days but not on other days, for example when the temperature is very high. It is vitally important for O&M specialists to have a thorough understanding of the medical conditions a student has and the implications of these conditions for that individual.

Persons with Cognitive Challenges

Depending on the functional level and age, some persons with cognitive challenges may learn to travel by rote on specific bus routes for which they have received O&M instruction, while other persons may use paratransit services for all trips. When working with children and adults with cognitive challenges, the O&M specialist needs to develop a productive relationship with the parents, caregivers, or service agency providers. The student, his family members, and the O&M specialist should collaborate about the person's ability to use fixed-route and demand response service.

Intensive instruction and repetition along the route comprise an effective teaching strategy for students with vision loss who have cognitive challenges. It is essential to develop a recovery strategy plan for when a person gets off the route, misses the stop, gets disoriented, the bus is delayed, or when other atypical or emergency situations occur. Input from the family or caregiver must be incorporated so that all parties involved know about and agree with the plan. If no atypical situations occur during O&M instruction, it may be necessary to create a situation such as purposely missing the bus due to arriving too late at the stop to evaluate the student's problem-solving skills and to provide an opportunity to practice the plan. Family members who are concerned or reluctant about their loved one using transit independently may want to observe transit lessons. See Chapter 19 for more information on O&M for this subpopulation of people with visual impairments.

Persons Who Are Deaf-Blind

Persons who are deaf-blind use fixed-route and demand response transit systems. Developing skills to communicate with transit system drivers and to solicit aid from the public, including other passengers, is crucial for individuals who do not use spoken English. It is important to decide beforehand if, when, and how the individual will solicit assistance for a transit task and to have backup plans for when the first attempt at communication fails (Sauerburger, 1993). O&M specialists should cover communication systems used by persons who are deaf-blind in their transit driver training programs, and make drivers aware that some of their passengers with vision loss may also be hard of hearing or deaf. Some cities, most notably Seattle, Washington, have organized methods and prefabricated kits of cards with bus route numbers for deaf-blind travelers. These cards inform the driver of what route the

passenger is seeking. O&M specialists should also teach drivers how to assist these persons in the event of an emergency.

When working with persons who are deaf-blind it is important to use the mode of communication preferred or required by the student (Lolli & Sauerburger, 1997). Deaf-blind individuals who use signed languages need to decide if they want a certified interpreter present during O&M instruction. O&M specialists may need to increase the time for transit lessons because of the logistical and communication needs. See Chapter 17 for additional information on communication strategies and use of public transportation.

SUMMARY

Many persons with visual impairments use public transportation to travel to places of employment, services, and social activities. O&M specialists should teach students how to utilize various modes of public transportation safely and efficiently, provide inservice training for transit drivers and customer service staff, and advocate for transit system accessibility. Because schedules, fares, policies, and security procedures change, it is important for O&M specialists to keep themselves updated regarding their local transit system's policies as well as federal regulations for transit. The United We Ride web site has resource information on funding, policies, useful practices, and links to federal agencies and transit regulations.

IMPLICATIONS FOR O&M PRACTICE

1. O&M specialists need to teach students how to utilize various modes of public transportation, including familiarization with transit vehicles, methods for planning trips,

locating the correct bus/train, boarding and exiting vehicles, paying fares, and soliciting information.

2. Students need to have a planned course of action to follow in the event that they miss their bus or train, get off at the wrong stop, or realize that the bus they are on is taking an alternate route. O&M instruction needs to provide opportunities to problem solve when unforeseen events occur, as well as incorporate strategies for emergency situations.

3. O&M specialists need to keep themselves updated regarding their local transit system's policies because schedules, fares, policies, and security procedures change.

4. Advocating for transit system accessibility is an important role of the O&M specialist. Participating on committees for accessible transit or transit system advisory boards is encouraged.

5. Inservice training for transit drivers and customer service staff should include strategies for providing complete, accurate information to persons with visual impairments; the importance of easy-to-understand stop announcements; the need to stop trains to line up with between-car-barriers and tactile indicators; federal regulations for passengers with disabilities, and how to assist visually impaired persons in emergency situations.

6. The ADA has regulations for stop announcements, priority seating for disabled passengers, lifts, paratransit eligibility and service, detectable warnings at train platforms, and between-car-barriers for trains. Discrimination by air carriers is covered by the Air Carrier Access Act. It is important for O&M specialists to know the regulations and to advocate for compliance in situations where transit systems are not meeting the regulations.

7. With the exception of metropolitan areas and small cities, bus service is the only type of fixed-route service available in most places.

8. Each public entity operating a fixed-route system is required by law to offer comparable ADA paratransit service to persons with disabilities who are not able to use fixed-route service (intercity bus, subway, light rail).

9. Technology such as audible real-time bus or train arrival information systems, remote infrared audible signage, mobile digital cameras, global positioning systems, online trip planning, and using virtual globe browsers have improved access to transit-related information. O&M specialists should keep abreast of this technology.

10. School-age children need to be introduced to the transit systems in their local areas long before they will be expected to ride alone. The decision about when someone is mature enough to ride alone needs to be made by that child's family, after input from the O&M specialist documenting that the child has mastered all transit-related skills consistently using safe travel practices.

11. Visually impaired persons with cognitive, medical, or physical challenges and those who are hard of hearing or deaf use public transportation. It is vitally important for O&M specialists to have a thorough understanding of the challenges and related implications for each individual.

12. There are many online resources available for O&M specialists in the area of public transportation including Easter Seals Project Action, United We Ride, the Transit Cooperative Research Board, the American Public Transportation Association, and the Federal Transit Authority.

LEARNING ACTIVITIES

1. Select an urban area from anywhere in the world. Find out what transportation modes are available in this area. Can trips be planned

online? What accommodations do these systems offer to persons with visual impairments (such as reduced fares, information in accessible formats, persons with disabilities on advisory boards or committees, and driver sensitivity training)? Plan a trip from a hotel in the center city area to the closest airport.

2. You are asked to conduct driver-training sessions for bus drivers from your local transit authority. What topics do you need to cover? Would these topics differ if you are training paratransit drivers? Create a training agenda for both groups that includes an outline, materials needed, and suggested time frame.

3. An adult who is totally blind contacts you as he wishes to appeal a decision made by the local paratransit agency. He would like you to provide input to paratransit staff regarding his abilities and his need to use paratransit for some trips. The applicant stated on his application that he uses fixed-route bus and rail service to some destinations. He has been turned down for paratransit services because the agency feels he is capable of using fixed-route services to all destinations. He is appealing this decision. You have never met this ap-

plicant. What kind of information would you collect to help him and what process would you use?

4. One of your student's parents is ready to allow her to ride buses by herself to the store in the central business district of her small city and to a friend's house in the suburbs. She is 17 years old and totally blind. Her parents want her to carry a written action plan for what to do if she gets lost, gets disoriented, misses her stop or bus, or is concerned that an adult is following her. How would you help her develop this plan? What recovery strategies does it need to include?

5. You need to teach a new client how to travel via subway to his new place of employment. Although he has advanced O&M skills, he has never traveled on a subway or negotiated a transit rail station as he recently moved from an area that did not have rail service. Develop lesson plans, skills checklists, and a sequence of instruction.

6. After evaluating your local bus and/or rail system, what steps could be taken to make the system more accessible for persons with visual impairments and how would you share this information with the transit system?

CHAPTER 14

Teaching the Use of Electronic Travel Aids and Electronic Orientation Aids

William M. Penrod, Daniel L. Smith, Rodney Haneline, and Michael P. Corbett

---

LEARNING QUESTIONS

- What are the two general categories of electronic travel aids (ETAs)?

- Why should secondary ETAs always be used in conjunction with a primary mobility system except in very specific and familiar circumstances?

- What are the three sources of energy that ETAs use for surface preview and obstacle detection?

- What impact may diabetes have upon the ETA user? What output (tactile or haptic, or auditory) is best for a prospective student with diabetes?

- How might ETAs be used with young children to promote concept development? How stringent would the controls be for a young student: should he or she take the device home or use it unsupervised?

- Besides concept development, what other measurable objectives may ETA training accomplish?

- What are some possible funding sources for ETAs?

- What characteristics should the initial training or evaluation site possess?

- The authors suggest that there are three basic methods used with secondary ETAs. What are they?

- What is meant by using an ETA "selectively"? When is this tactic advisable and under what circumstances? Give an example.

- Explain global positioning systems (GPS) and briefly describe their impact on wayfinding systems.

- Explain geographical information systems (GIS) and describe their impact on wayfinding systems.

- Identify three EOAs currently available. Describe each. What (if any) are their limitations?
- Explain how tall buildings, trees, and other overhead objects may affect the accuracy of EOAs.

This chapter provides O&M specialists with practical information on evaluation and curriculum suggestions for teaching many of the electronic travel aids (ETAs) and electronic orientation aids (EOAs) mentioned in Volume 1, Chapter 8. Whereas Chapter 8 in Volume 1 provides theoretical information on ETAs and EOAs, this chapter provides practical information on how to teach the use of these devices.

In the literature of the profession of orientation and mobility (O&M) much of the information useful to the O&M specialist regarding ETAs is technical and descriptive in nature (Blasch, LaGrow, and De l'Aune, 1996; Farmer & Smith, 1997; Penrod & Simmons, 2005; Penrod et al., 2006). There are also opinions regarding appropriateness of ETAs for specific segments of the legally blind population (Penrod & Blasch, 2005), and data regarding the usage of such devices (Blasch, Long, & Griffin-Shirley, 1989). Little has been written that offers teaching methodology and lesson sequencing for the O&M specialist (Penrod, Corbett, & Blasch, 2005). The intent of this chapter is to provide the O&M specialist with a resource for the design and implementation of orientation and mobility training for ETAs and EOAs. The authors' intent is to provide the O&M specialist with strategies and lesson sequencing that will generalize to new and emerging technologies as they become available.

OVERVIEW

Electronic travel aids (ETAs) are devices that are designed to give the student who is blind or is visually impaired, extended preview of the environment that would not be available if he is using a traditional primary mobility system alone (e.g., with a cane, human guide, or dog guide; Farmer & Smith, 1997). The device may be handheld, attached to the student's cane or wheelchair, or worn on the body. The ETA provides a display through signals that are audible, tactile-haptic or a combination of both. In this chapter this "display" is referred to as *output*, and it may be audible, tactile-haptic, or a combination of both.

Categories of ETAs

Because of renewed interest in ETAs and new interest in EOAs, terminology has been challenged to better describe these devices. While previously, ETAs were classified according to function and design—such as Type I, Type II, Type III, and Type IV devices (Farmer & Smith, 1997)—advances and new product designs have made that system obsolete. The authors have chosen to reestablish the original classification system of delineating only whether a device is a "primary" or "secondary" (Farmer, 1980) ETA.

There are two general categories of ETAs: primary and secondary (see Volume 1, Chapter 8). A primary ETA is one that provides surface preview and obstacle preview. At the present time the primary ETA devices integrate electronic sensors with the long cane. However, the Laser Cane and the UltraCane are no longer available. They are still being used by some persons who are blind. A secondary ETA must be used in conjunction with a separate cane, dog guide, or human guide to ensure the student's ability to detect drop-offs, stairs, and curbs. ETAs may use laser, infrared, or ultrasonic energy for this purpose. ETAs send energy out into the environment and receive the reflected energy for interpretation by the student. The device then displays its signal in the form of auditory or tactile-haptic feedback.

Each form of energy has its limitations. For example, laser light from the Nurion Laser Cane can be absorbed by the color black. This can give spurious signals on the down channel when contacting black baseboards or black and white floor tiles. This would give the student the information that a down step is ahead when in fact there is none. Ultrasonic sound can be reflected off smooth angled surfaces and not returned to the student. Fortunately, such occurrences are rare. The student should, however, understand how these energy forms operate and how these problems can occur. The ETA's main function is to detect obstacles and landmarks that the cane might miss and the dog guide would circumvent (Farmer & Smith, 1997).

While various ETAs have been marketed as primary ETAs, there are no primary ETAs on the market. As mentioned, the Laser Cane and the UltraCane (see Figure 14.1) are no longer available. The "K" Sonar is currently available, but it is not necessarily a primary ETA, and it may be dangerous to think of it as such, even though the manufacturer's manual for the "K" Sonar suggests that when the "K" Sonar is attached to the cane, it can also be considered a primary ETA. However, the American Printing House for the Blind (APH), which was the primary distributor for the device, refused to market the device as a primary ETA, and Terlau and Penrod (2008) refer to it as a secondary device in the APH manual.

Also regarding primary or secondary ETA status for the "K" Sonar, unlike the Laser Cane and the Ultra Cane, the "K" Sonar technology is not integrated into the cane but is attached to it. It is actually just the cane that is the primary system, not the integrated system. When attached, if the user holds the ETA rather than the cane and is positioned away from midline as the manufacturer suggests, the user's tactile sensations from the cane are negatively affected. Therefore, the "K" Sonar device is treated in this chapter as a secondary device.

Regarding secondary ETAs, three of the more popular ones are the Miniguide US, the

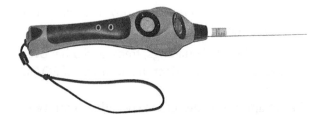

Figure 14.1. UltraCane primary electronic travel aid (ETA), top view

Hand Guide, and the K Sonar Device. The Miniguide US and the K Sonar Device both rely on sonar for obstacle detection, while the Handguide uses infrared light (see Figure 14.2).

The basic lesson sequence for teaching the use of ETAs that will be presented in this chapter is useful for teaching both primary and secondary ETAs. However, there are three special techniques for using secondary ETAs that will be presented first.

User Reactions

There are some general behaviors that have been observed and that have emerged from teaching the use of ETAs. Although these behaviors are not manifested in all students, they are mentioned here to alert the O&M specialist that they may occur during training.

1. Perhaps the most prevalent behavior when learning to use an ETA is the tendency for the student to devote almost complete attention to the device to the exclusion of other sensory information. This tendency may result in a temporary deterioration of mobility skills. Fortunately, as the student becomes more familiar with the device his mobility skills usually rapidly return. That is why it is critical that the student has a strong foundation in O&M skills. O&M specialists need to be aware that there is this initial period of adjustment associated with effective ETA use and allow for it.

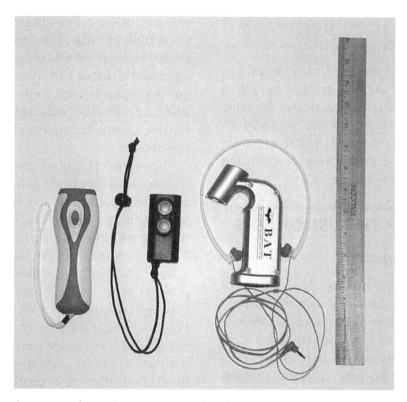

Figure 14.2. Popular secondary electronic travel aids (ETAs)
Left to right: Handguide by Guideline, Miniguide US, and K Sonar Device.

2. Initial instruction with an ETA, especially when the ETA has multiple channels or a sophisticated signal, can be quite tiring for the student as he is attending to the device as well as the usual sensory information provided by his cane or dog guide. The O&M specialist needs to be aware that some students may tire more quickly than others. The O&M specialist also needs to be cognizant of the impact of additional disabilities (e.g., diabetes) upon student fatigue. Diabetes may not only complicate O&M lessons in regard to fatigue, but also offer more serious and immediate health problems. The O&M specialist needs to be especially alert when working with "brittle diabetics" (Joffee & Rower, 1997). Diabetes may have a severe impact upon the user if neuropathy is an issue and the device relies solely on tactile-haptic output. Conversely, those learners who have significant hearing loss may be greatly challenged if the device has an auditory output (Penrod, Bauder, Simmons, & Brostek, 2009).

3. Another reaction frequently encountered is student frustration and confusion. This is usually the result of the student developing too much "dependence" upon the device rather than incorporating the information from the device into his repertoire of mobility skills. This could indicate that training has proceeded too fast. Learning to use an ETA may be likened to learning a foreign language in that it is difficult to grasp a lot of information initially and use it purposefully. It may take time for the student to integrate the ETA's information with his mobility skills,

particularly with ETAs that have multiple or complex signals.

One approach that is particularly helpful in ETA training is the use of a monitoring system so that the O&M specialist can receive the same auditory signals or vibrations that the student is receiving. The O&M specialist is then able to point out immediately the information to which the student needs to be attending.

TRAINING IN THE USE OF ETAS

Purpose of Instruction

One initial consideration in teaching the use of an ETA is to clarify for the student the purpose of the instruction. Specific purposes may include obstacle detection and avoidance, landmark identification, self-familiarization, alternate route determination, following other persons, straight-line travel, and trailing parallel surfaces (e.g., a wall, fence, or hedgerow). Another purpose is to facilitate concept development for younger students, which can be facilitated by using an ETA. The ETA may provide information about the world beyond the preview capability of the student's cane or dog guide, and also extend her knowledge of self-to-object and object-to-object relationships. The ETA can provide information that would never be available otherwise (i.e., an increased appreciation of the height and size of objects, such as trees, telephone poles, autos, fire trucks, and anything else that cannot be measured with outstretched arms). The ETA can bring this information to the student who is learning concepts. In all cases, the objectives need to be clear. An evaluation period may be needed so that the student can make an informed choice as to which ETA is most suitable for her needs.

Student Instruction

The O&M specialist needs to be aware of the student's mobility skills and any sensory, health,

physical, or mental conditions that might affect or preclude the use of the selected ETA. For example, a student with hearing loss might be a better candidate for an ETA with a tactile-haptic output than an ETA with an auditory output. The student needs to be responsible, motivated, and capable of maintaining and using the device selected.

Before a device is selected by a student, the training procedure needs to be discussed. In general, good motivation and success in past mobility training are good predictors for successful training with the ETA. It is always a good idea for the O&M specialist to have available an array of ETAs that can be used in the evaluation process. While this is a reasonable expectation for large organizations such as Veterans Affairs (VA) hospitals, residential schools, and state agencies, it is seldom a realistic expectation for private contractors or those O&M specialists employed in small school districts or small agencies.

The O&M specialist also needs to discuss potential funding sources for the purchase of the ETA. It is best to address this before training begins to avoid disappointment on the part of the student.

To this end, the O&M specialist should look at funding sources such as the following:

1. The student or her family
2. State agencies for the blind
3. Federal sources, such as the U.S. Department of Veterans Affairs
4. Service organizations, such as Lions Clubs
5. Private health insurance
6. Philanthropic organizations, such as Masonic charities and various foundations
7. School systems

The source of funding for the student's own ETA, if that is the objective, should be "locked in" before training starts to avoid frustration and confusion later. It is also best if the student's own ETA can be made available for the last stages of training so that it can be checked out thoroughly in real travel situations and any adjustments or repairs made before the end of training.

Training Areas

The selection of the initial training area is critical. It is extremely important to select an open area free of other sensory distractions for *initial* training or evaluation. An example would be a gymnasium or large room. Outdoor training areas need to be avoided, if possible, due to uncontrolled distractions such as traffic, construction, and other pedestrians.

For the beginning ETA student, receiving too many signals can be overwhelming. As an example, if training takes place in an average size furnished room the student will be receiving additional signals from furnishings and walls that may be confusing. This situation could be distracting to the student and an impediment to training. However, if a large room or gymnasium is not available, the O&M specialist needs to seek out a quiet open area outside.

The O&M specialist needs to set up environmental situations in this open area similar to that in Figure 14.3. Vertical movable poles are excellent for providing a variety of training situations. By using poles for initial training in a quiet environment, the O&M specialist can simulate many environmental situations and create a core of skills that the student can take out into the uncontrolled environment; this is because vertical poles simulate vertical obstacles that a student might encounter. These experiences will do much to ensure success by developing the student's confidence in the device and in her own capabilities in a safe, controlled setting and in a systematic manner. Some ETA manufacturers have their own prescribed training regimen for ETAs that need to be used. The poles, how-

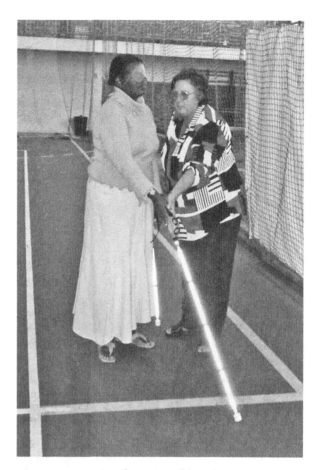

Figure 14.3. Students working in a gym

ever, are a good way to standardize initial training. Vertical poles make it easier to evaluate the student's problems and progress, and also greatly standardize situations in which a student is familiarized with several ETAs. Another advantage to using the poles is that they will always return a signal when in range of the particular device regardless of the angle of approach. Other environmental objects, depending on their size, angle, composition, and even color, may not always be detected depending on whether the device uses laser, infrared, or ultrasound, as each has its own capabilities and idiosyncrasies.

The O&M specialist can make his own set of poles or have them made with PVC pipe 2 to

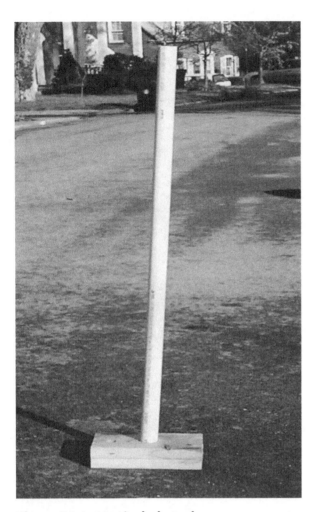

Figure 14.4. Vertical obstacle

2¹/₃ inches diameter and about 7 feet in length and with a square wood base 24 inches × 24 inches × 2 inches (see Figure 14.4). Six to eight poles should be considered a minimum, with 10 to 12 being ideal.

The poles may be arranged (at varying distances apart) to simulate any number of environmental situations, such as going through doors and trailing poles without making physical contact. Their uses are limited only by the O&M specialist's imagination.

A large, quiet, controlled area with no distractions and the training poles as described above

give the student the best setting and opportunity for learning the capabilities of the ETA. Only after the student is successful in this artificial setting does training need to move into natural and complex environments.

Training Preparation

Before preparing to teach the use of an ETA, it is recommended that all devices be checked to see that they are working properly. Fresh batteries should be used and extra ones kept on hand throughout training. It is also recommended that, when possible, an extra ETA of the type being taught be kept on hand in case of malfunction or breakage. These steps will ensure the continuity of the ETA training program.

The O&M specialist might wish to identify alternate training sites should circumstances change. All materials, including vertical poles, training manuals, and monitoring devices, need to be assembled beforehand. In the case of ETAs with replaceable batteries, it is important for students to carry extra batteries in case a long training session runs them down.

TECHNIQUES FOR USING A SECONDARY ETA

Basically, there are three methods for using a secondary ETA in conjunction with a standard long cane: the *scissors method*, the *forward and vertical method*, and the *trailing method*.

Scissors Method

The "scissors" method is arguably the most widely used technique in conjunction with a long cane. As its name implies, the device and the cane move in a scissors-like fashion where the axis of the device intersects with the shaft of the cane while walking and using the touch technique.

Important considerations while using this technique are that the student must always ensure that the ETA is positioned above the opposite wrist so it does not detect the user's hand and give a false signal (see Figure 14.5). It is also possible to walk and scan so fast that objects are not detected. So a slower walking pace is advisable when using this technique. With some devices, it is also important to incorporate a vertical motion at midline every few steps to detect head-height obstacles. The procedure is as follows:

1. Use the cane in traditional touch technique.

2. Holding the device slightly above the wrist of the hand holding the cane, the student

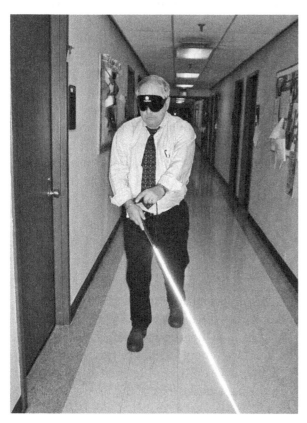

Figure 14.5. Scissors technique with Miniguide US

needs to make the cane and the ETA intersect while walking (e.g., when the student's left foot is forward the cane will be pointed to the right and the device will be pointed to the left, and when the student's right foot is forward the cane is pointed to the left and the device is pointed to the right).

Forward and Vertical Method

This technique can be invaluable and extremely efficient in the task of obstacle avoidance. The device is pointed straight ahead while using the touch technique. By including a vertical motion with the ETA every few steps, the student should benefit from extended preview to the front and overhead. For the student who is mainly concerned about overhanging objects, such as someone walking home from work through a residential area with overhanging bushes and tree branches, the device may be held stationary above the cane, angled slightly upward, providing the needed protection. The procedure is as follows (see Figure 14.6):

1. Use the cane in traditional touch technique.

2. Position the ETA at midline and hold stationary with the longitudinal axis of the device perpendicular with the student's frontal plane.

3. Move the ETA vertically every few steps in order to more efficiently detect overhead obstacles.

Trailing Method

This technique is useful to align and walk parallel to a wall or other vertical surface without making contact with the surface being trailed. It offers little benefit when the device is used in conjunction with a dog guide because trailing without making contact can be done by the dog guide. The procedure is as follows:

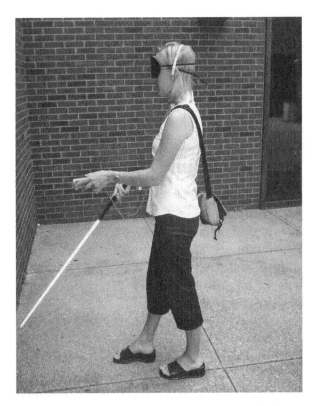

Figure 14.6. Forward and vertical method with K Sonar

1. Use the cane in traditional touch technique.

2. Have the ETA turned to "near-" or "short"-range setting. (Long-range settings may also be used in some circumstances.)

3. Position the ETA at midline and hold stationary with the longitudinal axis of the device pointed toward the wall being trailed.

4. Keeping the ETA beam at the limit of its range in contact with the object being trailed, the student will be able to stay within the maximum distance of the short-range setting from the object being trailed.

THE ETA CURRICULUM

Penrod, Corbett, and Blasch (2005) described a curriculum designed for Soundforesight, Ltd.,

to instruct students in the use of the Ultra-Cane. This curriculum has been used successfully for teaching students the use of the UltraCane and may be easily modified for teaching the use of other ETAs. This suggested curriculum serves as a basic model from which the O&M specialist may design a training curriculum specifically for the ETA and the individual being taught. Terlau and Penrod (2008) developed a "user's guide" for the "K" Sonar Device that provides suggestions for individual lessons.

The O&M specialist should be thoroughly familiar with the manufacturer's manual and training curriculum (if available) for the specific device being taught.

The following lesson sequence that follows is appropriate for primary and secondary ETAs, if modified to the peculiar, unique, and inherent characteristics of each device. Usually, the O&M specialist can plan lessons that range in time from a few minutes to more than an hour depending on the travel time to some of the outdoor lessons. The reader needs to be aware that this lesson sequence is not intended to be a complete curriculum. Instead, it is designed to be a guide for the O&M specialist in developing and tailoring lessons to different devices and the uniqueness of students (see Sidebar 14.1).

Lesson 1

Objective

The O&M specialist will demonstrate sonic, laser, or infrared fields. This is to be a familiarization lesson to demonstrate to the student the shape of the energy fields by examining them tactually or visually, and to increase familiarity with the control settings of the ETA.

Procedure

First, the student needs to be familiarized with the features of the ETA. Tactile and haptic pins

Key Points to Remember about Working with an ETA

- It is always a good idea to carry along extra batteries while on lessons.

- Always consider the weather when working outdoors with an ETA: Most are weather resistant, but seldom weatherproof!

- It is important to remember that traffic noise is different depending on the time of day that you plan your outdoor lesson.

- It is important to plan initial lessons indoors, in a quiet area with plenty of space.

- It is a good idea to prepare a "crib sheet" with notes to help you remember the important characteristics of the ETA. You may lose the confidence of your student if you can't remember ranges and characteristics of the device when asked!

and buttons need to be identified, the implications of different sounds identified, on-off switches need to be located, and range settings need to be explained. The student needs to become completely familiar with the location of transducers and other elements. Battery compartments and battery types need to be located and understood. Characteristics and limitations need to be explained at this time (i.e., resistance to moisture and other considerations).

Lesson 2

Objective

The student will become familiar with range settings of the forward channel. The purpose of this exercise is for the student to develop general proprioceptive awareness of the distance settings of the ETA.

Procedure

The student will turn the device on long range and will hold it at midline without moving it from side to side. Position the student squarely facing a wall at distances just outside that of the long-range setting. Allow her to walk forward and contact the wall. Repeat this exercise using other distances, all outside the long range of the device.

Repeat with the device set to short range, again starting outside of the long-range setting. Repeat as necessary to allow the student to learn the detection length of setting.

Lesson 3

Objective

The student will learn how to judge distance with an ETA using the variability of pulse or frequency information. The student will become familiar with the pulse or frequency aspect of the device and how it relates to distance, for example the vibrating pulses become faster or the auditory pitch changes as the student approaches the wall.

Procedure

The student is guided by the O&M specialist to a distance where the device is in close proximity (almost touching) a blank wall with the ETA turned on. The student is then guided away from the wall, turned 180 degrees and squared off, and asked to walk toward the wall and stop at the original beginning distance from the wall as identified by the pulse frequency. This lesson should be repeated using different distances from the wall. Repeat exercise using the remaining distance setting.

Lesson 4

Objective

The student will interpret pulse frequency as it relates to distances. The student will develop more familiarity and accuracy in relating pulse or frequency to distance.

Procedure

The O&M specialist will position the student at a distance from the wall within the long-range setting of the ETA. The student is asked to walk toward the wall and make contact with the cane tip. This exercise needs to be repeated at various starting distances. With a primary device, the O&M specialist needs to have the student hold the cane with the tip pointed toward the wall. With a secondary device, the student may either point the cane directly at the target with the tip on the floor or he may elect to use the cane in the traditional touch or diagonal technique (Hill & Ponder, 1976). The O&M specialist must ensure that the student realizes that a forward vertical obstacle such as a wall will become an overhead obstacle when the user of a device such as an UltraCane or Laser Cane approaches to within the range of the overhead beam.

Lesson 5

Objective

The student will use the ETA to "square off" or align perpendicularly with a wall. The student will learn to judge when the pulse or frequency is equal on both sides from midline.

Procedure

The O&M specialist places the student at an angle from a nearby wall within the range setting of the ETA. The student scans with the ETA to locate the wall and squares off facing the wall by scanning side to side with the device until the signal drops out equally on each side. Start at approximately five feet from the wall. Repeat the exercise from various angles and distances to the wall.

Lesson 6

Objective

The student will become familiar with range settings and incorporate the ETA using the touch technique (Hill & Ponder, 1976) or with a dog guide.

Procedure

The student will repeat Lesson 3, only moving the cane in the touch technique or while using his dog guide.

Lesson 7

Objective

This lesson is only for primary ETAs with more than one channel. The student will become familiar with the range of the upper channel when activated by a vertical or overhanging object. The upper channel emits energy to alert the user to impending overhead objects in contrast to the forward channel which alerts the user to objects in the user's path.

Procedure

This lesson is appropriate for primary ETAs only. The forward channel should be disregarded (may be occluded with tape or disabled if possible) at this point forcing the student to focus on one signal. The student will turn the ETA on and will center the device at midline without moving from side to side in the first stage of training. The student will walk to the wall until contact is made with the signal and then the cane tip. This lesson needs to be conducted in an area free of drop-offs and obstacles. Repeat several times.

Lesson 8

Objective

The student will become familiar with the upper channel while using the touch technique (Hill & Ponder, 1976). The student will gain more experience in using the signals from the ETA while traveling with a cane or while using a dog guide.

Procedure

The student will repeat the previous lesson, only using the touch technique or a dog guide. Some students may prefer using the constant contact technique. Students using secondary ETAs need to use a cane in conjunction with the device utilizing a scissors or forward and vertical method as described in more detail later in this chapter.

Lesson 9

Objective

The student will become familiar with detecting overhanging objects. When upper channel signals are received, the student will respond by changing direction and avoiding the overhang or using a modified upper-hand and forearm technique to deflect the obstacle while moving under it.

Procedure

The O&M specialist will hold a stick or cane with a piece of cardboard (cloth or magazine) suspended at head height and in the student's path. A magazine opened to the center and placed across a cane and held horizontally makes an excellent head-high object. This obstacle should be held at various heights and distances from the student. The student walks forward and is encouraged to use the upper-hand and forearm technique when the first signal is detected until the obstacle is contacted. Repeat this activity until the student responds appropriately and consistently by stopping just in front of the obstacle, using the upper-hand and forearm technique to deflect the obstacle while moving around or under the obstacle.

Lesson 10

Objective

The student will practice in travel situations that produce multiple channel signals. The student will become accustomed to interpreting multiple signals from primary devices or learn how to effectively scan using secondary devices to detect overhead obstacles. The student will simultaneously use his cane to detect drop-offs if using a secondary ETA. This lesson is not appropriate for a dog guide user.

Procedure

The O&M specialist places the student at varying distances from the wall. The student walks forward toward the wall. The student needs to stop when he is alerted to the forward channel and move forward until he detects the upper-channel vibration. Do this with various starting distances. Repeat this activity using the near and far ranges.

Lesson 11

Objective

The student will scan with the ETA to locate landmarks. The student will develop greater accuracy in finding and contacting objects.

Procedure

When placed in an open area where the O&M specialist has pre-placed chairs, poles, and other objects, the student will scan the area with the ETA and point to each object. Upon command, the student will approach the object using her preferred primary mobility system and make contact. The O&M specialist may then have the student return to the center of the room and locate the farthest and nearest of two objects. These activities are repeated until the O&M specialist is confident in the student's ability to determine distal relationships and the direction to nearby objects using the ETA.

Lesson 12

Objective

The student will detect simulated doorways. The student will use the ETA to pass through open doorways.

Procedure

When placed in an open area with two vertical PVC poles positioned within the range of the ETA, the student will locate the poles and while using his primary mobility system walk between the poles. This exercise is to prepare the student for finding open doorways and intersecting hallways.

Lesson 13

Objective

The student will use the ETA to parallel (trail) a wall without the cane or the body making contact with the wall.

Procedure

When the student is placed in a long quiet hallway in an (ideally) empty building, he will be asked to walk beside the hallway wall without making contact with the cane or his body. This task must be mastered before going on to Lesson 14.

Lesson 14

Objective

The student will detect doorways and intersecting hallways using the ETA.

Procedure

When using a human guide in a quiet hallway (preferably near an empty building), the student will be asked to parallel a wall and verbally indicate when open doors are detected using the ETA. If the device has a "gap-finding" feature, the O&M specialist needs to introduce that feature now.

Outdoor Lessons

The indoor lessons are designed to prepare the student for skills for more complex and less controlled outdoor environments. Initially, outdoor lessons need to be regimented and formalized to the extent that the student will be finding a particular landmark or trailing a particular wall, hedge, or tree line. Later, the student will be assigned to following specific routes, identifying salient features that may be used as landmarks; identifying and avoiding overhead and forward obstacles; detecting drop-offs, curbs, and steps; identifying and avoiding other pedestrians; and simultaneously maintaining safe travel techniques. After those skills are mastered, the student needs to be encouraged to use the ETA either exclusively if it is a primary device or selectively if it is a secondary device.

Lesson 15

Objective

The student will trail an outside wall, fence, or hedge line using the ETA and verbally indicate to the O&M specialist when gaps or open areas (e.g., walkways, alleys, or other open spaces) are encountered.

Procedure

Lesson 14 must be completed and mastered before Lesson 15 should be attempted by the student. Essentially, Lesson 14 is repeated, only in an outdoor setting. First the student needs to be exposed to a sidewalk with a wall or hedge row that can be trailed using the ETA. The student needs to be using his primary mobility system, but needs to take care not to make contact with his cane or body. During these initial lessons, the student needs to verbally identify walkways, driveways, and other "gaps" as encountered. These lessons need to be repeated until mastery is achieved.

Lesson 16

Objective

The student will trail an outside wall or building line in a downtown area using the ETA and verbally indicate to the O&M specialist when gaps or open areas (e.g., walkways, doorways, alleys, or other open spaces) are encountered.

Procedure

Essentially, Lesson 15 is repeated only this time in a downtown or light business setting. First the student needs to be exposed to a sidewalk with a wall or building line that can be trailed using the ETA. The student needs to be using his primary mobility system, but needs to take care not to make contact with his cane or body. During these initial lessons, the student needs to verbally identify walkways, doorways, driveways, and other "gaps" as encountered. These lessons need to be repeated until mastery is achieved (see Sidebar 14.2).

The authors wish to again emphasize that this lesson sequence guide has application potential for almost all primary ETAs and secondary ETAs. The O&M specialist is encouraged to modify or change the sequence of lessons, and add to or delete any portion of this guide, as appropriate, if working with persons who are multiply disabled, are cognitively impaired, or have physical limitations. The entire guide could be modified by the O&M specialist if the student intends only limited usage of the ETA (e.g., the older adult who will seldom travel away from her primary residence but may need assistance when traveling within a facility to the dining area or recreation room).

The "K" Sonar Device will require additional instruction because of its inherent qualitative characteristics, such as its differences in tone and pitch that indicate differences in texture and composition of objects that are detected (Terlau & Penrod, 2008). Another significant factor for consideration is that this ETA has a very audible "pulse" that may cause distraction to the student until mastery is determined. Even then, it may

---

SIDEBAR 14.2

More Key Points to Remember about Working with an ETA

- Secondary ETAs must be used with a primary mobility system, for example a cane, dog guide, or human guide.

- Primary ETAs do not require the use of a long cane, dog guide, or human guide to ensure the user's safety.

- To be an effective ETA user, you must have a solid foundation of O&M skills!

- Generally, secondary ETAs best serve the user when used selectively, like when

necessary to find a landmark or destination, when self-familiarizing, to avoid overhead obstacles, or to locate pedestrian controls at intersections.

- Never depend on any ETA to determine gaps in traffic to use for street crossings—*none have that capability!*

- When using ETAs with audible outputs, it is a good idea to remove the earphones when executing street crossings.

be advisable to remove the earphones before aligning oneself to cross the street. When the student reaches the other side of the street, the earphones may be replaced and usage resumed. However, after much practice many students wear the earphones continuously while traveling.

A Final Note on ETAs

All ETAs have their place among the array of ETAs available to persons who are blind. For instance, ETAs like the UltraCane, which uses tactile-haptic vibrations to alert the student to impending obstacles or landmarks, may be more suitable for a student who has a hearing loss but for whom neuropathy is not an issue. On the other hand, because the K Sonar Device uses audible pulses for similar purposes, it may be more suitable for the student who has problems with neuropathy but who does not have a hearing loss when used in conjunction with the user's primary mobility system. The lesson sequence was designed to serve as a basic model that the O&M specialist can modify when working with various ETA devices and diverse student groups.

ELECTRONIC ORIENTATION AIDS

Global positioning systems (GPS) use 24 satellites that orbit the earth to inform the user of his exact position on the earth's surface. Information may be given in terms of latitude, longitude, and elevation measured from sea level. It takes a minimum of four satellites providing input to the GPS system to provide the user with this degree of accuracy. GPS has been used for military applications for some time and proved invaluable to U.S. forces fighting in the desert with few landmarks to use for land navigation during the Persian Gulf War (Desert Storm).

Today, civilian use has increased GPS use tremendously. Outdoor enthusiasts and motorists use GPS with equal regularity and dependence. Now, persons who are blind have access to GPS

devices that provide audible detailed and adequate information needed to determine the answer to the two most pertinent questions in the field of orientation and mobility: where am I, and how do I get to where I want to go?

While GPS answers these questions with amazing accuracy and regularity, it is not perfect, nor is it without complications for the user who is blind or visually impaired. Tall trees, buildings, and mountains often interfere with GPS accuracy because the GPS requires a clear line of sight to the satellites. This "canyon effect" is the direct result of the GPS needing a clear view of the sky. In addition, most GPS devices require practice and instruction which may prove too difficult for some learners.

This section is designed to provide O&M specialists with sufficient information about the GPS systems that are available and to provide a generic curriculum that may be used to teach persons with vision loss. It is not the intent of this chapter to indicate a preference for one device over others.

Global positioning systems are positively changing the travel equation, but they are not an alternative for poor orientation and mobility skills. Assistive GPS products are an orientation complement to other mobility tools such as dog guides and long canes. With any of the GPS devices discussed, however, students can improve their travel planning and reduce travel time, and the travel anxiety related to the tasks of finding new places or soliciting orientation information. GPS travel is a useful tool in urban, rural and recreational environments. In North America and many other regions of the world, digital maps are available with complete street-level detail. Students experience the benefit of real-time intersection detection as well as local points of interest. Routes may be recorded or planned and guided by spoken instructions. Many students find GPS a handy contribution when traveling with a sighted companion or when public transportation or taxis are required. These simple to operate devices will facilitate orientation for people who are blind and visually impaired.

Students need to be taught when to listen to GPS, what to listen for, and how to use this new, independent source of information. This section highlights the important value of GPS-driven electronic orientation aids (EOAs) and serves as a model for learning how to use those devices for travel. Helping travelers who are blind use headings, route directions, and establish points of interest in a variety of travel environments is a new challenge for the profession. The Trekker is a good example of an electronic orientation aid that addresses the needs of travelers who are visually impaired. As such, it forms the nucleus of the EOA curriculum that is used in this chapter.

In the lesson sequence, students build skills with an EOA by performing simple tasks that are later combined into more complex mobility tasks. An important feature of this curriculum is the assignment of independent practice in between lessons.

Students require time to focus on the information from the GPS apart from the demands of the travel situation. Students also need time to practice lesson exercises with the GPS before trying to use it in conjunction with independent mobility.

Consumer Product Overview

Personal navigation devices are part of the most rapidly changing segments of the consumer electronics, recreation, transportation, law enforcement, military, and construction industries. Today, handheld GPS receivers are the most common electronic navigational devices and use low-level satellite signals to distinguish student location anywhere on the planet within a few yards. Continuous improvements in GIS mapping detail and location precision have driven GPS unit sales to record highs and pricing to all-time lows. For example, OnStar, a subsidiary of General Motors, provides voice guided turn-by-turn instructions to 5 million automobile subscribers. A by-product of

consumer popularity is the availability of inexpensive components (maps and receivers) that can be easily integrated into assistive technology form.

GPS receiver technology, adapted for access for students who are blind and visually impaired, has evolved parallel to consumer technology. Michael May, CEO of Sendero Group, is recognized as a front-runner and pioneer and began focusing on GPS starting in the early 1990s. His work culminated in the introduction of the Sendero GPS, also known as the BrailleNote GPS, in 2001. Today, the Sendero-Humanware Braille-Note GPS, the Humanware Trekker-Maestro GPS, and the Freedom Scientific PAC Mate StreetTalk GPS comprise the majority of adapted GPS devices used in North America (see Volume 1, Chapter 8).

These three products share GPS applications with similar features but, beyond that, differ significantly in form, complexity, access modality and price. Both the BrailleNote and PAC Mate products are commonly configured with text-to-speech output as well as refreshable braille output and students may choose either braille keyboards or QWERTY keyboards similar to those found on laptop computers. The integration of full-size keys and braille displays result in versions of these products being nearly as large as laptop computers and weighing over 4 pounds. In contrast, the Trekker-Maestro is a retrofitted personal digital assistant (PDA) and is subcompact, measuring less than a 3×5 inch card and weighing less than 6 ounces. In addition to text-to-speech output it also has subcompact buttons, similar to TV remote controls, for student interaction and data input. All three products use off-the-shelf, external, compact GPS receivers and have ports for headphones or compact speakers. In addition to GPS, they also have features consumers find valuable, including contact management, e-mail, Internet browsing, and media players. Manufacturers suggested pricing ranges from $1,700 to just under $7,000, depending on the product, model, and features. Students need to carefully weigh their preferences to determine which devices make the best travel companions. (The modified curriculum presented is based on a curriculum developed and used by Harold Abraham at Leader Dogs for the Blind.)

Lesson 1

Objective

The student will learn about the GPS network and GPS receiver technology (see Figure 11.23 in Chapter 11).

Procedure: Classroom Instruction

The O&M specialist describes the satellite system, military receivers, civilian receivers, using GPS outdoors, signal accuracy, and signal loss. A GPS receiver is not a two-way communication system and will not assist anyone else in knowing where the student is located. GPS will tell the student where he is located in the surrounding environment and where he has been. It also tells the traveler the routes he has just taken. Civilian GPS technology is limited to 30-foot accuracy, and is subject to signal loss when going under trees or next to tall buildings. The effect of tall buildings is sometimes referred to as the "urban canyon" effect.

The United States Coast Guard maintains a Navigational Center as a point of contact for civilian GPS students. This service can be accessed at www.navcen.uscg.gov and, along with NASA and the Federal Aviation Authority, is an excellent resource to learn the basics of GPS.

Lesson 2

Objective

The student will become familiar with the GPS physical unit.

Procedure: Classroom Instruction

Separate the GPS components. Each system will have a processor unit and a GPS receiver, gener-

ally in individual cases. Some systems will have headphones or a speaker. Attach each component to a charging unit or tip and layout the assembly in front of the student to begin the lesson. Demonstrate how to remove and reattach each charging tip.

Remove the processor unit from the charger and clearly identify all of the physical features. Features will include an on-off switch, an audio port, and other connector ports. Have the student become familiar with the device and thoroughly explore the device and components. It will require practice to remove and replace components like rechargeable batteries and memory cards or to attach and detach components. Each of these tasks is best demonstrated by starting the process for the student. Repeat each task several times.

It is important for the O&M specialist to perform the lesson exercises prior to working with students. As with most lessons, modify the examples to accommodate future versions.

Lesson 3

Objective

The student will learn to start the GPS system with the on-off and reset procedures.

Procedure: Classroom Instruction

The O&M specialist should instruct the student how to turn the unit on and off and to confirm that the GPS application software is running correctly.

If the GPS system fails to operate normally or will not respond, it will probably require resetting. Show the student the procedure to "soft" reset the system and repeat until memorized. If the system being used has a "hard" reset procedure, be careful that it does not remove any application software during the reset or require reconfiguration after the reset. Make a list of the procedures and keys used to start the GPS system.

Lesson 4

Objective

The student will learn to shift (raise or lower) the volume and control (increase or decrease) the speech rate.

Procedure: Classroom Instruction

Students will want to adjust the sound and speech rate for comfortable listening. The speech rate will have software controls and the speech volume may be either software or hardware depending on the system. Encourage the student to modify these settings as frequently as needed.

Lesson 5

Objective

The student will learn the names and positions of all the keys.

Procedure: Classroom Instruction

When students have mastered the on-off, reset, volume, and speech rate adjustments, they will be ready to learn the location, names, and functions of all the keys. Some GPS systems will have a built-in, context-sensitive feature to aid with key learning. If this feature is present, when turned on, the keys will speak their name and function when it is pressed. Teach the student the procedure for the key-learning feature.

Assign key practice as homework and quiz students on their keyboard skills before each lesson.

Lesson 6

Objective

The student will learn to adjust the GPS physical components for wearing on field exercises.

Procedure: Field Instruction

Clip the GPS receiver onto the GPS systems strap or a coat or jacket collar. Assist the student placing the GPS system strap over the shoulder opposite the hand they will use for GPS system operation. Guide the student on how to turn the GPS receiver on and off while it is being worn. Adjust the earphone or speaker if the GPS system has one.

Lesson 7

Objective

The student will learn to establish and check the GPS signal status.

Procedure: Field Instruction

With the strap and components properly adjusted, instruct the student to turn all the components on and make sure that the GPS software is running properly. Determine the strength of the GPS signal. When working properly, the GPS system will report the number of satellites in view and whether coverage is good or poor.

If the GPS system reports that the "GPS connection" is not active, check the receiver to make sure it is on, then use the system procedure or configuration to "bond" the receiver to the system. Some systems may require resetting or restarting.

Lesson 8

Objective

The student will learn to determine compass heading for the direction of travel.

Procedure: Field Instruction

It is a good idea to review compass headings at the beginning of this lesson and "brush up" students not accustomed to using them.

Instruct the student to tap the correct key whenever he wants to know where he is or in which direction he is traveling. This is the first exercise in which the GPS system will provide the student with travel information.

Instruct the student to walk away from the building entrance in one direction for about 30 to 40 feet and tap for direction. The GPS system will speak the compass direction of travel. Instruct the student to turn 90 degrees to the right or left and again walk 30 to 40 feet and tap for direction. Repeat this step twice more, each time turning in the same direction, until the student has returned approximately to the building entrance.

Modify this exercise for the work site. Try to conduct this lesson in an area where the student can walk in a 50-foot square adjacent to a building entrance but far enough away from an intersection to avoid automatic prompts. As with all field exercises, instructors need to try it themselves first so that the outcomes are consistent and predictable.

Lesson 9

Objective

The student will learn about points of interest (POIs) and how to create personal points of interest.

Procedure: Class and Field Instruction

Instruct the student that several million points of interest have already been created and stored on the map of the United States shipped with the GPS system. Each point of interest contains the name of a business or other public place along with street and city information. Students can search for POIs by category or other criteria and used as origins when browsing or creating routes, as well as destinations when planning routes. Points of interest may also be created anytime the student has an active GPS connection and wants to mark a specific location. Depend-

ing on the GPS system, points of interest may be created in the student's recorded voice and edited for title and other data.

To start this lesson go outdoors and establish an active GPS connection. Begin creating POIs to mark the entrances, landmarks leading to intersecting sidewalks, and intersections close to home base. Instruct the student to prepare what they would like to record first, such as "Polk residence revolving door." Next tap the key to mark or record a point of interest. Create 10 or more points of interest during this lesson.

Once points of interest have been created, the O&M specialist needs to instruct the student to retrace the original path. The GPS system will then automatically announce the recorded personal points of interest when approached within 30 feet (this may vary closer or farther). Assign point of interest creation as homework.

Lesson 10

Objective

The student will learn about travel modes and digital maps.

Procedure: Classroom and Field Instruction

Explain in detail pedestrian and motorized modes along with street segments and intersections or transition zones. Cover how the GPS system works when in an area where there are no streets. GPS systems generally contain maps with all the named streets in the United States (and even streets with no names). Streets are further classified as *segments*, a single street between two intersections. When the student is within 100 feet of a named segment, the GPS system will automatically switch to pedestrian mode and provide prompts that can easily be followed while walking, such as compass direction, points of interest, and next intersection. The student may also manually prompt for segment name, direction, and intersection. Any points of interest within the segment can easily be determined.

The Motorized mode is used for moving transportation and can be manually or automatically activated while in pedestrian mode. The GPS system will automatically prompt the student with intersection, and highway exit and entrance information. The student may also manually prompt for direction, next intersection, and speed by tapping the appropriate key.

Students need a solid understanding of the travel modes and prompting conventions to actively participate in higher number lessons. Prompt levels can be changed with the settings feature.

Lesson 11

Objective

The student will learn to locate personal POIs surrounding home base.

Procedure: Field Instruction

GPS systems will list points of interest within a short distance from the student's position when outdoors. Instruct the student to list the points of interest. Scroll through the list using the up and down arrows. Points of interest will be listed from closest to farthest and most systems will speak the distance and direction from the student. Conduct this lesson from different locations surrounding home base.

Lesson 12

Objective

The student will learn about GPS system virtual-browsing modes.

Procedure: Classroom and Field Instruction

GPS systems generally have two modes that students can use to take a "look" at maps either while indoors or when stationary outdoors. These virtual modes are helpful for learning new areas and planning travel activities.

Practice both browsing modes frequently during the GPS course and assign homework with various origins.

Lesson 13

Objective

The student will learn to identify traffic intersections.

Procedure: Field Instruction

Use a residential area for this exercise and begin in the middle of the block. Instruct the student to establish an active GPS connection, walk in one direction to determine compass direction and next intersection information, reverse direction, and determine the opposite compass direction and next intersection. When the student is confident about his location, direction of travel, and street side, instruct him to walk a route several blocks square, returning to the point of origin. The student needs to listen carefully to automatic prompts and manually prompt at mid-block intervals for reinforcement. Assist the student by also providing GPS system instruction at midblock, reserving intersections to focus on safe crossings. Use virtual browsing as part of the exercise.

Vary the pattern of the route until the student is comfortable exploring the area with GPS system prompts.

Lesson 14

Objective

The student will learn to use dialog box and to navigate menus—the beginning of software orientation and mobility.

Procedure: Classroom Instruction

Students need solid grounding in software orientation (know where they are) and mobility (set their objective and know how to navigate there) to complete lessons requiring menu and dialog box navigation. Begin this lesson by instructing the student to always start each process by first determining where he is within the application or by starting at a point with which he is familiar.

Instruct the student to extensively explore the application menus and submenus using arrow or direction keys.

Lesson 15

Objective

The student will learn to navigate and change information in dialog boxes.

Procedure: Classroom Instruction

Continue the foundation of software orientation and mobility by instructing the student to open a dialog box, such as the "searching for points of interest" dialog box. Explain to the student that dialog boxes are similar in purpose to print forms that are used to collect information. Each box on a print form, such as name, address, and so on, is equivalent to a dialog box field. Instruct the student to move from field to field using the Tab key and the Shift-Tab key to move backward a field. These keys will vary depending on the system.

Once students master the basics of software orientation and mobility, they can be introduced to performing advanced point of interest functions, such as searching and editing.

Lesson 16

Objective

The student will learn to edit points of interest.

Procedure: Classroom Instruction

Use the skills practiced in Lesson 15 to edit personal points of interest and rename the point of interest, and remove or re-record the voice note. As features vary system by system, substitute another feature as needed to conduct this lesson. Pay particular attention to movement between fields, movements within fields, how to save and exit dialog boxes, and how to return a dialog box.

Assign an exercise, such as editing personal points of interest, as homework.

The skills learned in this lesson can be applied to any dialog box in the Trekker application or System Bar. Experiment with editing route names at the end of the route lesson and changing the time and date from the Clock dialog box found on the System bar. Reinforce the rules of using Arrow keys to navigate menus, Tab and Shift-Tab to navigate dialog boxes, and Arrow keys to navigate combo and list box fields within dialog boxes.

Lesson 17

Objective

The student will learn to create pedestrian point to point routes.

Procedure: Classroom Exercise

Route creation is an important feature of the GPS application and will assist the student greatly in travel planning. Provide instructions for selecting the route origin and destination. The GPS system will create route directions and save the route using a specific naming convention.

Repeat this exercise with the student using various origins and destinations and assign route creation as homework.

The student will already be familiar with selecting points of interest and will find them easy to use as origins and destinations. Also use addresses as an origin or destination. The student will generally be able to select from city, street, and number "pick lists."

Use the GPS system to create a motorized route.

Instruct the student to virtually browse or "walk" the routes they have created. Step through the route one intersection at a time. Route browsing is a good form of preparation for route traveling and will improve route performance.

Lesson 18

Objective

The student will learn to walk point-to-point routes.

Procedure: Field Exercise

Start at the origin of a saved route and instruct the student to establish an active GPS connection and determine compass directions, adjacent intersections, and street side. Open the route activation dialog box and select the appropriate route. Once the route is activated, the GPS system will speak the route starting point and first instruction. This information can be manually repeated pressing the appropriate key. Instruct students to obtain the next instruction and route status at midblock intervals to avoid distraction while focusing on intersection crossing. Follow the route until the destination is announced and the route is automatically deactivated. Instruct the student to find the final objective, such as specific addresses and doorways, using orientation and mobility skills.

Repeat route exercises, chaining objectives with various destinations.

GPS accuracy will assist the student in arriving in close proximity to his final objective but will very seldom announce destinations with pinpoint precision. Routes may also not provide accurate directions for street side, and students should use their own skills to determine which street side to walk along and where best to cross. O&M specialists will benefit from performing this lesson themselves until they are comfortable with the outcomes.

Repeat this lesson, but modify the lesson for route reversal.

Lesson 19

Objective

The student will learn how to use the rerouting feature.

Procedure

Modify Lesson 18 to practice rerouting. Instruct the student to go several blocks or more off route, and then use the reroute feature to obtain new directions from their new location.

Lesson 20

Objective

The student will learn how to create quick routes.

Procedure: Field Instruction

Some GPS systems allow students to create quick routes. They are very similar to point-to-point routes. The origin will automatically be selected as the student's current location. Destination options will remain the same as point-to-point route creation.

After establishing an active GPS connection and determining the compass direction, street side, and adjacent intersection information, instruct the student to start the quick-route creation process. Once the route is created use the instructions in the previous lesson to complete the route activity.

Repeat quick-route exercises, chaining objective with various destinations, as well as exercises in rerouting and reversing routes.

Lesson 21

Objective

The student will learn how to change GPS system settings.

Procedure: Classroom Instruction

There are generally several settings that will change the way that GPS systems will prompt points of interest and provide other details while traveling or browsing. Instructors should experiment with these settings before instructing students. Determine how to change settings back to the factory defaults. It may be helpful with some students to initially reduce the GPS system "verbosity" to assist them in focusing on the new geographic data they are experiencing.

Lesson 22

Objective

The student will learn to maintain and update the GPS system.

Procedure: Classroom Instruction

GPS systems may require the updating of map or application software from time to time. Refer to the factory manual that comes with the GPS system to provide specific details and operations related to updating.

GPS system units may also include PDA features such as contact management, e-mail, and appointment scheduling. These features are independent of GPS operation and will likely require a separate course of instruction.

A Final Note on EOAs

Electronic orientation aids have much potential yet to be realized, and it is the authors' opinion that accuracy and functionality are limitless with new and emergent system improvements. The Trekker, Pac Mate, Trekker Breeze, and BrailleNote are all viable products on the market. They represent good examples of GPS systems and address the needs of travelers who are visually impaired. As with all competing systems, the decision of which system to use needs to be made by informed consumers who are blind.

CONCLUSION

No secondary ETA is capable of providing the student who is blind or visually impaired with adequate protection unless used in conjunction with a primary mobility system, for example a cane, dog guide, or human guide, except in very familiar indoor circumstances. In addition, to date there are no secondary or primary ETAs capable of safely determining gaps between moving vehicular traffic, so they should never be used for this purpose. However, when appropriately matched to a trained student they may offer a valuable supplement to the user's primary mobility system.

There are uses for primary and secondary ETAs that have yet to be explored and documented. For example, a secondary ETA might be useful in first-time job orientation, in school orientation, and playground orientation, or in helping learn complex or hazardous environments. Using an ETA in this ad hoc manner as a simple orientation aid might be accomplished with very little training.

Technology will continue to advance, and one trickle-down effect will mean more of the daily life needs of blind persons will be addressed by more accessible technology. As ETAs become less expensive, more compact, and more highly developed, it is hoped that also with them will come a more efficient way to disseminate the information on available ETAs to the field. Until more persons who are blind can learn and experience what this technology can do for them, ETAs will be helping a few, but be needed by many.

IMPLICATIONS FOR O&M PRACTICE

1. A primary ETA device is basically one that may be used independent of any other mobility system while offering the user a reasonable assurance of safety, for example a cane, dog guide, or human guide. A secondary device is one that must be used with a primary system to offer a reasonable assurance of safety.

2. It is important for the certified O&M specialist to convey to her students that no ETA will reliably determine gaps in traffic, and thus they should *never* be used for this purpose! No device currently on the market has the range or reliability for this purpose.

3. There are several comparatively new ETAs available to persons who are blind. Each has its own capabilities and each has its own limitations, thus some are appropriate for individuals who are only blind, while those same devices are completely inappropriate for the person with neuropathy. Other devices are inappropriate for individuals with hearing loss. The O&M specialist must recognize these variables and assist the potential user in informed and educated selection.

4. Each device mentioned in this chapter has its rightful place on the array of assistive technology available to persons who are blind for safe and efficient travel and wayfinding.

5. The advancements in GPS and GIS have revolutionized the field of orientation and mobility. Today, the traveler who is blind has at his fingertips more information than ever before. While not negating the need for traditional orientation skills, the person who is blind may travel independently in many unfamiliar locations without assistance. Further advancements will undoubtedly influence the field as devices become less costly.

LEARNING ACTIVITIES

1. Describe the attributes that one would look for in an adult who is considering an ETA. Compare to those of a prospective third grader. What would suitable learning objectives be for each?

2. Give your opinion as to which device(s) would be appropriate for an adult who travels well with his cane but occasionally has difficulty finding bus poles, bus shelters, mailboxes, and other landmarks. Consider the same person with the same needs but who also has a hearing loss. Consider the same person with the same needs who has diabetic neuropathy.

3. Determine a rationale for an appropriate ETA for the dog guide user with the same considerations as identified in activity 2. Will a dog guide user have a need for an ETA? Explain.

4. Describe an appropriate candidate for an EOA. Which are suitable for persons who have other considerations, for example those who are hearing impaired or have diabetic neuropathy.

5. Prepare an electronic notebook by going online of all currently available ETAs and EOAs. Be sure to include current costs. Keep the notebook updated periodically and it will be invaluable throughout your career.

6. The authors assert that many times the student has a tendency to attend completely to the signals emitted by the ETA to the exclusion of sensory input from other sources, including his primary mobility device. What would you suggest to minimize this occurrence?

7. Describe the meaning of *pulse* as it relates to ETA training.

CHAPTER 15

Teaching Orientation and Mobility for Adverse Weather Conditions

Julie-Anne Couturier and Agathe Ratelle

LEARNING QUESTIONS

1. What specific O&M problems are related to snow, ice, cold, rain, and wind, and can affect safety, efficiency, and comfort when traveling?

2. Which perceptual and cognitive skills facilitate successful travel in winter snowy conditions and which specific strategies, techniques, methods of travel, and equipment are found to be effective for traveling under snowy and icy conditions?

3. How can slips and falls on slippery surfaces be addressed? What contributing factors and intervention programs may reduce risks of fall events on icy surfaces?

4. How do adverse travel conditions interact with psychosocial, physical, and health issues? What precautions need to be taken under severe or extreme heat or cold?

5. What particular winter challenges are encountered by specific groups of students, for instance, persons with low vision, older adults, children, deaf-blind travelers, and dog guide users? How do fall prevalence and prevention issues relate to the aging population?

6. Which environmental adaptations would enhance safe and efficient travel in winter conditions? How can advanced technology contribute to more efficient winter travel?

Weather is the state of the atmosphere at a particular time and place. It includes such elements as temperature, humidity, precipitation, and wind. These elements act together and create favorable or adverse weather events, depending on their intensity. Rain, snow, wind, ice, and heat are events that may generate adverse conditions for pedestrians who are blind or visually impaired. They can greatly challenge or impair a person's perception and orientation, as well as his mobility.

To address issues and offer solutions for traveling under various adverse conditions, the intent of this chapter is twofold: to (1) present an extensive portrait of problems and strategies related to winter travel, such as mobility in cold, snowy, and icy conditions, which are of great concern for many people who are blind or visually impaired (Couturier, Ratelle, & Bilodeau, 2006; Dietrichson, Lund, Moe, & Saeter, 1998; Smith, De l'Aune, & Geruschat, 1992; Welsh &

Wiener, 1976); and (2) present specific strategies and adapted behaviors under other adverse weather conditions, such as extreme heat, when health may be at risk. Catastrophic events such as hail storms, severe thunderstorms, hurricanes, and floods are not covered by this chapter.

WINTER CONDITIONS AND GENERAL STRATEGIES

Winter climate embodies five basic elements which, together, can cause both psychological and physiological discomfort: (1) temperature—normally below freezing; (2) precipitation—often in the form of snow; (3) restricted hours of sunshine and daylight; (4) prolonged periods of the first three factors cited; and (5) seasonal variation within a same country (Pressman, 2004).

Winter is associated with cold, snow, wind, ice, and darkness during a considerable part of the year. Within some countries, such as Canada, Norway, Japan, or Russia, variations exist from one geographic region to another. In northern-latitude communities, such as those located above 60th parallel, winter can last up to eight months. In southern regions of these countries, weather may be less severe but difficult conditions still occur from November until the end of March. In Siberia, Y. Balashova, an O&M specialist (personal communication, September 12, 2006), stated that "November and March may be the worst with slippery travel surfaces, while January is the worst with –40°F (–40°C) frost."

As early as 1917, Canadian Phillip Layton, the treasurer of the Montreal Association for the Blind, who was himself blind, considered snow to be "one of the greatest obstacles to overcome when traveling alone" (Layton, 1917, p. 71). Many persons who are blind or visually impaired may, in fact, travel with more difficulty or less inde-

pendently in winter conditions. Yet, Rudkin (1971) states that winter travel is possible to achieve, even if it may be more difficult than summer travel. Many travelers with visual impairments can become very competent in these conditions.

In spite of the difficulty and importance of winter travel, there is a scarcity of literature and research pertaining to the subject. A report edited by Welsh and Wiener (1976) has provided substantial information that is still relevant today. This document compiled opinions and experiences shared by O&M specialists, faculty members from university programs, and travelers who were visually impaired, who had been brought together for a special national conference on winter travel, which was held in Minnesota. The conference design included discussion panels and field testing from which emerged numerous techniques and methods for dealing with winter traveling problems. Dietrichson, Lund, Moe, and Saeter (1998) also presented a thorough and integrated report following interviews and the videotaping of the outdoor travel of seven successful snow travelers. On their part, Rudkin (1971) and Morais et al. (1997) provided short practice summaries for snow or adverse weather travel. All these references highlighted substantial content that will be reviewed throughout the chapter.

More recent research studies, surveys, and other summaries of practice insights have also brought new significant information to the field. Couturier et al. (2006) conducted a pilot study with 33 experienced adult travelers who were blind, with the intention of updating some information on winter environments, such as icy conditions. A telephone interview with these participants sought to explore the most significant winter travel problems experienced by adults who are blind or visually impaired, as well as the most efficient winter travel strategies, including environmental adaptations, that would enhance winter traveling.

Varying and Unpredictable Environmental Conditions

A major feature of winter is the variability and unpredictability of its conditions (Dietrichson et al., 1998; Welsh & Wiener, 1976). Newly fallen snow, either powdery or wet, may produce a light, medium, or heavy cover, offering different challenges to winter travelers. Irregular obstacles are created, such as mounds of snow on sidewalks and at street corners. Snowfall may, at times, be accompanied by high winds, making travel even more difficult. Temperature can vary from above 32°F (0°C) to extremely cold weather. Some regions experience temperature changes that are sometimes drastic, even within a day, such as snowfall in the morning, rain at noon, and freezing rain overnight. Changing weather creates varying icy conditions on the sidewalk, while melting periods produce puddles of slush at street corners. Depending on temperature, pedestrian flow, and city maintenance services, environments may vary from block to block and frequently within the same block. Snow cover on one side of the street may have started to melt, while the other side has an icy surface.

Specific characteristics may also be found relating to urban, suburban, and rural areas. Urban areas may have snow clearance and removal processes better adapted to a larger population. In suburban areas, snow may be removed from one side of the street only, leaving big mounds of snow on the other side all through the winter. Rural areas are affected by high, howling winds, and snowdrifts that can block pathways and roads.

General Strategies for Winter Travel

The Winter Traveler Who Is Visually Impaired

In order to ensure safety and efficiency in winter travel, certain personal attitudes or behaviors are essential. Flexibility and perseverance are indicated for snow conditions. Cautious behaviors will be critical at street crossings and in extreme conditions of cold, wind, heavy snowfall, and freezing rain. Appropriate preparation for adverse weather conditions is primary and will initially rely on a good and thorough preparation for traveling in general (Dietrichson et al., 1998; Welsh & Wiener, 1976). In order to become a flexible traveler, one needs to first master the basics, such as the fundamentals of long cane use, auditory perception, the ability to cope with many ground covers, kinesthetic and distance awareness, and problem-solving ability. (For more information on these topics, see Chapters 1, 4, 5, and 12, and Volume 1, Chapters 4, 5, and 10.)

Changes in Travel Habits and Frequency

There has been little systematic research on how people who are visually impaired, including older adults, modify their travel habits in winter conditions. Wall (2001) conducted an exploratory study with 12 capable Canadian winter cane travelers, between the ages of 16 and 50, and sought to investigate how travelers with visual impairments modify their travel habits, procedures, and techniques in winter. Most respondents traveled less frequently in winter than in summer and only when circumstances required it. Respondents also tended to travel more within their neighborhoods, in both time and distance. In more difficult weather conditions, some used alternative transportation systems, such as taxis, buses, human guide, and door-to-door transportation (Couturier et al., 2006; Wall, 2001). Winter also reduces traveling for more vulnerable seniors.

Service Delivery System and Structure

If a general O&M training program has been provided during good weather conditions, additional training may be needed when winter arrives. In winter regions, outdoor instruction in O&M is, however, frequently initiated during winter. According to O&M specialists working in such climates, students receiving an initial outdoor training during winter, instead of summer, are likely to build better self-confidence in their overall travel habits. They will frequently express that traveling in warmer temperature seems easier. However, during winter conditions, O&M training may be postponed for more frail students, such as persons with health problems and some seniors, until milder weather prevails (Rockwitz, 2000).

O&M lesson planning needs to be flexible and adapted to winter conditions. Because of cold, lessons may be shortened or have more frequent pauses. The instructor may provide as much instruction as possible indoors prior to or after the lesson. During extreme conditions, travel skills may be practiced in university or school buildings, shopping malls, and subways, and include such skills as the use of tactile maps, intersection analysis, and low-vision skills.

O&M specialists require specific blindfold training for themselves in winter conditions, in order to better appreciate winter travel issues and related strategies. If such training has not been feasible during a student's university training program, special blindfold lessons may be done with another instructor or through inservice training following graduation.

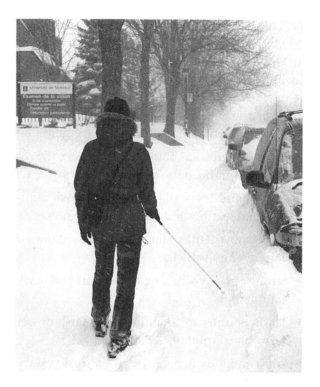

Winter creates a new physical environment.

SPECIFIC MOBILITY PROBLEMS AND STRATEGIES IN WINTER CONDITIONS

Access to Significant Sensory Information and Landmarks for the Traveler Who Is Visually Impaired

For the traveler who is visually impaired, winter creates a new physical environment that can deeply obscure significant sensory information that would be present in fair weather conditions. Usual tactile and auditory landmarks or cues

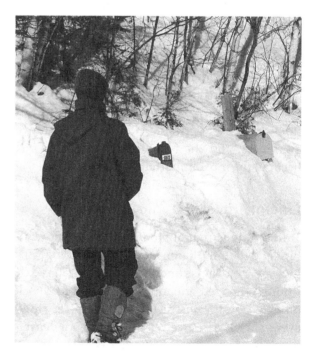

Snow obscures landmarks and destination points (mailbox).

are covered, changed, or lost (Dietrichson et al., 1998; Lundälv, 2001; Morais et al., 1997; Rudkin, 1971; Welsh & Wiener, 1976). These changes may include the following:

- With the first cold, hardened ground alters the differentiation of grass and pavement.
- Newly fallen snow absorbs and reduces the intensity of traffic noise or other usable sounds.
- Snowy and icy walking surfaces mask auditory and tactile cues, including cane noises.
- High snow banks along the streets dampen sounds from vehicles.
- Strong or gusty winds tend to distort and mask sounds.
- Traffic sounds are amplified with slush or wet snow on warmer days.
- Snow mounds may block access to necessary navigation points and impede street crossings.
- New clues may be found when melting occurs, such as running water in the gutter.

Travelers with visual impairments and O&M specialists agree that winter conditions necessitate less dependence on usual physical tactile clues and more reliance on other sensory inputs (Welsh & Wiener, 1976). In most winter conditions, the use of traffic, kinesthetic distance awareness, and the basic line of direction will become the most important orientation skills.

Line of Travel

Traffic sounds that are muffled during snowfall hinder dynamic alignment. Interpretation of various new traffic sounds can be reemphasized through directed attention, perceptual feedback provided by the instructor, and practice. However, travelers perceive sounds at increased distances in brisk cold weather (see Lawson & Wiener, Volume 1, Chapter 4). The pedestrian's

line of travel can also be disturbed by snow mounds of varying sizes on the sidewalk. When these are encountered, the traveler can determine consistency, height, and width of the mound by exploring it with the cane. He can check for packed snow, indicating a nearby pathway. In case of a low mound, he may walk through it.

Rudkin (1971), Welsh and Wiener (1976), and Graham (1998) have greatly emphasized concentration on the *basic or main line of direction* when traveling through different snow conditions. While walking through a light or medium cover of snow or when a mound of snow blocks the path of travel, the traveler needs to rely primarily on his line of direction and continue moving without stopping for minor distractions on the path. The traveler may also encounter misleading tactual information resulting from melting and refreezing snow or ice, and thus needs to concentrate more on traffic and his line of direction.

Additional training could be appropriate in refining the line of direction. This training might include the following:

- The student needs to be helped to constantly visualize walking on a sidewalk, parallel to the street, leading to a point farther ahead, such as the street corner. Even if an obstacle is encountered, the mental picture of the straight-line sidewalk needs to be kept clearly in mind. The overall mental picture of the environment needs to predominate over near surfaces.
- Practice in a large open space, such as a gym, a hall, or an auditorium. After squaring off at a starting point on one wall, the trainee walks directly to an objective (mental point) at the opposite wall, while the objective is continually kept in his mind's eye (Rudkin, 1971). Right angled and angular obstacles are placed along the line of travel and the trainee gets around them and yet retains his basic direction. A sound beacon can be placed at the objective.

- Spoken feedback from the instructor can be provided while veering, in order to recognize the proprioceptive cues (kinesthetic, vestibular) associated with walking a straight line (Guth & Rieser, 1997). Guérette and Zabihaylo (2000) suggest exercises in a long, open, and quiet outdoor area, free of obstacles and surface terrain changes. The trainee is instructed to walk naturally, without any travel device, in an attempt to maintain a straight line. A training sequence is followed, through which the instructor (1) walks in front of the trainee, gradually increasing the distance and decreasing the auditory cues; and (2) walks beside the trainee. During that sequence, the trainee uses auditory feedback, such as the voice of the instructor and echolocation cues, or tactual feedback when the instructor's body or a grass edge is encountered. Appropriate posture and gait components are reemphasized throughout the exercises.

Certain snow conditions may enhance a fluid and straight line of travel. Travelers can perceive the smoothness of the walking surface since cracks and ridges on the sidewalk get filled with packed snow. Following a snowfall, the snow removal process may leave mounds of snow on both sides of the sidewalk, creating a corridor or a physical guideline that can be trailed with the cane. Many inconvenient obstacles, such as poles, traffic signal control boxes, low-hanging signs, and overhangs, are surrounded by a mound of snow all through winter, which can serve as a buffer preventing undesired contacts. Packed paths of snow leading to a house entry or, in rural areas, to other farm buildings and sheds will help in maintaining a direction of travel. In residential, suburban, or rural areas, the traveler may have to walk in the street, but he can safely maintain his line of direction by shorelining the snowbank at the side of the street or the road. In using the latter technique, the traveler has to keep in mind that walking in the street can increase the danger from passing traffic. When traffic is approaching, the traveler should step aside and as far up onto the snowbank as is feasible without slipping and wait for the traffic to pass.

Walking in Winter Conditions with a Cane

Durability and sensitivity are important characteristics for a winter cane. The cane models most favored would be made of aluminum, carbon fiber, or graphite (Graham, 1998). Ambrose-Zaken (2005) conducted an extensive survey with 98 participants, relating to their knowledge of and preferences for long-cane components. In regard to travel in more difficult situations, such as rough terrain and unfamiliar environments, participants recommended a longer, rigid cane with a marshmallow tip. More specifically with adverse weather conditions, ethylene vinyl acetate foam grips and a solid tip were mentioned. The length of the cane could vary from 2 to 8 inches (5 to 20 cm) above xyphoid process at the bottom of the sternum.

The cane is a "powerful perceptual tool and allows perception of distal stimuli" necessary for travel preview (Guth & Rieser, 1997). Most exploratory behaviors of snow or ice terrain may be accomplished with *lateral motion* (or *sweep*) to determine more easily the texture of the terrain. A *pressure procedure* (*tapping a surface*), obtained with the touch technique, could be used to determine the hardness of the terrain (Guth & Rieser, 1997; see also Volume 1, Chapter 1). A relevant practice prior to winter traveling is poking or sweeping the cane into mounds or covers of fallen leaves during autumn.

Winter travelers may modify cane techniques, as long as safety is not sacrificed for convenience. Most of the following modifications have been found to be relevant by the following authors

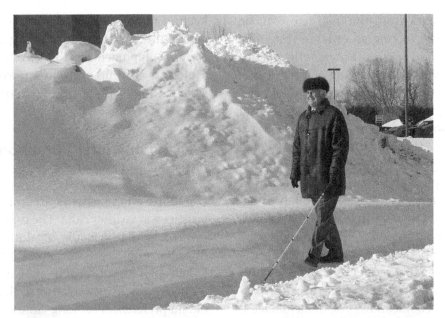

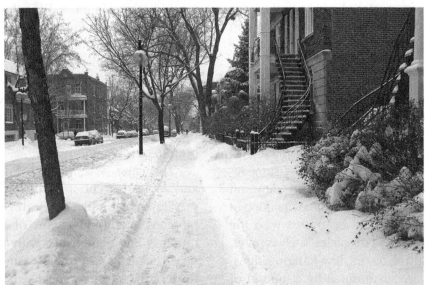

Mounds of snow create a corridor that facilitates a line of travel on sidewalk.

(Dietrichson et al., 1998; Rudkin, 1971; Wall, 2001; Welsh & Wiener, 1976):

- Use the constant contact technique more in general and in specific situations, such as walking on a light cover of snow or locating a shoreline.

- Use a heavier or a bouncing touch, with a higher arc, on a medium snow covered surface.

- A light touch is emphasized in heavier snow to prevent cane sticking in the snow.

- Use a reversed arc in powdered snow, where the cane is moved in such a way that the arc is

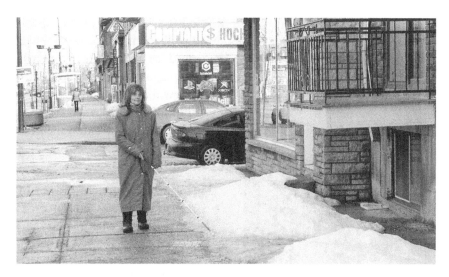

Pedestrian protected from overhangs during the winter period.

low in the middle and high at the sides. This technique avoids cane sticking in banks of snow while still offering protection.

- Permit the movement of the arm instead of just the wrist to provide more latitude in exploratory or trailing techniques.

- Vary the width of the arc, depending on the situation. Use a shortened arc when walking on a packed path of travel created with older existing snow.

- Experiment with different techniques that are best adapted to various situations: for example, poke the cane in the nearby snow in order to locate a hard-packed walking path, sweep the cane to determine the width of travel path, swing the cane higher to find landmarks or the top of snowbanks.

- When searching for landmarks, for example, a mailbox or a pole, trail the top of the snowbank by using a three-point touch technique.

Wall (2001) highlighted other procedures and cane techniques that are modified by winter travelers, such as using more force on touch and drag, traveling slower, exploring more, and depending on larger landmarks. Wall's study concluded that the amount of winter training received by the cane traveler does affect the number of modified techniques used; however, cane users who travel frequently will tend to modify their techniques more frequently for convenience and accessibility to fit all situations.

Maintaining Orientation

In winter, the traveler who is visually impaired may travel best in familiar areas (Dietrichson et al., 1998; Wall, 2001). If the traveler already knows the patterns and main information points of the environment, it is easier to measure and evaluate alternatives if significant information points are obscured, changed, or lost. However, unusual and unexpected situations occur regularly. One of the most frequent orientation struggles for a traveler during a snowfall is to know whether he is still on the sidewalk or if he has veered into the street (Couturier et al., 2006). As the traveler is likely to experience many recovery situations, he may need to use more problem-solving and decision-making skills during snow situations than during ordinary travel

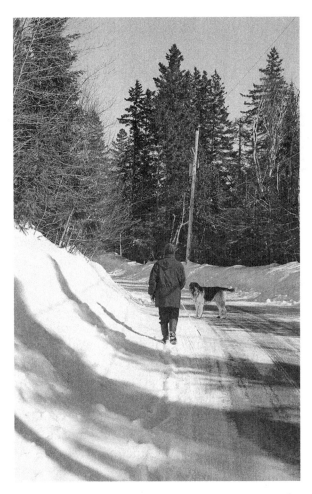

Shorelining snowbanks along rural roads makes traveling enjoyable.

(Dietrichson et al., 1998; Rudkin, 1971; Welsh & Wiener, 1976).

Efficient winter travelers need to continually anticipate the varying travel conditions they encounter, either within days, within a day, or within a short distance (Welsh & Wiener, 1976). To increase the ability to cope with adverse conditions, the following orientation guidelines might be of help.

- Develop knowledge of winter patterns and processes.

- Through experience, build a dependable knowledge base of the different environmental patterns and features of specific winter conditions. Identify *information points* that could be used for orientation on regular routes. For example, a large mound of snow adjacent to the sidewalk can indicate the proximity of a gas station area, or a traveler may shoreline a snowbank along the sidewalk in a residential area while counting openings to get to his home destination.

- Know the snow clearance or ice management procedures and sequence of a particular locality or area within a city.

- Plan travel carefully.

- Listen to the weather forecast every night in order to plan travel accordingly for the morning after (Will there be new snow? Will the sidewalks be icy? Will it be too dangerous to travel? Is walking the best solution? Does the weather forecast predict drastic changes within the next few days?). Through training, travelers may learn about situations in which safety could be threatened and the best travel strategy related to each situation. For more extreme conditions, the use of a human guide or door-to-door transportation may be preferable.

- Whenever needed, in the morning or throughout the day, use the help of a sighted person to update environmental conditions and plan traveling accordingly (How deep is the snow on the sidewalk now? What are the conditions at the street corner?).

- Whenever indicated, plan alternative routes on streets where the snow has already been removed.

- Travelers who rely on a more sequential route or linear approach in their orientation process are more likely to encounter substantial difficulty in winter conditions (Graham, 1998). As they may be unable to plan alternative routes, they may be advised to use paratransit transportation systems during the winter period or in the most severe weather conditions.

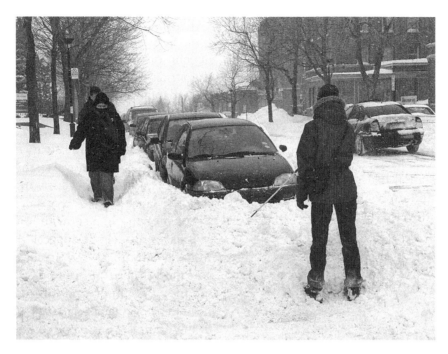

A sudden mound of snow encountered on the sidewalk may create disorientation.

- Use efficient recovery procedures.
- Use a specific problem-solving strategy. These processes are briefly illustrated through the following example of travel in snow conditions. When exposed to a new situation, such as a mound of snow on the sidewalk, a traveler needs to *explore* the environment in order to gather information about the significance of the change (Why is there a mound of snow? How big is it?). He then needs to *analyze and interpret* the environment with the cane and auditory sense (Is there a clearer path next to it? Where is the traffic? At what distance?). Then, the traveler *creates a hypothesis*, usually that he will find the sidewalk by turning and walking toward the sound of the traffic. Further he *confirms it* by walking toward the sound of the traffic (I have found a clear path again and can hear traffic on the street moving in a parallel direction; therefore, I am still walking on the sidewalk). If the hypothesis cannot be confirmed (traffic sounds appear farther away than they should or the street is found instead of the sidewalk), another hypothesis has to be constructed or assistance options need to be explored. Success in this process will build *self-efficacy* (see Volume 1, Chapter 6), an asset in future decision making.

- When experiencing disorientation, use the "spatial-framework" strategy that consists of imagining the surroundings as if they exist in a grid pattern and visualizing oneself standing within that framework, and tracking movements as they relate to the grid (Guth & Rieser, 1997).

- Solicit assistance when necessary. There may be fewer pedestrians on the street, or they may be in a hurry or concentrating on their own mobility because of adverse weather conditions. The use of a cell phone may be an alternative, as the traveler can immediately call a family member, a friend, or a policeman, and solicit his or her physical assistance at his actual location. While reducing stress, this strategy avoids unsafe decisions or actions and quickens the recovery process.

Street Crossings

Safety and orientation issues are interrelated at street crossings and especially so during winter conditions. The traveler needs to be constantly alert and cautious since all perceptual tasks may be affected. For all winter travelers having visual impairments, traffic will be a major source of information for street crossings (Welsh & Wiener, 1976).

Detection of Street Corners and Proper Waiting Position

Traffic sounds and kinesthetic distance awareness are the best cues for detection of street corners in typical winter conditions, where light packed snow covers the curb. Pole locators installed at intersections equipped with accessible pedestrian signalization (APS) may provide auditory cues about the proximity of the corner (see Barlow, Bentzen, & Franck, Volume 1, Chapter 11). On the other hand, judging the distance of vehicles will be more difficult during a snowfall. Traffic sounds are perceived to be farther away than they actually are, because of the reduced intensity of sounds (Wall, 2001). Cars on the perpendicular street may not be detected accurately by hearing, and warning tiles installed at specific street corners may not be noticeable when covered by snow. In order to determine one's proper position at a street corner or curb, one technique is suggested. As soon as the corner is anticipated and the decline of the blended curb perceived, the student needs to walk two to three steps toward the curb edge and stop. This strategy may limit disorientation from search movements to locate the curb and, most cru-

cially, may prevent the traveler from walking into the street. The number of steps taken will depend on the length of the blended curb and the stride of the person. Appropriate analysis and adaptation of this technique may be done with each student during training.

During some winter days, when obstacles at street corners are obvious (e.g., mounds of snow following snow removal), the traveler may adopt a checking procedure, in order to anticipate the safest way to negotiate such obstacles. In the presence of a snow mound at the corner, Morais et al. (1997) suggest that the traveler wait beyond the mound. In such cases, the traveler may either trail around or climb over the mound. Proximity and the danger of traffic need to be evaluated, and care needs to be taken to maintain the basic line of direction. Warmer days or late winter melting conditions generate large puddles of water and slush that can greatly alter one's direction. The traveler may be wise to step back to avoid being splashed by passing vehicles.

The traveler's visibility may be affected by winter conditions as the white cane easily blends in with white snow. Drivers' vision can be obscured by fog or snow partly covering car windows, or their attention may simply be focused on slippery road conditions. Visibility may be enhanced by wearing brighter colored clothes during winter travel (Y. Balashova, personal communication, September 12, 2006).

Alignment

When snow is falling, the reduced volume and intensity of traffic sounds may hinder the alignment task, since traffic cannot be heard at an appropriate distance. Auditory skills need to be practiced and reinforced. Most travelers with visual impairments choose to uncover their ears for better auditory perception at street crossings (Dietrichson et al., 1998; Morais et al., 1997; Wall, 2001; Welsh & Wiener, 1976).

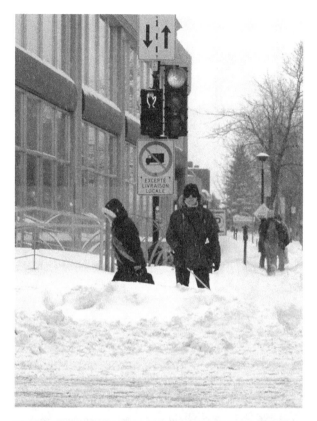

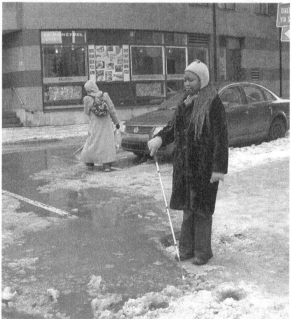

Street crossings are challenging for the winter traveler.

Recent snowfalls can create confusion, adding to the danger of misalignment. Pedestrians or snow removal machines produce paths that may lead diagonally toward the middle of the intersection. The traveler needs to be aware of such situations and concentrate on traffic and line of direction, or solicit assistance, if needed.

During very cold days, tolerance of low temperatures may be limited while waiting in a stationary position at a traffic light crossing. Travelers are more likely to make hasty, unsafe decisions to cross without appropriate alignment. The traveler may need to be reminded not to begin crossing until he is absolutely sure that it is safe to do so. He may plan an alternative route using busier streets, in order to obtain more consistent auditory information, as well as sighted assistance, if necessary.

APS provided with a beacon feature, such as a signal that alternates from one side of the street to the other, may facilitate alignment prior to crossing (Ratelle et al., 1998; see Barlow, Bentzen, & Franck, Volume 1, Chapter 11). Such systems could enhance safety and ease of travel in difficult winter conditions (Couturier et al., 2006).

Initiating Street Crossing

During a snowfall, traffic slowing or surging are not as distinct because drivers also move more slowly. In residential areas, the pedestrian's safety may be threatened by cars on the perpendicular street approaching the intersection and not able to stop because of slippery conditions (surfaces covered with icy snow or by a thin layer of fresh snow). At stop-sign crossings, the traveler may wait until the perpendicular traffic has gone through the intersection before initiating his crossing. When traffic sounds are absent or insufficient at street light crossings, the traveler may plan alternative routes by using busier intersections where sighted assistance is more accessible. APS, when available, offers necessary information to supplement crossing decisions.

Crossing the Street

During a snowfall, a pedestrian may encounter snow ruts while crossing and, as a result, may veer from his intended line of travel. The traveler needs to concentrate on his line of direction, maintaining dynamic alignment with traffic sounds and being alert to its proximity. In the presence of a mound of snow at the other corner, the traveler may explore with the cane and find a packed snow pathway through the fluffier mound.

In the springtime, the traveler also needs to be attentive to potholes as they are common in some cities (Couturier et al., 2006). Potholes are of various dimensions and depth and are usually unexpected. If not detected, they can cause falls or injuries in a zone (street) that is already life-threatening. To better detect them, the traveler should use good cane techniques, including constant contact with the surface terrain.

Walking on Ice and Balance Problems

Ice has been identified by 78 percent of survey respondents as one of the most difficult winter conditions (Couturier et al., 2006). Gao and Abeysekera (2004a) performed an extensive literature survey and presented a comprehensive review of slip-and-fall accidents on icy and snowy surfaces. They highlighted that winter conditions result in a significant increase of slip-and-fall accidents on icy surfaces among outdoor workers and the general population.

In many winter regions, a variety of icy conditions may occur throughout the winter season. Weather features that create icy conditions are freezing rain, rain followed by colder weather, or a snow-melting period generated by sun, pedestrian, or car traffic, followed by freezing overnight. Resulting surface conditions are varied: complete icy cover, varying icy spots, or ice covered by light powdered snow. These conditions

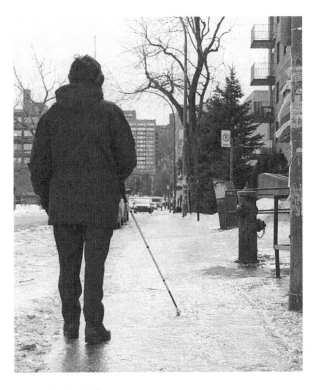

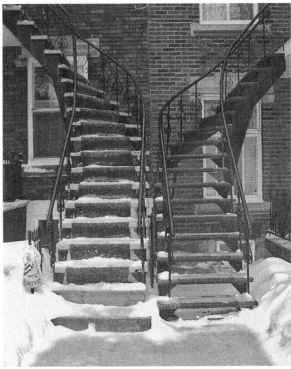

Icy surfaces may cause disorientation, slips, and falls.

are encountered on sidewalks, in driveways, at street corners, in building entrances, in shadowed areas, on steps going into buses or leading to houses, and when exiting cars or buses. Icy surfaces can be predictable following a freezing rain, but they can be unpredictable in many other situations, especially if icy conditions are due to improper maintenance services. Gao and Abeysekera (2004b) and Gao, Holmer, and Abeysekera (2008) found that fall events occurred mostly on "ice covered with snow," probably due to the inability to preview the hidden risk of slipperiness of the walking surface.

Slips and falls on icy and snowy surfaces have been a matter of research concern in Scandinavian countries for the last decade. Following a 3-year study of hospital-treated fractures in Norway, Ytterstad (1996) revealed that falls occurring in the public pedestrian traffic areas were five times more frequent during the seven winter months than during the "snow-free" months. Björnstig, Björnstig, and Dahlgren (1997) analyzed one year's injury data from the University Hospital of Northern Sweden and reported that slips and falls during winter caused 3.5 injuries per 1,000 inhabitants per year, the injury rate being the highest among elderly women. With regard to different wintry conditions, falls occurred more frequently on icy surfaces than on snowy surfaces. In fact, pedestrians had 14 times more injuries on high-risk days than during normal winter days (Grönqvist & Hirvonen, 1995). A high-risk day is characterized by a pronounced increase in temperature followed by a sharp fall of temperature.

Bruises, sprains, muscle pain, and fractures are common injuries resulting from slips and falls during winter and their related costs are also substantial (Gao et al., 2008). According to a Finnish study cited by Aschan et al. (2009), the costs due to slip-and-fall accidents are 10 times more than the costs related to winter maintenance services.

Contributing Factors to Slips and Falls

Gao and Abeysekera (2004a) present a systematic multifactorial analysis of slips and falls on icy and snowy surfaces. Besides *environmental climate factors* and *footwear properties* (see Winter Weather Clothing and Equipment), three other contributing factors to slips and falls are presented in this section.

Underfoot surface characteristics and friction. Low friction or poor traction between footwear and the underfoot surface has been identified as the primary risk factor contributing to slips and falls (Gao et al., 2008). Slipping occurs when the coefficient of friction (COF) between footwear and walkway surface provides insufficient resistance. Certain surfaces are likely to be more slippery than others. Melting ice, at 32°F (0°C), is more slippery than dry ice, found at less than 14°F (–10°C). A low COF (e.g., 0.01) indicates low resistance and that slipping can occur easily, such as on wet ice. A high COF (e.g., 0.2 or more) indicates more resistance to slipperiness, such as on dry ice. The lower COF on wet ice is explained by different ice properties, such as the formation of a liquid film on the icy surface that lowers adhesion friction. A water layer may also be formed by frictional heating caused by pedestrian traffic. Grönqvist (1995, cited in Aschan et al., 2009) validated a grading system which includes coefficient of friction measurements of surface slipperiness and their corresponding subjective values (see Table 15.1).

A minimal COF requirement of 0.2 has been identified for slip resistance on lubricated (water, oil) floors. In other words, friction values exceeding 0.2 are commonly regarded as safe when walking. (*Special note*: The reader needs to be aware that standards and measurements can vary between different countries. The reference system mentioned in this chapter is the one being used in Scandinavian countries.) According to

TABLE 15.1

Grading System of Coefficients of Friction and Subjective Values of Surface Slipperiness

Class	Explanation	Coefficient of Friction
1	Very slip-resistant	≥0.30
2	Slip-resistant	0.20–0.29
3	Unsure	0.15–0.19
4	Slippery	0.05–0.14
5	Very slippery	<0.05

Source: R. Grönqvist, *A Dynamic Method for Assessing Pedestrian Slip Resistance*, Ph.D. thesis, Finnish Institute of Occupational Health, Helsinki, 1995.

Grönqvist and Hirvonen (1995), a COF of 0.3 or more would be preferable for pedestrians' safety on winter surfaces. Older and disabled persons may even require higher level of friction (Aschan et al., 2009). In case of mobility disabled persons (e.g., amputees), Dura, Alcantara, Zamora, Balaguer, and Rosa (2005) demonstrated a COF requirement greater than 0.40.

Friction on ice can be improved by spreading abrasive material (sand or gravel) on pavement surfaces (Gao & Abeysekera, 2004a; Takahashi, Tokunaga, & Asano, 2007). Aschan et al. (2009) showed that friction was doubled on granulated surfaces, that is, when abrasive material was added. Although additional evidence is needed regarding the effect of anti-slip materials on icy surfaces, some research has revealed that sand could increase the COF up to 0.5 and more (Gao & Abeysekera, 2004a).

Most of the research pertaining to slips and falls on slippery surfaces has been conducted in the indoor or outdoor workplace. Little has been done in real-life situations, and more so, on icy

and snowy surfaces with the general population. In more recent years, a Portable Slip Simulator device was designed and constructed at the Finnish Institute of Occupational Health, with the objective of evaluating wintry surface conditions in situ, while taking into account human gait parameters (Aschan et al., 2009). Throughout their experiment, the researchers confirmed the usability and the validity of the device. It can be used to measure slipperiness of various walking surfaces under different weather conditions. It can also assess, under real wintry conditions, the slip resistance of different types of footwear found on the market. Consequently, the likelihood of measuring slip resistance on various wintry walking surfaces should provide opportunities to assess maintenance services, besides establishing models for predicting weather and pavement conditions for pedestrians. Research needs to be pursued because some icy conditions are more slippery than lubricated floors and a significant number of people in many countries are affected by wintry conditions.

Gait biomechanics. To guarantee dynamic stability during locomotion, the center of mass (COM) of the body must stay within the base of support (BOS) (Marigold & Patla, 2002). During walking, the COM passes outside the BOS twice every gait cycle—it passes in front of the trailing toe in early swing and is behind the leading heel in late swing (see Rosen, Volume 1, Chapter 5). These two phases in each gait cycle, during which there is instability, are particularly critical phases when falls might occur, that is, near the heelstrike and toe-off periods or where the COM is outside the BOS. On a slippery surface, Gard and Lundborg (2000) state that the heel strike causes a forward slip on the leading foot, which would very likely result in a backward fall. The toe-off period causes a backward slip on the trailing foot, which can be counterbalanced by stepping forwards with the leading foot. Gao and Abeysekera (2004a) further reported, "The forward slip (heel strike) is more dangerous and frequent. Whenever humans cannot counterbalance these slips, then loss of balance and fall will occur" (p. 573).

Researchers have found that proactive or more cautious gait strategies can be adopted when confronted with an impending slip-and-fall situation. Being able to anticipate (know) the slippery surface condition results in proactive adjustments, that is, step length and heel-contact velocity are reduced, while the contact area is increased (Marigold & Patla, 2002; Lockhart, Spaulding, & Park, 2007). Flat-foot landing, also called *gentle heel strike*, has indeed been demonstrated as a good adaptive strategy (Fong, Mao, Li, & Yong, 2008). However, older people may need an extra step in order to effectively adjust their gait before walking on a known slippery floor condition (Lockhart et al., 2007). More biomechanical research is needed on human gait changes on icy surfaces (Gao & Abeysekera, 2004a).

Human factors. Some researchers argue that "knowledge of the surface" is possibly the major determinant of postural adjustment on slippery surfaces; to some degree, this statement can explain why ice skaters can manage balance without falls, even under a COF value of 0.0046 (Gao & Abeysekera, 2004a). Knowledge is obtained through visual anticipation and relies on such functions as visual field, visual acuity, contrast sensitivity, and depth perception. Vision has an important role of planning movement. People who are blind or visually impaired may then be greatly disadvantaged on slippery surfaces. Due to reduction or absence of vision, they cannot preview the surface and its potential slipperiness and react in time, especially with unpredictable icy spots. Visual preview of a slippery surface needs to be made within a 10 to 16 feet (3 to 5 m) distance in order to allow sufficient reaction time (Gao & Abeysekera, 2004a).

A traveler with reduced visual acuity may use other environmental cues to detect changing surfaces, but his visual perception may be impaired by inadequate lighting, glare, and lack of contrast between the sidewalk and the icy spot. A person who is blind can use the cane as a probe to preview the environment, but perception through the cane hand may be limited. Detection with the foot will not allow enough time to react. Some research has, however, demonstrated that increased living experience in a winter climate reduces slips and falls on ice and snow (Gao & Abeysekera, 2004b). With anticipatory and preventive behaviors (see Strategies for Walking on Icy Surfaces), slipperiness may be successfully managed in some situations.

Certain clientele may particularly be at risk of slips and falls on wintry slippery surfaces because of age or health-related issues. In this respect, the O&M specialist needs to be concerned by the diabetic person with visual impairment. Diabetic peripheral neuropathy causes a loss of proprioception and distal sensation of the walking surface (see Rosen & Crawford, Chapter 18). Studies have reported that peripheral neuropathy reduces postural stability and increases the risks of falls (Simoneau, Ulbrecht, Derr, Becker, & Cavanagh, 1994). Simoneau et al. also reported that the deficit was greater when the condition was associated with loss of visual or vestibular cues. The loss of sensitivity reduces both underfoot detectability of slippery surfaces, as well as distal perception through the cane hand. Perception will also be lessened with frozen extremities, resulting from circulatory problems that occur frequently within this population.

Risks of Falls in Older Persons and Public Health Concern

Public health concern has significantly increased in the recent decades with regard to the high prevalence of falls and related injuries, especially hip fractures, among the aged population. Because this age group is projected to grow to almost 2 billion worldwide by 2050, the World

Health Organization (WHO) pinpoints an urgent need for preventive measures and continued research in all areas of fall prevention and treatment (WHO, 2007). A considerable amount of research and practice guides on the causes and treatments of falls in and around the home is currently available; however, slips and falls in winter conditions of community-dwelling older persons have received very modest attention. A two-year prospective study done in Minnesota with 263 women between 70 and 99 years old, reported slightly more falls during winter months; snow and ice accounted for only 6 percent of all falls. Most falls occurred indoors, while the yard was the most common location of outdoor falls (Nachreiner, Findorff, Wyman, & McCarthy, 2007).

Falls occur as a result of a complex interaction of biological factors with behavioral and environmental risks (WHO, 2007). While environmental and certain behavioral risk factors have not been assessed in depth, advanced age and related balance and gait impairment have continuously been demonstrated by the scientific community as risk factors for falls (American Geriatrics Society [AGS], British Geriatrics Society [BGS], and American Academy of Orthopaedic Surgeons Panel on Falls Prevention, 2001; Francophone Network for Injury Prevention and Safety Promotion [FNIPSP], 2004, [English version] 2008). In this respect, age-related physiological changes contribute to the increased injury rate on ice and snow for older adults (Gao & Abeysekera, 2004a). That is, declines in visual, vestibular, proprioceptive, and musculoskeletal functions make coordination and adapted postural strategies less effective, resulting in a lengthened reflex reaction time and a reduced capacity to recover balance in an incipient slip.

Fear of falling is also considered as a significant health problem (Li, Fisher, Harmer, & McAuley, 2005; Tinetti, Richman, & Powell, 1990). It leads not only to inappropriate balance control, due to muscles stiffening, but also to self-imposed restrictions in daily activity. Consequently, physi-

cal function may be reduced because of lower-body muscle weakening and restricted mobility. Fear of falling is among the factors that reduce winter outdoor travel by older adults.

Other behavioral risk factors include such aspects as the use of multiple or psychotropic medications, lack of exercise, and inappropriate footwear (WHO, 2007). Visual distraction or inattentiveness, rushing or hurrying behaviors, and carrying objects are also contributing factors to slips and falls (Gao & Abeysekera, 2008; Nachreiner et al., 2007). Except for medication, behavioral risk factors have been less documented scientifically, but under wintry slippery conditions, one may hypothesize their significant contribution to slips and falls.

In addition to the factors that contribute to falls within the older population, the O&M specialist needs to be fully aware of other issues pertaining to the older person living with a visual impairment. It seems essential to consider the interplay of three factors: (1) significant environmental hazards (prevalent and unpredictable icy surfaces), (2) age-related physiological impairments (including gait, strength, and balance), and (3) visual disabilities due to visual disorders (AMD, cataract, and glaucoma), such as loss of distance visual acuity and diminished contrast sensitivity related to the perception of low-contrast surface terrain (grayish icy surfaces). The compounding effect of these factors seems considerable, leading to the question of whether or not members of this group should go out during winter. Elsewhere in this chapter, solutions are suggested, such as avoidance of foot travel on high-risk days, use of appropriate footwear (see Winter Weather Clothing and Equipment), preventive and cautious behaviors, and appropriate city maintenance services (see Environmental Accessibility). Obviously, there is a strong need for research data related to safe and effective travel of visually impaired older individuals who live in a winter climate during 6 to 7 months per year.

Intervention Programs to Reduce Slips and Risks of Fall

A considerable body of evidence (including systematic research reviews and meta-analyses) has demonstrated the effectiveness of various preventive interventions of falls among older people (WHO, 2007). Multifactorial interventions are highlighted and include such aspects as (1) reduction of medications, especially psychotropic medication; (2) modification of environmental hazards in and around the home (e.g., anti-slip material in driveways, handrails on outdoors stairs); (3) appropriate footwear; and (4) balance and strength training and exercise (American Geriatrics Society [AGS] & British Geriatrics Society [BGS], 2006).

Physical exercises are among the most promising fall prevention strategies; they may improve balance, strength, reaction speed, and self-confidence, while preventing osteoporosis (a risk factor for fractures) (FNIPSP, 2008). Indeed, WHO (2007) emphasizes the need that all older people should participate in an exercise program that improves their strength and balance. Programs should, however, distinguish the needs of individuals at high risk for falls from the low-risk persons. In fact, the latter group can participate in a broad range of cost-effective physical activities, such as outdoor walking and indoor mall walking, while the high-risk group may receive an individually tailored program at home (WHO, 2007). In their guidelines for fall prevention, the AGS and BGS specify that although benefits of exercise programs have been proven, the optimal type, duration, frequency, and intensity of exercises remain unclear. It appears, however, that long-term, sustained exercises are recommended for sustained benefits. A recent study by Shumway-Cook et al. (2007) showed that participants who attended the 12-month exercise program on an average of 2.3 times per week had significantly fewer falls and a better performance on balance and mobility measures.

Among several suggested exercise programs, tai chi ch'uan has been viewed by the AGS and BGS as a promising type of balance exercise; it involves dynamic balance and relates more to walking. It consists of a gradual progression of slow, controlled movements that emphasize rotation of body and trunk, flexion of hips and knees, weight shifting, reciprocal arm movements, and balance (Miszko, Ramsey, & Blasch, 2004). An 8-week pilot study conducted by Miszko et al., with 10 older people who were visually impaired and practicing tai chi, also reported physiological and psychological benefits, including greater self-confidence during mobility.

Principles and methods of controlled fall may be found through different martial arts programs, such as judo and tae kwon do. There are six ways to fall: back or side (the two most common), front, back-rolling, front-rolling, and flip. During training, a progressive approach is used for each type of fall, that is, from sitting or kneeling positions to squatting and standing positions. During a fall, some tips or precautions may include the following: (1) stay relaxed to prevent injury, (2) spread the force of the fall evenly across as much of the body as possible and let the hands slap the ground as the body strikes it, (3) roll whenever possible, and (4) do not let the head hit the ground. Groen, Weerdesteyn, and Duysens (2007) demonstrated that martial art fall techniques decrease the impact forces at the hip of older persons during sideways falling.

Older people who are visually impaired may not be able to benefit from exercise programs because of a lack of transportation to such programs. Even if paratransit transportation is an alternative means for many older winter travelers, there is a lack of services in some regions or the existent services are limited to medical needs. Considering the increasing older population in the future and the negative effect of home confinement, isolation, and lack of exercise on mental and physical health, the issue of winter travel by older people with visual impairments will need to be addressed by governments, municipalities, and nonprofit service programs. Developing home-based programs could be a potential alternative.

Winter offers extremely pleasant activities and sports, such as downhill and cross-country skiing, ice hockey, and ice skating, that can also impact on physical well-being, fitness, endurance, and balance, all of which relate to O&M. These activities add to a person's ability to move in a snowy or icy environment (Willoughby & Monthei, 1998; Gao and Abeysekera, 2004b). Such activities can be experienced through special organized days or weekend groups or simply be integrated through O&M lessons.

Strategies for Walking on Icy Surfaces

In order to prevent fall events during winter months, pedestrians need to be continually aware of their surroundings and potential dangers. Preventive behaviors and safe walking strategies may also be adopted on slippery surfaces to reduce risks of slips and falls (Gao and Abeysekera, 2004a) (see Sidebar 15.1, "Strategies for Walking on Icy Surfaces," for more information).

There are some older people who are visually impaired and frequently travel by foot in their community in winter. During the winter season, a support white cane is often used, instead of a long cane, since it offers balance as well as good visibility. In very familiar environments, it can be safe enough for many older persons with low vision. In icy conditions, an ice spike can be fixed under the rubber tip of the cane, thus improving gripping on slippery surfaces. This special "flip up ice spike" is shaped like a ring, composed of several small spikes, mounted on a 4-inch shaft that can be fixed over the cane shaft. A flip-up mechanism arm allows placing the spike up, along the cane shaft, when unneeded. A support cane does not, however, ensure surface and foot placement preview. When indicated, a comprehensive functional O&M evalua-tion should be completed and include different trials with the long cane and the support cane separately and together.

Physical and Psychosocial Difficulties in Wintry Conditions

Travelers who are blind or visually impaired experience more uncertainty and less self-confidence in winter than in summer (Welsh & Wiener, 1976). Even capable travelers feel more unsafe (Wall, 2001). Frustration may be experienced with variable and unpredictable conditions. Anxiety can increase substantially when contact with a pathway is lost for any significant amount of time and distance (Graham, 1998). Extra attention and concentration are necessary during adverse weather travel, and mental effort is needed for performing more than one task at a time.

Exposure to extreme or severe cold conditions can be hazardous or even life threatening, The body and its extremities lose heat quickly. These weather conditions can cause frostnip (a mild form of frostbite where only the skin freezes), frostbite (a condition where both the skin and the underlying body tissues are frozen), or hypothermia (a drop in body temperature below 95°F or 37°C). Under severe cold conditions, the O&M specialist needs to be aware of recommendations issued by the weather services and heed warnings (see Table 15.2).

Diabetic persons, children, and older adults require closer attention by the O&M specialist in these conditions. Diabetic persons with peripheral neuropathy are at risk, as they may not be aware that their extremities are frozen due to a loss of peripheral sensation to cold. Long exposures to cold may be medically contraindicated. Older adults may have heart or respiratory problems or reduced physical resistance to extreme cold and winds that ought to be carefully evaluated and addressed, if necessary. Environment Canada's meteorological services have suggested

SIDEBAR 15.1

Strategies for Walking on Icy Surfaces

Information pertaining to preventive behaviors and walking strategies on ice has been collected through practice literature. The following is a list of some of the strategies that can be helpful for walking on icy surfaces and preventing falls.

- Plan ahead and get information about risky icy surfaces.

- Allow extra time for traveling.

- Use footwear with good traction (e.g., low heel, nonslip tread sole).

- Be alert, and walk s-l-o-w-l-y and cautiously.

- Spread feet apart side to side, about 30 cm (one foot) apart, to provide a wider base of support.

- Take smaller steps or shuffle feet.

- Walk nearly flat-footed, with knees slightly bent.

- Avoid carrying loads with the hands or use a backpack to free hands for balance, but keep in mind that a heavy backpack can increase balance problems.

- Be alert to ice under snow.

- Use alternative routes or walk on the less slippery side (sidewalk) of the street.

- Walk on the planter or furniture zone adjacent to the sidewalk, if it is less slippery than the sidewalk.

- Walk more cautiously when making a turn or going up and down slopes.

- Avoid shortcuts and walk on the more heavily traveled routes.

- Solicit physical assistance in high-risk situations.

- In cold temperatures, assume that all wet, dark areas on pavements are slippery.

- Use railings on stairs, and use a good grip on bus railings.

- Use special care when entering and exiting vehicles, use the vehicle for support, and always test the surface before making the first step out.

- Be cautious when entering buildings since melted ice or snow may create a slippery surface.

- Use "padding" for the hips or a bulky coat that will cushion the body.

Sources: R. W. Larson, "Mobility Strategies for Icy Conditions," *Journal of Visual Impairment and Blindness* 78, no. 8 (1984): 365–366; and web sites for the Environmental Health and Safety Department of the University of Montana and the Canada Safety Council (http://safety-council.org).

these behaviors to prevent cold injuries: listen to the weather forecast, plan ahead, dress warmly, seek shelter, stay dry, keep active, and know your own limits. Y. Balashova (personal communication, September 12, 2006) suggests pointing out locations of public places along travel routes that are available to stop in and warm up during cold days.

Experience of the Traveler with Low Vision

Smith, De l'Aune, and Geruschat (1992) report mobility problems in adverse weather for travelers with low vision. Glare is a major difficulty for many individuals because of white snow conditions or the combination of sun and snow.

TABLE 15.2

Wind Chill Hazards and Risk of Frostbite

Temperature (Include Wind Chill)	Risk of Frostbite	Health Concern
32 to 15°F (0 to −9°C)	Low	Slight increase in discomfort.
14 to −17°F (−10 to −27°C)	Low	Uncomfortable. Risk of hypothermia if outside for long periods without adequate protection.
−18 to −38°F (−28 to −39°C) Warning level for southern regions	Increasing risk: exposed skin can freeze in 10 to 30 minutes.	Cover exposed skin.
−39 to −52°F (−40 to −47°C) Warning level for northern regions	High risk: exposed skin can freeze in 5 to 10 minutes.	Cover all exposed skin.
−54 to −65°F (−48 to −54°C) Warning level for arctic regions	High risk: exposed skin can freeze in 2 to 5 minutes.	Be ready to cancel outdoor activities.

Source: Meteorological Service of Canada, Environment Canada, Government of Canada, *The Green Lane Brochure: humidity* (n.d.), Available from www.msc-smc.ec.gc.ca/cd/brochures/humidity_e.cfm, accessed October 7, 2006.

Discomfort and dazzling glare can be experienced (Lutd, 1997). A very thorough assessment is needed in various daytime conditions. Winter hats with visors may be very helpful, along with appropriate sunglasses. More than one filter may be necessary to meet all needs. Safety at street crossings can be compromised when the sun is low on the horizon, during early morning or late afternoon. For drivers and pedestrians, direct sunlight in front, at eye level, can be completely blinding. Street crossing alternatives may need to be explored for such situations. The student with low vision can visually track parallel cars or use the perpendicular red traffic light to determine the beginning of crossing on his parallel street. For more confidence, he may also be taught to interpret traffic surging sound cues to start crossing (see Barlow, Bentzen, Franck, & Sauerburger, Chapter 12).

Due to restricted hours of daylight throughout the winter, night blindness is experienced

for longer periods than during the summer. In southern Canadian regions, where darkness occurs as early as 4:00 P.M., especially around the Winter Solstice, night mobility lessons may be necessary with active persons, such as students and workers. Students mention that some night blindness problems are somewhat lessened with snow conditions, as white snow background heightens the low lighting level that may sometimes be seen at night from moonlight or residential streetlamps.

Decreased visual acuity reduces the distance at which relevant details pertaining to surface terrain will be seen and detected, for example, icy spots or other surface terrain changes, such as frozen ruts. Travelers with low vision may also be at risk in icy conditions because of lack of contrast on surface terrain. Ice may be completely covered by a thin coat of snow giving the appearance of a safe pathway. The traveler with a non-anticipatory attitude may not be prepared to react adequately to such situations. Many persons with low vision could benefit from the use of a cane to preview the environment in cases of unpredictable situations, for example, a puddle of water at the street corner. In such situations, an exploration technique of sweeping or poking the cane can be used whenever needed.

Visual perceptual distance detection training, similar to the V-Tech program described by Ludt and Goodrich (2002), could also build in visual strategies while walking, such as the use of perceptual and contextual cues and the up-and-down scanning technique. Considering the variable and unpredictable surface terrain that is typical to winter, systematic scanning and visual attention strategies that are usually taught in an unfamiliar environment could be replicated in winter. The V-Tech had significantly improved the distance detection of obstacles, but there exists no evidence of the effectiveness of this practice during winter conditions.

Typical visual landmarks, such as grass lines and colored objects, may be covered by snow. There can be a loss of contrast at intersections, as crosswalk lines have faded and cars and street asphalt have become grayish following salt coverings. Travelers may also experience loss of visual cues through dirty bus windows and steamed glasses that occur when entering a building. Assistance may be needed when visual landmarks normally used in bus transportation are obscured. Environmental color cues are much less frequent in winter, but there are black and white contrast cues that can be observed and used, such as a white mound of snow against a grayish pedestrian path on a business sidewalk.

Finally, low-vision devices, such as telescopes, may be difficult to use on very cold days. Gloves need to be taken off and fingers can get cold and numb. If viewing a sign or a pedestrian light at street crossing is impaired, other strategies such as soliciting assistance can be used.

Winter Weather Clothing and Equipment

Travelers in adverse weather conditions need to dress appropriately for comfort and protection. Hats and gloves may, however, impede perception of useful sensory information in snow travel. Some travelers will even avoid or delay wearing them.

Due to prevailing icy conditions during winter, footwear has a critical function in preventing slipping accidents. Footwear with good traction can provide multifold grip with the walking surface (Aschan et al., 2009). Out of nine different types of winter footwear purchased at the local shoe store, these researchers found that, on average, slip-resistant footwear had two times better grip than the slippery ones.

Overall research relating to anti-slip properties of winter footwear has evaluated different types of sole material, such as microcellular polyurethane, thermoplastic rubber, and crepe rubber (Gao & Abeysekera, 2004a). Soft sole materials have been found to offer the highest friction on hard ice and *crepe rubber* was the most recommended. In regard to wet ice, hard heels with sharp cleats were suggested, in combination with a softer base; cleats were able to scratch the soft ice. A study conducted in Japan recommended a rubber sole with an anti-slip glass fiber compound on the surface of the heel and the front of the sole (Gao & Abeysekera, 2004a). This type of footwear is commonly used and valued in Hokkaido, the northern-most island of Japan, where temperature averages 32°F (0°C) during the winter season (R. Tokunaga, personal communication, June 20, 2007). Nonetheless, designing the most appropriate footwear is challenging. Further investigation is needed, and many factors need to be considered, such as sole material, sole tread pattern, sole hardness, amount of wear and tear, and roughness (Gao & Abeysekera, 2004a).

On their part, Aschan et al. (2009) argue that no safety footwear soling provides an adequate grip on slippery icy conditions. And the situation is worse on wet ice. These authors specify that on "peak days" (i.e., hard and smooth ice covered by either a water layer or dry snow), footwear plays a minor role in gained friction. Anti-slip devices (worn over ordinary boots) can be used to provide extra traction. A study done in Wisconsin with 109 older community–dwelling persons confirmed that the Yaktrax Walker could prevent the risk of outdoor winter falls in fall-prone individuals, while increasing outdoor walking and the feeling of safety during walking (McKiernan, 2005).

Other research relating to anti-skid devices include three Swedish studies that evaluated devices currently found on the market (Gard & Lundborg, 2000, 2001; Gard & Berggard, 2006). *Whole-foot studs* were the preferred device in the first study, while a *fixed-heel device* obtained the highest score in the two other studies. However, some problems were reported in the last study, such as a change in gait pattern, instability, discomfort, and clumsiness. More research is needed and it should take into consideration stability, fitness, and ease of use of such devices, as many travelers often need to walk both indoors and outdoors during the same trip.

In terms of adverse weather clothing and equipment, the most common recommendations are as follows:

- *Head and ears.* Choose a hat that keeps head and ears warm but still permits sound transmission, such as a light knit woolen hat or a hat that only partly covers ears. Some people wear a hood that can be easily removed at street corners.

- *Coat and underwear.* Outdoor sporting stores offer highly specialized material (synthetic or down-filled) which combine both warmth and comfort criteria: insulation against cold and humidity, lightweight, windproof, and water-repellent. Underwear made of specialized fabrics, such as *merino wool*, *capilene*, or polar fabrics, are suggested for colder temperature and longer exposure to cold. Two layers of socks can be worn, the innermost made of synthetic material (e.g., polypropylene) and the outermost layer of polar or wool fabric. Wool and synthetic blended products are also available.

- *Gloves and mitts.* Some options offered are (1) a special mobility mitten through which the cane tip is inserted to cover the cane hand (Welsh & Wiener, 1976), and (2) a knitted convertible glove/mitten that consists of a fingerless glove tucked inside its own mitten, with the mitten opening to expose fingers and folding back to secure to the cuff with Velcro. Fingerless gloves are considered to be excellent for handling tools, while mittens may be put on to keep hands warm. This product is commonly found on the market. Overall, gloves may be preferred because of aesthetics, while providing ease in handling the cane. Outdoor sporting goods stores offer different models.

- *Boots and antiskid devices.* Footwear needs to be warm and waterproof, allow tactile foot perception, have a stable base of support, and offer slip resistance on slippery surfaces. Other factors to consider include weight, height, flexibility, ease of walking, and comfort (Gao and Abeysekera, 2004). High heels need to be avoided. There are also many types and models of anti-skid devices on the market. Common models are (1) whole-foot shoe cover (rubber sole device placed under the boot and covering the whole foot or critical parts such as heels and balls) with small steel spikes (such as Spiky), preferred for its aesthetics; and (2) whole-foot shoe cover with steel studs allowing high grip (such as Icer's or STABILicers), preferred for its additional traction in extreme icy conditions. There are other

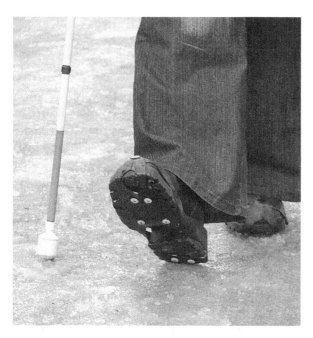

Anti-skid devices are useful on icy surfaces.

whole-foot, forefoot, or heel models (such as the whole-foot Yaktrax Walker or the Olang boots) composed of retractable ice picks placed on the heel and the foot blade.

- *Instructor equipment.* The O&M specialist needs to have extra equipment or clothing (hats, gloves, spikes, and scarf) for students who are not adequately prepared for adverse weather conditions. This may be especially helpful in school settings where children may come to school unprepared for the conditions or with adults who cannot afford the extra cost of good winter equipment.

Winter Issues Pertaining to Specific Students

Dog Guide Travel

The use of a dog guide may present some advantages during winter travel (see Whitstock, Franck, Haneline, & Brooks, Volume 1, Chapter 9; and Chapter 16, this volume). Some dog guide users may feel more confident in winter travel, as the dog guide can facilitate a straight line of travel, negotiate obstacles (snowbanks) on the path, as well as localize familiar destinations. The dog may also offer some counterbalance on icy surfaces. However, dog guides may encounter certain difficulties, such as locating curbs when the overall environment is covered by snow. While completing a street crossing, the dog may veer and stay in the parallel street in order to avoid obstacles (snowbanks). In case of disorientation and absence of auditory cues during a snowfall, the traveler with a dog guide will not be able to access tactual information for either exploring snow obstacles or finding landmarks. Among other problems, shorelining a snowbank while walking in the street may be more risky for the dog guide user, as the team may be walking too far away from the shoreline (Welsh & Wiener, 1976). Undoubtedly, specific winter follow-up may be appropriate so that both user and dog guide can master unusual and unpredictable situations.

The dog itself may have a limited resistance to cold, salt, and sand under the paws. It may be wise to rinse or wash the dog's paws when coming in from walks in the snow, particularly if the sidewalks were sanded and salted. Ice balls may also form on the dog's feet and some kind of dog boot may be needed. This condition can be minimized by trimming the hair between the dog's toes.

Environmental Concepts for Children

Environmental concepts relating to varying winter conditions need to be included in O&M curricula for children. Children need to be knowledgeable about subarctic and arctic climates and understand the formation of snow, rain, freezing rain, ice, and wind, including the effects of windchill (i.e., the combined effect of temperature and wind). They can learn how snowflakes vary, depending on the ambient temperature and humidity. Bernard Voyer, a famous world explorer who has walked to the North Pole, has stated that Inuits use 100 different expressions to describe winter and its snow crystals (Voyer, 2005).

Winter knowledge implies various motor and sensory experiences. By touching and exploring, children can become familiar with snowbanks, icicles, and different types of snow coverings (e.g., powder or wet snow). Learning should include listening to specific winter sounds, such as footsteps on cold crispy days and car tires on snowy or wet surfaces. Children need to have opportunities to play in the snow and experience different motor activities, like ice skating, tobogganing, and skiing. Building a snowman may help to reinforce body concepts.

For safety purposes, children need to be familiarized with winter maintenance machinery, such as snow removal machines on streets and sidewalks, snowblowers, and salt and sand spreaders. Familiarity with such machines helps to reduce fear that children may experience when they hear such machines during winter travel. Children need to be taught appropriate safety behaviors for when they encounter such machinery.

Travelers Who Are Deaf-Blind

The alteration or obliteration of important traffic auditory information will hamper travelers who are deaf-blind and increase their risks (see Lolli, Sauerburger, & Bourquin, Chapter 17). Hearing-aid users experience special problems, such as the amplification of wind through the aids. Sign language by hand-to-hand communication is limited during cold days when gloves are needed. O&M specialists need to anticipate these situations and provide as much information as possible indoors, prior to and after the lesson.

Environmental Accessibility

City Design, Maintenance Services, and Transportation

Norman Pressman, a Canadian professor, urban designer, and international consultant on the design of winter cities, urges such cities to acknowledge winter specifically, by planning for sustainable design and thinking in a "winter mode" when designing cities, public spaces, and transportation. To alleviate some of winter's negative aspects, he highlights such adaptations as (1) heated bus shelters; (2) transit scheduling based on more seasonal demand; (3) covered walkways or arcades in high-density pedestrian areas; (4) heated sidewalks in the busiest areas; (5) "winter-friendly" exterior public place designs, where sunlight is enhanced by short buildings that prevent shade, and wind effect is reduced by natural vegetation; (6) snow removal efficiency; (7) enhanced visual environment with colored houses; and (8) accommodation for the needs of the most vulnerable groups (Pressman, 2004).

Adequate city maintenance services have been reported as one of the major environmental adaptations that ought to be addressed for more efficient winter travel by persons who are blind or visually impaired (Couturier et al., 2006; Lundälv, 2001). This major issue has been reported by 48 percent of 33 respondents in Lundälv's study and by 85 percent of all respondents in Couturier's et al. study. Adequate services would need to include quick snow clearance and removal and spreading of anti-slip material (sand or gravel) on pedestrian icy areas. Indeed, Aschan et al. (2009) found that both slip-resistant and slippery footwear provided a good grip when friction values were measured on well-granulated surfaces.

City managers could establish a strategic maintenance program based on priorities, such as public spaces most frequented by older pedestrians (e.g., areas around hospitals, subway stations)

(Takahashi, Tokunaga, & Asano, 2007). Takahashi et al. proposed a management strategy in
Hokkaido (Japan) that involves a cycle of planning, implementing suitable operations, evaluating outcomes (e.g., frequency of pedestrian falls),
and reconsidering or further improving plans.
Travelers interviewed by Couturier et al. mentioned the need to address specific snow removal
requests to city managers that relate to individual
needs, such as snow removal on certain residential sidewalks. They also strongly recommended
public awareness campaigns that urge home owners not to throw their shoveled snow on sidewalks.
Snow clearance care may also be given to areas
surrounding traffic light poles requiring activation of a pushbutton. Finally, pedestrian notice
systems may need to be developed in order to give

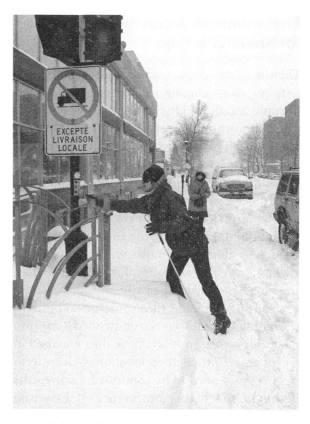

**Mound of snow blocking access to a pedestrian push-
button at a street crossing.**

warnings on very slippery days (i.e., peak in emergency units' admissions). The model developed in
Finland has been based on the Road Weather
Model and uses local radio, TV stations, or Internet to provide information about locations, time,
and reason for slipperiness (Aschan et al., 2009).

Efficient paratransit transportation during
extreme winter conditions is another environmental adaptation discussed by Couturier et al.
(2006). Under snowfall or freezing rain conditions, survey respondents would favor emergency
measures, such as an available volunteer network or a public door-to-door system that can be
requested the same day, which is not the way
paratransit systems usually work. Experience had
shown that such services were sometimes cancelled in severe winter conditions.

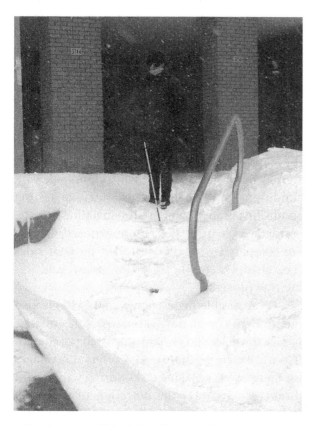

**Following snowfall, delayed snow clearance can im-
pede safety.**

Environmental Adaptations for Street Crossings

The use of detectable warning tiles at street corners in colder climate regions raises some important questions. One of the main concerns is the durability of products that can withstand the strong mechanical forces of snowplows. Earlier research in New Hampshire and Vermont evaluated different commonly used products and reported scraped-off, chipped, or broken domes, following one or two winters (Boisvert, 2003; Kaplan, 2004). An inset-tile installation procedure (i.e., domes are flush with the sidewalk surface) was found to be more effective than the glued-tile or stamped-tile procedures. And, with strong evidence, tiles constructed of high-strength materials were recommended. Cast iron or stainless steel products have thus emerged in recent years. Although observations of long-term performance need to be continued, two reports highlight the high performance of cast iron panels (Boisvert & Fowler, 2007; Kaplan, 2006).

On another hand, the effect of snow maintenance machinery on the durability of tiles has been tested in Alaska; machinery was adapted with a brush system in order to protect the domes, but data were not conclusive (McMillen, 2001). Present and other considerations may, finally, include the following aspects: the most appropriate type of snow maintenance machinery, the effect of deicing chemicals, such as salt or calcium chloride, on the warning tile material, and, lastly, maintenance problems related to the accumulation of debris on the tiles following winter months.

Other functional or clinical questions may be raised with regard to the value of warning tiles in winter. Do certain weather or surface conditions (e.g., light cover of snow, abrasive materials) have an effect on detectability of tiles? Is dynamic stability affected by wet conditions on such material as stainless steel? Do darker (black) tiles accelerate the snow and ice melting process, thus increasing detectability during winter? Landry, Ratelle, and Overbury (in press) conducted a semi-laboratory pilot study at the University of Montreal and evaluated foot detectability of eight different warning surfaces (two materials—stainless steel [Advantage] and polymere composite [Armor-Tile]—in four different colors). The experimental conditions included sunny February days, with a light cover of snow in the morning, and temperature varying between 32 and 14°F (0 and –10°C). Whenever needed, a gravel-salt mixture was spread on icy surfaces.

Conclusions from this study were (1) detectability rates varied from 64.24 percent at 24 inches (61 cm) (stopping on the tile) to 81.7 percent at 30 inches (76 cm) (stopping with the leading foot overstepping on the curb zone), suggesting that, under fair weather and adequate surface maintenance, detection of street corners equipped with warning tiles can be achieved during winter; (2) according to participants' subjective comments, gravel seemed to reduce the textural contrast between the tile and the adjacent surface; (3) both tile materials did not seem to affect dynamic stability during wet conditions; and (4) color did not seem to impact on the melting process and detectability. Research should be pursued in real wintry and sidewalk conditions and ought to also include testing conditions under which tiles installed on the east side of a street (i.e., more exposed to sun) are compared with tiles installed on west sides (i.e., shadows significantly slow snow- and ice-melting process).

An accessible pedestrian signal (APS) is also mentioned as a major factor that can enhance winter travel for the visually impaired population (Couturier et al., 2006). APS offers advantages for many street-crossing tasks during winter conditions, such as (1) the detection of the street corner through the pole locator, (2) help with alignment prior to and during crossing, when the system provides beaconing, and (3) improved departure time decisions (Williams, Van Houten,

Ferraro, & Blasch, 2005; see Barlow, Bentzen, Franck, & Sauerburger, Chapter 12). Respondents in Couturier's et al. study appreciated systems with a beacon, such as the "alternating signal system." This system provided auditory cues in absence of traffic sounds and reduced confusion as to the direction of crossing (forward or to the side). The fact that the beacon is centered within the crosswalk helped in maintaining a straight line of travel throughout the whole crossing and offered cues for localization of the opposite corner, which was especially helpful when snow mounds were present.

Advanced Technology

There is a scarcity of literature on the uses of electronic travel aids (ETAs) in adverse weather conditions. Some of the ETAs mentioned in the existing literature are no longer produced or have been replaced by other devices (see Smith and Penrod, Volume 1, Chapter 8). ETAs may have the potential to assist travel in winter conditions, by shorelining snow banks and searching for landmarks that are covered by snow. However, problems may also be associated with their use in adverse weather conditions (see Smith and Penrod, Volume 1, Chapter 8).

Adapted global positioning systems (GPS), such as the Sendero GPS, the Trekker, or the Trekker-Breeze, were mentioned as a good environmental facilitator for winter conditions by 10 functionally blind respondents in Couturier et al. (2006). Zabihaylo and Wanet (2006) conducted a focus group survey with eight adult travelers, in order to explore the benefits of the Trekker in winter. In general, the users of Trekker expressed greater confidence, better orientation, and more frequent travel, even in nonfamiliar environments. They found that the device is especially useful in various environmental conditions where landmarks are covered by snow, snow mounds, and ice. By using the points-of-interest function offered by the system, the traveler can locate landmarks and destinations, such as building entrances and residences. Other uses include recovery from disorientation caused by snow mounds at street corners and finding paths in cross-country skiing settings. The device works well in very cold weather. Its use may be limited by tall buildings and trees, and the auditory output may not be loud enough under some windy conditions (see Penrod, Smith, Haneline, & Corbett, Chapter 14).

OTHER PROBLEMS RELATED TO ADVERSE WEATHER CONDITIONS

Rain, Strong Winds, and Fog

Under windy conditions, it becomes difficult to hear traffic until it is very close (Welsh & Wiener, 1976). Winds will tend to distort and mask traffic sounds, thus hindering alignment and detection of traffic surge at street crossings. The cane may be harder to control and sideways wind may contribute to veering. On the other hand, rain increases intensity of traffic sounds, even up to 10 decibels (see Lawson & Wiener, Volume 1, Chapter 4). Specific auditory training may be necessary in order to interpret such traffic sounds effectively. Adequate rain gear would include a raincoat with a hood instead of an umbrella, which can harm other pedestrians and alter the quality of sounds. Some regions are more likely to be affected by fog. This condition mainly impacts on visibility for travelers with low vision and for drivers who may have difficulty seeing travelers who are visually impaired. Also, heavy fog may alter or slightly muffle sounds (Morais et al., 1997).

Extreme Heat and Hot Weather

Environmental Conditions

The O&M specialist cannot overlook the risks associated with extreme heat or hot weather.

Hot summer weather or heat waves are witnessed in southern-latitude regions just above and below the 40th parallel. Southwest regions of the United States, for example, may experience temperatures of 95–100°F (35–40°C) for 75 to 100 consecutive days (E. Siffermann, personal communication, October 10, 2006). Extreme heat is defined as "summertime temperatures that are substantially hotter and/or more humid than average for location at that time of year" (Centers for Disease Control and Prevention [CDC], 2009).

Under hot weather conditions, a person may suffer heat-related illnesses, as his or her body is unable to compensate and properly cool itself. Indeed, sweating is not enough under some conditions (e.g., humid weather) that cause a person's body temperature to rise rapidly. Even short periods of high temperatures can cause serious health problems (CDC, 2009). Hot weather conditions or overexposure to heat may cause *sunburn*, *heat rash* (a red or pink rash that can develop when the sweat ducts become blocked and swell), and *heat stress* (disturbance of the body's cooling system). Extreme or very severe conditions can provoke *heat cramps* (muscle contractions, usually in the hamstring muscles, that are forceful and painful), *heat exhaustion* (when people are physically active in a hot, humid environment and their body fluids are lost through sweating, causing the body to overheat), or life-threatening events like a *heat stroke* (when the body's cooling system stops working, and the internal temperature rises to the point where damage to the brain or internal organs may result). During extremely hot weather, some factors, such as high humidity, more intense exercise, and altitudes higher than 820 ft (2,500 m), further affect the effectiveness of the body's thermoregulation capacity (Mayo Clinic, 2006). Under extreme heat conditions, an O&M specialist needs to be aware of recommendations issued by the weather services and heed warnings (see Table 15.3). In some regions, the Humidex scale (computed value or scale used in a hot and humid environment that combines the temperature and humidity into one number to reflect the perceived temperature by the average person) can be a better measure of how stifling the air feels (comfort) than either temperature or humidity alone. An extremely high Humidex reading can be defined as one that is over 104°F (40°C), where great discomfort is felt. Unnecessary activity needs to be curtailed and exertion avoided (Meteorological Service of Canada, 1998).

Adaptive Strategies and Behaviors

According to the CDC, heat-related illness is preventable. Procedures and precautions are recommended when conducting outdoor O&M training under hot and extreme heat conditions (CDC, 2009; E. Sifferman, personal communication, October 10, 2006).

Physical health screening. Prior to an instruction session, determine if the student is prepared to safely participate in an O&M lesson. Conditions related to the increased risk of heat-related illnesses include age, obesity, pregnancy or breastfeeding, illnesses or health conditions (e.g., mental illness, heart disease, and high blood pressure), and alcohol or specific drug use (e.g., psychotropics, tranquilizers, and anti-Parkinson agents) (CDC, 2006, 2009). Age-related factors refer to infants, younger children, and elderly people who are at higher risks to heat illness. Essential measures for preventing heat stress or other heat-related illness with the aged population include avoiding sun exposure and reducing physical activity, such as gardening and taking long walks.

Clothing and sun protection. The sun's rays are stronger at higher altitudes and lower latitudes closer to the tropics. They are the strongest during the hours of 10:00 A.M. to 4:00 P.M. In order to protect oneself from the ultraviolet rays of

TABLE 15.3

Effects of Heat on the Body

Outside Temperature	Condition	Effect on Body
68°F (20°C)	Normal	Comfortable, normal heart rate.
77°F (25°C)	Normal	Normal heart rate and light sweating.
86°F (30°C)	Discomfort	Sweating helps blood cool, concentration is affected, and moderate sweating occurs.
95°F (35°C)	Heat cramps	Sweating is heavier, concentration is more difficult, heart rate increases, and muscle pains occur due to imbalance in body salts.
104°F (40°C)	Heat exhaustion	Heavy sweating, tiredness, rapid heart rate, and nausea.
113°F (45°C)	Heat stroke	Sweating stops; fainting may occur; danger of organ damage and death; hot, dry skin; and core temperature rises.

Source: BBC News (2009), *Hot Weather Risks*, available from http://news.bbc.co.uk/2/hi/health/medical_notes/5190094.stm, accessed March 22, 2010.

the sun, wear a wide-brimmed hat; wear lightweight, light-colored, and loose-fitting clothing; and cover the legs and arms. Wear sunglasses, and apply a sunscreen of SPF 15 or higher 30 minutes prior to going outside. Heavy-soled shoes with socks may be worn in order to protect the feet from sunburn and when stepping onto hot surfaces. For persons with low vision, an assessment of the most effective sunglasses or absorptive lenses needs to be done to maximize use of residual vision while protecting the eyes from the sun.

Preventing dehydration.   Water accounts for 60 to 70 percent of the body weight. Food provides about 20 percent of total water intake, while the remaining 80 percent comes from drinking water and beverages of all kinds. Men need more water intake than women. The following hydration calculator can be used to estimate the required daily liquid intake (i.e., drinking water and beverages) and takes into account that the person is having a normal diet and no medical

complications (e.g., fluid restriction or kidney disease). As a general rule, the daily liquid intake is 0.5 ounce (15 ml) of liquid for every 1 lb (0.45 kg) of body weight. This total daily liquid amount may be divided by 8 (i.e., an 8-ounce glass) to get the number of glasses of liquid to drink every day. For example, for a person weighing 120 lbs (54.5 kg), an amount of 60 ounces (1800 ml) of fluid is needed. Dividing this by 8 (i.e., 8 ounces per glass) or by 240 (i.e., 240 ml per glass) indicates that 7.5 glasses of liquid is needed per day (Griffin, 2007). Factors that influence increase of water needs are more intense exercise, hot and humid environments, overweight, pregnancy, health conditions (e.g., fever and diarrhea), and altitudes.

One of the biggest dangers of hot weather and extreme heat is the increased risk of dehydration. Preventive guidelines would include the following:

1. Increase fluid intake, regardless of the activity level (CDC, 2006).

2. Drink regularly, before getting thirsty. Drink slowly, by sipping instead of gulping.

3. Avoid liquids that contain alcohol or large amounts of sugar since they can cause more body fluid loss. If water is not available, non-carbonated soft drinks, such as fruit juice, may be a reasonable alternative. Very cold drinks can cause stomach cramps.

4. The O&M specialist needs to supply adequate amounts of water for himself and the student. Consider carrying a cooler with bottles of water in the car.

5. Insulated water bottle holders with shatter-resistant bottles are available at outdoor sporting goods and bike stores. Some have specific convenient traveling features, such as accommodating most 32-ounce (1000-ml) bottles, a zippered pocket for keys, cell phone, or other small items, a waist belt flap with hook and loop closure, or a shoulder strap for hand-free transport.

6. The O&M specialist needs to be aware of dehydration signs and symptoms, in order to provide appropriate intervention. These include mild to excessive thirst, fatigue, headache, dry mouth, little or no urination, muscle weakness, dizziness, and lightheadedness. Older people may also be less able to sense dehydration (CDC, 2006, 2009; Mayo Clinic, 2006).

Lesson scheduling and car transportation. Allow a flexible working schedule and conduct O&M lessons in the early morning and during evening hours. If the O&M specialist and the student are not accustomed to walking in a hot environment, start slowly by gradually increasing the pace and rest often in shady areas. All activities need to be stopped at the appearance of dehydration signs, as well as with heat exertion symptoms, such as heart pounding and gasping for breath. Indoor air-conditioned environments, like malls and school buildings, may be best suited for training

during conditions of extreme heat. Specific recommendations also pertain to the use of a car during lessons. Studies have shown that in an ambient outdoor temperature of 98.2°F (36.8°C), internal temperature of enclosed vehicles reached 124–153°F (51°C to 67°C) within 15 minutes (McLaren, Null, & Quinn, 2005). Even at a milder or cooler temperature (i.e., 72°F or 22.2°C), these authors reported rapid and significant heating (i.e., 117°F or 47.2°C) of the interior of vehicles. Cracking open windows is not an effective measure in decreasing either the rate of temperature elevation or the maximum temperature attained. During an O&M lesson, recommendations would then include this special warning: under no circumstances should the instructor leave a student alone in the car. Moreover, there may be damage (burns) caused by touching the hot metal on the car or holding a hot seat belt. Car maintenance is important and should include a reliable car emergency kit and checking the air-conditioning system.

CONCLUSION

Due to its prevalence in many regions of the world and during a major part of the year, winter needs to be specifically acknowledged. It may constitute one of the biggest environmental barriers for travelers with visual impairments.

There is a lack of evidence-based practice with regard to specific winter mobility problems and solutions encountered by all age groups having a visual impairment, including the growing aged population. Icy conditions that prevail in many winter regions have been regarded as a public health problem in many countries. The mobility problems related to wintry slippery sidewalks are very complex, include various factors, and need the involvement of other specialized fields, such as kinesiology and industrial engineering. There exist many unresolved issues and the need for future research is clearly identified.

Through training and practice, winter travelers can overcome some of the winter barriers. On another hand, city designers and managers can also alleviate specific winter travel problems for blind and visually impaired pedestrians. A multifaceted approach toward prevention should be envisioned and more collaborative work may need to be accomplished between visually impaired pedestrians, O&M specialists, engineers, researchers, and city and transit system managers, in order to better respond to the needs of more vulnerable travelers.

IMPLICATIONS FOR O&M PRACTICE

1. Winter travel is characterized by its variability and unpredictability. Variable conditions include cold, snow, wind, ice, and mixtures of two or more of these conditions. Conditions are hardly predictable since they may vary from day to day, within the same day, and from block to block.

2. Many O&M skills will be affected by winter conditions. Because of snow obstacles and lack of sensory information, problems commonly include loss of line of direction, disorientation, loss of landmarks, and ineffective street-crossing tasks. Cane techniques will vary according to different snow and ice conditions.

3. General strategies for snow travel require more problem-solving and decision-making processes that are gained through experience. Basic line of direction and more acute sensory perception, including kinesthetic distance awareness, need to be reemphasized. Street crossing tasks may be extremely challenging for the winter traveler, including finding the cleared pathway on the opposite side of a street following a crossing.

4. Ice introduces major mobility and safety issues, since it is a significant risk factor for falls and injuries. In order to prevent slipping and falling on ice, postural and gait adaptations need to be used. Slips and falls on icy and snowy surfaces need to be analyzed through a multifaceted system that includes the following factors: environmental (climate) factors, footwear properties, underfoot surface characteristics and mechanisms of friction between footwear sole and ice, human gait biomechanics, and intrinsic human factors.

5. The visual environment of the traveler with low vision changes under wintry conditions. Major mobility problems include increased glare, loss of the usual landmarks and cues, loss of contrast leading to undetected risky surface terrain like icy spots. Appropriate interventions include glare remediation, caution at street crossings, selective use of a long cane for surface preview, and visual strategies.

6. Many important issues pertaining to older people with visual impairments need to be addressed with regard to winter mobility. Due to physiological changes or decline and fear of falling, falls and injuries are increased on icy conditions.

7. Physical and psychosocial difficulties may be associated with winter travel and extreme heat conditions. People may experience uncertainty, increased mental effort due to more attention and concentration, anxiety, reduced physical endurance or fatigue, and isolation. The risks associated with certain health conditions can be increased under extreme weather conditions or can make travel in these conditions ill advised.

8. Special clothing, equipment, and precautions need to be used through severe cold and hot weather in order to ensure comfort and protection. Avoiding dehydration and heat exertion, as well as working or resting under cooler conditions, are advisable under

extreme heat and hot weather. Insulation against cold and humidity is one of the factors recommended for winter coats and boots.

9. Proper city maintenance services are a major environmental facilitator that could alleviate many winter mobility problems. Solutions are identified, such as proper snow removal and spreading abrasive material on icy surfaces. Other environmental adaptations could include efficient door-to-door public transportation services and more APS installations. The use of detectable warning tiles at street corners raises important questions of durability of products and detectability of tiles in specific winter conditions.

10. Service delivery systems need to consider specific adaptations to winter or hot weather mobility training. The O&M specialist needs to have appropriate preparation for winter travel.

LEARNING ACTIVITIES

1. Visit and interview a practitioner specialized in balance intervention programs or other related physical activities (tai chi or other martial art). Sort out preventive strategies and falling techniques that might be helpful for winter travel.

2. With a colleague, plan outdoor winter traveling activities with a blindfold and a decreased vision simulator, under varying winter conditions. Sort out problems and strategies related to each condition.

3. (a) Plan an inservice training on winter travel for city maintenance services employees, or (b) prepare a public awareness campaign that could emphasize preventive behaviors in more extreme winter conditions and appropriate civic behaviors to be adopted by citizens.

4. Within your working community, prepare a list of intersections that could benefit from an APS installation in order to improve safety at traffic light street crossings during winter.

5. Through various sources, including the Internet, develop a list of suggested clothing for hot or cold weather. The winter activity needs to include a visit to an outdoor sporting store to discuss the effectiveness of winter footwear and clothing for cold, wind, and ice.

CHAPTER **16**

Dog Guides and the Orientation and Mobility Specialist

Lukas Franck, Rodney Haneline, and Alan Brooks

LEARNING QUESTIONS

- Why is it necessary for applicants to a dog guide program to have completed a course in orientation and mobility?

- What criteria do dog guide schools set for accepting students?

- Why might a dog guide not be a good choice for older adults?

- What factors might argue for and against providing a dog to a high school student?

- What are the differences between dog guide and cane travel, and how might you go about preparing a cane travel student to get a dog guide?

- Is it necessary to use all three steps of the orientation, coaching, and solo (OCS) process when orienting a dog guide traveler to a new environment? Who makes the decisions about what to do?

- Where is the best place to stand when orienting a dog guide traveler?

This chapter addresses the skills that orientation and mobility (O&M) specialists use regarding dog guides. Some students may choose to use a dog guide, that is, to become dog guide "handlers." Handler is the term of choice for anyone working with a dog in any capacity, such as a police officer or a customs official. It is also used to refer to travelers who are blind working with their dog guides. Together, the dog guide and handler are referred to as a "unit." This chapter covers the learning process of a handler. The blind handler relies on much the same skill set as that of a cane traveler to remain safe and oriented. She uses the sound of traffic next to her to remain oriented. She listens for environmental information. She makes traffic judgments as those do when traveling with a cane. The skills taught in orientation and mobility continue to have value to the dog guide handler. An appendix at the end of the chapter gives dog guide resources.

However, there are some differences between how dog guide travelers gather information and how cane travelers do. The cane traveler will use tactile information more significantly than the dog guide handler and, as discussed in Volume 1, Chapter 9, the handler will assess his or her dog's actions and reactions—the behavior—and interpret it for orientation and other environmental information.

The O&M specialist typically comes into contact with potential dog guide handlers at two points in the rehabilitation process. As she educates her students, either children or adults, she assesses and advises students who are blind about mobility choices, and may answer their questions and provide them with information about dog guides during mobility training. Results of survey data (Seeing Eye Inc., 1992) indicate that the O&M specialist is a key source of motivation behind the person's choice to attend a dog guide school. She may even be asked to help prepare a student for dog guide training after the student has completed a course in cane travel. Second, many O&M specialists, at some point in their careers, are asked to provide orientation assistance to a dog guide handler, as discussed later in this chapter (Seeing Eye Inc., 1992). In so doing they may also see problems with a particular unit's work that they feel should be addressed.

The O&M specialist is the professional most likely to first discuss the possibility of dog guide mobility with visually impaired students. To advise a person who is blind in this area, the O&M specialist needs to recognize that the form of mobility which a person chooses is highly personal, and dog guides are not appropriate for all blind people. It has been estimated (Finestone, Lukoff, & Whiteman, 1960) that between 1 and 2 percent of the blind population in the United States use dog guides, and a similar figure occurs in Great Britain. A more up-to-date study is needed but has not been done.

ACCEPTANCE STANDARDS AMONG SCHOOLS

Each school sets its own criteria for acceptance of students. This is particularly evident in their consideration of applicants who have hearing losses and residual vision. As of this writing, several schools, among them Leader Dogs and Guid-ing Eyes in the United States, have specialized training programs for students who are deaf-blind. In Great Britain a small number of dogs have been specially trained for deaf-blind people. These dogs perform as dog guides on the street and hearing dogs when out of harness indoors.

Schools apply standards that have been developed internally and are implemented by their field evaluators and admissions staff. Schools that are members of the International Guide Dog Federation (see Volume 1, Chapter 9) also are required to have an appeals process.

Although an O&M instructor's report is very useful and an ophthalmologist's report may contribute valuable information, many schools also perform a functional on-site evaluation by school staff before acceptance. Information gathered on such a home visit is also invaluable to the dog guide school in the eventual making of the dog–human match. The success of the match may depend on information gathered during such an assessment.

There are several factors that must be taken into account by the individual who is visually impaired, by the O&M specialist who advises him or writes a report concerning the applicant, and the school considering them for training with a dog guide. These include personal preference, life circumstances and activity level, age, health and physical condition, hearing, amount of remaining vision (if any), and orientation skills.

A report by an O&M specialist to a dog guide school that addressed these factors would be highly valued by any school receiving it (see the section on Assessing the Potential Guide Dog Handler later in this chapter). Furthermore the specialist may be able to educate the prospective applicant who is unrealistic in his expectations of what a dog guide is, how one gets a dog, and what it will do. However, while there are those who are clearly inappropriate candidates—because of infirmity, for example—it is often best to leave admissions decisions to the several schools.

Personal Preference

Although it is not absolutely essential that the prospective dog guide handler love dogs, a strong dislike or fear of dogs will disqualify some. Dogs need to be fed, relieved, and groomed daily, and taken occasionally to visit the veterinarian. These things take time each day. For people who enjoy the companionship of dogs this will be a pleasure. Others may consider it a chore, but soon learn it is not difficult. The O&M specialist needs to take care not to discourage those who are unsure on this point, but remind them that this is one aspect of having a dog that needs to be considered.

Difficulties can also arise when a student has an interest in getting a dog guide, but the O&M specialist feels that a dog guide would be an inappropriate choice. Here the O&M specialist needs to use tact about expressing her opinion for this student and ultimately recognize that the decision to accept or not accept an indi-

vidual is ultimately made by the school to which the applicant applies. The input of the O&M specialist needs to be solicited and considered.

Life Circumstances and Activity Level

Dog guides need a certain amount of regular use and attention to be efficient mobility aids. Their work should average out to at least one outdoor mile per day, with more preferred. On some days, the dog might be used for several miles, while on another only sporadically; but likely candidates therefore either are, or desire to be, quite active. Employment, or the desire to be employed, is not a requirement, but may provide desirable routines. Many dog guide users work as volunteers; homemakers, with their busy routines, will benefit from dog guide mobility, as will active college students and retirees.

A properly working dog readily accepts the challenge of new situations, so dogs may be

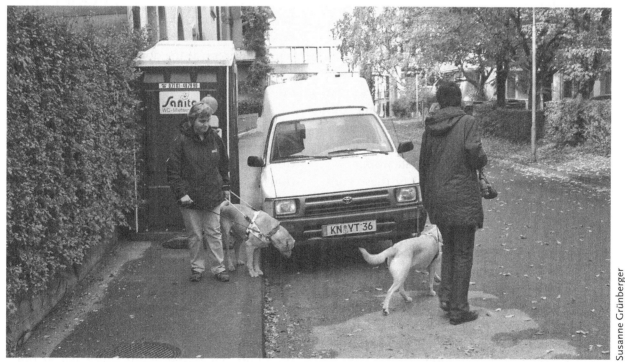

Susanne Grünberger

Two German handlers direct their dog guides around an obstacle on the sidewalk.

particularly valuable to the person who is blind who travels to new situations frequently. The dog's vision and memory, combined with the handler's understanding of sound orientation principles, supplements the student with his or her orientation. Travel, therefore, becomes less stressful. This may also be true for persons who travel frequently over complex routes that are always in transition, as is often the case in large cities.

Age

For many reasons, young people in high school are rarely considered as candidates for dog guides. One reason is that people under the age of 16 years old frequently lack the maturity and responsibility needed to give a dog the level of consistent care and handling that dog guides require. The high school environment itself has inherent difficulties, with large numbers of adolescents responding to peer pressure and focusing inappropriate attention on the dog and young handler.

In situations where a dog guide is considered, the young prospective dog guide handler must be in an environment where independent travel is possible. In suburban and rural settings, where school buses pick students up, deliver them to a school, and return them to their homes, other options should be available in the student's routine either in his or her home or school neighborhoods if the dog guide is to receive adequate work.

Younger applicants who satisfy these concerns are not infrequent, but will require careful evaluation by the schools. The schools also have individual policies concerning high school–age applicants. One school in Canada (Foundation MIRA) trains many high school-age (and younger) students. The school also provides or coordinates extensive O&M support to those students.

There is no upper age limit for dog guide handlers. However, the training is often physi-cally strenuous, and many older people will find it too exhausting. Older people who have a strong desire to continue a high level of independent activity, and have maintained good physical condition, may do well with a dog guide. The emphasis on maintaining physical fitness into the senior years may in the future make more older people who are visually impaired or blind eligible for dog guides.

Physical and Mental Health

Potential dog guide handlers need to be in good health. Not only is the training rigorous, but also once they return home, through their work with their dog, regular exercise will be a part of their life! The average dog guide walks at a brisk pace, although many walk more slowly.

The individual needs to have good coordination and balance, be of at least average intelligence, and be emotionally stable. Some attempts have been made to train visually impaired people with developmental delays to use dog guides, most notably by Guiding Eyes for the Blind (Zubrycki, 2009). These attempts have met with very limited success, as the dogs were not used extensively, and the students chose not to replace their original guides.

Dog guides may be especially well suited for students with diabetic retinopathy. Exercise is an important factor in keeping diabetes under control, and since dog guides need regular attention and exercise, they tend to help keep owners active. They may also help diabetics avoid bumps and bruises that can have especially serious consequences for them. Specific conditions such as controlled epilepsy, mild cerebral palsy, heart conditions, or other mild physical problems will not, of themselves, disqualify a person for consideration for a dog guide. The school in question will need to be especially thorough in the search for a dog appropriate for the person with the additional disability, and this may take time.

Several schools have undertaken to train dogs to guide blind travelers who are in wheelchairs. Generally power wheelchairs are suitable for this but manual chairs have also been used (Southeastern Guide Dogs, 2009).

Until the successful development of the antiretroviral drug therapies, persons with AIDS-related blindness had rarely been considered good candidates for dog guides. This is because the cytomegalovirus responsible for most AIDS vision loss struck late in the course of the disease, and the person was generally too weak to consider the use of a dog guide as an option for mobility. However, as a result of these new therapies, the increased life expectancy and greater stamina of people with AIDS has made it possible for some individuals to be considered good candidates for dog guides.

Hearing

Individuals with hearing loss that prevents them from accurately judging traffic in most situations are generally not good candidates for dog guide training. Their inability to accurately assess traffic leads to repeated incorrect commands, which put undue stress on a dog. However, exceptions may be made if they are willing to seek assistance at crossings, or their living conditions are such as to present a minimum of risk from vehicular traffic. Both Leader Dogs for the Blind and Guiding Eyes for the Blind in the United States, the Guide Dogs for the Blind Association of Great Britain, and other schools internationally have programs for deaf-blind travelers.

Individuals with hearing losses in the mild to moderate range can frequently do well with dogs. The dogs provide an additional margin of safety, a sense of security, and, through their behavior, information. Once again, this is an area in which individual schools have different standards for acceptance, and an individual home visit and assessment may be done. Advances in hearing aid technology suggest that schools need to regularly review their policies on training hearing-impaired students.

Amount of Remaining Vision

Most people with low vision have too much vision to be able to work effectively with a dog guide. In general, people who travel visually under many conditions while using the cane for identification and as an occasional probe, rather than as a true primary mobility device, will not benefit from dog guide mobility. The traveler will tend to anticipate stops or turns, and "steer" the dog around obstacles when vision is functioning at a high level. Then, when forced by lighting conditions to rely upon the highly skilled and responsible guide, he will find instead a dog whose skills are diminished and that is therefore less effective.

An exception may sometimes be made for people with degenerative eye conditions, who may be able to learn to use a dog to good effect, and establish good working patterns with a dog while they still have relatively effective vision. Usually this transition from depending on vision to no vision will be eased through the use of occluders in the training process. Individual schools vary in their policies concerning acceptance of applicants with residual vision, and some will consider low vision applicants if they meet the standard definition of legal blindness. Schools may also have their own staff assess these applicants.

Orientation Skills

As university-trained personnel and formal mobility instruction became available in the 1960s to people who were blind, the dog guide schools quickly saw the increased skills and confidence of applicants who had undergone mobility training. Therefore completion of a mobility training course, and some experience with independent travel, became increasingly important in selecting new applicants at all the dog guide schools.

It is best for dog guide handlers to have good mobility skills if they are to be effective travelers. It is still possible, however, for some people who have difficulty with spatial concepts to benefit from a dog guide. The dog guide selected must have an especially strong "work ethic" and a lack of distractibility, as distraction would throw the traveler off course. Once again, an independent evaluation by the dog guide school may be necessary.

ASSESSING THE POTENTIAL GUIDE DOG HANDLER

Schools take great care in evaluating individuals who apply. The O&M specialist has an important role in the assessment of a client's potential as a dog guide handler. Once a client has applied to a school, the specialist may well be asked to provide a mobility evaluation of the applicant.

The evaluation needs to include a description of the candidate's coordination, balance, and strength; orientation skills; ability to align with traffic sound; ability to recover when disoriented; and amount of mobility instruction already received.

Notes on the travel environment in which the student will be functioning, and something about her routines is helpful. Additional information about general abilities, personality, sense of responsibility, and capacity to make mature judgments is also important. If a candidate has vision, a description of how this vision is used in travel is helpful. Best and worst lighting conditions may also be noted. A sample evaluation form is included in this chapter.

The O&M specialist may be asked to recommend a specific school. If specialists feel uncomfortable with this, they may refer the client to the International Guide Dog Federation. In the United States and Canada, the American Foundation for the Blind publishes their *Directory of Services for Blind and Visually Impaired Persons in the United States and Canada*, or one may use the *Guide to Dog Guide Schools* prepared by Eames and Eames (1994), which lists most of the U.S. schools and facts about them. Also 13 U.S. schools participated in a 2006 survey created by Guide Dog Users Inc. (2006). Finally, please refer to this chapter's appendix for a list of dog guide schools in the United States and Canada.

Preparing the Prospective Dog Guide Handler

It is possible for the O&M specialist to help the prospective applicant to a dog guide program, or an accepted applicant, understand and prepare for the change in mobility and orientation. In the United States several dog guide programs including Leader Dogs for the Blind, Guiding Eyes, and Guide Dogs offer advanced seminars for O&M specialists. Many dog guide schools provide a basic introductory seminar that many university programs participate in.

The Institute Nazareth and Louis Braille in Quebec has an excellent video (now available in DVD) produced in cooperation with the dog guide program Fondation Mira (Guérette & Zabihaylo, 2001) that will give the specialist several useful tools and approaches.

An instructor at the Dutch dog guide school Koninklijk Nederlands Geleidehonden Fonds (KNGF; n.d.) developed DogSim, a dog guide simulator that will certainly help the prospective student prepare and understand the transitions. Information may be obtained at www.dogsim.com.

This device is pushed from behind by the O&M specialist. As a result, the student has the sensation of following the harness handle without either a real dog or a person ahead of him. It

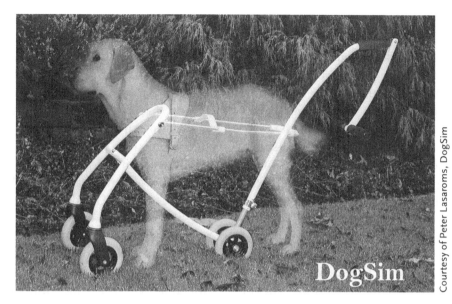

Courtesy of Peter Lasaroms, DogSim

An image of the DogSim, a dog guide simulator, illustrating how it simulates the experience of walking with a dog guide.

simulates the experience of working with a real dog guide quite accurately. DogSim can be used to help a trainee think about orientation without the level of tactile contact with the environment that cane travel affords.

THE O&M SPECIALIST'S ROLE IN THE TROUBLESHOOTING PROCESS

The O&M specialist may have several opportunities to observe a working dog guide unit. Some units will appear to be operating at a high level of efficiency, effectiveness, and safety. Others may not appear to enjoy the same level of smooth mobility. However at what point does a unit become problematic? Does the O&M specialist need to intervene? When and how? A dog guide user may request your assistance or observations. What are your responsibilities and obligations?

The work of the dog guide instructor and the work of the O&M specialist are similar in some ways and different in others. The dog guide instructor's education incorporates a great deal of information and experience relating to canine behavior, of course especially in relation to the use of dogs as guides (Harrison, 2006). While the O&M specialist can certainly assist in orientation, and may be able to spot a unit that is not functioning well, the O&M specialist's ability to resolve the issues they observe will be limited.

The O&M specialist needs to first be aware that criticisms of a working guide are best handled with considerable tact. It is likely that the handler may feel a nearly parental sense of loyalty to her dog guide, and a well-intentioned comment may generate a defensive reaction that seems extreme. This can be particularly true when "correction" is involved. *Corrections* are sharp leash tugs used to refocus a dog's attention when it is distracted. They should be administered quietly, quickly, and rarely. Even so they are often misunderstood by the general public, and sometimes are clumsily administered. The occasional correction is a standard part of dog handling. The O&M specialist needs to understand this, and not mistake normal correction for "abuse." Excessive correction, however, can indeed indicate a serious problem in the relationship and may make the O&M specialist feel that he needs to do something. A discussion in which the dog guide handler is told that she ought to call her school for suggestions may be appropriate.

A second caution involves "reporting" a dog guide user's problem to his school without the handler's knowledge. This tactic is ethically questionable—all the handlers are independent adults—and should your role become known it will certainly result in damage to your professional and personal relationship with the individual in question. The O&M specialist can certainly call a dog guide program for information while protecting a particular dog guide handler's anonymity. After discussing the situation in question with the handler, you might encourage him to contact the school. If the student is open to discussing the problem further, he may choose to call the school. Some students may welcome a conference call including the school and the O&M specialist. If you feel strongly that the individual's safety is at risk, and the individual will not take action on his own behalf, you may feel an obligation to call the school and discuss the situation.

With this caution, the O&M specialist may yet be able to help a dog guide handler become aware of and resolve some problems. The professional's skill and experience with dog guides will determine her comfort level. She may also feel more or less comfortable depending on which type of issue she is faced with. Frequently the issue will be one of orientation, and there one can easily assist. At other times the O&M specialist may be asked for detailed information about "What is my dog doing?" Here, too, one may be able to give a bit of information that clarifies or explains something—perhaps why a dog does something at a certain spot. For example, the handler may ask why her dog always pulls hard to the left as they approach a certain corner. The O&M specialist may notice that there is a grating there that the dog prefers to avoid and supply that information.

In other situations it may be possible to describe a problem that the handler may be unaware of (e.g., "The dog appears to be going into the street too quickly" or "The dog seems to be distracted"). It can be much harder to "diagnose" the cause of problems, and to come up with solutions for them. In the cases mentioned above, several possible causes and solutions come to mind, and these lists are far from exhaustive:

1. "The dog appears to be going into the street too quickly."

    a. The dog is tense.
    b. The person is tense and is rushing the dog (or has in the past).
    c. The dog is excited about going to a familiar destination.
    d. The dog is actually fine.
    e. The dog is not watching traffic.
    f. The dog is from a school that does not train traffic awareness.

2. "The dog seems to be distracted."

    a. The dog *is* distracted, but one of the following applies:
        i. The match is good, but the handler is not handling appropriately.
        ii. The match is bad.
        iii. The dog's temperament has "evolved" since "graduation," and the handler needs to learn new skills to cope with the changes.
        iv. The dog is overly energetic because the handler is not giving it enough work.

b. The dog is *not* distracted, but one of the following applies:

    i. The dog is fearful.

    ii. The dog is actually fine—a variant of normal.

The solutions for these problems are extremely variable and depend on multiple factors. The dog guide school and instructor have the expertise to play the key role in sorting out the possibilities and suggesting solutions. Once again, the O&M specialist is always welcome to contact a dog guide school with generic questions about proper work patterns and behavior.

PROVIDING ORIENTATION ASSISTANCE TO DOG GUIDE TRAVELERS

Students arriving at dog guide schools for training with their dogs have, for the most part, had at least some O&M training. Dog guide instructors are able to help the traveler transition between cane and dog and teach their students how to remain oriented when working with a dog. In the future, all instructors trained at International Guide Dog Federation–accredited schools will also have some background in orientation and mobility.

Dog guide travelers returning home with a new dog usually require no professional orientation assistance. They are able to manage their own transition using the instruction they received at their school. In some cases and situations, they may ask a friend or relative for help.

However, as travel becomes ever more complex travelers who are blind increasingly request orientation assistance from professionals. The O&M specialist needs to be aware that the dog guide handler's needs are somewhat different from those of the cane traveler. The sound of traffic, and auditory clues and landmarks of every kind, are important to both cane and dog

travelers. Although the speed of travel is often different for dog guide travelers compared to cane travelers, both rely heavily upon their sense of distance traveled over time to know they are close to a destination.

Dog guide handlers pay little attention to tactile information points and landmarks, as they are extremely difficult to locate without a cane. Also, since in general dogs view fixed objects as obstacles to clear or avoid, access to such landmarks is limited, although "sound shadows" are still available. However, underfoot landmarks, such as marked surface changes, ramps, and hills, are certainly accessible in many situations, and continue to be essential with a dog guide. Olfactory clues, sun, wind direction, and other clues that do not rely on physical contact may also be detected.

Dog guide handlers "read" their dog's behavior for its information value. They use their dog's desire to please, combined with the dog's intelligence and ability to see. In familiar environments dog guides will locate and indicate through "controlled anticipation" (see Volume 1, Chapter 9) places they recognize; these indications become landmarks or information points.

The task of the O&M specialist is to help the traveler put his dog's abilities and tendencies to work on his behalf. The specialist has two goals: (1) make sure the traveler has an overall orientation to the environment; and (2) if necessary, help the traveler teach his dog new goals and intermediate destinations. Later the dog's indication of these goals and destinations will be among the information points and landmarks the traveler uses. A three-step orientation, coaching, and solo (OCS) process is useful in whole or in part.

Orientation

An initial orientation to a complex environment is usually best accomplished while the O&M specialist serves as a sighted guide with the dog

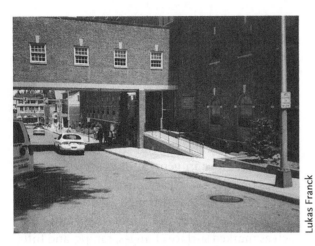

The orientation problem in this complex environment is to locate the ramp leading to the building when approaching from the right. The ramp in the middle of the block may not be available as a cue to the handler, who will be on the flatter top part of the ramp. Sound cues are available only in the form of an echo from the overhead passageway and nearby wall, once past the ramp.

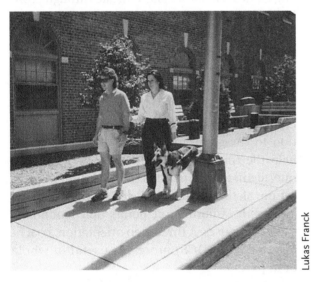

The O&M specialist initially walks the handler through the route one or more times as a sighted guide, with the dog at heel, while explaining the layout and any problems that might be anticipated. The handler praises the dog at key points on the route to help the dog learn those locations.

unit. The traveler may choose initially to leave his dog at home and to explore an area with a cane.

At specific points which the dog guide needs to indicate and which are devoid of other environmental clues—for example, the intersection of two pathways on a campus—the handler needs to put the dog at "sit," and make the point memorable to the dog with lavish praise, then repeat the approach to the spot. If the dog stops successfully, it needs to be praised. If not, a mild reprimand may be necessary.

Several walks through a complex route may be needed. It may be helpful to take a break at the destination after each walk-through. The handler's praise at the destination will facilitate the dog's learning.

Coaching

In this second step the O&M specialist needs to stay just behind the handler's right shoulder while the unit "works" the route. It is a good idea to prompt the handler to let her know she is approaching key points; otherwise, mistakes and variation may lead to confusion in the dog's mind. Review and narrate the route as you go, and point out time–distance ratios that become apparent as the unit works.

If the dog misses a turn on successive repetitions, the O&M specialist needs to suggest they take a break and come back later. Also, since dogs travel visually, once a dog has a clear destination in mind, and the handler trusts her dog to do it correctly, the handler may choose to allow the dog to skip an intermediate landmark that was created to allow the handler to be certain of her location and go directly and safely to the final goal. This is natural and acceptable.

Monitoring (or Solo Phase)

When necessary for the traveler's confidence, or to be sure that a complex route has been mastered, a monitoring phase may be added. If

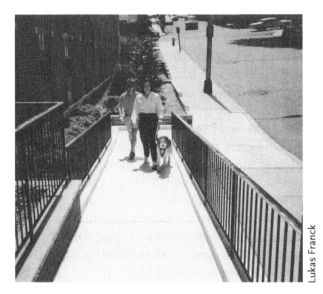

When coaching a team, the O&M specialist walks just behind the handler's right shoulder while the team works the route. The specialist alerts the handler when approaching key points on the route to avoid confusing the dog with wrong turns.

possible, observation needs to be conducted from a spot out of the dog's view. This can be quite difficult as dogs are extremely observant and have very sharp hearing and sense of smell in addition to vision. The best way is to have the client begin the trip at a prearranged time, or in response to a phone call. The observer needs to avoid intervening too quickly, but if necessary, the unit should calmly be directed to stop and return to the coaching phase.

The three-step process of orientation, coaching, and solo (OCS) is rarely used in its entirety. It may be necessary in complicated environments, or in situations which are so lacking in environmental information points that the traveler needs to rely exclusively on the dog's behavior for information. It may also be useful with travelers who have very poor orientation skills or a poor sense of direction. Otherwise, most travelers need little or no assistance.

Depending on the individual and the setting, a verbal orientation to a situation may be all

that is necessary before the traveler has a complete and confident grasp of the new situation. In more difficult situations, a single walk-through either with a human guide or with the O&M specialist in a coaching position, may give travelers enough information and experience to make them safe and confident. A few repetitions without a true solo trip may also be just the answer.

Another method for orienting a handler to a new environment, in particular in environments that are poor in available environmental information such as mall parking lots, is what is called a *backchain*. Here the route is learned from the destination backwards to the beginning. For example, if the route began at a bus stop and required crossing a large parking lot with the destination being a door into a mall, orientation and teaching would begin at the door, and going into the mall would be the first step. The next step would be to begin at the curb out of the parking lot, and go to the door into the mall and then into the mall (where the dog would receive a lot of praise!). Step 3 would begin a few steps into the parking lot, across the perimeter road, to the curb, and then to the door and into the mall, and so on. Work back to the bus stop as the last step in the chain. The advantage of a backchain is that one is always working from weakness into strength, from least familiar to most familiar.

The instructor and the handler should establish a partnership from the beginning to determine what the handler wants to do, and to review the teaching–learning and travel options that are available. Often the handler will be able to tell the specialist how best to provide information to the unit.

Self-Familiarization

Typically dog guide handlers will familiarize themselves with an unfamiliar hallway or classroom by initially working the length of the hallway or the perimeter of the room to ascertain that there are no unexpected steps or other hazards. Then the handler will drop the harness, putting the dog off duty, and further explore the room, using standard self-protective hand techniques and a systematic exploration pattern.

When traveling in a strange neighborhood or town, the ability to solicit quality information is critical. It is the exception to the rule (i.e., the offset crossing with traffic islands, or the major construction site) that causes problems for both dog guide and cane travelers.

To become familiar with the sequence of shops on a block, the handler uses *moving turns*, which are also known as *suggested commands*. Somewhat similar to trailing in function, these commands enlist the dog's vision and initiative to seek out likely looking destinations. If given the command "Right" in the middle of a block, an experienced dog guide will seek out the door of a building or shop. If this turns out to be wrong, another set of commands will bring the traveler to the shop next door. Shops that have actually been visited will likely become memorable in the dog's mind. The dog will then indicate the shop on the next passing, giving the handler location information through anticipatory behavior and requiring the handler to employ "controlled anticipation" to pass them.

DOG GUIDES, CANES, AND ELECTRONIC TRAVEL TECHNIQUES

In the early days of The Seeing Eye, during the 1930s, probably following the German model that Dorothy Harrison Eustis observed in Potsdam in 1927 (see Volume 1, Chapter 9), students were trained to use a short cane in the right hand in conjunction with the dog guide in their left. The short cane, while ineffective as a primary mobility device, was recognized as a symbol of blindness, while the dog guide initially was not. It was also felt that a probe might be of some value. It was inconvenient to have both hands

occupied and experience proved that the cane was rarely used. Within a decade the cane was phased out in the United States, although it is still used in some European dog guide programs, probably because of the prevalence of older infrastructure that is less systematic and predictable than that in the United States and Canada.

The cane can still be used in certain situations if the traveler prefers; please also see Volume 2, Chapter 1, which reviews the long cane technique in depth. For example, some travelers who are blind may choose to familiarize themselves with new areas using a cane. This may be done either before or after traveling through it with the dog. The long cane should never be used while the dog is guiding. When using the cane, the dog must be in the "heel" position. With this in mind, we can see that the only acceptable cane for this arrangement is the collapsible cane. It can be put away and does not present a problem when not in use.

Self-familiarization to a new environment would be the most likely use for the cane in conjunction with the dog guide. An office building or college campus can offer some real challenges when attempting to locate certain objects. One may know the layout and general area where an office or classroom should be, but one cannot expect the dog to locate the exact door to that area. If the traveler were to repeatedly ask the dog to "find the door," only to find it is the wrong door, both the handler and the dog can become confused. However, if the dog is placed at the "heel" position and the cane is used in a diagonal position or modified touch technique to trail the wall, the traveler has a good chance of finding the room quickly and with little confusion to the dog. These techniques also offer more protection from the waist down than simply trailing the wall with one's hands.

If the objectives remain constant over a period of time the preceding practice may serve to "pattern" the dog to the specific objective. The practical application for self-familiarization to a new environment is as follows. The handler should do the following:

1. Solicit information prior to arrival at the building or objective.

2. Once in the area, and having ascertained either by prior inquiry or by working the dog through the space, that there are no drop-offs, make use of the collapsible cane in a diagonal technique to trail the wall and locate the objective. Remember the dog should be in the heel position.

3. Upon locating the objective, the handler needs to tap the door or objective to focus the dog's attention, *move into the room or area*, and give the dog lavish praise.

4. Next he needs to put the cane away and work the dog back to where they started. While working he needs to keep in mind *time*, *distance*, and *rate*. That is to say, the traveler needs to work to develop a sense of how long it will take them to go a certain distance at the dog's speed. Then, when the traveler tries the route again, he will know when they are approaching their goal, and she will be able to give a "suggested command." Asking the dog to locate the now-known destination, the dog will be motivated to return to the objective for the praise it knows it will receive.

5. If the dog does not locate the objective, the handler needs to locate it with his cane once again and repeat the process. If a guide dog is taken to an objective and praised a few times, it will locate the same objective within a short time.

All dog guide schools encourage students to keep up their cane skills in order to be prepared for all contingencies. Dogs are not always required in certain settings such as sporting events in large arenas, where the handler will likely be accompanied by sighted friends. When waiting for a replacement dog, or if the dog becomes ill,

the traveler will need to use the cane to maintain independence.

Little research has been conducted into the use of various electronic travel aids (ETAs) in conjunction with dog guides. Experimentation has occurred at the dog guide schools themselves, under the auspices of ETA manufacturers, and by individual blind travelers. Of particular interest are the MiniGuide, and GPS systems as described in Volume 1, Chapter 8, and Chapter 14 of this volume. These systems hold exceptional promise for dog guide travelers.

The additional information and spatial awareness gained through the proper use of an ETA may enhance travel through the environment (Seeing Eye Inc., 1984). By extending sensory range, an ETA may allow either a cane or dog guide traveler in an unfamiliar environment to accurately locate destinations, and to more effectively interpret landmarks and information points. For this reason, it may be useful for teaching potential destinations to a dog in a new environment.

For example, it may initially be easier to locate a recessed entrance using an ETA rather than a cane or dog alone. Once it has been located, the dog guide handler praises her dog. Having learned this door as a potential destination, the dog will likely indicate it by pausing there when next in the area, making future use of the ETA unnecessary.

There are potential problems with both the ETA and the GPS from the point of view of good dog guide use. Dog guide use entails fluid motion and rapid mutual responsiveness between dog and handler. Unless additional information provided by the ETA or GPS is processed instantaneously, it may disrupt the otherwise smooth functioning of the unit (Kay, 1980). With ETAs, the dog guide handler must take care not to use the ETA to do the dog's job and diminish "guide responsibility." The handler must not "steer" or cue the dog when encountering objects detected in or around the travel path. Another common tendency when using the ETA to search for information laterally is to lean away from the dog to extend still further the range of the ETA. This is unsafe and needs to be avoided.

Training with an ETA or GPS needs to begin separately from work with a dog, and should only be integrated into travel with the dog guide when the traveler has reached a reasonable level of proficiency. As an intermediate step, it may be possible to simulate the effect of dog guide travel through the use of the empty harness without the dog (a Juno harness). At the point of integrating the two modes of travel it is essential to involve a dog guide instructor as an advisor.

Dog guide handlers with hearing impairments may benefit from ETA use as a means of receiving additional information from the environment. ETAs that provide tactile feedback are obviously required. The MiniGuide has been used experimentally in this capacity. Skillful use of an ETA has been achieved by some students when working on routes with few available clues and landmarks. The ETA can be used to identify objects outside the normal line of travel. An example would be a post or tree placed just off the path in a park or campus area. The response to the ETA from such an object may provide a landmark on a new or unfamiliar route. However the dog's tendency to anticipate ("controlled anticipation") will soon render the use of the ETA redundant as the dog becomes familiar with the route.

There is some innovative work being undertaken at various dog guide schools using the new generation of GPS navigation devices which many guide dog users find beneficial. Courses in the use of GPS are often better undertaken after guide dog mobility becomes familiar and routine. To undertake training in the use of GPS and dog concurrently would involve many stoppages to the dog's work and this may be counterproductive. With GPS, the handler runs the risk of becoming distracted by the technology, and neglecting his dog handling skills. However, the fluent GPS user who is also a good dog guide handler has a tremendous mobility advantage.

One way of minimizing this interference is by using the "virtual mode" that GPS systems have to explore the route thoroughly before actually walking the route. This will minimize the amount of interaction required with the GPS device on the actual route.

CONCLUSION

Mobility is the shared goal of the dog guide programs and O&M specialists. Each specialty needs to understand something about the other. The O&M specialist may act as an advisor and assistant to a blind person in regard to dog guide mobility. Dog guides are not for everyone, but for some the dog guide will enrich the travel experience of a blind person profoundly. The O&M specialist's information and encouragement may be a turning point for that individual.

When orienting a dog guide handler to a new area, remember that the handler has expertise with the dog that you, as an orientation and mobility specialist, do not. Your input on safety and route choice can help make learning a new area with a dog guide pleasant and efficient for the handler.

IMPLICATIONS FOR O&M PRACTICE

1. The O&M specialist may assist the dog guide handler at two points. She may advise the handler about getting a dog guide, and may help to prepare the traveler for the transition between cane and dog. She may assist the dog guide handler in orientation to new environments.

2. Factors that dog guide schools take into account in deciding to accept an applicant for a dog include: personal preference, life circumstances and activity level, age, health and physical condition, hearing, amount of remaining vision (if any), and orientation skills.

3. Life circumstances may dictate the amount of use a dog gets, as well as what type and where.

4. Helping a cane traveler transition to dog guide use involves encouraging the traveler to rely less on tactile information, and more on acoustic information and time–distance relationships as well as their dogs' behavior for information.

5. When a dog guide handler is having trouble, O&M specialists need to be careful not to offend the student with negative comments. They should provide information but be careful not to get in over their heads. The dog guide school is the first resource the O&M specialist should refer to.

6. When orienting a dog guide traveler to a new environment, the O&M specialist can use the orientation, coaching, and solo (OCS) process in whole or in part.

7. Electronic travel aids (ETAs) including GPS can be used with a dog guide, but care needs to be taken not to interfere with the dog guide's work. The handler can be distracted by technology at times. GPS can be very effective with dog guide travelers. It may be best to master the GPS without the dog guide present, to achieve a fluent skill with a GPS before reintegrating the dog guide.

LEARNING ACTIVITIES

1. Look at a complex environment and identify a destination that you would need to develop a route to. Think how you would orient someone to it using a cane. Now think how you would do it with a dog guide traveler. Remember: dogs have vision, and memory! Where would the handler be able to accurately direct the dog?

2. Using vision loss simulators, make a determination about where *you* believe vision loss would reach a functional level where the in-dividual might benefit from dog guide travel. Keep acuity and field loss and a combination of both in mind. Add a hearing loss to the experiment.

3. Discuss the thought process a dog handler needs to go through before giving the "Forward" command to his dog at the down curb. Keep in mind orientation, safety, and handling requirements. (Is the dog paying attention?)

4. A 45-year-old female with RP and cataracts (20/400, 10 degrees remaining field) and a mild hearing loss is interested in discussing dog guides with you. She is doing very well with her cane, is employed, and is very active; in fact, many of her acquaintances do not think she is "really blind." What would you think, and what would you tell her?

5. How is it possible that Morris Frank (Volume 1, Chapter 9) and many other early dog guide travelers were successful without O&M training?

6. One of your students although working hard with you, is adamant about applying for a dog guide. You don't feel she is a good candidate—at least not now, but maybe not ever! What do you do?

APPENDIX: DOG GUIDE SCHOOLS IN THE UNITED STATES AND CANADA

* Indicates schools accredited as of 2009 by the International Guide Dog Federation.

American Guide Dog Schools

*Fidelco Guide Dog Foundation, Inc.
P.O. Box 142
Bloomfield, CT 06002
(203) 243-5200

*Freedom Guide Dogs
1210 Hardscrabble Rd.
Cassville, NY 13318
(315) 822-5132

*Guide Dogs for the Blind, Inc.
P.O. Box 1200
San Rafael, CA 94915
(415) 499-4000

*Guide Dog Foundation for the Blind, Inc.
371 East Jericho Turnpike
Smithtown, NY 11787
(516) 265-2121

*Guide Dogs of America
13445 Glenoaks Boulevard
Sylmar, CA 91342
(818) 362-5834

*Guide Dogs of the Desert, Inc.
P.O. Box 1692
Palm Springs, CA 92263
(619) 329-6257

*Guiding Eyes for the Blind, Inc.
611 Granite Springs Road
Yorktown Heights, NY 10598
(914) 245-4024

*Leader Dogs for the Blind
1039 South Rochester Road
Rochester Hills, MI 48307
(248) 651-9011

Pilot Dogs, Inc.
625 West Town Street
Columbus, OH 43215
(614) 221-6367

*Southeastern Guide Dogs
4120 77th Street East

Palmetto, FL 33561
(941) 729-5665

*The Seeing Eye, Inc.
P.O. Box 375
Morristown, NJ 07963-0375
(973) 539-4425

Canadian Dog Guide Schools

*BC Guide Dog Services
6050 44th Avenue, Delta,
BC V4K 3X7
(604) 940-4504

*Canadian Guide Dogs for the Blind
P.O. Box 280,
4120 Rideau Valley Drive North
Manotick, ON K4M 1A3
(613) 692-7777

*Canine Vision Canada
P.O. Box 907, 152 Wilson St.
Oakville, ON L6K 3H2
(905) 845-8225

La Fondation Mira Inc (MIRA)
1820 Rang Nord-Ouest
Sante-Madeleine, QC J0H 1S0
(514) 875-6668

Other

The International Guide Dog Federation
Hillfields, Burgfield Common
Reading RG7 3YG
United Kingdom
+44 1189 833572
www.igdf.org.uk

PART FOUR

Orientation and Mobility and Different Disabilities

CHAPTER 17

Teaching Orientation and Mobility to Students with Vision and Hearing Loss

Dennis Lolli, Dona Sauerburger, and Eugene A. Bourquin

LEARNING QUESTIONS

- What is the range of communication modes available for working with a student who is deaf-blind?

- How can a traveler who is deaf-blind get across a street?

- What skills does the traveler who is deaf-blind need to effectively use public transportation?

- How can a traveler who is deaf-blind communicate with the public?

- What are the major areas of modification to the traditional O&M curriculum for travelers who are deaf-blind?

This chapter addresses the special challenges to orientation and mobility (O&M) specialists when teaching people who are visually impaired and also have a hearing loss; these individuals are often referred to as *deaf-blind* or *dual sensory impaired.* It addresses available communication modes, travel issues, and useful skills for the deaf-blind person.

According to the National Center for Health Statistics, the population of people who have a significant hearing loss in the United States is greater than 20 million (approximately 8.6 percent). The number of people who are *functionally* deaf, who cannot hear normal conversation even with hearing aids, is estimated at 1 million people according to the National Center for Health Statistics (Gallaudet University, 2004). The Gallaudet Research Institute (Gallaudet University is the world's only liberal arts college for individuals who are deaf or hard of hearing) reports 37,500 children and youth who are deaf or hard of hearing in the United States (Gallaudet University, 2005), and the National Technical Consortium for Children and Youth Who Are Deaf-Blind maintains a census which reported approximately 11,000 individuals who had dual sensory impairment between birth and age 22 (2004). According to the Helen Keller National Center for Deaf-Blind Youths and Adults ("Frequently Asked," 2005), the adult population of individuals who are deaf-blind is approximately 70,000; this estimate does not include a significant number of older Americans who have both vision and hearing losses.

OVERVIEW OF DEAF-BLINDNESS

The Deaf-Blind Population

Individuals with combined hearing and visual impairments encompass a full range of personal qualities. People who are both blind and deaf use many of the same travel techniques as do people who are blind and have normal hearing. They can achieve a high level of independence; many use public transportation, commute to work, shop and run errands, and travel alone across the country and around the world. The deaf-blind population is heterogeneous. The O&M specialist needs to determine the adventitious versus congenital nature of the sensory loss, whether there is a syndrome causing the dual sensory loss, and the extent of remaining sensory abilities (Lolli, 2006). These variations of when and how deaf-blindness occurred may suggest ways to approach the person's O&M needs.

By focusing on the distinct qualities of their students who are deaf-blind, O&M specialists will open themselves to rich professional experiences. In some respects, teaching O&M skills and techniques to people who are deaf-blind is not that different from teaching people who are solely visually impaired. The primary distinctions, which need to be considered throughout the program of students who are deaf-blind, are the communication methods used by the student; the need to modify techniques to accommodate the hearing loss; the need to consider the student's conceptual understanding of environments; and the need to understand and accommodate cultural differences, especially Deaf culture as described in the section Cultural Issues of Deaf-Blindness later in this chapter (note that the word *Deaf* is often capitalized when it refers to what is considered a separate culture or community). Each of these issues is addressed in this chapter.

Generally, as with individuals who are blind, the nature of how and when the disability occurred needs to be considered. Hearing children normally acquire the spoken language of their culture; those who are born deaf will also acquire language if they are exposed to communication in a modality that they can perceive, such as sign language (discussed later in this chapter). Often, however, this communication environment is not provided, resulting in impaired development of language, conceptual understanding, and interpersonal relationships. This potentially profound impact of congenital deafness is multiplied when the person is blind as well. Conversely, people who have good language skills and conceptual understanding and who lose their hearing and vision adventitiously need to usually learn new ways to communicate and learn about the world around them. For example, people who had relied on spoken language may need to learn such skills as speechreading (understanding spoken words by using information from the lips, facial movement and expression, body language, and other clues to meaning), signing, or having words spelled to them when they become deaf. Those who had relied on speechreading or sign language may need to learn to perceive language and learn new concepts by tactile methods when they become blind. Even after learning these skills, difficulties may continue because their friends, family, colleagues, and others are not willing or able to accommodate to their new methods of communication.

Effects of Hearing and Vision Loss

When sensory input is limited, the ability to know what is happening in the environment is also limited. It is understood how this affects the concept development and environmental awareness of children and adults who are blind, but for people who are deaf-blind this effect is more than the combination of deafness and blindness together. This combination loss can remove a person from both their social and situational contexts.

The disconnection of the deaf-blind person with his/her environment is present in all of his/her movements: i.e., although he/she may be well trained, there is always a risk that something may happen which he/she may be incapable of grasping or controlling. Things happen around one in which one feels implicated but will never know exactly how they happened. One needs to have a great sense of self-control and a sense of calm, the ability to deduce and resolve problems and a strong practical sense. (Alvarez, 1993)

In addition, when people have diminished communication, regardless of the cause, they may be insulated from their environment and isolated from others. Their ability to express themselves, be aware of what is happening around them or understand what they experience, comprehend which options are available, and make choices can be severely restricted. This difficulty with understanding the content or meaning of the communication can lead to inappropriate and unexpected behavior. The real source of the behavior may rest with the person's difficulty to respond to his circumstance.

As a result, many individuals who are deaf-blind struggle to understand their world. A great deal of the incidental learning that takes place during everyday experiences by children and adults with normal vision and hearing is not available for those who are deaf-blind. Thus it is critical that O&M specialists routinely provide information about and discuss the events within environments for their students who are deaf-blind. Without this opportunity to discuss things with others, even those who have a variety of experiences can be experientially deprived because they are not aware of, or do not understand, what is happening. This is particularly true of children who are deaf-blind. Early on, these children will need guided activities to assist in developing their concepts of people, relationships, home life, school and other environments they encounter. For children who are deaf-blind, experiences are most meaningful when they are presented in an organized way and have context.

Often, decisions are made for people who are deaf-blind, without their even being aware of or involved with the choices, because of their dual sensory impairment. Frequently, they will need to learn how to assert themselves, make decisions, and gather the information needed to do so. The instructor facilitates this development, and does not make decisions for students or assume that because they are deaf-blind they need to use certain procedures. Students (or their guardians, if appropriate) can make informed decisions about which procedure to use when the instructor provides them with information and feedback about the effectiveness of the strategies and techniques.

Those who cannot see or hear sufficiently to communicate and learn through hearing and vision need to communicate and learn about their world primarily through touch, resulting in a need for physical contact, which makes some people uncomfortable. It can be difficult for students and instructors to attend to learning when there is discomfort or uncertainty about what is acceptable, and others may take advantage of students who don't know what is appropriate. The instructor and the student can reduce the uncertainty by discussing this issue frankly and clarifying each of their levels of comfort with touching, and consider what kinds of physical contact are appropriate and acceptable with others. Interaction with the public can also be difficult because of social concerns about touching strangers and the reluctance of some people to touch or be touched by others. Some methods of communication that are effective with the public require less physical contact than others, and students need to choose those with which they are comfortable. By being aware that some people are uneasy about touching, students can be patient when the public seems reluctant or unable to communicate with them, and flexible about trying alternative methods.

Cultural Issues of Deaf-Blindness

The specialist working with people who are deaf-blind needs to take into account cultural and community considerations. No statement about a group of people applies to each member, and this is certainly true regarding people who are deaf or deaf-blind. However, there are factors that social patterns bring to bear on the practice of O&M. The O&M specialist needs to be aware that some deaf people identify with a culture and set of norms that differ from their non-deaf (hearing) peers. The Deaf community is composed of a diverse group of people who share a common social and educational history, a language, and mutual circumstances in relationship to the population at large (Gannon, 1981). "For people in the Deaf community, deafness has a social rather than an audiological meaning. To be Deaf is to be a member of a special group, to claim one's culture and community as one's own" (Glickman & Harvey, 1996, p. 127). Many people who are deaf do not approach their hearing loss as a medical-pathological issue, and have a high regard and appreciation for sign language (Padden & Humphries, 1998). As seen in the examples to follow, this may sometimes influence the specialist's approach to instruction.

Deaf culture and language are visually based, and the loss of sight can have a profound effect on the individual. The relatively smaller size of the community can intensify the need or desire for privacy. The instructor can anticipate that some consumers who are deaf will be especially resistant to practices that may alter the ways they travel or communicate. Using a long cane or learning tactile methods of communication brings significant psychosocial issues to the forefront. As symbols of vision loss in a visually based culture, these adaptations may be emotionally charged and effect barriers between members of the Deaf community who are blind and those who are sighted. Sensitivity and respect toward these concerns will increase the chances of successful interaction (Smith, 2002, p. 80).

Cross-cultural considerations among deaf, deaf-blind, and hearing communities are critical when instruction is provided to people who are not members of the majority population. Cultural and linguistic appropriateness can be achieved when the specialist considers social differences in her lesson planning. For example, because signed communication can be observed and understood from a distance, O&M lessons might be planned to take place off the campus of the student's residential school for reasons of privacy, or signed communication regarding O&M instruction can be conducted discreetly out of view from others. Interaction between the student who is deaf-blind and the instructor may involve different "rules" and manners, which come from "an evolving Deaf-Blind culture" (Smith, 2002, p. 39). Examples of differing group norms might include: how to begin a conversation with a person who is deaf-blind, what types of touching are appropriate, and the use of humor in discourse. The specialist can follow the lead of the individual who is deaf-blind and ask questions in an open and respectful way.

Etiology of Deaf-Blindness

With such a heterogeneous population there are a number of etiologies that are linked to deaf-blindness. DB-Link in their *Overview of Deaf-Blindness* monograph (Miles, 2005), describes the most common causes, adapted from *Etiologies and Characteristics of Deaf-Blindness* (Heller & Kennedy, 1994).

There are a number of syndromes that may result in a combined hearing and vision loss such as Down, Usher, and Trisomy 13 syndromes. Another clustering of etiologies of hearing and vision loss is associated with multiple congenital anomalies: CHARGE association, hydrocephaly, fetal alcohol syndrome, and maternal drug abuse. Prenatal and postnatal conditions additionally can result in hearing and vision loss. Examples of this are rubella, toxoplasmosis, AIDS, herpes and syphilis, as well as asphyxia, head injury, stroke, encephalitis, and meningitis.

The O&M specialist needs to feel comfortable learning about these various conditions on an as-needed basis. It is typical that she may also consult with families and early intervention teachers about ways to stimulate self-awareness and environmental awareness. Frequently the home environment can be made more appropriate and stimulating by information the O&M specialist passes along to parents and family members.

COMMUNICATION

Because it is crucial that the instructor and student have clear, meaningful communication, the instructor's first priority is to determine the most effective ways to communicate with the student. Students who are deaf use various communication methods, including manual signing systems. In order to effectively teach O&M skills, the instructor must arrange to use a shared language or communication system that best matches the preference and skills of the consumer. If the instructor is not fluent in that language or communication system, she arranges for whatever consultation, assistance, and interpretation are required to achieve comfortable, comprehensive communication.

The most common languages used by people who are deaf-blind in the United States are spoken and written English and American Sign Language (ASL). Most people who are deaf-blind have some hearing or some vision or both and therefore can rely on a combination of inputs, so specialists can expect that one or a combination of auditory, visual, and tactile modes will be present when communicating with their students who have a hearing loss. In addition to spoken, signed, or spelled-out language, communication can consist of gestures, demonstration, behaviors, and symbols. Many people who are deaf-blind use

several methods of communication—one for regular communication and others to use with the uninitiated public (Bourquin & Sauerburger, 2005).

Sign Language

A common misconception is that the instructor can effectively communicate with students who use a signed language by signing vocabulary found in an ASL book or dictionary. However, because of the significant differences in grammatical structure and production, expressing individual signs in English word order is usually ineffective for communication. Likewise, written messages may not be fully understood by students whose first language is not English.

In 1960, William C. Stokoe published the seminal *Sign Language Structure: An Outline of Visual Communication Systems of the American Deaf*, becoming the father of the linguistics of American Sign Language. Since then, volumes regarding this topic have appeared in the professional and popular literature. American Sign Language is used among deaf people, and is a separate and distinct language which has its own grammar, semantics, lexicon, and mode of production; it is not constructed by producing signs which match words in spoken English. Although ASL shares the linguistic characteristics of other languages (for example, phonology and morphology), it does not share an exact equivalent vocabulary or word order with spoken English. ASL components include signs, classifiers (which function like spoken language pronouns), use of space (for example, for verb inflection and nominal referencing), facial grammar (such as temporal information), and a degree of gesture and iconicity (Lucas & Bayley, 2005; McNeill & Duncan, 2005). There are other derivative forms of manual communication, such as *signed English*, which are based on ASL but do not constitute distinct languages. Despite the common misconception, sign language is not universal. For example, England and the United States share a common spoken language but *not* the same signed language.

Most developed countries or regions around the world have their own signed languages. American Sign Language is the prevalent language in the North American Deaf communities. Estimates on the number of people who use ASL vary widely; the most reliable demographics are from the 1970s, when estimates indicated up to 500,000 people used ASL at home (Mitchell, Young, Bachleda, & Karchmer, 2006). Certainly, the contemporary use of ASL and other sign systems is ubiquitous throughout the United States, and O&M specialists can anticipate working with sign language users during their careers.

Tactile and Low-Vision Signing

Students who utilize a manual language typically express themselves visually to people who are sighted; their receptive language modes may vary according to their visual functioning and preferences, and can include any of the following:

- Visual reception with restricted visual fields or diminished acuities, where the person who is signing adjusts the distance from the student, and may limit the space where she produces signs and relays grammatical information.

- Reception with tracking, when the student maintains physical contact with the arm, wrist, or hand of the signer, in order to access and augment information that is not fully available visually.

- Tactile signing, when vision is not effective for receiving language. In this modality, the student places her hand or hands on top of the signer's and receives all or most of the linguistic information tactually. This involves additional physical and mental effort, and involves specific modifications in the signed language (Collins & Petronio, 1998; Frankel, 2002).

English

Most people who lost their hearing after they learned to speak or who have remaining functional hearing continue to use the language that is spoken in their community, such as English in the United States. English is also preferred by some people who are congenitally deaf who were raised using the "oral" method of communication. Most people who became deaf after learning to speak, as well as a few people who are congenitally deaf and had extensive training, can speak well enough to be understood readily. To communicate verbally with the public, some people who are deaf-blind play recorded messages using a tape or digital recorder or a device that can record and play messages repeatedly with the push of a button or buttons.

English can be conveyed to people who have a hearing loss through one or more of the following approaches:

1. Residual hearing, with or without amplification from assistive listening devices.

2. Speechreading, which is sometimes augmented with "cued speech," in which sounds that cannot be discerned by speechreading are conveyed with accompanying hand shapes and placements.

3. Signed English, which is a system of modified signs presented in English word order. This is sometimes referred to as *total communication* when paired with spoken language, and often used in education settings with children who are deaf. Other terms referring to this communication strategy are *contact language*, *simultaneous communication*, and *pidgin signed English* (PSE).

4. Printed, scripted, or typed English on readily available media such as paper or computer terminals. For students with low vision, a thick felt pen on paper, large font on a laptop display,

or dry-erase white board can serve as the communication instrument.

5. Spelling out of words, using techniques such as fingerspelling, print-on-palm, and specialized communication devices. Fingerspelling is the representation of English words, letter by letter, produced visually or into the hands of the person who is deaf-blind. Print-on-palm (P-O-P) is a technique of forming blocked letters into the hand, using the index finger. Each word is spelled out using capital letters (except for the letter *i*). Alphabet cards or plates with raised characters or braille, used by moving the person's finger over the character, is another method. Technology-savvy students may use computerized refreshable braille displays in order to receive typed messages through portable electronic devices such as the screen braille communicator (see Figure 17.1).

Often the easiest way to explain a technique, whether the student has normal hearing or is deaf, is to demonstrate it, either by having the student see or feel the instructor use the technique, or by positioning the student and giving feedback while she tries it. For example, while the student tries to use the cane correctly, the instructor can place a hand over the student's hand and move the cane; the instructor can position the student's arm in upper-hand and forearm technique while the student approaches an overhanging obstacle, and so forth.

Demonstrations and Gestures

People who are deaf-blind can use gestures and demonstrations to communicate with others, such as pointing to what they want, or gesturing to a salesperson that they want to buy an item that they found. To explain to another person how to communicate with them, for example, they might demonstrate how to print on their palm.

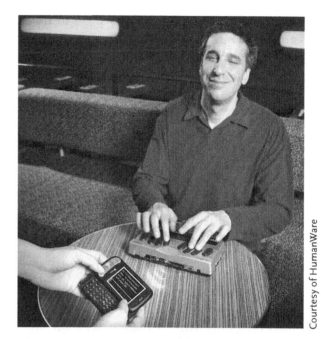

Courtesy of HumanWare

Figure 17.1. The DB Companion
This communication device enables conversations between an individual who is deaf-blind and a sighted person. A message input on the braille notetaker by the person who is deaf-blind will appear in print in the window of the communicator. The message here reads, "Hi, I'm blind and I can't hear. To communicate with me, type a message on this keyboard and press [the return key]." Whatever the sighted person types in print is displayed in refreshable braille on the notetaker for the deaf-blind person to read.

Signals and Symbols

Communication can often be expedited by signals that are universally understood, such as a "yes" or "no" shake of the head. Signals can also be established as needed, such as by arranging to tap students a certain way to indicate corrections that are needed in their technique ("two taps on your elbow means you're out of step"), or by making up a signal to indicate that they are approaching a door when the instructor is guiding them. When people who are deaf-blind ask others a question, they can show a note or say, "Please tap me twice to signal 'yes' and once for 'no,'" or vice versa. O&M specialists also need to use a signal to identify themselves each time they approach students who cannot see or hear them. Each person who is deaf-blind needs to learn the signal to indicate an emergency, made by using a finger to trace an *X* on his back or arm.

Minimal Language

Some students who are deaf-blind have minimal language skills or no formal language. This may be due to cognitive delays that impact on language acquisition, or due to a life situation that has prevented the individual from exposure to any natural signed or spoken language, or both. For example, some individuals who are deaf-blind have been raised in settings that do not have educational programs with sign language, some children who are deaf-blind were raised exclusively at home where visual or tactile language did not occur, and some children have been placed within institutions that afforded no opportunity to acquire language.

Students with minimal language skills might communicate with gestures and body language, or facial and vocal expressions. Techniques that may be effective for communicating with these students are gestures, expressions, and demonstrations, and using signs and symbols which can be taught to represent objects, destinations, or concepts. When working with students who have multiple disabilities, the O&M specialist often works as a member of a team that includes caregivers and family and other educational and rehabilitation professionals such as physical and occupational specialists, and communication specialists (professionals who work with people who have communication disabilities, which can include speech therapists and audiologists who are experienced and knowledgeable about working individuals with developmental disabilities). When appropriate, the O&M specialist needs to work with the communication specialist and team to develop communication that is appropriate to the stu-

dent's needs, and encourage others to communicate as fully as possible with the student. The authors have observed adults who are deaf-blind with minimal communication skills improve their ability to express themselves, make choices, and understand others after they were exposed to consistent, frequent communication in a mode that they could perceive (tactile, visual, auditory, or a combination). An excellent resource about enhancing communication with students whose language is undeveloped is Baumgart, Johnson, and Helmstetter (1990), and readers are referred to the chapter on learners with cognitive delays, and Gee, Harold, and Rosenberg (1987), who address O&M with severely disabled learners who have dual sensory impairments.

When working with students whose communication skills are minimal, the O&M specialist needs to help develop strategies to allow the students to anticipate what is happening; understand the intent of the O&M sessions; and make choices. These students can best learn to anticipate each activity if activities are scheduled consistently and regularly. Instruction of O&M techniques for students with minimal language ideally needs to occur when the students normally would use those techniques to travel from one location to another.

Use of Symbols

Symbols or *object cues* (the use of an object to represent a concept, such as a spoon representing eating), which are often used with people with limited language skills, can indicate specific things (such as juice or a coat), destinations (such as the student's desk, playground, or woodworking shop), or concepts (such as time to prepare for bed, feelings and desires such as anger or happiness, wanting to rest or take a walk, etc.). For example, students with limited language skills may request juice by showing the caregiver a certain cup, and an instructor might ask them to get their coats by handing them a symbolic square of fabric. Because it is so important for students to understand the purpose of O&M lessons and strategies, destinations need to be consistently and clearly explained to them each time a route is initiated, and this can also be done with symbols or object cues. For example, they might be given a spoon whenever they are going to the cafeteria, a seat belt buckle each time they go to the car, and a piece of sandpaper to indicate that they are going to the woodworking shop.

Photographs or pictures may be used for such purposes as to provide students with a way to indicate their frustration, boredom, or satisfaction, or to order food, such as "hamburger" and "french fries with ketchup." For students without sufficient vision, these communication tools would need to be identified tactilely. Some students may learn best if the symbols initially are actual items, such as a piece of cereal to represent breakfast, a plastic cup to represent drink, or scissors to represent crafts class. Once understood, these symbols are then paired with and eventually replaced by increasingly abstract symbols, such as ASL signs, textured squares or forms, or drawings. Other students may be able to learn abstract symbols or signs without first learning concrete symbols.

Unless the signal or symbol that the instructor teaches the student is intended for limited use between them, it needs to be as universally understood as possible, such as ASL signs—which many people recognize—or symbols which are labeled so that people who are new to the student, as well as salespeople and other strangers, can understand them. According to Baumgart et al. (1990), whatever is chosen to augment communication needs to be appropriate for the student's age and social interaction and, most important, meet the student's needs to communicate and understand.

Calendar Boxes

For individuals who require a concrete system of communication, including some individuals who are deaf-blind, a *calendar box* can be used to convey the student's schedule or progression of activities (see Figure 17.2). A calendar box usually consists of a row of boxes, or a long box with dividers forming separate cubicles into which symbols are placed, using a symbol for each activity. The student reaches into the first box to retrieve, for example, a cup to signify that it is time for a snack; after snack time he returns the cup to the empty bin and checks the next bin to find perhaps a ball, which is understood by that student to symbolize time for gym. The symbols are not generic, but are individually designed for each student to be most easily associated with the activity by that individual. For example, for students whose main mode of exploring the world is tactile, swimming could be symbolized by a swatch from the locker room carpet or a piece of Styrofoam from a float; time to get ready to go home could be symbolized by a seat belt clasp, a piece of coat fabric, or the like. The symbol can be carried to the activity, perhaps in a backpack or waist pack, as a reminder of what the student is doing, and then if the activity takes place in a special location that the student needs to find, a matching symbol can be placed at the site in a place where the student is likely to find it, such as on the back of the chair or, if the student is in another room, on the doorjamb where he enters the room. At the end of the activity, the student returns the symbol to the bin in such a way that indicates that the activity is finished, such as placing it in a "finished" box designated to receive symbols from completed activities or having a lid to each bin which is open before each activity and closed once the activity is completed and the symbol returned.

Once the object symbol is returned, the next bin is checked for the next object. An excellent resource about calendar box systems is *Calendars for Students with Multiple Impairments Including Deafblindness*, available through the Texas School for the Blind and Visually Impaired (Blaha, 2001).

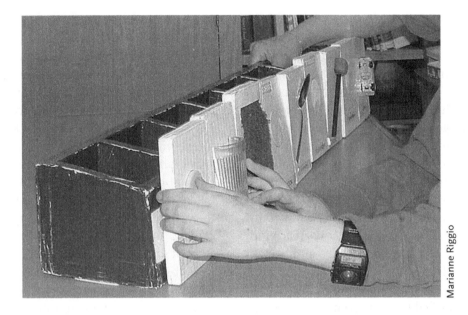

Marianne Riggio

Figure 17.2.
A calendar box organizes tactile symbols of daily activities to help students understand and anticipate the schedule. This calendar box starts the day with each symbol in front of its bin. A student can locate the symbol that indicates the next activity, carry it to the activity, and place it in the bin when the activity is finished.

CONSIDERATIONS FOR COMMUNICATION

Many people who are deaf-blind retain enough vision or hearing to understand spoken English by speechreading, or listening, or both. Those who rely on hearing need to be asked whether they prefer high or low tones and at what distance the instructor should speak. Background noises need to be avoided. An assistive listening device can help by enabling the O&M specialist to speak into a microphone that transmits the voice (by wire or broadcast) to the listener's receiver or hearing device, reducing interference from other sounds. If the student is reading the instructor's lips, the instructor needs to speak clearly without exaggerating and have good lighting on her face.

Visual and Tactile Communication

If the student will receive messages visually, the hand movements, print, or objects being used to convey the communication need to be the appropriate size, contrast, and distance from the student. Suitable lighting conditions are also very important. For example, if the O&M specialist is signing to the student, the light needs to be in front of the specialist (bright light from behind needs to be avoided); the specialist needs to wear clothes of a solid color that contrasts with the color of her skin; and the signs need to be made from a distance that is comfortable for the student. For students with restricted visual fields, the signs need to fit within the area that they can see, which increases the farther the specialist is from the student. When writing notes, the specialist needs to use letters of the size, thickness, and contrast that the student can see easily, perhaps using magnifiers, lights, or other equipment. When using objects as symbols, the O&M specialist needs to choose and position them so that the student can see them readily.

When O&M specialists approach students who receive communication tactilely, they need to touch them on the hand, arm, or shoulder to avoid startling them, and establish a signal or *name sign* with which they can identify themselves. The specialist's fingernails need to be smooth and short to avoid scratching the student. In hot conditions, powder can be sprinkled onto the hands to make the contact less sticky, and to communicate in cold weather, the specialist and the student can each put their hands into a muff to keep warm (see Figure 17.3).

Many people who are deaf-blind use various modes of communication because their vision or hearing fluctuates or is deteriorating (see Sidebar 17.1, "Communication within the Community"). For instance, some people need to switch to a different mode when circumstances are noisy or poorly lit, such as those who normally can see signs or symbols well, but need to perceive by touch in certain lighting conditions. Others who are blind and losing their hearing may be in the process of changing from communicating auditorily to learning to use signs or braille devices. Some deaf people who are losing their vision adjust to communicating tactilely by feeling others' signs. It is important to be flexible and use whichever mode is most effective in that situation for a specific student.

Concepts and techniques can be explained using representative models and tactile maps and graphics, as well as by drawing shapes on the student's hand or back, or using the instructor's hands (preferably in standard ASL handshapes, such as the ASL signs that represent *vehicle, chair, person,* and *wall*) to represent the position or movement of objects or people. For example, a person can be represented by a raised index finger or by the entire hand with two fingers pointing down to represent the legs. One of the instructor's hands can represent a chair, a wall, or the landing of a stair, while the other hand represents the person moving toward the chair or parallel to the wall, or leaning back while standing at the edge of the landing, and so forth. The instructor's finger could also represent a cane moving in the technique being described, the instructor's hands can represent vehicles moving to illustrate traffic patterns, and so on. The instructor's hand movements can be observed by students either visually or tactilely by placing their hands on those of the instructor.

Using Telecommunications

During O&M training, people who are deaf-blind learn to communicate to use taxis and call for directions and bus information. This can be done using technology that enables people who are deaf-blind to use a telephone and recognize when someone is at their door. A variety of pagers that are developed for deaf people will alert them to such sounds as telephones, doorbells, alarm clocks, and smoke alarms; some are installed or wired at the source, and others are portable and can be used when visiting hotels or other places. These pagers or *alerting devices* can provide output that people who are deaf-blind can use, such as flashing lights, loud buzzers, air from fans, or vibrating receivers that can be carried, worn, placed under pillows, or attached to beds.

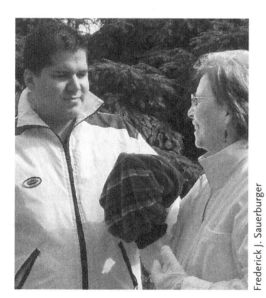

Frederick J. Sauerburger

Figure 17.3.
A muff can be used for tactile communication in cold weather.

Communication within the Community

People who are deaf-blind can use many different approaches to communicate with the public. Often, initiating contact and eliciting necessary information or assistance from strangers require incorporating one or more strategies. Some examples to effectively solicit people's attention, communicate the traveler's need, and explain how the public needs to respond are as follows:

A traveler enters an unfamiliar store and stands near the door while tapping his white cane and holding up a card saying, "Please help me find a SALESPERSON. TAP ME if you understand. You can print letters on my palm—I am DEAF *and* BLIND." Someone touches him hesitantly, and he shows the person how to print on his palm. The person doesn't respond, so he writes another note saying, "Please use your finger to print on my palm; I am looking for a salesperson," again shows how to print, then extends his palm and waits. The person prints, "I am a saleslady. Can I help you?" The traveler hands her a typewritten note with a list of items and the message, "I would like to buy these items. Please get them while I wait here, and print in my palm the names of any items which you do not have. Thank you." The woman goes and fills a basket with the items, then shows them to him, and he nods in approval. He takes out his wallet and again demonstrates that he wants her to print the price in his palm. She

does so, he pays, and she places the items in a bag. He thanks her with a smile and a nod, and turns to leave with the bag. When he doesn't find the door immediately, she pulls him toward it. He takes her arm and follows her outside, thanks her again, and walks back to his bus stop.

———

A traveler stands near a corner, and whenever she sees movement of people passing by she says, "Excuse me—please tell me where Matthew's Drug Store is." She finally notices that one person has stopped, and says, "Please write on this paper whether it is on this block or across the street—use very large letters because I am deaf and can't see well." She hands the person the paper and a thick marker; after he hands it back to her, she holds it close to her face and reads, "It is on this block." She asks him how many doors from the corner it is, hands him the paper and marker, and he writes, "6 doors." She points first to her right and says, "Is it this way . . ." then to her left ". . . or that way? Please move my hand to point toward the store." He doesn't comply, but she can see he is moving his arms. "I can't see you," she explains, "please either point my hand toward the store, or guide me to it." He takes her by the arm, she uses the Hines break to take his arm, and they walk toward the store. When he stops, she thanks him, finds the door, and enters.

Telephone communication is accessible to people who are deaf or deaf-blind through various options. Using a TTY (telecommunication device for the deaf), they can call directly to any office or individual who also has a TTY. People who are

deaf-blind can access TTYs that have large visual displays or refreshable braille output. In countries that offer this service, people with normal hearing who have no TTY can communicate with people who are deaf by using a relay service. This service is available without charge throughout the United States; dialing 711 will access this service in many locales.

The relay service can be used either with text using a TTY or, as is now becoming ubiquitous in the United States among people who are deaf and have sufficient vision, through video relay service (VRS) using a video camera attached to the deaf person's television or computer monitor. For text relay service, the communication assistant will transliterate the conversation back and forth between the hearing and deaf callers through TTY. VRS provides professional interpreters to facilitate calls between deaf and hearing people, and many services also provide VRS with spoken Spanish. Besides telephone communication, O&M specialists will find that personal computers and portable devices can effect easy communication with people who are deaf or deaf-blind through e-mail and instant messaging. As technology advances, the O&M specialist can expect easier and more effective communication methods with consumers who are deaf or deaf-blind.

THE USE OF QUALIFIED INTERPRETING SERVICES

The O&M specialist faces the challenge of effective communication when she does not share a language or communication modality with a student. This may often be the situation when working with people who are deaf or hard of hearing. The specialist needs to be certain to effect the best possible communication strategies by using the language and communication mode of the student to facilitate instruction. When the O&M specialist works with a student whose first language is ASL, she will often collaborate with another professional, a sign language interpreter. This collaboration focuses on language and communication; issues related to teaching or O&M are the domain of the O&M specialist. The level of proficiency in ASL required to effectively impart the

complex concepts of O&M will often be beyond the skills of the O&M specialist. While O&M specialists are encouraged to learn as much as they can of the language and mode of the student in order to enhance rapport, instructors must use the best possible interpretation for their O&M student during instruction.

Interpreters are bilingual individuals who provide professional services for people who do not share a language. Producing translation between ASL and spoken English is referred to as *interpreting*; when it is done with English-like sign systems, the attempt to match specific signs for words in English word order is specifically called *transliteration*. The rest of this chapter will use the term interpreting to mean either. Also note that the term *interpreter* is preferred for this role; other terms such as *translator*, *transcriber*, and *signer* designate other language-related roles and tasks.

The O&M specialist is cautioned not to use the students' family members or friends as interpreters; the interpreters' job requires them to be neutral parties in the role of communication facilitator. Professional interpreters follow a code of ethics and conduct which ensures the O&M specialist that all utterances will be accurately conveyed between the instructor and the student. As well, the interpreter will generally interpret everything spoken or signed during a lesson. Conversations directly with an interpreter, to the greatest extent possible, need to occur before or after lessons.

The interpreting *process* is a complex mental and physical set of tasks, which strives to convey the meaning from utterances in one language, into equivalence in another. The interpreter receives the source language (for example, spoken English) and determines the meaning, drops the form (the spoken words), re-creates the message into the target language (signs), and produces the equivalence message. When this process involves signers who are deaf-blind there is additional complexity. According to Jacobs (2005), "Deaf-Blind interpreting takes the task of interpreting to the

Nth degree . . . [and] there are the added elements of visual information, phonological, morphological, syntactic and lexical modifications, pacing, modality and tactile feedback mechanism."

Communication Strategies

Interpretation can occur between the instructor and the student using various strategies, depending on the ease of communication and the complexity of the message. Often the interpreter will work in a *simultaneous* mode, meaning that as the instructor speaks, the interpreter produces an equivalent message in the target signed language. Likewise, when the student who is deaf signs, the interpreter will voice into spoken English. The instructor may notice a lag between signs and spoken words, known as *processing time*, when the interpreter is mentally working to find meaning in the speaker's message and equivalence in the target (receiver's) language. This simultaneous mode is the most typical manner of sign language interpretation, but not always the appropriate or most successful strategy available to the specialist and the interpreter.

Interpretation can also occur in a *consecutive* mode, which can often result in better communication. In this model of *communication turn taking*, the instructor imparts a certain amount of logically connected information or idea. The speaker then stops, the interpreter considers the meaning of what was conveyed, and then produces the message in ASL. When the student responds, the interpreter follows the same pattern of sequential communication. Because of the flexibility and additional available time in consecutive interpreting, the instructor may find that complex material is processed and understood better following this model.

The instructor will be more effective when she reserves time with the interpreter before and after instruction (sometimes called *pre-conferencing* and *post-conferencing*). To prepare for the lesson, the instructor can inform the interpreter of the goals of the lesson, specialized vocabulary she may be using, and other information that may be particular or unusual. For example, the instructor might let the interpreter know that she will be discussing *shorelining techniques* (a term the uninitiated interpreter may not be familiar with), that her goal is for the student to properly effect a specific cane movement (a technique which may be unfamiliar), and that the interpreter needs to be aware that the working environment may include locations with moving vehicles such as streets and driveways. The instructor is mindful that she is responsible for the safe placement of the interpreter during the O&M lesson, away from traffic or other dangers. After the student has completed the lesson, the instructor and interpreter may again meet alone to discuss the efficacy of the communication.

Interpreters for People Who Are Deaf-Blind

O&M specialists need to always employ professional and qualified interpreters. This is not always an easy task, especially when seeking interpreters for people who are deaf-blind; according to Moss (in Jacobs, 2005), only about 1 percent of interpreting programs in the United States offer a required course in interpreting for consumers who are deaf-blind. The Registry of Interpreters for the Deaf, Inc. (in a system developed in cooperation with the National Association of the Deaf), grants national certification for interpreters, usually considered the highest standard in the field, through a rigorous testing system. Many states also offer gradational certification or licensing programs, known as *quality assurance systems*.

Often interpreting agencies or programs for people who are deaf in the local community are the best place for finding and hiring qualified interpreters. The instructor needs to impart as much appropriate information and specifics regarding the consumer who is deaf-blind as possible to the interpreter or interpreting entity, such as language preference, communication mode, time and duration, and location for an assignment. Interpreters also need to be informed if they need to come prepared with appropriate shoes and clothing to walk long distances or be outside. Payment for interpreters is typically the responsibility of the agency, institution, school, or business which is providing the instruction. Rates for interpreting services vary by region of the country.

It may be helpful to arrange for the same interpreter to provide services for a series of ongoing lessons. Not all interpreters are knowledgeable or comfortable working with consumers who are deaf-blind. There are elements of working with individuals who are deaf-blind that are not common to many interpreters, such as increased physical contact, making accommodations to differing visual functioning and impairment, communicating environmental visual information, and accepting ancillary responsibilities such as acting as a human guide. The O&M specialist needs to approach the interpreting situation with an open mind, address the interpreter as she would any other professional, and feel free to communicate information and questions at the appropriate times.

MODIFICATIONS OF THE O&M CURRICULUM FOR STUDENTS WHO ARE DEAF-BLIND

The instructor needs to be flexible, and adapt techniques when needed for the specific needs of the student, as the hearing loss and other considerations associated with some of the syndromes that cause deaf-blindness necessitate a modification of the O&M curriculum for students who are deaf-blind. For example, syndromes such as Ushers I are associated with vestibular or balance difficulties, which often become exaggerated with vision loss or blindfolding because the only remaining sensory input available for balance is

from proprioception. With practice, the traveler who is deaf-blind usually learns to react more quickly to proprioceptive information, and develop compensatory strategies (see Chapter 5, which deals with balance difficulty).

For orientation, people who have no functional hearing as well as no vision may rely on information such as their understanding of the layout of their environment (their cognitive map), kinesthetic and tactile information, vibrations, air movements and temperature, the sun, and smells. For example, the student might know that the instructor is nearby from the slight vibration of the floor made by the instructor's footsteps, or the air the instructor stirs when walking by. Electronic travel aids (ETAs; see Chapter 14) can be helpful to people who are deaf-blind for orientation, not only for tasks such as finding overhanging obstacles and objects in open space such as poles and doorways, but also for augmenting information that is normally available to people who are blind and who have normal hearing. For example, a person who is deaf-blind can maintain alignment through open spaces by using an ETA to shoreline nearby lines such as buildings or hedges (which can often be done using echolocation by people with normal hearing) or by using the ETA to locate and walk toward an object ahead, including vehicles that are waiting on the street being crossed (E. Gervasoni, personal communication, March 10, 2007). A large percentage of individuals who are deaf-blind have useful residual vision or hearing or both, which needs to be assessed and utilized fully for orientation (see Volume 1, Chapters 3 and 4).

Most O&M techniques can be used by people who are deaf-blind with a few modifications and considerations related to communication issues, the inability to hear, and/or the balance difficulties inherent in syndromes of deaf-blindness such as Ushers I. For example, traditional O&M techniques as varied as human guide, street crossings, finding dropped objects, and sidewalk recovery use hearing (Hill & Ponder, 1976), so when teaching these skills to travelers who are deaf-blind, the O&M specialist will consider alternative techniques and strategies which alleviate the need for audition, straddle communication barriers, or address the unique travel needs of people who are deaf-blind. Some examples follow:

- Students who are deaf-blind benefit from learning to shoreline without becoming disoriented in driveways and openings. This is because students who are blind and have normal hearing are traditionally taught to maintain a mid-sidewalk orientation by using auditory clues from parallel traffic sounds and echolocation information, and an effective strategy for maintaining orientation along the sidewalk without this auditory information is to shoreline along a building, curb, grass line, or other natural boundary.

- Human guide techniques may need to be modified in order to facilitate communication with a student who is deaf-blind, for example when the guide and the person who is deaf-blind need to pass through closed doors. One such technique is for the guide to control the door himself or, if the door opens on the side of the student, place the student's hand on the door for him to hold as they pass through without the need for verbal explanation or instruction (Bourquin, 2002, 2005).

- Many travelers who are deaf-blind prefer *constant contact* (when the cane tip maintains contact with the ground surface ahead of the traveler) as their default cane technique, as they are unable to benefit from the sound of the cane tapping on the surface of the ground, and the constant-contact cane technique offers greater surface tactual information. Many tips are now available that glide well on various surfaces.

- Because they cannot hear environmental sounds and therefore are less aware of the surroundings, many travelers who are deaf-blind prefer to extend their reach by using a longer cane or an arc that is wider than normal. This modification of widening the arc provides travelers with more environmental information but, unless the cane tip touches the ground as it passes in front of them (as it does when using constant-contact cane technique), it may not provide sufficient warning of upcoming drop-offs.

- Some instructors find that students with a hearing loss and a corresponding vestibular problem experience balance problems that are exacerbated by the standard midline hand placement while using a cane. These students may prefer to offset the advantages of centering the cane by learning a strategy for maintaining an appropriate arc while holding the cane off-center.

These are but a few examples that demonstrate the need for the O&M specialist to be flexible when considering the standard curriculum for O&M, and willing to work with the traveler who is deaf-blind in considering and implementing appropriate but unconventional strategies when necessary.

Communication and learning styles need to be considered when planning the O&M program. The length of the program or individual sessions for people with whom communication is slow or cumbersome will need to be longer than it is for other people. Individuals who are deaf-blind and cognitively impaired often require an approach that allows for presenting skills and concepts first by describing them, then presenting them experientially, and finally reviewing them. Throughout this process, the instructor needs to keep in mind whether the student is conceptualizing either by sequential memorization of landmarks, understanding the interrelationship among the parts of the route, or understanding the spatial layout and the relationship of objects and landmarks within the area, and thereby being able to plan multiple routes through it (see Volume 1, Chapter 2).

Traveling in the Community

In order to travel independently in the community, people must know how to communicate and interact with the public, be able to make decisions, and be aware of the environment and safety issues. Although these are important to include in O&M programs for people who are blind, their importance is multiplied for blind people who are also deaf.

Because it is virtually impossible for any person to travel within a community without interacting with people, travelers need to consider how to do so effectively, and be aware of their effect on the public. Although this is somewhat difficult for people who cannot see others, the difficulty is magnified for people who also cannot hear, which makes this one of the most crucial issues for the O&M specialist to address with students who are deaf-blind. Many people with visual and hearing impairments assume that others recognize that they can not hear or that others know how to communicate with them. Yet, not only is the public typically unaware of their disability, even when people who are deaf-blind write or say that they are deaf-blind and explain how to communicate, people usually do not understand or are too startled to respond appropriately. When this happens, the person who is deaf-blind often misconstrues people's reaction and assumes that they are calloused, intentionally rude, afraid, or have an aversion to people who are deaf-blind. When this happens repeatedly, the person who is deaf-blind can become reluctant to interact with the public further. To alleviate this situation, the O&M instructor can (1) prepare the student with successful strategies to communicate with the public (communication strategies are described in the next section), (2) help the student realize that people will be confused and uninformed and will require patience and repeated explanations of exactly how to communicate with or help him, and (3) describe how others reacted when they interacted with the student. When providing this feedback, the instructor gives details and is honest.

Because access to pedestrians may be difficult or undependable for travelers who are deaf-blind once they are in the community, it is usually best if they gather relevant information and plan their trips as much as possible ahead of time. For example, they will want to know about community characteristics, general business hours, locations that are likely to have pedestrian traffic, how safe or dangerous the area is, and whether there are particular areas within the community that need to be avoided.

Communication Strategies with the Public

Travelers who are deaf-blind need to be able to communicate with the public for such tasks as finding a salesperson and making a purchase, or getting information or assistance when they are lost or need to plan alternative routes because of construction or bus changes. Because people often do not respond to the first approach or explanation, the traveler who is deaf-blind needs to be skilled at several communication methods that can be used with the public. For example, one person may use gestures, prepared cards, and pictures labeled tactilely; another uses spoken English, printing on the palm, and gestures. Travelers whose communication skills are limited need to learn to recognize when they need assistance and be familiar with strategies to get it.

To communicate with others, the traveler first needs to get their attention using such strategies as the following:

- Gestures, such as tapping the cane or appearing to look around for help.

- Sounds, such as spoken voice, recorded messages, or a whistle.

- Notes, cards, or signs held where others can see them. These need to be legible and, if being held up for others to see, have key words visible from a distance. To avoid showing the wrong message or holding it upside down, the notes and cards need to be organized (perhaps putting them on a ring or in a notebook to keep them in order), and easily identifiable to the traveler using such techniques as clipped corners, staples, hole punches, color coding, and special notations in large print or braille.

Regardless of the method used, the traveler's message needs to provide information in the following order:

- First: The assistance being requested

- Second: How others can offer assistance or communicate

- Last: The traveler's visual and hearing impairment

For example, an effective message might be, "Can you please tell me if this is the 90 bus? Please nod your head 'yes' or 'no' because I am deaf and can't see well." Typical cards may be worded as shown in Figure 17.4.

The traveler who is deaf-blind needs to specify to others exactly how they can communicate or assist; the method chosen will depend on the situation and the traveler's skills. Some suggestions are for the traveler to ask the public to

- tap the traveler to indicate their presence or willingness to help (the traveler might then give more specific instructions);

- write or spell to the traveler in a specified manner, such as print in large letters with a marker that the traveler provides, print on the traveler's palm, type into a device that has a keyboard for the speaker, and a braille or print display for the receiver (such as a screen braille communicator, as already mentioned);

- speak to the traveler in a specified manner, such as in a place where the traveler can speechread

> Please help me to
> CROSS STREET.
> TAP ME if you can help because
> I am DEAF and BLIND.
> Thank you.

> Please HELP ME get some
> INFORMATION
> so I can find where I am going.
> TAP ME if you can help because I am both
> DEAF and BLIND.
> You can print letters in my palm with your finger. THANK YOU.

Dona Sauerburger

Figure 17.4.
Samples of typical cards that can be used by individuals who are deaf-blind to communicate with members of the public.

well, or into the microphone of the traveler's assistive listening device, or close to the traveler's ear;

- signal "yes" or "no" by nodding one's head, or tapping twice for "yes" and once for "no"; or

- do something specific, such as point to (or turn the traveler to face toward) the destination or guide her to it, make a phone call, or draw a map. A traveler who wants to expedite communication or whose limited understanding of English makes it difficult to understand statements written by others might instead plan the communication to structure their response. For example, the traveler might ask others to check items from a multiple-choice list or fill in blanks in a form prepared ahead of time (with assistance if needed), or point (with their own or the traveler's finger) to the appropriate place on a tactile, braille, or large-print list, map, or form.

Public Transportation

Because communication with the public is difficult for many travelers who are deaf-blind, it is essential that they plan ahead as much as possible when using public transportation. Accurate background information will be needed relating to schedules, route numbers or names, and fares. When using buses, trains, or taxis, there needs to be an awareness of the form of assistance that will be needed. A plan needs to include how to communicate to obtain assistance and then prepare whatever notes, cards, recorded messages, equipment, maps, or drawings will be needed. To get some of this information by telephone, travelers may use amplifiers, text or video relay services, or an interpreter (see the earlier section in this chapter, Considerations for Communication, for information about how people who are deaf-blind can communicate by telephone). Once the communication cards are prepared, the traveler needs to organize them in a fashion that allows them to identify their message, and how they need to be oriented for presentation to the public.

Travelers who cannot see, hear, or reliably feel the air movement when the bus or train approaches can detect it using an electronic travel aid (ETA) or vibrotactile device which changes sound into vibration, or solicit aid using strategies already described. If there are usually no other people where the traveler waits for the bus, she can hold up a card or sign informing drivers which bus she desires, asking to be guided to it when it arrives, and explaining that she is deaf and blind. Taxi passengers need to inform the dispatcher how the driver needs to announce and identify himself (for example, ring the doorbell and hand the traveler his identification when the door opens; or look in the lobby for a tall woman with blond hair and a white cane and tap her on the shoulder; or ask the dispatcher to call the traveler and inform her that the taxi is in front of the house; and so forth). When the driver arrives, the traveler needs to inform him how to communicate, and repeat the explanation if needed (especially when the driver needs to inform the traveler of the fare).

Travelers need to use an appropriate communication method to inform the bus or taxi driver where they want to get off. Giving the driver a note, even if the communication is verbal, helps avoid misunderstandings as well as awkward situations when the driver forgets the destination and tries to ask the traveler to repeat it. Travelers who cannot recognize when they have arrived at their destination need to ask the driver to inform them by a specified method (tap or wave at them, hand them their note back, or whatever is most appropriate). Bus drivers may see the travelers and be less likely to forget about them if they sit near the door or directly in back of the driver. This location has typically been set aside for passengers with disabilities, and students need to be familiarized with it. Holding a note with the name of their stop on their lap also helps others remember to inform them when to get off.

Train and subway passengers often can recognize their station by counting how many times the train stops and opens its doors (as the doors open, passengers who are deaf-blind may feel a breeze or check with their cane or hand to feel the opening, and sometimes they can feel the vibrations of the opening door in the wall next to it) or noting such cues as which stations are far apart, crowded, aboveground or below, and so forth.

Crossing Streets and Driveways

When teaching skills and concepts for crossing streets, driveways, or lanes to people who are blind or visually impaired, regardless of their hearing ability, O&M specialists can consider (and teach their students to consider) the following issues:

- Strategies for crossing each given situation, using whatever information (sensory or otherwise) is available

- Risks of crossing in a given situation
- Strategies to reduce those risks
- Whether the risks are acceptable
- Alternatives when the risks of crossing alone are not acceptable

Students who have functional hearing or vision are taught to use that hearing and vision and tactile and kinesthetic information as efficiently as possible to determine the intersection's geometry, traffic control and traffic patterns, alignment, and appropriate time to initiate the crossing. Additional street-crossing information can sometimes be gained from sources such as accessible pedestrian signals (APS), electronic travel aids (ETAs), and devices such as a Tactaid, which vibrates in response to sounds. Unfamiliar intersections need to be analyzed to determine such features as the geometry of the intersection and its traffic control as well as the traffic volume that is typical for various times of the day. People who don't have the ability to perceive and process sufficient visual or auditory information to perform this analysis need to know how to use the assistance of people with vision or hearing to get enough information to do so. The assistant can describe the intersection geometry (width of streets and the angle of the intersection) effectively by using a tactile map or drawing the design on the person's back or hand, and can describe the pattern, volume, and speed of traffic by pointing to the vehicles as they pass (with the hand of the person who is deaf-blind on the assistant's pointing hand) or drawing their movement on the person's back or hand. Since traffic often varies according to the time of day and week, the observation of the traffic needs to be done at various times to enable the person who is deaf-blind to understand the typical situations at that intersection throughout the day or at the time of day she is likely to travel there.

Using Functional Vision or Hearing

At signalized intersections, people who are deaf-blind and have sufficient functional vision can scan for dangers at the appropriate time in correct sequence (see the section on Analyzing Signalized Intersections in Chapter 12). For visual scanning and assessing the speed and distance of vehicles at crossings with no traffic control, see the section on Assessment of Crossings and Detection of Gaps and Uncertainty in Chapter 12.

For suggestions to facilitate and augment functional hearing, see Volume 1, Chapter 4. Skills such as localizing traffic surges and using the sound of traffic for alignment can be taught by having the consumer first experience the sounds with feedback, then try to apply the use of those sounds.

For example, to learn the use of traffic sounds for alignment, the student needs to listen to the traffic when he's aligned, then change positions to be slightly misaligned and distinguish the difference. If he detects no difference, he can exaggerate the misalignment until he can distinguish it. If he can make the distinction, he can practice using the sounds to align.

To learn to localize the sounds of traffic surges, the student can stand at a four-way stop-sign intersection, where the sources of traffic surges are unpredictable. The instructor identifies from where the sound of each vehicular surge is coming, and when the student seems able to differentiate the sources, he can practice identifying where each surge is coming from.

These exercises need to be done not only during initial training, but also whenever people lose any hearing. Unilateral or asymmetrical hearing losses often distort sounds, and people need to understand how the traffic sounds with their current hearing.

Using Devices to Gain Information

At signalized intersections, accessible pedestrian signals (APS) with vibrotactile output can enable people who are deaf-blind to recognize the onset of the walk or green signal; regulations are being proposed that all APS have vibrotactile output, and many APS have it now. However it is important that the person who is deaf-blind: realize the risks of vehicles turning into his path; knows how to reduce those risks; and makes decisions as to whether the risks are acceptable (see Chapter 12). Also, the vibration of the pedestrian signal caused by rumbling trucks has sometimes been mistaken for that of the signal, so it is important that the person who is deaf-blind be able to reliably identify the signal's vibration and distinguish it from other environmental vibrations. Modern APS that require pedestrians to push a button may have a locator tone to enable blind pedestrians to find the button (again, see Chapter 12), but blind pedestrians who cannot hear the locator tone can use a systematic searching pattern to find it (see Chapter 12 for conditions that might indicate the need to search for a pedestrian pushbutton).

People who are deaf-blind have used ETAs at signalized intersections to augment awareness of traffic movement and position (E. Gervasoni, personal communication, March 10, 2007). In the early 1980s, trainers at The Seeing Eye tried using a specially modified extended-range ETA with several graduates with moderate to severe hearing losses to detect patterns of vehicles moving in the intersection. This effort didn't succeed, at least in part because of technical problems with the device (Lukas Franck, personal correspondence, January 2007). As with all street-crossing tasks, the strategy of using an ETA as well as the skill to use it should be dependable in order to be considered a reliable strategy.

Devices which transform sounds into vibrotactile output, such as the Tactaid, have been used to detect approaching vehicles in quiet situations (Sauerburger, 1987). In most situations the detection of vehicles with this device is insufficient to be certain that there is a gap long enough to cross. However, when the person who is deaf-blind has decided that the risk of undetected approaching vehicles is acceptable at a given situation because of the low volume or slow speed of the traffic there, the vibrotactile device may provide additional security, and help avoid walking into a moving vehicle.

When There's Not Enough Information

Sometimes all available sensory input and technological resources are not sufficient to obtain all the information needed to determine where, how, and when to cross, as well as how much risk is involved in crossing. For example, the person who has no functional vision or hearing may be able to use assistance to determine an intersection's geometry to know where to stand and how to align to cross, and an APS to determine when to start crossing and an ETA to determine if any vehicles are nearby, but may not be able to determine whether a vehicle is turning left into the crosswalk from the other side of the street or approaching to make a right-turn-on-red too fast to stop for the pedestrian.

If the risk is too great, travelers who are deaf-blind can consider alternatives to independent crossing, such as the following:

1. Getting assistance to cross

2. Crossing where they can hear or see better, or are more expected by and visible to the drivers

3. Crossing at a different intersection with more effective traffic control

4. Avoiding the crossing (take the bus to end of line; have food or merchandise delivered; use rides and taxis, bus/paratransit, and so forth)

5. Requesting engineering alterations such as APS; leading pedestrian intervals which reduce conflicting traffic by providing a walk signal to pedestrians a few seconds before

vehicles; providing bulbouts (curbing extensions into the street on opposite outside shorelines) resulting in a shortened street-crossing distance and narrowing the street to slow the traffic. (See Chapter 12 and Volume 1, Chapter 11 on accessibility and complex environments.)

Getting Assistance to Cross

People can get assistance to cross from passersby or, in places where there are few or no other pedestrians, from drivers or people in the community.

To get assistance from a passerby, people who are deaf-blind need to capture his attention and convey not only that they want to cross the street but also that they need assistance to do so. To capture attention, the person who is deaf-blind can make sure to be visible and not hidden behind poles, bushes, or parked vehicles, and can go to places where there are likely to be people, such as busy corners, bus stops, and business entrances. Devices such as ETAs can be used to indicate the presence of pedestrians.

The desire to cross the street can be conveyed to the public by standing at the curb and facing the street, but this does not convey the need for assistance. According to a survey of several dozen passersby (Sauerburger & Jones, 1997), some people who see a person standing at the curb with a white cane or dog guide will assume that she needs no assistance, and pass by. Thus the person who is deaf-blind must convey not only the desire to cross, but also the need for assistance, for example with body language and gestures, a card, voice, recorded message, or the like. The O&M specialist can help the person who is deaf-blind evaluate which strategies are most effective for that person in that situation by observing the public's reactions and reporting them to the person who is deaf-blind.

When assistance is offered, the person who is deaf-blind needs to immediately indicate which street she wants to cross, for example by pointing to that street when tapped. The person who is deaf-blind needs to learn to recognize when she is being guided across the wrong street, and be able to indicate to the guide that she wants to cross the other street.

Using Cards

People who are deaf-blind have been soliciting assistance to cross streets using communication cards for at least 65 years (Bourquin & Moon, 2008). The effectiveness of using a card to obtain assistance has been studied since 1988, when DeFiore and Silver (1988) observed that enlarging the size of key words on the card decreased the average time required for someone to obtain assistance. Florence and LaGrow (1989) observed that very few passersby would help a woman when she tried to hand them a card which said she is deaf-blind and needed assistance to cross. Further studies (Franklin & Bourquin, 2000; Sauerburger & Jones, 1997) demonstrated greater success when holding the card up near the shoulder where it can be seen from the front and back, rather than trying to hand people the card. Sauerburger and Jones (1997) learned that the card first needs to indicate the need for help to cross the street, then ask the public to tap the person who is deaf-blind, and finally explain that the person is deaf and blind.

Franklin and Bourquin (2000) added graphics to the design of the communication card illustrating human guide technique to increase recognition and comprehension by the public. In two subsequent investigations, a pilot study at the Helen Keller National Center and a dissertation research project (Bourquin, 2007; Bourquin & Moon, 2008), variables such as intersection type, the gender of the traveler who is deaf-blind and the helper, and other environmental factors were possible influences on the effectiveness of cards. Results of the regression analysis showed that larger communication cards solicited assis-

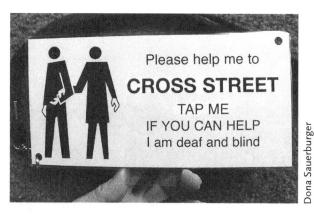

Figure 17.5.

A 4-×8-inch card for obtaining help with street crossings.

tance from the public at statistically significant quicker rates for travelers who are deaf-blind. In experiments in suburban and urban settings, travelers received help with a street crossing card sized 4×8 inches in a mean wait time of about 30 seconds, or on average until two or three pedestrians passed by the person who is deaf-blind (see Figures 17.5 and 17.6).

Drivers will get out of their vehicles and guide people across if they are aware of the need, for example if they see a person holding up a small sign with words such as "Help Cross Street" written large enough for the drivers to see easily. The sign can have more text, such as "Please tap me if you can help; I am both deaf and blind" written in smaller print to be read when someone approaches. This strategy seems to work well when drivers have a place to pull over conveniently, and when the traffic has a stop sign or signal or if it is moving slowly enough that drivers can read the sign, although drivers seem reluctant to get out of their vehicle in inclement weather. People who are deaf-blind can experiment to see how likely they will get assistance from the drivers at a given location and circumstances, and brainstorm with the O&M specialist to improve the sign or their position and posture if needed.

Often, people in the community are also willing to assist people who are deaf-blind to cross the street. For example the person who is deaf-blind can ask for assistance from customers and staff inside nearby stores or businesses (Gervasoni, 1996), or make arrangements with residents or businesspeople near the intersection (Sauerburger, 1993). One woman who is deaf-blind had to cross an intersection to get to the subway to work. She used her braille TTY and the relay service to telephone a 7-11 convenience store that was across that street. They agreed to watch for her, and she would then go to the corner and wait for their assistance. Other people make arrangements when they schedule an appointment with their hairdressers, such that the staff will watch for them to get off the bus and then will go over to help them get across the street.

When being guided across the street, the person who is deaf-blind needs to have the arm of the guide in order to be in control and ensure that he is not abandoned before reaching the other side. The public will often be concerned about and follow or accompany or try to guide the person who is deaf-blind after the crossing, so when they reach the other side, unless the person who is deaf-blind wants assistance to cross the other street, he needs to clearly indicate that he is fine and needs no more assistance—a "thumbs-up" sign is often effective for this purpose.

Some people who are deaf-blind who feel comfortable with the risks of unexpected or turning vehicles do not want people to guide them across, but only to inform them when it is time to start crossing. In this case, it is important that clear, unambiguous communication be established for the other person to indicate the time to cross. Some examples of this type of communication could be asking the other person to give a unique signal that is not commonly used such as squeezing the hand of the deaf-blind person or, if the person who is deaf-blind has enough vision or hearing, having the other person indicate

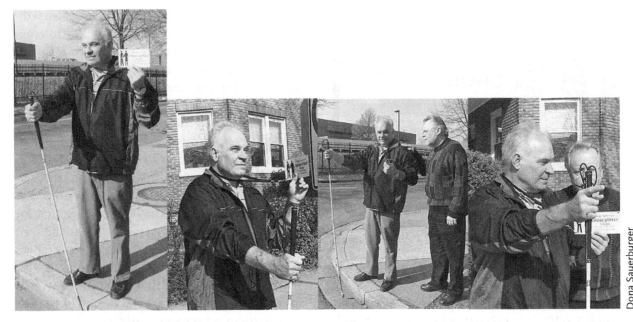

Dona Sauerburger

Figure 17.6
To get assistance to cross a street, the person who is deaf-blind stands at the curb facing the street to be crossed, holding the street-crossing card over the shoulder where it can be seen from behind as well as in front, and periodically turning the card 90 degrees to be seen from the sides. When tapped, the deaf-blind person points toward the street that he desires to cross.

crossing time verbally or by pointing. Having a stranger simply tap the person who is deaf-blind to indicate it is time to cross can too easily be miscommunicated.

DOG GUIDES

Some people who are deaf-blind choose to use dog guides for many of the same reasons as do people who are blind and can hear, and they can utilize the dog guide just as effectively (see Chapter 16 and Volume 1, Chapter 9). Like any dog guide user, travelers who are deaf-blind need to know where they are going. They also need to recognize when the dog needs correction (for example, when it is distracted and reaches to sniff something or veers the wrong way), which is normally accomplished by noting the dog's movement, not by hearing. Those who are unable to give the dog appropriate verbal commands

can use a dog guide trained to recognize hand signals or gestures. For more detail on using dog guides see Chapter 16.

SUMMARY

The purpose of this chapter is to encourage the O&M specialist to become knowledgeable about and professionally involved with the deaf-blind population. While individuals who are deaf-blind may be different from other O&M students, they will offer the O&M specialist an opportunity to be imaginative and creative. Working with these individuals will offer a chance for O&M specialists to expand their knowledge base and develop practical learning applications in a variety of domains. For example, there will be the need to learn about effective communication modes, become aware of relevant technical support equipment; evaluate the pros and cons of modifications in cane techniques, and become sensitized to environmental modifications for someone with hearing and vision losses. Two of the more critical areas for travelers who are deaf-blind are the abilities to negotiate street crossings and solicit assistance for travel-related needs. These critical skill areas are linked to the success your students will achieve in traveling comfortably within their environments.

This chapter discusses the full range of the deaf-blind population. Whether the O&M specialist is working with preschool or school-age children, working-age adults in the community, or older individuals, there is background material within this chapter to get started. It is our conviction that, once understood, this material best serves your students as you apply and, when needed, adapt it to their particular travel needs.

IMPLICATIONS FOR O&M PRACTICE

1. The O&M specialist does not need to be reluctant to work with people who are deaf-blind because, with the exception of communication, most of the training and O&M strategies will be the same as they are for hearing blind people.

2. Because limited sensory input results in limited incidental learning and knowledge of what is happening, it is critical that O&M specialists provide information about and discuss the events and qualities within environments for their students who are deaf-blind. Without this opportunity to discuss things with others, even those who have a variety of experiences can be experientially deprived because they aren't aware of or don't understand what is happening.

3. For people whose communication is minimal, one of the priorities of the O&M specialist is to help develop strategies to enable them to anticipate what is happening, understand the intent of their O&M sessions, and make choices.

4. Because people who cannot see or hear need to communicate and learn about their world primarily through touch, there is a need for physical contact, which makes some people uncomfortable, and this can make it difficult for them to attend to learning. The instructor and the student can reduce the uncertainty by discussing this issue frankly, clarifying each of their levels of comfort with touching, and considering what kinds of physical contact are appropriate and acceptable with others.

5. Clear, comfortable communication is necessary for learning to take place, so an O&M specialist's first priority is to determine how she can communicate most proficiently with students and arrange for whatever interpreters or communication systems are needed. The O&M specialist should be aware of the common communication techniques and tips for using them, which are explained in this chapter. The O&M specialist should also realize that each person who is deaf-blind is unique, and, in order to learn effectively, the O&M specialist will need to use communication methods that are appropriate and comfortable for that person.

6. American Sign Language (ASL) is a distinct language, and not the English language conveyed with signs. Thus when the O&M specialist is working with students whose language is ASL, it would be inappropriate and ineffective to teach by using English, even if it is spelled out or signed for the student. If the O&M specialist is not fluent in ASL, an interpreter is needed to teach these students.

7. The O&M specialist needs to establish a way to quickly identify herself, such as creating a special signal or sign, and use it whenever approaching the student who is deaf-blind.

8. The O&M specialist can teach students who are deaf-blind how to phone for directions, bus information, and taxis, just as she does for students who are blind and have normal hearing, because there are devices and relay services by which people who are deaf-blind can use the telephone to call other people. People who are deaf-blind can also be alerted to the ringing telephone, doorbell, and smoke alarm by using pagers that are marketed for people who are deaf.

9. Individuals who are deaf-blind and multiply impaired often require an approach which allows for skills and concepts to first be presented in a descriptive way, then presented experientially, and finally presented and reviewed descriptively again.

10. O&M programs for students who are deaf-blind place more emphasis on teaching how to communicate and interact with the public, be able to make decisions, and be aware of the environment and safety issues than do O&M programs for students who are blind and have normal hearing.

11. One of the crucial issues for the O&M specialist to address when teaching people who are deaf-blind is how to interact with the public. The O&M instructor should (a) prepare the student with successful strategies to communicate with the public, (b) help the student realize that people will need to be informed (often repeatedly) exactly how to communicate with or help the person who is deaf-blind, and (c) describe how others reacted when they interacted with the student.

12. Because the public often does not respond to the first approach or explanation of a person who is deaf-blind, travelers who are deaf-blind need to be skilled at several communication methods that can be used with the public. Regardless of the method used, the traveler's message should provide information in the following order: what assistance is being requested, how others can offer assistance or communicate, and the traveler's visual and hearing impairment.

13. O&M specialists teach students who have functional vision or hearing how to use it most effectively to cross streets, including where and how to scan for vehicles that might cross their path. They also teach them how to recognize those situations in which they are unable to detect vehicles or traffic signals well enough to know when is the appropriate time to cross a given intersection or driveway, and to make decisions concerning which of these situations are too risky to cross independently. The O&M specialist provides them with enough information to make these decisions (such as frequency of moving vehicles, the likelihood that drivers will see and stop for them, and so forth), and alternative strategies such as how to solicit assistance and plan alternative routes.

LEARNING ACTIVITIES

1. It is possible for students who are deaf-blind who have a variety of experiences to be experientially deprived. How can this happen and how can it be avoided?

2. Explain the O&M instructor's first priority when meeting a student who is deaf-blind.

3. Describe how an O&M instructor who is not fluent in American Sign Language (ASL) should communicate with a student whose primary language is ASL.

4. Discuss whether O&M instructors can rely on spelling (fingerspelling, writing notes, Teletouch, and so forth) to communicate with students who are deaf-blind and whose language is ASL.

5. Describe how people who are deaf-blind should communicate with the public. What

information does their message need to convey, and in what order?

6. When people who are deaf-blind communicate with the public, they need to explain how the other person can respond. What are some ways that the public can respond to people who are deaf-blind?

7. Without proper intervention and training, many people who are deaf-blind become reluctant to interact with the public. Why does this happen, and what can the O&M specialist do to prevent it?

8. Explain how people who are deaf-blind can call bus companies for information.

9. Explain how people who are deaf-blind can use taxis.

10. Describe how people who are deaf with functional vision can cross at intersections with traffic signals when they cannot see the signal.

11. Explain the choices available to people in situations where their hearing and vision is insufficient to identify the appropriate time to cross a street.

12. For some students, deafness has a social rather than an audiological meaning. Discuss how this might impact the lesson planning of the mobility specialist.

CHAPTER 18

Teaching Orientation and Mobility to Learners with Visual, Physical, and Health Impairments

Sandra Rosen and James S. Crawford

LEARNING QUESTIONS

- Why is it important for O&M specialists to be knowledgeable about physical or health impairments and about the use of ambulatory aids?

- What do O&M specialists need to know about physical and health impairments and about ambulatory aids?

- What neurological, orthopedic, and health impairments (that can impact mobility) are common in children? Adults? Which do, or can, have a related visual impairment?

- How do these physical or health impairments affect physical functioning, and in turn, mobility?

- What are the basic types of ambulatory aids used by people with physical or health impairments?

- How can standard mobility techniques be modified for students who use ambulatory aids?

One purpose of this chapter is to provide a brief overview of common physical and health impair-

ments. While it is impossible to cover all conditions in one chapter, we focus on some of the most common physical and health impairments that O&M specialists serving students with visual impairments may encounter. Some of these conditions have associated visual impairments; others do not, yet are sufficiently prevalent in the population that teachers are likely to serve students who have such conditions at some time in their careers (see Sidebar 18.1). A brief explanation of the medical nature of each condition will be given to provide an understanding of its unique impact on O&M. The rest of this chapter deals with the use of ambulatory aids and explores modifications of mobility techniques and techniques for O&M instruction for people with both visual and other disabilities.

The number of people who have health concerns in addition to visual impairment is increasing. Medical technology has increased the survival rate of at-risk neonates (Hintz, Kendrick, Vohr, Poole, & Higgins, 2005), although often with serious medical complications. In addition,

Physical Disabilities Frequently Accompanying Vision Loss

A basic understanding of the causes and effects of physical disabilities that can accompany vision loss is necessary in the management of students with multiple impairments, in program planning, and in the provision of high-quality, comprehensive service.

The following list includes three basic categories of disability. It is by no means comprehensive, but it is an overview of conditions that, when occurring together with vision loss, can directly affect the education and rehabilitation of people with visual impairments.

1. Conditions that occur independent of visual impairment and that are found in the visually impaired population to the same degree as in the general population

   a. Rheumatoid arthritis

   b. Amputation or orthopedic impairment

   c. Cardiovascular disorder (e.g., heart disease or high blood pressure)

   d. Selected neurological disorders (e.g., seizure disorders)

   e. Hearing loss

   f. Osteoarthritis

2. Conditions that may occur as a direct or indirect result of vision loss or that may be intensified secondary to visual impairment

   a. Vertebral and postural deformities

   b. Poor sensory development and awareness

3. Conditions that frequently have an associated visual impairment

   a. Diabetes mellitus

   b. Cerebrovascular accident (i.e., stroke)

   c. Cerebral palsy

   d. Multiple sclerosis

   e. Acquired brain injury

---

as people live longer, they are subject to many of the physical conditions and impairments associated with aging (see Chapter 10).

Unlike students who are solely visually impaired, students who also have physical disabilities and/or health impairments come with a vast array of different conditions and needs. Some students have conditions affecting their neurological systems; some their bones and muscles; others have conditions affecting their lungs, heart, digestive system, and even their skin.

Each condition potentially affects mobility in different ways. It can easily be said that no two students with physical disabilities and/or health impairments are the same. Information on a student's medical condition can usually be found in school records, from the rehabilitation counselor, or sometimes from the student himself. When information is not automatically available to the O&M specialist, the adult student, or parent or guardian of a younger student, may sign a release form to allow the O&M specialist to obtain information from medical records provided by a doctor or other health care provider. Orientation and mobility specialists need to check with their employers on specific procedures for obtaining information about an individual's physical and medical conditions. Employers may also have regulations on how that information can be shared and with whom it can be shared. The procedures for intervening in medical emergencies will also vary from employer to employer.

ORTHOPEDIC IMPAIRMENTS

Orthopedic impairments are those that affect primarily the muscles, bones, and joints. Two of the most common orthopedic conditions are arthritis and osteoporosis.

Arthritis

With regard to arthritis, there are two general categories—rheumatoid arthritis and osteoarthritis. Rheumatoid arthritis is an autoimmune process that can affect children (known as Still's disease) as well as adults, causing pain and damage to affected joints. Osteoarthritis is more commonly seen in adults and generally results from long-term wear and tear on the joints (most often the hips and knees).

Rheumatoid Arthritis

Rheumatoid arthritis (RA) is an autoimmune condition, meaning that the body forms antibodies against some of its own tissues. RA affects small joints in a bilateral and symmetrical manner. The severity of the symptoms can fluctuate from day to day or even from morning to evening, although muscle and joint stiffness are usually notable in the morning and after periods of inactivity. Symptoms may increase in cold temperatures, or with overexercise or fatigue.

In advanced cases of RA there is a characteristic joint deformity of the fingers and toes called *subluxation with ulnar deviation*, which means that the joints between the fingers and hand, for example, degenerate and the fingers begin to deviate toward the little finger side. When the person bends his fingers (as in holding a cane), the fingers tend to pull further toward the little finger side, adding stress and discomfort at the joints. This can cause pain when holding the cane. Lastly, people who have RA may be taking anti-inflammatory medications such as aspirin. It is always important for the O&M specialist to know what medications a

student is taking and any potential side effects of those medications (see the section on Medications for Health Conditions later in this chapter). Many people who take long-term aspirin therapy, for example, can develop high-tone hearing losses that disappear when treatment is stopped.

As already mentioned, RA is not just a disease of adults or of the elderly. There is a form of RA that affects children and is called by many names, including *juvenile rheumatoid arthritis* (JRA), *Still's disease*, or *juvenile chronic polyarthritis*. In addition to the typical symptoms of RA described, it needs to be noted that some students with JRA can develop iritis (inflammation of the iris). This condition can give students photophobia (hypersensitivity to light) and blurred vision. As a result, these students will often wear UV-protectant sunglasses if sunlight causes discomfort.

Osteoarthritis

The symptoms of osteoarthritis are similar to those of rheumatoid arthritis, but people are not as greatly affected by cold temperatures. Although any joint can be affected, osteoarthritis most notably affects the large, primarily weight-bearing joints and may or may not be either bilateral or symmetrical.

Implications for O&M Training

When working with a student who has arthritis, one of the most important things to keep in mind is to minimize pain and stress on arthritic joints and thereby help to prevent further joint damage. A rule to always observe is "If it hurts, don't do it"! Some sample modifications and tips to reduce stress on the joints are as follows:

- If grasping the handle of a cane increases pain in the finger joints, build up the diameter of the cane grip to ease the stress on the finger joints. This can be done by simply wrapping some sort of padding around the grip. Pipe insulation or several layers of the tape that bicyclists use to wrap bicycle handlebars work well for this purpose.

- Have the student use a lightweight cane to reduce the stress placed on hand and wrist joints.

- There are many commercially available creams that advertise providing a temporary reduction in joint discomfort. Also, wrapping painful joint(s) in 7–13 layers of thick, dry towels for 20–30 minutes before a lesson can sometimes reduce pain sufficiently to allow more comfortable participation in an O&M lesson. Wrapping the joint(s) in towels works by concentrating the body's heat in the joint(s) where the additional warmth helps to alleviate discomfort.

- Plan lessons to avoid overexercise or fatigue, which can exacerbate symptoms. Occasional rest periods can also be very effective in prolonging productivity.

- Be aware that symptoms may increase in cold temperatures—the traveler needs to dress warmly and wear warm gloves when needed.

Osteoporosis

Osteoporosis is a chronic condition in which the bones thin, becoming brittle and weak. While there is a variation of the condition called *osteogenesis imperfecta* that affects children, most cases of osteoporosis are seen in the elderly. Whenever the condition exists, however, it increases the potential for broken bones from falls, or in severe cases, from even seemingly harmless bumps. Extra caution is needed on O&M lessons to ensure that a traveler with osteoporosis does not stumble or fall and proper cane technique can become critical to ensure that the traveler will detect all obstacles with the cane and not her body. If a traveler is prone to falling (for example, has impaired balance or travels on uneven terrain such as unpaved roads or broken sidewalks), a physical therapist can be consulted to determine if a support cane or walker would help provide additional support to help prevent serious falls during travel.

Use of Prostheses

Prostheses are used to replace missing body parts such as hands, arms, feet, and legs. Body parts may be missing because of injury, congenital birth defects, or following amputation necessitated by complications from certain medical conditions such as diabetes or cancer.

The most important considerations when working with a student who uses a prosthesis is to know what motions can and cannot be performed using the prosthesis. For example, students who have an above-knee prosthesis will generally go up a step or curb with their other leg first, and down with the prosthetic leg first. Some students who have a below-the-knee prosthesis will do the same. Students who have two arm prostheses may benefit from a special holder to attach the cane to one of the prostheses. The cane techniques will, of course, need to be modified so that the student can perform them within the functional limitations of the prostheses. Ask the student to show you what he can do with his prosthesis and any modifications he uses to perform tasks. Also, remember that prostheses don't transmit sensation. So the student will not be able to discern texture differences underfoot or to receive tactile information through the cane.

One of the biggest concerns to students who use prostheses, especially leg prostheses, can be skin breakdown caused by rubbing between the student's residual limb and the socket of the prosthesis. Depending on the student's medical condition, he may or may not feel pain or discomfort when this happens. See the subsection entitled Pressure Sores under the Diabetes section later in this chapter for information on what to watch out for and how to handle any situations in which there is skin irritation caused by a poorly fitting prosthesis.

Use of Orthoses

Orthoses are splints or braces that are designed to either support joints during motion or to help maintain alignment of joints and prevent deformity. Orthoses worn on the leg might serve to prevent foot drop (the inability to lift the forefoot to prevent dragging the toe on the ground when taking a step), or they might support the knee to keep it from buckling or hyperextending during weight bearing. Orthoses worn on the arm most commonly serve to support hand and wrist joints in the presence of conditions such as severe rheumatoid arthritis that can lead to deformities.

Orthoses are generally made by professionals called *orthotists*. Occupational therapists also make some orthoses to support specific hand and arm functions. If a student complains of discomfort from an orthosis or the O&M specialist notes an unexplained change in gait pattern, it might signify that the orthosis is not fitting properly. Check for skin breakdown (see the subsection entitled Pressure Sores later in the chapter under the Diabetes section). The student will often be referred to an occupational therapist or doctor to check the fit of an orthosis.

NEUROLOGICAL IMPAIRMENTS

Neurological impairments encompass a wide range of conditions affecting the brain, spinal cord, and the peripheral nerves that connect the spinal cord to the skin and muscles of the body. Some conditions are progressive, but others are not. This section provides an overview of some of the most prevalent neurological conditions that have unique implications for O&M: brain injury, seizure disorders, and multiple sclerosis.

Brain Injury

Although they share many of the same symptoms, there are actually two different classifications of brain injury: traumatic brain injury (TBI) and acquired brain injury (ABI).

Traumatic brain injury is caused by an external physical force that is hard enough to cause the brain to move within the skull, or to break the skull and directly injure the brain. It can occur from such things as automobile accidents, falls, sporting injuries, and shaken baby syndrome.

Acquired brain injury is caused by a disruption in oxygen to the brain. Stroke, aneurysm, heart attack, tumors, infectious disease, toxic exposure, and drug abuse are some common causes.

As a special note, cerebral palsy is a form of brain injury (either TBI or ABI) that occurs prenatally, at birth, or during the first few years of life. There are many types of cerebral palsy which are classified by characteristics of muscle tone and distribution of involved extremities (see Sidebar 18.2).

Brain injury can occur at any age. The brain is divided into several sections, each with a primary purpose (for example, language, vision, emotion, sensory, motor, and cognition). Because of the brain's central role in how the body and mind operate, an injury to the brain can lead to any number of functional impairments: speech and language; memory; attention; reasoning; abstract thinking; concentration; judgment; problem solving; sensory, perceptual and motor abilities; psychosocial behavior; physical functions; as well as information processing and speech (Brain Injury, June 10, 2006). Brain injury in itself rarely presents with a single impairment, but often results in a variety of additional functional disabilities. The following sections focus on the sensory and motor aspects of brain injury. Cognitive, behavioral, and other implications are discussed in Chapter 19, "Teaching Orientation and Mobility to Students with Cognitive Impairments and Vision Loss."

Sensory Implications of Brain Injury

Brain injury can affect any or all of the sensory systems. These effects can be mild or severe, and can occur throughout, or in isolated parts of, the body. Many will have a significant impact on learning for students with visual impairment. This section will focus on those sensory systems

Cerebral Palsy: Classifications

Cerebral palsy is one of the most common additional disabilities found in children with visual impairments and constitutes 33 percent of the nonvisual disabilities associated with visual impairment (Flanagan, Jackson, & Hill, 2003).

Specific types of cerebral palsy are often classified on the basis of which part(s) of the body are affected and the impact of brain damage on motor functioning (specifically muscle tone). The most common classifications are as follows:

- *Hypotonic*: characterized by hypotonia (low muscle tone) throughout the body

- *Spastic*: characterized by hypertonia (high muscle tone). The tone is usually high in the affected extremities. Tone in the trunk may be either high or low.

- *Athetoid*: characterized by athetosis (fluctuating muscle tone). The student has abnormal shifts of muscle tone in which she assumes and retains abnormal and distorted postures. Facial movements, tongue, lip, and breath control are often involved, leading to problems in speech and eating. Involuntary, jerking, and irregular (*choreoathetoid*) movements may also be present.

- *Mixed*: characterized by hypertonia in some parts of the body and athetosis in other parts of the body. A common situation, for example, involves athetosis above the waist and spasticity below the waist. This is often called *spastic-athetoid*.

With regard to classification based on the part(s) of the body affected, the hypotonic, athetoid, and mixed forms of CP affect all four extremities; therefore, a classification of cerebral palsy related to the number of limbs involved is made only in the presence of spastic cerebral palsy:

- *Monoplegia*: weakness or paralysis of one extremity.

- *Hemiplegia*: weakness or paralysis of either the left or right side of the body, but not both. The arm and leg on the affected side generally have increased muscle tone, the arm typically being more involved than the leg. Symptoms of increased tone include difficulty lowering heel to the ground (excessive muscle tone in the calf) and holding the arm with the elbow bent. Because motor tracts cross at the brain stem, damage on right side of the brain causes left hemiplegia and vice versa.

- *Diplegia*: weakness or paralysis of all four extremities with only minimal involvement of the arms. Depending on the severity of involvement, the knees may tend to come tightly together or the legs may cross over one another ("scissoring"); due to high muscle tone in the calf muscles, the student may walk on tiptoes.

- *Paraplegia*: weakness or paralysis of the legs.

- *Triplegia*: weakness or paralysis of three extremities.

- *Quadriplegia*: weakness or paralysis of all four extremities with the legs more involved than the arms. The trunk and face may also be involved.

that most directly impact O&M: vision, hearing, touch, and proprioception.

Vision

Vision problems occur when structures of eye, eye tracts (optic nerve and optical pathways), or portions of the optical cortex are damaged. Visual skills that can be affected by brain injury include tracking, fixation, focusing, depth perception, peripheral vision, binocularity, maintaining attention, visualization, near vision acuity, distance acuity, and visual perception (Dutton, 2002; Thomas, 1994). See Chapters 3 and 20 for more information.

Tactile and Proprioceptive Sensation

Loss of tactile and proprioceptive sensation is not uncommon in brain injury, especially in some forms of cerebral palsy. Proprioceptive sensation tells a student the position of a body part in space. Poor proprioceptive feedback is one factor leading to the impaired balance and coordination seen in students with brain injury. With regard to tactile sensation, there are actually six types, any of which can be impaired in the presence of brain injury: deep touch (awareness of touch), light touch (texture discrimination), two-point touch (ability to differentiate between one and two points of contact under the fingertip—an essential ingredient to reading braille), vibration, pain, and temperature. Stereognosis (the ability to tactually identify an object in the hand) is a combination of tactile and proprioceptive inputs. While is it not always possible to improve tactile sensitivity or awareness when it is decreased due to brain injury, it is important for the O&M specialist to know what, if any, impairment a student might have. When tactile awareness cannot be improved, it becomes necessary to modify learning activities to de-emphasize (or, if necessary, eliminate) the need for tactile input. An occupational therapist or physical therapist can perform an easy assessment to determine the exact nature and extent of any tactile or proprioceptive impairment and can give suggestions for proprioceptive and tactile awareness activities that might be recommended for an individual student. Before deciding that the inability of a student with a brain injury to perform specific motor tasks is due to cognitive or motivational factors, have his sensation tested, if possible—this can save much time and frustration on the part of both the student and mobility specialist.

Hearing

Although not seen as commonly as visual impairments, hearing impairments can occur in the presence of brain injury. See Chapter 17 for more information on working with students who have both visual and hearing impairments.

Motor Implications of Brain Injury

Motor impairments can include abnormal muscle tone with reduced motor speed and loss of coordination, depending on the area of the brain involved and the severity of the injury.

Muscle Tone

Muscles work together in groups to effect movement. One set of muscles flexes (bends) a joint while another extends (straightens) it. Normally, when one group contracts, the other relaxes in a delicate balance of tone and controlled movement (see Volume 1, Chapter 5 for an additional discussion of muscle tone). In brain injury, the balance of this mechanism is disrupted and one of three things occurs: (1) excessive neural impulses are sent to some or all of the muscles resulting in excessive stiffness, (2) insufficient neural impulses are sent resulting in a lack of movement readiness, or (3) inconsistent neural impulses are sent resulting in fluctuating muscle tone (see Figure 18.1).

As mentioned earlier, muscle tone can be either low or high. A student with low muscle tone may appear "generally weak," but this is not the case. The "apparent weakness" is an artifact of the increased neurological effort to bring the muscle tone to baseline before movement can occur as well as the increased neurological input needed to give strength to that movement. Many students with hypotonia fatigue more quickly than those without hypotonia due to the increased neurological demands of sustained movement. While some students may be diagnosed as having *hypotonic cerebral palsy*, hypotonia is more truly a symptom characteristic of delayed development than a true diagnosis of its own. Mild forms of hypotonia are often seen in students who are congenitally blind (having light perception or less) but who do not have cerebral palsy.

The most common form of high muscle tone (hypertonia) is spasticity. Spasticity is usually categorized by the muscle group(s), flexors or extensors that are hypertonic. When one group of muscles is hypertonic, their reciprocal (opposite) muscles will often appear "weak" due to the fact that the neurological input to the hypertonic muscles is so great that the reciprocal muscles cannot overcome the pull of their hypertonic counterparts. Table 18.1 shows which joints are flexed and which are extended in the student's normal resting position with the varying types of spasticity.

Table 18.2 lists several effective strategies to minimize the stimulation of abnormal tone whenever possible. Physical therapists are also excellent resources for questions or assistance in identifying synergies and isolating motions.

When there is an imbalance in muscle tone, problems in both posture and visual functioning can occur. For example, a learner whose head is always turned to one side will have difficulty focusing on objects in front. He will also have difficulty maintaining a straight line of travel and holding his cane hand in midline. Similarly, a learner whose body is in constant motion (athetosis) will often have difficulty controlling his line of travel and the movement of the cane. When muscle tone is high, voluntary movements tend to be slow because before effective movement can occur, the brain must work to inhibit muscle tone in hypertonic muscles while activating their hypotonic counterparts. When spasticity is severe, it may not be possible to inhibit hypertonia

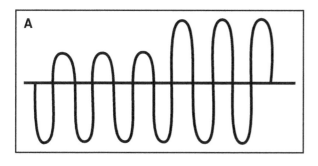

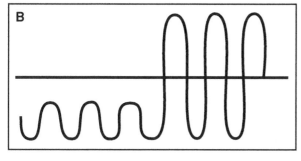

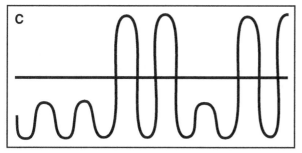

Figure 18.1.

(A) Excessive neural impulses are sent to some or all of the muscles, resulting in excessive stiffness; (B) insufficient impulses are sent, resulting in a lack of movement readiness; and (C) inconsistent impulses are sent, resulting in fluctuating muscle tone.

TABLE 18.1

Resting Positions of the Limbs in the Presence of Spasticity

Flexor Spasticity	Position of Limbs
In the arm	Upper arm is slightly forward and out to the side. Elbow is bent. Forearm is rotated to face palm downward, but occasionally upward. Wrist is bent. Fingers are bent.
In the leg	Hip and knee are bent. Foot may point upward. Foot may be rotated to face the sole toward midline.
Extensor Spasticity	
In the arm	Upper arm is drawn toward midline. Elbow is straight. Forearm is rotated to face palm downward. Wrist is straight. Fingers are bent or straight.
In the leg	Hip and knee are straight. Foot is pointed downward. Foot may be rotated to face the sole toward midline.

TABLE 18.2

Strategies for Minimizing Excessive Muscle Tone

Contributing Factors	Strategies to Try
Loud noises	Avoid sudden, loud noises when possible.
Sudden movements	Move slowly and methodically when handling students. Tell them what you are going to do before you do it.
Fatigue	Pace the day's activities, allowing for rest breaks as needed.
Illness	Understand the impact of the illness and pace the activities.
Temperature	Keep temperature comfortable—wear appropriate clothing for the weather, keep in the shade as much as possible in very hot weather, and keep hydrated.
Effort	Modify the task to make it physically easier.
Stress, emotions	Minimize frustration and negative stress. In the case of positive emotion, just understand and accept its impact on muscle tone.
Touching hypertonic muscles	Check with an occupational or physical therapist for techniques that can be used with a specific student to help maintain muscle tone as close to normal as possible.

sufficiently to allow effective movement. In addition, excessive muscle tone can often be aggravated by internal and external factors. For example, stress, cold temperatures, fatigue, and emotions such as fear, anger, frustration, or even excitement can increase the abnormal tone. When this is the case, it can interfere with a student's comfort, balance, coordination, and ability to focus, concentrate, and sometimes even learn. For this reason, it is essential to minimize the effects of abnormal muscle tone on O&M whenever possible.

With specific regard to cerebral palsy and posture, some students develop secondary orthopedic deformities such as hip dislocation, kyphosis (forward rounding of the upper spine), lordosis (swayback of the lower spine), and scoliosis (sideways curve of the spine) due to the unequal pull of hypertonic and hypotonic muscles on the spine. In addition, hypertonic muscles can also develop contractures. This reduces the range of available motion at a joint and hence a student's ability to move a limb fully. To maintain flexibility, some students use orthoses (braces and splints) and receive daily "range-of-motion" exercises designed to keep muscles and joints flexible. Some students also take medication to control excessive muscle tone and to promote muscle relaxation although some of these medications may also have such side effects as drowsiness. If this is the case, adjusting instruction to take advantage of the times of day when the student is most alert is essential. If side effects are excessive and interfere with learning, the student's parents can check with the doctor to see if modifying the dosage or times the medication is taken can relieve any side effects. (See the section on Medications for Health Conditions later in this chapter.)

Coordination

In addition to abnormal muscle tone, brain injury can also impact coordination (see Volume 1, Chapter 5 for a brief description of coordination).

Some of the coordination problems are the result of impaired proprioception. There are specific types of coordination problems, however, that can occur in the presence of brain injury:

- *Ataxia* (impaired coordination of muscular action due to disturbance of sense of balance): This generally results from injury to the cerebellum. Students with ataxia are especially prone to poor balance and equilibrium. Students walk with a wide-based gait (feet wide apart), trunk weaving back and forth, and arms held out to the side. They appear to walk as if on a rolling boat or as if intoxicated. Pure ataxia is rare among people with cerebral palsy, but it may be present together with athetosis or spasticity. It is more commonly seen in later-onset TBI or ABI.

- *Athetosis* (slow, writhing movements): This is a result of fluctuating tone. Movements are characterized by "overshooting" and "undershooting" a target, resulting in "flailing" motions. When a student begins a movement, activation of one muscle groups leads to the unwanted activation of others. The limb writhes (rotating back and forth, extending and flexing) and slowly makes its way to the intended destination. As an example, the hand may have an alternating grasp and then reflexive involuntary release (*avoiding reaction*); the trunk and head may rotate, and the arms may appear to flail in wide motions before they land on the item for which the student is reaching. As the student continues to perform the movement, the mere effort of doing so gradually increases the baseline muscle tone so that the degree of fluctuations between low and high tone diminishes and the student is eventually able to perform the movement or "reach the target."

- *Tremor* (involuntary shaking movements that are regular and rhythmical):

- *Intention tremor*: occurs upon movement, is silent when the limb is at rest.

- *Postural tremor*: greatest when a limb or the whole body moves against gravity. For example, a person who has a postural tremor will shake while sitting or standing, but not while lying down.

- *Resting tremor*: generally is greatest when the body part is at rest and diminishes when the student moves the part.

- *Apraxia* (difficulties in motor planning): The limb is not paralyzed, but in severe cases, the student may be unable to perform a motion on command, yet will be able to do so spontaneously at another time. In less severe cases, apraxia may take the form of difficulty in coordinating the hand and finger positions to execute motor tasks efficiently.

As a special note, children with cerebral palsy may also have coordination difficulties due to the retention of primitive neurological reflex activity that normally becomes integrated during the first year of life. Sidebar 18.3 describes some of these reflexes and their implications in O&M.

Regardless of the type of coordination difficulty that a student might show, stress and efforts to rush or move more quickly can exacerbate coordination problems. For this reason, patience and allowing extra time to perform motor activities are very important.

Seizure Disorders

Seizures are, in fact, one of the most common neurological disorders affecting children. All students, regardless of age, however, who have seizures should wear a Medic Alert bracelet stating the student has a seizure disorder and listing medications being taken. Some students will even wear a protective helmet if they have frequently occurring seizures that result in falls.

In general, seizures result from an abnormal discharge of electrical activity in certain brain cells (Adams & Vicar, 1993, cited in Agnew, Nystul, & Conner, 1998). Seizures can last only a few seconds or for several minutes; they can occur every few minutes, or only once a year. Sometimes impending seizures can be sensed by students; other times seizures occur without warning. Many seizures can be controlled fully or partially by medication. The nature of the seizure depends on the location of the discharge and how far it spreads. This abnormal discharge is characterized by changes in consciousness, motor activity, sensory phenomena, or inappropriate behavior (Agnew, Nystul, & Conner, 1998). Seizures may occur as part of a larger disorder or as a neurological condition of its own. A single seizure in itself does not indicate epilepsy; however, when chronic, this condition is known as a *seizure disorder* or *epilepsy*.

Some seizures, referred to as *reflex seizures*, can occur in response to either internal or external stimuli (Xue & Ritaccio, 2006). Depending on the individual student, internal stimuli include such things as stress, excess fatigue, lack of sleep, illness, fever, electrolyte imbalance, excess fluid or salt intake, or withdrawal from antiepileptic medication (Dreifuss, 1983). External stimuli can include somatosensory stimuli; visual stimuli such as bright or flashing lights, or visual patterns (for example, reflecting geometric designs); auditory (for example, a fire alarm), vestibular, and olfactory stimuli; high-level processes such as cognitive, emotional, and decision-making tasks; and other complex stimuli (Dreifuss, 1983; Panayiotopoulos, 2002, cited in Xue, 2006). While external stimuli, however, only trigger or exacerbate seizure activity in a small percentage of people, it is still essential that O&M specialists be aware of this possibility and avoid stimuli (for example, avoid flashing lights when doing visual functioning activities) that might evoke a seizure in a student.

The International Classification of Epileptic Seizures (Holmes, 2004) categorizes seizures as partial, generalized, and unclassified. Following are the most common forms of seizures.

Cerebral Palsy: Coordination Problems Caused by Reflex Activity

Cerebral palsy is uniquely characterized by the persistence of primitive reflexes, especially the asymmetrical tonic neck reflex (ATNR). In normal neonatal development, early movement is characterized by primitive reflexes which are then integrated during the first year of life and replaced by mature neurological reactions. These mature reactions support voluntary functional motor activities such as rolling, sitting, standing, and walking. When, due to brain injury, the primitive reflexes do not properly integrate, motor development can lag or become impaired. The strength and persistence of the retained reflex will depend on the classification and severity of the cerebral palsy. Some of the more common reflexes which can be retained in students with cerebral palsy and which can impact O&M include the following:

- *Asymmetrical tonic neck reflex (ATNR)*: Extension of the arm and leg on the side toward which the head turns; flexion of the arm and leg on the opposite side. Depending on its strength, it can interfere with midline activities such as bilateral hand usage, eating, rolling over, walking, and using a cane. Continual positioning of the head turned to one side often interferes with the development of eye–hand coordination and can lead to the development of scoliosis and hip dislocation in some students who are severely involved. One strategy to limit the impact of the ATNR on a student's ability to perform mobility skills is to "break the pattern." Just as "breaking the pattern" can often inhibit a synergy, the same principle applies here. For example, the ATNR greatly interferes with midline activities. By asking the student to perform a skill in such a way that at least one hand is held in midline, the influence of the reflex on the entire skill can be reduced. An example of this would be to have the student hold onto a map at midline with one hand while using his other hand to read it.

- *Symmetrical tonic neck reflex (STNR)*: Flexion of arms and neck with extension of legs; extension of arms and neck with flexion of legs. It interferes with crawling and walking.

- *Tonic labyrinthine reflex*: Increased flexor tone in the prone (stomach-lying) position; increased extensor tone in the supine (back-lying) position. It interferes with hand and arm usage, crawling, and walking.

- *Palmar reflex*: Closing of hand around an object which touches the palm; grasp remains as long as the object contacts the palm. It interferes with the development of release and many types of voluntary grasps. For students who have a strong palmar reflex, use utensils with a hard handle to help inhibit the strength of the reflex.

- *Startle reflex*: Sudden flexion, extension, and repeated flexion of the body in response to a sudden noise or movement. It can cause a momentary increase in muscle tone and loss of concentration. Moving slowly, speaking in a soft, modulated voice, and verbally preparing a student for an activity can go a long way to avoid inadvertently stimulating a startle reflex.

Partial Seizures

Partial refers to the fact that these seizures have a localized onset, are focused in one particular area of the brain, and are restricted to specific areas of the body. Partial seizures can last several minutes and are often followed by confusion and decreased ability to remember, understand language, or concentrate. If the student is walking, guide her gently to a safe place. Stay close until the seizure has ended and the student is completely aware of where she is and can respond normally when spoken to. But, remember, if confronted or restrained after the seizure, the student may react with negative behaviors such as verbal or physical aggression. During the seizure, the student may lash out instinctively if grabbed or held down.

Partial seizures may be subdivided into several types: (1) simple partial, (2) complex partial, and (3) complex partial with secondary generalization (Holmes, 2004).

Simple partial seizures. Simple partial seizures usually last about 10–30 seconds, during which time the student is awake and alert. Although simple partial seizures can produce sensory (somatosensory), autonomic, or psychic responses, they most commonly produce motor symptoms. The arm or leg may make a jerking motion; even very small muscles such as those in the finger or face can be affected. Simple partial seizures may involve one select area, such as the hand or foot, or may spread to other motor areas along the limb. Somatosensory symptoms can include numbness or tingling in the affected body part (or nearby body parts), certain odors or tastes, visual hallucinations (for example, lights or colors), and sometimes a feeling of falling or floating. Other symptoms can include a faster heart rate, dilation of the pupils, and, very rarely, abdominal pain. Although psychic symptoms are more often associated with complex seizures, they can occur with a simple partial seizure. Psychic symptoms can include certain emotions, hallucinations, or other disturbances in cognitive functioning. Of interest is the fact that all of these simple partial seizure effects may also occur as an "aura," or warning, which precedes a more complex or generalized seizure (Devinsky, 1994; Epilepsy Foundation of America, 1994).

Complex partial seizures. Also known as a *temporal lobe seizure* or a *psychomotor seizure*, the complex partial seizure generally lasts from 30 seconds to several minutes. It is often multisymptomatic and usually involves certain motor behaviors and psychic symptoms. The child may demonstrate involuntary motor activity such as spasmodic movements of the hand or face. She may appear to be conscious, but she will be in an altered state of consciousness, an almost trance-like state (Mayo Clinic, March 11, 2007). During a complex partial seizure, the child loses contact with her surroundings and may wander around as though sleepwalking, pick at clothing, mumble, laugh, gesture, make chewing movements, cry out, speak the same words over and over, or run away in apparent fear. Whatever form of automatic movement the student performs, the same behavior will generally be repeated with each seizure. Psychic symptoms such as fear, joy, or embarrassment may also occur, as well as illusions and hallucinations. Feelings of déjà vu (memory flashbacks) may also occur. When the seizure is over, the student may feel confused about what has taken place and may be tired or even sleep during this time. This is known as the *postictal phase*. This type of seizure tends to show an increase in adolescence and adulthood. A child who has experienced neonatal convulsions, cerebral palsy, or head trauma may be at increased risk of developing such seizures.

Complex partial seizures with secondary generalization. According to the Mayo Clinic (2007), partial nonconvulsive seizures originate in and usually stay confined to one part of the brain, although they can secondarily generalize to cause a convulsive seizure.

Generalized Seizures

Generalized seizures occur in both hemispheres, or begin in one area and then move to involve both hemispheres. There are many different types of generalized seizures ranging from *absence seizures* to *convulsive seizures.*

Absence seizures. In absence seizures (formerly known as *petit-mal seizures*), the student will suddenly lose consciousness, stop what he is doing, and either stare straight ahead or roll the eyes upward. There may be some small, involuntary movements such as eye blinking or mouth twitching, chewing, or brief aimless movements of the hands or limbs; there is no other movement. Unlike daydreaming, it is not possible to bring a student out of an absence seizure by touching or speaking to him. Absence seizures usually last less than 10 seconds, and rarely more than 30 seconds. When the seizure finishes, the student will often resume activity unaware that anything has occurred. An absence seizure is the most common type of childhood epilepsy. It tends to become less frequent during adolescence and rarely continues into adulthood (Mayo Clinic, 2007).

Convulsive seizures. Generalized tonic-clonic seizures (formerly known as *grand-mal seizures*) are characterized by an aura which occurs minutes or seconds before the onset of the seizure. An *aura* is a "subjective sensation or motor phenomena that precedes and marks the onset of a paroxysmal attack, as of an epileptic attack." Some examples of an aura might include a foul taste or strange odor immediately before a seizure. Students can also have a *prodrome*, which manifests itself as a headache, a mood change, irritability, difficulty sleeping, or a change in appetite and which can occur hours or days before a seizure. For some students, the onset of a generalized tonic-clonic seizure comes without warning. A generalized tonic-clonic seizure begins with a sudden loss of consciousness. The student may emit a brief cry. This cry does not indicate pain or discomfort, but is just the sound made by air being forced out of the lungs as the chest and abdominal muscles contract. The tonic (rigid) phase occurs first and usually lasts less than a minute. In the tonic phase, the muscles will be rigid with the arms and legs extended and the back arched; the student's eyes may roll upward and she may have a blueness of the lips, nail beds, and sometimes the skin due to irregular or shallow respiration. The clonic (jerking) phase follows in which the body exhibits rhythmic, jerking motions that gradually decrease in frequency. After this phase ends, the student may lose bladder or bowel control. Throughout the seizure, saliva may pool in the mouth and breathing may be noisy. The student can aspirate saliva, bite her tongue, and vomit during the seizure. The entire seizure usually lasts 2 to 5 minutes. Following a seizure, the student may be unable to remember that anything happened. Typically, students will wake up from the seizure confused and tired. They will often sleep for one-half hour to two hours.

There is little that the O&M specialist can do during a tonic-clonic seizure. Some common sense procedures, however, include loosening any tight shirt collar and moving any potentially dangerous or fragile objects out of the way. If possible, place a pillow under the student's head. Do *not* insert any objects into the student's mouth, and don't resist or attempt to restrain the student while he is having a seizure because this can result in injury. After the seizure ends, let the student lay on his side to maintain an open airway and prevent fluids in the mouth from entering his lungs. Stay with the student as he may be confused for a period of time.

Absence and convulsive seizures are the two types of generalized seizures most common in school-age students. Others include those that have just a tonic phase in which the person becomes rigid and falls to the ground (tonic seizures); clonic phase (clonic seizures); sudden, brief muscle jerks (myoclonic seizures); or a sudden and complete loss of muscle tone in which the person will collapse to the ground (atonic seizures). Some students may have more than one type of seizure disorder. Students with multiple disabilities and neurological impairments are more likely to have several types, sometimes taking the form of a syndrome such as Lennox-Gastaut syndrome, which involves tonic-clonic, atonic, and myoclonic seizures (Heller et al., 1996).

It is not always possible to tell what causes a particular seizure episode in a student. Some factors that can facilitate the occurrence of a seizure, however, include emotional stress, fatigue and lack of sleep, constipation, a cold or the flu, and lack of regularity in taking antiseizure medication.

Seizure Medications

A variety of antiepileptic drugs (AEDs) are now available for treating seizure disorders. Some drugs are more effective than others, and so the correct drug and dosage are necessary for optimal effect. While two-thirds of patients with epilepsy have their seizures controlled by AEDs (Agnew, Nystul, & Conner, 1998) there are side effects to these drugs (for example, a sedative effect), which can adversely affect cognitive and behavioral functioning in children. A student with epilepsy may therefore be drowsy at times. As a result, he may have difficulty concentrating or performing complex tasks such as analyzing traffic patterns. The O&M specialist may be asked to observe the student and to note if any side effects, such as drowsiness or a rash, occur. This information can be quite important to the doctor in adjusting the dosage.

Response to Seizures

The first rule of thumb is to be prepared. The O&M specialist needs to obtain as much baseline information about the student as possible, including the type of seizure that the student typically exhibits and a description of what it looks like, typical frequency or duration, any known factors that can stimulate a seizure in that student, whether or not the student has auras or prodromes that might indicate an impending seizure, and the student's typical behavior following the seizure. In addition, the O&M specialist needs to have information on any medications that the student takes as well as their side effects, and any limitations on activity.

When a student does have a seizure, it is important to record a detailed description of the seizure, including its time and length, whether or not a prodrome or aura occurred, whether or not the student lost consciousness, how the student acted following the seizure (for example, alertness, fatigue), whether or not the student was injured (for example, from a fall), and what first aid was given (including by whom). A sample form for recording information following a seizure is shown in Figure 18.2.

It may not be necessary to summon medical assistance each time that a student has a seizure. The general guidelines for summoning emergency medical attention include the following:

- The seizure lasts more than 5 minutes or does not abate within a reasonable time (determined by the individual student's doctor).

- Another seizure starts right after the first. Continuous seizures (that is, status epilepticus) can cause permanent brain damage or death and can occur in students who have either partial or generalized seizures.

- The student can't be awakened after the seizure ends.

- The student has several seizures and doesn't regain consciousness between them.

- The student is pregnant or has another condition such as heart disease or diabetes.

SEIZURE OBSERVATION RECORD

Student's name and age: _____ Name of O&M Specialist: _____

Time, place, and date of seizure: _____

Directions: In the chart below, mark any symptoms a student exhibits during any point(s) in the seizure. Describe any unlisted symptoms under "Other."

	Before seizure	During seizure	After seizure
Behavioral Symptoms			
Behaves normally			
Agitated			
Combative			
Hyperactive			
Fatigued			
Lethargic			
Withdrawn			
Other:			
Cognitive Symptoms			
Alert			
Awake but not responsive			
Confused			
Shows memory loss			
Talks illogically			
Unaware of surroundings			
Unconscious			
Other:			
Emotional symptoms			
Angry			
Anxious			
Depressed			
Excited			
Fearful			
Happy			
Irritated			
Other:			

Anecdotal Description of Seizure Events
What was the sequence of events? What happened first, next, etc.?
How long did the seizure last?
What sides/parts of the body were affected? How were they affected?
Were there any triggers (e.g., flashing lights, temperature changes, illness, or stress)?
Was the student injured (e.g., from a fall)?
What first aid was given? By whom?
How long after the seizure did the student take to return to normal functioning? Describe the recovery.

Figure 18.2. Sample Form for Recording Seizures

- The student is injured during the seizure.
- The seizure happens in the water, or you think this might be the student's first seizure.

The O&M specialist, however, always needs to consult with the school or agency, the student and the family (depending on the age of the student), or the student's doctor to determine how potential seizure episodes need to be handled.

Multiple Sclerosis

Multiple sclerosis (MS) is an inflammatory disease of the central nervous system (CNS), which consists of the brain and optic nerves and spinal cord. MS is usually a slowly progressing disease characterized by periods of relapse (known as *exacerbations*) and partial recovery (known as *remissions*). MS can affect multiple body functions including sensory-motor functioning, speech, and cognitive functioning. Symptoms can be unpredictable and vary from student to student and from time to time in the same student. Following are some of the primary effects of MS.

Sensory Functioning

MS can affect all of the sensory systems including vision. Difficulties with vision are often one of the first symptoms of MS. These symptoms can range from nystagmus, double vision, and eye discomfort to total blindness. Other sensory symptoms can include decreased proprioception and decreased tactile sensation. Numbness in the face, arms or legs is, in fact, one of the most common symptoms of MS and is often an early symptom. The numbness may be mild or so severe that it interferes with the ability to use the affected body part. For example, a student with decreased feeling in her feet may have difficulty walking. Decreased tactile sensation in the hands may impact writing or holding objects safely. Additionally, some people who have MS also experience abnormal sensations such as pain without apparent cause, burning, itching, tingling, and pins and needles. Although hearing loss may take place during an acute exacerbation, it is generally an uncommon symptom of MS.

Motor Functioning

Muscle weakness, muscle spasms, and spasticity are motor problems common to MS. In addition, many people with MS can experience some degree of tremor, or uncontrollable shaking. Tremors can occur in various parts of the body. The most common form of tremor in MS is the *intention tremor*, which occurs during movement; there is no shaking when the person is at rest. The tremor develops and becomes more pronounced as the person tries to grasp or reach for something, or move a hand or a foot to a precise spot.

People with MS who have tremors may also have associated symptoms such as difficulty in speaking clearly (*dysarthria*) or difficulty in swallowing (*dysphagia*)—activities that are governed by many of the same pathways involved in coordinating movement.

It is often difficulties in gait (walking) that pose the most common mobility limitations in MS. Gait problems are usually related to several factors (National Multiple Sclerosis Society, 2003).

Gait problems are generally due to the following reasons:

- *Weakness*: Weakness can cause problems such as toe drag, foot drop (inability to lift the toes with each step), or other gait abnormalities such as *vaulting* (a compensatory technique that involves raising the heel on the stronger leg to make it easier to swing the weaker leg through), compensatory hip hike, trunk lean, or circumduction (swinging leg out to the side). People can compensate for such weakness with the use of appropriate exercises and assistive devices, including braces, canes, or walkers.

- *Spasticity*: Muscle tightness or spasticity can also interfere with gait. Antispasticity medications may help some in treating this symptom. Stretching exercises can also be helpful.

- *Loss of balance*: Balance problems typically result in a swaying and "drunken" type of gait known as *ataxia*. People with severe ataxia often benefit from the use of an ambulatory aid.

- *Neuropathy*: Some people with MS have such severe numbness in their feet that they cannot feel the floor or know where their feet are. This is referred to as a *sensory ataxia*.

- *Fatigue*: Many people will experience increased gait abnormalities or difficulties when fatigue increases.

- *Dizziness*: Dizziness is a common symptom of MS. People with MS may feel off balance or lightheaded, or less frequently they have the sensation that they or their surroundings are spinning—a condition known as *vertigo*. These symptoms are due to damage in the complex pathways that coordinate visual, spatial, and other input to the brain that is needed for balance.

Cognitive Functioning

Approximately 50 percent of people with MS will develop some degree of cognitive dysfunction, affecting the ability to think, reason, concentrate, or remember. However, only 5–10 percent of people with MS develop problems that are severe enough to interfere in a significant way with everyday activities (National Multiple Sclerosis Society, 2006). Cognitive changes can vary considerably from person to person and are generally mild. It is also common for certain functions to be unaffected while others are more involved. Memory is the cognitive function that is most likely to be affected. Other cognitive functions frequently affected include speed of information processing, executive functions (planning, prioritizing, and judgment), visuospatial functions (impairment in visual perception and constructional abilities), abstract reasoning and problem

solving, and attention and concentration—especially the ability to maintain attention and to divide attention between separate tasks.

Speech and Language

Speech disorders are fairly common in more advanced cases of MS and range from mild to severe. One pattern that is commonly associated with MS is "scanning" speech. This occurs when the normal "melody" or speech pattern is disrupted with abnormally long pauses between words or individual syllables of words. Another common speech difficulty is that of "slurred" speech. This is usually the result of weakness and/or incoordination of the muscles of the tongue, lips, cheeks, and mouth. Other speech problems include nasal speech, which sounds as though the person has a cold or nasal obstruction. Last, one of the most frustrating deficits for some with MS is word-finding difficulty—the experience of having a word on the tip of one's tongue but not being able to remember it.

Fatigue

Fatigue is one of the most common symptoms of MS, occurring in about 80 percent of people. In addition to typical causes for fatigue that anyone might experience, there is, however, another kind of fatigue specific to MS (National Multiple Sclerosis Society, 2005). Researchers are beginning to outline the characteristics of this so-called MS fatigue.

- Generally occurs on a daily basis
- May occur early in the morning, even after a restful night's sleep
- Tends to worsen as the day progresses
- Tends to be aggravated by heat and humidity
- Can come on easily and suddenly
- Is generally more severe than normal fatigue
- Is more likely to interfere with daily responsibilities

Temperature Sensitivity

The symptoms of MS will often increase in severity when the temperature is hot. For this reason it is important to plan lessons at times of day when the heat is not extreme and to have an array of backup indoor lessons available for use on exceedingly hot days.

CHRONIC HEALTH IMPAIRMENTS

Chronic health impairments that students might have can affect any organ system—the heart and circulatory system, lungs, and other internal organs. It is not possible to cover all health conditions in this chapter. This section is intended to cover only those conditions that have the greatest implications for O&M: diabetes, heart disease, hemophilia, asthma, HIV and AIDS, and sickle cell anemia.

Diabetes

Diabetic retinopathy is one of the leading causes of adult visual impairment in the United States. Diabetes mellitus is a disorder of carbohydrate, protein, and fat metabolism that may become apparent anytime between early infancy and old age. As we eat, specialized cells in the pancreas, known as beta cells (in the Islet of Langerhans located within the pancreas) produce a hormone called *insulin*. Insulin is a hormone that allows the body to burn glucose (a form of sugar produced when starches and sugars are digested). When we eat, the amount of glucose in the blood rises and signals the pancreas to release an appropriate amount of insulin into the bloodstream. All body tissues, including the muscles, brain, heart, liver, and kidneys, use glucose for energy. Without insulin, glucose does not enter tissue cells, but builds up in the blood and eventually overflows into the urine. As a result, body tissues are deprived of their energy source.

There are several different "types" of diabetes, differentiated largely by the amount of pancreatic functioning and occasionally by the age of onset. Type 1, also known as *insulin-dependent diabetes* (IDDM) and *juvenile diabetes*, occurs when the pancreas produces little or no insulin. This type of diabetes usually begins in childhood or young adulthood. The cause of Type 1 diabetes is not completely known, however it is believed that the body's own immune system destroys the insulin-producing cells in the pancreas. There appears to be a heredity influence, but the degree to which genetics gives one a susceptibility to developing Type 1 diabetes is not known. Viral factors are also suspected of playing a potential role.

Type 2 diabetes, also called *non-insulin-dependent diabetes* (NIDDM) or *adult-onset diabetes*, usually affects people age 40 years and older, although children in the United States are being diagnosed more and more frequently with this type of diabetes (National Center for Chronic Disease Prevention and Health Promotion, 2005). Type 2 diabetes, is in fact, the most common form of diabetes. Unlike people with Type 1 diabetes, people with Type 2 diabetes do produce insulin. Their insulin, however, is either insufficient, or the body is unable to use the insulin properly. They use oral medication to stimulate insulin production or to enhance the cells' reception of insulin.

It is important to monitor blood sugar and to maintain it at a normal level as much as possible. This will enable the student to feel better and will help prevent diabetic emergencies (see Hyperglycemic and Hypoglycemic Reactions later in this chapter). It can also reduce some of the long-term complications of diabetes such as vascular damage arising from diabetes-induced arteriosclerosis in which high levels of sugar in the blood damage blood vessels (Merck Manuals, 2003). Even with the best control, however, complications do arise. In addition to visual impairment, these complications include renal (kidney) failure and premature heart attacks. Renal failure and heart attack are in fact, among the primary causes of death in many people with Type 1 diabetes, many of whom live only into their third or fourth decade of life. Other common complications are decreased tolerance of extremes in temperature, peripheral neuropathy (loss of sensation in hands and feet), susceptibility to infection, and poor healing of wounds that can, in turn, lead to amputation.

Visual Impairment Secondary to Diabetes

A unique aspect of diabetic retinopathy is that a student's functional vision can fluctuate from day to day or even hour to hour. This fluctuation can be due to a number of causes, the most critical one perhaps being connected to a hypoglycemic (excessively low blood sugar levels) attack. On their "good" days, many students, such as those who easily pick up drop-offs visually in good lighting, may use a cane only for identification. However, on their "bad" days or at night, they need to be able to use a long cane for mobility purposes. Therefore, a student should not be evaluated just on her "best vision" days. If fluctuation is frequent or varied, it may be necessary to work with other members of the student's health care team to stabilize the student's blood glucose level.

Nephropathy

Diabetes is the leading cause of kidney failure in the United States (Centers for Disease Control and Prevention, 2005). The disease will often progress to the point that the student will need a kidney transplant. When working with a student who has had a kidney transplant, there are several critical precautions that O&M specialists must follow (Ponchillia, 1993).

• Because the new kidney is placed in front of the body, collisions need to be avoided at all costs.

• A person who has had a kidney transplant is required to take immunosuppressants and is therefore highly susceptible to germs. The O&M specialist, therefore, needs to take all precautions to minimize possible infection, including not working with such a student if he has even a mild cold.

Peripheral Neuropathy

Peripheral neuropathy generally begins between 10 and 20 years after the onset of the disease. The hands and feet are most susceptible to peripheral neuropathy due to the smaller size and therefore greater vulnerability of blood vessels. Neuropathy in the feet and legs may make it more difficult to detect drop-offs, inclines, and declines. Students who have had amputations and use prosthetic legs may have the same difficulties. Peripheral neuropathy may also result in an uncontrollable foot drop that may alter the student's normal gait, limit her endurance, and compromise safety. In such cases, the student may wear an ankle–foot orthosis (a plastic brace that fits inside his shoe) to restrain the foot drop.

Neuropathy in the hands may make it difficult to detect changes in surface textures through the cane. For this reason, using cane techniques such as touch-and-slide and constant-contact techniques that convey more information about the walking surface can be helpful for people who have peripheral neuropathy. Similarly, using a lighter weight cane and learning to use the cane lightly will often allow stronger vibrations to be transmitted through it.

Because peripheral neuropathy causes people with diabetes not to feel pain, they are at greatly increased risk of injury and infection, especially in the feet, even from wounds that began as minor cuts or bruises. In fact, peripheral neuropathy increases the risk of amputation substantially—one-half of all amputations in the United States involve patients with diabetes (Birrer & Sedaghat, 2003).

Pressure Sores

A pressure sore is caused when circulation to a specific spot of the body (most commonly the feet) is sufficiently impaired to cause *tissue necrosis* (tissue death). This is most often caused by either continuous pressure or concentrated high pressure. Concentrated high pressure is usually the result of a sudden, unexpected accident such as stepping barefoot on a stone. To avoid injury from concentrated high pressure, some good rules of thumb include never walking barefoot and always shaking out shoes before putting them on (and checking them for tears in the lining, or any other rough spots that might cause a spot of concentrated pressure on the skin). If using a cane causes pressure areas on the fingers, it might help to wrap the grip in a soft material, take breaks, or even switch hands to use the cane. Continuous pressure, on the other hand, can be caused by repetitive mechanical stress which leads to inflammation and then eventually to necrosis. The most common culprits are shoes that are too tight. In this case, the pressure sore will generally be found on the side edge of the foot, sometimes on top of the toes, or on the inside edge of the sole. When working with a student who has diabetes, it is important for the O&M specialist to always be alert to even the slightest change in a student's gait that could indicate an improperly fitting shoe, a blister, or even an ingrown toenail (Joffee, 1997).

There are a number of strategies that people with diabetes can use to minimize injury to their hands and feet. These strategies center on facilitating the circulation to the hands and especially the feet to the maximum degree possible. To avoid injury due to repetitive mechanical stress, it often helps for the student to wear athletic shoes with cushioned midsoles (silica gel or air cells) that are "broken in" and polyester or blend (cotton–polyester) socks that reduce shear forces and moisture buildup. These steps minimize trauma and blisters. Walking shorter distances and resting more often also help—it takes only 15–30 seconds

of rest to restore circulation. In addition, a good rule of thumb is to never wear new shoes for more than 2 hours at a time, and then check the feet for pressure areas (they will appear as red spots). If the skin looks okay, the student can wear the shoes longer the next time. Many people with diabetes will make a practice of changing shoes frequently throughout the day, perhaps using 5-hour intervals such as from 7:00 a.m. to noon, from noon to 5:00 p.m., and from 5:00 p.m. to 10:00 P.M. When taking off one's shoes, it is always good practice to check the socks for any wrinkles or wet spots that may correspond to the site of an injury.

People with diabetes should check their feet on a regular basis to spot pressure areas before they turn into pressure "sores" which can cause serious medical complications. If the student is unable to check his feet independently, or does not have a family member or friend who can assist him, he may ask the O&M specialist to assist him in this effort. What does a pressure sore look like? There are distinct warning signs of a potential pressure sore of which the student and the O&M specialist should be aware. These include pain (which the student may not feel if the peripheral neuropathy is severe), swelling, bruising, or blistering, deep tenderness, redness or gray–black discoloration of the skin (an inflamed area is also generally hot to the touch before it breaks down), groin pain (indicates possible inflammation occurring in an insensitive foot), and an open sore which may have an odor.

But what if a pressure sore does develop? The immediate treatment for any pressure area, whether it is just a mild "red spot" on the skin, or an open sore, is to immediately remove all pressure. If the sore is open, place a sterile bandage over the sore and refer the student for immediate medical attention. It is critical to refrain from putting any pressure on an area in which a pressure sore may be forming. This may mean canceling O&M instruction (or doing lessons that do not require weight bearing on a sore foot) until the area is healed. The good news is that if the area is rested and, if caught early, the process reverses and the tissue heals.

Controlling Blood Sugar Levels

The key word in diabetes management is *control*. That is, maintaining the delicate balance between sugar intake, exercise, and insulin. There are many types of insulin, each of which have different absorption peaks. This peak time is predictable and differs for the types of insulin used. Regular insulin, for example, normally peaks in three to four hours; other types of insulin have a 5–8-hour peak or a 24-hour steady timed-release absorption. A new type of insulin absorbs in about 15 minutes. Many people take combinations of regular and longer-acting insulin. These facts can be pieced together to formulate the best times for walking, the amounts of insulin needed, or the use of supplemental snacks to help regulate blood sugar levels.

Because the body's use of insulin is affected by exercise, this can also have a significant impact on the ideal scheduling of O&M instruction. Blood glucose levels rise after eating and so the best time for exercise is to coincide with these rising levels. Conversely, if exercise is done when the insulin action is peaking, there is an increased risk of a hypoglycemia (low blood sugar) reaction which can be life threatening. For this reason, it is often best to plan lessons to take place soon after meals whenever possible.

Hyperglycemic reaction. Also called *ketoacidosis*, this reaction occurs when the level of insulin in the bloodstream is insufficient to metabolize enough sugar for the body tissues to use. This can occur from too little exercise, or from eating too much in relation to the amount of insulin taken. Stress, hormonal fluctuations, illness, or foods that are absorbed in the bloodstream more quickly than expected, common colds, viruses, and high stress can throw off the system because they cause blood sugar levels to be elevated. Also

when levels are high, the student becomes susceptible to other infections such as sore throats.

Symptoms of hyperglycemic reactions include dry, hot skin; excessive urination; excessive thirst; drowsiness and lethargy; deep and/or labored breathing; fruity-smelling breath; and blurry vision. In essence, since the body needs sugar for energy, it steals energy from fats stored in the body. When the fats are broken down, ketones are released. Too many ketones become poisonous, and without proper treatment the student may fall into coma requiring hospitalization. This is a gradual process that generally develops over a period of days. For this reason, it is not an emergency, but the student needs to consult a doctor to see if her medication needs adjustment.

Hypoglycemic reaction. Also called an *insulin reaction*, this reaction occurs when the level of insulin in the bloodstream exceeds the required amount of sugar to balance its effect. An insulin reaction can be caused by eating too little in relation to the amount of insulin taken, or from waiting too long to eat after taking insulin. This reaction most commonly occurs before meals. Hypoglycemic reactions can also be caused by an increase in exercise. Exercise helps the body to metabolize glucose more efficiently so that the body may suddenly have an imbalance between its insulin and available glucose. Another potential cause of hypoglycemia has to do with the injection site on the body. Insulin can be injected in a number of sites, including the arms, legs, abdomen, and buttocks. Not only does the absorption time from each site vary (the fastest from the abdomen and the slowest from the buttocks), but exercising the injection site increases the speed of absorption, making the peak time earlier (Kozel, 1995). The type of walking done in a mobility lesson may create these types of problems in some individuals. For these reasons, it is critical that a student's insulin dosage be adjusted to account for any changes in her daily exercise regime.

Unlike a hyperglycemic reaction, an insulin reaction can be life threatening. Each person may experience different symptoms signaling the onset of an insulin reaction (American Association of Diabetes Educators, 1998). Some people are aware that they are having a reaction; others become desensitized to insulin reactions, causing their bodies not to provide any symptoms to indicate the onset of a reaction. This latter situation is called *hypoglycemic unawareness*. It is critical, therefore, that the O&M specialist be able to recognize the symptoms and react, especially if a student is having a hypoglycemic episode, but is unaware that it is happening. The symptoms of hypoglycemia are varied and may differ significantly between children and adults who use insulin. Symptoms can occur suddenly and can include: inappropriate responses, confusion and inattention, drowsiness, pale complexion, perspiration, headache, crankiness, lack of coordination, loss of judgment, trembling, perspiration, sudden hunger, rapid pulse, nausea, vomiting, and dizziness. Untreated reactions can be fatal. It is important that instructors understand procedures established by their employers for handling medical emergencies. Students need to be encouraged to have with them what they will need to treat their medical needs. Instructors may need to have releases signed by the student and/or their parents giving the instructors permission to, and instructions on how to, treat the situation.

The treatment for hypoglycemia is to provide a form of sugar immediately. One of the best sources of sugar which can be absorbed quickly into the bloodstream are glucose tablets or a gel that comes in a small tube and is used by unscrewing the cap and squeezing a small amount of the paste onto the inside of the student's cheek. Both are easy to use, do not need to be refrigerated, and are small enough to be carried conveniently. They are available in some pharmacies and are also sold by some local offices of the American Diabetes Association. Other sources of sugar which are readily available include fruit juice, sugar cubes, regular (non-diet) soda, honey, cake icing, and lifesavers (only if the student is alert enough to avoid choking). Chocolate is not an optimum choice because it has a high fat content and fat is harder than sugar for the body to metabolize.

The student should begin to feel better within 10 minutes of taking sugar. If so, give the student some additional food (for example, milk, bread, and crackers) and let him resume normal activities. If the student does not begin to feel better immediately, give more sugar. If the student still does not improve within 10–15 minutes, it might be necessary to seek medical assistance. Continue to administer sugar. If the student becomes unconscious, rub some liquid sugar, jam, honey, or syrup on the inside of the cheek where it can be absorbed without risk of choking. Regardless of how mild a reaction might seem, it is important not to leave the student unattended until the reaction is over.

It is vitally important for the O&M specialist to watch for behaviors that might mean a reaction is beginning, and to act appropriately. This means always keeping sugar available for emergencies. If a reaction occurs, but it is unclear as to whether it is a hypoglycemic or hyperglycemic reaction, the rule of thumb is to still administer sugar. The reasoning behind this is if the student is having a hyperglycemic reaction, the effects will take days to build and a little excess sugar will not seriously add to the problem. On the other hand, if the student is having an insulin or hypoglycemic reaction, a lack of sugar can be fatal.

In all cases, it is important to note specific information including time of day, symptoms, how much and what type of sugar was administered, and whether or not the sugar had an effect. This information is vital to doctors as they monitor and adjust dosages of insulin and prescribe diets. One recommendation is to keep a diabetic information sheet including the following information:

- The student's name, address, and phone number
- School or agency name, address, and phone number
- Physician's name and phone number
- Person to notify in case of emergency
- Type of insulin, amount taken, and time of day injections given
- Symptoms that the student typically experiences and how the student wants reactions to be handled
- What time of day reactions are most likely to occur

Heart and Blood Pressure Disease

Heart disease can affect people of all ages, from birth through the senior years. Some heart conditions affect the valves within the heart or the rhythm of the heart. Others cause clogging of the arteries that feed the heart or simply weaken it. The most common conditions are described here.

Congestive Heart Failure

Congestive heart failure is due to the inability of the heart to pump blood with its usual efficiency. Much as a water balloon expands when filled with water, the heart enlarges and due to its large size, it presses on the lungs which are next to it. As a result, people who have congestive heart failure will generally have poor endurance, shortness of breath, and chest pain if they overexert. At times they may also experience dizziness if the heart is not pumping sufficient blood to the head at that moment. The O&M specialist needs to be alert for signs of dizziness or shortness of breath during a lesson and allow the student sufficient opportunities to sit and rest as needed.

Angina Pectoris

Angina pectoris is a condition, commonly due to atherosclerosis (clogging of the arteries), in which the blood and oxygen supply to the heart are impaired. Symptoms of an angina episode are very similar to those of a heart attack and include chest pain which is often described as a constrictive, strangling sensation or severe indigestion; a heaviness, tightness, or pressure on the chest; a choking or burning sensation; and shortness of breath. Other symptoms may include pain that radiates to the neck, jaw, back of the neck, area between the shoulder blades, left shoulder, or abdomen. Many people with angina carry nitroglycerin tablets. Nitroglycerin works by causing the blood vessels around the heart to open, allowing more blood to get to the heart muscle. A student will put a tablet under his tongue. People generally carry the tablet in a purse or a right-hand pocket (it is easier to reach into a right-hand pocket if there is pain in the left arm). Pain may occur after, rather than during, exercise and generally lasts less than 5 minutes. It will generally subside with rest, and the student will recover quickly if he sits or stands quietly. If it does not subside, the O&M specialist needs to call for medical assistance.

An understanding of these major heart conditions is important so that the O&M specialist can be alert to signs of stress and can take cardiac needs into consideration in planning lessons. Minimizing undue stress to the heart is critical to avoid a heart attack. Some basic principles to keep in mind when working with a student who has a heart condition include the following:

- *Assessing exercise tolerance*: Determine if problems occur while performing specific activities or while experiencing strong emotions; have the student describe conditions that might cause pain and the type of pain or symptoms usually experienced.
- Keep a list of medications being taken and be aware of all side effects and precautions.
- Minimize undue stress, both emotional and physical. If the student tires, sit down for a few minutes, then continue the lesson.

- *Things to remember*
  - Cardiac status may vary from day to day.
  - Extremes in hot or cold temperatures can increase cardiac stress.

Classic Heart Attack

The symptoms of a heart attack are similar to those of angina, but are much more severe. Common symptoms in men consist of a severe, steady pain in the chest, often described as a feeling of a vise-like squeezing or crushing weight. The pain may begin during activity, rest, or even sleep, and does not subside. The student may have shortness of breath or exhibit wheezing. His skin may be pale, moist, and cool, and even have bluish tint. He may feel nausea and may perspire. His pulse will be fast, slow, weak, or irregular and he may feel faint or weak. He may exhibit mental confusion or even loss of consciousness. Women may experience any of these same symptoms, but the symptoms often tend to be much less pronounced.

If a student exhibits the symptoms of angina or of a heart attack, he needs to sit down immediately. If possible, a chair with the back and arms supported is best. Arm support actually lessens strain on the heart. The O&M specialist needs to monitor the heart rate and obtain medical assistance if necessary. The O&M specialist needs to know CPR and be prepared to administer it, if necessary

As a note, children rarely have sudden heart attacks as do adults, but it is still important to monitor a student's physical activity if he has a heart condition. If a student's activity level exceeds his cardiac tolerance, symptoms may still include shortness of breath, chest pain, cyanosis (blue coloration of lips and fingertips), very rapid or irregular heartbeat, and unusual fatigue. If any of these symptoms occur, the student needs to sit down, with his arms and back supported, and rest. If the symptoms are severe, or do not disappear within a few minutes, it will be necessary to obtain medical assistance. The O&M specialist

needs to talk with the student's parents about procedures to follow and needs to be very familiar with school policy on handling medical emergencies.

Blood Pressure

Hypertension. High blood pressure, also called *hypertension*, is a chronic condition, usually managed by medication, diet, or both. Some medications used to control hypertension are diuretics which means that they serve to reduce the fluid levels in the bloodstream. Students who are taking diuretics may need more frequent bathroom breaks.

Certain conditions such as stress, anxiety, strong emotions, excessive fatigue, or illness, however, can cause even controlled blood pressure to rise to unsafe levels. An unsafe rise in blood pressure can lead to serious complications including a stroke. The symptoms of an unsafe rise in blood pressure include a headache, unexplained irritability, and even a reddening of the face.

Hypotension. During an O&M lesson, an unsafe drop in blood pressure, called *hypotension*, would most likely be caused by overexertion (as in the case of congestive heart failure). The primary symptom of low blood pressure is dizziness. Some heart medications called *beta blockers* are designed to reduce the heart rate and blood pressure. They can, however, cause dizziness and other symptoms of hypotension such as fatigue, drowsiness, lightheadedness, and decreased blood flow to the hands and feet. Other medications, also designed to reduce excessively high blood pressure, are called *diuretics*. When taking these medications, a person must have an adequate intake of fluid or the medications can cause dehydration that, in turn, can also lead to low blood pressure (Hemmila, 2007). A hint for dealing with hypotension is to remember that blood pressure is normally highest when a person is lying down, lower when sitting, and lowest yet when standing. Therefore, if a person feels dizzy, having that person sit down immediately can not only prevent a fall but also work to help return the blood pressure to normal.

Asthma

People with asthma are sensitive to certain materials or conditions that cause an inflammation or swelling of the inner lining of the lungs. When an asthma attack occurs, the lining of the lungs quickly becomes swollen. The air passages fill up with thick mucus and the muscles around the bronchial tubes can also tighten abnormally resulting in further narrowing of the air passages. This narrowing of the air passages causes a characteristic wheezing sound as the student exhales. An asthma attack can potentially be life threatening.

Some asthma attacks have obvious precipitating factors, while others can appear to occur without cause. Some people with asthma will carry a peak-flow meter, which is a handheld device for measuring their airflow to determine if an attack is imminent. Factors which serve to stimulate attacks in some people include the following (Centers for Disease Control and Prevention, 2006):

- Inhaled allergens such as grass, trees, weeds, and pollens.

- Dust, wool, feathers, molds, tobacco smoke, chalk dust, hair spray, perfume, odors from cleaning supplies or other aerosols, and animal hair or secretions.

- Extreme conditions, such as very cold or very hot weather. In some people, barometric changes, dampness, wind, or very low indoor humidity have also been known to set off asthma attacks. Others are affected by high humidity as dust mites and molds pose more of a problem to people who are sensitive to them.

- Strenuous exercise, and exposure to smog and particles in the air from car exhaust or other pollution.

- Respiratory infections.

- Medications that are sometimes used to treat other diseases can aggravate asthma. For example, strong beta blocker eyedrops taken for glaucoma might enhance an asthma response. A beta blocker or an ACE inhibitor that some people take for blood pressure can provoke a cough. Food additives, such as sulfites found in wine, can also trigger an asthma attack.

Contrary to popular belief, asthma is not caused by emotions. Emotional upset, however, can trigger an attack in some students, particularly when accompanied by shouting, crying, or rapid breathing.

Acute attacks can either begin dramatically with multiple, severe symptoms occurring simultaneously, or they can begin slowly, with gradually increasing respiratory distress. Mild attacks can often be controlled by having the student simply sit down, rest, and breathe easily. Relaxing and focusing on diaphragmatic breathing can also be helpful in alleviating mild attacks. More significant attacks are often treated with medicine that relaxes the muscles of the bronchial tree. This medicine is often taken in the form of an aerosol inhalant which the student carries at all times and self-administers. If the student's condition does not improve, or if it worsens, it will be necessary to obtain immediate medical assistance. It is important to remember that whether mild or severe, the loss of breath can be terrifying. Most students are helped by reassurance that the teacher will help them and that the episode will pass.

While it is impossible to prevent all asthma attacks, there are a number of things that O&M specialists can do to minimize the potential for their occurrence. For example, it is always helpful to eliminate as many substances as possible from the environment that might trigger an attack. At times it may be better to do activities in a warm environment rather than outside in cold, dry air. During strenuous activity, some people tend to breathe through their mouths, allowing the cold or dry air to reach the lower airways without passing through the warming, humidifying effect of the nose. In addition to mouth breathing, air pollutants, high pollen counts, and viral respiratory tract infections can also increase the severity of wheezing with exercise. If it is necessary to work outside in very cold weather, some students find it helpful to wear a scarf over the face to limit lung exposure to cold air.

When working with a student who has asthma, it is always good to have the following information immediately available in case of an asthma attack:

- Brief history of the student's asthma and symptoms of an attack
- List of factors that make student's asthma worse
- List of student's asthma medications
- Contact information for the student's health care provider and for the parent, the guardian, or a close relative
- Description of the student's treatment plan, including recommended actions to help handle asthma episodes

HIV and AIDS

Acquired immunodeficiency syndrome (AIDS) is the result of infection with the human immunodeficiency virus (HIV). This virus gradually weakens the body's immune system and opens the way for other diseases to successfully attack the body. Not all students who are infected with HIV have AIDS. It is only when the immune system is so weakened that it cannot fight serious infections and certain types of cancer that the student is said to have AIDS.

In addition to primary infections, the decreased functioning of the immune system can lead to a variety of neurological complications including nerve damage (for example, neuropathy that can cause pain, tingling, and numbness in the feet and legs and sometimes in the hands and fingers). This pain may be the result of medications, but regardless, it can be severe and can make walking difficult. Brain damage can lead to dementia, strokes, headaches, and behavioral changes. Confusion, seizures, vision loss, and memory and cognitive deficits may also be seen (National Institute of Neurological Disorders and Stroke, 2007). Neurological symptoms are generally mild in the early stages of AIDS but can increase in severity in the later stages.

It should be noted that the symptoms in children differ from those experienced by infected adults. Children often experience progressive encephalopathy (brain dysfunction). They often have problems of growth and development, losing many developmental milestones as the encephalopathy progresses.

At the time that this chapter is written, there is no known cure for AIDS. Although considered a terminal illness, death is not from the virus itself, but rather from various opportunistic infections (those notably seen only when immune systems are weakened) and other conditions.

Eye Diseases Associated with AIDS

It is estimated that about 75 percent of AIDS patients develop eye problems of some sort (University of Michigan Kellogg Eye Center, 2006). The retina is most commonly affected. The following list mentions only a few of the opportunistic infections and other conditions that may cause visual impairment in students with AIDS:

- The cytomegalovirus (CMV), a member of the herpes family, is the most common cause of serious visual impairment associated with HIV infection and is the one most likely to lead to blindness. Clinically, CMV appears as lesions on the retina with varying amounts of hemorrhage. Swelling of the optic nerve and vessel closure may also occur. Changes can occur in one or both eyes. CMV may cause blurry vision or visual field loss, and also has been known to cause total blindness related to damage to the retina. Normally, CMV disease that affects the eye occurs only in the developing fetus or individuals whose immune system is severely compromised. Visual changes associated with CMV affect approximately 20 percent of persons living with AIDS (PLWA). CMV also affects the gastrointestinal system, the brain, and the adrenal glands.

- Kaposi's sarcoma is a vascular tumor that may cause purple-red growths on the eyelid or conjunctiva. Although the tumors do not invade the eye, they may block part of the visual field as they grow.

- Uveitis, an infection in the uveal tract of the eye that affects visual function by degrading or compromising acuity. This visual complication may be the first sign of several chronic infections for HIV-positive individuals. These infections may include tuberculosis, syphilis, histoplasmosis, coccidiomycosis, and toxoplasmosis.

- Toxoplasmosis, a protozoan parasite, is another opportunistic infection that can lead to retinal inflammation or can produce spots of retinal destruction due to the formation of toxoplasmosis cysts.

- Cryptococcal meningitis damages the optic nerve and other centers in the brain.

- Central nervous system infections are the second most common cause of visual impairment in people with AIDS. Both toxoplasmosis and cryptococcal meningitis may be involved. Similarly, CMV can cause encephalitis of the brain stem. Any of these may lead to diploplia, blurred vision, or difficulties in movement of the eyes.

- HIV retinopathy is a microvascular disorder that is characterized by the presence of *cotton-wool spots*, microaneurysms, retinal hemorrhages, telangiectatic vascular changes, and areas of capillary nonperfusion. Functionally, these in-

dividuals can suffer from field losses and even retinal detachments.

Transmission of HIV

HIV is a fragile virus that does not survive long outside of body fluids, or in fluids that have left the body and are no longer at body temperature. Therefore, HIV cannot be transmitted through casual contact such as sharing air, water, food, a bathroom, or a water fountain, all of which may take place between the student and instructor during lessons.

The most common routes by which HIV enters an individual's bloodstream are direct entry into a vein or through a break in the skin or mucous linings such as those found in the eyes, mouth, and nose.

HIV has been found in blood, semen, human breast milk, vaginal secretions, and cerebrospinal fluid. Other body fluids, such as urine, saliva, and vomit, do not pose the risk of transmitting HIV unless blood is visibly present in these fluids. In fact, there are no anecdotal reports involving transmission through urine, tears, saliva, or mosquito or human bites. In essence, repeated studies have failed to show any risk from "casual contact." There is no evidence that HIV can be contracted from being bitten by mosquitoes or other bugs; being bitten by animals; eating food handled, prepared, or served by somebody with HIV infection; sharing toilets, telephones, or clothes; sharing forks, spoons, knives, or drinking glasses; touching, hugging, or kissing a person with HIV; or attending school, church, shopping malls, or other public places with HIV-infected people.

The major concerns for the O&M specialist with regard to these infections are to prevent oneself from becoming infected through contact with blood or body fluids that might carry the virus, and similarly, to protect the student, to the maximum degree possible, from contracting infections that might be transmitted to him unwittingly. To this end, it is important to have all involved, teachers and students alike, practice good hygiene skills such as hand washing throughout the day. The O&M specialist needs to reschedule lessons with these students if the specialist has a contagious illness which would otherwise not preclude working (for example, a cold) and needs to comply with a set of procedures known as "universal health precautions" (see Sidebar 18.4). Universal health precautions outline procedures that can be taken to achieve both of these ends. In fact, because they minimize the potential for transmission of infection, universal health precautions are actually important to follow at all times, whether or not one is working with a student who has HIV or AIDS.

Privacy Issues

Despite the fact that HIV cannot be contracted through casual contact, there remains some misinformation and fear among the public. As a result, since 1980, when children with AIDS began to be identified, they and their families have been the victims of discrimination (U.S. Department of Health and Human Services, 1987). To prevent discrimination, many states have decided that since AIDS cannot be transmitted by casual contact, the risks to others are not sufficiently great to warrant violating a person's or family's privacy. Organizational, local, and federal policies and statutes ensuring nondiscrimination and confidentiality prohibit certain clinical and educational records and personnel files from including potentially discriminatory information about HIV and AIDS without either parental consent or age-appropriate assent of the student (Committee on Pediatric AIDS, 2000). The O&M specialist may therefore be unaware if he is teaching a student who is HIV-positive or who has AIDS. The importance of following universal health precautions cannot be overemphasized.

Implications for O&M Training

In light of recurrent infections or an increasing physical debilitation that the student may be ex-periencing, a student's ability to participate in instruction can vary from day to day or even hour to hour. This may be particularly true for students who are experiencing severe pain, or even a cognitive deterioration that can be associated with AIDS-related dementia. It is therefore always a good idea to confirm all meetings with the student several hours before scheduled appointments, because the student's health and capacity to participate in an O&M session can change significantly from lesson to lesson. Furthermore, goals and instructional programs will need to be reassessed and modified as the student's physical condition changes. An unwanted side effect of the privacy legislation mentioned above, however, is that the O&M specialist may not know that he is working with a student who is HIV-positive or who has AIDS. Without such knowledge, it is often difficult to plan lessons for students and to determine appropriate long-term goals.

Because visual impairment often does not occur until the later stages of AIDS, it may also coincide with the time in which the student may be dealing with issues of his own mortality. Such issues can affect people in highly personal and individual ways, and in some cases can greatly impact a student's motivation to participate in O&M instruction. Frequently a student's level of motivation is reflected by his perception of "time" (Joffee, 1997). Some students may be highly motivated to complete O&M instruction, feeling that time is of the essence so they can resume their normal level of mobility for daily living needs. Other students, however, may see their vision loss as the beginning of the end. Perceiving that time is not on their side, they may exhibit a low level of motivation to learn O&M skills (Joffee, 1997).

Sickle Cell Disease

Sickle cell disease is transmitted through an autosomal recessive inheritance pattern, characterized by an abnormality of hemoglobin (a pro-

Universal Health Precautions

Universal precautions refer to the steps professionals need to take in order to reduce their risk of infection with HIV and all other blood-borne organisms (for example, the hepatitis B virus). These precautions are *universal* because they need to be followed at all times, not only when an O&M specialist is dealing with a student who is known to be HIV-positive.

In response to the serious nature of hepatitis B and human immunodeficiency virus (HIV) infections, the U.S. Centers for Disease Control have recommended "universal blood and body-fluid precautions." These measures are intended to prevent transmission of these and other infections. Because it is not always possible to know if a specific student has a communicable infection, these precautions need to be used with every student, regardless of her medical diagnosis.

The purpose of the procedures outlined herein is to establish basic guidelines intended to assist students who may suddenly have a personal hygiene emergency. Instances of such emergencies may include, but not be limited to, a bleeding nose, sneezing, coughing, vomiting, uncontrollable urinating, sudden bowel movement, and serious scrapes and cuts.

ACCIDENTAL EXPOSURE

Accidental exposure to blood, body products, or body fluids places the exposed individual at risk of infection. The single most important step in preventing exposure to and transmission of any infection is anticipating contact with infectious materials in routine as well as emergency situations. Diligent and proper hand washing, the use of barriers, appropriate disposal of waste products, and proper decontamination measures will enhance protection of both the O&M specialist and the student.

HAND WASHING AND GLOVES

If hands (or other skin) become soiled with blood or body fluids, they need to be washed immediately before touching anything else. Proper hand washing is critical in preventing the spread of infection. Use running water, lather with soap, and use friction to clean all surfaces of hands (including any hand jewelry). Rinse well with running water, and dry hands with paper towels. If soap and water are unavailable, wet towelettes, hand sanitizer, or "hand-wipes" may be used.

CLEANUP

Spills of blood and body fluids that are covered under universal precautions need to be cleaned up immediately. Recommended procedures from the Centers for Disease Control and Prevention (1996) include:

- Wearing disposable gloves as a minimum measure of protection. The use of this barrier is intended to reduce the risk of contact with blood and body fluids for the O&M specialist as well as to control the spread of infectious agents from student to student.

- Mopping up spills with paper towels or other absorbent material.

- Using a solution of one part household bleach (sodium hypochlorite) in 10 parts of water, wash the area well.

- Disposing of gloves, soiled towels, and other waste in a sealed double plastic bag, and throw it in the garbage out of the reach of children.

tein) in the red blood cell. The disease gets its name from the sickle shape of the (normally round) red blood cells.

A primary function of red blood cells is to carry oxygen to the tissues. When red blood cells become sickled in shape, they do not flow through blood vessels as smoothly, and can stick to the vessel walls, blocking blood flow through smaller vessels. The tissue beyond the blockage does not receive sufficient oxygen and dies. This can cause irreparable damage, especially if the blood flow is to a vital organ (for example, eyes, brain, heart, or kidneys). A second consequence of sickling is anemia, which leads to the common name, *sickle cell anemia* (SCA). Chronic anemia can lead to retardation of growth and other developmental problems.

Some students with SCA who have had an injury to the brain may have a visual impairment such as optic nerve damage or cortical visual impairment in addition to other consequences of brain injury. The visual impairment can take the form of decreased acuity, decreased field, and problems of visual perception. Students with SCA will often have short attention spans, tire easily, and may have frequent absences from school due to anemia. These absences may last several days or longer, and may increase in frequency during the adolescent years.

Students with SCA are prone to "sickle cell crises" at irregular intervals. Sickle cell crisis can last for hours or weeks and may occur several times per year. It can be precipitated by dehydration, infection, and occasionally stress. In turn, they can cause pain and serious health complications as blood flow to vital organs and tissues is compromised. The symptoms of a sickle cell crisis can be numerous and vary, depending on where in the body the blockage to blood flow occurs. In general, symptoms can include severe pain, nausea, headache, unexplained abnormal behavior, sleepiness or lethargy, urinary bleeding, relative weakness of one side of the body, cough, fever, pallor, or shortness of breath.

There are things that teachers can do, however, to minimize situations that might precipitate a sickling crisis. For example, avoiding situations of extreme emotional stress, physical exercise, dehydration, chilling, infection, and altitude change are important. If a crisis does occur, the teacher can provide simple first aid procedures which focus on improving blood flow. These procedures include applying warm compresses to the painful area, covering the student with a blanket, loosening tight clothing, and letting the student rest. Teachers working with these students should watch for the signs of a crisis, be prepared to provide first aid, and should notify the student's parents and school nurse or other medical personnel when a crisis occurs.

Medications for Health Conditions

People take medications for a variety of health reasons including such conditions as high blood pressure, seizure disorders, and diabetes. While this chapter has discussed a few medications specific to certain conditions, one of the most important issues for the O&M specialist to be aware of is that sometimes medications have side effects that can impact instruction. For example, some medications taken to control seizures can make the student sleepy. Some blood pressure medications, if not taken correctly can cause the student's blood pressure to rise too high or drop too low. Students with certain heart conditions may carry nitroglycerin tablets that they need to take in case of a cardiac emergency. Some anticancer medications, antihistamines, diuretics, antidepressants, and even some acne medications can make students photosensitive. For students taking these medications, sunscreen is a must. Some medications can have side effects that even affect vision. For example, some antianxiety medications such as valium can cause blurred vision in some students; others such as dilantin (taken for some cardiac and circulatory disorders) can cause nystagmus; others such as prednisone (a steroid used to treat conditions such as some cases of asthma) can cause cataracts or increased ocular pressure.

Implications for O&M Training

It is always important to know what medications a student may be taking, their purpose, any potential side effects, and any precautions that need to be taken. For example, using sunscreen is a must for a student who takes medications that can increase photosensitivity.

There are several ways to learn more about medications. The student or student's family may be able to give information about any side effects that the student typically experiences from medication. The information sheets that come with medications also give this information. Additionally, pharmacists are excellent resources for learning about the purposes and potential side effects of a given medication. Pharmacists refer to the *Physician's Desk Reference* for this information. The information is generally written in medical terminology, but the book is available in some libraries and many pharmacies will let you look up information in the book if you ask.

When working with a student who is taking medication, it is important to watch for side effects and to note what they are and when they occur. Sometimes unwanted side effects can be avoided by changing medications. Other times, side effects can be handled by modifying the lesson. For example, if a student who is taking blood pressure medicine suddenly feels dizzy, he can sit down for a minute; a student who is photosensitive (especially if he is visually photosensitive) may wish to wear sunglasses or a visor, even on cloudy days. Sometimes side effects can be minimized by scheduling lessons for a time of day when the side effects tend to be less noticeable.

Up to this point we have examined some of the more common medical conditions that O&M

specialists may encounter when working with students. The next section will focus on another aspect of physical and health disabilities—working with students who use ambulatory aids.

AMBULATORY AIDS

Some people with medical conditions such as those just described rely on ambulatory aids for physical support to move in their environments. *Ambulatory aids* include wheelchairs, scooters, orthopedic canes, crutches, and walkers. While wheelchairs or scooters may not be "ambulatory" aids in the strictest sense of the word, they do provide some people with ambulation difficulties a means of mobility, and in that regard they can also be considered ambulatory aids.

Most ambulatory aids fall into four common categories: wheelchairs and scooters, walkers, crutches, and canes. Although this chapter cannot provide a comprehensive treatment of the topic of ambulatory aids, it provides an overview of devices that are commonly used by people who, because of physical impairments, require physical support for mobility. In general, people use wheelchairs or scooters when they are unable to walk or when they have medical conditions that, when severe, limit endurance in walking. Health conditions that limit walking include heart diseases such as angina pectoris and congestive heart disease. These conditions often impair the heart's ability to keep up with the increased circulatory demands of exercise. People with these conditions generally limit their physical activity; some may use a wheelchair or scooter if they need to travel long distances. In the latter instance, the wheelchair is generally pushed by another person unless it is motorized, because manually propelling a wheelchair actually places even greater physical demands on the heart than does walking. Common lung diseases such as emphysema (which causes shortness of breath when overexerting) also limit a student's ability to exercise. People with severe emphysema may also use a wheelchair (again, generally either motorized or propelled by another person) for traveling long distances. Lastly, circulatory problems such as intermittent claudication can limit a student's ability to walk long distances. *Intermittent claudication* is characterized by an inability of the circulatory system to pump sufficient blood (into the legs, for example) to keep up with the muscles' metabolic needs when exercising. With this condition, a student may experience leg pain when walking long distances; therefore a student who is subject to intermittent claudication might not need an ambulatory aid when walking short distances, but would perhaps use a wheelchair to travel longer distances.

Others, who need physical support to walk, may use walkers, crutches, or canes. The choice of aids depends on factors such as the student's medical condition, the terrain to be traversed, social situations, or even the student's level of fatigue on a given day. Some people may even use a variety of aids over time if their physical condition is such that they either experience an improvement as a result of healing or the benefits of therapy, or experience a decrease in function due to the effects of a progressive disorder.

There are three basic elements of travel for all people, whether sighted or visually impaired, whether ambulatory or not. They are orientation, the negotiation of obstacles in the travel path, and the detection and avoidance of hazards. Inherent in these elements are factors such as safety, quality, and efficiency of movement. However, for the individual who is visually impaired and who also needs an ambulatory aid, there are special and unique considerations for support as well as for environmental preview. Although the approaches presented here by no means represent the entire spectrum of equipment possibilities or even mobility skills, it is hoped that they will stimulate thought and creative approaches to mobility for users of ambulatory aids who have visual impairments.

Mobility for People with Visual Impairments Who Use Wheelchairs or Scooters

Of all the ambulatory aids wheelchairs and scooters provide the most physical support to the user. There are many different types of wheelchairs, from standard models to models designed especially for extra physical support, to "sport" models designed for speed. Some wheelchairs are manually propelled (commonly referred to as *manual wheelchairs*). Other wheelchairs are motorized (sometimes called *power* or *electric wheelchairs*). Procedures for maneuvering a manual wheelchair in various environments are outlined in Sidebar 18.5.

All wheelchairs need to be individually measured and prescribed for the user in order to provide proper support and maximum efficiency of movement. In addition, depending on the user's physical abilities and needs, wheelchairs can be equipped with special features such as extended headrests (for people who require head support), elevating leg rests (for people who must keep one or both legs elevated), anti-tip bars that prevent the wheelchair from tipping over backwards, removable armrests, and wheel adaptations (for people who can use only one arm or who are unable to grasp the hand rim easily when propelling a manual wheelchair). In addition, there are a number of accessories that can be special ordered to make the use of wheelchairs safer and easier. Such accessories include wheelchair trays and baskets to hold items, and specially designed brakes that prevent wheelchairs from rolling backward unexpectedly on inclines. Accessories and aids can generally be purchased at medical supply stores. Cane holders and holsters are available through medical supply stores and some O&M professional organizations, and can even be homemade.

Motorized wheelchairs are most commonly used by people who lack the endurance or upper arm strength to propel a wheelchair manually, or

Procedures for Maneuvering a Manual Wheelchair

SIGHTED GUIDE TECHNIQUE
Participating in basic travel

- Guide pushes wheelchair, providing information about the route as necessary.
- Alternatively, guide gives verbal directions while walking beside the chair while a traveler wheels herself.

Negotiating doorways

- Guide holds door open as traveler maneuvers wheelchair through doorway.
- Alternatively, traveler holds door open with appropriate hand while guide pushes wheelchair through doorway. (Note: In certain situations, going through backward may be more efficient.)

Negotiating curbs

Up curb

- Guide pushes wheelchair so that front wheels are directly in front of curb.
- Guide tilts chair backward by stepping down on tilt bar (located between big wheels) and moves forward until front wheels pass over top of curb and rear wheels contact curb.
- Guide gently lowers front of chair so that front wheels contact ground; guide then pushes chair forward until big wheels contact the side of the curb.
- Guide leans forward and lifts or rolls the chair up and over the curb.

Down curb

Method Number 1

- Guide pushes wheelchair so that front wheels are directly in front of curb.
- Guide tilts chair backward by stepping down on tilt bar (located between big wheels).
- Guide moves forward until front wheels pass over top of curb, gently lowering chair down the curb, and making sure that both rear wheels contact pavement at the same time.
- Guide gently lowers front of chair so that front wheels contact ground.

Method Number 2

- Guide turns wheelchair around to face away from the curb.
- Guide lowers big wheels down the curb, making sure that both rear wheels contact pavement at same time.
- Guide pulls wheelchair backward, gently lowering front wheels down the curb.

INDEPENDENT TRAVEL

Negotiating doorways

Doors that push open

- Traveler maneuvers wheelchair up to door and positions it at a slight angle to allow one hand to contact the door.
- Traveler leans slightly forward in the chair and pushes door open, using the other hand to propel the wheelchair through the doorway.
- As soon as footrests clear the door, the traveler releases the door and uses both hands to propel the wheelchair forward out of the doorway. (Note: If the door is not heavy, the traveler can push it open with the footrests.)

Doors that pull open

- Traveler positions wheelchair in front of, and at a slight angle to, the door, but far enough away so that door will not contact footrests as it opens.
- Using one hand to pull the door open, the traveler propels the wheelchair through the doorway with the other hand. (Note: Sometimes it helps to pull the door open quickly so that it has a slight swing. This allows the traveler to move the wheelchair into the doorway while the door swings closed. The traveler can then continue through the doorway without needing to hold the door open.)

for those who travel long distances. Some people also prefer them because they require almost no physical effort to propel. The user propels the wheelchair forward or backward, or turns it by using a joystick mounted on the frame next to the armrest. For users who lack sufficient arm use to operate a joystick, motorized wheelchairs can be operated using controls that are activated by head movement, eye control, or even mouth. The speed of the wheelchair can be preset at slow, medium, or fast, or can be set to allow the user to accelerate to any desired speed within an available range (up to 6.5 mph) depending on the user's preference and ability to efficiently control the chair's direction of movement.

Motorized wheelchairs consist of a sturdy wheelchair frame with a battery-operated motor enclosed in a case that is generally housed in the back of the wheelchair between the large wheels. The motor works in part on a gear system to also prevent runaways when on an incline or decline. The battery requires regular recharging. This battery generally allows an average of 20 miles (ranging from 15 to 25 miles) of continuous use depending on such factors as the kind of motorized wheelchair, the weight of the user, and the type of terrain being traversed. Also, extremes of hot and cold temperatures will reduce the amount of time the battery will remain charged. A common indication that the battery power is running low is an undesired decrease in speed. Some wheelchairs are equipped with a gauge or panel displaying a series of lights that light up in succession, indicating the amount of charge remaining in a battery. On some models these lights will flash when the battery needs to be recharged. If the battery loses power, the wheelchair can be pushed manually by another person, although it will be necessary to disconnect the gears in the motor, and the wheelchair may still be physically difficult to push. Motorized wheelchairs are also very heavy and therefore difficult to load into vehicles for transport. While there are some experimental wheelchairs designed to travel safely up or down some curbs and over uneven terrain, most

motorized wheelchairs used today must negotiate level differences via curb ramps, driveways, blended curbs, or curb cuts.

Obstacle Detection

One of the great challenges in travel encountered by wheelchair users who are visually impaired is the quick avoidance of obstacles, hazards, and drop-offs in the travel path. If users do not have sufficient warning of obstacles, hazards, or drop-offs, or reaction time for stopping the wheelchair safely, they can inadvertently contact these things—with the potential for injury. In such a case, it may be necessary to recommend a decrease in available speed of the wheelchair. Such a change can be done at any medical supply store with a simple adjustment. A possible additional alternative would be to provide users with an electronic travel device, a long cane, or both to enable them to be aware of such things sooner.

For obstacle or hazard detection, the list of innovative solutions is endless. To warn students of an approaching down step, raised, or colored strips (often rubber, metal, or vinyl tape) can be placed on the floor sufficiently in advance of the down step to allow wheelchair users time to stop safely. In order to avoid unexpected and potentially painful contacts with walls, up steps, garbage cans, furniture, and other objects, one can purchase footrests that are longer than the user's foot. Longer footrests can avoid many stubbed toes. These footrests can be purchased from dealers who sell wheelchairs. To detect obstacles at waist height, a lap tray provides an effective bumper. As a note, if a lap tray is used, it needs to be clear for students with low vision so that they can see through the tray for preview of the terrain in front of them.

Collisions with objects on the side such as walls, doors, counters, and so on can cause scrapes, bruises, and painful bumps when a hand is unexpectedly caught between the metal pushing rim of the wheel and the object. One solution is to place flexible curb feelers (available at auto supply stores) or semi-flexible wire on the post of the

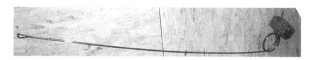

Figure 18.3.
When attached to a wheelchair, this curb feeler scrapes against nearby objects, warning the user of obstacles.

front wheel or on the vertical post at the front of the armrest (see Figure 18.3). The feeler will gently scrape an obstacle alongside the wheelchair before the user is close enough to contact it with his hand. The curb feeler also makes an audible signal as it contacts an object, letting people know that they are very close to it. Curb feelers, when positioned at a 45-degree angle backward (rather than perpendicular to the student's path) will gently slide along a surface without scratching it and will bend backward when traversing doorways, thereby not blocking passage.

People who are visually impaired and use wheelchairs have the same training needs as their counterparts who do not use wheelchairs. For the wheelchair user, the travel considerations and techniques may be different. For example, the techniques used to maneuver a wheelchair through a doorway depend on several factors. Does the door open toward the person or away? Does it open to the right or left? How much space is to either side of the door? How heavy is the door? Is it spring-loaded or free-swinging? How high is the threshold? Are there other environmental factors like wind that may make the door harder to open than at normal times? There are too many variables to accurately predict what problems each individual wheelchair user may have or how O&M techniques may have to be modified. The following are samples of modifications of O&M techniques.

Human Guide

Perhaps the easiest way to "guide" a student who uses a wheelchair would be for the guide to push the wheelchair. Most power wheelchairs have

mechanisms to release the automatic brakes that keep the chair from rolling when it is not being driven. The students need to be able to either disengage the mechanism themselves or be able to describe the process to their guide. In many cases, however, this is not the best answer. For example, if the guide is a cane user, the position behind the chair makes it impossible to reach far enough forward with the cane to clear the path and have adequate advance warning of obstacles or hazards. It is also very difficult to push scooters or power wheelchairs. Many ultralight wheelchairs don't have back frames to push from. For some people, pushing themselves is a matter of pride, dignity, and self-respect. Being pushed can feel humiliating. If the guide is going to push the wheelchair, they always need to ask for permission first. To avoid injuring the wheelchair user, the guide needs to make certain that the student's hands are clear of the wheels.

Some wheelchair users are able to hold onto a guide's arm. While some may not have the physical ability to hold on safely, maintain the grasp, or feel and respond to subtle movements from the guide's arm, others do have adequate arm strength, flexibility, and proprioception to do so successfully. While holding the guide's elbow is one way to be guided, it is easier for many people to put their hand on top of the guide's forearm, which is held parallel to the floor. This allows the guide to point in the direction of the desired turn. Especially for turns toward the wheelchair user, this facilitates smooth turns. For manual chairs, the forearm position also allows the guide to help propel the chair. As the guide pulls his grasped arm forward, the student pushes the opposite side wheel with her other hand. If the chair unintentionally turns away from the guide, the guide needs to slow down so that the student can keep up with her free hand. If the guide is visually impaired and uses a cane, he needs to modify his cane technique and pace to ensure that his is adequately covering both himself and the far side of the wheelchair.

Some people who use electric chairs or scooters don't mind having another person operate the controls of the chair and to help steer. When doing so, the guide needs to turn the power or speed control to a low setting. The chair controls are very sensitive and are more difficult to control from the side than they are from the seat. Especially at first, the guide should not operate the chair from in front.

Some wheelchair users choose to follow the guide visually instead of maintaining physical contact. In order to do this safely, the wheelchair user also needs to be able to detect drop-offs independently, either by spotting the drop-off visually, using a cane in conjunction with being guided, or by visually noticing subtle level changes in the guide's movement. Visually tracking transition points on the guide, such as from a light shirt to dark pants, can make it easier for the person being guided to detect level changes.

Navigating Doors with a Guide

When pushing someone in a wheelchair, it is often awkward navigating doors, especially when the doors are self-closing. Students who can use their arms can often assist with doors. If the door is a pull door and there is adequate space on the handle side of the door, the guide needs to push the wheelchair up to the wall to the handle side of the door. The student can reach up and grab the door; then, as the guide pulls the wheelchair backward, the student pulls the door open. If the door opens away from the student, the guide can push the chair up to the center of the doorway. The student can then reach up and work the door handle. The student holds the door open while the guide then pushes the chair forward and then is able to take the weight of the door from the student.

With a power chair or scooter, whether the guide is controlling the chair or the student is holding the guide's arm, the guide can pass through the door first. It is often easier for the guide to turn

around and back through the doorway. Again, if the student has use of her arms, she can assist with the door as they pass through.

Trailing

Two additional challenges facing wheelchair users who are visually impaired are maintaining orientation to the environment and following a straight line of travel. Straight-line travel is especially problematic for many wheelchair users who do not have sufficient vision to aid them in this task. When using a wheelchair, one does not have the degree of proprioceptive feedback of direction that is available when walking, and it is much harder to monitor one's movement through space. Also, many neurological conditions such as a stroke, cerebral palsy, and traumatic brain injury can impair the proprioceptive sensory system, making it even harder for a student to monitor her position in space. For some students, practice in pushing equally with both arms can be helpful in increasing proprioceptive awareness of straight-line travel.

Orientation to the environment, use of landmarks, and, when necessary, assistance with travel in a straight line can be accomplished through trailing a wall or other parallel surface. Many people who use wheelchairs can trail walls in the same way as people who do not use wheelchairs—they can either use their hands or a cane. Using one's hand to trail, however, does not allow for detection of drop-offs or obstacles in front of the chair. The footplate of the chair usually extends beyond the student's reach, causing her to bump the intersecting wall or other obstacle with the footplate instead of contacting it with her hand. For students without adequate vision to see obstacles and drop-offs, hand trailing needs to be done only in safe, familiar environments.

When hand trailing with a power chair or scooter, a patting method may be preferable, instead of a dragging method. If sliding one's hand along the wall, the person in the chair needs to watch hand positioning very closely. With the power chair or scooter, jamming fingers can be more painful due to speed, the reaction time for stopping, and the braking distance of the chair. Also, people's arms are often in a less flexible position than they are when they are standing. If the joystick is on the side of the wall to be trailed, they may not be able to use their hands. They may need to use a cane or other method. Some people have used a folded or short cane to maintain contact with a wall.

When using the hand to trail with a manual chair, there are several possible methods:

1. The student propels the wheelchair using the outside hand (one furthest from the wall or trailing surface). She holds her arm nearest the wall forward as far as possible and exerts pressure on the wall to help with propulsion and to keep the chair pointed straight ahead (pushing forward on the opposite wheel rim turns the foot plate forward with each push). If the student needs to, she can bend the elbow of her arm nearest the wall in time with the push of her outside hand, then re-extend her hand on the wall as she reaches back for a new push with the outside hand.

2. If the student's arm is too weak to keep the chair from turning into the wall, she may have to use both hands to push the chair forward one push, then reach up to check the wall. The student does not need to give more than one or two forward pushes before checking the wall.

3. Some people have learned to use both hands to push the chair, while extending their elbow, pinky, or side of the hand to contact the wall.

For those who can't use a cane or their hands to trail, some have successfully used curb feelers from a car to trail a wall or curb. Trailing can be done in a quiet environment by listening to the sound of a curb feeler gently scraping across the parallel surface. When contacting surfaces of different materials, the sound made will change. In this way a student in school, for example, can differentiate between tile walls, metal lockers, wood or brick, or glass surfaces. Similarly, the number of openings, whether doorways or intersecting hallways, can be identified by the cessation of sound from the curb feeler. While the sound of curb feelers indicate when the wheelchair moves away from the wall (or there is an opening), they do not let the student know when she gets too close.

Use of Electronic Travel Aids

Electronic travel aids (ETAs) provide another means of travel without unwanted encounters with obstacles or hazards (see Chapter 14, "Teaching the Use of Electronic Travel Aids and Electronic Orientation Aids"). The MiniGuide, placed on its side and clamped to a wheelchair tray, or otherwise secured in a position at the user's midline, provides an arc of ultrasound that covers body and wheelchair width quite well. It may also be placed on a swivel bracket for scanning.

Head-mounted devices can provide similar coverage. The use of these devices, however, requires the user to keep his head up at all times so the device will not detect the user's lap unintentionally. This can be difficult in the presence of certain physical impairments. One disadvantage of most devices, however, is that they will not detect down curbs or descending stairs. A solution to this problem is the use of a long cane.

Cane Techniques

The use of the long cane by the wheelchair user is really not as complicated and formidable a task as one might imagine. It may require the use of a motorized wheelchair, a scooter, or a means of propelling a manual wheelchair with one arm, although some students have found success by using the cane both as a propeller and an environmental sensor. When doing so, the student first places the cane tip at her side and "pushes off" with it in the same way that a skier pushes off with a ski pole. The student then quickly moves the cane to a forward position to clear the next area in front of her wheelchair while propelling forward with her other hand on the wheel. The sequence then repeats itself. This technique requires great trunk, shoulder, and arm strength as well as coordination, but for some students, even some without low vision, this technique works. Another method of propelling a wheelchair with one arm is often used by people who have hemiplegia (paralysis on one side of the body). They propel forward (and consequently to the opposite side) by pushing on the rim of the large wheel with their stronger arm, and then correct their direction by pushing against the ground with their foot, much as one does when sitting on a scooter or wheeled office chair and turning or rolling from one desk to another. For people who are able to use one foot for steering, this method frees one hand to use a cane or ETA, or to trail.

Another option for propelling a wheelchair using only one arm is to use a wheelchair equipped with a one-arm drive mechanism or to use a monodrive wheelchair. The one-arm drive mechanism consists of two concentric rims on one of the large wheels. To turn left, one rim is pushed; to turn right, the other rim is pushed. To move forward or backward, both rims are pushed or pulled simultaneously. Use of the one-arm drive, however, requires a high level of strength and motor control to use, and it is difficult to move forward in a perfectly straight line without periodic veer correction.

Similarly, the monodrive wheelchair is one that is manually propelled by pumping a hand lever back and forth. To turn, the user turns the hand grip of the lever left or right. To brake, the user pushes the lever fully forward. Although the monodrive wheelchair has been shown to maneuver fairly easily over rough terrain, its

pump mechanism can make it difficult to identify veering.

Last, motorized scooters and chairs are becoming increasingly popular, especially by the elderly and by people who have limited endurance. Some motorized scooters, however, have a steering bar (tiller) located directly in front of the body at midline. Most people can reach around the scooter's tiller with the long white cane. As an alternative, the hand holding the cane can rest on the handle of the tiller. The tiller can be leaned back toward the user to make it easier to reach around or over. Some scooters of this type also require two hands to steer. Many newer models offer controls at a student's side, much like a motorized wheelchair, and make it much easier to use a long cane. When using a scooter, it should be noted that three-wheeled scooter models can tip over more easily than a wheelchair or four-wheeled scooter when encountering uneven terrain.

Students need to learn all of the standard cane techniques including two-point touch, constant contact, three-point touch, and touch and drag. Sidebar 18.6 offers a few quick tips on canes for wheelchair users.

When using a long cane, the tip remains in contact with the ground at all times. Doing so increases detection of even subtle terrain changes such as slight drop-offs, bumps, slopes, or grass that can impact the stability or maneuverability of the wheelchair. Many people using two-point touch are unable to detect such small level changes and a drop-off of just two inches is enough to tip over a wheelchair. Using a constant-contact technique also minimizes the physical effort of using a cane for people who have limited arm strength.

Cane tips with a large surface (for example, a jumbo roller tip, marshmallow tip, or ball tip) are recommended to minimize chances of the cane tip sticking in sidewalk cracks or rough surfaces. These tips also do not wear down as readily as standard nylon tips, and many students find that

Tips on Canes for Wheelchair Users

- Adjust the length of the cane to the person's speed. Usually, the longer the cane, the faster the person can go. The cane needs to be as long as needed to allow sufficient reaction time to stop the wheelchair, yet not so long that the student cannot maneuver it safely and fluidly.

- The student can hold the cane either with the hand centered or to the side with one's arm supported on the armrest. This choice generally depends on physical ability, need, and student preference. Similarly, one can choose to use either the handshake or pencil grip, again depending on student preference. For students who prefer to hold the cane in midline, it is often recommended to use a pencil grip because it allows the student to hold the cane at a higher angle. In this way, if the cane tip contacts an object abruptly, the cane grip will tend to move upward rather than impact the student's stomach should she continue to move forward any distance before stopping. Roller tips are often preferred. Jumbo rollers or roller ball tips (the latter the size of a pool cue ball) should be tried.

- It is recommended that the wheelchair user not use a telescoping cane, or use it with caution, because the added momentum often present in the movement of the wheelchair can cause some canes to collapse rather than remain extended when contacting obstacles in front of the user.

- Rigid canes are ideal, but they are hard to put away when not in use. One idea is to purchase a clip or clamp designed to hold reachers. The cane can be placed in the clamp when not in use. It will also help to identify the person as being visually impaired. Make sure the clamp will hold the cane tight so that it doesn't slip down and touch the ground. Also make sure that the clamp is positioned so that the student can reach the cane. The cane sticking up may also help with visibility.

- Rigid fiberglass canes have some flex to them. When a rigid fiberglass cane hits an obstacle, it gives the user less of a jolt. It also tends to bend (up to a point before splitting) and frees the tip when it gets caught in a crack.

- For power chairs and scooters, primarily teach use of the cane in the nondominant hand. The dominant hand is needed for driving.

- For scooters, teach students to be able to use either hand to drive the chair, so they can in turn use the cane in either hand. This is especially important for navigating doorways.

- Remove baskets, lap trays, or other interfering attachments from the front of chairs. Many people like the baskets on the front of their chairs, but get one that is easily removable so that the cane can be used at night, in unfamiliar areas or as needed. People who choose to reach around their baskets tend to be less accurate with or responsive to their canes. Many lap desks have to be removed completely to get them out of the way. Lap trays that are hinged on one side can be moved out of the way when not needed, and then swung back when needed.

the jumbo roller tip rolls most easily over ground surfaces.

The student will also make a wider than normal arc with the cane, because it is important to cover the width of the wheelchair in addition to the body width (an additional 4–8 inches). Also, just as it is important to clear the area in front of oneself before proceeding forward, it is important to carefully clear to the side before turning in order to detect any obstacles, hazards, or level changes that the front casters of the wheelchair or footrests might encounter during the turning process. In fact, side drop-offs are more dangerous than front drop-offs in that a wheelchair is more likely to tip over when going over a side drop-off. The instructor needs to make sure that the person is using a wide-enough arc that he has time to detect the drop-off and either stop or correct the line of travel before the front wheel hits the drop-off.

An effective method of helping a student learn to react quickly to cane contacts while using residual vision to navigate is to use a blindfold or lower field occluder while practicing reaction to cane contacts. Lay out obstacle courses or random low obstacles for the student to hit with her cane and see if she reacts in time to keep from rolling over the obstacles. If she doesn't learn to stop in time, the speed on the chair or the length of the cane may need to be adjusted.

For students using manual chairs, if they can place one foot on the ground, it will help maintain the straight line of travel and free one hand up to use the cane. The student propels the wheelchair with one hand (which will tend to turn the wheelchair toward the opposite side with each push of the wheel rim) and uses his foot as an anchor to return the chair to a straight forward direction. The line of travel will be straightest if the hand pushing the wheelchair is on the side opposite the foot being used to propel or guide the chair. The student's leg does not need to be strong enough to pull the chair, just strong enough

to reach forward and give a new anchor point for the chair to move forward.

Some people are unable to visually determine the height of drop-offs. By locating the drop-off with the cane, then pulling up to it (just like finding the top of stairs), the cane can be raised until the tip clears the top of the drop-off. This gives the person the height of the drop. By starting with the cane held as close to vertical as possible, then resting the cane against a solid object (handlebars, joystick box, lap desk, knee etc.) slide the hand holding the cane to the top of the solid object. Next, lift the hand and cane together until the tip clears the top of the drop-off. The new distance between the hand and the top of the solid object is the height of the curb. The height that a chair can safely drive off of or climb over is determined by the make of the chair, the position of the wheelie bars, and the individual's ability to drive off the drop-off in a straight line.

Controlling a Power Chair

For a person to drive a power chair or scooter, it is critical that they not move faster than they can preview the path in front of them and react to potential obstacles or hazards. Most power chairs and scooters have controls to adjust the speed at which they move. Some have an adjustment for the sensitivity level of the joystick. For indoor travel, turning the power control to half speed is usually sufficient for maintaining control. Outdoors and especially at street crossings, the person may want to turn the power back up to full speed.

One method to determine if the person has adequate control of her chair is to have the person drive down the hall at top speed, then yell stop. Measure the distance that the chair rolls after the joystick or power lever has been released. If this distance is greater than the distance at which the person can detect obstacles, drop-offs, or hazards, then the speed is not safe and she needs to keep her chair at a lower power or speed setting.

A second way to check is to place something that the person can see on the floor at a random place in the hall. Have her drive down the hall at full speed and stop as soon as she sees the obstacle. If the chair fails to stop before reaching the obstacle, the speed is too high. If she cannot see the obstacle, place something that she can feel with her cane and have her stop when she feels the cane contact the obstacle.

A third method is to walk in front of the student with a cane pointed back toward her, but just out of reach. Randomly plant the cane on the floor so that the student will hit it with her own cane. Without moving the instructor's cane, check to see if the student can stop before running into it with the wheelchair. If not, then she is going too fast. The instructor needs to be ready to drop his cane to avoid breaking it, just in case the student does not stop.

For some people, the factory speed settings are too fast for them to control. The dealer can adjust the power settings for various actions. In particular, turning speed may need to be adjusted. Often, the turning speed is preset at 75–80 percent of full power. Many students may need to reduce their turning speed to 50 percent of full power. Reducing turning speed gives the student more control over her turns. If she frequently turns too far, then reducing the speed of the turns is in order. In the chairs with multiple modes, each mode can be set individually for a specific type of environment.

It is critical that the instructor has a means to stop a student's momentum. Depending on the situation and the student's reaction time, simply saying, "Stop," may not allow the student to stop in time. Before doing any outdoor assessment or instruction, the instructor needs to work out with the student how he will stop the student should she start to head into a dangerous situation. The procedure for stopping the student needs to be practiced in a clear, safe open area before proceed-

ing. Options to stop the wheelchair in an emergency situation include such things as attaching an "attendant control" device to the wheelchair. These devices can be purchased at wheelchair supply stores and allow the O&M specialist to override the student's control of the wheelchair at any time. In this way, the O&M specialist can stop, start, or turn the chair in any way necessary for safety. Another option is for the instructor to walk on the side of the chair nearest the joystick. If it is necessary to intervene, he can simply reach over and take control of the joystick.

Visibility

An additional problem commonly faced by wheelchair users is visibility. Because a wheelchair can be quieter than a cane, it may be a silent-moving obstacle to other students who are blind. Some wheelchair users place a playing card in the spokes of the large wheel to give an auditory indicator of their movement. This is most commonly done in schools or centers where there are large numbers of people with visual impairments moving about. As the card wears and softens, the sound becomes quieter, so users replace the card periodically. If users wish to begin with a quieter sound, they can soften the card slightly before use.

Visibility to traffic is another concern of wheelchair users. Because users are lower to the ground than people who are standing and because they might show up in unexpected places (for example, moving along a road edge, or entering a road from a driveway in areas where there are no curb ramps), there is the concern that they will not be seen readily by drivers. This is critical in street crossings and areas without sidewalks where the wheelchair user might need to travel on the road edge. In response to this concern, some wheelchair users attach a red bicycle flag on a tall pole to the handle of their wheelchair to draw drivers' attention to them when they are crossing streets (see Figure 18.4). Other students choose

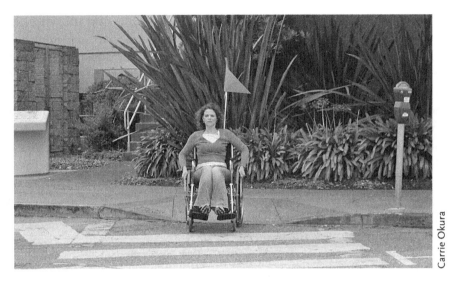

Carrie Okura

Figure 18.4.
This traveler has attached a bicycle flag to her wheelchair to enable drivers to see her more easily in traffic.

not to use a flag in order to avoid drawing undue attention to themselves. If a student chooses to use a flag, bicycle dealers can often provide custom brackets to attach flags to the wheelchair.

A special consideration in providing O&M instruction to people who use wheelchairs is that of transferring from a manual wheelchair to another sitting surface, such as the seat of a car. Depending on the student's medical condition, strength, and weight; the model of wheelchair used; environmental considerations; and student preference, this transfer can be accomplished in one of several ways. Sometimes wheelchair users are able to transfer in and out of the wheelchair without assistance. Sometimes they will use special equipment such as a sliding board (see Figure 18.5). At times, the O&M specialist may need to provide assistance during the transfer process. If the planned program of O&M instruction requires that the student transfer in or out of the wheelchair, the O&M specialist needs to become familiar with the technique(s) used by that student and how to safely and effectively assist, if necessary. The specialist can do this by simply

asking the student and a family member for information (or even a demonstration, if appropriate). Additionally, physical therapists, occupational therapists, and other medical personnel can provide general information and guidelines on safe and effective transfer techniques.

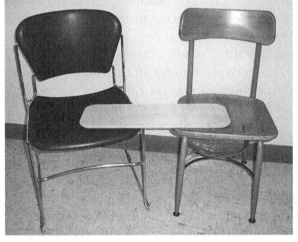

Sandy Rosen

Figure 18.5.
Sliding boards form a bridge to slide from one surface to another.

Negotiating Ramps at Buildings

For manual wheelchairs, ascending ramps into buildings are often too steep for a person to negotiate independently without rolling backward between pushes on the wheel rims. In this case, the person can solicit assistance or if handrails are available, use them to help pull herself up the ramp. The following sequence is for situations where the ramp is too steep for a person to navigate using just the wheel rims to move forward.

- *Up*: (1) With one hand on the rail, and the other on the wheel, at the same time, the hand on the rail pulls, while the hand on the wheel pushes forward. Try to remain straight in the process. (2) Release with the hand on the handrail and quickly reach forward to a new grasp. (3) Release the hand on the wheel and quickly establish a new grasp. (4) Repeat the procedure.

- *Down*: Basically, going down is the same procedure. (1) Allow the chair to drop with both hands at the same time. (2) Quickly readjust the grip on the handrail side. (3) Quickly readjust the grasp on the wheel. (4) Repeat the procedure. Note that other users will control the downward momentum of the manual wheelchair by using the hand brakes to apply varying amounts of "resistance" to the large wheels.

- *Hill climbers*: An accessory called hill climbers allow the wheels to roll forward, but not backward. Hill climbers are essentially unidirectional brakes. They are attached above the wheel. When the lever is pushed back, the hill climber doesn't touch the tire. When the lever is pushed forward, a ridged half circle glides over the forward moving tire. When the tire moves backward, the ridges grip and the hill climber rolls down to apply pressure, breaking the regress of the tire. The cli-

ent has to be able to flip the hill climber on or off. If it is left on, the person cannot back up from a desk, obstacle, or make a backward pivot turn.

Sidewalk Travel

Several suggestions may make it easier for students to safely navigate the sidewalk.

1. Stay to the inside shoreline. It is often flatter than the outside shoreline. The edges of driveways often have severe slopes, sometimes steep enough to tip a wheelchair.

2. Watch out for lateral slopes. Some chairs will swing out of control on steep side slopes. Some people lose control because they become frightened. Some scooters will tip if the slope is steep enough.

3. People, who trail walls auditorily or visually when indoors, may have a very difficult time without those walls to follow.

4. Some people may need to reduce their traveling speed. Often, the student doesn't realize the potential dangers outdoors that were not present in familiar indoor environments.

5. Match the pace of the other pedestrians. For the student with low vision, weaving in and out of pedestrian traffic can lead to accidents.

6. Don't forget to look up for overhangs. If students focus too much on the ground, they may miss overhanging limbs or the like.

7. Avoid driving off the side of the sidewalk into the grass. In some cases it is okay, but in some, there is a severe level change, which can tip the chair.

8. Recheck the cane skills to see if changes need to be made. For a wide variety of reasons, a student's cane skills can deteriorate in the transition from indoor to outdoor travel.

9. Due to hills, cracks, and distances to be traveled, some people who use manual chairs indoors will need to switch to power chairs outdoors.

Negotiating Curb Ramps at Street Corners

Negotiating a curb ramp at a street corner can sometimes pose a challenge for the wheelchair user who has a visual impairment. Curb ramps can face either straight across the perpendicular street, be oriented perpendicular to the line of travel, point diagonally across the intersection, or take up the entire corner. Students need to demonstrate the ability to safely navigate a wide variety of ramp types.

The following safety tips can make the trip easier. Once the student locates the corner, she can use her cane to locate the center of the ramp and the direction of the downward slope. By reaching to both sides of the ramp with the cane, the student should be able to detect the beveled sides of the ramp (where the ramp rises to the height of the curb). The center of the ramp should then be the midpoint between the two sides. Some people can detect the two sides by swinging their cane back and forth across the ramp. Others need to reach out with their cane as far as they can, then draw it back to the chair to determine if there is a drop-off in that direction. Using the clock face, they should reach out at 10, 11, 12, 1, and 2 o'clock to search for the drop-off. Once they think that they have found the ramp, they should face the ramp and repeat the process. When they repeat the process, they may find that the center is not where they initially thought it was. If the wheelchair is not centered in the ramp, it could list sideways on the ramp or come down with an uncomfortable and potentially dangerous bump when the wheelchair rolls forward over the beveled ramp edge onto the street.

Street Crossings

With curb ramps. The student negotiates the curb ramp first, and then stops to wait when the front wheels reach the bottom of the ramp and waits at the bottom of the curb ramp to initiate the street crossing. Once the center is established, the person needs to descend the ramp as close to the center as possible and parallel to the decline of the ramp. She does this by entering the downward slope of the ramp slowly, and stopping the wheelchair before the front wheels cross the lip of the ramp and go into the street. Using the cane in constant-contact technique is one way to monitor the location of the wheelchair relative to the street edge of the ramp and the beveled sides. Once positioned at the edge of the ramp, the wheelchair user positions the cane in the waiting position and crosses at the appropriate time. She then positions the wheelchair to go up the center of the wheelchair ramp on the other side of the street. If she veers during the crossing, she can locate the upward ramp on the other side of the street using standard street-crossing recovery skills.

It is also important to note that a downward slope of a curb ramp may be angled kitty-corner rather than directly across the street. Because it may be necessary to enter the street on an angle rather than aligned for a straight crossing, the student needs to be able to realign in order to complete the crossing. Some students may find this difficult to do quickly enough to complete the crossing safely. The safety and effectiveness with which a student can negotiate curb ramps needs to be determined by the wheelchair user and the O&M specialist on a case-by-case basis.

If the student might have trouble crossing the street in adequate time, crossing on the left side of the street may allow the perpendicular traffic on the last half of the crossing a better view of the student trying to finish the crossing.

On streets with steep cambers, the chair may not be able to climb the hill quickly enough. The student can turn slightly away from the parallel street to see if the chair climbs more easily when moving across the incline, rather than directly up the hill. If it does, she can turn back toward the parallel traffic and zigzag up the hill. Sometimes this is only needed to get started and the first zig will be adequate to get the chair moving. The student needs to be able to reestablish her line of travel after the turns.

Without curb ramps or in areas without sidewalks. If the intersection doesn't have curb ramps, the student can travel along the quieter of the two streets and locate the nearest driveway. She can access the sidewalk from the driveway and handle the intersection as if it didn't have sidewalks.

If there are no sidewalks and the student needs to travel in the street along the curb edge, the manner in which a student positions herself for the crossing can vary. In areas with an adequate shoulder, a student who cannot see the far side of the intersection can drive around the corner onto the perpendicular street and, when the edge straightens out, square off the back of the wheelchair to the edge. If the student can see the far side of the intersection, or if there is not an adequate shoulder on which to wait, she needs to wait at the point of the corner and not continue around it. The person who can see the far side may want to keep her chair parallel to the curb, taking up as little space as possible. Safety in completing such crossings needs to be determined individually by the O&M instructor and the student for each crossing location. Safety will be determined by the student's travel skills, visibility to traffic, ability to use residual vision, size of the intersection and of any shoulder or safety zone near the curb, and traffic flow at the intersection. These procedures should not be used in unfamiliar areas or areas where there is heavy traffic.

Mobility for People with Visual Impairments Who Use Walkers

While there are many different types of walkers, they all consist of four legs and a handle (or two) with which the user maneuvers. Most walkers will fit into the back of a car or a large trunk, and some are designed to fold for easier transport. Some are equipped with tips especially designed to grip the ground securely with suction-cup action when weight is placed on the walker. Others have special tips called "glide tips" that let the walker literally glide along almost any surface. If the walker does not come with glide tips, the student can purchase them at a medical supply store; some people even cut tennis balls and place them on the legs to allow the walker to glide on smooth indoor surfaces. Due to safety considerations, however, these modifications always need the prior approval of a qualified health professional such as a physician or physical therapist.

Other walkers come with wheels. Some walkers have wheels only on the front two legs; others have wheels on all four legs. Some have hand brakes and others do not. Walkers with wheels are used by people who do not have sufficient strength, coordination, or balance to lift the walker during ambulation. The user simply rolls the walker forward or lifts the two back legs and rolls the walker forward on the front two wheels. With the latter model, if the user places any weight on the walker, the back legs contact the ground automatically and provide a stable support.

Some walkers are held in front of the student (see Figure 18.6A); some are held on the side (see Figure 18.6B); others are placed behind the student, and pulled forward with each step. These latter walkers are often used by children who need support from behind to maintain an erect posture while walking. Some walkers are designed for use with one hand. Some walkers even come with fold-down seats for people who may have limited endurance and need to travel distances longer

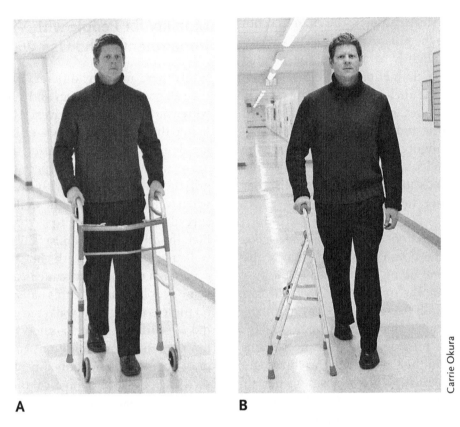

A   B

Carrie Okura

Figure 18.6.
(A) Some walkers are held in front of the student; and (B) some walkers are held on the side.

than their endurance allows. In addition to these basic types of walkers, there are a variety of modifications for children depending on age, physical size, and physical impairment. Last, there are a variety of accessories available such as carrying baskets that fit on the front or sides of walkers.

It is generally the role of the physical therapist to prescribe and fit a walker to a student. The height of the walker needs to be such that when the student stands erect and about halfway into the walker and holds the handrails, his elbow will be bent to 30 degrees from the vertical (see Figure 18.7). Another way to measure the proper height is to have the student stand with his arms hanging comfortably at his sides and note that the height of the walker comes up to the bony protrusion on the side of the wrist. As a note,

this latter approach will not work for people who have conditions in which their arms are proportionally too short or too long compared to their height (for example, Marfan's syndrome). The proper elbow position (30 degrees of flexion) places the triceps muscle in the arm (the one that straightens and stabilizes the elbow) at an optimum amount of stretch to contract quickly and strongly if the student suddenly places weight on his arms in an effort to support himself or catch his balance. When using the walker it is important that the student walk halfway into the walker with each step. Walking further into the walker can make it unstable, and walking further behind the walker can cause the front of the walker to tip up and slide out from under the student if he stumbles. Walking too

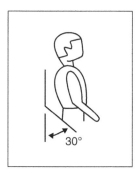

Figure 18.7. Proper Elbow Position for Using a Walker
A bend of 30 degrees at the elbow positions the arm to provide optimum support when using a walker.

far behind the walker also sacrifices lateral support for the student.

Human Guide with a Walker

One of the most effective ways to serve as a human guide for a student who uses a walker is to perform *reverse sighted guide*. This can be done in one of three ways:

1. The guide can hold the student's elbow and apply light pressure to let the student know to turn right or left. The guide needs to maintain light pressure and avoid pushing the student's elbow forward in order to not interfere with the student's balance or place uncomfortable pressure on the student's arm. If they need to stop, the guide can use additional pressure on the elbow as a signal to stop or pull lightly back on the elbow.

2. Alternatively, the guide can lightly place one hand on the student's back, between the shoulder blades. No forward pressure is applied when walking straight ahead. By giving light pressure on either the left or right shoulder blade, the guide can tell the student when and how much to turn when needed. To stop, the guide simply tells the student to stop or can place one hand on top of the nearest shoulder as a signal to stop.

3. As another option, the guide can place his hand on top of the student's hand as they walk and give gentle prearranged tactile signals for stopping, starting, or turning.

While some students may be uncomfortable with tactile signals on their back, arm, or hand, these techniques are extremely efficient means of conveying directional information and allow for conversation while traveling. For students who prefer to not have the guide make physical contact with them, the guide can simply provide verbal instructions.

Some students who have four-wheeled walkers with seats may choose to sit on the seat while the guide pushes the walker. While riding, the student can pick up his feet and place them on the bars coming up from the back wheels. Some walkers actually come with footrests for use while sitting on the walker. Not all walkers with seats, however, are sturdy enough to be pushed forward while the user is sitting. Some walkers will collapse if they suddenly contact a large crack (including tactile warning strips). In addition, some walkers may not easily roll over cracks or thresholds when the student's weight is in the seat. If the student is able to put his feet down and lift his weight slightly, however, the front wheels will often go ahead and hop the crack or threshold.

Orientation and Trailing

Adapted mobility for those who use a walker follows many of the same principles as for those who use a wheelchair. With regard to orientation, straight-line travel can be as difficult for people who use walkers as it is for those who use wheelchairs. Practice in extending both arms forward equidistantly with each step may help some people to improve proprioceptive awareness of straight-line travel. With specific regard to trailing, there are many ways in which a student can follow a wall, for example, when using a walker. He might be able to simply walk near the wall and either reach out with his hand, or even just reach an elbow out to contact the wall with each step. Another option is to hold a folded (or telescoped) cane in the hand nearest the wall, and trail the wall with the end of the cane.

Similarly, some have used curb feelers mounted on the front leg of the walker (about 2 inches off the ground, and facing backward at a 45-degree angle) to trail vertical surfaces. Ideally, curb feelers provide information about objects on the user's side before any unwanted contact with the hand (although some students do find it difficult to tell when they are too close to the wall and inadvertently still contact the wall with their hand). Mounting the feelers at about 2 inches off the ground is recommended, because at this height they will be low enough to detect steps, curbs, or similar low objects. Mounting them backward at a 45-degree angle positions the feelers to bend backward when going through doorways instead of catching on the door frame.

Obstacle Detection

Early obstacle detection is extremely important for people who use walkers. Due to the effects of impaired balance, sudden changes in terrain can sometimes present serious challenges to balance, even when one is using an ambulatory aid. While walkers do not safely detect drop-offs, some walkers do provide limited obstacle detection. Those that are held in front of the user provide a ready-made forward bumper to indicate contact with an obstacle in the student's path. Adding a ribbon or light PVC tubing that stretches between the front legs at knee height can provide additional object detection without interfering with the student's gait or safety. Walkers held on the side will detect obstacles on the side. Walkers held behind the user, however, provide no forward obstacle detection. In this latter situation, it may be pos-

sible to adapt the walker by placing a removable bar or strap across the front opening to detect obstacles before the user contacts them with his body. Homemade devices can be easily fabricated to serve this function—such devices, however, must be attached so they do not interfere with foot placement during ambulation or become a hazard to the student when getting into and out of the walker. A physical therapist can be of assistance in determining the best type and location of such a device for a specific user.

Using the Long Cane with a Walker

As is true when using a wheelchair or scooter, the long cane provides an excellent means of obstacle detection when using a walker. While it may, at first, appear impossible to use a long cane when both hands are needed to maneuver a walker, there are actually several ways in which this can be done. One solution is to push the walker forward with one hand while using the long cane in the other hand (see Figure 18.8). Depending on the terrain, the weight of the walker, and the student's strength, this can be surprisingly easy to do. If the student is using a walker with wheels or glide tips, it may be possible for him to hold the walker with one hand and hold the cane and walker simultaneously with the other hand. In this case, the palm of the cane hand presses on either the walker handle or on the center bar. The student holds the cane in a pencil grasp and uses the constant contact technique as he walks. Some students prefer a cane with a roller tip or one that is very lightweight (for example, fiberglass) to do this most easily. The diagonal technique is, of course, not recommended because it will not reliably pick up many low obstacles or side drop-offs.

If the student does not have the agility to hold the walker and use the cane at the same time, or does not have the balance or strength to hold on with just one hand, he may be able to perform the following three-step approach: from a standing

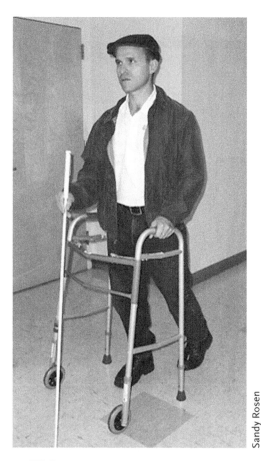

Sandy Rosen

Figure 18.8.
This traveler is pushing the walker forward with one hand while using the long cane in his other hand.

position, the student uses the cane to clear the path, then grasps the walker and moves the walker forward. He then steps up into the walker, reestablishes his balance, and repeats the process. This is a very slow process, but it can work in unfamiliar areas, on sidewalks, or when the student knows that he is approaching a drop-off or obstacle.

Another option is to use a walker designed specifically for use with one hand. One model is held on a student's side. It may provide slightly less support than a front model, but it will free the use of one hand for the long cane. Another model is a front model with a small handle that protrudes from the center bar of the walker (see Figure 18.9). The handle is angled slightly to the

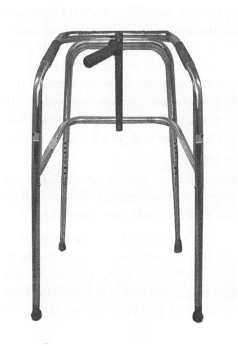

Figure 18.9.
A walker designed for use with one hand.

right for right-handed users, and to the left for left-handed users. The walker either can be lifted with one hand and moved forward or, if glide tips are placed on the feet, can be slid forward for each succeeding step. Although designed for use by people with only one functional hand, it can be successfully used by people who have two hands but need one hand free to trail a wall or use a long cane without sacrificing the support of a walker.

Negotiating Curbs and Ramps

Curbs often pose a challenge for people who use walkers. If the student has sufficient strength and balance, it is possible to safely negotiate curbs using the following techniques:

1. Standing halfway into the walker, the student places all of his weight on his legs and places no weight on the walker.

2. He moves the walker forward (not moving forward himself) until the front legs or wheels of the walker detect the edge of the curb. If the walker does not detect the edge of the curb without moving so far forward that the student's balance is compromised, he should bring the walker back to the normal walking position, take one step forward, and repeat the process.

3. When the curb edge is detected, the student places the front legs at the edge of the curb and walks halfway into the walker.

4. He then lowers (or lifts) the walker over the curb and ensures that all four legs are stable. If the walker has hand brakes, the student must engage the brakes to stabilize the walker. He can then step up or down safely.

Mobility for People Who Use Crutches or Canes

Crutches provide slightly less physical support than walkers, but more support than canes. There are two basic types of crutches—*underarm* and *lofstrand* (also called *forearm* or *Canadian crutches*) (see Figure 18.10)—and people may use either one or two crutches depending on their need for physical support. Lofstrand crutches, made of metal, provide slightly less support than underarm crutches, but require less coordination to use and allow users much greater flexibility of movement. The metal forearm cuff allows people to lift their arms up or forward to open doors or handle objects (such as money when paying for items at a store) without the crutch falling away. Similarly, there are several kinds of support canes such as quad canes and straight canes (see Figure 18.11). Quad canes provide the greatest amount of support due to their relatively large base of support, but some students find them awkward to use, finding that they must slow their pace considerably in order to place all four feet of the cane on the

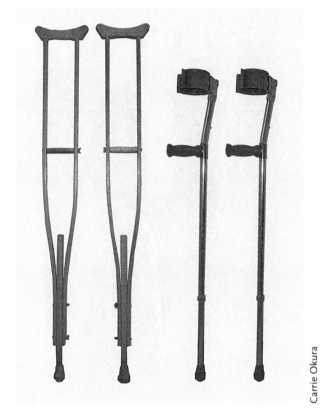

Figure 18.10.
Underarm crutches (left) and forearm crutches (right).

Carrie Okura

ground simultaneously with each step as required in order for the cane to provide proper support.

As with walkers, it is the role of the physical therapist to prescribe and fit crutches or canes to a student. The height of the crutch or cane handle needs to be such that when the student stands erect and with the tip of the device about 2″ in front of and 2″ to the side of his near foot, his elbow will be bent to 30 degrees from the vertical (see Figure 18.7). There are several different gait patterns that people use when walking with crutches or canes, and they are determined by a physical therapist based upon a student's strength, coordination, and stamina. When walking with only one crutch or cane, however, it is almost always held on the side opposite the weaker leg.

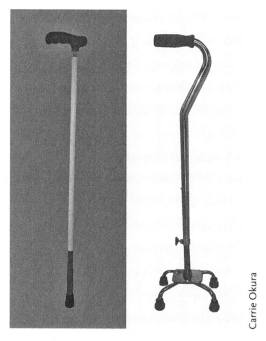

Figure 18.11.
Examples of support canes: straight cane and quad cane.

Carrie Okura

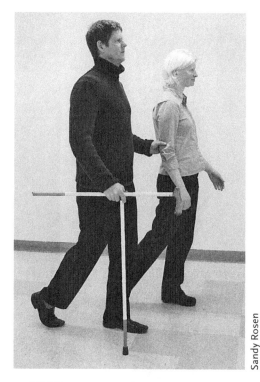

Sandy Rosen

Figure 18.12.
Carrying second support cane while walking with a guide.

Doing so increases the base of support for the student when he lifts his good foot to step forward and momentarily places maximum weight on his weaker leg.

Using a Human Guide with Crutches or Canes

Methods 1 and 2 described under the Mobility for People with Visual Impairments Who Use Walkers section may work as well for people who use crutches or canes. Many people, however, find it more comfortable to use the traditional human guide technique. If the student uses only one crutch or cane, he can hold the guide's arm with his free hand. If he is using two crutches or canes, however, he may prefer to hold the guide's arm with one hand and either carry the device in his other hand (see Figure 18.12), or have the guide carry the device. If the student needs physical support from the guide while walking, the guide can bend his elbow to place his forearm horizontal

and the student can interlink his arm for support while walking (see Figure 18.13).

Orientation and Trailing

Some students will have sufficient balance to be able to use the crutch or cane to trail a vertical surface. To do so, the student simply taps the vertical surface on his side with the near device and then places it forward to take his next step. This process is repeated every second step.

Obstacle Detection

As was seen for those who use walkers, people who use two crutches or canes can be faced with the difficult challenge of detecting obstacles with sufficient warning to avoid collisions

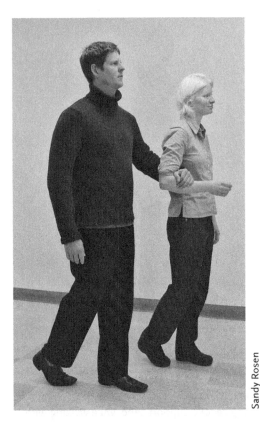

Sandy Rosen

Figure 18.13.
In this position, the guide's arm provides physical support to the student while walking.

(and sometimes a subsequent loss of balance). There are some solutions, however, each with varying degrees of effectiveness and ease of use, depending on the student's physical abilities and travel needs. One solution is to use ETAs to obtain advance warning of obstacles (other than down steps) in one's path. Another solution is to use the ambulatory aid(s) to trail and clear the path in front. This latter solution can be used by those who possess sufficient strength, coordination, and balance to support themselves on one crutch or cane while using the other as a probe. To do so, the student places her weight on one crutch while placing the tip of the other crutch across her body, then sliding it in an arc in front of back to its original resting point (see Figure 18.14). This

clears a one-step distance ahead (as a note, a student who does not have sufficient vision to preview the area ahead should always step only up to where the crutches have cleared, never beyond). Teaching a student with a visual impairment to use an ambulatory aid to clear a path and to trail needs to be done with the advice of, or in conjunction with, a physical therapist to ensure that this procedure can be done safely without causing excessive physical strain or potentially aggravating an existing medical condition.

Using the Long Cane with Crutches or Canes

Another method of clearing a path and trailing is to use a long cane. If people use only one crutch or support cane for walking, they can often use a long cane easily. In this situation, they hold and use the crutch or support cane in the hand dictated by their support needs and hold the long cane in the other hand. This is true whether they are left- or right-handed. A longer cane than usual may be helpful if additional reaction time is needed when balance is impaired. They walk using the standard gait pattern for using one crutch or support cane: the aid, followed by the weaker leg, then the stronger leg. Some people will move the aid and the weaker leg forward together for increased speed. The long cane is also used in a traditional manner, with the hand and arm position remaining the same as when using the long cane alone. The users keep "in step" with the long cane as they walk, contacting the cane tip to the ground on one side as the foot on the opposite side steps down. In this way (assuming the aid is held in the left hand), the crutch or support cane and the tip of the long cane will touch the ground on the left as the right heel steps down. Then the long cane will touch down on the right as the student steps forward with his left foot. The process is then repeated. Using an ambulatory aid and a long cane together takes coordination and prac-

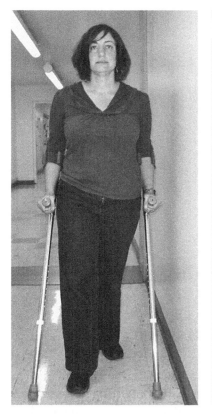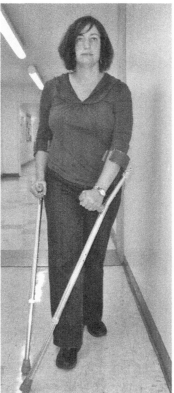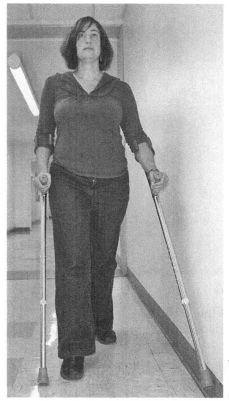

Carrie Okura

Figure 18.14.
Using a crutch to clear the path and to trail.

tice but it is an effective and efficient means of independent travel for people who need to use both devices.

Negotiating Stairs with Crutches or Canes

To ascend stairs, people can walk up to the first riser, so that their toes are 2–3 inches away from it. They then step up with their stronger leg, followed by the weaker leg and the crutch(es) or cane(s). To descend stairs, people can walk up to the edge of the first step and lower the crutch(es) or cane(s) and the weaker leg to the next step at the same time. They then bring the stronger leg down. They repeat the process for each successive step (see Figure 18.15A–C). People who use quad canes may find at times, that the stairs are too

narrow to safely support all four feet of the quad cane. In this case, the cane may be turned sideways to fit all four feet on the next step.

Travel on stairs takes a lot of strength and coordination. People who do not have sufficient strength or coordination to do this may choose to use the handrail. If there is a handrail on each side, most students will choose to use the handrail on the side opposite the weaker leg, in order to gain a wider base of support and more stability, although this can vary by student preference. To do this, they place the crutch or cane nearest the handrail in their other hand and hold it sideways (see Figure 18.15D) by grasping the shaft of the crutch just below the hand grip. The procedure for ascending or descending stairs is then performed as above.

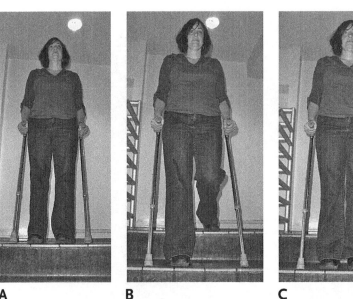
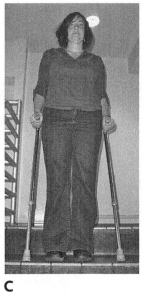
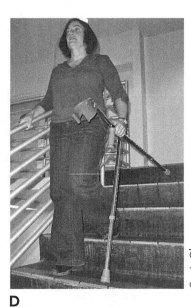

A   B   C   D

Figure 18.15.
Descending stairs when using crutches (A–C); and (D) holding crutches when descending stairs and using a railing.

Some students who do not have sufficient strength to negotiate stairs in this manner may turn sideways as they go up and down. Walking down sideways shifts much of the demands for knee stability to the strong ligaments on the side of the knee, lessening demand on the weak leg muscles. If there is a railing available, the student faces the railing and holds it with both hands for greater stability as he walks up or down sideways, one step at a time. Again, it is generally advisable to go up leading with the stronger leg and down leading with the weaker leg for maximum stability.

If the traveler does not need to hold the handrail for stability when ascending or descending stairs, he can use the aid and the long cane together by combining the standard procedures for using each on stairs.

Spotting by the O&M Specialist

No discussion of ambulatory aids used by people with visual impairments would be complete without addressing techniques the O&M specialist can use to ensure students' physical safety while they learn independent travel skills. When people using ambulatory aids walk on uneven terrain, ice, or wet or slippery surfaces; ascend or descend stairs or curbs; or become fatigued, balance can become much more precarious than under ordinary circumstances. In these situations, careful spotting is even more necessary to assist students to maintain balance, or avoid serious injury if they lose balance and fall. *Spotting* refers to the procedure by which an O&M specialist carefully positions himself next to a student, watches for signs indicating that the student is about to lose balance, and responds instantly in order to provide physical support or to break a fall. The best position for spotting is to stand slightly behind and to the side of the student on level ground. When ascending stairs, it is important to stand behind and below the student. When descending stairs, the O&M specialist needs to stand in front of and below the student. A trick used by physical therapists to enable them to most effectively and safely stabilize a student who has started to fall, or to lessen the impact of the fall, is to hold onto the student's belt when walking down stairs, or in other situations where balance may be unsure. The O&M specialist holds

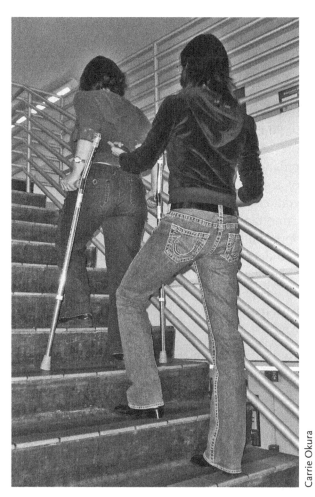

Figure 18.16.
Using a belt in spotting.

onto the belt in a palm-up position (see Figure 18.16). Holding onto a student's belt needs to be done with the student's permission but it provides excellent leverage for the O&M specialist to break a fall if the student loses his balance. The O&M specialist may also wish to carry a spare belt with him for students who do not have their own. Gait belts with handles are commercially available at medical supply stores. A man's leather belt, at least 2 inches wide, also works well. Women's belts, elastic or cloth belts, or narrower belts are generally not strong enough for spotting purposes. By purchasing a man's belt (the largest size possible), and drilling holes in the belt at 1-inch intervals (done inexpensively at shoe repair

shops), the O&M specialist will have a belt available that fits all students. The belt should be as snug a fit as the student can comfortably tolerate in order to provide optimum leverage for the instructor to prevent a fall if the situation arises.

Using Ambulatory Aids on Mass Transit

Most cities equip buses with driver-operated lifts that raise wheelchair users in and out of the bus. To use a lift, the user generally backs onto the lift, facing the curb. It is important that she move completely onto the lift so that the gate can close on the sidewalk side. Some scooters have difficulty fitting on lifts because of their size. If using a manual wheelchair, the student locks the brakes (motorized wheelchairs lock automatically when the joystick is not in the "drive" position). Wheelchair users who are unable to look behind them will often attach mirrors to the sides of the wheelchair to assist them in backing up. When the lift is raised to the height of the bus floor, the wheelchair user rolls backward and takes a place alongside the window at the front of the bus. If the bus has a ramp instead of a lift, the student simply rolls up and down the ramp in a forward direction. While not always the case, some bus aisles are large enough for a student to enter in a forward direction and then turn around.

Once in place, the brakes of manual wheelchairs then need to be locked to keep the wheelchair from rolling as the bus starts, stops, and turns. Some buses are equipped with special clamps or tie-downs to secure the wheels and prevent rolling when the bus is in motion. Not all buses are so equipped, however, and the clamps do not fit all wheelchairs. For added protection against rolling during a sudden stop, some wheelchair users choose to hold onto a nearby vertical pole. To exit the bus, the wheelchair user will move forward onto the lift, which is then lowered to the curb. Lifts generally have handrails that wheelchair users can hold for extra stability during the raising and lowering process. Public

Carrie Okura

transportation agencies across the country have worked hard to make buses and trains wheelchair accessible. It may still be necessary, however, to contact the bus company prior to travel for information on the times or routes such buses run or request that an accessible bus be used on a given route at a given time.

Subway trains are generally accessible to people using wheelchairs or ambulatory aids as the floor of the train car is level with the platform in most stations. It is important to be very careful of the gap between the subway car and platform when boarding or exiting, however, as the tips of walkers, crutches, or support canes can catch in the gap, as can some very small wheels on wheelchairs. Most wheelchairs have front wheels that are large enough to move smoothly over the gap, but if the wheels are small, users will generally move quickly over the gap to "bridge it" before the wheel can slip down. If the small wheels stop while over the crack, they can turn sideways and drop between the railcar and the platform. Users also can make a point of entering the door from either a "straight-on" direction, or backward (if they can see behind them for safe navigation) in order to minimize the chances of a wheel catching in the gap.

Buses and subways generally have seating next to the door for people with mobility problems. In some cases, seats are removed immediately next to the door to leave space for wheelchairs or scooters, or the front seats fold away to allow room for them. Crutches and support canes, as well as long canes, are held vertically, out of the aisle when the user is seated, to avoid tripping nearby passengers.

Choice of Equipment

It is generally the role of the physical or occupational therapist to determine the type of wheelchair or scooter (including accessories) that a student will use. Therapists are also responsible for fitting the wheelchair or scooter to the user to ensure that it is the proper size, and teaching the student how to use it. Physical therapists additionally prescribe, fit, and teach people how to use other ambulatory aids such as walkers, crutches, and support canes. The choice of aids for a given student is made based on several interrelated factors such as the student's age, balance, coordination, muscle tone, need for postural support, presence of sensory impairment, diagnosis or prognosis of medical condition, endurance, level of activity, and sometimes even financial considerations, such as insurance coverage. This decision can often be based on factors that are not always apparent to nonmedical personnel. For example, a student who appears to be able to walk with fair balance when not using a cane at all might actually be given two canes. This might be a student with fragile bones or fragile circulation in the feet who has impaired balance and can be seriously hurt if he steps down hard on one foot when catching his balance. Furthermore, the aids prescribed can change as a student's medical situation improves or worsens, or as children mature or people age. For this reason it is important that the aids used by a student are prescribed by a physical therapist or physician, and that no changes are made without consulting a physical therapist or physician.

At the same time, however, the requirements of O&M, such as reaction time when encountering obstacles, the effect on balance of unexpected collisions with objects, and early detection of steps and changes in terrain may not be factors that physical therapists consider when prescribing ambulatory aids. It is therefore vital for O&M specialists and physical therapists to work in concert, whenever possible, to initially prescribe aids or to revise a system to meet both the physical support and independent mobility needs of the student with a visual impairment.

Maintenance of Equipment

The need for regular maintenance of wheelchairs can range from minimal to significant. Wheelchairs need to be kept clean, dry, and rust-free.

They need to be inspected periodically for loose and worn parts. Pneumatic tires need to be properly inflated at all times. The motor of a motorized wheelchair will need regular maintenance to adjust drive belt tensions, inspect wires for worn insulation, and maintain battery terminals free from corrosion. It is not the role of the O&M specialist to maintain the equipment, but in noticing problems early the O&M specialist can not only alert the student to problems but can perhaps avoid an equipment breakdown in the middle of a lesson.

Very little maintenance is required of walkers, crutches, and canes. Basically maintenance consists of inspecting the crutch or cane tips for signs of wear and cracking. Over time, the rubber may dry through exposure to heat and sun, and may crack. When this occurs, it is best to replace the tips before they crack completely open and fall off. Similarly, the bottoms of the tips need regular inspection. When new, the bottom of a tip has a series of concentric rings that form a ridged suction cup. This provides a mild suction with the ground when weight is applied to the aid, providing increased traction and increased stability. When the tip begins to wear, the ridges wear down and the bottom of the tip becomes smoother, much the same way that the tread on a tire wears through use. When this happens, traction provided by the cane tip is decreased, just as it is for automobile tires. The cane is then more likely to slide out from underneath the student when on wet or slippery surfaces such as wet pavement or a waxed floor. When the ridges are worn, it is time to replace the tip. Replacement tips can be purchased inexpensively from any medical supply store and some drugstores.

Summary

As in the general population, the number of people who have additional health concerns is growing. O&M specialists are increasingly being called upon to work with students who have a wide variety of additional medical conditions and even some who use ambulatory aids. It can easily be said that no two students with physical disabilities are the same. For these students, O&M takes on new and fascinating challenges. Addressing the physical and health concerns during the O&M program, however, does not need to be as much of a challenge as it first may seem.

While the number and nature of additional conditions seem endless, there are several universal principles that form the foundation for serving all students. These principles first include understanding the nature of the condition and its symptoms. Be aware of any potential health-related problems that can arise during instruction and know the warning signs. Have an action plan prepared to deal with any problems. Second, look at the specific physical activities that a student can do and note which activities pose challenges. Third, modify the technique or activity (for example, modify the cane, cane technique, or length of lessons), modify the environment (for example, work in an air-conditioned area if the weather is too hot for the student's health to tolerate), or modify the teaching approach (for example, have multiple lesson plans available for days when the student is not feeling up to par or break lessons into short segments, allowing for short breaks as needed, use universal health precautions as necessary).

Following the above principles; seeking out informational resources and useful devices, equipment, and products; and working collaboratively with education and rehabilitation professionals, city officials, and others can go a long way to making a seemingly impossible task become both fun and successful.

Working with students who have additional physical and health concerns provides an exciting challenge and opportunity for O&M specialists to teach safe and effective travel skills to people who may once have thought they could never travel because they could not hold a long cane while using an ambulatory aid, or to whom services had been denied because of the "limitations" of their physical impairment. Furthermore, O&M

specialists have the unique opportunity to teach other professionals about the need, value, and possibilities of independent travel by people with visual impairments.

IMPLICATIONS FOR O&M PRACTICE

1. Extra caution is needed on O&M lessons for those with osteoporosis to avoid falls, and proper cane technique can become critical to ensure that the traveler will detect all obstacles with the cane and not her body.

2. Brain injury can affect many areas of functioning, including cognitive, motor, and sensory abilities as well as speech, language, and behavior.

3. Seizures can occur in response to stimuli that originate either inside or outside of the body. While external stimuli only trigger or exacerbate seizure activity in a small percentage of people, it is still essential that teachers be aware of this possibility and avoid stimuli (for example, avoid flashing lights when doing visual functioning activities) that might evoke a seizure in a student.

4. Students who are diabetic are at high risk of serious infection, even from small lesions. O&M specialists need to monitor students for injuries, such as cuts, bruises, or blisters that may occur during lessons, and note whether students' footwear or prosthetic devices fit properly.

5. Before beginning to work with a student who has a heart condition, the O&M specialist needs to identify the condition, learn when problems occur, ask the student to describe the condition, and identify medications, along with side effects and precautions.

6. Students can carry a health care card with contact information; information on the med-

ical condition, history and symptoms; and other information related to the condition and its treatment as appropriate. The O&M specialist always needs to have similar information readily available for his or her own use in case of emergency

7. O&M specialists may be unaware or unsure if individuals they are teaching are HIV-positive or have AIDS or have other blood-borne pathogens. Therefore, O&M specialists need to follow current public health practices and appropriate infection control procedures when providing services to all individuals.. O&M specialists need to initiate O&M services, schedule, and pace lessons with students who have AIDS, while considering the varying state of the student's health. It may be necessary to reevaluate and change instructional goals and strategies during the instructional period.

8. Ambulatory devices include walkers, crutches, canes, and other ambulatory devices. O&M specialists and physical or occupational therapists can work together to meet both the physical support and independent mobility needs of the student with a visual impairment.

LEARNING ACTIVITIES

1. Do an Internet search to learn more about specific medical conditions that students may have.

2. Contact organizations such as the Heart Association or American Diabetes Association for information and pamphlets.

3. Contact support groups that focus on specific medical conditions (for example, brain injury and multiple sclerosis) and talk with members about their experiences and what personal pointers or advice they might give to service providers.

4. Visit the physical therapy department at a local hospital to observe people being fit with ambulatory devices and instructed in their use. Talk with physical and occupational therapists about ways that they and O&M specialists can work together.

5. Contact medical equipment specialists to find out what kinds of equipment and accessories might be available for your student.

6. Talk to people who use ambulatory devices to learn about tips for use in specific environments, as well as the pros and cons of each type of device and accessories.

7. Rent or borrow a wheelchair or other ambulatory device(s) and spend a day using them to give you a sense of what students experience and how the use of device(s) impacts mobility.

CHAPTER 19

Teaching Orientation and Mobility to Students with Cognitive Impairments and Vision Loss

Grace Ambrose-Zaken, Colleen Rae Calhoon, and James R. Keim

LEARNING QUESTIONS

- What impacts on orientation and mobility (O&M) instruction do memory deficits have on students with visual impairments and learning disabilities? What strategies would you incorporate into your teaching to address these needs?

- How can you employ a student's use of tactile symbols to make the student aware of the sequence of the upcoming lesson?

- List and describe the three design elements needed in a lesson plan. What guidelines need to be followed when creating a task analysis for teaching a student who has visual impairments and cognitive impairments?

- What are the least to most restrictive prompt types used to teach a student with visual and cognitive impairments a new skill, and what elements of social interactions are needed to travel?

- What strategies can be used to promote a student's on-task behavior during an O&M lesson?

The purpose of this chapter is to describe six classifications of cognitive impairments that sometimes occur in children who are also blind or visually impaired. These combinations of impairments can have a significant impact on the orientation and mobility of the students who experience them. This chapter describes 10 general program strategies (teamwork, communication, planning and record keeping, time considerations, task analysis, sequenced instruction, environment, motivation, prompting, and choice making) that can be helpful in addressing 10 skill areas (attention, sensory integration, behavior, memory, concept development, generalization, problem solving, social skills, orientation, and mobility) for students who have both visual and cognitive impairments.

David was a healthy 54-year-old man who was involved in an automobile accident. David sustained minor physical injuries and irreversible vision and cognitive impairments. Since the accident, David's vision is 20/200 (OD) and 20/800 (OS). His brain injury impaired his ability to think and reason, understand words, remember things, pay attention, solve problems, talk, and learn new skills. David has worked together with his family, a licensed occupational therapist (OT), and a licensed physical therapist (PT) to map out a rehabilitation plan that would enable him to return to the activities important to him prior to the accident.

When David began O&M instruction, his current level of travel was described in the O&M report as "able to follow a guide visually. He travels only when accompanied; has limited ability to speak; and demonstrates slow response times to verbal requests." O&M instruction will focus on "use of functional language to complete activities, evaluation and instruction techniques for oriented travel, and instruction in mobility techniques."

David, now 57, has consistently made progress in learning both orientation and mobility skills. He is now able to travel inside his home unaccompanied, using a long cane. He has demonstrated consistency over time with safe travel in his residential neighborhood. At this time, David is learning how to analyze and cross at lighted intersections. Further, his route planning has become less and less dependent on family.

The progress David has made since his head injury suggests that his appropriate long-term goal is independent travel in complex environments, with multiple transportation options, and using intermittent to limited supports such as a job coach.

———————

Tameka is 11 years old and was born autistic and totally blind. She began O&M instruction at the age of 3. Her first O&M assessment showed that her language, social, and travel skills were severely delayed. She traveled with an escort within her school building, had a limited ability to follow one-step directions, and would bite, scratch, and hit others during transitions.

Tameka's O&M specialist worked together with Tameka's educational and behavioral team to implement a system of prompts and rewards designed to teach her language, travel, and social skills. In the beginning, her O&M goals were to travel her daily routine within the school (e.g., school bus, bathroom, cafeteria, gymnasium, playground, main office, and speech therapist's office), as safely, efficiently, gracefully, and independently as possible. At 11 years old, Tameka is currently able to travel the six routes she uses every day with no assistance. Tameka is always trailed by a staff member. Based on her progress, the goals set for Tameka did expand to include learning a route in her residential neighborhood. Tameka will always require an O&M specialist to learn new indoor and outdoor routes. Tameka's long-term travel goal of independent travel in familiar environments and multiple transportation systems with limited to extensive supports is a realistic one. While Tameka will never be cleared to travel alone outside, her lessons traveling outdoors are providing experiences in interacting appropriately with the world outside her school.

The combination of blindness or severe visual impairment and cognitive impairment impacts development and use of O&M skills. Appropriately timed, accurately planned, intensive intervention can increase a student's control over and participation in daily travel needs. The continuum of skills taught by O&M specialists are important for students who have both visual and cognitive impairments because (1) safe movement through the environment creates opportunities for learning; (2) traveling as independently as possible is important to all aspects of cognitive, sensorimotor, and affective development; and (3) the greater control a student who has visual and cognitive impairments gains over her travel, the more choices she will have as an adult.

According to the 27th Annual Report to Congress (2005), specific learning disabilities, mental retardation, emotional disturbance, autism spectrum disorders, developmental delay, and traumatic brain injury account for 69 percent of students age 6 through 21 served under the Individuals with Disabilities Education Act (IDEA). The learning disability category represents almost half (47.4 percent) of all students served, with mental retardation (9.6 percent), emotional disturbance (8 percent), autism spectrum disorders (2.3 percent), developmental delay (1.15 percent), and traumatic brain injury (0.4 percent) making up the remaining total (U.S. Department of Education, 2005).

Students for whom visual impairment is one of several identified disabilities are typically counted within other disability categories such as multiple disabilities. This means the number of children in the United States who are blind or visually impaired overall is severely underreported by federal and state entities (Erin, Daugherty, Dignan, & Pearson, 1990; Pogrund, Fazzi, & Lampert, 1992).

Estimates of prevalence of the population of children who are blind and visually impaired vary from 1 per 1,000 (Erin, 2003) to 25 per 1,000 children (Cotch & Janiszewski, 2002). A study conducted by the Centers for Disease Control and Prevention (CDC) found that nearly three-quarters of children with visual impairments in their sample of almost 1,300 students also had one or more other developmental disabilities such as mental retardation (1996).

A dual diagnosis of visual impairment and cognitive impairments may result from a genetic abnormality, a sustained injury (e.g., chemical, oxygen deprivation, or physical) or may be of unknown origin (Jones, 2002). While it is understood that an injured brain can shift functions to different parts of the brain by creating new pathways and allowing a substantial recovery of lost function, the addition of blindness or visual impairment introduces greater complexity to this process (Sousa, 2001).

OVERVIEW OF SIX CLASSIFICATIONS OF COGNITIVE IMPAIRMENTS

Learning Disabilities

A learning disability is "a disorder in one or more of the basic psychological processes involved in understanding or in using language, spoken or written, that may manifest itself in an imperfect ability to listen, think, speak, read, write, spell, or do mathematical calculations. This can include conditions such as perceptual disabilities," but is not related to another disability such as visual impairment (Department of Education, *34* Code of Federal Regulations §300.7(c)(10), Assistance to States for the Education of Children with Disabilities, Federal Register, March 12, 1999).

A student who is blind or visually impaired and has a learning disability presents a unique challenge to O&M specialists because the delays associated with learning disabilities are similar to the impact that vision impairment has on development (Layton & Lock, 2001). When instructing the student who is visually impaired and has a learning disability, O&M specialists may find that the attempts to instruct students through sensory perceptual channels traditionally used for O&M are met with less success or cause the student discomfort.

Thus, a student with a learning disability who has *auditory perceptual problems* has difficulty distinguishing differences between sounds and localizing a sound. These students may have difficulty following verbal directions or instructions and learning or remembering information given verbally. Students with learning disabilities who have *body and spatial relationship problems* may be easily disoriented even in familiar environments, confuse basic positional concepts such as up with down and right with left, or exhibit directionality problems. Students with learning disabilities who have *conceptual deficits* may have difficulty making connections within similar learning constructs; for example, understanding that addresses that go up sequentially by two when traveling north, then go down sequentially by two when the route is reversed. These students may have difficulty with context prediction, defined as being able to predict the future such as the ability to make safety or orientation decisions based on current contextual clues, or answering comprehension-type questions. Students with learning disabilities who have related *memory deficits* may have trouble remembering what was seen, heard, or shown; may have difficulty remembering sequences in directions or instructions; and may have difficulty with memorization of facts, routes, or destinations. These students may appear forgetful, may have weak expressive and receptive language skills, and rarely use appropriate nouns, substituting instead "that thing" or "you know." Students with learning disabilities may make the same errors over and over again. As a result of *behavior deficits*, a student may struggle to sit still, may demonstrate impulsivity and may not consider the consequences before acting. Students with learning disabilities often have a "short fuse" or have a low frustration level, which may impact lesson length and/or the degree to which an O&M specialist allows frustration into the O&M lesson. Students with learning disabilities may have difficulty finishing activities and be easily distracted and fidget. Some students exhibit negative or oppositional behavior and have trouble following rules; they are often disorganized and lose things. *Visual perceptual problems* are seen in a student's difficulty with fluent reading such as frequent letter reversals (Kinsbourne & Graf, 2001).

Intellectual Disability

Mental retardation is a term that continues to be used in diagnostic, legal, and public policy arenas; however, within the educational community the term *intellectual disability* is preferred by the American Association on Intellectual and Development Disabilities (formerly AAMR; see AAIDD 2003; ARC 2004). IDEA defines *mental retardation* as "significantly subaverage general intellectual functioning, existing concurrently with deficits in adaptive behavior and manifested during the developmental period, that adversely affects a child's educational performance" [*34* Code of Federal Regulations $300.7(c)(6)]. Thus, by definition, deficits in adaptive behavior or ability to cope with the demands of everyday life are as important as the numeric measure of IQ when identifying persons with cognitive impairments (AAMR, 2002; Greenspan, 1999).

IQ has long been found to be as limited in its usefulness as an accurate predictor of O&M ability as the acuity measure is in predicting one's visual functioning (Corn, 1987; Joffee & Erhesman, 1997). Like visual acuity measures, traditional IQ tests only measure a narrow aspect of one's ability. While certain aspects of independent travel require higher order thinking and reasoning skills, it is also true that functional travel skills are learned via sensorimotor domains (knowledge from sensory input or motor actions) and affective domains (knowledge from emotional input or interactions). Both sensorimotor and affective experiences are believed to make important contributions to one's ability to travel (Long & Hill, 1997).

The U.S. Department of Education (2002) uses the term *mental retardation* and defines students who are cognitively impaired as those who demonstrate global delays in the areas of cognition, speech and language, gross and fine motor activities, activities of daily living (ADLs), and social and personal activities. A student with *cognitive delays* may exhibit limitations in concept development, attention span, memory, abstract thinking, and generalization of skills across environments and problem solving. Students with *speech and/or language delays* may be nonverbal, have limited receptive and expressive language, demonstrate echolalic language, and/or have language-processing problems. Students with *gross and/or fine motor delays* may have poor balance, posture, flexibility, and eye–hand and eye–foot coordination. Students with *ADL delays* may have difficulty performing basic self-care routines (e.g., bathing, dressing, and eating). Students with *social and/or personal delays* may exhibit a limited ability to interact appropriately within social situations.

Developmental Delay

IDEA established a developmental delay categorical option for use with students age 3 to 9 [*34* Code of Federal Regulations §300.7(b)(1)]. Developmental delay is an *ongoing, major delay in the process of development* that may be due to a genetic disorder, due to complications at birth, or of unknown origin. Developmental delay is estimated to affect 5 to 10 percent of children (Shevell et al., 2003). Developmental delay is defined as significant delay in two or more of the following developmental domains: gross/fine motor, speech/language, cognition, social/personal, and activities of daily living when compared with the skills attainment of chronological peers (Kinsbourne & Graf, 2001).

The term *developmental delay* is usually reserved for younger children (i.e., those typically younger than 5 years of age), whereas the term *mental retardation* is usually applied to older children when IQ testing is more valid and reliable. A child who is blind or visually impaired with a developmental delay is not necessarily destined to be labeled cognitively impaired after early identification enables professionals to provide early intervention and instruction (Shevell et al., 2003).

Autism Spectrum Disorders

Autism spectrum disorder is the general term for the continuum of diagnoses related to autism, including Asperger's syndrome, childhood disintegrative disorder, fragile X disorder, hyperlexis, and pervasive developmental delay. Within the autism spectrum disorder designation, cognitive abilities can range from intellectually gifted to severe impairments, with cognitive impairment present in about 70 percent of individuals with an autism spectrum disorder (Gense & Gense, 2005).

The Office of Special Education Programs only began reporting the category *autism* during the 1991–1992 school year (U.S. Department of Education, 2002). Since 1992, reporting in this category has increased dramatically, growing from approximately 5,500 students age 6–21 served under IDEA to almost 79,000 (1.4 percent) in 2000–2001 and 2.3 percent in 2003 (U.S. Department of Education, 2005). There is no estimate of statistical prevalence of autism spectrum disorders in children who are blind and visually impaired (Gense & Gense, 2005).

Individuals with an autism spectrum disorder are often described as being asocial, have a tendency to perseverate on an idea or engage in repetitive behaviors, and may excel at visual spatial skills but perform poorly on verbal, generalization, memory, and conceptual tasks. Often these students exhibit extreme sensitivity to sensory input such as fluorescent lighting, odors from cleaning agents, being touched by others, and sounds, such as lawn mowers in the distance (Gense & Gense, 2005). Behaviors frequently seen in students with an autism spectrum disorder include a lack of impulse control, heightened frustration level, and difficulty with transitions. As illustrated in the Tameka vignette, the child with an autism spectrum disorder and visual impairment can develop functional travel skills through systematic intervention by an O&M specialist.

Children who are blind and visually impaired may exhibit similar tendencies even if they are not autistic, and they may sometimes be described as having autistic tendencies. The difference is children who are blind can be redirected into activities that are meaningful and provide sensory feedback, but in children with an autism spectrum disorder, these behaviors increase when they are anxious and/or stressed, making them difficult to redirect (Cross, Frazeur, Traub, Hutter-Pishgahi, & Shelton, 2004). When working with "students with autism spectrum disorders *and* visual impairment (ASDVI), both the content of and methodology for instruction need to be different from those for students who have only one of these disabilities" (Gense & Gense, 2005, p. 47) as evidenced in the examples provided under the section of this chapter titled Ten Skill Areas.

Emotional Disturbance

Federal regulations define *emotional disturbance* as a condition in which a "child's educational performance is adversely affected by an inability to build or maintain satisfactory interpersonal relationships with peers and teachers and exhibits inappropriate types of behavior or feelings under normal circumstances" [34 Code of Federal Regulations §300.7(c)(4)]. Various factors such as heredity, brain disorder, diet, stress, and family functioning have been suggested as possible causes, while no one cause has been directly linked to all behavior or emotional problems. Children who have emotional disturbances may have the following characteristics and behaviors: hyperactivity (short attention span, impulsiveness), aggression or self-injurious behavior (acting out, fighting), withdrawal (failure to initiate interaction with others, retreat from exchanges of social interaction, excessive fear or anxiety), immaturity (inappropriate crying, temper tantrums, poor coping skills), and learning difficulties (academically performing below grade level) (NICHY, 2004).

Children with serious mental illness such as borderline personality disorder, bipolar disorder, or schizophrenia may exhibit distorted thinking, excessive anxiety, bizarre motor acts, and unusual mood swings. In children who have mental illness, these behaviors may continue over long periods of time. Their behavior is a signal that they are not coping with their environment or peers (Greene, 2001).

Traumatic Brain Injury

Federal regulations define traumatic brain injury as an acquired injury to the brain caused by an external physical force, resulting in total or partial functional disability, psychosocial impairment, or both, that adversely affects a child's educational performance. The term applies to open or closed head injuries resulting in impairments in one or more areas, such as cognition; language; memory; attention; reasoning; abstract thinking; judgment; problem solving; sensory, perceptual, and motor abilities; psychosocial behavior; physical functions; information processing; and speech [34 Code of Federal Regulations §300.7(c)(12)]. As illustrated in the opening vignette of David, when an individual has traumatic brain injury and a visual impairment, O&M specialists are a vital part of the rehabilitation team. They work closely with families, physicians, occupational and physical therapists, communication specialists, psychologists, and other related health service providers to design and implement a program to address the student's impairments.

Common visual disorders found in students with traumatic brain injury include field loss, reduced acuity, double vision, field anomalies, cortical visual impairment, low vision, or total blindness. Functional vision loss may also result from perceptual deficits. For both cortical visual impairment (CVI) and functional vision loss, the eyes and the optic nerves may function normally; however, the brain may not be able to process or interpret visual information (for more information on CVI, see Chapter 20).

An O&M specialist who plans to work with children with traumatic brain injury will benefit from an understanding of the brain and the strategies that are successful when instructing this diverse group of students. This brief overview of the brain anatomy will serve to facilitate a better understanding of how injuries to different areas of the brain may predict student functioning post injury.

The new age of brain research has brought a greater understanding to the amazing adaptability or plasticity of the brain. Where once it was thought that the adult brain is "hard-wired" with fixed and immutable neuronal circuits that could not be repaired after injury, this is no longer considered the case. Instead, it has been shown that there is no fixed period of time after which brain plasticity or the ability for the brain to change is blocked or lost. It is now understood that with new learning comes new connections within the brain throughout one's lifetime (Barkovich, 2005; Goldberg, 2001).

While current research supports the idea of the brain functioning on a cognitive continuum (Goldberg, 2001), there is still an advantage to using these well-known divisions of the brain

to describe brain function and behavior that neurologists continue to use (Barkovich, 2005). This section will provide an overview of the brain in order to aid O&M specialists' ability to assess and plan instruction for students who have visual and cognitive impairments.

The brain consists of the cerebrum, brain stem, and cerebellum (see Figure 19.1). The cerebrum, Latin for "brain," is the newest (evolutionarily speaking) and largest part of the brain. It controls perception, imagination, thought, judgment, and decision making. The brain stem is the oldest part of the brain. It controls various autonomic functions such as respiration and the regulation of heart rhythms as well as perceptual functions such as the primary aspects of sound localization. The cerebellum governs coordination and control of voluntary movement.

The brain appears divided into two hemispheres, right and left, with nerves from the right side of the body crossing to the left hemisphere and nerves from the left side of the body crossing to the right brain hemisphere. In a typically developing brain each hemisphere controls different functions as illustrated in Table 19.1.

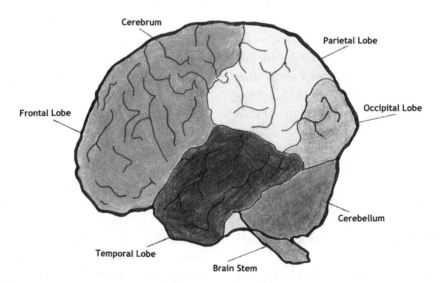

Figure 19.1. Exterior of the Cerebrum from the Left Side

TABLE 19.1

The Dominant Functions of Right and Left Brain

Left Brain	Right Brain
Controls logic	Controls emotions
Controls words	Controls pictures
Controls parts and specifics	Controls wholes and relationships among the parts
Controls analysis (breaking apart)	Controls synthesis (putting together)
Controls sequential thinking	Controls simultaneous and holistic thinking
Is time-bound, has a sense of time and goals and your position in relation to those goals	Is time free, might lose a sense of time altogether
Governs the right side of your body	Governs the left side of your body

Each half (hemisphere) of the cerebrum is divided into four lobes (frontal, temporal, parietal, and occipital). The right and left frontal lobes, called the *executive center of the brain*, are important to impulse control, judgment, memory, problem solving, socialization, and spontaneity. Frontal lobes assist in planning, coordinating, controlling, and executing behavior. People who have damaged frontal lobes may experience problems with these aspects of cognitive function, being at times impulsive and impaired in their ability to plan and execute complex sequences of actions, and perhaps persisting with one course of action or pattern of behavior when a change would be appropriate (perseveration) (Goldberg, 2001).

The *temporal lobe* is located above the ears and controls hearing, speech, and memory. The temporal lobe is very important for language. The brain has two temporal lobes, one on each side of the brain, located near the ears. Damage to the right temporal lobe tends to impair memory for sounds and shapes. Damage to the left temporal lobe can drastically impair memory for words as well as the ability to understand language (Jones, 2002).

The *occipital lobe* is the main center for processing visual information. Damage to the front part of the occipital lobe can impair the ability

to recognize familiar objects and faces and to accurately interpret what is seen (Jones, 2002).

The *parietal lobe* is directly on top of the brain and deals with calculation, orientation, and perception of stimuli related to touch, pressure, temperature, and pain. Damage to the front part of the parietal lobe on one side causes numbness and impairs sensation on the opposite side of the body. Damage to the back part of the parietal lobe causes right–left disorientation and problems with calculations and drawing.

Both visual and cognitive impairments impede the brain's ability to gather information, and a cognitive impairment can impede one's ability to assimilate and use information effectively. The previous descriptions of common cognitive impairments and the impact of intellectual disability, developmental delay, learning disabilities, autism spectrum disorders, emotional disturbance, and traumatic brain injury on the functions vital to the instruction and use of orientation and mobility by students who are also blind or visually impaired lead to the question "Where do we go from here?" The next two sections of this chapter will attempt to answer that question by describing 10 general program strategies that O&M specialists use when teaching the 10 priority skill areas for students with visual and cognitive impairments.

TEN GENERAL PROGRAM STRATEGIES

Ten general program strategies for teaching students who have visual and cognitive impairments are teamwork, communication, planning and record keeping, time considerations, task analysis, sequenced instruction, environment, motivation, prompting, and choice making. The strategies were ordered to match the sequence of events that occur when adding a student who is visually and cognitively impaired on to your caseload. Each of these common strategies has been framed to specifically address how they may be applied to meet the 10 ability (skill) areas addressed later in this chapter.

Teamwork

The complex needs of students who have visual and cognitive impairments suggest that no single discipline has the breadth and depth of expertise and resources necessary to solely provide for these students. Individuals who have visual and cognitive impairments typically will have multiple professionals providing specialized services. For example, Tameka has an assigned classroom teacher and a one-to-one paraeducator for the entire day, every day. Other professionals such as the speech and language therapist, physical therapist, occupational therapist, O&M specialist and teacher of visually impaired students provide pull-out or integrated therapy services at appropriate intervals during the week. Some professionals, such as physicians, psychiatrists, and social workers may have limited contact with the student. The use of *teamwork* strategies, also known as *interdisciplinary collaboration*, enables professionals to coordinate efforts and involve the family (Drew & Hardman, 2004). For school-age children the team consists of the members of the student's individualized education program (IEP) team, and in adults the team

is made up of professionals, staff, and members of the student's family. Teams are used to develop programs and strategies as well as identify responsibilities, priorities, and future directions (Pierce & Everington, 2002).

Professional challenges are found in daily interactions between professionals in contact with students who have visual and cognitive impairments. The classroom teacher has a need for O&M specialists to provide opportune information to aid travel in and around the school building. O&M specialists need to be able to communicate with the teacher, to make the information useful, and to obtain data on their experiences with the student. Communication is a two-way interaction and, in fact, multidimensional when one considers the information flow between the families and various service providers (Drew & Hardman, 2004).

During the extended evaluation process needed when assessing students who have visual and cognitive impairments, the more efficiently the team works together via a collaborative model, one that is multidirectional and dynamic (Fazzi, 2001; Forney & Heller, 2004), the better the flow of information will be for evaluation, planning, and program implementation on behalf of the shared student. In the teamwork model, new ideas may be generated through group interaction that may not be generated when professionals isolate themselves from the group (Giangreco, Cloninger, Dennis, & Edelman, 2000).

The goal for O&M specialists in collaborating with the team is to enhance each student's daily travel experiences. Methods include allowing team members to observe O&M lessons, providing inservice trainings, conducting home visits, and working closely with the one-to-one aids and other support personnel. Observation of O&M lessons gives opportunities for the other team members to see how a student travels and to provide their own insights (Hamill & Everington, 2002). Inservice trainings are used to inform small or large groups about specific travel needs of a particular student or specific mobility techniques. Home visits support the development and implementation of a more consistent travel program by providing insight into how the client travels, and how he communicates his feelings, wants, and needs. The family knows what makes the student happy, what irritates him, and how to soothe him.

Tables 19.2–19.11 (later in the chapter) give numerous examples of using teamwork as an instructional strategy; one example of using teamwork during instruction can be found in Table 19.6. It is estimated that 290,000 paraprofessionals work in special education alone (Likins, 2002). Paraprofessionals often assume a large role in daily activities of students who have visual and cognitive impairments. Thus, these students may travel more frequently with a paraprofessional than any other staff member. The relationship that develops between an instructional assistant and a student has the potential to promote or hinder the O&M goals of that student. Thus, another aspect of teamwork is the O&M specialist's careful, measured instruction and support of the paraprofessional to develop her ability to support the student's travel goals (Pickett, 2002; Wiener et al., 1990). For example, O&M specialists may work on having the instructional assistant travel discreetly during change of classes. This means that the assistant becomes comfortable with the idea of having the student walk at a distance from her, rather than in direct contact with or next to her. One example of using teamwork during instruction can be found in Table 19.7 (later in the chapter).

Communication

Communication is an "interactive exchange between two or more people to convey needs, feelings, or ideas" (Gense & Gense, 2005, p. 133). Students who have visual and cognitive impairments may have expressive and receptive lan-

guage disorders and/or a language-processing disability. There are a number of effective methods that O&M specialists can use to communicate with the student with language impairments.

By collaborating with team members and observing their interactions with the student, O&M specialists can identify appropriate verbal and nonverbal communication strategies currently in use. In addition, information regarding alternative communication methods and a student's personal communication system can be obtained from the assistive technology specialist or the speech and language pathologist. Some of the options include spoken word (vocal language), sign language, symbolic systems, tactile systems, written communication, and/or augmentative communication devices.

The assistive technology specialist or speech and language pathologist can assist O&M specialists with integrating the use of alternative communication systems. For some students the most effective method for communicating information about their schedule, order of tasks, or travel destination involves the use of a symbol system. Symbols used for communication are actual objects used to represent people, places, things, or activities (Knott, 2002; van Dijk, 2006). For example, when Tameka is given a spoon,

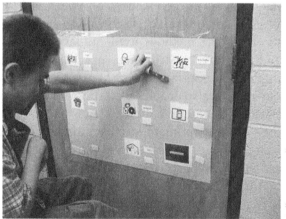

Colleen Rae Calhoun

A student using a tactile symbol system.

this action communicates to her that it is time to travel to the cafeteria for lunch (see also Chapter 17).

Symbol systems can be expanded and used as schedule systems. A schedule system is a series of symbols arranged in a sequence representative of the student's day (Silberman, Bruce, & Nelson, 2004). Calendar systems are a tangible, nonverbal method for the student to anticipate which activity will occur first, next, and last (van Dijk, 2006). They can also be used to indicate the sequence of a lesson.

Speaking in social interactions may be difficult for the student who has visual and cognitive impairments to manage effectively, particularly the student with an autism spectrum disorder. A student's ability to solicit assistance, make a purchase, advocate for her needs, and problem-solve may hinge on her ability to communicate with others. The use of prepared "scripts," written and rehearsed dialogue, is a method that enables students to gain success in situations that require speech. One example of using communication during instruction is found in Table 19.8 (later in the chapter).

Planning and Record Keeping

As an O&M specialist, it is important to develop the discipline of writing and maintaining accurate records on each student on your caseload. Written documentation is the O&M specialist's record of the methods used, student response, and any travel restrictions, concerns, or issues that are appropriate for use by the team. Accurate records also enable O&M specialists to keep track of the multiple threads of instruction that they are attempting to teach simultaneously, to chart student progress, and to produce accurate assessment reports, lesson plans, and progress reports.

The diversity and low incidence of students who have visual and cognitive impairments mean there are neither standardized forms nor assessment protocols readily available to chart a student's progress against a norm. When teaching such students in the classroom setting, special education teachers use alternative assessments that are rooted in general education standards and are usually combined with life skill standards (Kleinert & Kearns, 2004). "A memorandum from the U.S. Department of Education Office of Special Education and Rehabilitation Services makes clear the U.S. Department of Education's position: Alternate assessments need to be aligned with the general curriculum standards set for all students" (Kleinert & Kearns, 2004, p. 121). In this spirit, O&M specialists, when creating O&M assessments and instructional plans for students with visual and cognitive impairments also need to draw assessment items and modify instructional goals found in the traditional O&M curriculum.

After assessment reports, O&M specialists' written lesson plans, lesson summaries, and progress reports are the most important documents needed for planning and record keeping. Lesson plans are created prior to a teaching session. The process of creating a lesson plan aids O&M specialists in staying focused on each student's unique needs. Though a planned lesson may not go "according to plan," the exercise of creating a lesson plan reminds O&M specialists of the prompt levels, behavior plan, schedule of reinforcement, as well as concepts and skills being worked on by the student prior to the lesson (see also Chapter 8; and Volume 1, Chapter 12).

There are many different lesson plan forms that are useful (see Figure 19.2 for one example). The following three elements are important components of any lesson plan:

1. It has a consistent format that is professional in look and in tone, and includes a consistent header that contains relevant student information, the long-term objective, and the lesson objective;

LESSON PLAN: ROUTE TO GROCERY STORE

Provider:	Maryland School for the Blind	Case # 1713	
O&M Specialist:	Jane Doe	Date: 08/01/10	Time: 10 AM–12 PM

Consumer Name: Tameka Barnes	Age: 10
Visual Impairment: NLP	Autism, Mental Retardation, Lang. 4 years
Mobility Tool: Ambutech, 52", folding, rolling marshmallow tip, aluminum	

Long-Term Goal:
Upon completion of high school, Tameka will use a cane to travel using the appropriate sensory, environmental, social and mobility skills for the task independently in familiar environments and in unfamiliar environments, with appropriate adult supervision.

Lesson Goal:
Tameka will travel to her local grocery store with adult supervision within 20–30 feet to monitor for safety during block travel and within 5 feet of student when crossing Mars & Alley 3 and while walking along Parkville Shopping Center. On-task behavior prompts will occur immediately with a partial verbal cue, "Look and listen."

Lesson Objectives:
1. After review of route and crossing script, Tameka will demonstrate safe street crossings at two stop sign-controlled intersections. At each crossing, Tameka will verbally state street crossing script (clear area, position cane, look/listen left, right, left, safe to cross or not safe to cross, tap tap, and go) while performing the listed activity with minimal to no partial verbal prompts.
2. After debrief, Tameka will locate and confirm the entrance to the grocery store by tactiley identifying landmarks or independently choosing to solicit assistance from a stranger with partial verbal prompt 1 minute after Tameka starts walking in wrong direction.
3. After preview of soliciting aid script, Tameka will locate the Customer Service Desk within the grocery store by knowing the route or seeking assistance from a stranger after full verbal prompt.
4. Using script, Tameka will independently solicit information at the Customer Service Desk regarding cost of oatmeal.

Materials:
Written scripts for lesson preview & review, ID card, emergency contact information, cane

Environment:
Home community. Starting point—Tameka's house. Route: Travel along Taylor Ave. making "all quiet" street crossings at two stop sign-controlled intersections (Mars and Alley 3). Turn left into the Parkville Shopping Center. Travel straight past the cart corral and exit doors to locate the entrance to the grocery store. Ending points: store entrance and customer service desk

Skills	Time	Eval	Activities
Rapport and set up	3		Review necessary materials with Tameka (T) with verbal and physical prompts as needed—fluency level

(continued on next page)

Figure 19.2. Sample O&M Lesson Plan for a Student with Vision Loss

Skills	Time	Eval	Activities
Review	3		Review last lesson accomplishments (verbal prompts to obtain recall) and give lesson objective.
Preview: Memorize crossing script	10		Have student state street crossing script (verbal prompt to remember steps).
Street-crossing technique	12		Ask T to travel to Mars St. and to stop after crossing Mars St.
	2–5		Observe T cross Mars St. (fluency level)
Debrief: street-crossing technique	2		Debrief and give "high 5" after crossing
Street-crossing technique	15		Ask T to travel to Alley 3 and to stop after she crosses Alley 3
	2–5		Observe T cross Alley 3 (fluency level)
Debrief: street crossing technique	2		Debrief and give "high 5" after crossing Alley 3. Ask T to continue to Parkville Shopping Center and stop when she reaches the cart corral.
Orientation skills	2		Observe T make left turn into Parkville Shopping Center (generalization level)
Identify auditory landmarks: recognize automatic door of the grocery store; indicates arrival at destination **Debrief**	5		If T continues past cart corral for more than 2 minutes use full physical prompt paired with verbal prompt to stop T and indicate the cart corral. Debrief overall travel (verbal prompt- recall information)
Preview: Route and Customer Service Script: "Excuse me, can you tell me how much the oatmeal is? Thank you."	2		Have T point to the sound of the automatic door (reward). Preview route to Customer Service Desk (CSD) and have student say script.
Uses Customer Service Script	15		Have T travel independently to CSD and give nonverbal signal when done.
	2–5		Approach T at CSD. Check information; human guide to debrief area.
Debrief	7		Review lesson successes and challenges, work toward T being able to identify one thing she liked/didn't like...or one thing that was easy/hard.

Comments: Were there safety concerns? Did they meet the objectives? Environmental lesson influences? Learner behaviors? Prompting levels? Next lesson idea?

Services Provided by:	Date:

Figure 19.2. (Continued)

2. It is broken into steps and corresponding activities with an estimate of the amount of time the lesson will focus on each step; and

3. It provides space for performance ratings and notes where O&M specialists can make comments on student performance immediately following the lesson including any changes to the lesson that occurred.

Lesson summaries are informal notes about the lesson that are written shortly after teaching the student. Lesson summaries in planning the next lesson and writing progress reports. Progress reports are written at established intervals for the family and the student to have a record of the student's progress. Beginning with the passage of IDEA in 1997, each IEP must state how families of students with an IEP will be informed of the progress their child is making toward annual IEP goals, and the extent to which that progress is sufficient to enable the child to achieve the goals by the end of the year (WAC 392-172-160). One example of using record keeping and program planning during instruction is found in Table 19.5 (later in the chapter).

Time Considerations

Time considerations for the student include scheduling: for example, the best time of the day for learning, the most functional time of the day for learning, length of the lesson, the lesson frequency, student fatigue, and program duration (the time span needed for a student to achieve mastery of long-term goals). When creating a schedule, O&M specialists need to consider the student's goals and objectives first.

When it is vital that the student be alert for a lesson, O&M specialists can attempt to garner the best time of day with respect to the student's endurance or "freshness" for a lesson. Best time of day may be the first class in the morning; just before, midway, or just after medication has been

administered; before physical education; at lunch time; or even on a certain day of the week. When the most important aspect of the lesson is that it takes place during the most functional time of day, then the O&M specialist will fit her schedule to the student's schedule.

It is up to the professionals to be creative and flexible to meet the needs of all students based on their goals. Students with visual and cognitive impairments may require time to adjust to a new instructor. The instructor can facilitate rapport building by participating in the familiar classroom activities for a few days or weeks before starting separate O&M lessons. Thus, to achieve the goal of changing classes or walking to meet the paratransit bus, a combination of best time of day and best functional time of day may be needed. In all environments, there are "rush hour" times within a day. Thus, with the goal of walking the route during "rush hour" in mind, O&M specialists might opt to teach a route during a quiet time of day when the student is most alert, and later have the student work to tolerate completing the route during rush hour.

With some creativity, O&M specialists can manipulate lesson frequency to take best advantage of student characteristics and support repetitive learning in functional environments. Options to choose from include scheduling multiple short lessons every day or daily lessons that fit into the student's routine. When the O&M specialist's schedule can accommodate lessons only once or twice a week, train related staff to provide practice on selected skills (as recommended by the Association for Education and Rehabilitation of the Blind and Visually Impaired O&M Division position paper "Model Program for Use of Orientation and Mobility Assistants" [2004] and limited by the O&M Division position paper "Orientation and Mobility Specialist Roles, Responsibilities, and Qualifications" [2004]) on her "off days."

The student who has visual and cognitive impairments often takes longer to attain specific skills; and each time he changes settings (from school to a workplace or parent's home to an assisted living facility), additional O&M instruction is needed. Even with repetition and consistent carryover of skills, it may take a student months or years to learn a specific skill or set of travel directions. With this population of students, the length, frequency, and duration of O&M lessons will be determined by the student's performance and progress. One example of using time considerations as an instructional strategy can be found in Table 19.2 (later in the chapter).

Task Analysis

Task analysis is a system for refining curriculum by breaking down whole skills and concepts into their action sequence, parts, or steps. The purpose of task analysis is to simplify and reduce the demands on the student during instruction by teaching attainable units of a skill. Once a task analysis has been written, it can also be used for planning the level and type of prompts to be used during instruction, conducting curriculum-based assessment of student progress (Drew & Hardman, 2004), and using forward and backward chaining techniques (Chapter 8; Fazzi & Petersmeyer, 2001; Scheuermann & Webber, 2002).

The number of steps in a task analysis depends on the student's current response time in completing each step and his ability to generalize behaviors across tasks. Wehman and Kregel (1997) recommended the following guidelines for developing a task analysis:

1. Each step should be listed in specific behavioral terms so that mastery can be observed.

2. Write each step so that it can become a prompt for the next step.

3. If the step has the word "and" in it, determine if the student can achieve it or whether it needs to be broken down further.

4. Pilot-test the task analysis with the student before finalizing it for instruction.

A task analysis (see Sidebar 19.1) can become an assessment tool to track progress. Student achievement is evaluated by observing which steps need to be taught at the *acquisition level* (student intermittently or does not attempt to complete the step after prompt or response time is severely delayed), which at the *fluency level* (student completes the step after a prompt, with slow response time), and which at the *maintenance level* (student completes step with intermittent prompts or no prompt, and response time is appropriate to the task) and the *generalization level* (student completes steps without prompts and with an appropriate response time across environments) (Scheuermann & Webber, 2002).

Task analysis, paired with either forward or backward chaining, is a useful technique for teaching routes. In chaining, O&M specialists first select the route to the destination; second, designate attainable or "teachable" sections along the route; and third, write the steps in order from start point to destination. Teachable sections are manageable travel distances (manageable in relation to a student's physical stamina, behavior plan, motivation, and cognitive ability) between unique and permanent landmarks or choice points. The process of task analysis involves listing the landmarks and natural choice points sequentially along the route (see Sidebar 19.1).

In forward chaining, each time the student who has visual and cognitive impairments travels the route, she will work on skills for completing part of the route independently. Instruction starts at the same point or home base, and each step is taught sequentially. A modification of forward chaining is to teach the student the first and last sections of the route; once mastered sequentially, introduce the remaining "middle" sections. Backward or reverse chaining is teaching the last section of the route first. One example of applying task analysis in

SIDEBAR 19.1

Sample Task Analysis of a Route for Derrick: From the Front Door of His Job Site to Inside His Office

FRONT DOOR OF JOB SITE TO INSIDE HIS OFFICE

1. Enter front door (partial physical prompt), and confirm by visually locating reception desk and saying hello to receptionist (full verbal prompt).

2. Travel green carpet until it ends at the intersecting hallway (human guide).

4. Turn left into the hallway (human guide).

5. Travel to the end of the hallway until reaching and locating the red metal fire door (human guide).

6. Go through the door, cross the open space in the stairwell, and locate the stairs using the constant-contact touch technique (human guide).

7. Locate the ascending stairs with a cane (human guide).

8. Use the cane to ascend one flight of stairs to the red fire door and identify 2 on the door (human guide).

9. Exit the stairwell door and locate the green carpet (backward chaining begins here—intermittent need for a partial physical prompt).

10. Traverse the carpet using constant contact, touch the trail, and visually locate the first room on the right, room #207 (demonstrates fluency).

11. Confirm the room number with braille and an augmentative device to enter the office (demonstrates fluency).

---

forward chaining is found in Table 19.10 (later in the chapter).

Sequenced Instruction

The term *sequencing* or *sequenced instruction* may describe the order in which a set of short-term objectives are taught so as to achieve a long-range goal. Sequence may also be used to describe a series of events within a single activity, such as is found in a task analysis. The instructional sequence for teaching students who demonstrate difficulty learning new skills is narrower in scope and focused on meeting a student's most immediate travel needs using the most appropriate mobility skills for the task.

An effective model for sequential instruction in these specific tasks such as learning the constant-contact technique on a functional route is having the student repeat the same behavior or skill in the same way, in the same location each lesson, within the critical skills model (CSM) (Ehresman, 1994; Fazzi & Petersmeyer, 2001). The CSM asks the instructor to prioritize and select the most critical skill to teach first, select the essential parts of the skill to be taught, and choose the location where it is most needed (Fazzi & Petersmeyer, 2001). Critical skill selection is based on two principles: (1) the technique or skill is the most appropriate to complete this task, and (2) the lesson is functional and will enable the student to travel to a destination that is vital to her everyday routine. One example of using sequenced instruction within a lesson can be found in Table 19.4 (later in the chapter).

Environment

In this section, *environment* is used in reference to place, such as an elementary school classroom, congested hallway, or residential block. Each of these environments indicate different travel demands and sensory stimuli. When working with students who have visual and cognitive impairments, O&M specialists need to be aware of the interplay between the environment and the student's behavior and ability to learn.

When something within the environment is causing the student distress or to become distracted from travel activities, the questions to ask are as follows: what stimuli are causing distress or distraction? Can the stimulus (e.g., noise, sight, odor, or activity) be changed or not? If not, will the student be able to learn to tolerate the noise, sight, odor, or activity in the environment? Does a recommendation need to be made that the student be prevented from having to encounter the offending stimulus or stimuli?

In the student's home or classroom, the environment can and needs to be altered to accommodate specific needs of the student. In public spaces, modification of the environment may be feasible and might require special permission before changes are made. However, there will be environments where it is either inappropriate or not feasible to make changes, such as a privately owned business or a grocery store. In such cases, a student's behavior and ability to tolerate the space may make avoidance of the space altogether an appropriate solution. One example of considering environment during instruction is found in Table 19.3 (later in the chapter).

Motivation

For students who have visual and cognitive impairments, the interest and desire to learn orientation and mobility may need to be developed through the skilled use of a rewards-based system. O&M lessons have the advantage that there are many fun and rewarding destinations to travel to and there are physical and psychological benefits associated with sustained activity, such as walking. However, for some students, intrinsic motivation or the engagement in the activity as an end in itself, needs to be taught. In these cases, O&M specialists can use external reinforcers such as praise or a token system to encourage students to engage in O&M lessons (see Jacobson & Bradley, Volume 1, Chapter 7). The plan is for the students to be externally motivated into having experiences that build an internal motivation to travel.

In order to use a reward system successfully, it is vital to discover what motivates the student. With students who have visual and cognitive impairments, finding the extrinsic motivators requires a collective team effort. Finding appropriate motivators is more challenging with students who have difficulty expressing themselves. One example of using motivation when teaching can be found in Table 19.10.

It is important to note that novel experiences, like getting to push all of the elevator buttons or saying "echo" inside the gymnasium to hear the sound reverberate, can be motivating ends to a lesson. However, these experiences can get out of control and become a learned inappropriate behavior. Students who have visual and cognitive impairments may have an avid interest in one subject. For example, a student might be fixated on listening to "oldies" music. On the surface, the promise of getting to listen to his favorite music may seem to be a strong motivator, but often the fixation is so strong that mention of the activity at the start of the lesson distracts the student from attending to the lesson.

A primary consideration in motivating students who have visual and cognitive impairments to complete the learning activities designed by O&M specialists is the careful development of rapport. Such students may be slow to accept a new O&M specialist. Therefore, O&M specialists need to be patient and not attempt to push a student to work on orientation and mobility goals before trust and acceptance has been gained. In students with visual and cognitive impairments, building trust and rapport may take several weeks or even months. O&M specialists begin by taking part in activities, spending time with and relating to the student and support personnel in non-O&M-related capacities and then introduce O&M activities within those familiar routines prior to attempting to remove the student from the classroom.

Prompting

Providing an additional cue after an initial directive has been given to a student is called *prompting*. Students with visual and cognitive impairments generally benefit from more frequent prompting to achieve a correct response. Prompting is a more effective tool when it is carefully designed, controlled, and measured (Fazzi & Petersmeyer, 2002; Gense & Gense, 2005; Scheuermann & Webber, 2002). When the goal for instruction is that the student will initiate a desired behavior after a natural cue, O&M specialists should consider prompt type, delivery interval, and level of intensity.

Prompt types (from least to most restrictive) are as follows:

- *Natural cue*: Defined as a naturally occurring sensory event within the environment with no additional instructor prompt. For example, the elevator door opens and the student clears the floor before entering.

- *Position of student to objective*: The O&M specialist pairs a physical or verbal cue to locate the student within reach to respond to a natural cue. A student is given a verbal cue, "Meet me at the door to begin our bus lesson"; the proximity of the door to the student's locker should cue her to gather her needed materials for the lesson (e.g., bus pass and cane).

- *Visual gesture or auditory cue*: The O&M specialist uses an abbreviated visual or auditory message to signal the student to initiate or continue an action: pointing at a sign or tapping on a table.

- *Verbal or symbol cue*: The O&M specialist uses a full word or statement or physical interaction with a symbol to signal the student to initiate or continue an action: "Stop and square off," and/or has the student place his hand on the classroom symbol outside the classroom door.

- *Modeling*: The demonstration of the desired behavior. The O&M specialist demonstrates upper- and lower-hand protection for the student to see and/or touch.

- *Physical cue*: The O&M specialist uses an appropriate touch varying in duration (brief touch to full physical assistance) to signal the student to initiate or continue an action.

A natural cue would be when the student's cane drops into a descending stair. Positioning the student so that her cane is on the lip of the stair might be enough to trigger the appropriate response needed to begin the stair sequence. A visual gesture to a student with low vision might be for the O&M specialist to hold up her hand to signal stop. A verbal cue could be a leading question prior to the event, such as "What do you do when your cane falls off the edge?" Modeling could include the O&M specialist or a peer demonstrating the correct behavior. A physical prompt is when the O&M specialist shapes student behavior using appropriate physical contact.

With the exception of the natural cue, each of the prompt types can be regulated by changing the response interval for the delivery of the prompt (from immediate to a longer and longer delay), and engaging in the appropriate level of prompt intrusiveness (from full to partial) (Gense & Gense, 2005; Scheuermann & Webber, 2002). The response interval or time delay (Kaiser, 1993; Scheuermann & Weber, 2001) is a procedure whereby O&M specialists wait for a student-initiated response after a stimulus has occurred before giving a prompt. The purpose of a time delay is to decrease the student's dependence on teacher instructions and models and to encourage the student to act independently (Scheuermann & Weber, 2002).

Intrusiveness (full or partial) is related to the intensity of the prompt given. A full or partial prompt can be expressed across all prompt types. *Full prompt* means that the entire cue is provided; *partial prompt* indicates a shorthanded version of the cue is being employed. It is important to select prompts appropriate for the student.

Fading is a term for using less intrusive prompt types, increasing the response time, or reducing the level of prompt intensity. An example of fading would be O&M specialists beginning with the use of a hand-over-hand full physical prompt and full verbal prompt to have the student maintain contact with the wall during trailing. In using hand-over-hand prompting, an O&M specialist places his hands over the student's hands to guide them through the action. As the student's resistance to this position decreases, O&M specialists begin to lessen the physical prompt, perhaps keeping only a finger on the back of the student's hand, and then only touching the back of the student's hand (paired with the verbal cue "Keep trailing") when he pulls away from the wall. O&M specialists fade verbal prompts to "trail" or "T" and finally to using no prompts at all.

Choice Making

Self-regulated learning refers to the process whereby students direct their thoughts, feelings, and actions toward the attainment of their goals (Zimmerman & Schunk, 2001). When students have

few if any choices, their behaviors are externally regulated (Schunk, 2004). For the student with visual and cognitive impairments opportunities for personal choice are important because much of the time he may need to be assisted by others.

Here are some guidelines for giving the student choices:

1. Allow the student to make choices and make sure those choices can be carried out. Do not give the student the option to do something that cannot be granted, such as traveling to see a movie during school hours.

2. Use choices that can easily be part of the pre-planned lesson. For example, have the student decide which activity he wants to do first or let him arrange the order in which he will complete a set of activities for that lesson. Remember to put out only the activities that are the choices available for that lesson.

3. Present choices in a way that allows the student to give an accurate answer. If he always chooses the last thing you say, word or picture cards may help him make his own preference known (Hamill & Everington, 2002). Another way to alleviate this problem may be to repeat the question after giving all the choices. For example, "Which cane tip would you like to try today, the roller or the marshmallow? Which cane tip would you like to use today?"

Examples for providing choice in mobility lessons include the following: choose between a motor task and a cognitive task, or pick between two route options. Use strategies such as a "yes" and "no" board or a board with photographs of the actions or activities to choose from to support choice making. Remember to present choices in a way that the student can be successful in answering.

TEN SKILL AREAS

Ten skills that are needed by students who have visual and cognitive impairments to participate in and succeed in O&M instruction are attention, sensory integration, behavior, memory, concept development, generalization, problem solving, social skills, orientation strategies, and mobility techniques. The skill areas were ordered to suggest a sequence: first, gain a student's attention, and support his or her sensory needs, behavior plan, and memory triggers; and, second, teach concepts and ability to generalize, solve problems, and use social skills, orientation strategies, and mobility techniques. Each of the skill areas is defined, and three levels of instructional goals are provided to match the student's present level of performance. Students who have visual and cognitive impairments cannot be fit neatly into an ability level, and students will be working toward different goal levels across skill areas. Tables of teaching strategies for addressing the ability levels in each skill area are found throughout the following pages.

The goal statements are offered as high, medium, and low targets, or goal levels, for each skill area. These are long-term goals, and as such are written with the idea that when mastered, O&M instruction will end. Often students who have visual and cognitive impairments will have a lifetime of support personnel with whom they will travel. The role of support personnel (family, friends, and paid staff) then needs to be included in the end goal of O&M instruction.

Attention

Attention span is the length of time a student is able to stay on task using appropriate behavior with and without supervision (Sacks & Silberman, 1998). It is a cognitive skill that impacts nearly all learning tasks. Examples of O&M-related attention goals for students who have visual and cognitive impairments include attend-

ing to instructions, staying focused on travel until the destination is reached, or shifting attention from a favorite hobby to a learning activity. The ability of such students to maintain or shift attention while completing O&M tasks may need direct intervention.

O&M specialists should measure and record the student's attention span and plan lessons that actively engage the student within that time frame. A student's attention span may be impacted by a variety of factors including her ability to process sensory and environmental information, and her age and level of travel experience, motivation, distractibility, and perseveration.

- *Level-1 attention goal.* To attend to directions and prompts of support personnel when traveling.
- *Level-2 attention goals.* To attend to multiple sensory stimuli and remain focused to demonstrate oriented and safe travel in familiar indoor and outdoor settings, and will attend to directions and prompts when traveling with support personnel to unfamiliar indoor and outdoor environments.
- *Level-3 attention goal.* To attend to multiple sensory stimuli and remain focused to demonstrate oriented and safe travel within the community using public transportation independently.

Table 19.2 suggests a number of strategies for reaching all three levels of attention goals. Some strategies can be used for more than one level.

Sensory Integration

Sensory integration is the ability to interpret, filter, and combine sensory messages from the body and the surroundings. Sensory stimuli are "passed back and forth between the central nervous system (CNS) and nerves in the brain and spinal cord, and the peripheral nervous system with the nerves that are outside the CNS"

TABLE 19.2

Instructional Strategies for Teaching Attention Skills

Strategies	Goal Level		
I. General Strategies	1	2	3
a. Position self in front of the student when talking.	x		
b. Step into student's space to gain his attention.	x		
c. Remove unnecessary distractions (e.g., unneeded materials).	x		
d. When exiting a room, close the door to help the student shift attention.	x	x	
e. Provide an initial prompt to begin the lesson (lesson preview).	x	x	x
f. Develop a list of steps for students to use to complete a task.		x	x
g. Decrease distractions by using a study carrel or quiet room.		x	x
h. Limit the amount of verbal, auditory, and environmental information presented at one time.		x	x
i. Use voice (songs, rhythmic talking, or a sing-song cadence) to gain and keep attention.		x	x
j. Use an enthusiastic, happy, and inviting voice to maintain student attention.		x	x
l. Enable student to redirect himself back to task by carrying a destination object.		x	x
m. Simplify language: use key words to prompt or communicate an idea or direction.		x	x
n. Teach students to focus on travel tasks by limiting self-imposed distractions (e.g., listening to headphones, daydreaming, and being too social or drowsy).			x
o. Plan short "mini"-lessons (10–15 minutes) that focus on one skill or activity within a functional activity or setting.			x
p. Use a timer with students to agree on how long an activity will last, and work to increase the time.			x
q. Prompt and redirect the student's attention back to task using his personal communication system.			x
r. Use engaging materials and play activities.			x
s. Introduce new skills in a small, highly controlled environment, and slowly introduce distractions (anything that challenges the specific student's attention to task such as sound, size of environment, and obstacles).			x

(Kranowitz, 2003). Sensory stimuli include visual, auditory, olfactory, and touch, movement, gravity (vestibular), and body position (proprioceptive). Approximately 42 percent of children and youth with autism and Asperger' syndrome have sensory integration disorders (Anzalone & Williamson, 2000; National Research Council, 2001, Turnbull, Turnbull, & Wehmeyer, 2007).

Students who have visual and cognitive impairments students who have an autism spectrum disorder and/or other cognitive impairments may have either under- or overresponsiveness to sensory stimuli, although overresponsiveness or hypersensitivity is more common (Gense & Gense, 2005). These students may, as a result, have difficulty interpreting sensory information and identifying its meaning so that it can be used to complete functional travel tasks. Some sensory stimuli may cause adverse reactions in students.

- *Level-1 sensory goal.* To tolerate aversive sensory information during travel with intermittent to extensive prompts from support personnel.

- *Level-2 sensory goals.* To identify and manage sensory information to travel safely in familiar indoor and outdoor environments and in unfamiliar indoor and outdoor environments with intermittent to no prompts from support personnel.

- *Level-3 sensory goal.* To integrate sensory information to travel safely and independently in familiar and unfamiliar indoor and outdoor environments.

Table 19.3 offers instructional strategies for addressing various levels of sensory integration goals.

Behavior

The student who has visual and cognitive impairments may exhibit interfering behaviors or behavior problems such as being quick to anger, being in a state of agitation, unpredictability, impulsivity, inattention, severe mood swings, total resistance to O&M (or to instruction), self-stimulating repetitive actions, as well as verbal and physical aggression during O&M lessons. Behavioral theorists suggest that aggressive and interfering behaviors may be attempts by the student to communicate about an environment, person, or activity (van Dijk, 2006). It is important to document any behavioral incidents that occur in an attempt to better anticipate or reduce interfer-

ing behaviors. When appropriate, O&M specialists need to seek support from a behavior specialist to understand and employ recommended behavior management strategies.

- *Level-1 behavior goal.* To respond to the efforts of O&M specialists and support personnel to reduce behavioral outbursts when traveling.

- *Level-2 behavior goals.* To maintain control of one's emotions and behave in a consistent, predictable manner in familiar indoor and outdoor settings and in unfamiliar indoor and outdoor environments and respond to the efforts of O&M specialists or support personnel to reduce behavioral outbursts.

- *Level-3 behavior goal.* To maintain control of one's emotions and behave in a consistent, predictable manner in challenging environments and situations.

Table 19.4 presents strategies for teaching behavioral skills for all three goal levels.

Memory

Learning involves forming associations between stimuli (e.g., visual, tactile) and responses (reflexive, planned action). Once a stimulus is attended to and perceived, the input is transferred to short-term (working) memory for a brief time. If the stimulus or response is not perceived or if a cognitive impairment prevents, limits, or alters how the brain gathers and interprets the stimuli, the transition from short-term memory to long-term memory is not completed (Schunk, 2004). The memory is lost.

Encoding describes the process of new (incoming) information moving from short-term to long-term memory. Encoding is accomplished by making new information meaningful. Simply attending to and perceiving stimuli does not ensure that learning will occur. When a student who has visual and cognitive impairments

TABLE 19.3

Instructional Strategies for Teaching Sensory Integration Skills

Strategies	Goal Level		
I. General Strategies	1	2	3
a. Consider how the student processes and responds to auditory information and directions. The student may benefit from a multisensory approach where orientation and mobility (O&M) specialists provide a combination of tactile, visual, and auditory information when identifying objects (e.g., hearing, touching, and tasting the "water fountain").	x	x	
b. Develop lesson plans that gradually lengthen the time a student is exposed to aversive sensory stimuli. When possible, students should determine the proximity and duration of the experience as they work toward tolerating the offensive stimulus.	x	x	
II. Auditory			
a. Offer sound occluders (earplugs or headphones) to muffle sound and reduce aversive stimuli.	x		
b. Modifications to reduce sound include hanging pads on walls, turning off electrical appliances (heaters, fans), changing lights from fluorescent to incandescent, carpeting floors, teaching in a study carrel, placing tennis balls on chair legs, and drawing blinds or curtains.	x		
c. Use a human guide to reduce the duration of exposure to aversive sound. Control the exposure by walking fast or slow.	x	x	
d. Build tolerance of environments that contain the offensive sounds by gradual, controlled exposure over numerous lessons.	x	x	
e. Create "sound tapes" of nonpreferred sounds. These tapes can be used to isolate sounds for identification or be reviewed in increments to build tolerance.		x	
f. Use structured activities when teaching sound identification, localization, and tracking skills. A remote-controlled doorbell gives students the ability to control the frequency and duration of a sound as they practice these skills.		x	x
g. Teach the student to filter extraneous sounds and focus on the relevant auditory information. Direct the student to focus on the sound of the cash register when looking for assistance in a store. Redirect saying, "We are listening for the cash register."		x	x
h. Provide a script for lengthening the period of time a student can tolerate an aversive sound. Here is an example script for walking past construction sounds: (1) "Those are construction sounds," (2) "A little bit more sounds," (3) "Almost finished with sounds," and (4) "Finished with sounds . . . good job!"		x	x

(continued on next page)

Strategies	Goal Level		
III. Tactile			
a. Follow the occupational therapist's recommendations for preparing the student's tactile senses. For example, just prior to the student gripping a cane, apply a hand massage or squeeze a therapy ball	x	x	
b. Student may prefer to face a blank wall rather than the speaker when listening to verbal directions.	x	x	
c. Acknowledge student's comments and body language after touching a texture. Remove aversive stimuli.	x	x	x
d. Consider hand-under-hand prompting. Place the O&M specialist's hand on the activity with the student's hand on top. Incrementally remove the specialist's hand, allowing the student to have increased contact with the material.	x	x	x
IV. Visual			
a. Assess the effects of movement, congestion, and student stamina on student's visual perception.	x	x	
b. Gradually introduce a variety of visual environments that offer simple and complex levels of sensory information. Experiment with lighting conditions (bright versus cloudy) or the amount of pedestrian traffic the student encounters at different times of the day.	x	x	x

TABLE 19.3 *(Continued)*

shows limited ability to encode new concepts and skills, O&M specialists need to employ organization, elaboration, and schema structures in their teaching.

Gestalt theory suggests that the use of well-organized material is easier to learn and recall: that learning is enhanced by classifying and grouping bits of information into organized chunks. "Organized material improves memory because items are linked to one another systematically" (Schunk, 2004, p. 160). In practice, *chunking* is teaching students to identify a multisensory sequence of steps by a key word. In other words, *cafeteria* means the following: leave the class, turn right, traverse the stairs to the second floor, and trail the wall on your right to the cafeteria door. Chunking is also an effective tool that will eventually enable O&M specialists and students to communicate the steps of lengthy routes

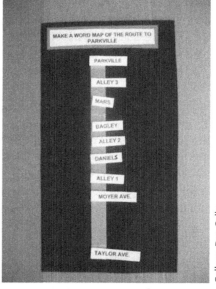

A "sequence card" system or word map used as a memory aid to order the street names along a particular route.

Colleen Rae Calhoun

TABLE 19.4

Instructional Strategies for Teaching Behavior Skills

Behavior	Goal Level		
I. General Strategies	1	2	3
a. Review behavioral expectations and responsibilities prior to the start of a lesson.	x	x	
b. Develop behavior contracts and reward systems with the student.	x	x	
c. Make use of student's communication strategy to give choices.	x	x	x
d. Focus praise and attention on positive behaviors.	x	x	x
e. Provide time at the beginning and end of activities to students who have difficulty transitioning.	x	x	x
f. Take a structured break. This consists of a planned, non–orientation and mobility (O&M) activity such as listening to music or taking a few seconds to jump and clap.	x	x	x
g. Use a predictable lesson structure to introduce "change" into the lesson. The lesson starts the same each time: step 1—communicate the lesson goal or plan; step 2—warm-up activity; step 3—practice activity; step 4—new (change) activity; step 5—break; step 6—practice; and step 7—end-of-lesson activity.	x	x	x
h. Use the student's communication device and/or tangible schedule system in O&M activities.		x	x
i. Use key words, colored cue cards, nonverbal signals, or tactile symbols as prompts for the student to modify his or her behavior.		x	x
j. Teach the lesson in a preferred environment.		x	x
k. Participate with the student in the activity that precedes and follows the O&M lesson to support the student's ability to make transitions easier.		x	x
l. Use the student's communication system to prepare for schedule changes.		x	x
m. Modify the environment to avoid triggering an interfering behavior.			x
n. If a student has a difficult time adjusting to new people, try having the parent or a staff member co-teach the lesson. This co-teaching model also benefits O&M specialists as the familiar staff person or parent can assist in learning how best to work with the student.			x
o. Employ an object cue to signal the beginning or end of a task.			x
p. Identify supports in place to help the student monitor and self-regulate his own behavior.			x
q. Let the student make choices on reinforcements and the reinforcement schedule.			x
r. Use note cards or a checklist to convey lesson expectations. This system shifts the demand from the O&M specialist to the card system.			x

using a three- or four-step sequence (e.g., bench, water fountain, and bus stop).

Elaboration is the process of expanding upon what a student already knows. Elaborations assist encoding and retrieval because it links information to be remembered with an understood concept. The more often an idea is encountered, the stronger its representation in memory. A schema (plural, *schemata*) is a structure that organizes large amounts of multisensory information into a meaningful system. Any well-ordered sequence can be represented as a schema. One type of schema is "taking the bus to school." The steps consist of activities such as waiting for the bus, climbing the high metal stairs, finding a seat, staying upright against the bus motion, and exiting (Schunk, 2004). Schemata are important because they indicate what to expect in a situation.

When the student is provided multiple rehearsal opportunities throughout the day, learning is optimized. O&M specialists can create materials which enable other professionals to provide students who have visual and cognitive impairments practice and rehearsal opportunities including: recorded step by step audiotapes, memory books, flash cards, written or recorded social scripts, cue card systems, word maps, tactile maps, and checklists (Downing, 2004).

- *Level-1 memory goal.* To use memory aids (tapes, books, scripts) to complete routes in familiar environments with intermittent to extensive prompts from support personnel.

- *Level-2 memory goals.* To make limited use of memory aids to travel routes in familiar environments with intermittent to no prompts from support personnel. Each new route will be acquired via direct instruction.

- *Level-3 memory goal.* To travel routes in familiar environments with limited or no use of memory aids without prompts from support personnel. New routes may be learned through indirect instruction.

Table 19.5 presents strategies for teaching memory skills for all levels of memory goals.

Concept Development

Conceptual knowledge describes a student's ability to form mental representations of people, places, things, physical properties, events, actions, and reactions (Fazzi & Petersmeyer, 2001). Individuals who have visual and cognitive impairments may have limited experience directly interacting with the environment and may have a limited ability to employ incidental learning strategies to acquire age-appropriate knowledge of body concepts, spatial and positional concepts, laterality, time–distance relationships, and environmental concepts.

It is not uncommon for a student who has visual and cognitive impairments to demonstrate particular concepts and skills at a higher level than their overall abilities and functional performance would suggest. These "scattered skills" are an important instructional building block for identifying the student's strengths in the area of concept development. Careful observation across home, work, school, and leisure environments will aid O&M specialists in identifying what concepts are in place for the student and what concepts need to be developed.

- *Level-1 concept goal.* To develop an understanding of basic body and spatial concepts, to follow simple one- or two-step directions en route with intermittent to extensive prompts from support personnel.

- *Level-2 concept goals.* To acquire and use concepts in familiar settings with limited ability to generalize concepts in familiar settings given intermittent to no prompts from support personnel. Each new route will be acquired via direct instruction.

- *Level-3 concept goal.* To acquire and use concepts and to generalize learned concepts for

TABLE 19.5

Instructional Strategies for Teaching Memory Skills

Strategies	Goal Level		
I. General Strategies	1	2	3
a. For students who forget their destination en route, try single-message augmentative communication devices.	x		
b. For students who have difficulty unlearning behaviors, use "errorless learning" to guide them through a route or assist them to perform a skill correctly the first time, every time.	x	x	
c. Present information using a multisensory approach: graphs, pictures, tactile, or visual cues.	x	x	x
d. Include fun and motivating experiences en route.	x	x	x
e. For students who forget their destination en route, have them carry a simple object cue or symbol from their schedule system.	x	x	
f. Use rhymes and rhythmic phrases. For squaring off, "Bottom to the wall, back to the wall, head nice and tall; square off, cross the hall."	x	x	
g. Teach student to sing directions using the beat of a familiar song (e.g., a nursery rhyme, rap tune, or holiday chorus).	x	x	
h. Have student review the audiotape of social scripts before a social interaction.		x	
i. Introduce new routes using full prompts to enable the student to complete the entire route each lesson.		x	
j. Have student answer, "Who, what, where, when, and how?" before engaging in soliciting aid.		x	x
k. Use "fill-in-the-blank" statements: "To get a drink of water, I'm going to the __."		x	x
l. Organize information to be memorized by creating a script.		x	x
m. Have students use assistive communication devices en route.		x	x
n. Use forward- and backward-chaining strategies to teach routes.		x	x
o. Organize by numbering the steps of a task.		x	x
p. Use checklists that begin as tangible memory aids (braille, print, or audio list); the goal is for the student to complete the task without it.			x
r. Have the student tape-record as he moves through the route and include information that is meaningful and memorable to him.			x
s. Teach student the use of commercially available recording devices to record information obtained by soliciting aid (phone numbers, addresses, bus schedule information, etc.).			x
t. Organize information to be memorized by developing a mnemonic sequence. For example: mnemonics for a street crossing might be OAR=orientation, analyze, and ready to go; or ACACAC=align, clear, analyze, check for cars, and cross.			x
u. Use route shapes (e.g., I, L, U, and Z) to identify routes.			x

the purpose of travel in familiar and unfamiliar environments.

Table 19.6 presents strategies for teaching concepts at all levels of concept goals.

Generalization

Generalization is the student's ability to make use of a concept or skill learned in one setting in a variety of settings (Scheuermann & Webber, 2002). Students with cognitive impairments, particularly autism spectrm disorders and visual impairments and intellectual disabilities, demonstrate difficulty with generalization (Gense & Gense, 2005; Turnbull, Turnbull, & Wehmeyer, 2007). Through systematic instruction, the O&M instructor can develop the student's ability to

apply environmental concepts (hallway layout, intersection shapes), techniques (trailing, cane skills, and street-crossing strategies), and related O&M skills (stranger danger, phone usage, and money skills) across travel settings.

- *Level-1 generalization goals.* The consistent use of a human guide, self-protective techniques, and selected cane techniques in familiar indoor environments with intermittent to extensive prompts across a variety of support personnel.

- *Level-2 generalization goals.* The ability to consistently demonstrate learned concepts and skills when traveling in familiar indoor and outdoor settings, and in unfamiliar indoor and outdoor environments generalize critical safety

(continued on next page)

TABLE 19.6

Instructional Strategies for Teaching Concepts

Strategies	Goal Level		
I. General Strategies	1	2	3
a. Employ the same concepts, actions, and activities in a variety of settings. For example, the positional concepts associated with body–object relationships are needed in every environment. A verbal prompt ("Find the chair in front") paired with an auditory cue (e.g., physically tapping the chair) can be used across settings.	x	x	
b. Teach concepts, like donning winter coats, in a group setting.	x	x	
c. Coordinate the instruction and use of concepts across instructional environments. For example, a discussion of even and odd numbers in math can be carried over to lessons on the use of numbering systems or money skills in a grocery store.	x	x	
d. Give students hands-on tactile experiences such as encouraging the student to sit, kneel, or lay down on the ground to feel the environmental object being discussed (e.g., corner, or curb cut).	x	x	
e. Use repetition of actions, words, and routines.	x	x	
f. Movement and body concepts can be taught through playing games (e.g., Red Rover; Duck, Duck, Goose; and catch; and on playground equipment).	x	x	
g. Use consistent labels and terminology.	x	x	

TABLE 19.6 (*Continued*)

Strategies	Goal Level		
I. General Strategies	1	2	3
h. When students use a form of echolalia, confirm what they say to determine understanding.	x	x	
i. Use real activities to reinforce position concepts (e.g., "The juice is *next to* your hand," "Pick *up* the juice," and "Put the juice *on* the tray").	x	x	
j. Use current weather conditions to practice travel preparation concepts. Have students step outside before the lesson to determine the appropriate apparel (rain, winter, and sun).	x	x	
k. Teach concepts in the actual location where they are needed.	x	x	
l. Capitalize on "teachable moments."	x	x	x
m. A popular game is called Where Is It? The O&M specialist places a student in a stationary chair in the middle of four objects (e.g., a keyboard, Elmo, a large tactile doll, and a ball) positioned front, back, right, and left. The student describes how her movement changes the position of the objects in relation to her body.	x	x	x
n. Obstacle courses are a method for O&M specialists to isolate and develop both spatial and positional concepts. The course itself can be a series of mats, chairs, tumble bolsters, ladders, swings, trash cans, or any other available materials against a wall to go over, under, and around.	x	x	x
o. Take advantage of environmental features that change. When it rains, snows, and ices, use the cane to learn about the puddles and to deal with the puddles, snow, and so on.	x	x	x
p. Play Scavenger Hunt and hide objects at familiar landmarks. The student uses the Scavenger Hunt list to locate destinations.		x	x
q. When students use verbal shorthand, saying "this" or "it," ask them to use "the word."		x	x
r. The Freeze Game: As the student walks in the hallways or to an intersection, say, "Freeze." The student reaches out to locate the closest landmark. The student then points and identifies what should be in front of, behind, to the right of, and to the left of him.			x
s. Use simple models to develop abstract concepts. These models can be used to preview an activity or referred to at the actual training site.			x
t. Use a table to represent a block, have the student label streets, and add landmarks. Students can plan and alternate routes around the block table.			x
u. Use the long cane or folding cane as a tangible reference. The long cane can be held along the side of the student's body to emphasize parallel or moved in front of his body to show perpendicular. The folding cane can be used to create right angles and rectangles that suggest the traveler's relationship to a city block.			x

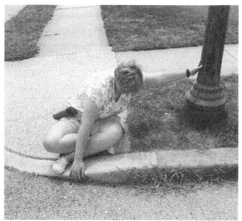

This student's hands-on tactile exploration of the street corner allows her to physically feel the relationship of her body to the curb and the lamppost in order to create a spatial understanding of her position.

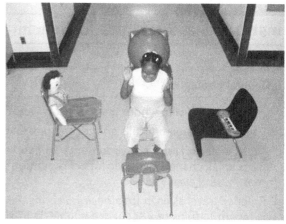

A student with visual and cognitive impairments playing the O&M game "Where is it?" to learn basic spatial concepts (left, right, back, and front).

skills (such as stranger danger and phoning for help) when separated from support personnel.

- *Level-3 generalization goal.* The ability to consistently demonstrate learned concepts and skills when traveling in familiar and unfamiliar environments.

Table 19.7 presents strategies for teaching generalization skills at all three levels.

Problem Solving

During travel, when a problem is encountered a solution is needed. It is not uncommon for a student who has visual and cognitive impairments to be unable to recognize when there is a problem or respond effectively to a problematic situation. Thus, *problem solving* is an important aspect of orientation and mobility instruction.

Instruction begins by developing a student's ability to recognize feelings of fear, pain, confusion, discomfort, or desire. The common types of problems the student will likely face are social skills, orientation, mobility, and personal needs; students need opportunities to experi-

ence and to learn strategies to resolve these problems.

1. *Social skills problems*: Stranger danger, personal space, and interpersonal skills.
2. *Orientation problems*: Recognize being lost, recover from being lost, and correct veer.
3. *Mobility problems*: Cane malfunction, accepting or rejecting assistance, and weather.
4. *Personal needs issues*: Student needs (sustenance, bathroom, and to end activity).

Problem-solving strategies are either general or specific. General strategies can be applied to problems in several domains regardless of content; specific strategies are applied only to particular situations. For students who have visual and cognitive impairments, strategies that are more situation specific may need to be the focus of instruction (Perla & O'Donnell, 2004).

- *Level-1 problem-solving goal.* To solve all problems by using rote problem-solving techniques to request assistance from a supervising adult.

Instructional Strategies for Teaching Generalization Skills

Strategies	Goal Level		
I. General Strategies	1	2	3
a. Alternate staff with whom the student travels on daily routes.	x		
b. Focus instruction on skills and techniques that are vital to safety.	x	x	x
c. Teach skills in familiar environments for extended periods of time, and track small changes. Provide lots of repetition and practice over months and even years.	x	x	x
d. Practice travel skills in unfamiliar locations. For example, the student is taught to think of a sequence of objects in an obstacle course numerically. In one direction, the obstacles are numbered 1, 2, and 3. The student is then taught to reverse the numbers when he returns in the other direction (3, 2, and 1). Employ the technique of numbering objects encountered on an obstacle course to landmarks encountered along a residential route and reversing the numbers upon return.	x	x	x
e. Use concepts and skills mastered in familiar settings across other settings.	x	x	x
f. Have students use "social scripts" in the community.		x	x
g. Vary the time when the student travels.		x	x
h. Apply the student's understanding of object relationships to landmarks on daily routes: for example, "Stand facing the chair," and "keep the wall on your left."		x	x
i. Have students use orientation and mobility (O&M) skills (room familiarization) in unfamiliar buildings.			x

- *Level-2 problem-solving goals.* To solve problems by asking for assistance from a supervising adult or following a prescribed and practiced sequence of problem-solving steps which target specific problem situations.

- *Level-3 problem-solving goal.* To apply general strategies to familiar problems and follow a prescribed list of steps in a variety of environments.

Table 19.8 presents strategies for teaching problem solving at all three levels.

Social Skills

Social skills enable the student who has visual and cognitive impairments to develop relation-ships and seek support needed for travel activities. These students often must be taught the basic elements of social interaction (Wolffe, 1998). The basic elements of social interactions needed for O&M are interpreting and using nonverbal communication, turn taking, initiating an interaction, maintaining an appropriate topic of discussion, and understanding or dealing with another person's perspective. O&M specialists along with the speech and language pathologist and other team members can create structured learning opportunities to support the development of the student's social skills and their use during functional travel activities.

TABLE 19.8

Strategies for Teaching Problem-Solving Skills

Strategies	Goal Level		
I. Solving Social Problems	1	2	3
a. Teach the student to face others when soliciting aid.	x	x	x
b. Teach the words *stranger* and *danger*.		x	x
c. Teach the student to confirm driver information before entering a vehicle and practice not entering if the wrong information is given.		x	x
d. Model appropriate and inappropriate positioning. Teach the student exceptions: for example, one is allowed to stand closer on the elevator and in crowds (on public transit).		x	x
e. Teach the student how to react when his cane inadvertently contacts someone.		x	x
f. Teach students where and when to make personal adjustments to clothing or body.		x	x
g. Through modeling and role-play, teach students how to match their body language and body positioning with the intent of their communication (frown and move away to avoid someone who persistently invades their personal space).			x
h. Ask a known staff person or a community worker to attempt to obtain personal information or money from the student.			x
i. Teach the student to seek immediate assistance from a community worker (e.g., a bus driver or store employee) if there is a physical safety concern.			x
II. Solving Orientation Problems	1	2	3
a. Teach the student to label the feeling when lost: for example, *butterflies*.		x	x
b. Teach the student solution scripts to recover from being lost (e.g., paratransit drops student off at the wrong location): (1) solicit aid; and (2) if no aid is available, call the emergency contact number on cell phone.		x	x
c. Use drop-off lesson within a familiar indoor environment to simulate getting lost.		x	x
d. Teach cell phone skills including the operation of the phone and pre-program emergency number or employ voice-activated dialing systems.			x
e. Use walkie-talkies for students who have difficulty with cell phones or students who benefit from more frequent contact.			x
III. Solving Mobility Problems	1	2	3
a. Students who are especially hard on their canes need to use rigid canes only.		x	

(continued on next page)

T A B L E   1 9 . 8   *(Continued)*

Strategies	Goal Level		
b. Teach the student a specific procedure to follow when his cane breaks (e.g., use a cell phone to seek assistance).			x
c. Teach the bus traveler to use alternative transportation in adverse weather.			x
IV. Personal Needs	1	2	3
a. Have students bring their symbol communication system to express their basic needs (help, bathroom, drink) on every orientation and mobility (O&M) lesson.	x		
b. Teach the student scripted questions to ask for something.	x	x	
c. Program augmentative communication devices to ask for help (devices can be clipped on the student's pocket, carried in a waist pack, or fastened to a neck strap).	x	x	
d. Establish a signal for getting help from a supervising adult.	x	x	x
e. Teach students to recognize their personal feelings of fear, pain, confusion, frustration, and desire by labeling emotions when they occur on lessons.	x	x	x
f. Teach coping strategies (students should put in earplugs when they hear construction).		x	
g. Teach students personal scripts.		x	
h. Create problem-solving opportunities around motivating tasks or environments: "How do you locate the music store and find your favorite CD?"		x	x

- *Level-1 social goal.* To respond to social routines during travel with intermittent to extensive prompts from support personnel.

- *Level-2 social goal.* To interact during travel in familiar indoor and outdoor environments and unfamiliar indoor and outdoor environments with intermittent to no prompts from support personnel.

- *Level-3 social goal.* To acquire and use social skills for the purpose of interacting while traveling in familiar and unfamiliar environments.

Table 19.9 presents strategies for teaching social skills at all three levels.

Orientation

Orientation can be as complex as using a compass and a topographical map to orienteer in the wilderness or as simple as walking a familiar route via rote memory. For students who are blind or visually impaired, "orientation is the knowledge of one's distance and direction relative to things observed or remembered in the surroundings and keeping track of these spatial relationships as they change during locomotion" (Blasch, Wiener, & Welsh, 1997). For the student who has visual and cognitive impairments, oriented travel is the use of landmarks, following specific routes, and soliciting assistance to travel as safely and independently as possible.

TABLE 19.9

Examples of General Strategies for Teaching Social Skills

Strategies	Goal Level		
I. General Strategies	1	2	3
a. Use games such as Simon Says, Red Light Green Light, Mother May I, and rolling a ball from one person to another to develop turn taking.	x	x	x
b. Use social stories to preview social expectations at the start of travel tasks.		x	
c. Use key word prompts to redirect students who perseverate on personal topics of interest.		x	
d. Set aside a specific time in the lesson to discuss the student's topic of interest.		x	
e. Isolate and role-play elements of social interactions during individual and group social activities.		x	x
f. Teach the student to use nonverbal communication (e.g., turn head to speaker, make eye contact, and use serious facial expression and head shaking) when declining unwanted assistance.		x	x
g. Teach students the reciprocal pattern of conversation (wait their turn before speaking at the service desk).		x	x
h. Provide and practice with specific scripts to begin, interrupt, or make conversation.		x	x
i. Teach the student to interpret facial and body language to identify and respond appropriately.			x
j. Play games to give the student the opportunity to interpret and practice gestures.			x
k. Give the student concrete examples of how his social interactions make other people feel.			x

Using landmarks enables students to name, identify, and associate place. Landmarks are unique and permanent, are perceived by one or more senses, and indicate a specific place. Learning routes using memory enables students to focus travel demands on completing essential routes as independently as possible. The ability to solicit aid supports travel by enabling the traveler to request help from known and unknown persons.

Students who have visual and cognitive impairments fall within a continuum of oriented travel ability; with some students requiring full physical assistance during travel and others demonstrating oriented travel in familiar and unfamiliar environments.

Renowned scholar in the field of autism spectrum disorders Lyndall Hendrickson wrote of her experiences with students who experienced an autism spectrum disorder and exhibited "savant-type memory for location" (Hendrickson, 1996). She wrote that Patrick, a student with an autism spectrum disorder and with delayed speech and intellectual ability, at 8 years old was able to retrace a complex route one week after his first visit.

Hendrickson remarked that he made his way through a "noisy, busy city which was not familiar to him ... [though] he could not talk, read or write." She continued, "I tried to confuse him on the third trip by altering the route across city blocks but his sense of direction was so strong that it still enabled him to reach the University" (1996, p. 8).

In the case of an *orientation savant*, the student who is visually impaired and has an autism spectrum disorder is able to remain oriented in simple and complex familiar and unfamiliar environments, but may have difficulty with concepts (e.g., use of numbering systems), exhibit communication delays, and exhibit unsafe travel practices (e.g., improper cane technique).

- *Level-1 orientation goal*. To attend to directions and intermittent to extensive prompts of support personnel when traveling.

- *Level-2 orientation goals*. To use landmarks, follow routes, and solicit assistance to safely and independently travel in familiar indoor and outdoor settings, and the ability to follow directions and prompts when traveling with support personnel to unfamiliar indoor and outdoor environments.

- *Level-3 orientation goal*. To use landmarks, follow routes, and solicit assistance to safely and independently travel in familiar and unfamiliar indoor and outdoor environments.

Table 19.10 presents strategies for teaching orientation skills at all three goal levels.

TABLE 19.10

Instructional Strategies for Teaching Orientation

Strategies	Goal Level		
I. General Strategies	1	2	3
a. Keep orientation lessons short to reflect a student's attention span or stamina.	x	x	x
b. Develop the ability of teachers, families, and paraprofessionals to reinforce basic orientation tasks (e.g., make right-angled turns when traveling with human guide).	x	x	x
c. Have students use a fixed-card system that is presequenced in a book format.		x	
d. Ask leading questions to prompt the student through stating the travel plan.		x	
e. Have students participate in making a route cue card system.		x	x
f. Students with low vision can create and use a sequential picture book of the landmarks encountered along a route.		x	x
g. Students who are blind can create and use an audio recorder or "key word" booklets to sequence landmarks.		x	x
h. Help students develop "travel plans" prior to executing the route.		x	x
i. Ask student to state directions prior to traveling route.		x	x
j. The orientation and mobility (O&M) specialist and student sing a "route song" before traveling. A route song is simply putting the steps of the route to a familiar tune to aid memory.		x	x

(continued on next page)

TABLE 19.10 (Continued)

Strategies	Goal Level		
k. Have students sequence their "card" system prior to executing each route.			x
l. Use the student's card system (auditory, visual, or tactile cards) to promote memory. For practice, (1) shuffle the cards and have the student sequence them, (2) take out a card and have the student identify what step of the route is missing, and (3) use the cards to plan the reverse route or alternate routes.			x
m. Have the student use a notebook system with scripts, maps, and directions.			x
n. Give students orientation homework (meet me at the snack bar after school).			x
II. Landmarks	1	2	3
a. Create accessible landmarks: affix pictures or other object cues at consistent, safe locations on doorways.	x	x	
b. When students have limited communication skills, observe what they pay attention to along a route. The student may consistently stop and rub a specific bump on the wall or react to a light in the ceiling. Attempt to have the student name this location and incorporate it into route-planning lessons.		x	
c. Teach students to use landmarks that are meaningful to them.	x	x	x
d. Identify types of sensory stimuli the student attends to (e.g., overhead heating and air conditioning vent, red fire door, or a brightly lit or low-lit area).	x	x	x
e. Teach students to attend to the meaning of, and response to specific, existing landmarks and information points; loud chatter in the cafeteria during mealtimes, or the sound of automatic doors at the grocery store are locations toward which they can travel.	x	x	x
f. Give students the opportunity to explore various "echo" sounds such as in a gym, hallway, or stairwell, and ask students to name that location.	x	x	x
g. Challenge students to use the names of hallways and buildings within their travel environments. Initially students can name locations in a manner that is meaningful to them such as the "echo hallway" or the "quiet hallway," and later begin incorporating standardized labels within a building.		x	x
h. The Spin Game: the student identifies a location and is then spun by the O&M specialist; the student has to reorient.			x
III. Routes	1	2	3
a. Assign a "start point" and "destination" to each route. The start location serves as a reference point and needs to be stationary/permanent and connected to the destination. Actual location names are preferred over "made up" names.	x	x	x

(continued on next page)

TABLE 19.10 (Continued)			
Strategies		**Goal Level**	
b. Teach student to locate start point landmark at the beginning and end of route lesson.	x	x	x
c. Be consistent when communicating route information. Name landmarks, hallways, buildings, and streets within travel environments and consistently use those names.	x	x	x
d. A route "to" a destination needs to be taught separately from the "return" trip.	x	x	x
e. Teach route one step at a time until mastered when using reverse chaining technique.		x	
f. Teach routes to destinations that motivate the student.		x	x
g. Residential block, use a consistent start location until the student has oriented to the 4 sides of the block and has developed a basic understanding of the block concept.		x	x
h. When initially teaching new building, begin with the shortest route (desk to front door). Each successive route can add on to that route (desk to bathroom; desk to gym).		x	x
i. Teach route two or three steps at a time when using forward chaining technique.			x
j. Use graphic materials (e.g., APH Picture Maker: Wheatley Tactile Diagramming Kit and light box, or homemade objects) to create route diagrams.			x
IV. Soliciting Assistance	**1**	**2**	**3**
a. Teach the student to use a script to solicit aid.		x	x
b. Have students locate destinations by seeking aid.			x
c. Teach places to go to obtain aid.			x
d. Provide practice soliciting aid en route: known and unknown people/places.			x
e. Provide experiences with incorrect directions, partial information, or unfriendly assistance to teach correct response.			x

Mobility Skills

This mobility skills section presents strategies for teaching the unique content that is the M in O&M. Mobility skills encompass four areas: human guide, self-protection, use of adaptive mobility devices and cane skills, and outdoor travel. The instructional considerations for teaching students who have visual and cognitive impairments described in this chapter are effective strategies for

teaching them select mobility skills. Instructional emphasis is on the ability to design a program that meets the most pressing travel needs of the student with techniques that will provide long-term mobility solutions.

The challenge to every O&M specialist who works with students who have visual and cognitive impairments is to be strict when evaluating a student's mobility skill performance. *Performance* needs to meet both the criteria for mastery and consistency needed in the particular skill to benefit from employing it. *Mastery* is the level at which the student can demonstrate a skill precisely as instructed. *Consistency* is the frequency with which the student is able to perform a skill at mastery level when it is needed on the travel route.

O&M specialists are integral in clearing students to cross streets independently or restricting independent outdoor travel for the purpose of safety. The restrictions on outdoor travel may include limiting street crossing to specific intersections or requiring that the student always travel accompanied. When students are restricted in some way from independent outdoor travel, then mobility goals must include the role support personnel will have in supporting interdependent completion of mobility tasks.

The same standard can be applied to cane coverage. When a student who has visual and cognitive impairments does not demonstrate an appropriate level of mastery or consistency with arc width or ability to stop at a surface level change, independent travel will not be recommended; instead, O&M specialists can work toward integrating the student's support systems into his long-range travel goals. O&M lessons can now focus on increasing the predictability of a student while traveling and the distance the student can walk apart from his support personnel.

- *Level-1 mobility goal.* To demonstrate mobility skills with directions and intermittent to extensive prompts from support personnel.

- *Level-2 mobility goals.* The student will demonstrate mobility skills safely, efficiently, and consistently in familiar indoor and outdoor settings with minimal to no supports and the ability to travel at a short distance from formal supports when traveling with support personnel to unfamiliar indoor and outdoor environments.

- *Level-3 mobility goal.* The student will demonstrate mobility skills safely, efficiently, and

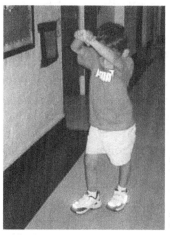

A student with cognitive impairments using the two-handed upper hand and forearm protective technique, a basic self-protective mobility skill.

consistently across familiar and unfamiliar environments with minimal to no supports.

Table 19.11 presents strategies for teaching mobility skills at all three goal levels.

SUMMARY

Developing an appropriate program in O&M for students who have visual and cognitive impairments requires, first and foremost, functional knowledge of the impact the combination of a visual impairment and cognitive impairment has on a student's ability to acquire travel skills incidentally. Second, it requires the knowledge of general program strategies that enable quality O&M instruction. Third, it requires knowledge of skill areas that are needed to acquire travel skills through structured instruction.

The population of students who have visual and cognitive impairments is diverse. This diversity led to the organizational framework of this chapter. Within each classification of cognitive impairment there are clear definitions

TABLE 19.11

Instructional Strategies for Teaching Mobility Skills

Strategies	Goal Level		
I. General Strategies	1	2	3
a. Initially, accept and praise all efforts toward demonstration of the skill.	x	x	
b. Introduce new mobility techniques employing prompts and methods of full and partial participation to prompt positioning and motor patterning.	x	x	
c. The instructor may need to position herself in front of the student and use a combination of voice and physical prompts to entice the student to move.	x	x	
II. Working with a Physical Therapist (PT) or Occupational Therapist (OT)	1	2	3
a. Make use of gross motor strategies used by PTs when teaching skills that require balance and coordination (stairs, uneven surfaces).	x		
b. Make use of PT suggestions and equipment such as the use of bolsters to promote hip shift and ladders to promote alternating hand and leg movements.	x		
c. Make use of PT physical cueing for stairs and surface changes.	x		
d. Make use of OT suggestions to adapt the adaptive mobility device (AMD) or cane grip, modify hand position and cane grasp, and promote hand strength and wrist movement.	x	x	x
III. Games	1	2	3
a. Use obstacle courses to teach mobility skills.	x	x	x
b. Use Shake Em Up game to practice grip as a lesson warm-up. (1) the orientation and mobility (O&M) specialist yells, "Shake em up"; (2) student switches hands with the cane and shakes his hands; (3) someone yells, "Stop"; (4) the student quickly reestablishes grip; and (5) review the grip script (pointer finger flat, thumb on top, fingers curled, and arm in front).		x	x
IV. Basic Skills	1	2	3
a. Student's physical stamina may limit the amount of time he can maintain a static position; try two-handed upper-hand and forearm technique.	x		
b. Teach self-protective techniques while seated on floor or in chair.	x		
c. Begin trailing using human guide while trailing.	x		
d. Place tactile markers on trailing surface to help the student maintain contact.	x		
e. Use a tactile prompt on the student's fingers (feather duster) as he trails to promote forward movement and arm extension.	x		
f. Affix a tactile marker at specific square-off points.	x	x	
g. Physically assist student into position.	x	x	

(continued on next page)

Strategies	Goal Level		
h. A student may prefer to grasp an arm that is covered with a shirt.	x		
i. Student can sit on the floor when locating dropped objects.	x		
j. Add weight (small beanbag) to the student's forearm to increase the proprioceptive awareness needed to refine arm placement.		x	
k. When negotiating narrow passageways, the student places a free hand on the guide's shoulder and walks in single file.		x	
V. Adaptive Mobility Device (AMD) and Cane Skills	1	2	3
a. Use a durable rigid cane for instruction.	x		
b. Change the cane tip if the student perseverates on it.	x		
c. A student may need to spend seconds or minutes daily touching the cane grip to build tolerance before holding it.	x		
d. A student who throws his cane may be communicating a desire to end the lesson. Have the student search, locate, and pick up the cane. Redirect the student to continue using the cane for a short distance. Provide the student with a "script" to express "finished." Reinforce the appropriate request and shift the lesson focus.	x		
e. Provide hand-over-hand assistance to establish and maintain grip.	x	x	
f. To teach grip, attach small tactile markers at the hand location on the AMD or cane grip (e.g., velcro, moleskin, or tape on a large paper clip).	x	x	
g. Remove rubber cane grip and replace with a non-aversive texture if needed.	x	x	
h. Make up songs to develop the coordinated movement of the long cane.	x	x	
i. To narrow and direct erratic arc width, have the student walk along the wall while the O&M specialist uses another cane to give boundary to opposite side.	x	x	
j. To maintain cane tip on the ground add weight (insert and stabilize BBs in the shaft).	x	x	
k. Teach the student to store cane in the same location at school, at work, at home, in the car, and on public transit.		x	x
l. Teach the student skills for locating and picking up a dropped cane.	x	x	x
m. Teach only two cane skills: constant contact touch technique (CCTT), and trailing.	x	x	x
n. Have the student do cane movement "warm-ups" before the lesson while sitting in a chair or standing against a wall.	x	x	x
VI. Street Crossing	1	2	3
a. Before teaching street-crossing techniques, the student needs to demonstrate consistent response to a "stop" prompt within one step.		x	x
b. Teach the student each specific street-crossing element for mastery (e.g., a series of lessons focusing only on alignment techniques).		x	x

(continued on next page)

TABLE 19.11 *(Continued)*

Strategies	Goal Level		
c. Use an auditory sound source on the opposite curb to serve as a beacon for the student's alignment (e.g., clicker, remote door chime, and hand clapping).		x	x
d. Use the cane as a physical reference to check body alignment: "nose, waist and toes in one straight line."		x	x
e. Teach crossing scripts: for example, (1) stop at corner, (2) align, (3) listen for cars, (4) last look left, (5) no cars and all quiet, and (6) cross.		x	
f. Isolate the first footstep off the curb, by placing a target (6"×6" piece of carpet) on the street where the student's first step needs to land.			x
g. Develop routes that contain similar intersections where the student can cross multiple times with the same rules.			x
h. For auditory students, teach counterclockwise (CCW) street crossings until the student demonstrates success, and then introduce clockwise (CW) crossings.			x
i. For visual students, teach CW street crossings until the student demonstrates success, and then introduce CCW crossings.			x
j. Some students can cross secondary streets only at traffic light–controlled intersections, which may affect the route design.			x
k. Teach recognizing when to interact with others or seek aid to cross a street.			x
l. Teach and practice gaining aid by the use of social scripts to (1) ask a passerby to help cross the street, and (2) enter a nearby business establishment and ask for help to cross.			x
m. Teach procedure for getting aid: (1) prearrange aid at a business, and (2) use a "help" signal to request aid from the job coach.			x
VII. Vehicle Transit	1	2	3
a. Provide opportunities to practice in cars (entering and exiting, seat belts, and storing the cane).	x	x	
b. Teach students concepts of personal space, transit scripts, and stranger awareness.		x	x
c. Use checklists and scripts to assist the student in completing routine taxi, carpool, fixed-line, and paratransit travel tasks.		x	x
d. Preview the vehicle and transportation system the student will be using (e.g., taxi, paratransit, bus, train, or subway). Identify procedural and environmental triggers that may challenge the student. For example, a student may need to be desensitized to the sound of bus air brakes.		x	x
e. Teach the use of memory devices to obtain and manage route information such as a recorded phone conversation: a phone-recording device (such as Telephone Pick Up, available from Radio Shack), digital recorder, loop tape, direction book, and picture book.		x	x

and there are gradations of involvement. Thus, the skill area sections offer small units of learning activities for 10 skills that attempt to respond to those gradations in an organized manner. This chapter serves to equip O&M specialists with the understanding of how important it is to be prepared before the student walks in the door, to measure outcomes, and to work toward clearly defined goals.

There is still a need for scientific study of the impact that these suggested O&M strategies have on the long-term travel abilities of students who have visual and cognitive impairments. The 10 general program strategies (teamwork, communication, planning and record keeping, time considerations, task analysis, sequenced instruction, environment, motivation, prompting, and choice making) and 10 skill areas (attention, sensory integration, behavior, memory, concept development, generalization, problem solving, social skills, orientation, and mobility) are well-established approaches for working with the student who has visual and cognitive disabilities that will continue to prove useful well into the future.

IMPLICATIONS FOR O&M PRACTICE

1. According to the 27th Annual Report to Congress (2005), specific learning disabilities, mental retardation, emotional disturbance, autism spectrum disorder, developmental delay, and traumatic brain injury account for 71 percent of students age 6 to 21 served under IDEA. The learning disability category represents half of all students served, with mental retardation (10.6 percent), emotional disturbance (8.2 percent) autism spectrum disorder (1.4 percent), developmental delay (0.5 percent), and traumatic brain injury (0.3 percent) making up the remaining total (U.S. Department of Education, 2002).

2. While certain aspects of independent travel require higher-order thinking and reasoning skills, it is also true that functional travel skills are learned via sensorimotor domains, knowledge from sensory input or motor actions and affective domains, and knowledge from emotional input or interactions. Both sensorimotor and affective experiences are believed to make important contributions to one's ability to travel (Long & Hill, 1997).

3. It has been shown that there is no fixed period of time after which brain plasticity or the ability for the brain to change is blocked or lost. It is now understood that with new learning comes new connections within the brain throughout one's lifetime (Barkovich, 2005; Goldberg, 2001).

4. Task analysis, paired with either forward or backward chaining, is a useful technique for teaching routes.

5. The critical skills model of instruction asks the instructor to prioritize and select the most critical skill to teach first, then select the essential parts of the skill to be taught and the location where it is most needed (Fazzi & Petersmeyer, 2001).

6. In students with visual and cognitive disabilities, building trust and rapport may take several weeks or even months. O&M specialists begin by taking part in activities, spending time, and relating to the student and support personnel in non-O&M-related capacities and then introducing O&M activities within those familiar routines prior to attempting to remove the student from the classroom.

7. During the O&M lesson allow the student to make choices, and make sure those choices can be carried out.

8. Behavioral theorists suggest that aggressive and interfering behaviors may be attempts by the student to communicate about an

environment, person, or activity (van Dijk, 2006).

9. It is not uncommon for a student who has visual and cognitive disabilities to demonstrate particular concepts and skills at a higher level than their overall abilities and functional performance would suggest.

10. Through systematic instruction, the O&M instructor can develop the student's ability to apply environmental concepts (hallway layout, intersection shapes), techniques (trailing, cane skills, street crossing strategies), and related O&M skills (stranger danger, phone usage, money skills) across travel settings.

LEARNING ACTIVITIES

1. Observe O&M specialists teaching indoor and outdoor travel skills to students who have visual and cognitive impairments.

2. Read current literature, attend conferences and lecture series to stay aware of new technologies and insights into working with students who have visual and cognitive impairments.

3. Interview adults who have cognitive impairments about their experiences.

4. Familiarize yourself with a student's tactile communication system. Observe how it is used during the day and across settings.

5. Evaluate your daily routes. How often do you travel the same way to the same location at the same time and in the same manner? What is predictable in that route? Have you ever encountered an unexpected detour on a familiar route that required the ability to read or comprehend verbal directions to complete? Explore the implications of that occurrence on students who have visual and cognitive impairments who were cleared to travel independently on one specific daily route.

Teaching Orientation and Mobility to Students with Cortical Visual Impairment

Christine Roman-Lantzy

LEARNING QUESTIONS

- Why is cortical visual impairment (CVI) the leading cause of visual impairment in children in developed nations?

- How are the causes of CVI different from the causes of ocular visual impairments?

- What are the unique visual and behavioral characteristics of individuals with CVI that distinguish CVI from ocular visual impairments?

- What is the purpose of the CVI Range?

- How can results of the CVI Range and use of the CVI Orientation and Mobility Resolution Chart be used to guide O&M lesson planning?

- Why is it critical to use the principles of CVI to guide O&M instruction?

This chapter begins with short summaries of the O&M experiences of three students. All three of these students experience visual difficulties because of cortical visual impairment (CVI). They all have three elements that indicate this diagnosis: (1) an eye exam that is either normal or cannot explain the degree of diminished functional vision, (2) a history of a significant congenital or acquired brain injury or neurologic disorder, and (3) the presence of the unique visual behaviors associated with CVI. Some of these behaviors include attraction to specific colors, difficulties with visual fields, difficulties with visually complex arrays, the inability to visually attend to novel targets, and difficulties with viewing targets at a distance. Although the visual behaviors observed in Sally, Miles, and Stan may seem confusing, these behaviors are in fact common in infants, children, and adolescents who are diagnosed with CVI. The challenge for teachers of students with visual impairments and O&M specialists is to become familiar with the principles and methods for teaching students who have visual impairment because of injury to the visual pathways and visual processing centers of the brain. Students who have CVI have needs that are uniquely distinct from students who have ocular forms of visual impairment. The approach offered in this chapter is based on these unique concepts intended to help students with CVI improve their vision by addressing the CVI visual and behavioral characteristics and then applying these principles to traditional O&M instruction

(Roman-Lantzy, 2007). An awareness of important CVI-related behaviors is the key to providing instruction for orientation in space and safe, efficient travel.

Sally is a 6-year-old student who was referred for an O&M evaluation. She is in a self-contained special education classroom for students who have significant and multiple disabilities. Sally spends much of her day staring at overhead lights or the ceiling fan. Sally can walk but prefers to move through her classroom by crawling or scooting on her behind. When she does walk independently, she frequently falls over toys or furnishings in the room. Sally does not look into the faces of the children or adults in the room and she only seems to look consistently at the few red objects sent from home by her mother. Sally has esotropia in her right eye but has an otherwise normal eye exam. Her medical records include a history of 25-week gestation prematurity and periventricular leukomalacia.

––––––––

Miles has received services from a teacher of the visually impaired and an O&M specialist since his return to third grade after a near drowning accident. According to his doctors, Miles has made a remarkable recovery and has only one residual difficulty, CVI. He has a normal eye exam but struggles with both near and distance tasks throughout the school day. The teacher finds some of Miles's behaviors quite confusing. He is able to read familiar words when they are presented in isolation but cannot recognize the same words when they appear in a phrase or sentence. Miles is unable to describe what he sees in illustrations although he can recount the events of a story in precise detail. Miles moves around the classroom without difficulty but he becomes fearful on the playground preferring to remain close to the adults who monitor during recess. He can locate a rolling yellow ball during gym class but cannot find his spoon

when it falls on the floor of the cafeteria during lunchtime.

––––––––

Stan has spastic quadriplegia, expressive language difficulties, and CVI as a result of meningitis that occurred in infancy. His cognitive skills seem typical of his classmates, average ninth graders, and Stan has been successful learning to use technology to help him access information and to complete assignments. Stan recently learned to operate a power wheelchair although the teachers in Stan's high school have concerns regarding his safety. Stan has never worn glasses but the teachers have trouble understanding how this is possible. Stan cannot identify people or features of the environment at distances beyond 10 feet. Stan does not recognize steps or other drop-offs, and he regularly runs into other students or teachers with his chair in the busy corridors.

The focus of this chapter is on helping O&M specialists understand how best to help students as varied as these three learn how to travel through their environments as independently as possible.

DEFINING CORTICAL VISUAL IMPAIRMENT

Visual impairment caused by injury or structural differences in the brain is not a new phenomenon. As early as 329 B.C., Alexander the Great suffered a transient form of blindness after being injured in the head by a stone from a catapult during the siege of Cyropolis (Lascaratos, 1998). Since the 1950s an unexpected and generally short-term form of vision loss in individuals who have had heart attacks or cardiac surgery has been identified as cortical blindness. Cortical blindness is a phenomenon caused by lack of oxygen to the brain. And although it has been recorded in humans for thousands of years, it was rarely diagnosed in children until the 1980s.

Prior to 1980, few infants or children who had significant brain injury survived. However, as medical technology and expertise improved, infants and children with neurological problems who once rarely survived began surviving in greater numbers. In 1974 neonatology became a subspecialty in the field of pediatrics and with medical advances came a marked progression in infant survival rates. According to Woodrum (1998), 90 percent of infants weighing 900–999 grams at birth, and at 26–27 weeks gestation survived but in 1970 there was a less than 10 percent survival rate of infants with the same birth weight and gestational age. However, with increased survivability came an increased number of long-term disabilities, including CVI.

Cortical visual impairment (CVI) is a term used to describe a visual impairment that is due to damage to the visual pathways and visual processing centers of the brain (Jan, Groenveld, Skynda, & Hoyt , 1987). Once known as cortical blindness, CVI is a diagnosis used with both children and adults. Although the term *cortical visual impairment* will be used in this chapter, it is important to recognize that other terms are also used to describe visual impairment due to brain injury or structural abnormalities in the brain. Cortical visual impairment is most commonly used in North America but cerebral or neurological visual impairment are more commonly applied in Europe (Dutton, personal communication, 2006; Jan, 2006). Attempts are being made to clarify the terminology used to describe brain-related visual impairment and to distinguish the important differences between students who have visual processing disorders often associated with learning disabilities from those who have visual impairment (see Chapter 19).

Dr. James Jan (2003) offers medical and educational definitions of CVI. The medical definition describes CVI as follows: "Bilaterally diminished visual acuity caused by damage to the occipital lobes and or to the geniculostriate visual pathway. CVI is almost invariably associated with an inefficient, disturbed visual sense because of the widespread brain disturbance." The educational definition offered by Dr. Jan is that "CVI is a neurological disorder which results in unique visual responses to people, to educational materials, and to the environment. When students with these visual/behavioral characteristics are shown to have a loss of acuity or judged by their performance to be visually impaired, they are considered to have CVI." The effect of CVI can be mild, moderate, or severe, and it can occur in students who have diverse levels of cognitive and motor functioning. CVI can occur as a congenital condition, or it can occur in an infant, child, adolescent, or adult as a result of neurological trauma.

One of the major differences between cortical and ocular forms of visual impairment is that CVI, because it is caused by injury or structural differences in the brain, has the potential to improve or, in some cases, even resolve.

MEDICAL CAUSES OF CVI

Professionals who work with individuals who have ocular forms of visual impairment are obligated to become familiar with the eye conditions that cause visual problems. The conditions that cause CVI are not problems that occur in the eye; they are brain problems. O&M professionals are similarly obligated to be knowledgeable about both eye and brain conditions that may result in visual impairment.

The diagnosis of CVI is indicated by the occurrence of three factors: (1) a typical eye exam (or an ocular condition that cannot account for the significant loss of vision), (2) the presence of an atypical neurological condition, and (3) the presence of a unique combination of visual and behavioral characteristics. It is critical that O&M specialists become familiar with the medical causes of CVI. The medical conditions associated with CVI include both congenital and acquired causes. Congenital conditions are those that occur before or around the time of birth. Acquired causes include trauma or medical problems that lead to brain damage that occur after the perinatal period. Whether congenital or acquired, CVI is caused by injury or damage to the visual centers of the brain (Jan & Groenveld, 1993). While some individuals with CVI may have coexisting ocular disorders, in general the structures of the eyes are normal or the eye disorder cannot explain the significant loss of visual function (Skoczenski & Good, 2004). The medical causes that represent conditions commonly associated with CVI are asphyxia, perinatal hypoxia-ischemic encephalopathy, cerebral vascular accident, intraventricular hemorrhage, periventricular leukomalacia, central nervous system infection, structural abnormalities, and trauma (Huo, Burden, Hoyt, & Good, 1999; Jan & Groenveld, 1993; Teplin, 1995).

Asphyxia

Asphyxia occurs when the brain is deprived of oxygen and abnormal levels of carbon dioxide and acid are present. If this condition persists, brain cells can die and disabilities such as cerebral palsy, seizures, hearing loss, and CVI can occur (Rivkin, 1997).

Hypoxia-Ischemic Encephalopathy

Hypoxia-ischemic encephalopathy (HIE) is a term used to describe the clinical condition that occurs after reduced oxygen or blood flow to the brain. HIE is distinct from asphyxia because of the reduced blood flow to the brain. Even though HIE frequently results from asphyxia, not all individuals who experience reduced oxygen to the brain will also have reduced blood flow to the brain. Like asphyxia, the more severe forms of HIE result in long-term disability, including CVI.

Perinatal Cerebral Vascular Accident

Perinatal cerebral vascular accident (CVA) or infant stroke is generally a condition that occurs in full-term infants; it is rarely associated with prematurity (de Vries, Dubowitz, Dubowitz, & Pennock, 1990). The causes of cerebral vascular accident in infants are unclear (Rivkin, 1997). This type of brain bleed occurs when blood vessels rupture primarily in the left hemisphere. The extent of damage depends on the degree and location of the bleed. Infant stroke may result in cerebral palsy, developmental delay, and visual impairment (Volpe, 1987).

Intraventricular Hemorrhage

The type of brain bleed associated with prematurity is intraventricular hemorrhage (IVH). IVH occurs in premature infants who are born at the earliest gestational age and of the lowest birth weights (Ment, Scott, & Ehrenkranz, 1987). Severity of IVH is classified by a grading system ranging from least severe (Grade I) to most severe (Grade IV). In Grade I and II IVH, a small amount of blood occurs either outside or inside the lateral ventricles but without associated long-term damage to the brain. Grade III and IV bleeds result in larger amounts of blood leaking into the ventricles or engulfing brain tissue outside the ventricle. These more significant bleeds are associated with an increased risk of cerebral palsy or CVI (Perlman, 2001; Volpe, 1997).

Periventricular Leukomalacia

Periventricular leukomalacia (PVL) is destruction of white matter in particular areas of the brain near the ventricles as a result of decreased blood flow in an especially vulnerable area of the brain (Vaucher, 1988). PVL is associated with spastic diplegia and often involves both optic and acoustic radiations resulting in central vision and hearing impairment (Volpe, 1997). Of all the brain conditions associated with CVI, PVL is the most common (Perlman, 2001).

Central Nervous System Infections

Congenital and acquired infections also place an infant or child at risk of CVI (Jan & Groenveld, 1993). Williamson & Demmler (1992) state that infections affect at least 40,000 newborns each year, and some of these infections have long-term effects in the visual system. Both bacterial and viral infections place the infant or child at risk. Two infectious conditions associated with CVI are meningitis and cytomegalic inclusion disease (CMV).

Structural Abnormalities

A number of structural malformations of the brain can result in CVI. Interruptions to the development of the structures of the brain may result in developmental and sensory difficulties. Although some structural differences occur because of chromosome abnormalities or specific syndromes (Volpe, 1987), other structural problems occur without obvious cause (Nickel, 1992). Examples of structural brain malformations include congenital hydrocephalus, microcephaly, agensis of the corpus collosum, and lissencephaly (smooth brain syndrome).

Trauma

Acquired causes of CVI occur because of trauma to the brain after the perinatal period (Huo et al., 1999). This type of trauma may result from a number of conditions including near sudden infant death syndrome (SIDS), near drowning, shaken baby syndrome, auto accidents, and brain tumors. In all cases, trauma may result in injury to the visual pathways or visual-processing centers of the brain and, therefore, may result in CVI (Arditi, 2000).

VISUAL AND BEHAVIORAL CHARACTERISTICS OF INDIVIDUALS WITH CVI

The diagnosis of CVI is associated with a unique set of visual and behavioral characteristics typically exhibited by individuals with this condition (Jan & Groenveld, 1993). These characteristics, together with a history of neurological problems and an eye exam that is either normal or cannot explain the degree of vision loss, are used as a formula that guides physicians, educators, and O&M specialists in diagnosis and intervention. These characteristic include color preference, attraction to movement, visual field preferences, difficulties with visual complexity, atypical visual reflex responses, difficulties with visual novelty, atypical distance viewing, light-gazing behaviors, visual latency, and atypical visual motor patterns.

Color Preference

Individuals with CVI often have a preferential response to targets of a particular color (Jan & Groenveld, 1993). The most common color preferences are red or yellow but any color could potentially be the "favorite." Parents are often reliable reporters of their child's color preference (Roman, 1996) and some individuals will be able to report this information for themselves. The CVI trait of color preference should not be confused with someone declaring pink as their favorite color because they like to wear pink and own a number of pink items. The CVI characteristic is one in which the individual with CVI may respond only to red targets. Targets of all other colors may be ignored. The preferred color serves as a sort of visual "anchor," drawing the individual's visual attention to objects or materials of that particular color. It is unclear exactly how color preference develops in individuals with CVI; it may be related to experience or to some other phenomenon. Regardless of the reason, it is important for O&M specialists to identify the student's preferred color and use it to highlight visual targets.

Attraction to Movement

The CVI characteristic of attraction to movement is one in which the individual is visually attracted to targets that have the physical properties of movement or that have shiny or reflective surfaces, thus simulating movement. The attraction is so strong that the individual may only notice things that move and ignore other, nonmoving targets. This has a particularly important effect on orientation and mobility. The O&M specialist can use movement features of environments to facilitate orientation or even mobility but it is critical to remember that the individual with CVI may notice *only* the moving elements and disregard the stationary ones, as in the following example.

> A gentleman who has CVI because of a head injury uses a cane when in unfamiliar or congested areas and uses movement information points to guide his route. He believed he could safely jog as long as he ran along the side of the road with the flow of traffic. Clearly he wasn't safe. One day there was a parked car on the side of the road that he did not perceive at all until he ran directly into it, breaking his leg in several places. This same individual is able to work out using a punching bag without missing contact with the bag, but he is unable to locate or identify common stationary objects that are placed on a table in front of him.

Visual Field Preferences

Jan and Groenveld (1993) state that visual field problems are almost always present in individuals with CVI. These field differences exist in in-

dividuals who may have normal structures of the eye and whose visual impairment is caused by injury to the visual pathways or processing areas of the brain. Dutton (2001) describes lower field losses to be a common occurrence with CVI. Lateral peripheral function appears to be most intact, and this finding may help explain the strong attraction to moving or reflective targets. Visual field problems are especially significant in an individual's ability to become oriented and to move safely in an environment. Drop-offs, unexpected obstacles in peripheral fields, and moving targets may all become potential threats to the safety of individuals who have CVI. An O&M specialist will need to carefully assess field function and determine whether a cane or other mobility device is indicated. (See also Geruschat & Smith, Chapter 3; and Volume 1, Chapter 3.)

Difficulties with Visual Complexity

Difficulties with visual complexity is the CVI characteristic in which individuals have difficulty "sorting" or locating a symbol or object when it is surrounded by other targets. This phenomenon occurs in the three-dimensional world as well as with two-dimensional materials. There are three specific ways in which difficulties with complexity interfere with visual functioning. The first consideration is the complexity of the target. Highly patterned objects may be ignored while those made of a single and especially the preferred color will be more likely to elicit visual attention. Second, it is important to consider the visual array. Single targets presented against a plain background are more easily located whereas objects placed against a patterned or cluttered background may fail to be located. For many individuals who have CVI, busy environments or visually cluttered arrays may be perceived as "hidden picture" displays in which individual objects become "lost" in the background of other objects or images. O&M specialists need to be alert to the possibility that landmarks identified in isolation or in low complexity settings may not be recognized if the visual conditions of the environment change or if the landmark or information point occurs in a visually complex or cluttered area. For example, if a student is being oriented to a school during the summer months when hallways are devoid of decorations, the student may have little difficulty locating the drinking fountain that serves as a landmark that helps locate the restroom. However, the same landmark may be far more difficult to identify when the school year starts and teachers have filled the hallways with back-to-school decorations. It is critical to remember that variation in visual ability may be more a function of changes in the environment than changes in the visual capacity of the student who has CVI.

The third component of the CVI characteristic of complexity refers to the degree of complexity of the sensory environment. Although many students who don't have CVI benefit from instruction presented with multisensory inputs, the student with CVI is generally less able to use vision when there is competition from other sensory stimuli such as sounds, environmental textures, and smells. Certain environments may therefore pose a great challenge for the student with CVI. The school lunchroom and the playground are settings in which there are numerous visual, auditory, and even tactual inputs occurring simultaneously. Under these conditions the student who has CVI may be unable to process the visual information in the presence of the other stimuli. The student may require human guide assistance, or may use a cane or other mobility device to be safe in these highly complex settings.

Atypical Visual Reflex Responses

There are two visual reflexes that may be atypical in students who have CVI even when they have a normal eye exam. The first is the visual blink reflex in which an individual blinks at the moment they are touched between their eyes. This is a reflex that is present from birth (Volpe, 1987) and is a sign of intact visual and neurological systems. Many children with CVI do not blink when touched on the bridge of the nose. The other reflex that is often atypical in students with CVI is the visual threat reflex. This reflex causes an individual to blink in anticipation of an incoming target moving toward the face. It is tested by swiftly moving an open hand toward the face on midline. This reflex is dependent on the development of binocular fusion and therefore is tested after 6 months of age. Students with CVI may fail to blink or have a delayed or latent blink. The main impact of this characteristic for O&M specialists is that students with CVI may not be able to protect themselves from objects moving quickly toward their faces. A moving swing on the playground and a propelled ball are examples of possible threats to a student who has atypical visual reflex responses.

Difficulties with Visual Novelty

The visual system is highly sensitive to information that is unfamiliar. In fact, the more novel the target, the more quickly the brain responds to examine it (Hubel, 1995). Forced-choice preferential-looking tests of visual acuity are based on the novelty principle. Preferential looking assumes that when a typically developing infant is presented with both a gray pattern and a striped pattern, the infant will look first and for the longest time at the striped, more visually discrepant or novel pattern. Students with CVI generally have a counterintuitive response to novelty. They often avoid looking at new targets, looking primarily only at things previously viewed. Preferred objects may be those items that have been consistently present and that meet other CVI characteristic criteria of simplicity, preferred color, or movement. This occurrence has major implications for O&M. The student with CVI who has difficulty recognizing novel features of the environment is at significant risk and may not be able to travel independently in new places. It is important for the O&M specialist to select landmarks that are either familiar or that share characteristics of color and complexity with the previously used landmarks.

Atypical Distance Viewing

The CVI characteristic of difficulties with distance viewing is especially important in consideration of O&M. Students with CVI often bring targets very close to their faces or move within inches of a target to examine it. This behavior may be anticipated in individuals who have ocular forms of visual impairment but it seems confusing to observe this close viewing behavior in students who have a normal or near-normal eye exam. Distance viewing difficulties are linked to the CVI characteristic of complexity. Reducing the distance between the target and the individual can reduce complexity by lessening the amount of background information the student sees and thus making a target more visually accessible. O&M specialists will need to evaluate the student's distance vision abilities and the amount of complexity in specific environments in order to determine whether the student is able to travel safely and independently. It is important to acknowledge that some individuals who have CVI may be able to detect targets at greater distances when the environment is simple or without many visual elements of form, color, or movement. The more complex a setting, the closer the individual will need to be in order to identify the salient feature of a target, information point, or landmark.

Light-Gazing Behaviors

Light gazing is the CVI characteristic used to describe prolonged periods of attention to primary sources of indoor or occasionally, out-

door light. Although Good (2001) and others have reported photophobia in some individuals with CVI, many students with CVI will seek and gaze at light as a primitive form of visual input. It is common to observe light gazing when students with CVI are in overly complex settings, or when they are overstimulated, tired, or ill. Students who light gaze may be able to use light information points to guide independent or assisted O&M. These may include light emanating from doorways, lighted signs, or traffic light signals.

Visual Latency

Visual latency refers to a delay between the time a target is presented and the time the student visually notices it. This delay can be seconds or in some cases, minutes long. Responses can include eye contact with the target, turning in the direction of the target, becoming quiet, or smiling. When presented with an object, students with CVI may appear inattentive unless they are provided with ample wait time. Latency time may be decreased if moving, shiny, familiar, favorite-color objects are presented in the preferred visual field. There are obvious safety considerations for individuals who experience the CVI characteristic of visual latency. A delay in visually noticing a moving car or the presence of an open door can result in injury. Again, the O&M specialist may need to evaluate whether a mobility device is needed or in some cases, the individual who experiences significant visual latency may need to travel with a human guide.

Absence of Visually Guided Reach

This characteristic refers to a specific look–reach pattern associated with students who have CVI. This pattern is one in which the individual with CVI typically looks toward a target, looks away, and then reaches for the object without looking at it. This CVI characteristic results in difficulties completing tasks that require visually guided reach. Some individuals with CVI may appear to search for a target first with their eyes, and then look away and continue the reach and grasp tactilely. The visual-motor difficulties associated with this CVI characteristic may be related to the individual's inability to process visual responses simultaneously with other sensory stimuli, in this case, touch. For example, an individual with this characteristic may visually locate a red elevator button but glance away from the target as their hand moves in the direction of the up or down indicator button.

ASSESSMENT AND PROGRAM PLANNING

Traditional functional vision assessment for students with ocular forms of visual impairment follows a protocol in which the guiding question is "How does damage to the eye affect vision?" Evaluating near and distance visual acuities, visual fields, color discrimination abilities, binocularity, and lighting requirements helps resolve this question. The protocol for assessing the functional vision of students with CVI is fundamentally different and is guided by the question "How does injury to the brain affect vision?" The protocol for answering this guiding question must be unique and based on the visual and behavioral characteristics associated with CVI. Unlike other types of visual impairment, CVI has the potential to improve or even resolve. This raises the stakes on being precise in understanding exactly what the student can and cannot see so that activities in which vision is used are targeted to be as effective as possible. It is also important to recognize that cortical and ocular impairments may occur together and therefore, it is critical that the teacher of students with visual impairments, O&M professional, and entire educational team work closely together. This in-

cludes a thorough record review of medical and educational reports, as well as an in-depth parent interview.

The CVI Range

Teachers of students with visual impairments and O&M specialists can assess the extent of effect of CVI and which characteristics are present using a specialized evaluation designed for individuals with CVI known as the CVI Range (see Figure 20.1). The CVI Range is to be completed by one or more members of the educational team. It is not necessary for both the teacher and O&M specialist to conduct a CVI Range assessment although it is helpful if they have the opportunity to assess together. The CVI Range (Roman-Lantzy, 2007) is an instrument developed for use by teachers of students with visual impairments and O&M specialists. The CVI Range was systematically used in five-year training programs in eight states. Interrater reliability for those using the CVI Range is approximately 0.94. In a study conducted by Newcomb (2009), the CVI Range was found to have a significant degree of interrater reliability, test–retest reliability, and content validity.

The score derived from this assessment is based on a 0-to-10 scale where 0 = no functional vision and 10 = near-typical or typical functional vision. The score is used to guide the development of precise interventions that reflect the student's CVI status. As with any intervention, it is critical that the program planning match, not exceed or underestimate, the student's visual functioning level.

There are two methods used in the CVI Range to determine the extent of effect of CVI. The first method, known as the Across–Characteristics Assessment Method, presents a variety of statements that describe typical behaviors of students with CVI at specific levels. Each level on the form incorporates a number of the CVI characteristics and is meant to be a snapshot of how CVI traits

THE CVI RANGE
Christine Roman-Lantzy

Student/child's name:_____ Age:_____

Evaluator(s):_____ Evaluation Date: _____

This assessment protocol is intended for multiple evaluations over a period of time. Suggested scoring (no less than 3 times per school year):

   a. Initial assessment (red)
   b. Second assessment (blue)
   c. Third assessment (green)
   Further assessments will require a new form.

Totals:	Evaluation 1 (red)	Evaluation 2 (blue)	Evaluation 3 (green)
1. Range for Rating 1			
2. Total for Rating 2			

0	1	2	3	4	5	6	7	8	9	10

No functional
vision

Typical or
near-typical
visual functioning

(continued on next page)

Figure 20.1. The CVI Range

Source: Adapted from Christine Roman-Lantzy, *Cortical Visual Impairment: An Approach to Assessment and Intervention* (New York: AFB Press, 2007).

Rating I

Rate the following statements as related to the student/child's visual behaviors by marking the appropriate column to indicate the methods need to support the scores:

O = information obtained through observation of the child/student
I = information obtained through interview regarding the child/student
D = information obtained through direct contact with the child/student

In the remaining columns, indicate the assessed degree of the CVI characteristic:

- R   The statement represents a resolved visual behavior
- +   Describes current functioning of student/child
- +/– Partially describes student/child
- –   Does not apply to student/child

CVI Range 1–2: Student functions with minimal visual response

O	I	D	R	+	+/–	–	
							May localize but no appropriate fixations of objects or faces
							Consistently attentive to lights or perhaps ceiling fans
							Prolonged periods of latency in visual tasks
							Responds only in strictly controlled environments
							Objects viewed are a single color
							Objects viewed have movement and/or reflective properties
							Visually attends in near space only
							No blink in response to touch and/or visual threat
							No regard of the human face

(continued on next page)

Figure 20.1. *(Continued)*

CVI Range 3–4: Student functions with more consistent visual response

O	I	D	R	+	+/−	−	
							Visually fixates when the environment is controlled
							Less attracted to lights, can be redirected
							Latency slightly decreases after periods of consistent viewing
							May look at novel objects if the novel objects share characteristics of the familiar objects
							Blinks in response to touch and/or visual threat but the responses may be latent or are inconsistent
							Has a "favorite" color
							Shows strong visual field preferences
							May notice movement objects at 2–3 feet
							Look and touch completed as separate events

CVI Range 5–6: Student uses vision for functional tasks

O	I	D	R	+	+/−	−	
							Objects viewed may have two to three colors
							Light is no longer a distractor
							Latency present only when the student is tired, stressed, or overstimulated
							Movement continues to be an important factor for visual attention
							Student tolerates low levels of background noise
							Blink response to touch is consistently present
							Blink response to visual threat is intermittently present
							Visual attention now extends beyond near space, up to 4 to 6 feet
							May regard familiar faces when voice does not compete

(continued on next page)

Figure 20.1. (Continued)

CVI Range 7–8: Student demonstrates visual curiosity

O	I	D	R	+	+/–	–	
							Selection of toys/objects is less restricted, requires one to two sessions of "warm up"
							Competing auditory stimuli tolerated during periods of viewing—the student may now maintain visual attention on objects that produce music
							Blink response to visual threat consistently present
							Latency rarely present
							Visual attention extends to 10 feet with targets that produce movement
							Movement not required for attention at near
							Smiles at or regards familiar and new faces
							May enjoy regarding self in mirror
							Most high-contrast colors and/or familiar patterns regarded
							Simple books, picture cards, or symbols regarded

(continued on next page)

Figure 20.1. (*Continued*)

CVI Range 9–10: Student spontaneously uses vision for most functional activities

O	I	D	R	+	+/−	−	
							Selection of toys/objects not restricted
							Only the most complex environments affect visual response
							Latency resolved
							No color or pattern preferences
							Visual attention extends beyond 20 feet
							Views books or other two-dimensional materials, simple images
							Uses vision to imitate actions
							Demonstrates memory of visual events
							Displays typical visual-social responses
							Visual fields unrestricted
							Look and reach completed as a single action
							Attends to two-dimensional images against complex background

(continued on next page)

Figure 20.1. (*Continued*)

The CVI Range: Within–CVI Characteristics Assessment Method

Rating II

Determine the level of CVI present or resolved in the 10 categories below and add to obtain total score. Rate the following CVI categories as related to the student/child's visual behaviors by circling the appropriate number (the CVI Resolution Chart may be useful as a scoring guide):

- 0 Not resolved, usually or always a factor affecting visual functioning
- .25 Resolving
- .5 Resolving, sometimes a factor affecting visual functioning
- .75 Resolving
- 1 Resolved, not a factor affecting visual functioning

	Not Resolved		Resolving		Resolved
1. Color preference	0	.25	.5	.75	1
Comments:					
2. Attraction to movement	0	.25	.5	.75	1
Comments:					
3. Visual latency	0	.25	.5	.75	1
Comments:					
4. Visual field preferences	0	.25	.5	.75	1
Comments:					
5. Difficulty with visual complexity	0	.25	.5	.75	1
Comments:					
6. Light gazing	0	.25	.5	.75	1
Comments:					
7. Difficulty with distance viewing	0	.25	.5	.75	1
Comments:					

(continued on next page)

Figure 20.1. (*Continued*)

8. Atypical visual reflex responses	0	.25	.5	.75	1
Comments:					

9. Difficulty with visual novelty	0	.25	.5	.75	1
Comments:					

10. Absence of visually guided reach	0	.25	.5	.75	1
Comments:					

Figure 20.1. (*Continued*)

present at increasing levels of functional vision. Level 1–2 represents a minimal level of vision; Level 9–10 represents near normal levels of functional vision. A score is derived when a ceiling effect occurs; that is, when the individual statements are no longer describing a behavior that is true of the student. The CVI Range Scoring Guide provides examples of behaviors associated with each item in the Across-Characteristics Method. (See Appendix 20A); for more information on the CVI Range Scoring Guide, see Roman-Lantzy, 2007.

The second method used in the CVI Range, the Within–CVI Characteristics Method, is meant to determine the extent of the effect of CVI within individual characteristics. The evaluator now rates the effect of all 10 CVI characteristics individually, and potential scores of 0, .25, .5, .75, or 1 are assigned for each characteristic, where 0 represents no resolution of the effect of the characteristic and 1 represents complete resolution. After a value or degree of effect has been determined for each characteristic, all values are added together, and that total is the student's CVI score using the second method.

The CVI Orientation and Mobility Resolution Chart (Roman-Lantzy, 2007) can be used to assist in scoring the Within–Characteristic Method (see Figure 20.2). Both scores are recorded on the cover sheet of the CVI Range. The two scores are rarely identical, and thus the lower and the higher scores are marked on the 0–10 number line, and the span between these values becomes the CVI Range. This range score represents the overall level of effect of CVI as well as the degree of effect of individual CVI characteristics.

Using the CVI Range score, the O&M specialist can refer to the CVI O&M Resolution Chart to begin program planning. The Resolution Chart has two main functions. First, it can be used as a working document to track progress. Second, the Resolution Chart can be used to consider the possible confound of ocular visual impairment. Starting at the far left of the chart, the O&M specialist can mark an X through any statement that represents a resolved behavior. Boxes with statements that represent current behaviors need to be outlined or highlighted, and any statement that may never resolve because of a coexisting

CVI ORIENTATION AND MOBILITY RESOLUTION CHART

CVI Characteristics	Phase I Building Visual Behavior Level I Environmental Considerations Range 1–2	Range 3–4	Phase II Integrating Vision with Function Level II Environmental Considerations Range 5–6	Range 7–8	Phase III Resolution of CVI Characteristics Level III Environmental Considerations Range 9–10
Color preference	Single-color environmental features may be attended to in near space	Strong single-color preference persists	Objects or environmental features that have 2–3 colors may now be attended to within 4–6 feet	More colors, high-contrast areas may elicit visual attention	Safe travel not dependent on color cues
Attraction to movement	Targets viewed have movement and/or reflective properties; may be attentive to ceiling fans	Movement in the environment may distract from primary target	Movement may be needed to establish attention on target/destination	Movement not required for attention within 3–4 feet, may be necessary beyond	Movement not necessary for near or distant visual attention
Visual latency	Prolonged periods of visual latency	Latency slightly decreases after periods of consistent viewing	Latency present only when student is tired, stressed, or overstimulated	Latency rarely present	Latency resolved
Visual field preferences	Distinct field preferences; may use one eye for peripheral vision, the other eye for central vision	Visual field preferences; peripheral fields dominate	Visual field preferences persist	Increasing use of right and left fields for near and distance activities	Visual fields unrestricted

(continued on next page)

Figure 20.2. CVI Orientation and Mobility Resolution Chart

Source: Adapted from Christine Roman-Lantzy, *Cortical Visual Impairment: An Approach to Assessment and Intervention* (New York: AFB Press, 2007).

Difficulty with visual complexity	Visually attends only in strictly controlled environments—those without sensory distractions Engages in rote, assisted travel	Visually attends to or fixates on simple targets at near (within 3 feet), with environment controlled for sensory distractors	May be able to tolerate low levels of familiar background noise while maintaining visual attention on familiar targets Engages in rote or route travel with adapted visual cues	Competing auditory stimuli tolerated during periods of viewing May travel familiar routes using naturally occurring, simple landmarks or cues	Only the most complex environments affect independent travel Environmental or traffic signs may now be useful for independent travel
Light gazing	Is overly attentive to lights Room light may have to be reduced	Is less attracted to lights; can be redirected to other targets Lighted areas continue to distract the student	Light may be paired with signs or landmarks to increase visual attention	Light may be used to initiate visual attention on a target location or a landmark	Light is no longer a source of distraction and responses to light are typical. Some students may experience photophobia in natural light
Difficulty with distance viewing	Visually attends in near space only	Occasionally attends visually to familiar, moving or large targets in simple or familiar settings, up to 3–4 feet	Visual attention extends beyond near space, up to 4–6 feet Complexity in the environment may reduce this distance	Visual attention extends to 10 feet with targets that produce movement Color cues, movement and size of target may be factors in visual attention	Visual attention extends beyond 20 feet Student demonstrates memory of routes, cues or landmarks and may now be able to travel independently

Atypical visual reflex responses	No blink in response to touch and/or visual threat	Blinks in response to touch but response may be latent	Blink response to touch is consistently present Blink to visual threat is intermittently present	Blink response to visual threat is present. May now anticipate approaching obstacles, but latency may occur in high-complexity environments	Blink response to visual threat consistently present
Difficulty with visual novelty	Responds only to familiar objects	May visually attend to objects or environmental features if they share characteristics with the familiar objects	Visually attends to landmarks or cues that are highlighted with familiar color or pattern	Selection of objects or environmental and route cues remembered after several sessions of familiarization	Selection of objects and environments not restricted or specially adapted
Absence of visually guided reach	Reach, touch, and look occur as separate functions	Reach, touch, and look occur briefly but inconsistently	Visually guided reach is used with familiar materials, simple configurations, and "favorite" color	Look and reach occur in sequence but not always together	Look and reach occur as a single action

Key:

- Draw an X through boxes that represent resolved visual behaviors
- Use highlighter to outline boxes describing current visual functioning
- Draw an "O" in boxes describing visual skills that may never resolve because of coexisting ocular conditions

Figure 20.2. *(Continued)*

CVI ORIENTATION AND MOBILITY RESOLUTION CHART

CVI Characteristics	Phase I Building Visual Behavior Level I Environmental Considerations		Phase II Integrating Vision with Function Level II Environmental Considerations		Phase III Resolution of CVI Characteristics Level III Environmental Considerations
	Range 1–2	Range 3–4	Range 5–6	Range 7–8	Range 9–10
Color preference	Single color environmental features may be attended to in near space	Strong single color preference persists	Objects or environmental features that have 2–3 colors may now be attended to within 4–6 feet	More colors, high contrast areas may elicit visual attention	Safe travel not dependent on color cues
Attraction to movement	Targets viewed have movement and/or reflective properties; may be attentive to ceiling fans	Movement in the environment may distract from primary target	Movement may be needed to establish attention on target/destination	Movement not required for attention within 3–4 feet, may be necessary beyond	Movement not necessary for near or distant visual attention
Visual latency	Prolonged periods of visual latency	Latency slightly decreases after periods of consistent viewing	Latency present only when student is tired, stressed, or over-stimulated	Latency rarely present	Latency resolved
Visual field preferences	Distinct field preferences: may use one eye for peripheral vision, the other eye for central vision	Visual field preferences; peripheral fields dominate	Visual field preferences persist	Increasing use of right & left fields for near & distance activities	Visual fields unrestricted
Difficulty with visual complexity	Visually attends only in strictly controlled environments—those without sensory distractions Engages in rote, assisted travel	Visually attends to or fixates on simple targets at near (within 3 feet), with environment controlled for sensory distractors	May be able to tolerate low levels of familiar background noise while maintaining visual attention on familiar targets Engages in rote or route travel with adapted visual cues	Competing auditory stimuli tolerated during periods of viewing May travel familiar routes using naturally occurring, simple landmarks or cues	Only the most complex environments affect independent travel Environmental or traffic signs may now be useful for independent travel

Light gazing	Is overly attentive to lights. Room light may have to be reduced	Is less attracted to lights; can be redirected to other targets. Lighted areas continue to distract the student	Light may be paired with signs or landmarks to increase visual attention	Light may be used to initiate visual attention on a target location or a landmark	Light is no longer a source of distraction and responses to light are typical. Some students may experience photophobia in natural light
Difficulty with distance viewing	Visually attends in near space only	Occasionally attends visually to familiar moving or large targets in simple or familiar settings, up to 3–4 feet	Visual attention extends beyond near space, up to 4–6 feet. Complexity in the environment may reduce this distance	Visual attention extends to 10 feet with targets that produce movement. Color cues, movement and size of target may be factors in visual attention	Visual attention extends beyond 20 feet. Student demonstrates memory of routes, cues or landmarks and may now be able to travel independently
Atypical visual reflex responses	No blink in response to touch and/or visual threat	Blinks in response to touch but response may be latent	Blink response to touch is consistently present. Blink to visual threat is intermittently present	Blink response to visual threat is present. May now anticipate approaching obstacles, but latency may occur in high-complexity environments	Blink response to visual threat consistently present
Difficulty with visual novelty	Responds only to familiar objects	May visually attend to objects or environmental features if they share characteristics with the familiar objects	Visually attends to landmarks or cues that are highlighted with familiar color or pattern	Selection of objects or environmental/route cues remembered after several sessions of familiarization	Selection of objects and environments not restricted or specially adapted
Absence of visually guided reach	Reach, touch, look occur as separate functions	Reach, touch, look occur briefly but inconsistently	Visually guided reach is used with familiar materials, simple configurations, and "favorite" color	Look and reach occur in sequence but not always together	Look and reach occur as a single action

Key:

- Draw an X through boxes that represent resolved visual behaviors
- Use highlighter to outline boxes describing current visual functioning
- Draw an "O" in boxes describing visual skills that may never resolve because of coexisting ocular conditions

Figure 20.3. Sample Completed CVI Orientation and Mobility Resolution Chart

ocular condition needs to be marked with an *O*. Figure 20.3 provides examples of these markings on the CVI O&M Resolution Chart.

If a coexisting eye condition occurs, the boxes marked with an *O* will be monitored and if after time, all or most other boxes on the chart are marked with an *X* except the *O* boxes then the O&M specialist can conclude that the primary cause of visual impairment can be considered ocular rather than cortical. Interventions should then be based on the principles and methods used with individuals who have ocular visual impairment because the CVI will have essentially been resolved.

Using the CVI Range to Guide O&M Instruction

The basic strategies and techniques for O&M instruction should not differ for those students who have CVI. The major difference lies in the integration with standard O&M techniques of the student's assessed CVI needs, as indicated by the CVI Range score and the highlighted boxes on the CVI O&M Resolution Chart. In other words, the CVI characteristics are applied as an overlay to the goals for O&M. Several examples may help illustrate this.

Joey

Joey is a 5-year-old student who has CVI as a result of hypoxic ischemic encephalopathy (HIE). He has seizures throughout the day and receives his nutrition by g-tube inserted into his stomach. Joey has head control and is able to maintain sitting balance in his wheelchair. His classroom paraprofessional wheels him from the bus to the classroom and then from room to room throughout the school building during the day. He receives services from a teacher of the visually impaired and an O&M specialist who together assessed Joey using the CVI Range. Joey's CVI Range score was 2. His scores revealed the presence of the CVI characteristics. For Joey's scores, see Table 20.1.

Joey's CVI Range score indicates he has inconsistent use of vision and that his visual functioning is dependent on a number of very specific factors. Joey uses his vision only when the environment is free of visual complexity and when there are no auditory, tactual, or olfactory distractions. He may be able to use red, moving features that are within 3 feet of Joey's body as visual information points to assist him in becoming oriented or moving systematically through an environment. Clearly, as first indicated by the CVI Range scores and then by marking the CVI O&M Resolution Chart, independent travel is not a safe or realistic option for Joey (see Figure 20.4). Joey's overriding goal is to develop consistent visual attention on targets that match Joey's specific CVI needs. It is critical that the teacher of visually impaired students and the O&M specialist provide information to Joey's teachers and family to emphasize the need for consistent adaptations and, therefore, opportunities for Joey to increase use of functional vision. Adaptations for Joey include the use of red rope lighting attached to the edges of his classroom door and a red plug-in light positioned in Joey's peripheral field of view at the changing table in the bathroom.

Anna

Anna has CVI as a result of a head injury she suffered in a car accident. In addition to her visual impairment, Anna has been diagnosed with spastic diplegia, left esotropia, and difficulties with speech. Her cognitive abilities appear to be nearly normal as evidenced by her receptive language and her ability to use augmentative communication devices. Anna is able to walk independently with the assistance of ankle-foot orthoses and a walker. Her O&M specialist and

TABLE 20.1

Joey's CVI Range Scores

CVI Characteristic	Score	Comment
Color preference	0	Joey orients most frequently to objects that are red.
Difficulty with novelty	0	Joey primarily looks at his red light-up toy, a red pinwheel, and a red slinky.
Visual latency	0	Joey has a long delay to look toward an object, even favorite and red objects, every time an object is presented.
Visual field preference	.25	Joey rarely fixates on objects but will turn in the direction of a moving, shiny, red object at his right and occasionally at his left.
Difficulty with complexity	.25	Joey will localize on and occasionally fixate on single color (red), objects presented against a plain background and only when there are no sound or touch distractions.
Light gazing	.25	Joey stares at primary sources of light when the environment is complex.
Difficulty with distance viewing	.25	Joey views familiar, moving, red targets when they are presented within 3 feet of his body.
Atypical visual reflex responses	.5	Joey blinks when touched at the bridge of the nose but not in response to visual threat.
Attraction to movement	.25	Joey primarily looks at his slinky, red pinwheel or occasionally at simple red nonmoving objects.
Absence of visually guided reach	.25	Joey primarily looks away while reaching except when objects are highly familiar and placed on a simple background.

her teacher of visually impaired students use information derived from her CVI Range scores to help program planning. Anna's CVI Range score was 5. Her scores revealed the presence of CVI characteristics. (See Table 20.2 for Anna's scores.)

Anna's CVI Range score indicates that she is able to use her vision more consistently than Joey. Unlike Joey, Anna is able to tolerate a greater degree of sensory competition while using her vision and she can now incorporate vision and functional tasks. Anna's level of usable vision now makes it possible for her to learn to travel simple routes in familiar settings. However, in order for Anna to best use her vision her CVI O&M Reso-

lution Chart (Figure 20.5) suggests that it will be necessary for the O&M specialist to select landmarks and possibly create information points based on her individual CVI needs in order to assist Anna in both orientation to the route and in safe travel through it.

Examples for both are provided in the following list:

• Place bright yellow, reflective, Mylar targets (incorporating the CVI characteristics of color, movement, and low complexity) on landmarks and information points including drinking fountains, doorway edges, Anna's chair and desk, door knobs or openers, wall corners at

CVI ORIENTATION AND MOBILITY RESOLUTION CHART

JOEY

CVI Characteristics	Phase I — Building Visual Behavior / Level I Environmental Considerations — Range 1–2	Phase II — Integrating Vision with Function / Level II Environmental Considerations — Range 3–4	Range 5–6	Phase III — Resolution of CVI Characteristics / Level III Environmental Considerations — Range 7–8	Range 9–10
Color preference	Single color environmental features may be attended to in near space	Strong single color preference persists	Objects or environmental features that have 2–3 colors may now be attended to within 4–6 feet	More colors, high contrast areas may elicit visual attention	Safe travel not dependent on color cues
Attraction to movement	Targets viewed have movement and/or reflective properties; may be attentive to ceiling fans	Movement in the environment may distract from primary target	Movement may be needed to establish attention on target/destination	Movement not required for attention within 3–4 feet, may be necessary beyond	Movement not necessary for near or distant visual attention
Visual latency	Prolonged periods of visual latency	Latency slightly decreases after periods of consistent viewing	Latency present only when student is tired, stressed, or overstimulated	Latency rarely present	Latency resolved
Visual field preferences	Distinct field preferences: may use one eye for peripheral vision, the other eye for central vision	Visual field preferences; peripheral fields dominate	Visual field preferences persist	Increasing use of right and left fields for near and distance activities	Visual fields unrestricted
Difficulty with visual complexity	Visually attends only in strictly controlled environments—those without sensory distractions Engages in rote, assisted travel	Visually attends to or fixates on simple targets at near (within 3 feet), with environment controlled for sensory distractors	May be able to tolerate low levels of familiar background noise while maintaining visual attention on familiar targets Engages in rote or route travel with adapted visual cues	Competing auditory stimuli tolerated during periods of viewing May travel familiar routes using naturally occurring, simple landmarks or cues	Only the most complex environments affect independent travel Environmental or traffic signs may now be useful for independent travel

Light gazing	Is overly attentive to lights; Room light may have to be reduced	Is less attracted to lights; can be redirected to other targets; Lighted areas continue to distract the student	Light may be paired with signs or landmarks to increase visual attention	Light may be used to initiate visual attention on a target location or a landmark	Light is no longer a source of distraction and responses to light are typical; Some students may experience photophobia in natural light
Difficulty with distance viewing	Visually attends in near space only	Occasionally attends visually to familiar, moving or large targets in simple or familiar settings, up to 3–4 feet	Visual attention extends beyond near space, up to 4–6 feet; Complexity in the environment may reduce this distance	Visual attention extends to 10 feet with targets that produce movement; Color cues, movement and size of target may be factors in visual attention	Visual attention extends beyond 20 feet; Student demonstrates memory of routes, cues or landmarks and may now be able to travel independently
Atypical visual reflex responses	No blink in response to touch and/or visual threat	Blinks in response to touch but response may be latent	Blink response to touch is consistently present; Blink to visual threat is intermittently present	Blink response to visual threat is present; May now anticipate approaching obstacles, but latency may occur in high complexity environments	Blink response to visual threat consistently present
Difficulty with visual novelty	Responds only to familiar objects	May visually attend to objects or environmental features if they share characteristics with the familiar objects	Visually attends to landmarks or cues that are highlighted with familiar color or pattern	Selection of objects or environmental/route cues remembered after several sessions of familiarization	Selection of objects and environments not restricted or specially adapted
Absence of visually guided reach	Reach, touch, look occur as separate functions	Reach, touch, look occur briefly but inconsistently	Visually guided reach is used with familiar materials, simple configurations, and "favorite" color	Look and reach occur in sequence but not always together	Look and reach occur as a single action

Key:

- Draw an X through boxes that represent resolved visual behaviors
- Use highlighter to outline boxes describing current visual functioning
- Draw an "O" in boxes describing visual skills that may never resolve because of coexisting ocular conditions

Figure 20.4. CVI O&M Resolution Chart Completed for Joey

TABLE 20.2

Anna's CVI Range Scores

Characteristic	Score	Comment
Color preference	.5	Anna most consistently notices objects, landmarks, or information points that are yellow but will also occasionally alert to other bright colors.
Difficulty with novelty	.5	Anna looks at any new objects, landmarks, or information points that share characteristics of color, simplicity, or movement of her original "preferred" objects.
Visual latency	.75	Anna occasionally demonstrates a delay in locating and/or fixating on targets; complex environments increase latency response.
Visual field preference	.5	Anna notices targets most quickly when they approach from her right, peripheral field; she also frequently fails to detect objects or drop-offs, or surface changes in her lower field.
Difficulty with complexity	.5	Anna visually locates objects, landmarks, or information points when they are yellow or single colored and when they are placed against a background with little additional information.
Light gazing	.5	Anna will at times gaze at primary sources of light; light gazing increases if there is a significant amount of noise or visual complexity.
Difficulty with distance viewing	.5	Anna is able to visually locate objects, landmarks, or information points at distances as great as 6 to 8 feet from her body.
Atypical visual reflex responses	.5	Anna consistently blinks when touched at the bridge of the nose; she does not blink in response to a target moving quickly toward her face.
Attraction to movement	.5	Anna is both attracted to and distracted by objects, landmarks, and information points that move in space or that have a shiny or reflective surface; she can occasionally visually locate familiar, single-color targets in low-complexity environments.
Absence of visually guided reach	.25	Anna is able to pair looking and reaching in low-complexity settings, and generally with familiar objects.

hallway intersections, or any surfaces associated with destinations in Anna's daily travel routines.

- When using bright yellow targets at specific distances along the route to be learned it is critical that the flags be positioned at eye level (CVI characteristic of visual fields) and that they be positioned in areas that are free from decorations or patterned backgrounds (CVI characteristics of preferred color and complexity of array).

- During instruction, prompt Anna to look for the specially adapted CVI information point when she is within 3 to 5 feet of it (CVI characteristic of distance viewing).

CVI ORIENTATION AND MOBILITY RESOLUTION CHART

ANNA

CVI Characteristics	Phase I Building Visual Behavior Level I Environmental Considerations		Phase II Integrating Vision with Function Level II Environmental Considerations		Phase III Resolution of CVI Characteristics Level III Environmental Considerations
	Range 1–2	Range 3–4	Range 5–6	Range 7–8	Range 9–10
Color preference	Single color environmental features may be attended to in near space	Strong single color preference persists	Objects or environmental features that have 2–3 colors may now be attended to within 4–6 feet	More colors, high contrast areas may elicit visual attention	Safe travel not dependent on color cues
Attraction to movement	Targets viewed have movement and/or reflective properties; may be attentive to ceiling fans	Movement in the environment may distract from primary target	Movement may be needed to establish attention on target/destination	Movement not required for attention within 3–4 feet, may be necessary beyond	Movement not necessary for near or distant visual attention
Visual latency	Prolonged periods of visual latency	Latency slightly decreases after periods of consistent viewing	Latency present only when student is tired, stressed, or over-stimulated	Latency rarely present	Latency resolved
Visual field preferences	Distinct field preferences; may use one eye for peripheral vision, the other eye for central vision	Visual field preferences; peripheral fields dominate	Visual field preferences persist	Increasing use of right and left fields for near and distance activities	Visual fields unrestricted
Difficulty with visual complexity	Visually attends only in strictly controlled environments—those without sensory distractions; Engages in route, assisted travel	Visually attends to or fixates on simple targets at near (within 3 feet), with environment controlled for sensory distractors	May be able to tolerate low levels of familiar background noise while maintaining visual attention on familiar targets; Engages in rote or route travel with adapted visual cues	Competing auditory stimuli tolerated during periods of viewing; May travel familiar routes using naturally occurring, simple landmarks or cues	Only the most complex environments affect independent travel; Environmental or traffic signs may now be useful for independent travel

(continued on next page)

Figure 20.5. CVI O&M Resolution Chart Completed for Anna

Light gazing	Is overly attentive to lights / Room light may have to be reduced	Is less attracted to lights, can be redirected to other targets / Lighted areas continue to distract the student	Light may be paired with signs or landmarks to increase visual attention	Light may be used to initiate visual attention on a target location or a landmark	Light is no longer a source of distraction and re-sponses to light are typical / Some students may experience photophobia in natural light
Difficulty with distance viewing	Visually attends in near space only	Occasionally attends visually to familiar, moving or large targets in simple or familiar settings, up to 3–4 feet	Visual attention extends beyond near space, up to 4–6 feet / Complexity in the environment may reduce this distance	Visual attention extends to 10 feet with targets that produce movement / Color cues, movement and size of target may be factors in visual attention	Visual attention extends beyond 20 feet / Student demonstrates memory of routes, cues or landmarks and may now be able to travel independently
Atypical visual reflex responses	No blink in response to touch and/or visual threat	Blinks in response to touch but response may be latent	Blink response to touch is consistently present / Blink to visual threat is intermittently present	Blink response to visual threat is present / May now anticipate approaching obstacles, but latency may occur in high-complexity environments	Blink response to visual threat consistently present
Difficulty with visual novelty	Responds only to familiar objects	May visually attend to objects or environmental features if they share characteristics with the familiar objects	Visually attends to landmarks or cues that are highlighted with familiar color or pattern	Selection of objects or environmental and route cues remembered after several sessions of familiarization	Selection of objects and environments not restricted or specially adapted
Absence of visually guided reach	Reach, touch, look occur as separate functions	Reach, touch, look occur briefly but inconsistently	Visually guided reach is used with familiar materials, simple configurations, and "favorite" color	Look and reach occur in sequence but not always together	Look and reach occur as a single action

Key:

- Draw an X through boxes that represent resolved visual behaviors
- Use highlighter to outline boxes describing current visual functioning
- Draw an "O" in boxes describing visual skills that may never resolve because of coexisting ocular conditions

Figure 20.5. (*Continued*)

- When planning adaptations the O&M specialist should attempt to pair the specially adapted information point with a naturally occurring landmark. By doing this, Anna will be learning the placement of environmental features she will eventually use if the CVI adaptations are no longer necessary.

- In consideration of Anna's CVI characteristic of light gazing, plan initial lessons in areas where Anna will be positioned with her back to major sources of light. Otherwise she is likely to gaze at the light source over other visual information.

- Plan initial lessons during times when there is low student activity in the hallway in order to help Anna cope with her CVI characteristics of attraction to movement and difficulty coping with complexity of array and the distractions of high-sensory-laden environments.

- When planning simple outdoor routes, select visual information points that are appropriate for Anna's level of CVI. Select yellow, simple, and moving targets as visual targets. This may include looking for the school bus, using bright yellow traffic posts, curb highlighting, or outdoor benches. Anna may require adult assistance depending on the degree of visual and auditory complexity in the setting.

It is critical that the O&M specialist and teacher of visually impaired students provide Anna's teacher and family with information regarding her visual abilities and challenges. Depending on the situation and the degree of adaptation provided, Anna may function with relative visual efficiency. However, when adaptations or the environment are not compatible with her CVI, Anna may appear to be nonvisual. The seeming contradiction can be best understood when Anna's visual functioning is considered in the context of the unique visual and behavioral characteristics of CVI.

Max

Max has CVI as a result of nearly drowning. He was a typically developing 16 year old when the incident occurred. As a result of asphyxia caused by the accident, Max has learning difficulties, and although the structures of his eyes were found to be healthy, the ophthalmologist diagnosed Max with CVI. He has received services from a teacher of visually impaired students and an O&M specialist for two years since his accident, and his functional vision has improved markedly as documented by assessments using the CVI Range. His initial CVI Range score was 3 out of 10. His latest CVI Range score was 8.25 out of 10. Max's scores showed the presence of the CVI characteristics as shown in Table 20.3.

Max's CVI Range scores indicate significant improvement in functional vision and resolution of the CVI characteristics of color, novelty, latency, light gazing, and visual reflex responses. The CVI characteristics that continue to interfere with typical visual functioning are visual fields, visual complexity, distance viewing, movement, and visual motor. Based on Max's CVI O&M Resolution Chart (Figure 20.6), his teacher of visually impaired students adapts educational materials to make them less complex and assists Max in learning to identify salient features in print, illustrations, charts, or maps found in Max's textbooks.

Max's O&M specialist provides instruction to help Max be more safe and independent in indoor and outdoor environments. Some suggested interventions for O&M include the following:

- It is critical that the O&M specialist provide all of Max's teachers and his family with information regarding Max's visual abilities and challenges. In many situations, Max no longer acts like an individual with low vision or blindness and his visual limitations may not

TABLE 20.3

Max's CVI Range Scores

Characteristic	Score	Comment
Color preference	1	Max no longer demonstrates a visual preference for targets of a specific color.
Difficulty with novelty	1	Max visually alerts to new targets over those that are familiar.
Visual latency	1	Max no longer demonstrates a delay in visual response when targets or objects are presented.
Visual field preferences	.5	Max most frequently notices targets that approach from his left peripheral field; he frequently fails to detect objects, drop-offs, or surface changes in his lower field. Max uses a long cane for outdoor and unfamiliar indoor travel.
Difficulty with complexity	.75	Max is able to read two-dimensional symbols and signs when presented against a simple background; he can maintain visual attention while voices, traffic sounds, or music are present, and he can identify targets that have two- or three-color multicolor or pattern surfaces. Highly complex settings like shopping malls, busy outdoor environments, or concerts require adult assistance.
Light gazing	1	Max is no longer distracted by primary sources of indoor or outdoor light.
Difficulty with distance viewing	.75	Max can detect two- or three-color landmarks or information points from distances up to 10 to 15 feet depending on the degree of environmental complexity.
Atypical visual reflex responses	1	Both the blink and visual threat reflex are normal.
Attraction to movement	.75	Max continues to be distracted by targets that produce movement or that are made of shiny or reflective surfaces.
Absence of visually guided reach	.5	While reaching for objects, Max looks at the object, looks away, and then reaches without looking at the target approximately 50 percent of the time.

be obvious. In fact, Max may be able to move through familiar environments without assistance. However, in novel surroundings or in settings where there is a great deal of environmental complexity, Max may need assistance from either a human guide or he may choose to use his cane.

- Max continues to need his cane to detect drop-offs, especially in unfamiliar or crowded areas of his school and community. He is quicker at locating both pedestrian and vehicular traffic that approach from his left side than from his right side.

- Max will benefit from O&M instruction in areas of his community that are high in visual complexity. Map skill instruction will help reinforce Max's understanding of routes and alternative approaches to specific destinations.

CVI ORIENTATION AND MOBILITY RESOLUTION CHART

MAX

CVI Characteristics	Phase I Building Visual Behavior Level I Environmental Considerations		Phase II Integrating Vision with Function Level II Environmental Considerations		Phase III Resolution of CVI Characteristics Level III Environmental Considerations
	Range 1–2	Range 3–4	Range 5–6	Range 7–8	Range 9–10
Color preference	Single color environmental features may be attended to in near space	Strong single color preference persists	Objects or environmental features that have 2–3 colors may now be attended to within 4–6 feet	More colors, high contrast areas may elicit visual attention	Safe travel not dependent on color cues
Attraction to movement	Targets viewed have movement and/or reflective properties; may be attentive to ceiling fans	Movement in the environment may distract from primary target	Movement may be needed to establish attention on target/destination	Movement not required for attention within 3–4 feet, may be necessary beyond	Movement not necessary for near or distant visual attention
Visual latency	Prolonged periods of visual latency	Latency slightly decreases after periods of consistent viewing	Latency present only when student is tired, stressed, or over-stimulated	Latency rarely present	Latency resolved
Visual field preferences	Distinct field preferences; may use one eye for peripheral vision, the other eye for central vision	Visual field preferences; peripheral fields dominate	Visual field preferences persist	Increasing use of right and left fields for near and distance activities	Visual fields unrestricted
Difficulty with visual complexity	Visually attends only in strictly controlled environments-those without sensory distractions. Engages in rote, assisted travel	Visually attends to or fixates on simple targets at near (within 3 feet), with environment controlled for sensory distractors	May be able to tolerate low levels of familiar background noise while maintaining visual attention on familiar targets. Engages in rote or route travel with adapted visual cues	Competing auditory stimuli tolerated during periods of viewing. May travel familiar routes using naturally occurring, simple landmarks or cues	Only the most complex environments affect independent travel. Environmental or traffic signs may now be useful for independent travel

(continued on next page)

Figure 20.6. CVI O&M Resolution Chart Completed for Max

Light gazing	Is overly attentive to lights; Room light may have to be reduced	Is less attracted to lights; can be redirected to other targets. Lighted areas continue to distract the student	Light may be paired with signs or landmarks to increase visual attention	Light may be used to initiate visual attention on a target location or a landmark	Light is no longer a source of distraction and responses to light are typical. Some students may experience photophobia in natural light
Difficulty with distance viewing	Visually attends in near space only	Occasionally attends visually to familiar, moving or large targets in simple or familiar settings, up to 3–4 feet	Visual attention extends beyond near space, up to 4–6 feet. Complexity in the environment may reduce this distance	Visual attention extends to 10 feet with targets that produce movement. Color cues, movement and size of target may be factors in visual attention	Visual attention extends beyond 20 feet. Student demonstrates memory of routes, cues or landmarks and may now be able to travel independently
Atypical visual reflex responses	No blink in response to touch and/or visual threat	Blinks in response to touch but response may be latent	Blink response to touch is consistently present. Blink to visual threat is intermittently present	Blink response to visual threat is present. May now anticipate approaching obstacles, but latency may occur in high complexity environments	Blink response to visual threat consistently present
Difficulty with visual novelty	Responds only to familiar objects	May visually attend to objects or environmental features if they share characteristics with the familiar objects	Visually attends to landmarks or cues that are highlighted with familiar color or pattern	Selection of objects or environmental/route cues remembered after several sessions of familiarization	Selection of objects and environments not restricted or specially adapted
Absence of visually guided reach	Reach, touch, look occur as separate functions	Reach, touch, look occur briefly but inconsistently	Visually guided reach is used with familiar materials, simple configurations, and "favorite" color	Look and reach occur in sequence but not always together	Look and reach occur as a single action

Key:
- Draw an X through boxes that represent resolved visual behaviors
- Use highlighter to outline boxes describing current visual functioning
- Draw an "O" in boxes describing visual skills that may never resolve because of coexisting ocular conditions

Figure 20.6. *(Continued)*

- Signs that have color and that are presented against simple backgrounds will be easier for Max to see. When a known sign is presented in an array of three or more signs, Max may not be able to locate the sign because of the degree of visual complexity.

- Max can locate landmarks, information points, or familiar people at distances up to 15 feet in most settings. When the environment is novel or visually complicated, his ability to detect salient features will occur at significantly shorter distances. Max should not be expected to travel independently during school field trips, or in new communities. Max will need extensive O&M instruction at his future college campus.

- Max continues to have difficulty using print materials for in-class and homework assignments. He is able to read enlarged print on the CCTV and he uses audiobooks to access information in high-content classes such as literature, history, and psychology. Color coding should be used to highlight salient features of graphs, charts, and maps.

- Max uses the movement of people or objects to help establish attention and to maintain attention on specific visual features of the environment. It is important to recognize that incidental movement may distract Max. He has been known to follow the movements of pedestrians into a street he does not intend to cross. Max needs to double-check his position by using landmarks rather than simply following the movements of people or a line of vehicular traffic.

CONCLUSION

These three CVI-student profiles represent three different levels of the effect of CVI. Students with CVI have a broad range of abilities and needs, including the need for O&M instruction. O&M specialists need to recognize that students with CVI have unique needs that can best be

met by considering the essential characteristics that make it different from ocular forms of visual impairment.

IMPLICATIONS FOR O&M PRACTICE

1. CVI is the leading cause of visual impairment in children in all first world nations.

2. Individuals with CVI have a medical history of neurological impairment.

3. CVI can be a congenital or acquired condition.

4. The functional vision of children with CVI can improve.

5. CVI is most reliably identified by unique visual and behavioral characteristics.

6. The CVI Range is used to assess the functional vision of individuals with CVI.

7. The CVI O&M Resolution Chart is used to record both visual progress and O&M skills to indicate the degree of effect that CVI is having on a student.

8. O&M program planning for individuals with CVI should integrate O&M principles with the assessed levels of the unique CVI characteristics.

LEARNING ACTIVITIES

1. Review the medical records of students who have CVI. Identify the neurological condition that is the cause of the student's diagnosis of CVI.

2. Observe a student who has CVI in living and learning settings. Record observations regarding behaviors associated with CVI.

3. Conduct the CVI Range assessment with a student who has CVI. Use the range scores to complete the CVI O&M Resolution Chart.

4. Identify indoor and outdoor environmental landmarks based on preferred color, attraction to movement, visual novelty, and environmental complexity for an individual who has CVI.

5. Create a map of an indoor or outdoor route traveled by an individual who has CVI. Adapt the map according to scores for individual CVI characteristics obtained from the CVI Range.

CVI Range Scoring Guide

This Scoring Guide is used to help assign scores to a student during assessment. For each statement in the CVI Range assessment form, it indicates which CVI characteristics the statement encompasses and provides examples of visual behaviors that correspond to each possible score of R, +, +/−. or −.

Phase	Range	Statement	CVI Characteristic	R	+	+/−	−
I	1–2	**May localize, but no appropriate fixations on objects or faces**	Color, movement latency, visual fields, complexity, novelty	Fixates on objects or faces	May occasionally glance in the direction of an object or face, but attention is intermittent and eye-to-object attention occurs rarely	Gives brief, inconsistent attention toward an object or face (may be determined by report only, not observation)	No attention in the direction of any object or face, either by report or observation
I	1–2	**Consistently attentive to lights or perhaps ceiling fans**	Movement, complexity, light-gazing	Able to look at targets in the presence of primary sources of light	Stares into sources of indoor or outdoor light and is unable to attend to other targets unless the lights are turned off or the student is positioned away from the light	Occasionally able to attend to nonlighted targets, even in the presence of primary sources of light	No attention to light or any other target
I	1–2	**Prolonged periods of latency in visual tasks**	Latency	Little or no delay in directing vision to a target	Demonstrates a delay in directing vision to a target every time or nearly every time a new object is presented or a new activity begins	Delay in directing vision to a target occurs only when tired, stressed, ill, hungry, or overstimulated	Profound delay in directing vision to a target; only rarely seems to view a target
I	1–2	**Responds only in strictly controlled environments**	Complexity	Attends to visual targets in the presence of more than one visual target, sound, or touch	Attends to visual targets only when there are no visual, auditory, or tactile distractions	Occasional attention to visual targets in the presence of certain or familiar visual, auditory, or tactile distractions	No consistent visual attention to any visual targets

(continued on next page)

Phase	Range	Statement	CVI Characteristic	R	+	+/-	-
I	1–2	Objects viewed are a single color	Color, complexity, novelty	Looks at objects that are any color and/or more than a single color	Glances at or briefly fixates on single-color objects; may be reported to be a favorite color	Glances at or briefly fixates on objects of favorite color, and occasionally on objects of other colors. May also glance at or briefly fixate on objects that have more than a single color	No consistent visual attention to visual targets of any particular color
I	1–2	Objects viewed have movement and/or shiny or reflective properties	Movement	Looks at objects that are neither moving nor shiny or reflective	Only looks at objects that move, have moving parts, or are made of shiny or reflective materials	May need movement and/or shiny or reflective objects to initiate visual attention. Occasionally attends to objects without movement properties	No consistent visual attention to moving or nonmoving targets
I	1–2	Visually attends in near space only*	Complexity, distance viewing	Looks at objects that are beyond 18 inches away	Glances at or briefly fixates on objects only when they are presented within 18 inches	Occasional glances at or fixates on objects beyond 18 inches	No consistent visual attention to objects at any distance
I	1–2	No blink in response to touch or visual threat*	Visual reflexes	Blinks when touched at bridge of the nose or in response to a target moving on midline toward the face	Fails to blink	Occasionally blinks in response to touch or threat	Eyes not open
I	1–2	No regard of the human face*	Complexity, novelty	Looks directly into faces, even if briefly or inconsistently	No attention to human faces, may seem to "look through" people	Occasionally glances into faces, even if without eye-to-eye contact	No consistent attention to targets of any kind

I–II	3–4						
I–II	3–4	**Visually fixates when the environment is controlled**	Complexity	Establishes eye-to-object contact with familiar or novel objects or human faces, even in the presence of visual or other sensory stimuli	Intermittent eye-to-object contact, but only when visual, auditory, and tactile distractors are reduced or eliminated / A small degree of additional sensory input may be tolerated while viewing	Occasional eye-to-object contact, but conditions for fixations may vary	May turn in the direction of a target, but no eye-to-object contact
I–II	3–4	**Less attracted to lights; can be redirected**	Light-gazing	Does not stare at primary sources of light	May stare at lights, but is able to shift attention from lights when appropriate visual targets are presented in controlled environments	Primary sources of light must be eliminated only on rare occasions for visual attention to a target to occur	All primary sources of light must be eliminated for visual attention to a target to occur
I–II	3–4	**Latency slightly decreases after periods of consistent viewing**	Latency	A delay in directing vision toward a familiar object is rarely, if ever, present	Demonstrates a delay in directing vision to a target some of the time or for shorter durations of time / Latency may fade as vision is used more consistently	Delay in directing vision toward a target occurs frequently, but not every time a familiar target is presented	Delay in directing vision toward a target is always present
I–II	3–4	**May look at novel objects if they share characteristics of familiar objects**	Novelty	Is able to glance toward or have eye-to-object contact with objects never previously seen that may or may not resemble "favorite" objects	Is able to glance toward or have eye-to-object contact with new objects if they have matching features of color, movement, or low complexity	Is able to glance toward or have eye-to-object contact with objects that have few similar traits, but may share at least one matching element of color, movement, or complexity	Is able to glance toward or have eye-to-object contact only with a small set of highly familiar objects

(continued on next page)

Phase	Range	Statement	CVI Characteristic	R	+	+/-	-
I–II	3–4	Blinks in response to touch and/or visual threat, but responses may be latent and/or inconsistent	Visual reflexes	Blinks immediately when touched at the bridge of the nose and/or when a target moves quickly toward face	Blinks to touch at bridge of the nose and possibly to the quick movement of a target toward the face, but responses may be delayed or slightly inconsistent	Blinks to touch, but not to a target moving quickly toward the face	Does not blink consistently to either touch at the bridge of the nose or to a target moving quickly toward the face
I–II	3–4	Has a "favorite" color	Color	Visual attention to objects is not dependent on a particular color	Continues to most consistently glance toward or have eye-to-object contact with targets made of a single, preferred color, over objects of all other colors	Favorite color may be necessary to initiate looking. Some part of the target may be made of the "favorite" or preferred color for visual attention to occur	No consistent attention to objects
I–II	3–4	Shows strong visual field preferences*	Visual field preferences	Visual attention occurs equally in all fields	Glances toward or has eye-to-object contact with targets when presented in specific positions of peripheral and/or central viewing fields. Preferences not as rigid as in Range 1–2	Glances toward or has eye-to-object contact with targets in most viewing positions, with a slight preference for the original preferred position	Glances toward or has eye-to-object contact in one viewing field only
I–II	3–4	May notice movement objects at 2 to 3 feet	Movement, complexity	Pays visual attention to objects that do not move or have reflective properties at distances up to 3 feet or beyond	Glances toward or has eye-to-object contact with objects that move in space or are made of shiny or reflective materials and are at distances up to 3 feet	Movement or reflective properties are required to initiate visual attention. One element of the object may be moving, shiny, or reflective for visual attention to occur	Movement or reflective materials are necessary for visual attention, and viewing distance is within 18 inches of face

		Behavior	Category				
I–II	3–4	**Look and touch completed as separate events**	Visually guided reach	Reach and touch occur simultaneously, even if used inconsistently	Attempts to reach or swat at a target, but does not use a visually guided reach / Look, look away, then reach pattern is used	Occasionally uses visually guided reach	Makes no attempts to reach or swat at targets
II	5–6	**Objects viewed may have two to three colors**	Color, complexity	Pays visual attention to multicolor or multipattern objects, with or without preferred color	Looks directly at targets that have a pattern of two to three colors / Preferred color is at least one element of the pattern	Looks directly at targets that have two and occasionally three colors / Preferred color is always one of the colors	Pays visual attention only to objects of a single preferred color
II	5–6	**Light is no longer a distractor⁎**	Light-gazing	Normal responses to high and low levels of light	No light-gazing behavior	Occasional gazing at primary sources of light	Light-gazing occurs consistently
II	5–6	**Latency present only when the student is tired, stressed, or overstimulated**	Latency, complexity	No delay in directing visual attention to a familiar or noncomplex target	Delay in directing visual attention toward a target only when experiencing fatigue or inappropriate levels of multisensory input	Occasional delay in directing visual attention to a target	Consistent delay in directing visual attention to a target
II	5–6	**Movement continues to be an important factor for visual attention**	Movement	Moving, shiny, or reflective materials are not required for visual attention at near or up to 6 feet away	Visual attention most consistent with materials that move or are shiny or reflective / Some element of movement of entire target does not have to be moving, shiny, or reflective for visual attention to occur	A small element of movement may help establish or maintain visual attention	Only materials with elements of movement establish or maintain visual attention

(continued on next page)

Phase	Range	Statement	CVI Characteristic	R	+	+/−	−
II	5–6	**Student tolerates low levels of background noise**	Complexity	Visual attention established and maintained in typical multisensory environments	Visual attention is maintained even in the presence of low-volume sound, familiar voices, or familiar environmental sounds	Occasionally is able to maintain visual attention in the presence of sound One or two particular sounds are tolerated during viewing; many are not tolerated	No or little visual attention in the presence of other sensory inputs
II	5–6	**Blink response to touch is consistently present**	Visual reflexes	Blink-to-touch response present; blink-to-visual-threat response (when target moves quickly toward face) inconsistently present	Blinks simultaneous to touch at bridge of nose consistently	Emerging pattern of blink-to-touch response present	Occasional or absent blink-to-touch response
II	5–6	**Blink response to visual threat is intermittently present**	Visual reflexes	Blink-to-visual-threat response consistently present	Blink-to-visual-threat response present in 50 percent of attempts	Blink-to-threat response occurs, but in fewer than 50 percent of attempts	No blink-to-visual-threat response present
II	5–6	**Visual attention now extends beyond near space, up to 4 to 6 feet**	Complexity, distance viewing	Visual attention or eye-to-object contact with targets beyond a distance of 6 feet	Can visually locate or fixate on certain targets at distances as far as 6 feet Ability to detect objects or movement at 4 to 6 feet may depend on the degree of environmental complexity	Occasional ability to locate or fixate on targets as far as 6 feet away, even when the background is visually noncomplex	Visual attention or eye-to-object contact within 3 feet

II	5–6	**May regard familiar faces when voices do not compete**	Complexity, novelty	Makes eye-to-face contact, even if inconsistent, and maybe simultaneously with speech	Glances at or looks directly into faces of familiar people, but only when the familiar person is not speaking	Glances at or looks directly into faces, but responses are inconsistent or fleeting	No regard of the human face
III	7–8	**Selection of toys or objects is less restricted; requires one to two sessions of "warm up"**	Complexity, novelty	Novel objects that match complexity requirements are visually regarded	Looks at new objects that have attributes of familiar objects Recognizes new object immediately after one to two presentations	Look at new objects that have attributes of familiar ones, but requires more than two presentations before object is recognized immediately	Looks at familiar objects; novel objects must closely resemble familiar ones
III	7–8	**Competing auditory stimuli tolerated during periods of viewing; may now maintain visual attention on objects that produce music**	Complexity	No amount of sensory information interferes with visual attention	Is able to look at objects that simultaneously produce music or other sounds	Occasionally is able to maintain visual attention while other sensory input competes Particular types of sensory inputs may continue to interfere with visual attention	Visual attention depends on low or no additional sensory input
III	7–8	**Blink response to visual threat consistently present**	Visual reflexes	Blinks to approach of unexpected inputs within a complex environment	Blinks simultaneous to the approach of an object or open hand moving quickly on midline toward the face	Occasionally blinks to the approach of an object or hand moving quickly on midline toward the face	No blink-to-threat response
III	7–8	**Latency rarely present**	Latency	Delayed response to visual input never occurs	Seldom demonstrates a delay in detecting a target after it is presented	Novel objects, complex environments, or fatigue may increase degree of delayed response	Delayed response to new and familiar targets continues to exist

(continued on next page)

APPENDIX 20A (Continued)

Phase	Range	Statement	CVI Characteristic	R	+	+/−	−
III	7–8	Visual attention extends to 10 feet with targets that produce movement*	Movement, complexity, distance viewing	Visual attention even beyond 10 feet and/or visual attention up to 10 feet with targets that are stable	Is able to visually locate and/or fixate on certain targets at distances as far as 10 feet away, especially with targets that produce movement Attention at this distance may depend on the degree of complexity of the environment	Occasionally gives visual attention to targets at 10 feet, generally when the environment is controlled for other sensory inputs	No visual attention to any targets at distances as far as 10 feet
III	7–8	Movement not required for attention at near	Movement, complexity	Is able to detect targets that do not have moving, shiny, or reflective properties beyond near distance	Is able to visually detect and attend to objects or visual targets that do not move or are not made of shiny or reflective materials within 18 to 24 inches	Occasionally is able to detect and attend to visual targets beyond 2 feet	Is not able to detect or attend to nonmoving targets beyond 2 feet
III	7–8	Smiles at/regards familiar and new faces*	Complexity, novelty	Has eye-to-eye contact with most faces; discriminates new from known people	Glances at and/or has eye-to-eye contact with familiar and new faces	Occasionally glances toward and/or makes eye contact with familiar faces	Gives no attention to faces
III	7–8	May enjoy regarding self in mirror*	Complexity, novelty	Maintains consistent eye-to-eye contact with self in mirror	Consistently glances and/or looks directly at mirror image even though eye-to-eye contact may not occur	Inconsistently glances at own image in mirror	Mirror primarily serves as a light-gazing device
III	7–8	Most high-contrast colors and/or familiar patterns regarded	Color, complexity, novelty	Is able to visually attend to materials that have more than two to three colors that may not include the preferred color	Is able to visually attend to objects of any bright color or objects that have simple, multicolor patterns	Is able to visually attend to some simple patterns, especially familiar ones or those that are highlighted with the preferred color	Preferred color continues to be necessary as an element of an object

III	7–8	**Simple books, picture cards, or symbols regarded**✲	Complexity, novelty	Is able to visually identify elements of age-appropriate books or other two-dimensional materials	Visually attends to two-dimensional materials that have little complexity and that include one- to two-color images	Visually attends to a small set of two-dimensional materials; is not able to generalize the images to new contexts May use lightbox and lightbox pictures to facilitate attention to two-dimensional details	Is visually inattentive to two-dimensional materials
III	9–10	**Selection of objects not restricted**	Complexity, novelty	Demonstrates visual curiosity and seeks out novel objects or materials	Is able to visually examine and/or interact with objects of any color and of any surface pattern, even if they are novel	Recognizes and/or attends to visually novel objects with a single previous experience	Visually attends to objects that share elements of familiar objects
III	9–10	**Only the most complex environments affect visual response**	Complexity, novelty	Demonstrates visual curiosity in complex environments, identifies or attends to novel elements within 20 feet	Demonstrates visual curiosity in familiar and novel environments, except those with an extreme degree of visual and other sensory complexity	Demonstrates visual curiosity in familiar environments that have low degrees of sensory complexity	Does not demonstrate visual curiosity
III	9–10	**Latency resolved**	Latency	Directs vision to indicate wants or needs	Demonstrates no delay in visually detecting a target after it is presented	Rarely demonstrates a delayed visual response to a target	Demonstrates a delayed visual response to targets when tired or overstimulated
III	9–10	**No color or pattern preferences**	Color	Demonstrates typical abilities to attend to colors or patterns	Color highlighting or pattern adjustment or highlighting is not required for visual attention	Some novel patterns or symbols require color highlighting for visual attention	Color highlighting of salient features or details is required for visual attention

(continued on next page)

APPENDIX 20A (Continued)

Phase	Range	Statement	CVI Characteristic	R	+	+/-	-
III	9–10	**Visual attention extends beyond 20 feet**✶	Distance viewing	Is able to visually locate and/or fixate on targets at distances commensurate with peers	Is able to visually locate and/or fixate on certain targets at distances up to and possibly beyond 20 feet away	Is able to visually locate and/or fixate on targets that produce movement or are shiny or reflective at distances of 20 feet / Is able to visually locate and/or fixate on targets without movement 10 to 19 feet away; complexity of environment will continue to affect distance	Is able to visually locate and/or fixate on targets up to 10 feet away
III	9–10	**Views books or other two-dimensional materials, simple images**	Complexity	Identifies salient features of two-dimensional materials with no adjustment or adaptation	Detects or identifies pictures or symbols in books with simple configurations	Detects or identifies familiar elements in familiar two-dimensional, simple materials	Is visually inattentive to two-dimensional materials
III	9–10	**Uses vision to imitate actions**✶	Complexity	Repeats actions in response to an indirect, incidental model	Repeats actions in response to a direct model	Repeats actions in response to a visual and physical prompt model	Does not imitate visual actions
III	9–10	**Demonstrates memory of visual events**✶	Complexity, distance viewing	Anticipates an action or event based on environmental visual cues	Demonstrates recognition of a person, place, or event that has occurred in the past	Demonstrates recognition of a person, place, or event that occurs in a rote routine	Demonstrates no recognition of actions or events that occur as a rote routine

III	9–10	**Displays typical visual-social responses**✳	Complexity	Initials social contact or demonstrates withdrawal from unfamiliar individuals	Demonstrates appropriate affective social responses to input from facial expressions or gestures of adults or peers	Demonstrates appropriate affective social responses with familiar people	Demonstrates no reliable affective or social responses to peers or adults
III	9–10	**Visual fields unrestricted**✳	Visual fields	Has full use of both central and peripheral visual fields	Has full functional use of peripheral visual fields; some central visual difficulties related to complexity	Demonstrates greater reliance on peripheral fields; may continue to use near viewing for two-dimensional materials	Demonstrates visual field preferences
III	9–10	**Look and reach completed as a single action**	Visually guided reach	Consistently uses visually guided reach, regardless of the size of target or complexity of background	Uses visually guided reach, but may be affected by size of target or complexity of background	Uses visually guided reach only when the background complexity is reduced	Rarely uses visually guided reach
III	9–10	**Attends to two-dimensional images against complex backgrounds**✳	Complexity	Is able to identify salient features and additional details in unadapted, two-dimensional materials with backgrounds of high visual complexity	Is able to identify salient features and additional details in age-appropriate two-dimensional materials with minor or no adaptations	Is able to identify salient features in adapted two-dimensional materials with backgrounds of low complexity	Is not able to identify salient features in two-dimensional materials

✳An asterisk after a statement in column 3 indicates that the CVI characteristic associated with the statement may not resolve if the student has a co-existing ocular visual impairment.

Source: Reprinted from Christine Roman-Lantzy, Cortical Visual Impairment: An Approach to Assessment and Intervention (New York: AFB Press, 2007).

CHAPTER 21

Travel Instruction for Individuals with Nonvisual Disabilities

Bruce B. Blasch, William R. Wiener, Patricia J. Voorhees, Barbara Minick, and Jay Furlong

LEARNING QUESTIONS

- What are the similarities and differences between orientation and mobility (O&M) training and travel instruction?

- What are the fundamental principles that are shared by orientation and mobility for individuals with a visual impairment and travel instruction for sighted individuals with disabilities?

- What conditions might affect mobility and produce a functional limitation in independent travel?

- What are some of the social and environmental constraints that restrict an individual's mobility?

This chapter presents an expanded perspective on mobility training for people with a variety of disabilities, similar to the model of serving all disabilities that is prevalent within physical therapy and occupational therapy. In view of the current trends such as the need to be more cost-effective with the instructional time of the orientation and mobility (O&M) specialist, increasing budgetary limitations, and the increasing cost of gas, the future may bring an increasing demand for O&M specialists who can provide independent mobility training in a local area to both the small population of persons with visual impairment and the larger number of sighted individuals with functional mobility problems.

This chapter briefly summarizes the history of travel instruction (TI) programs for teaching independent travel to individuals with functional mobility limitations, reviews the similarities and differences between O&M and TI, and proposes a model containing principles that are fundamental to both. It also describes techniques routinely used in TI and the travel needs of people with specific disabilities.

It is inspiring to reflect upon the impact that O&M instruction, which began at the Hines VA Hospital, has had upon programs for individuals with visual impairment across the United States and in other countries around the world, as detailed in Chapters 13, 14, and 15 in Volume 1 of this book. The success of O&M instruction has also inspired the development of similar training for people with nonvisual disabilities. For a long time there was a tendency to ignore the needs of individuals who had other disabilities that lead to restrictions in independent mobility and who would benefit from mobility training (Blasch, 1994). More recently, travel training for individuals with intellectual disabilities began to appear in various locations, in most cases as either a direct or indirect spin-off from O&M programs (Wiener & Siffermann, 1999).

The term *travel instruction* has come to be applied to "one-to-one instruction provided to people with disabilities other than blindness or visual impairments whose purpose is to enable safe and independent travel in unprotected environments, including on public transit" (Competencies for the Practice of Travel Instruction and Travel Training, n.d.). This type of instruction, while similar to O&M, has some specific differences, as explained later in this chapter. This type of training first sprang up in an unorganized fashion in different parts of the United States. In many cases, families of sighted children with functional mobility problems who witnessed the success of children and adults with visual impairment in achieving independent mobility began to want the same mobility independence for their family members. Out of necessity, since there were no formalized programs to prepare travel instructors at that time, people with as little as a high school education and very limited training began providing what became known as *travel training* or *travel instruction* for individuals with disabilities other than blindness. With

the advent of IDEA and the inclusion of travel instruction (2004) as a component of special education, there began a growing demand to provide training in independent mobility for all individuals with mobility limitations.

Currently, no existing university preparation programs provide professionally trained travel instructors. However, some O&M specialists provide travel instruction for sighted individuals with functional mobility problems. Some of these professionals are in private practice and some are already employed by school systems to teach both students with visual impairments and sighted students with other disabilities.

TRAVEL INSTRUCTION TO DATE

What would be the outcome if an O&M specialist had additional training to teach independent travel to individuals with nonvisual disabilities? In one attempt to find out, the Wisconsin Council of Developmental Disabilities funded a project (Blasch, 1982) to employ an O&M specialist with training in travel instruction for individuals with nonvisual disabilities, to provide mobility instruction to individuals with a broad range of disabilities. The individuals served had the following disabilities and diseases: cognitive, communication, hearing, behavioral, and learning disabilities, and specific physical disabilities such as cerebral palsy, cardiopulmonary pathology, muscular dystrophy, emphysema, and epilepsy. In 7 percent of the students, visual impairment was listed as a secondary impairment. While there are many reasons for providing this service, one of the outcome measures used in this study was cost savings. Cost savings reflected the difference between the costs for specialized transportation provided prior to the implementation of this TI program and the costs for public transportation required after TI had been provided. A cost savings of $117,540 was realized in its first year of operation, based on 36 participants, after the costs of the O&M specialists were deducted (Blasch, 1982). An even more telling measure of the perceived value of this program, however, may be the fact that at the end of the project, Milwaukee County (Wisconsin) Department of Public Works hired the O&M instructor involved to continue providing a comprehensive mobility program for visually impaired and sighted individuals with disabilities.

In addition to the University of Wisconsin master's degree program (1977–1981) funded by the Rehabilitation Services Administration, a baccalaureate program in travel instruction was funded by the U.S. Office of Education at Western Michigan University in the fall of 1999. The purpose of the program was to graduate 8 to 10 students per year who would teach people with disabilities other than blindness to travel independently. After 5 years of operation, the program graduated 40 students as travel instructors. Of that number, 24 went on to study orientation and mobility at the master's level and practice both travel instruction and orientation and mobility. One went on to study rehabilitation teaching and rehabilitation counseling, and three became occupational therapists. The remainder continued to practice within the field of travel instruction with people who had nonvisual disabilities (Helen Lee, personal communication, 1999). Those who integrated travel instruction with orientation and mobility were described by their supervisors as being more knowledgeable about disabilities than the typical orientation and mobility specialist. They were appreciated by their employers for their broad knowledge and have shown that the integration of travel instruction with orientation and mobility establishes a valued professional.

Similar comprehensive programs have been carried out by Pittsburgh Public Schools (Laus, 1974, 1977), Montgomery County (Norristown, PA) Intermediate Unit No. 23 (Williams, Hoff, Millaway, & Cassidy, 1982), Wayne County (Dear-

born Heights, MI) Associations for the Retarded (Brambila-Hickman & Denniston, 1984), and Allegheny County (Homestead, PA) Intermediate Unit No. 3 (Holsopple & Beigay, 1998–present). These programs have demonstrated the success and effectiveness of providing TI to individuals with disabilities other than visual impairment. In many of these situations, it was an O&M specialist with additional preparation who provided the travel instruction. Programs in the state of Pennsylvania (such as the Allegheny Intermediate Unit) employ special education certified teachers with specialized, comprehensive additional training in travel instruction.

There are also professionally staffed programs available to assist persons with certain physical impairments to learn to use prosthetic devices or other equipment such as wheelchairs and orthopedic canes, to assist in locomotion, or to relearn the use of muscles needed for ambulation (Blasch & Welsh, 1980). There are also programs to teach cognitively impaired individuals specific routes, methods for crossing streets, or bus-riding skills (LaGrow, Wiener, & LaDuke, 1990).

In terms of the need for TI programs, a study published in *Critical Issues in Special Education* (Sorrells, Rieth, & Sindelar, 2004) indicated that only 29.4 percent of individuals with mental retardation and 32.5 percent of those who were orthopedically impaired were reported as having "High Community Living Skills," which includes, among other things, independent mobility skills, bus travel, and the like. By comparison, persons who were visually impaired had a higher rating of 41.2 percent. In a comparative study (Sheppard-Jones, Prout, & Kleinert, 2005), "Results indicate that when a significant disability is present, a lack of transportation is an even greater problem, which could further explain the discrepancies found in employment." A survey conducted in Maryland (Conley, 2003) reported that transportation issues created employment difficulties for 75 percent or more of the individuals needing vocational supports.

SIMILARITIES AND DIFFERENCES BETWEEN O&M AND TI

TI is a close relative of O&M. While there are differences that separate the two disciplines, there are many more similarities than differences. TI for students who have disabilities other than visual impairment is generally a short-term program of instruction that culminates with the use of public transportation to reach objectives. In contrast O&M is a more comprehensive program of instruction that can take many months when comprehensive services are required. The basic structures of the two professions, however, are much the same. The model of TI for children unfolds with a sequence of fundamental skills, pre-TI, and transportation training (Wiener & Siffermann, 1999). In contrast, O&M for children consists of basic skills, indoor travel, and residential, rural, business, downtown, and public transportation. The elements of concept development, spatial concepts, cognitive mapping, spatial updating, memorization, public interaction, problem solving, decision making, and psychosocial functioning are common to both.

Fundamental Skills

In the fundamental skills portion of TI, the consumer often requires basic concepts before independent travel is possible. These concepts include such items as telling time (although not a necessary skill for independence in travel), dialing the phone (both a public telephone and a cell phone) and communicating, using a self-identification system, and handling money. Many of these fundamental skills are taught in the early years by classroom teachers (both special education and regular education) but often need to be taught or reinforced by travel instructors. O&M specialists, of course, teach concept development but concentrate more on the concepts relating to body awareness and spatial awareness

(see Chapter 7 and Volume 1, Chapter 5). The O&M specialist often teaches students about their bodies and how they move through space. The travel instructor spends more time on the basics of personal organization, interacting with others, problem solving, and decision-making and fundamental orientation skills.

Pre-TI Skills

Travel instruction programs within a school facility can begin with developing some fundamental skills prior to independent travel. These can include increasing basic pedestrian concepts, recognizing landmarks, using signage, communication with others, and general rules of safety. These skills can be developed in the community surrounding the school the student may attend, or within the student's neighborhood. This is accomplished by walking routes and locating objectives. In this process there is much similarity between elements of O&M and TI. The main differences revolve around the techniques that are used to facilitate independent travel. Travelers without visual impairment are taught to depend on their vision to ensure their safety as they walk along the block and make street crossings. While O&M specialists teach the use of vision to students with low vision, they also teach a comprehensive system of nonvisual techniques to permit safe travel using sensory substitution relying in part on hearing and the sense of touch through the cane.

Transportation Training and Independent Travel

Independent travel instruction typically is taught to a specific destination. The average instructional time for an individual receiving TI is 4–5 weeks (20 to 25 round-trip instructional sessions). Each morning the instructor accompanies the student on a trip to a planned destination, oftentimes a work site or a school, and returns with that student at the end of the day. As part of this instruction, the student learns a specific travel route. Competency must be demonstrated in the street-crossing skills specific to the route, transit, and related travel skills. The type of disability that the individual experiences determines the instruction given. Individuals with intellectual disabilities need to reach full competency levels to identify the route, recognize landmarks along the route, choose the correct bus by reading or matching numbers or words, identify the correct bus coinage, identify a landmark for exiting the bus, interact appropriately with others along the travel route and on the bus, and make timely and appropriate decisions. Individuals who use wheelchairs or other ambulatory devices need to learn how to best use their equipment to travel in a challenging environment and to board the bus and demonstrate an understanding of the securement features and how they are applied to their wheelchair. Individuals with forms of autism and other disabilities may need to learn how to find appropriate information in an environment loaded with distracting information. The list of requirements will vary greatly depending on the disability or combination of disabilities. While the O&M specialist needs to keep some of these same considerations in mind when working with individuals with multiple impairments, this is not the case for students who have no disabilities other than blindness.

When examining the two professions, there appear to be many similarities between travel instruction and O&M. In O&M the order and length of how these skills are introduced may be different from TI and the use of public transportation may be included at different points from TI. While TI is oftentimes not introduced until during the transitional years of education, there can be an argument made for introducing pre-travel skills at a younger age similar to O&M. Students with the most severe disabilities often require instruction on pre-travel skill concepts, which could be integrated into the special educa-

tion classroom curricula. Individuals with more significant disabilities oftentimes will require more intensive instruction during the independent TI process in order to ensure success. Even with these differences, the functions and the goals are the same.

There is also a striking similarity between the competencies that are required for the effective practice of TI and for O&M. The following competencies in TI were identified and listed according to instructor ranking of importance (Wiener and Siffermann 1999):

- Environmental analysis
- Assessment, instructional methods, and strategies
- Travel concepts
- Travel skills and techniques
- Psychosocial aspects of disability
- Systems of transportation
- Legal and ethical issues
- Administration and supervision
- History and philosophy
- Sensory motor functioning
- Human growth and development
- Professional information
- Medical aspects of disability
- Mobility-related devices

This list was assembled after a thorough job analysis of travel training practitioners at four schools and agencies that had comprehensive programs of instruction. The list is nearly identical in content to O&M competencies and also similar in order of importance. Therefore the two professions share many of the same academic domains and have related functions, although modifications of those functions would occur as a result of the nature of the clientele. Following are some of the most obvious differences.

Differences between TI & O&M

Location Identification

In O&M, the drop-off lesson plays an integral part in building confidence of the student and testing his ability to resolve lost situations. The student is typically dropped off within an area that is familiar and then is expected to gather information while traveling that will result in identification of his location and to travel to a specified objective. In contrast, travel instructors provide an assignment called *location identification*. Travel instructors make this part of the later stages of the training and often tie it in with public transportation. Instead of dropping someone off in a familiar area, they have the student continue travel on a transit vehicle into a new area beyond which they are familiar. Accompanied by the travel instructor, the student is required to identify her location, find a public telephone to contact a family member, and supply specific information as to her whereabouts. Often this is accomplished by visually identifying the name of the streets at the closest corner or by the student entering a store and asking the storekeeper the location of the shop. The student may then plan a trip back or use the phone in the store to contact someone who can help. This difference in approach between O&M and TI is due to the differences between categories of students. TI students with the ability to function visually cannot be dropped off in familiar areas. They instead need to be exposed to new situations and, in the case of lower functioning students without sophisticated problem-solving skills, need to demonstrate safe problem-solving strategies.

Soliciting Aid

A useful technique in O&M is the act of soliciting aid. At times when a student needs further information, she is taught how to approach a stranger and ask questions that will result in useful information about the location of a destination. In contrast, most students of TI are discouraged from soliciting aid from just anyone. This is due to the vulnerability of a person with developmental disabilities who could be manipulated by an unscrupulous person. TI students therefore are taught how to identify and approach uniformed or respected employees such as community workers, store clerks, bank tellers, or uniformed workers such as police or postal service people.

Independent Lessons versus Following

The independent or solo lesson is a part of many O&M programs. Students, once they have reached a specific level of independence, may be asked to travel to an objective without the assistance of an instructor and then return to the starting point. During the exercise, many instructors tell their students that they will be observing to learn how the student uses the information available and to ensure safety. In a similar fashion when teaching independence, TI uses an exercise called a *following* to evaluate the student's ability to travel independently. This is a critical component of TI because it is sometimes a characteristic of students with developmental disabilities to follow the rules when accompanied by an instructor but then to disregard them when observation is withdrawn, or (in the case of an individual, for example, with autism) become overly anxious, which may result in impulsive and unsafe behavior. Anecdotal information has shown that students will sometimes cross on the red light or in the middle of the block when the instructor is not watching. Therefore a "following" is established where the student is told that he will not be observed by the instructor and will be asked to travel independently. In these cases a travel instructor who has not worked with the student is assigned to follow while the student believes that he is traveling independently. This allows the instructor to gain essential information on the safety of the student. While O&M specialists may consider such deception as unethical, travel instructors report that it is essential to gain the information needed for safety, final documentation of achieved competencies, and reassurance to the school system or agency, families, and guardians.

Stranger Approach

As mentioned earlier, many students with developmental disabilities may be vulnerable when traveling independently. Some may be gullible and easily convinced to accept a ride from strangers who may have an unethical motive. To avoid this possibility, students are taught neither to share information with strangers nor to accept rides. One way of assessing the success of this training is to set up an artificial situation where someone perceived as a stranger will offer a ride to a student. Working collaboratively with the local police departments, the travel instructor will arrange for someone such as a plainclothes police officer or detective in an unmarked vehicle to drive by and try to coax the student into his car. If the student accepts, the officer will identify himself, and the instructor who is clandestinely observing will intervene. A collective discussion is held by the travel instructor with the police officer, the student, and the family or guardian to discuss the importance of avoiding potentially unsafe situations. The instructor will then resume instruction regarding the avoidance of strangers or in conjunction with the families or guardian, and reevaluate the student's emotional readiness for independent travel. While O&M specialists have not seen the need for this kind of practice and instead tend to use role-playing to convey this information, travel instructors insist that it is essential to ensure the safety of their students.

Similarities between the Two Models

It is evident that O&M and TI have much in common. The competencies needed for effective practice are similar between the two disciplines. Travel instructors have the need for similar academic competencies but do not have the benefit of university preparation in their discipline. Therefore, the backgrounds of travel instructors ranges from a high school graduate to a master's degree in a related field. Educational agencies are beginning to recognize the need for certified special education teachers with additional competencies in the teaching of travel instruction to school-age children. It is the authors' belief that travel instructors need to have a baccalaureate degree with additional demonstrated competencies in the teaching of travel skills to persons with disabilities. Both O&M and TI services stress independence and gradually require their students to take on more responsibilities for their actions. While the concepts taught may be somewhat different, the need to teach them as preparation for independent travel is essential to both. The length of training is different between the disciplines, with intensive one-on-one TI being shorter and more concentrated but the achievement of independence for an individual with disabilities is recognized after a longer period of instruction on basic skills for travel readiness and the development of travel-related skills. The goal of independent mobility, however, remains the same for both O&M and travel instructors. Based on these commonalities, a model of principles fundamental to both O&M and TI is discussed in some detail in the section that follows.

A FUNDAMENTAL MODEL FOR O&M AND TI

Independent Travel

Independence in mobility involves a number of skills including those required for ambulation or movement, environmental negotiation, and effective social interaction (Blasch & Welsh, 1980). *Independent movement* refers to the act of moving through the environment in a safe and efficient manner (LaGrow & Weessies, 1994), while *environmental negotiation*, or *wayfinding*, refers to the act of moving through the environment with purpose (i.e., to reach a destination) (Passini, Duprae, & Langlois, 1986). Social interaction is essential to the cooperative act of travel required by complex environments (e.g., acquiring assistance or directions, using public transportation, and interacting with others during travel) and is generally a part of the ultimate reason for traveling (i.e., interacting with those at the destination of travel). Deficiency in any of these aspects of independent travel may result in a functional mobility limitation.

Functional Limitations

Any number of conditions may affect mobility. Visual impairment and blindness are among the more obvious of these conditions. The field of blindness and visual impairment has developed the most systematic and comprehensive programs of mobility instruction. The specific mobility consequences of these conditions are well known (Long, McNeal, & Griffin-Shirley, 1990; Smith, De l'Aune, & Geruschat, 1992; Uslan, 1990; Hill & Ponder, 1976; Jacobson, 1993; LaGrow & Weessies, 1994; Welsh & Blasch, 1980). Other conditions are less obvious and often have more subtle effects on one's ability to travel. A hearing impairment, for example, would not necessarily restrict one's ability to get about in an environment. Yet, like a visual impairment, it results in a reduction in the amount and range of information available to the traveler. Those with significant hearing impairments may not benefit from auditory signals, warnings, and environmental or route descriptors, nor may they rely upon public address announcements concerning the arrival, departure, location, destination, or upcoming stop when using public transportation. Most significant, however, they may have difficulty interacting with others throughout every stage of the travel process.

Other individuals with disabilities encounter problems when planning or carrying out routes of travel for different reasons. Mobility skills require the traveler to possess accurate spatial, directional, and environmental concepts; store and recall information from memory; make decisions; and solve problems (Hill & Blasch, 1980). Problems may arise as the result of a number of conditions, including intellectual disabilities, specific learning disabilities, attention deficits, traumatic brain injury (TBI), mental illness, dementia and experiential deficits (Welsh, 1972; Hughes, Smith, & Benitz, 1977; Blasch & Welsh, 1980).

The person with intellectual disabilities may, like the person who is hearing impaired, experience communication problems and, like the person who is congenitally blind, lack certain basic concepts about the environment (Laus, 1977). He is likely to be unable to understand the general layout of the environment sufficiently to solve orientation problems and take alternative routes. He may be stigmatized by certain visible aspects of his disability or inappropriate behaviors in public. Many individuals with intellectual disabilities also have basic posture and gait deficiencies and lack basic skills such as those necessary in money exchanges and safety procedures in negotiating street crossings. All of these difficulties can create mobility problems for the person and make his family strongly resist his traveling alone. The person with intellectual disabilities may, like the person who is hearing impaired, experience communication problems and, like the person who is congenitally blind, lack certain basic concepts about the environment (Laus, 1977). Since those early years of mobility instruction, the societal movements toward mainstreaming and inclusion have caused teachers, rehabilitation counselors, and society at large to focus on an individual's abilities and strengths. Over the years, much time and attention have been dedicated to assisting persons with intellectual disabilities to develop a repertoire of productive and socially adaptive behavior (Beirne-Smith, Ittenback, & Patton, 2002).

A person who has severe behavior and emotional problems may also have travel difficulties. She may lack confidence in her ability to handle the complexity and confusion of large-city environments. In some cases distinctive postures and gait patterns result from institutionalization (e.g., a shuffle or pacing may be caused by being in a confined space, lack of exercise, lack of opportunity for rapid movement, to mention a few; in some cases it is a stereotypical mannerism or modeling of other individuals' gait), while in others an individual's unusual gait may be modeled by other individuals. Therefore, the individual may have developed what has been referred to as an "institutional gait" or pacing behavior that may stigmatize the individual on the street (Haring & Schiefelbusch, 1967). She may exhibit inappropriate, challenging, and stigmatizing behaviors that cause interaction problems with others. Difficulties with crowded areas and crowds in general may produce great anxiety or trigger aggressive reactions. She may have difficulty with impulse control and may be attracted to unsafe neighborhood situations while waiting for transportation. She may become distracted by traffic and crowded streets. Orientation problems and crossing busy streets can cause stress and discourage travel. She may have difficulty planning trips and allowing sufficient time to get to appointments, or may allow too much time and arrive inappropriately early for job interviews or work.

Individuals with certain learning disabilities may also have travel problems. Some are unable to sort out the complex stimuli of the urban environment and become disoriented, particularly if they are away from a frequently traveled route or are required to take a unique route in a familiar area. They may be unable to read street signs and the names of stores or businesses, and therefore have to develop other strategies to maintain orientation and locate objectives. Some persons with learning disabilities are unable to use the numbering systems in large buildings and thus have orientation difficulties. They may have other

difficulties, such as time and money concepts, and coordination deficiencies that make driving difficult or impossible.

Vestibular defects, physical disabilities, heart disease, impairments of the central nervous system, arthritis, emphysema, obesity, and frailty or poor health may reduce one's ability to travel any distance and even the range or speed of movement within an environment. Problems with gait and stability make it difficult to deal with uneven terrain, steps and stairs without railings, and deep curbs and obstacles in the path of travel that must be stepped over. The individual who uses orthopedic or other mobility aids to counter these difficulties (e.g., canes, walkers, wheelchairs, and electric scooters) may not fit through tight spaces, remain stable on lateral tilts, be capable of traversing curbs and steps, or fit on public transport. Furthermore, the speed at which the individual travels, with or without aids, may not be sufficient to allow for safe crossings at some intersections. Similar problems may be faced by elderly or frail travelers as well.

Elderly persons have a number of mobility problems associated with diseases and disabilities that frequently accompany the aging process (see Chapter 10). They may be unable to pass a driver's test, or they may have a restricted driver's license. If elderly people can no longer drive, they may become "passive passengers" and consequently pay less attention to the environment and their orientation. They also may not be able to walk long distances and have difficulty on stairs and inclines. They may fear falling and the complications that come with injury, and they may not be able to cross streets quickly enough to guarantee their safety. Some older persons have their mobility further limited by their environment, especially where they feel vulnerable to attacks and muggings.

Functional mobility limitations can arise for a number of reasons. One cannot predict the difficulties an individual may face with travel by simply identifying a disorder or diagnostic category (Blasch & Welsh, 1980). An analysis of a number of factors is necessary (Blasch, 1994b).

Factors Affecting Independent Mobility

The potential for independent mobility is affected by the interaction between one's personal abilities (Pa), which is in turn affected by type of impairment or condition, illness, and age, and the environmental demands of travel (Ed). As the environmental demand increases, the potential for independence decreases. This interaction may be mediated or modified through an intervention (I). This intervention may be designed to reduce environmental demand or provide the traveler with the skills needed to deal with the environment, or both. Thus, one's potential for mobility independence (Mi) can be conceptualized using the following formula: $Mi = (Pa - Ed) + I$. The following sections, Personal Abilities and Environmental Demands, are presented in relation to factors that limit functional abilities. The sections Intervention and Providing Mobility Instruction to Sighted Individuals with Disabilities present some of the positive approaches to enhance mobility independence.

Personal Abilities

Personal abilities are affected by the presence of impairments, illnesses, and other conditions affecting one's sensory, cognitive, motor, and psychosocial ability. These functional limitations may interact in a manner or degree that subsequently affects the individual's ability to gather, process, or act upon environmental information for the purpose of travel. The degree, type, and number of disabilities affecting the individual interact with other personal variables, including self-concept, motivation, experience, and knowledge, to affect one's overall performance (Blasch & Welsh, 1980; see Chapter 6 in Volumes 1 and 2). The range of disabilities that have affected in-

dependent mobility and have been successfully addressed by an O&M specialist include intellectual, communication, hearing, behavioral, and learning disabilities; cerebral palsy; cardiopulmonary pathology; muscular dystrophy; emphysema; epilepsy; and mental illness (Blasch, 1982). This listing of disabilities is certainly not exhaustive, but serves as a sample of impairments affecting independent mobility. For a listing of personal abilities that relate to one's independent mobility, see Sidebar 21.1.

Sensory Abilities

Safe and purposeful movement through the environment requires the traveler to take in, interpret, and react to information about the environment through which she is moving. Movement can take place without this environmental information, but the movement will be neither oriented nor necessarily safe. Many people have difficulty with independent travel because of deficiencies in their ability to receive or interpret environmental information.

Environmental information is gathered through the visual, auditory, vestibular, tactile, olfactory, proprioceptive, and gustatory senses. Vision is the most efficient of these and provides one with varied and rich information concerning the environment of travel, including traffic and traffic patterns, the path of travel, and obstacles and drop-offs within that path, as well as information that can be gained from signs (e.g., street and store names, the location of exits and restrooms, transit information, and the time to cross streets), maps, and models. The auditory sense also provides long-range information concerning the environment, traffic patterns, and when it is safe to cross a street, in addition to information which may be gained from public address announcements (e.g., transit information or emergency evacuation procedures) or through direct conversation. Other, more direct information may be gained from the vestibular

Personal Abilities That Relate to One's Independent Mobility

I. Sensory

    A. Visual

    B. Auditory

    C. Vestibular

    D. Tactile

    E. Proprioceptive

    F. Olfactory

    G. Gustatory

II. Cognitive

    A. Concept development

    B. Problem-solving and decision-making abilities

    C. Information-gathering and -processing abilities

    D. Short- and long-term memory

III. Motor and psychomotor

    A. Perceptual abilities

    B. Body awareness

    C. Posture

    D. Balance and gait

    E. Speed

    F. Endurance and stamina

    G. Strength

    H. Flexibility

    I. Agility

    J. Perceptual and motor coordination

IV. Psychosocial characteristics

    A. Self-concept

    B. Motivation

    C. Experience

    D. Personality

---

proprioceptive–kinesthetic systems, and from the tactile and olfactory senses as well.

The information gained from the senses needs to be processed before it is usable. Deficiencies in the information-processing system may be caused by single or multiple impairments of the sense systems themselves or by problems in the perceptual mechanisms through which the person interprets the information picked up and delivered by the senses. Deficiencies in either system may pose barriers to travel, as can other conditions that affect one's ability to gain or process information.

Cognitive Abilities

The information gained needs to be turned into usable concepts (i.e., spatial and environmental)

before it can be acted upon (Hill & Blasch, 1980; see Volume 1, Chapter 1). Individuals with intellectual disabilities and those who have specific learning disabilities or other cognitive impairments, especially if these are present from birth, are more likely to experience difficulty in developing adequate body, spatial, and environmental concepts. These concepts are very important to orientation and subsequent environmental negotiation or wayfinding.

Purposeful negotiation of an environment requires the individual to establish and maintain orientation while traveling (see Chapter 2 and Volume 1, Chapter 2). To do this, the individual needs to understand the environment well enough to plan and execute routes, reverse routes, and use alternate routes when necessary. This requires an ability to store and recall information, solve problems, and make decisions, all of which may be difficult for persons with cognitive problems. Related to these skills is the ability to read maps or other representations of the environment as aids in planning a route or understanding an area. Problems with these skills may not pose insurmountable barriers to travel, but do pose limitations or a need for alternative solutions. Communication deficits often associated with cognitive problems (i.e., reading, aural comprehension, and oral–aural interaction) may limit the amount and type of information that may be available to the individual during the mobility process (see Chapter 17).

Deficiencies in the ability to solve problems that arise during travel may be due to the lack of appropriate concepts for doing so, failure to attend to relevant stimuli, problems with the process involved in reasoning and decision making, or the lack of efficient strategies for doing so (see Chapter 12). Some impairments, especially those that directly affect cognitive functioning, obviously affect a person's reasoning powers and therefore his problem-solving abilities. For others, difficulties with reasoning and problem solving are related more to their lack of opportunity to be responsible for themselves, often resulting from a pattern of social interaction in which the person with the disability is never allowed to make decisions and suffer the consequences of wrong decisions. Without such experiences, a problem-solving skill does not generally develop (Hughes et al., 1977; National Research Council, 2000).

Motor and Psychomotor Abilities

Purposeful negotiation of the environment requires more than the skills involved in orientation; it also depends on the ability to move within and through the environment. One's ability to move may be affected by a number of factors, including the actual ability to do so (e.g., posture, balance, gait, speed, endurance, strength,

flexibility, agility, and motor control). Some individuals may be unable to move due to paralysis, while others may have difficulty in their ability to direct their movement based upon the sensory information they receive. In the former, the problem does not exist in the receptive mechanisms, but rather in the person's ability to produce accurate movements based upon the information received or because of neural disruption. This can cause difficulties in locomotion as well as in driving a vehicle (Bardoch, 1970). Others have problems negotiating various aspects of the physical environment (e.g., dealing with uneven terrain, stepping up curbs, and traversing stairs without handrails).

Some physical and neurological impairments involve the skeletal and neuromuscular components of the body that are responsible for a person's ability to stand upright and ambulate with an erect posture. Other impairments affect posture and gait indirectly through the difficulties a person has in perceiving correct posture and making changes in his own stance in relation to the vertical, or as a result of the reluctance of families and teachers to expect and reinforce correct posture in children with disabilities.

Poor posture and gait can make movement through the environment inefficient, uncomfortable, or even impossible (see Volume 1, Chapter 5). Some posture and gait deficiencies make movement more precarious since they impair the reflexes through which the individual draws back from danger. Others make reactions slower and movements less precise (Aust, 1980; Rosen, 1997). Reductions in strength, flexibility, and agility pose similar problems for the individual when dealing with terrain changes, steps, and curbs. Thus the individual's mobility may be limited by physical demands that the environment places on the traveler (see Chapter 12). Similar restrictions may be imposed by reduced endurance and speed, especially as it affects the range of travel (see Chapters 5 and 18, and Volume 1, Chapter 5).

Psychosocial Characteristics

Psychosocial factors refer to the social and psychological variables that affect the way an individual relates to the social and physical environment in which he lives and travels (see Chapter 6, Volumes 1 and 2). These variables affect one's expectations of self in terms of the types of behaviors that can or need to be carried out, and the likelihood of successfully doing so. The latter is referred to as the *sense of self-efficacy*: "Efficacy expectations determine how much effort people will expend and how long they will persist in the face of obstacles and aversive experiences" (Bandura, 1977, p. 194). They are affected most of all by the cumulative effects of one's efforts and may be altered by one's experiences and interactions with others (Bandura, 1977). For a recent national study relating to psychosocial characteristics, refer to the National Longitudinal Transition Study—2 (NLTS2), funded by the National Center for Special Education Research at the Institute of Education Sciences, U.S. Department of Education, and initiated in 2001. This study provides a national picture of the self-concept of youth with disabilities as they moved into adulthood and includes self-representations of themselves, their schooling, their personal relationships, and their hopes for the future. For a complete treatment of psychosocial factors, see Chapter 6, Volumes 1 and 2.

Consideration of Other Factors

The degree to which any of the disabling conditions will affect one's performance is dependent on a number of factors. The first is the history of the impairment or health problem experienced and the effect it has on personality, self-concept, and sensory, cognitive, and motor abilities. The second is the number of disabilities experienced and the interactive effect they have on performance. One need only examine the potentially disabling conditions and their causes to appreci-

ate the possibilities for different effects across individuals (see Sidebar 21.2).

The third consideration to keep in mind is that the effects of a disability associated with an impairment or illness vary for each individual in relation to type, location, extent, stability, and age of onset (LaGrow, 1992). And finally, it seems that disability has a variable effect on performance across individuals due to differences in self-concept, motivation, experience, and knowledge (Blasch & Welsh, 1980).

Environmental Demands or Constraints

Personal ability and the degree of environmental accessibility interact to produce functional mobility limitations. Constraints may arise from one's social environment, while demands are usually placed on the traveler by the physical environment. The social environment consists of those people whose actions affect the individual, including family members, rule and policy makers, environmental planners, service providers, the public in general, and others using the environment (see Sidebar 21.3).

Social Environment

Family members and others in authority (e.g., teachers, principals, and supervisors of day or residential facilities) may restrict an individual's opportunities for, and therefore experience with, travel in an attempt to protect that person from the perceived dangerous and embarrassing aspects of travel. They may also do so because of a misconception, due to either ignorance or prejudice, of the individual's ability or potential for travel (see Chapter 6, Volumes 1 and 2). Rule makers (e.g., principals, superintendents, lawmakers, and people responsible for instruction) may wish to protect themselves or their employees (or constituents if in government) from potential environmental hazards, or they simply

Potentially Disabling Conditions and Their Causes

I. Sensory disabilities

   A. Visual impairment

   B. Hearing impairment

   C. Vestibular and kinesthetic dysfunction

II. Circulatory disorders

   A. Arteriosclerosis

   B. Heart disease

III. Orthopedic disorders

   A. Amputations

   B. Arthritis

   C. Muscular dystrophy

IV. Disorders of the central nervous system

   A. Stroke

      1. Spasticity

      2. Rigidity

      3. Hemiplegia

   B. Neoplasm—tumors

   C. Epilepsy and other seizure disorders

   D. Cerebral palsy

      1. Spasticity

      2. Athetosis

      3. Ataxia

      4. Tremor and rigidity

      5. Mixed types

   E. Multiple sclerosis

   F. Parkinson's disease

   G. Spinal cord dysfunction

      1. Paraplegia

      2. Quadriplegia

   H. Spina bifida

   I. Traumatic brain injury (TBI)

V. Respiratory disorders

   A. Emphysema

   B. Asthma and allergies

VI. Behavioral disability

   A. Attention deficit disorder (ADD)

   B. Attention deficit hyperactivity disorder (ADHD)

VII. Intellectual and perceptual disabilities

   A. Specific learning disabilities (SLD)

   B. Intellectual disabilities—mild (ID-Mi)

   C. Intellectual disabilities—moderate (ID-Mo)

   D. Intellectual disabilities—severe (ID-Severe)

   E. Intellectual disabilities—profound (ID-Profound)

   F. Emotional disability and mental illness

VIII. Geriatric disorders (pathologies associated with aging)

IX. Endocrine disorders

   A. Obesity

   B. Body disproportion

   C. Diabetes

   D. Body structural disorders

      1. Gigantism

      2. Dwarfism

X. Communicative disorders

   A. Articulation

   B. Delayed speech development

   C. Aphasia

XI. Genetic disorders

   A. Trisomy 21

   B. Fragile X

   C. Prader-Willi syndrome

   D. Williams syndrome

   E. Mitochondrial myopathy

XII. Neurological disabilities

   A. Autism

   B. Asperger's syndrome

(continued on next page)

Environmental Factors Affecting Functional Mobility

I. Social factors

   A. Family responses

      1. Overprotectiveness versus support

      2. Realistic versus idealistic expectations

      3. Flexibility versus inflexibility

   B. General public

      1. Understanding versus ignorance

      2. Supportive assistance (as necessary) versus prejudice or fear

II. Physical factors

   A. Buildings

      1. Public

         a. Entrances, doors, doorways, and door handles

         b. Stairs, ramps, and handrails

         c. Hallways, corridors, and aisles

         d. Floors and floor coverings

         e. Toilet facilities

         f. Furniture

         g. Elevators and escalators

         h. Telephone locations

         i. Drinking fountains

         j. Suspended objects and projections

         k. Display islands

         l. Signage (e.g., directional arrows, universal signs, and raised numbers)

         m. Concessions and vending machines

         n. Coatracks and cloakrooms

         o. Lighting, including neon, strobe, and fluorescent

         p. Isolated areas

      2. Commercial

         a. Counters and aisles

         b. Seating

         c. Cafeteria lines—ordering and utensils

         d. Box office

         e. Turnstiles

         f. Ticket machines and kiosks

      3. Residential

         a. Furnishings

         b. Key locks and keypads

         c. Controls (e.g., light and heat)

         d. Kitchen counters, cupboards, and appliances

   B. Residential neighborhoods

      a. Curbs, curb cuts, curb ramps, and gutters

      b. Crosswalks

      c. Traffic signals and intersection design

      d. Parking lots

      e. Signage

      f. Sidewalks and footpaths

      g. Driveways

      h. Manhole covers and gratings

      i. Mailboxes, fire hydrants, and trash receptacles

      j. Overhanging branches, shrubbery, and fences

      k. Public telephones

      l. Drinking fountains

   C. Business and shopping districts

      a. Parking and passenger loading zones

      b. Barricades

      c. Outdoor steps and stairs

      d. Projections, control boxes, and poles

(continued on next page)

e. Parking meters

f. Vending machines

g. Furniture

h. Landscaping, outdoor planters, and ornamental structures

i. Sidewalks and footpaths

D. Metropolitan areas

  a. Street widths

  b. Crowd congestion

  c. Masking noises

  d. Safety islands

  e. Roundabouts

  f. Open excavation sites

  g. Intersection design, traffic flow, and traffic patterns

E. Manufacturing and industrial sites

  a. Entrances

  b. Gates

  c. Platforms and loading docks

  d. Industrial machines and equipment

F. Transportation systems

  1. Bus and trolley

    a. Steps

    b. Railings

    c. Seating

    d. Crowd congestion

    e. Shelters

    f. Fare boxes and systems of payment

    g. Ramps and lifts

    h. Securements

  2. Subways and elevated trains

    a. Turnstiles

    b. Platforms

    c. Gaps

    d. High-level platforms

    e. Bridge plates

    f. Elevators

    g. Escalators

    h. Moving sidewalks

  3. Airplanes and trains

    a. Terminals

    b. Stations

    c. Airports

  4. Cars, taxis, and vans, including accessible features

  5. Paratransit

G. Recreational facilities

  1. Parks, monuments, historic sites, and trails

    a. Width of walkways

    b. Surface of walkways

    c. Access to swimming facilities

    d. Recreation equipment

    e. Access to information and directions

  2. Amusement parks

  3. Athletic centers

  4. Movie theaters

  5. Malls

  6. Parking lots

  7. Public announcements

III. Climatic factors

A. Weather

  1. Cold, including wind chill factor

  2. Rain, snow, and hail

  3. Heat and humidity, including heat index

  4. Wind

B. Air quality

  1. Pollution—pollen and car fumes

  2. Altitude—high and low

may not be concerned enough to fully consider the needs of anyone "outside of the norm." Environmental planners (e.g., architects, engineers, and governmental planners) now need to take into account the Americans with Disabilities Act (ADA) to make certain that new and existing structures are in compliance with the law. ADA requirements extend to all public spaces and include buildings, malls, streets, campuses, neighborhoods, and transit systems (see Chapter 12 and Volume 1, Chapter 11).

Service providers (e.g., information and transit personnel; clerks in stores, offices, and hotels; waiters and waitresses; and sales personnel) also need to be aware of and be in compliance with the ADA law. In years past accessibility may have been limited due to ignorance, embarrassment, or prejudice. However, the traveler with a disability is less stigmatized due to inclusion within the schools and modifications to the community, which allow for accessibility to provide a venue to pursue everyday activities.

Physical Environment

The physical structure of the environment may place demands on people to perform at a level that is beyond their capacity. All people have limits in terms of the types of terrain they can traverse; however, some have real difficulties with environments that have been constructed with the able-bodied traveler in mind (Morgan, 1976). This may be true even after environmental modification. Those persons may only be able to travel safely and efficiently in low-demand environments (e.g., a single-story building with no stairs and easily opened doors) or those specifically designed to enhance accessibility (e.g., those with ramps and elevators provided for access, quality lighting and signage, accessible toilets and drinking fountains, removed or modified turnstiles, and revolving doors) (see Chapter 12 and Volume 1, Chapter 11). Many factors must be

considered when evaluating the potential effect of the environment on travel.

The demands that environments (this includes work, education, and the health system) place on travel have a varying effect on individual performance. Some may be too complex or require too much memory, while others demand too much agility, speed, or endurance. Wide-open spaces may prove to be troublesome for visually impaired individuals (Smith et al., 1992), while areas with tight passages may be impossible to traverse for persons in wheelchairs, and those without sidewalks restrict the elderly to their homes and yards (Long et al., 1990). The effect of the interaction between personal ability and environmental demands and constraints may be mediated through intervention.

Intervention

Interventions may involve a number of strategies carried out on both a personal and societal level. These strategies include modifying the environments, advocating for the rights of the traveler, educating the public, and providing formalized and comprehensive TI to individuals with functional limitations. The first two aim to reduce the demands of the physical environment on the traveler. The third seeks to remove undue constraints imposed by the social environment, and the last is designed to enable the individual to circumvent those that remain. (See Sidebar 21.4.)

Environmental Modification

Environments may be physically modified to enhance their accessibility, reduce the demand they impose on performance levels, and make travel easier. Many of these modifications are relatively simple and inexpensive (e.g., physical barriers may be removed, ramps or handrails may be installed, lighting added, signage improved, route markers added, and memory cues

---

SIDEBAR 21.4

Intervention Strategies to Promote Independent Mobility

I. Environmental modification

   A. Societal

   B. Task and environmentally specific

II. Advocacy

   A. Institutional or societal advocacy

   B. Personal advocacy

III. Education and instruction

   A. Public education

   B. Direct individual instruction

---

provided). They may be done to improve the accessibility of environments in general. The ADA, which is federal law, now requires state and local municipalities to meet standards of accessibility in all public places (see Chapter 12 and Volume 1, Chapter 11). As such, barriers to safe travel are being removed and accessibility to public places is being improved. Newly constructed environments are being built with these regulations in mind. Standards have been set for all public places. However, general modifications for accessibility (i.e., braille markings in elevators and curb cuts at intersections) are not yet in place in every environment, nor can they be expected for years to come. Furthermore, mandated modifications are not appropriate or sufficient for every need, since they are indeed general standards and cannot hope to account for the specific abilities or disabilities of every individual. Thus, some personal solutions may be required as well.

These solutions tend to be both task and environment specific. Where possible, they may be made by the traveler, an instructor, or a family member (e.g., those made around the home, school, or place of work). In other cases, appropriate authorities (e.g., transit or municipal) may have to be approached for action. In many instances, modifying the immediate environment may be the most effective intervention available.

Advocacy

Advocacy by and on behalf of persons with disabilities is a key to their successful integration in society. It was through large-scale advocacy that disabled persons' rights to equal opportunity, education, and access were recognized and protected by the law. Groups of and for people with disabilities continue to lobby to ensure that gains made in the Architectural Barriers Act of 1968, the Rehabilitation Act of 1973 (with the 1992 amendments), and the ADA of 1990 (PL 101–336) are enforced and continue to be improved upon (see Volume 1, Chapter 12). Institutional or societal advocacy is often required to get system-wide changes made. Yet, a more direct approach with local authorities is also required to meet individual needs.

In this case, specific barriers to an individual's independence and possible solutions for their travel may be addressed. The local transit authority, for example, may be approached directly to get a particular bus stop added or changed along a route to accommodate the needs of a given traveler by lowering demands for performance that may block her successful participation in everyday life. A street sign posing a hazard to an individual may be moved to ensure safety, or a business may be asked to comply with a local ordinance banning delivery vehicles from parking on the crosswalk. This may be done by the individual, a travel instructor, an O&M specialist, a professional advocate, or a consumer group, or through the organized efforts of associations.

Public Education

Educational programs may be provided for the public or to targeted groups (e.g., teachers, nurses, police, and architects) as another form of advocacy to reduce some of the social barriers or constraints that limit the individual's opportunity to travel. Programs may be designed to raise awareness of the abilities and needs of disabled travelers or provide specific instruction to those who are expected to meet those needs. For example each transit agency is responsible for training its operators. Although instruction can vary, the primary focus is on the safe operation of the vehicle and with learning the myriad of routes. However, the ADA requires sensitivity and awareness training for operators of both mass transit and paratransit. Operators learn how to use the wheelchair lift and how to apply the securements to the passenger and his wheelchair. This provides a valuable and meaningful opportunity for travel instructors and O&M specialists to present at these sessions. It may also be valuable to include students to discuss some of the strategies they have learned in using public transportation.

Individual Instruction

Direct individual instruction is required to teach the individual with functional mobility limitations the skills and strategies needed to cope with the demands of the environment, establish and maintain orientation, plan routes to reach destinations while circumventing obstacles, use public transit systems, and interact with the public and service providers during travel (Laus, 1977).

Ideally, these services are individualized to meet the traveler's specific needs, provided on a one-to-one basis in the actual environments of travel and delivered by a qualified instructor (Blasch, 1994b; Blasch & Welsh, 1980; LaGrow et al., 1990; Welsh, 1972).

Mobility instruction, as discussed in other chapters of this volume, encompasses many components; however, there is a primary focus on three general areas: devices, skills, and strategies. There are many mobility devices, such as wheelchairs, crutches, support canes, and walkers, as well as long canes, electronic travel aids (ETAs), and dog guides. These devices range from the very simple to the very sophisticated.

The second area involves the acquisition of skills. Basically a skill as such is proficiency or mastery in the performance of some task. The task may be using a compass, reading a map, taking a direction, or using a mobility device. The skills that are taught in mobility instruction are predominantly cognitive and motor.

Finally, the area in which O&M and TI instruction is exemplary in the fields of rehabilitation and special education is the use of strategies. Strategies are generally thought of as an ingenious plan, method, or effective way of getting a result. Many times individuals are forced to use their ingenuity to try some innovative or alternative behavior to circumvent some obstacle, or it may be the strategy of employing the use of a specific device such as a cane or walker. One specific example of an effective strategy is using assistance and taking charge of the situation. It is the strategies of how to ask for assistance, formulating the questions, repeating the answer, and possibly explaining to a pedestrian the best way to provide physical assistance. Once the strategies have been taught through a systematic curriculum of instruction, the individual then develops skill and proficiency in the application of these strategies. With the increase in skill level, there is also an increase in self-confidence and self-efficacy.

There are several key factors to the intervention component of O&M and TI that have proven extremely effective. One critical factor is providing individualized instruction. Teaching in independent travel requires individualized instruction. Because of the variety of components that are involved, it is unlikely that any two students will be able to proceed at the same rate. Attempting to teach two students at one time will result in danger for the students and inefficient instruction. Because part of the focus of O&M and TI needs to be on independence and individual problem solving, teaching more than one person deprives one or the other of the students of the opportunity to learn to make decisions on his or her own and bear their consequences, which the student will have to do when traveling independently. Individualized instruction also enables the O&M specialist and travel instructor to structure the situation to reflect the level of complexity that is most needed by a particular student at that time in the learning process (Welsh, 1972).

Another critical instructional component is that instruction can be adequately provided only in natural environments similar to those in which the student will later travel. Although teaching in simulated and protected environments may be necessary for beginning instruction, it is not sufficient for the development of all needed skills. Natural or ecologically relevant environments are qualitatively different from the hallways of institutions such as schools and hospitals. In the students' routine environment there is a bombardment of stimuli and a variety of competing concerns such as existing dangers, the reactions of pedestrians, the possibility of getting lost, and the preoccupation with the actual business of the trip. The method that has proven to be the best way to prepare for such situations is instruction and practice in the real environment (Welsh, 1972). The importance of this concept for O&M instruction for multiply impaired individuals has been rediscovered and given great prominence (Bailey & Head, 1993; Gee, Harrell, & Rosenberg, 1987; Joffee & Rikhye, 1991).

Since TI and O&M instruction have concentrated on teaching in the real environment, the O&M specialist and travel instructor have developed a unique knowledge and expertise in teaching environmental problem solving. Examples of specific environmental problem situations include what to do when confronted with a detour or barrier; if the elevator is not functioning; if veering occurs on a street crossing or in a parking lot; recovery from veering into a driveway or a street; and establishing one's location on a drop-off lesson, "lost situations," and stranger approach, to mention a few. Aspects of this environmental problem-solving knowledge base are similar to those used by the person who participates in the sport of orienteering.

Traditionally, orienteering is a timed cross-country race in which the participants use a map and compass to plan the most efficient route between controls (checkpoints) on an unfamiliar course set in a large, wooded area. However, for the purposes of teaching environmental problem solving, courses can be set up anywhere—classrooms, playgrounds, and neighborhoods, and events can be held for a variety of purposes: to learn new settings, exercise, teach independent mobility (Blasch, 1981a, 1981b, 1984; Langbain, et al., 1981), promote inclusion (Blasch, 1994), and provide enjoyable activity. This activity, like O&M instruction, TI and independent mobility, may be designed to improve the following skills: map-reading skills and orientation; landmark identification and use, distance estimation, use of compass directions for orientation, route following and planning, development of problem-solving and decision-making strategies, and practice in taking precautions against becoming lost or disoriented (Blasch, 1994b).

Another important teaching component in TI and O&M instruction is the need for lessons of graduated difficulty and responsibility. Various components have to be broken out of the total mobility task and presented sequentially. It is important to develop certain basic skills before the student can be expected to deal with other people in travel situations. For example, the student needs to be able to handle less congested areas of travel before proceeding to more complicated areas. A student also needs to develop confidence in her own travel abilities before she works on the skills of soliciting and using assistance. Although the particular sequence or approach may differ somewhat for individual students, and the approach used for persons with different disabilities may vary from that which has been most helpful for visually impaired persons, O&M specialists need to be expert in planning sequenced lessons of graduated difficulty and responsibility. Such skill is necessary for work with persons with all types of mobility limitations, particularly as it relates to the development of the person's self-confidence in her travel abilities and the overcoming of any fears and anxieties that may exist.

Another common factor that has emerged in mobility instruction for people who are visually impaired is the synthesis of skills (self-efficacy and self-confidence). The synthesis of skills may be viewed as the whole of independent travel being greater than the sum of its parts (Volume 1, Chapter 7). No matter how expertly the student performs the various subskills in isolation, the various components frequently do not come together as smoothly as expected. Unless the student gets an opportunity to put it all together in practice situations with an O&M specialist available for feedback and assistance, it is likely that the student will not be able to learn to travel to full potential, at least not as soon as she might with such professional training.

Finally, one of the more important elements of mobility instruction is the designation of mobility instruction as the primary responsibility of one or more full-time staff members of an agency or program (Welsh, 1972). This is best done by the O&M specialist or travel instructor (Laus, 1974, 1977; Blasch, 1982; Williams et al., 1982; Brambila-Hickman & Denniston, 1984). Where mobility instruction of some sort is offered in programs for persons with limitations other than visual impairment, many times it is done by someone whose main responsibility lies elsewhere and who provides TI only when time permits or when the need is so obvious and pressing that other duties must be put aside. Giving specific staff members full-time responsibility for TI is an important step in the recognition and development of this service as an essential part of the program. The presence of an O&M specialist or travel instructor in a program also indicates that someone in the organization, who has a professional responsibility, will focus attention on this area and on the literature to learn how to improve the service. A designated person is able to devote full attention to this service without the distractions of other responsibilities, or resulting conflicts, which may arise.

The strategies involved in the instruction of persons with functional mobility limitations are essentially the same as those used with persons who are visually impaired (Welsh, 1972; Blasch & Welsh, 1977; Blasch, 1981a). The program is individualized to account for the traveler's personal abilities and meet his specific needs (which may be even more varied than those presented by the visually impaired population, if this is possible) and is provided on a one-to-one basis.

Less emphasis, however, is placed on teaching the basics in the use of travel devices (if a travel device is necessary), since this is the responsibility of others (i.e., occupational and physical therapists) and is usually done before TI in the outdoor or natural environment begins. On the other hand, more emphasis is placed on working and cooperating with other professionals. Less emphasis may be placed on sensory training and more on the development of safe street-crossing skills, routes and recovery techniques for those with cognitive impairments, and route planning to circumvent physical barriers for others. Similar attention is given to the use of public transportation and interaction with the public. These points are illustrated in some brief examples of providing TI to sighted individuals with disabilities. The following section discusses some of the routinely used techniques and presents case histories.

TRAVEL INSTRUCTION: A MODEL FOR INSTRUCTION

Environmental Assessments

This model for instruction includes assessing the environment, conducting an assessment of the individual's travel skills and abilities, including a functional assessment, and a four-phase instructional process. Travel instructors view the environmental conditions in conjunction with the abilities of the person who is to be instructed. The environmental situation is considered in light of the characteristics of the individual and his ability to navigate the complexity of the travel situation, including such factors as noise, traffic, crossing patterns, time of day for travel, and variability of the traffic situations. An environmental assessment is performed once information is gathered regarding the unique needs of the individual and the nature of the necessary travel.

For many individuals with a cognitive disability, the environmental assessment is typically route specific to one intended destination from their residence, and in most instances travel is to a school, rehabilitation facility, or job location. Travel instructors will subsequently look at the usual considerations found in most ecological surveys (i.e., studying the relationship of the individual and the environment), which include such factors as traffic lights, stop signs, restrooms, shopping areas, and the responsible use of cell phones or the location of public telephones.

Individuals with a cognitive disability frequently obtain work in areas that are service related such as in restaurants, hotels, and establishments such as nursing homes or hospitals. These locations have shift hours, and travel may be required during off-peak hours, weekends, and holidays. Environmental considerations must include factors such as whether the individual will be traveling in daylight or dark. Intersections need to be timed and viewed during the actual hours of travel, as the light cycle and flow of traffic could be significantly different at 5:00 p.m. versus 1:00 p.m. The instructor needs to assess whether the student may be at risk traveling during periods when many areas would be isolated.

Observing the environment with an understanding of the student's disability is an integral component of the environmental assessment. Individuals with autism may experience difficulty if traveling during peak hours when the noise level in a public transit facility may be high, or when needing to cross heavily traveled intersections with the sounds of traffic congestion and high levels of visual distractions. Individuals with Williams syndrome can be extremely social and may enjoy crowds as they provide numerous opportunities for conversations. Yet a transit terminal may not be the best transferring point as it raises a person's risk level to interact with total strangers. And a person with Down syndrome may not be the best candidate for a work location that requires walking up a steep hill due to the tendency for weak ankles, heart problems, and poor stamina. This does not imply that the person needs to be excluded for consideration, but the instructor needs to be alert for possible difficulties and therefore consider alternate routes or strategies.

When assessing a route for the potential independent traveler, the instructor needs to thoroughly evaluate the travel contingencies, which need to be taught. Is there a possibility that the student may board the wrong bus? If riding a rail line, what are the transit agencies' contingency plans? Could the student possibly exit at the wrong location? Is more than one fare payment required? What if the student lost his money or arrived home to an empty house and had forgotten his key? All of these aspects need to be thought out, and the instructor needs to incorporate the potential problems into the training program.

In many programs, job coordinators will ask a travel instructor to perform an environmental assessment to determine if a route is not only feasible for travel, but practical as well. Travel instructors view the various options and choose the safest route, which may not always be the most expeditious route. A street crossing at a traffic light may be safer even though it is two blocks away from the intended destination. Considerations for travel may include learning to travel to work, but the return trip may require the person to use paratransit due to a complex intersection that he may be unable to cross for the outbound bus. A properly performed environmental assessment is critical for the ultimate success of the student in independent travel.

Assessments of the Individual

When assessing an individual with a disability, transit agencies, community agencies, and educators will often use a method of assessment that evaluates a client's ability in a familiar or simulated setting. This form of assessment is referred to as performance assessment and is defined as "testing methods that require students to create an answer product that demonstrates their knowledge of skills" (U.S. Office of Technology Assessment, 1992, p. 16). These assessments typically occur in a classroom setting or office. As an example of what is evaluated, individuals are asked to provide information about their schedule or routine, to relay personal information such as name and address, to show recognition or understanding of safe travel techniques (stranger danger), and are tested on their ability to read functional words or traffic signs. Individuals are asked to perform tasks that assess their functional reading, math, receptive and expressive language, and means of communication. Behavioral assessments or reports are also gathered from family, teachers, and other involved professionals.

The performance-based assessment serves a purpose in instances when determining basic skill readiness. This is helpful in situations such as when transit agencies need to determine some minimal readiness level for a person's capability for using the fixed-route system versus paratransit. This assessment may also provide information for educators to use for determining basic prerequisite skills prior to referring a student for TI.

The weakness and danger of using this method as the *only* criteria for demonstration are that it lacks application of skill ability in the actual community setting with the multiple distractions and natural environmental risk factors. The community as an assessment environment is not stagnant and therefore provides a more accurate evaluation of the individual's skill level and ability.

Professionals who will be providing actual instruction in travel and mobility also need to conduct a functional assessment in order to produce a thorough and realistic evaluation of a client's ability to travel in the natural environment (see Volume 1, Chapter 12). A person's capabilities for travel rely on factors such as, but not limited to, the following:

- Orientation in unfamiliar settings
- Visual perception and auditory motor integration
- Problem solving and decision making in the environment where they will travel
- Basic functional life skills
- Awareness of and appropriate response to possible signs of danger
- Safe and proper interactions with strangers and community members
- Physical stamina and basic movement

One area which is critical for evaluation is the area of visual perception and integration.

Many individuals with cognitive impairments may have other impairments which would affect their ability to safely navigate the environment. When reviewing the student's records, the instructor needs to determine if there are any perceptual deficits such as visual inattention (which would include the possibility of any visual field loss), visual-scanning difficulties, spatial and perceptual organization, and the ability to ignore visual interference or distractions. Although travel instructors cannot medically diagnose conditions, there are certain informal tests that can be completed as part of an assessment process (see Chapter 3).

In addition, during the assessment process, one needs to provide opportunities to informally evaluate an individual's ability to problem solve, that is, to be able to "shift perceptual organization, train of thought, or ongoing behavior" (Lezak, 1995) to meet the varying needs of the moment:

> Conceptual inflexibility appears in concrete or rigid approaches to understanding and problem solving . . . and [one] cannot dissociate their response or pull their attention away from whatever is in their perceptual field or current thoughts . . . there is an inability to shift behavior readily, to conform behavior to rapidly changing demands on the person. (Lezak, 1995, p. 666)

During the functional evaluation, there may be other concerns discovered (see Sidebar 21.5). For example, during the assessment the travel instructor may note that individuals with traumatic brain injury (TBI) may appear to notice turning cars *only while in motion*. They may not see motorists who are waiting to turn at a traffic light, but once the vehicle begins to move, they are able to visually notice the car. There are certain neurological conditions such as the Riddoch phenomenon, where individuals can perceive moving objects, but not stationary ones (Lue, Volpe, & Galetta, 2001, p. 315). Without the functional evaluation, this travel problem may not be detected.

Instructional Process

Teaching students with disabilities to travel independently may be viewed as a four-phase instructional process. For those who are school-age, many of the fundamental skills (or pre-travel skills) have oftentimes been integrated into the school's curriculum and are taught by a special education classroom teacher, frequently in consultation with the travel instructor. Once the student has been determined (as a result of the assessment process) ready for independent travel, instruction is provided as outlined later in this chapter. In the case of adults who have not already attained these skills, the travel instructor will be responsible for teaching these fundamental pre-travel skills.

The four-phase instructional process incorporates fundamental skills and travel skills, frequently route specific, to the intended destination. For many school-age children, the fundamental skills are oftentimes introduced within a classroom environment. These can include, but are not limited to, time and time management, demonstration of understanding of functional travel-related words, money, communication skills, and basic orientation concepts. The travel instructor evaluates the student's capability in those functional skills essential for travel in the community and instructs as necessary until mastery occurs. "The fact that learners construct new understandings based on their current knowledge highlights some of the dangers in teaching by telling" (Schwartz & Bransford, 1998). It is not enough to have students say that they ought to look both ways before crossing a street; the travel instructor must also be sure that students actually look both ways before crossing streets they encounter on their lessons.

Case Study: Charles

At age 19, Charles, a young man with mild cerebral palsy, attended high school in a major metropolitan area. Charles used crutches to ambulate within the school building. Although most of his school career focused on his educational program, emphasizing academic skill development, at his transitional Individualized Education Program (IEP), the family requested travel instruction. Given the metropolitan area where he resided, using public transportation was the most practical and economical means for his personal travel needs. Charles intended to pursue postsecondary education; however, he had limited exposure to traveling within the community.

During the internal school assessment, it was observed that Charles was able to negotiate the school building as well as the stairs within the school independently. Despite the crowded hallways when classes were in session, Charles was able to navigate without difficulty.

The functional assessment in the community included the use of public transportation as well as Charles' pedestrian skills at intersections. The most significant concern noted was Charles'

inconsistency in identifying oncoming traffic. At times, he moved forward as if to cross when a turning car was immediately in front of him. In addition, Charles had difficulty ambulating across the street within the amount of time allotted during the pedestrian walk segment. Although prior to the external assessment Charles' pace had been pre-tested within the school building (in a hallway between classes), it was noted during the functional evaluation that his performance was significantly different. When in the community, Charles demonstrated a decreased ability with his stamina to cross streets within the pedestrian cycle as well as his ability to filter out the essential stimuli.

The results of the assessment were shared with the IEP team. With consultation from the travel instructor, the occupational and physical therapist developed a program to build Charles' stamina within the community. This included a measured-off distance simulating a road span within the school and working to increase his walking speed to travel this distance within a specified time.

Depending on the complexity of the trip, as well as the individual's disability, the four-phase travel instruction may require 20 to 25 round-trip training sessions. The specific destination is typically to a work site or school location. The instructional process includes Phase I (direct instruction), Phase II (observation), Phase III (problem-solving instruction, and Phase IV (unknown observation and final documentation).

Phase I provides direct instruction in the specifics of the travel route including the street crossings essential for travel, the specific transit route (if applicable), and the related travel skills

such as fare costs, a system for organizing personal belongings, and fundamental skills such as time and money management. Phase II provides an opportunity for the student to continue to demonstrate mastery of the skills as the instructor observes from a short distance. Intervention occurs only if the student's safety is at risk. Problem-solving opportunities are allowed to be resolved by the student as they arise without instructor intervention, unless there is a safety risk. Phase III provides instruction in the problem-solving components which are specific to the travel route. At this point the student experiences and demonstrates to competency levels, through actual simulations (e.g., the boarding of a wrong transit vehicle, missing one's stop, losing one's fare, and a blocked sidewalk). During this phase, *location identification exercises* are conducted as explained earlier in the chapter. Phase IV involves obtaining the final documentation of the student's travel capabilities by a travel instructor whom the student does not know. It is recommended that this instructor be observed by the student at some point during the training walking in the area and utilizing the transportation at the same time. This avoids potential concerns by the student that they are being "followed."

During all aspects of training, the travel instructor is emphasizing communication skills, basic orientation concepts, as well as appropriate interaction with strangers and community workers. Training is conducted in an unobtrusive manner, so that attention is not directed to the individual. Other safety concepts, such as being discreet with one's money and personal information, including not wearing identifying logos such as school name or place of business (including name tags), are taught.

During the course of instruction, travel instructors are writing daily reports that are shared with the family. This documentation serves the purpose of providing not only a record of the student's progress, but also detailed information about the student's needs as well as his successes in the development of independence. Oftentimes families need to be integral "partners" and may need to provide encouragement. This encouragement can come in many different ways such as offering support, allowing for the continued independent travel instruction (especially in families that may be fearful), or assisting in the development of organizational skills such as being prepared, waking up on time by using an alarm clock, or making one's lunch in advance.

TRAVEL INSTRUCTION FOR SPECIFIC DISABILITIES

Working in the field of travel instruction requires an understanding of a large number of disabilities and strategies. The following sections focus on a few of the populations that receive travel instruction.

Cognitive Disabilities

Cognitive disabilities can be acquired as a result of a genetic disability such as Down syndrome, fragile X syndrome, Williams syndrome, Tourette syndrome, and Prader-Willi syndrome. Other causes can include a traumatic brain injury, defects acquired prenatally such as fetal alcohol syndrome, or agenesis of the corpus collosum, as well as neurological impairments such as autism or a learning disability (see Chapter 19).

When working with an individual who has a cognitive disability, it is important to familiarize oneself with some of the common characteristics of the specific impairment. Although professionals should never pre-judge or make assumptions regarding an individual's capabilities, instructors need to be aware of some traits that may exist, and instruction needs to be modified to meet the needs of the individual. For the purposes of this chapter, it would not be feasible to discuss in detail the causes or possible instructional strategies for all of the different travel skills with which individuals with cognitive disabilities may have difficulty. A few of the areas are briefly discussed later in this chapter to provide the reader with some fundamental information and recommendations.

Many students with cognitive disabilities may have difficulties with reading (e.g., street signs or names of stores), memory, and verbal communication. One technique to circumvent this limitation is to use index cards (flash cards) with hand-drawn or photographed landmarks that can be laminated to protect against weather conditions. These cards can be used on a key ring or in a book form and sequenced for a specific route, or used to solicit assistance from the public. A specific lesson would be to have the student go into a store (prearranged with the store staff by the travel instructor) and ask for stationery or an advertisement with the store name and logo. Then the student can cut out the information and affix it to a flash card for future use as a visual reminder. Another helpful orientation tool is the use of an auditory cassette tape that gives a verbal step-by-step sequence of a route.

These activities also help to reinforce the use of appropriate landmarks (see Chapter 2, Volumes 1 and 2). Often students with intellectual disabilities have not been taught to use primary landmarks, or they select inappropriate secondary landmarks such as a car or a seasonal window display in a store. Instruction in the selection of stationary landmarks becomes an important aspect of TI. One unique method involved a necklace like a charm bracelet, made by the student with significant objects representing sequential landmarks. This allowed the student to focus on meaningful landmarks and the necklace served as a mnemonic to remember the route sequence. When traveling in a car, families can be encouraged to have their child give the directions when going to the store (e.g., turn right—or point—at Burger King). Although an individual may have an intellectual disability, this does not mean that student has trouble with orientation. It is not uncommon for students who cannot read to develop other strategies when they are traveling on a new route in an unfamiliar area.

Map reading is another task that is often not taught because of preconceived expectations about individuals with intellectual disabilities. If the individual is unaware that maps are comprised of symbols representing the environment, start with pictures, photographs, or drawings of actual environments such as a classroom. Have the student point to the chair that she is sitting on in the picture. Then point to the window in the picture and have the student walk to the window. Gradually progress from the picture to symbolic representations on a map. If successful, progress to maps of the school, playground, home, neighborhood, and so on. Teaching the use of maps in this way is something that family members may also reinforce.

Another important aspect of the instruction is to teach an individual how to ask for information. This may begin with whom to ask. Generally, there is a great concern on the part of the families of a student with intellectual disabilities regarding the student's ability to make good judgments; for example, about "stranger danger." There is a concern that the student may be vulnerable to abuse or inappropriate requests. Therefore, it is important to do role-playing and teach the student how to identify a "safe stranger." A safe stranger may be described as someone who is easily identified by a uniform or name tag (e.g., bank tellers, police, and bus drivers). TI provides opportunities for the student to role-play and demonstrate the ability to solve common travel problems, such as being approached by a stranger or getting lost. In the role-play, it is important to rehearse information-gathering questions and getting useful directions. In some cases, the student may have a card with the address to show to the bus driver and a card of a different color with the return address to show to the bus driver when returning.

Crossing streets is frequently a challenge for many of these students. The most effective teaching strategy is one-on-one instruction and consistent practice at street crossings in the student's community where they are likely to travel. The student may not be able to tell the instructor what type of street crossing he is making, but he needs to be able to demonstrate proficiency 100 percent of the time before the mobility instructor signs off on traveling alone.

One method used in the St. Paul, Minnesota, public schools is to videotape the student crossing streets and review the videotape in a classroom setting. Some students respond well when they observe their instructor making good or poor street crossings and are asked to evaluate. It is not uncommon for the student to be able to stand at a corner and accurately assess the street crossing and indicate when it is safe to cross. However, the student may never have been allowed to implement the decision, so he waits for a verbal cue from the parent or family member to verify his decision. Therefore, the travel instructor may have to teach the student environmental decision making and implementation. This may be accomplished by the behavioral procedure of fading. The travel instructor may start with the student (who may be extremely fearful) holding on to the instructor in the sighted guide technique (as opposed to holding hands), but with the student making the decision when to cross. The student continues to make the decision when to cross, but the progression of fading then has the travel instructor standing next to him, directly behind, then 6 feet behind, and so on. This is an extremely important learning concept. This may be the first time some individuals are allowed to make such decisions and act on them.

For those students who have trouble with problem solving, repetitive community-based travel experience seems to build a foundation upon which they can draw information that they later are able to transfer to new and previously frustrating situations. The pivotal teaching tool on which students rely and base their problem-solving strategies is the "emergency information card." The emergency information card is a laminated card with emergency telephone numbers, names, addresses, a picture, and even pertinent medical information that the student keeps in his wallet. Reconstructing actual problems that the student has experienced while using the emergency information card in the community in a safe classroom setting provides opportunities for role-playing solutions. Videotaping these role-playing situations becomes a useful tool for future students as well. Overall, the use of the emergency information card helps students develop a sense of self-assurance that enables them to learn how to solve problems. It is also valuable for the mobility instructor to have a copy of the same card. This is a safety precaution in case the student is lost and the mobility instructor has to ask people if they have seen the student. It is helpful to have a picture of the student. Also, for those students who have a state issued non–driver's license identification (which is recommended for those learning independent travel), it is helpful to know that police departments are able to access the photo image in the event of an emergency.

Families or caretakers may unintentionally foster dependence in the life of a person with an intellectual disability. It is important, therefore, to involve the families or caretakers very early in the travel program. Instructors may choose to invite families and students to express their concerns and jointly strategize approaches to the instructional sequence that will satisfy everyone. The instructor may also choose to invite families or caretakers to observe lessons or help create the next lesson plan. Some of the families' fears may be based on a limited knowledge of public transportation or their limited knowledge of problem-solving strategies. Other parental fears may be based on years of witnessing the student's high level of vulnerability. An effective teaching strategy is to teach the student the strategies for "what to do if . . . ." For example, when the student is able to tell the instructor what he would do if a stranger approached, the support of the parents or caretakers is enlisted to role-play the "stranger approach." Some police community outreach programs may be willing to assist the mobility instructor in creating a "setup" where a students is approached by a policeman out of uniform. The policeman offers the student a ride or candy, or tests whatever his particular area of vulnerability happens to be. The student's reaction to the undercover policeman is one measure of the student's ability to avoid dangerous situations.

Some students may exhibit inappropriate social behaviors. Some of these behaviors may keep store clerks or others from offering assistance or cause a bus driver to keep a student off a bus. Videotaping a student in a community setting and subsequently showing the videotape to the student may have a profound effect on his choice of community behaviors. Many of these same teaching procedures may be applicable to individuals with other disabilities.

Persons with autism spectrum disorders (see Sidebar 21.6) vary greatly in their abilities and functional limitations. One frequently noted characteristic is difficulty with changes in routine. Research has occurred in the area of autism, and there are numerous books available that can provide professionals with information on introducing social skills, communication, and learning how to teach flexibility—all essential components for travel in the community (Gense & Gense, 2005; Grandin, 2006; Stillman, 2003).

Traumatic Brain Injury

Travel instructors who receive a referral for a person with traumatic brain injury (TBI) need to make certain that they have access to the individual's neurological report. The location of the brain injury will provide critical information that the instructor needs to have to evaluate the person's abilities for travel. For example, damage to a person's frontal lobe could affect areas such as judgment, moods, and inhibitions, expressive language skills as well as other executive functions. Injury to the parietal lobe could impact visual attention as well as the ability to focus on more than one task. Injuries to the occipital lobe could create visual field loss (Lue, Volpe, & Galetta, 2001).

Problems with visual processing, short-term memory, maintaining orientation, map reading, and fear of independent travel may also be frequent outcomes of TBI. The role of the travel instructor is to assist the student with reentry into the community as an independent traveler after a probable long stint in a rehabilitation setting.

In addition to providing intensive instruction with street-crossing skills, teaching strategies also focus on giving the person with TBI some tangible ways to maintain orientation. Examples of this may be in the form of a mnemonic such as a written list of landmarks and turns. This strategy compensates for the three remaining problems that affect travel efficiency: short-term memory problems, map-reading problems, and fear of independent travel.

Instruction needs to begin with the student making a checklist of things to bring with him while traveling (e.g., wallet, identification, a cell phone or change for a phone call, flip chart, or an information book of the route). Start with familiar locations and ask the student to select a route that he would like to master, such as the route to work or the grocery store. Develop a sequenced flip chart (such as small index cards which are easily transportable and can be readily changed if the travel route is altered) of written travel instructions or photographs of sequential landmarks to help stay oriented. If this route is a walking route, the student can hold the device. If the student is a driver the circular file flip chart may be mounted on the dashboard of the car.

The performance of students recovering from TBI may vary from day to day. Build in recovery strategies that students may use to help themselves if they become disoriented. Have students practice soliciting assistance, making a phone call on a cell phone or pay phone, and providing the location where they became disoriented or their current location.

For students who want to advance their travel skills to unfamiliar indoor and outdoor areas, equip them with strategies that will help them

Case History: Gregory

At age 20, Gregory, a student with autism, was referred for a travel instruction assessment to evaluate his potential to learn to travel from his home to his college program, as he was dependent on family members for all his travel needs. The evaluation indicated that Gregory was able to obtain information from maps, transit schedules, and other resources, and he was able to manage both money and time resources. Gregory's biggest problem was in the area of problem solving.

As an example of this difficulty, one day Gregory approached an automated door on the college campus. This presented a problem as Gregory was uncertain if he could open the door manually as with most other doors. After waiting outside the door for several minutes, he then looked in the direction of the travel instructor (TI) hoping for assistance. The TI prompted Gregory to examine the signage and observe other individuals as they used the door. Again, several minutes passed before Gregory asked if he was allowed to open the door by pulling on the handle or pressing the button. He was encouraged to try and, after pushing the button, was rewarded by the successful opening of the door.

To develop Gregory's functional independence and ability to problem solve, an instructional program was developed around the pedestrian and public transit trip to and from his college program. The structure of the program included opportunities for problem solving, both simulated and naturally occurring. Gregory traveled between home and school five times a week and practiced, with the travel instructor, problem solving around situations that could possibly occur during this particular travel route. These included missing a bus, boarding the wrong bus, losing his transit fare, and identifying his location in unfamiliar environments.

During one of the problem-solving lessons, the student practiced boarding a wrong bus route. Gregory rode until the end of the line, where he disembarked and then needed to determine another bus route which would transport him in the direction of his school program. This was difficult for Gregory as he was approaching the school from a different direction, and although he appeared to recognize his stop, he did not initiate an action to disembark. Continued problem-solving lessons were provided until Gregory was able to make safe and independent decisions without guiding questions or instructional intervention. Gradually, Gregory gained confidence in his decision-making ability, which enabled him to initiate action in resolving problems.

As a result, Gregory learned to adjust his plan of action when outside forces intervened to alter his normal course of action. He completed the independent travel to his school program and continued with his postsecondary career goals. Later, the family shared that his confidence continued to grow as he felt comfortable independently, adjusting his travel time to meet any changes in his schedule. For example, if Gregory needed to remain at school to work on a class project, he was able to determine a later time for travel. For many persons with autism, change in routine can be difficult. However, the problem-solving opportunities allowed Gregory to build on his strengths.

stay oriented. Walk or drive through the new route, and teach them to use and carry, if applicable to the traveler, a compass and tape recorder. Have the students describe the route they are taking on an audiotape. Subsequent lessons include observing students completing the route while they are listening to the tape, and eventually fading the student from using the tape if this is feasible. Another option for some individuals with TBI would be to use personal digital assistants (PDAs) which have satellite navigation systems. The range and level of travel complexity can best be mutually determined by the travel instructor and the student, frequently discussing the student's readiness for more complex travel. If the student would like to work toward driving long distances to unfamiliar destinations, map-reading skills are helpful but not mandatory. Some of the pocket computers that sequentially list the routes, interstate services, and directions are very affordable. The traveler can also request that complex maps be simplified for easier reading or put on an audiotape. However, travel instructors need to make certain that the individual does demonstrate consistency in his ability to safely travel and negotiate the environment. For people who cannot read a map because of difficulty using cardinal directions, mounting a compass on the car dashboard and adjusting the modified map so its directional arrow matches that of the car compass may prove helpful.

Also, persons with TBI who may be interested in learning to drive need to be referred to a rehabilitation center that specializes in teaching driver's education to individuals with disabilities. These locations have certified instructors, specialize in adaptive driving, will perform an intensive evaluation of the individual's capabilities in this skill, and provide instruction if the individual is determined capable. In other situations the damage may be to such an extent that an area of the brain that governs one's inhibitions, long-term memory, or ability to safely cross streets on a consistent basis is impacted, af-

fecting the individual's ability to travel safely. In this case, paratransit may be the best solution to handle transportation needs, and the travel instructor needs to write a report to include in the individual's application for paratransit to the local transit authority.

Hearing and Communication Impairments

For the travel instructor who is teaching a student who is deaf or hard of hearing, it is important to learn sign language or enlist the services of a sign language interpreter. One of the first critical areas to evaluate is in the use and understanding of the language common to travel in the community. For example, the word *corner* can have more than one meaning. To be effective, it is important to break down the lessons into concrete parts and translate this information so it is understood. Similarly, it is important to have the mobility lessons in the natural environment. Present the lesson in its entirety first. The use of photographs prior to the lesson can help to illustrate what is to be expected for the day. Go through the entire route with the student without too much detail or explanation at first. Allow the student to visually absorb as much of the route as possible. Subsequent lessons will involve taking notes (by the student or the travel instructor) of any unusual or permanent circumstances that the student has not noted previously (e.g., one-way streets) and pointing these out.

As noted earlier, functional limitations may show up in many individuals with nonvisual disabilities. Teaching the student how to solve travel problems includes social awareness as well as challenges with the environment. If the student seems to have problems with social graces (sitting too close to other passengers on the bus, signing to a fellow student inside another passenger's "space," taking a seat on a bus that was designated for the elderly), videotape the student in action and then view the tape and reenact these situations in a classroom or the student's home. Illustrate how the student intrudes upon another passenger and then strategize with the student in a more polite way to handle herself in the community. This may be accomplished through role-playing.

However (to reiterate what was discussed earlier in the chapter), solving travel problems is much more effective if it is done on the spot, at the time of the problem, in the community. As with any type of mobility instruction, the instructor needs to develop a sense of when it is appropriate to intervene and when it is appropriate to allow the student to struggle a bit. However, some students may not know they have a problem. They may be unaware they are lost and continue traveling as if all is well. To allow a student to continue traveling in the wrong direction indefinitely will not necessarily serve a learning goal. It is better to allow the student to become slightly disoriented, but not too far from what is visually familiar. In later lessons when the student's visual scope of "what's familiar" broadens and she begins to connect whole blocks together in a cognitive map, the mobility instructor may find it of educational value to allow the student to travel in the wrong direction for a greater distance (see Chapter 2, Volumes 1 and 2).

Making needs and wants known or asking directions involves preparing the student for an actual experience of being lost. Continually putting the student in a contrived situation will not make the experience meaningful. Wait for a "teachable moment" when students really need assistance, and then allow them to practice what they have learned and ask for help. For students who are deaf or hard of hearing, carrying a pad of paper and a pencil becomes as important as a wallet or billfold. For the student who is also intellectually disabled, the challenge may be how to clearly get a message across to a hearing person. Most likely, the initial experience will not be enough. But this experience can be role-

played over and over again in the classroom or at home, and written phrases memorized for different situations. The other half of this challenge is the response the student receives from a clerk, security guard, or the general public. Persons offering assistance may give a verbal response instead of writing it down, or they may write the response down using words that are not understood. The student needs to be prepared to express what he needs from the person as clearly as possible. When the student is unable to write in an emergency, body movements and gesturing may be useful. The mobility instructor can expect that this type of instruction may take several years or more to complete with weekly practice before the student is a safe and efficient independent traveler.

The person with a communication disorder has similar problems to the individual who is deaf or hard of hearing, and the solutions may be exactly the same. The main difference is that the individual can hear but is not able to articulate his needs. Persons with autism may frequently confuse their pronouns, for example. The problem-solving and soliciting assistance strategies are much the same, with the exception that this person may use an augmentative communication device or communication system with which the general public is probably not familiar. It is often valuable to role-play interactions with the public. The travel instructor needs to work closely with the student's augmentative communication specialist or a speech and language pathologist to develop strategies for using the correct communication device or communication system in public. For more information on working with individuals with hearing impairments, see Chapter 17.

SUMMARY

O&M for individuals with a visual impairment and TI for sighted individuals with disabilities share more similarities than differences. Some of the terminology and areas of emphasis may differ somewhat; however, many of the mobility strategies and teaching techniques are the same. This chapter described a model of principles fundamental to O&M and TI. This model provides a process of determining a person's functional limitations that may inhibit independent mobility. An individual's disability and/or the environmental demands may determine functional limitations to independent mobility.

This chapter illustrated some examples of teaching strategies and techniques for providing TI to sighted individuals with various disabling conditions. The intent is to provide the O&M specialist with a number of applied examples, but not an exhaustive teaching curriculum for each disability, and to demonstrate that the similar teaching and strategies routinely used in O&M directly transfer to TI. The examples and solutions cited for a specific disability are certainly not restricted to use with that particular disability, but may indeed be applied to any individual with a similar functional mobility problem.

As one would expect for travel instruction, less emphasis is placed on vision or the lack of it, with more attention placed on the consequences, causes, and treatment of other disabilities. The instructor needs to be familiar with the mobility strategies used for coping with various conditions. As a result, the O&M specialist, with additional training, is more of a specialist in "mobility" when it comes to dealing with sighted disability groups, and is therefore more versatile. This is not so different from the demands currently placed on the O&M specialists who are increasingly teaching more individuals with multiple impairments and low vision, rather than totally blind travelers (Uslan, Hill, & Peck, 1989).

Currently, travel instructors and some O&M specialists have emerged to provide mobility instruction to those with functional mobility limi-

tations. Travel instructors have the need for similar academic competencies but do not have the benefit of university preparation in their discipline. Therefore, the backgrounds of travel instructors range from a high school diploma to a master's degree in a related field.

O&M programs were originally designed to meet the needs of veterans who were adventitiously blinded during and immediately following World War II. Numerous modifications have been made since then to make O&M instruction more appropriate for persons of diverse ages, needs, and abilities (e.g., preschoolers, the very old, those with low vision, and the multiply impaired). It seems compelling that the profession of O&M take the initiative and coordinate with travel instructors to expand to include all persons with functional mobility limitations. The sharing of knowledge and experience between O&M specialists and travel instructors would provide the best possibilities for quality mobility and TI in the future for students with other mobility limitations.

IMPLICATIONS FOR O&M PRACTICE

1. Mobility services are available to other individuals with a variety of functional mobility limitations; however, these programs are generally limited in focus and thus fail to recognize the comprehensive nature of mobility as a skill area and the myriad of subtle factors involved in independent travel.

2. Independence in mobility involves a number of skills, including those required for ambulation or movement, environmental negotiation, effective social interaction, and problem solving.

3. The potential for independent mobility is affected by the interaction among one's personal abilities, which is in turn affected

by impairment, illness, age, and the environmental demands of travel. As the environmental demand increases, the potential for independence decreases. This interaction may be mediated or modified through an intervention. This intervention may be designed to reduce environmental demand or provide the traveler with the skills needed to deal with the environment, or both. There are a number of factors that contribute to the degree to which any disabling condition will affect one's mobility.

5. The physical structure of the environment may place demands on people to perform at a level that is beyond their capacity. Accessibility reduces this environmental demand.

6. Interventions for independent mobility may involve a number of strategies carried out on both a personal and societal level.

7. Mobility instruction, as discussed in other chapters of this volume, encompasses many components; however, there is a primary focus on three general areas: devices, skills, and strategies.

8. There are several unique intervention components to mobility instruction, including individualized instruction; teaching in the natural environments; teaching environmental problem solving; lessons of graduated difficulty and responsibility; and the synthesis of mobility skills.

9. It is essential that one or more full-time staff members of an agency or program have primary responsibility for the mobility instruction.

LEARNING ACTIVITIES

1. Develop a case for teaching mobility to disabled individuals other than the visually impaired. Has this been done before?

2. List the conditions that may affect mobility and produce a functional limitation in independent travel.

3. Describe the meaning of the formula: $Mi = (Pa - Ed) + I$, and give a specific example.

4. Describe some of the social environmental constraints that restrict an individual's mobility.

5. Describe specific personal and societal interventions for independent mobility.

6. Describe a specific mobility device, skill, and strategy (not something for a visually impaired individual).

7. Describe orienteering and how it could be used to teach individuals with different functional mobility limitations.

8. Map-reading problems are common to individuals with some types of impairments. Define these impairments. How would you teach map reading differently?

9. Observe individuals with disabilities and evaluate their mobility skills. Are there any similarities with the mobility problems of individuals with a visual impairment?

10. Discuss if teaching O&M to individuals other than those with a visual impairment would detract from services for individuals who are blind or visually impaired.

EPILOGUE

Although the future of orientation and mobility is bright, the profession also faces many challenges. Funding for university training programs continues the downward slide that was discussed in the Epilogue of the second edition of *Foundations of Orientation and Mobility*. "Doing more with less" is still the theme for these programs. The need for intensive blindfold and low vision simulation training has made university programs very expensive and has required investment on the part of the federal government to ensure their availability. The sustained growth of university programs will require increasing investment in their development.

The shortage of qualified practitioners in orientation and mobility also persists. This has been the case throughout the history of the profession, and efforts to increase the numbers have resulted in only small increases. With the possibility of eventually increasing third-party reimbursement, the need for additional instructors will become critical. Increases in the numbers of university programs will be needed, as will more efficient means to educate additional personnel. Most of the university O&M programs have already shifted to include more online or distance-education courses. The need to increase the number of graduates may require new models within university programs and increasing reliance on quality distance-learning methods without reducing the high standards that have made the graduates of these programs highly employable.

Additional challenges and opportunities may result as we serve more people with multiple disabilities. Education for professionals must continue to expand preparation to serve individuals who experience a number of concomitant disabilities. Instruction in these areas will require expanded curricula and teaming with other professionals. Eventually this may lead to broadening the profession to include the provision of travel instruction to persons who have disabilities other than blindness.

Technology and the environment will certainly play a role in the future development of O&M. It is already clear that quiet cars are presenting challenges to travelers. The expanding use of roundabouts, channelized intersections, and unusual geometric configurations of intersections will require new approaches. The increasing complexity of the environment is coupled with the blossoming of technology. Continued development of global positioning systems and accessible pedestrian signals will provide a means for O&M specialists to assist their students to expand their horizons and overcome barriers. Continued research will be needed into new technologies and methods that will make independent travel as safe and efficient as possible

The O&M profession will continue to grow and prosper as it continues to provide an essential service. Healthy growth will depend on continued efforts to expand the research and knowledge base. It is hoped that the current edition of *Foundations of Orientation and Mobility* will stimulate new research and add to the development of the profession, and that future editions will continue to do so as well.

REFERENCES

Access Board. (undated). *Pedestrian access to modern roundabouts: Design and operational issues for pedestrians who are blind*. Washington, DC: U.S. Architectural and Transportation Barriers Compliance Board. Available from www.access-board.gov/research/roundabouts/bulletin.htm, accessed August 18, 2007.

Access Board. (1998). *Americans with disabilities act accessibility guidelines for transportation vehicles*. Available from www.access-board.gov/transit/html/vguide.htm, accessed April 21, 2010.

Access Board. (2004). *Americans with disabilities act and architectural barriers act accessibility guidelines* (ADA-ABA-AG). Washington, DC: U.S. Architectural and Transportation Barriers Compliance Board.)

Access Board. (2005). *Draft guidelines for accessible public rights-of-way (Draft PROWAG)*. Washington, DC: U.S. Architectural and Transportation Barriers Compliance Board.

ADA Regulations, guidance, and procedures. (2007). Available from www.fta.dot.gov/civilrights/ada/civil_rights_13884.html, accessed May 12, 2010.

Adelson, E., & Fraiberg, S. (1974). Gross motor development in infants blind from birth. *Child Development*, 45(1), 114–126.

Adelson, E., & Fraiberg, S. (1976). Sensory deficit and motor development in infants blind from birth. In Z. S. Jastnzembska (Ed.), *The effects of blindness and other impairments on early development*. New York: American Foundation for the Blind.

Advanced Bionics Corporation. Images. Available from www.bionicear.com/professionals/photolib.asp, accessed July 17, 2006.

Agnew, C. M., Nystul, M. S., & Conner, M. C. (1998). Seizure disorders: An alternative explanation for students' inattention. *Professional School Counseling*, 2(1), 1096–2409.

Ahmed, K., McCallum, D., & Sheldon, D. (2005). Multiphase micro-drop interaction in inkjet printing of 3d structures for tactile maps. *Modern Physics Letters B*, 19(28–29), 1699–1702.

Air Carrier Access Act. (1986). Nondiscrimination on the basis of disability in air travel. Available from http://airconsumer.ost.dot.gov/rules/382/SHORT.htm, accessed March 29, 2007.

Allen, K. E., & Marotz, L. (1994). *Developmental profiles: Pre-birth through eight*. Albany, NY: Delmar.

Allen, W., Courtney-Barbier, A., Griffith, A., Kern, T., & Shaw, C. (1997). *Orientation and mobility teaching manual* (2nd ed.). New York: CIL Publications.

Altman, J., & Cutter, J. (2004). Structured discovery cane travel. *29th institute on rehabilitation issues: contemporary issues in orientation and mobility*. Washington, DC: Rehabilitation Services Administration, U.S. Department of Education.

Alvarez, R. D. (1993). Deaf-blind education: Access to context. *Journal of the International Association for the Education of Deaf-Blind People*, 2, 5–9.

Ambrose, G. V. (2000). Sighted children's knowledge of environmental concepts and ability to orient in an unfamiliar residential environment. *Journal of Visual Impairment & Blindness, 94*(8), 509–521.

Ambrose-Zaken, G. (2005). Knowledge of and preferences for long cane components: A qualitative and quantitative study. *Journal of Visual Impairment & Blindness, 99*(10), 633–645.

American Academy of Opthalmology and Otolaryngology (1969). American Academy of Opthalmology and Otolaryngology guide for conservation of hearing. New York: AAOO.

American Association of Retired Persons. (1990). *A profile of older Americans.* Washington, DC: Author.

American Association of State Highway and Transportation Officials [AASHTO]. (2004a). *A policy on geometric design of highways and streets* (5th ed.). Washington, DC: Author.

American Association of State Highway and Transportation Officials [AASHTO]. (2004b). *Guide for the planning, design, and operation of pedestrian facilities.* Washington, DC: Author.

American Association on Mental Retardation. (2002). *Mental retardation: Definition, classification, and systems of supports* (10th ed.). Washington, DC: Author.

American Diabetes Association. (2007). Eye complications. Available from www.diabetes.org/type-1-diabetes/eye-complications.jsp, accessed May 17, 2007.

American Foundation for the Blind. (2000). *What do you do when you see a blind person?* (Video). New York: Author.

American Geriatrics Society (AGS) & British Geriatrics Society (BGS). (2006). *Updated practice guideline for the prevention of falls in older persons from the AGS and BGS.* Expert panel, American Geriatrics Society 2006 Annual Meeting, Session "Evidence-based practice guideline for the prevention of falls in older persons." Available from http://medscape.com/viewarticle/532942, accessed March 3, 2009.

American Geriatrics Society (AGS), British Geriatrics Society (BGS), & American Academy of Orthopaedic Surgeons Panel on Falls Prevention. (2001). Guidelines for the prevention of falls in older persons. *Journal of the American Geriatrics Society, 49*(5), 664–672.

American Medical Association (1947). American Medical Association Council on Physical Medicine

Tentative standard procedure for evaluating the percentage of hearing in medicolegal cases. *Journal of the American Medical Association, 133,* 396–397.

American National Standards Institute (ANSI). (2003). *Specification of hearing aid characteristics* (ANSI S3.22–2003). Melville, NY: Author.

American Psychiatric Association. (2000). *Diagnostic and statistical manual of mental disorders, DSM-IV-TR* (4th ed.). Arlington, VA: Author.

American Public Transportation Association. (2006a). Available from www.apta.com/research/stats/bus/definitions.cfm, accessed May 13, 2006.

American Public Transportation Association. (2006b). Available from www.apta.com/research/stats/rail/definitions.cfm, accessed May 17, 2006.

American Public Transportation Association. (2007). Available from www.publictransportation.org/facts/, accessed August 14, 2007.

American Public Transportation Association. (2009). Available from www.apta.com/media/releases/090309_ridership.cfm, accessed March 22, 2009.

Andrews, R., & Wyver, S. (2005). Autistic tendencies: Are there different pathways for blindness and Autism Spectrum Disorder? *British Journal of Visual Impairment, 23*(2), 52–57.

Andrews, S. K. (1985). The use of capsule papers in producing tactual maps. *Journal of Visual Impairment & Blindness, 79*(9), 396–399.

Angwin, J. P. B. (1968a). Maps for mobility—1. *New Beacon, 52,* 115–119.

Angwin, J. P. B. (1968b). Maps for mobility—2. *New Beacon, 52,* 143–145.

Anthony, T. (1993). Orientation and mobility skill development. In Blind Childrens Center (Ed.), *First steps: A handbook for teaching young children who are visually impaired* (pp. 115–138). Los Angeles: Blind Childrens Center.

Anthony, T., & Lowry, S. (2004). Sensory development. In T. L. Anthony, S. S. Lowry, C. J. Brown, & D. D. Hatton (Eds.), *Developmentally appropriate orientation & mobility* (pp. 123–240). Chapel Hill: FPG Child Development Institute, University of North Carolina at Chapel Hill.

Anthony, T. L., Bleier, H., Fazzi, D. L., Kish, D., & Pogrund, R. L. (2002). Mobility focus: Developing early skills for orientation and mobility. In R. L. Pogrund & D. L. Fazzi (Eds.), *Early focus: Working* with young children who are blind or visually impaired and their families (2nd ed., pp. 326–355). New York: AFB Press.

Anthony, T. L., Lowry, S. S., Brown, C. J., & Hatton, D. D. (2004). *Developmentally appropriate orientation and mobility*. Chapel Hill: FPG Child Development Institute, University of North Carolina at Chapel Hill.

Anzalone, M. E., & Williamson, G. G. (2000). *Sensory processing and motor performance in autism spectrum disorders* (Vol. 9). Baltimore: Brookes.

Apple, L. E. (1962). Factors in mobility rehabilitation which experience has proven useful. *Proceedings of the Mobility Research Conference*. New York: American Foundation for the Blind.

Architectural and Transportation Barriers Compliance Board. (1991). *Americans with disabilities act accessibility guidelines for buildings and facilities*. Washington, DC: Author.

Arditi, A., & Zihl, J. (2000). Functional aspects of visual neural disorders of eye and brain. In B. Silverstone, M. A. Lang, B. P. Rosenthal, & E. E. Faye (Eds.), *The Lighthouse handbook on vision impairment and rehabilitation* (pp. 263–286). New York: Oxford University Press.

Arizona Department of Education. (1997). Arizona Academic Standards. Phoenix, AZ: State Board of Education.

Armstrong, J. D. (Ed.). (1973). *The design and production of maps for the visually handicapped*. Mobility Monograph No. 1. University of Nottingham, UK.

Arnoldi, K., Pendarvis, L., Jackson, J., & Batra, N. (2006). Cerebral palsy for the pediatric eye care team—Part III: Diagnosis and management of associated visual and sensory disorders. *American Orthoptic Journal, 56*, 97–107.

Aschan, C., Hirvonen, M., Rajamäki, E., Mannelin, T., & Ruotsalainen, R. R., & Ruuhela, R. (2009). Performance of slippery and slip-resistant footwear in different wintry weather conditions measured *in situ*. *Safety Science, 47*(8), 1195–1200.

Ashmead, D., Guth, D., Wall, R., Long, R., & Ponchillia, P. (2005). Street crossing by sighted and blind pedestrians at a modern roundabout. *Journal of Transportation Engineering, 131*, 812–821.

Ashmead, D., & Wall, R. (1999). Auditory perception of walls via spectral variations in the ambient sound field. *Journal of Rehabilitation Research and Development, 36*, 313–332.

Association for Education and Rehabilitation of the Blind and Visually Impaired, Orientation and Mobility Division (AER O&M Division). (2006). Teaching street crossing at signalized intersections. Available from http://oandm.aerbvi.org/position_paper3.htm, accessed March 14, 2009.

Association for Education and Rehabilitation of the Blind and Visually Impaired, Orientation and Mobility Division (AER O&M Division). (2008). Teaching street crossing at streets and lanes where there is no traffic control. Available from http://oandm.aerbvi.org/PositionPaper_TeachingStreetCrossings2008.htm, accessed March 14, 2009.

Association for Education and Rehabilitation of the Blind and Visually Impaired, Orientation and Mobility Division (AER O&M Division). (2010). Position papers and resolutions. Available from http://oandm.aerbvi.org/position_papers.htm, accessed March 31, 2010.

Aust, A. M. D. (1980). Kinesiology. In R. L. Welsh & B. B. Blasch (Eds.), *Foundations of orientation and mobility* (pp. 37–71). New York: American Foundation for the Blind.

Austin, T., & Sleight, R. (1952). Accuracy of tactual discrimination of letters, numerals, and geometric forms. *Journal of Experimental Psychology, 43*, 239–249.

Ayres, A. (1979). *Sensory integration and the child*. Los Angeles: Western Psychological Services.

Ayres, A. J. (1989). *Sensory integration and praxis tests* (p. 11). Los Angeles: Western Psychological Services.

Azusa Unified School District. (1984). *Priority goals checklist for orientation and mobility*. Azusa, CA: Author.

Bachman, J. E., & Fuqua, R. W. (1983). Management of inappropriate behaviors of trainable mentally impaired students using antecedent exercise. *Journal of Applied Behavior Analysis, 16*, 477–484.

Bachman, J. E., & Sluyter, D. (1988). Reducing inappropriate behaviors of developmentally disabled adults using antecedent aerobic dance exercises. *Research in Developmental Disabilities, 9*, 73–83.

Bagley, M. (1994). *Confident living program facilitator manual*. Sands Point, NY: Helen Keller National Center for Youths and Adults with Deaf-Blindness.

Bailey, B. R., & Head, D. (1993). Orientation and mobility services to children and youth with multiple disabilities. *RE:view, 25*(2), 57–64.

Baird, A. A., & Goldie, D. (1979). Activities and experiences develop spatial and sensory understanding. *Teaching Exceptional Children, 11,* 116–119.

Baker, L. D. (1973). Blindness and social behavior: A need for research. *New Outlook for the Blind, 67*(7), 315–318.

Baldwin, D. (2003). Wayfinding technology: A road map to the future. *Journal of Visual Impairment & Blindness, 97*(10), 612–620.

Bambara, J. K., Wadley, V., Owsley, C., Martin, R. C., Porter, C., & Dreer, L. E. (2009). Family functioning and low vision: A systematic review. *Journal of Visual Impairment & Blindness, 103*(3), 137–149.

Bandura, A. (1977). *Social learning theory* (2nd ed.). Englewood Cliffs, NJ: Prentice-Hall.

Bandura, A. (1982). Self-efficacy mechanism in human agency. *American Psychologist, 37,* 122–147.

Bandura, A. (1986). *Social foundations of thought and action: A social cognitive theory.* Englewood Cliffs, NJ: Prentice Hall.

Bandura, A. (1997). *Self-efficacy: The exercise of control.* New York: W. H. Freeman and Company.

Bandura, A., & Adams, N. E. (1977). Analysis of self-efficacy theory of behavioral change. *Cognitive Therapy and Research, 1,* 287–308.

Banja, J. D. (1994). The determination of risks in orientation and mobility services: Ethical and professional issues. *Journal of Visual Impairment & Blindness, 88,* 401–409.

Bardach, Joan L. (1970). Psychological factors in the handicapped driver. *Psychological Aspects of Disability, 17* (1), 10–13.

Barkovich, J. A. (2005). *Pediatric neuroimaging* (4th ed.). Philadelphia: Lippincott, Williams & Wilkins.

Barlow, J. M. (2004). Orientation and alignment for street crossing: Pedestrians who are blind or visually impaired. In *Proceedings of the Wayfinding at Intersections Workshop.* Washington, DC: Institute of Transportation Engineers/U.S. Access Board.

Barlow, J. M., & Bentzen, B. L. (1994). *Cues blind travelers use to detect streets.* Cambridge, MA: Volpe National Transportation Systems Center, Federal Transit Administration.

Barlow, J. M., Bentzen, B. L., & Bond, T. (2005). Blind pedestrians and the changing technology and geometry of signalized intersections: Safety, orientation and independence. *Journal of Visual Impairment & Blindness, 99*(10), 587–598.

Barlow, J. M., Bentzen, B. L., Bond, T., & Gubbe, D. (2006). Accessible pedestrian signals: Effect on safety and independence of pedestrians who are blind. Transportation Research Board 85th annual meeting compendium of papers. Washington, DC: CD-Rom, Transportation Research Board.

Barlow, J. M., & Franck, L. (2005). Crossroads: Modern interactive intersections and accessible pedestrian signals. *Journal of Visual Impairment & Blindness, 99,* 599–610.

Barlow, J. M., Franck, L., Bentzen, B. L., & Sauerburger, D. (2001). Pedestrian clearance intervals at modern intersections: Implications for the safety of pedestrians who are visually impaired. *Journal of Visual Impairment & Blindness, 95,* 663–667.

Barraga, N. C., & Erin, J. N. (1992). *Visual handicaps & learning.* (3rd ed.). Austin, TX: PRO-ED.

Barraga, N. C., & Morris, J. E. (1980). *Program to develop efficiency in visual functioning: Sourcebook on low vision.* Louisville, KY: American Printing House for the Blind.

Barth, J. L. (1982). The development and evaluation of a tactile graphics kit. *Journal of Visual Impairment & Blindness, 76*(6), 269–273.

Baumgart, D., Brown, L., Pumpian, I., Nisbet, J., Ford, A., Sweet, M., Messina, R., & Schroeder, J. (1982). Principle of partial participation and individualized adaptations in educational programs for severely handicapped students. Available from www.mncdd.org/parallels2/pdf/82-WIP-TAS.pdf, accessed November 19, 2007.

Baumgart, D., Johnson, J., & Helmstetter, E. (1990). *Augmentative and alternative communication systems for persons with moderate and severe disabilities.* Baltimore, MD: Paul H. Brooks.

BBC News. (2009). Hot weather risks. Available from http://news.bbc.co.uk/2/hi/health/medical_notes/5190094.stm, accessed March 22, 2010.

Beirne-Smith, M., Ittenbach, R. F., & Patton, J. R. (2002). *Mental retardation.* (6th ed.). Upper Saddle River, NJ: Merrill.

Beleveau, M., & Smith, A. J. (Eds). (1980). *The interdisciplinary approach to low vision rehabilitation*. Stillwater: Oklahoma State University, National Clearinghouse on Rehabilitation Information.

Benjamin, A. (2001). *The helping interview with case illustrations*. Boston: Houghton-Mifflin.

Bentzen, B. L. (1977). Orientation maps for visually impaired persons. *Journal of Visual Impairment & Blindness, 71*, 193–196.

Bentzen, B. L. (1983). Tactile specifications of route configurations. In J. Wiedel (Ed.), *Proceedings of the First International Symposium on Maps and Graphics for the Visually Handicapped*. Washington, DC.

Bentzen, B. L. (1989). Considerations in the design of tactile maps for use by visually impaired travelers on rail rapid transit. *Enhancing the use of rail rapid transit by visually impaired travelers* (Vol. 7, Report No. UMTA-MA-06-0141-88-7). Washington, DC: U.S. Department of Transportation.

Bentzen, B. L. (1997). Orientation aids. In B. B. Blasch, W. R. Wiener, & R. L. Welsh (Eds.), *Foundations of orientation and mobility*. (2nd ed., pp. 284–316) New York: AFB Press.

Bentzen, B. L., & Barlow, J. (1995). Impact of curb ramps on safety of persons who are blind. *Journal of Visual Impairment & Blindness, 89*, 319–328.

Bentzen, B. L., Barlow, J. M., & Bond, T. (2004a). Challenges of unfamiliar signalized intersections for pedestrians who are blind: Research on safety. *Transportation Research Record: Journal of the Transportation Research Board, No. 1878*, pp. 51–57.

Bentzen, B. L., Barlow, J. M., & Franck, L. (2000). Addressing barriers to blind pedestrians at signalized intersections. *ITE Journal, 70*(9), 32–35.

Bentzen, B. L., & Peck, A. (1979). Factors affecting traceability of lines for tactile graphics. *Journal of Visual Impairment & Blindness, 71*, 264–269.

Bentzen, B. L., Scott, A. C., & Barlow, J. M. (2006). Accessible pedestrian signals: Effect of device features. *Transportation Research Record: Journal of the Transportation Research Board, No. 1982*, pp. 30–37.

Berg, R. V., Jose, R. T., & Carter, K. (1983). Distance training techniques. In R. T. Jose (Ed.), *Understanding low vision* (pp. 277–316). New York: American Foundation for the Blind.

Bergman, M. (1957). Binaural hearing. *Archives of Otolaryngology, 66*, 572–578.

Berlá, E. P. (1972). Behavioral strategies and problems in scanning and interpreting tactual displays. *New Outlook for the Blind, 66*, 272–286.

Berlá, E. P. (1973). Strategies in scanning a tactual pseudomap. *Education of the Visually Handicapped, 5*, 8–19.

Berlá, E. P., & Butterfield, L. H. (1977). Tactile political maps: Two experimental designs. *Journal of Visual Impairment & Blindness, 71*, 262–264.

Berlá, E. P., & Murr, M. J. (1975). The effects of noise on the location of point symbols and tracing a line on a tactile pseudomap. *Journal of Special Education, 9*, 183–190.

Berlin, L. J., Brooks-Gunn, J., McCarton, C., & McCormick, M. C. (1998). The effectiveness of early intervention: Examining risk factors and pathways to enhanced development. *Preventive Medicine, 27*, 238–245.

Berube, L. (1991). *Terminolgie de neuropsychologie et de neurologie du comportement*. Montréal: Les Éditons de la Cheneliie'ree Inc.

Birren, J. (1959). *Handbook of aging and the individual*. Chicago: University of Chicago Press.

Birrer, R. B., & Sedaghat, V. (2003). Exercise and diabetes mellitus: Optimizing performance in patients who have Type 1 diabetes. *Physician & Sportsmedicine, 31*(5), 29–33, 37–41.

Bishop, M., Hobson, R. P., & Lee, A. (2005). Symbolic play in congenitally blind children. *Development and Psychopathology, 17*(2), 447–465.

Björnstig, U., Björnstig, J., & Dahlgren, A. (1997). Slipping on ice and snow—Elderly women and young men are typical victims. *Accident Analysis and Prevention, 29*(2), 211–215.

Blasch, B. (1994). *Spatial orientation and wayfinding in elderly persons*. Final report.

Blasch, B. B. (1981a). Foundations for mobility instruction: A mobility model. *Proceedings of the Second International Mobility Conference*. Paris: IMC2.

Blasch, B. B. (1981b). *Independent mobility training to increase the activities of independent living for disabled individuals* (Project No. 19132). Madison: Wisconsin Division of Vocational Rehabilitation.

Blasch, B. B. (1982). *Mobility training for use of existing public transportation services. Final report* (Grant

Proposal No. 19935 [ICI]). Madison: Wisconsin Council of Developmental Disabilities.

Blasch, B. B. (1994a). *Orienteering for persons with developmental disabilities* (Project No. ADD# 07DD0273/13). Madison, WI: Department of Health and Human Services, Office of Human Development Services.

Blasch, B. B. (1994b). The mobility therapist and the non-exclusive mobility model. Paper presented at the Seventh International Mobility Conference, Melbourne, Australia.

Blasch, B. B. (1994c). The non-exclusive model of mobility and the mobility therapist. *Visions in Mobility: Proceedings of the Seventh International Mobility Conference.* Melbourne: Royal Guide Dogs Associations of Australia.

Blasch, B. B., & Brouwer, O. (1983). Innovative uses and content of maps for persons with visual impairment. In J. Wiedel (Ed.), *Proceedings of the First International Symposium on Maps and Graphics for the Visually Handicapped.* Washington, DC.

Blasch, B. B., & De l'Aune, W. R. (1992). A computer profile of mobility coverage and a safety index. *Journal of Visual Impairment & Blindness, 86*(6), 249–254.

Blasch, B. B., LaGrow, S. J., & De l'Aune, W. R. (1996). Three aspects of coverage provided by the long cane: Object, surface, and foot-placement preview. *Journal of Visual Impairment & Blindness, 90,* 295–301.

Blasch, B. B., Long, R. G., & Griffin-Shirley, N. (1989). Results of a national survey of electronic travel aid use. *Journal of Visual Impairment & Blindness, 83,* 449–453.

Blasch, B. B., & Penrod, W. (2006). Orienteering for people with visual impairments. Presentation at O&M Division Day, International Conference, Snowbird, Utah: Association for Education and Rehabilitation of the Blind and Visually Impaired.

Blasch, B. B., & Welsh, R. (1977). Orientation and mobility training for persons from all handicapped groups. In *Proceedings of the Biennial Convention.* Portland, OR: American Association of Workers for the Blind.

Blasch, B. B., & Welsh, R. L. (Eds.) (1980). Training for persons with functional mobility limitations. In

Foundations of orientation and mobility (pp. 461–476). New York: American Foundation for the Blind.

Blasch, B. B., Welsh, R. L., & Davidson, T. (1973). Auditory maps: An orientation aid for visually handicapped persons. *New Outlook for the Blind, 67*(4), 145–158.

Blasch, B. B., Wiener, W. R., & Welsh, R. L. (Eds.). (1997). *Foundations of orientation and mobility* (2nd ed.). New York: AFB Press.

Blasch, D., & Kaarlela, R. (1971). Orientation and mobility fans out. *Blindness Annual, 1971* (pp. 9–18). Washington, DC: American Association of Workers for the Blind.

Bledsoe, C. W. (1980). Originators of orientation and mobility training. In R. L. Welsh & B. B. Blasch (Eds.), *Foundations of orientation and mobility* (pp. 581–624). New York: American Foundation for the Blind.

Blind Childrens Center. (1986). *Move with me: A parents' guide to movement development for visually impaired babies.* Los Angeles: Author.

Blind Childrens Center. (1995). *Starting points: Instructional practices for young children whose multiple disabilities include visual impairment.* Los Angeles: Author.

Bloom, B., Englehart, M., Furst, E., Hill, W., & Krathwohl, D. (1956). *Taxonomy of educational objectives. Handbook 1: Cognitive domain.* New York: David McKay.

Blyskal, J. (1996). 2 old 2 drive. *Good Housekeeping,* June, p. 90.

Boekaerts, M. (2002). *Motivation to learn.* Educational Practices series 10. Geneva: UNESCO, International Academy of Education and the International Bureau of Education.

Boisvert, D. M. (2003). *Durability of truncated dome systems (a.k.a. detectable warning surfaces): Evaluation report.* Report No. FHWA-NH-RD-MPS2002-2. Concord, NH: Materials & Research Bureau, New Hampshire Department of Transportation and Federal Highway Transportation.

Boisvert, D. M., & Fowler, J. (2007). *Durability of truncated dome systems: Interim evaluation report, fall 2007.* Concord, NH: Materials & Research Bureau of the Hew Hampshire Department of Transportation. Available from www.nh.gov/dot//org/pro

jectdevelopment/materials/research/projects/documents/mps2002-2_report2.pdf.

Bond, T. L. (2006). Accuracy, errors and illusions in unimodal and bimodal vehicular motion tracking: An ecologically based evaluation of multimodal enhancement and the dynamic capture effect. Doctoral dissertation, Boston College.

Bourquin, E. (2002). Sighted guide technique for deafblind travelers. In *National interpreter curriculum for deaf-blind interpreting* (Video). San Diego: Dawn Sign Media.

Bourquin, E. (2005). Guiding tasks for interpreters working with deaf-blind travelers. *Registry of Interpreters for the Deaf Views, 22,* 17–19.

Bourquin, E. (2007). Travelers who are deafblind: A correlational study of influences on assistance-gaining for street crossings. PhD diss. University of Phoenix, Phoenix, AZ.

Bourquin, E., & Moon, J. (2008). Studies on obtaining assistance by travelers who are deaf-blind. *Journal of Visual Impairment & Blindness, 102*(6), 352–361.

Bourquin, E., & Sauerburger, D. (2005). Teaching deaf-blind people to communicate and interact with the public: Critical issues for travelers who are deaf-blind. *RE:view, 37*(3), 109–116.

Bradette, M., Couturier, J., & Rousseau, J. (2005). Impact on night vision aid on orientation and mobility and daily activities. *International Congress Series, 1282,* 71–74.

Brain Injury. (n.d.). Symptoms of brain injury. Available from www.braininjury.com, accessed March 10, 2006.

Brain Injury Association of America. (n.d.). About brain injury. Available from www.biausa.org/aboutbi.htm, accessed March 11, 2007.

Brain Injury Association of America. (n.d.). Types of brain injury. Available from www.biausa.org/Pages/types_of_brain_injury.html, accessed June 10, 2006.

Brambila-Hickman, B., & Denniston, K. (1984). *Mobility training curriculum for developmentally disabled adults.* Dearborn Heights, MI: Wayne County Associations for the Retarded.

Branch, L. G., Horowitz, A., & Carr, C. (1989). The implications for everyday life of incident self-reported visual decline among people over age 65. *The Gerontologist, 29*(3), 359–365.

Bransford, J. D., Brown, A. L., & Cocking, R. R. (Eds.) (2000). *How people learn: Brain, mind, experience, and school.* Washington, D.C.: Committee on Developments in the Science of Learning. National Research Council, National Academy Press.

Brown, C., & Bour, B. (1986). *Volume V-K: Movement analysis and curriculum for visually impaired preschoolers.* Tallahassee: State of Florida Department of Education Bureau of Education for Exceptional Students.

Buchner, D. M., & de Lateur, B. J. (1991). The importance of skeletal muscle strength to physical function in older adults. *Behavioral Medical Annals, 13,* 91–98.

Burlingham, D. (1965). Some problems of ego development in blind children. *Psychoanalytic Study of the Child, 19,* 95–112.

Butler, R., & Lewis, M. (1973). *Aging and mental health.* St. Louis: C.V. Mosby Co.

Byers-Lang, R. E., & McCall, R. A. (1993). Peer support groups: Rehabilitation in action. *RE:view, 25*(1), 32–37.

California State Board of Education. (1997a). *Mathematics content standards for California public schools: Kindergarten through grade twelve.* Sacramento: Author.

California State Board of Education. (1997b). *Physical education guidelines for kindergarten through grade twelve.* Sacramento: Author.

California State Board of Education. (1998). *Science content standards for California public schools: Kindergarten through grade twelve.* Sacramento: Author.

California State Board of Education. (2005). *Visual and performing arts: Dance content standards for California public schools: Kindergarten through grade twelve.* Sacramento: Author.

Campbell, A. J., Robertson, M. C., LaGrow, S. J., Kerse, N. M., Sanderson, G. F., Jacobs, R. J., et al. (2005). Randomized controlled trial of prevention of falls in people aged ≥75 with severe visual impairment: The VIP trial. *British Medical Journal, 331,* 817–820.

Canada Safety Council. (2006). Safety tips for winter walking. Available from www.safety-council

.org/info/seniors/winter.html, accessed October 2, 2006.

Capezuti, E., Boltz, M., Renz, S., Hoffman, D., & Norman, R. (2006). Nursing home involuntary relocation: Clinical outcomes and perceptions of residents and families. *Journal of the American Medical Directors Association, 7*(8), 486–492.

Carhart, R. (1960). Auditory training. In H. Davis & R. Silverman (Eds.), *Hearing and deafness* (2nd ed.). New York: Holt, Rinehart & Winston.

Carkhuff, R. R. (1969). *Helping and human relations.* New York: Holt, Rinehart & Winston.

Carkhuff, R. R. (2000). *The art of helping in the 21st century.* Amherst, MA: Human Resources Development Press.

Carroll, J., & Bentzen, B. L. (2000). American Council of the Blind survey of intersection accessibility. *The Braille Forum, 38*(7), 11–15.

Carroll, T. J. (1961). *Blindness: What it is, what it does, and how to live with it.* Boston: Little, Brown.

Casten, R., & Rovner, B. (2008). Depression in age-related macular degeneration. *Journal of Visual Impairment & Blindness, 102*(10), 591–599.

Casten, R., Rovner, B., & Edmonds, S. (2002). The impact of depression in older adults with age-related macular degeneration. *Journal of Visual Impairment & Blindness, 96*(6), 399–415.

Centers for Disease Control and Prevention (CDC). (n.d.). Important asthma triggers. Available from www.cdc.gov/asthma/faqs.htm, accessed May 17, 2007.

Centers for Disease Control and Prevention (CDC). (1996). Prevalence of selected developmental disabilities in children 3–10 years of age: The metropolitan Atlanta developmental disabilities surveillance program, 45(No. SS-2), 1–13.

Centers for Disease Control and Prevention (CDC). (2003). National Center for Health Statistics. Available from www.cdc.gov/nchs/nhis.htm, accessed March 24, 2005.

Centers for Disease Control and Prevention (CDC). (2005). *National diabetes fact sheet: General information and national estimates on diabetes in the United States, 2005.* Atlanta, GA: U.S. Department of Health and Human Services, Centers for Disease Control and Prevention.

Centers for Disease Control and Prevention (CDC). (2006). Frequently asked questions (FAQ) about extreme heat. U.S. Department of Health and Human Services. Available from www.bt.cdc.gov/disasters/extremeheat/faq.asp, accessed July 14, 2007.

Centers for Disease Control and Prevention (CDC). (2009). Extreme heat: A prevention guide to promote your personal health and safety. U.S. Department of Health and Human Services. Available from www.bt.cdc.gov/disasters/extremeheat/heat_guide.asp, accessed March 23, 2010.

Chad, K. E., Reeder, B. A., Harrison, E. L., Ashworth, N. L., Sheppard, S. M., Schultz, S. L. et al (2005). Profile of physical activity levels in community-dwelling older adults. *Medicine and Science in Sports and Exercise, 37*(10), 1774–1784.

Chalkley, T. (2000). *Your eyes* (4th ed.). Springfield, IL: Charles C Thomas.

Chapman, E. K. (1978). *Visually handicapped children and young people.* London: Routledge.

Chen, D (Ed.). (1999). *Essential elements in early intervention.* New York: AFB Press.

Chew, S. (1986). The use of traffic sounds by blind pedestrians (Ph.D. diss., University of Minnesota, 1986). *Dissertation Abstracts International, 47,* 08B.

Children's Hospital Boston. (n.d.). Leg length discrepancy. Available from www.childrenshospital.org, accessed February 25, 2008.

Choi, S.-W., Peek-Asa, C., Zwerling, C., Sprince, N. L., Rautiainen, R. H., Whitten, P. S., et al. (2006). A comparison of self-reported hearing and pure tone threshold average in the Iowa Farm Family Health and Hazard Survey. *Journal of Agromedicine, 10*(3), 31–39.

Chow, D., Kwok, M., Au-Yang, A., Holmes, A., Cheng, J., Yao, F., & Wong, M.S. (2005). The effect of backpack load on the gait of normal adolescent girls (electronic version). *Ergonomics, 48*(6), 642–656.

Cimarolli, V., Sussman-Skalka, C., & Goodman, C. (2004). Programs for partners: Support groups for partners of adults with visual impairments. *Journal of Visual Impairment & Blindness, 98*(2), 90–98.

Cimarolli, V. R., Reinhardt, J. P., & Horowitz, A. (2006). Perceived overprotection: Support gone bad? *The Journals of Gerontology Series B: Psychological Sciences and Social Sciences, 61,* S18–S23.

Clarke, K. (1988). Barriers or enablers? Mobility devices for visually impaired multihandicapped infants and preschoolers. *Education of the Visually Handicapped, 20,* 115–132.

Clarke, K. L., Sainato, D. M., & Ward, M. E. (1994). Travel performance of preschoolers: The effects of mobility training with long cane versus a precane. *Journal of Visual Impairment & Blindness, 88,* 19–30.

Cleveland Clinic Health Information Center. Recognizing and treating heat-related illness. Available from www.clevelandclinic.org/health/health-info/docs/3000/3097.asp?index=10872.

Clifton, K. J. (2003). Independent mobility among teenagers: An exploration of travel to after-school activities. *Transportation Research Record: Journal of the Transportation Research Board,* 74–80.

Colby Trott, M., Laurel, M., & Windeck, S. (1993). *Senseabilities: Understanding sensory integration.* San Antonio, TX: Therapy Skill Builder.

Colcombe, S. J., Kramer, A. F., Erickson, K. I., Scalf, P., McAuley, E., Cohen, N. J., et al. (2004). Cardiovascular fitness, cortical plasticity, and aging. *Proceedings of the National Academy of Sciences of the United States of America, 101*(9), 3316–3321.

Collins, S., & Petronio, K. (1998). What happens in tactile ASL? In C. Lucas (Ed.), *Pinky extension and eye gaze: Language use in deaf communities* (pp. 18–37). Washington, DC: Gallaudet University Press.

Committee on Pediatric AIDS. (2000). Education of children with human immunodeficiency virus infection. *Pediatrics, 105*(6), 1358–1360.

Coren, S., & Hakstian, A. R. (1992). The development and cross validation of a self-report inventory to assess pure-tone threshold hearing sensitivity. *Journal of Speech and Hearing Research, 35,* 921–928.

Corn, A. L. (1987). Socialization and the child with low vision. Keynote Address to the Sixth Canadian Interdisciplinary Conference on the Blind Child, Nova Scotia.

Corn, A. L., Bell, J. K., Anderson, E., Bachofer, C., Jose, R., & Perez, A. (2003). Providing access to the visual environment: A model of comprehensive low vision services for children. *Journal of Visual Impairment & Blindness, 97,* 261–272.

Corn, A. L., & Sacks, S. Z. (1994). The impact of nondriving on adults with visual impairments. *Journal of Visual Impairment & Blindness, 88*(1), 53–68.

Cotch, M. F., & Janiszewski, D. R. (2002). *National Health Interview Survey (NHIS).* Hyattsville, MD: U.S. Department of Health and Human Services.

Couturier, J. A., Ratelle, A., & Bilodeau, E. (November 2006). Orientation and mobility issues related to winter conditions: Opinions of functionally blind experienced travelers. Paper presented at the NE/AER Conference 2006, Montréal, Québec.

Cowen, C., & Shepler, R. (2000). Activities and games for teaching children to use magnifiers. In M. D'Andrea & C. Farrenkopf (Eds.), *Looking to Learn* (pp. 167-188). New York: AFB Press.

Crandall, W., Bentzen, B. L., & Myers, L. (1998). Remote signage development to address current and emerging access problems for blind individuals. *Part I. Smith-Kettlewell research on the use of Talking Signs at light controlled street crossings.* Report to National Institute on Disability and Rehabilitation Research, Washington, DC.

Cratty, B. J. (1965). *Perceptual thresholds of nonvisual locomotion (Part 1).* Los Angeles: University of California.

Cratty, B. J., & Sams, T. A. (1968). *The body image of blind children.* New York: American Foundation for the Blind.

Cratty, B. J., & Williams, H. (1966). *Perceptual thresholds of nonvisual locomotion (part 2).* Los Angeles: University of California.

Crews, J. (1991). Strategic planning and independent living for elders who are blind. *Journal of Visual Impairment & Blindness, 85*(2), 52–57.

Crews, J. E., & Campbell, V. A. (2001). Health conditions, activity limitations, and participation restrictions among older people with visual impairments. *Journal of Visual Impairment & Blindness, 95*(8), 453–457.

Crews, J. E., Jones, G. C., & Kim, J. H. (2006). The effects of comorbid conditions among older persons with vision loss. *Journal of Visual Impairment & Blindness, 100*(Special Supplement), 842–848.

Crone, K., & McKinney, B. (2004). *Program in low vision therapy.* Houston: Region 4 Education Service Center.

Cross, A., Frazeur, T., Traub, E. K., Hutter-Pishgahi, L., & Shelton, G. (2004). Elements of successful inclusion for children with significant disabilities. *Topics in Early Childhood Special Education, 24*(3), 169–184.

Crouse, R. J., & Bina, M. J. (1997). The administration of orientation and mobility programs for children and adults. In B. B. Blasch, W. R. Wiener, & R. L. Welsh (Eds.), *Foundations of orientation and mobility.* (2nd ed., pp. 646–659) New York: AFB Press.

Current Estimates. (2004). How many deaf people are there in the U.S.? Gallaudet University. Available from http://gri.gallaudet.edu/Demographics/deaf-US.php, accessed March 3, 2007.

Dacen-Hagel, D. L., & Coulson, M. R. C. (1990). Tactual mobility maps—A comparative study. *Cartographica, 27*(2), 47–63.

Darken, R., & Peterson, B. (2002). Spatial orientation, wayfinding and representation. In K. M. Stanney (Ed.), *Handbook of virtual environments design, implementation and applications* (pp. 493–518). Hillsdale, NJ: Erlbaum.

Dauterman, W. L. (1972). *Stanford multi-modality imagery test.* New York: American Foundation for the Blind.

DeFiore, E. N., & Silver, R. (1988). A redesigned assistance card for the deaf-blind traveler. *Journal of Visual Impairment & Blindness, 82*(5), 175–177.

De l'Aune, W., Lewis, C., Dolan, M., Grimmelsman, T., & Needham, W. (1976, April). Two sensory aids having profound effects on the blind. Paper presented at the IEE International Conference on Acoustics, Philadelphia, PA.

De l'Aune, W. R., Welsh, R. L., & Williams, M. D. (2000). A national outcomes assessment of the rehabilitation of adults with visual impairments. *Journal of Visual Impairment & Blindness, 94*(5), 281–291.

DeLoache, J. S. (1991). Symbolic functioning in very young children: Understanding of pictures and models. *Child Development, 62*, 736–752.

Denham, J., Leventhal, J., & McComas, H. (2004). Getting from point A to point B: A review of two GPS systems. *AccessWorld, 5*(6), available from www.afb.org/afbpress/pub.asp?DocID=aw050605, accessed April 21, 2010.

Department of Health and Human Services. (2002). *The management of sickle cell disease* (NIH Publication No. 02-2117). Washington, DC: Author.

Dettmer, P., Dyck, N., & Thurston, L. P. (2002). *Consultation, collaboration, and teamwork for students with special needs* (3rd ed.). Boston: Allyn & Bacon.

de Vries, L., Dubowitz, L., Dubowitz, V., & Pennock, J. (1990). *Brain disorders in the newborn.* London: Wolfe Medical Publications Ltd.

Dietrichson, J., Lund, R., Moe, C., & Saeter, E. (1998, July). Mobility in the snow. Paper presented at the 9th International Mobility Conference, Atlanta, GA.

Dodds, A., Ferguson, E., Ng, L., Flannigan, H., Hawes, G., & Yates, L. (1994). The concept of adjustment: A structural model. *Journal of Visual Impairment & Blindness, 88*, 487–497.

Dodds, A. G. (1989). Motivation reconsidered: The importance of self-efficacy in rehabilitation. *British Journal of Visual Impairment, 7*, 11–15.

Dodson-Burk, B., & Hill, E. W. (1989). *An orientation and mobility primer for families.* New York: American Foundation for the Blind.

Doolittle, P. E. (1997). Vygotsky's Zone of Proximal Development as a theoretical foundation for cooperative learning. *Journal on Excellence in College Teaching, 8*(1), 83–103.

Dote-Kwan, J. (1995). Instructional strategies. In D. Chen & J. Dote-Kwan (Eds.), *Starting points: Instructional practices for young children whose multiple disabilities include visual impairment* (pp. 43–56). Los Angeles: Blind Childrens Center.

Downing, J. E. (2004). Communication skills. In F. P. Orelove, D. Sobsey, & R. K. Silberman (Eds.), *Educating children with multiple disabilities: A collaborative approach* (4th ed., pp. 529–562). Baltimore: Paul H. Brookes Publishing, Co.

Drew, C. J., & Hardman, M. L. (2004). *Mental retardation: A lifespan approach to people with intellectual disabilities* (8th ed.). Columbus, OH: Pearson Merrill Prentice Hall.

Duffy, M. (2005). *Making life more livable: Simple adaptations for the homes of blind and visually impaired older people* (rev. ed.). New York: AFB Press.

Dunham-Sims, F. (2005). Orientation and mobility and the itinerant teacher. In J. E. Olmstead (Ed.), *Itinerant teaching: Tricks of the trade for teachers of students with visual impairments* (pp. 125–159). New York: AFB Press.

Dura, J. V., Alcantara, E., Zamora, T., Balaguer, E., & Rosa, D. (2005). Identification of floor friction safety level for public buildings considering mobility disabled people needs. *Safety Science, 43*(7), 407–423.

Dutton, G. (2002). Visual problems in children with damage to the brain. *Visual Impairment Research, 4*(2), 113–121.

Dutton, G. N. (2001). Cerebral visual impairment in children. *Seminars in Neonatology, 6*(6), 477–485.

Dykes, J. (1992). Opinions of orientation and mobility instructors about using the long cane with preschool-age children. *RE:view, 24*(2), 85–92.

Eames, E., & Eames, T. (1994). *A guide to the dog guide schools* (2nd ed.). New York: Baruch College Guide Dog Book Fund.

Easter Seals Project ACTION. (2003). *Accessible pedestrian signals: A curriculum development project draft final report.* Washington, DC: Project ACTION.

Easter Seals Project ACTION. (2006). Toolkit for the assessment of bus stop accessibility and safety. Available from http://projectaction.easterseals .com, accessed May 18, 2006.

Easton, R. D., & Bentzen, B. L. (1980). Perception of tactile route configurations by blind and sighted observers. *Journal of Visual Impairment & Blindness, 74,* 254–257, 261–264.

Edman, P. K. (1992). *Tactile graphics.* New York: American Foundation for the Blind.

Ehresman, P. (1994). Facilitating successful outdoor O&M instruction of multihandicapped blind travelers. *RE:view, 25*(4), 179–184.

Ellis, M. J., MacLean, W. E., Jr., & Gazdag, G. (1990). The effects of exercise and cardiovascular fitness on stereotyped body rocking. *Journal of Behavior Therapy and Experimental Psychiatry, 20,* 251–256.

Engel, R., Welsh, R., & Lewis, L. (2000). Improving the well-being of vision-impaired older adults through orientation and mobility training and rehabilitation: An evaluation. *RE:view, 32*(2), 67–76.

Engelman, K. K., Altus, D. E., Mosier, M. C., & Mathews, R. M. (2003). Brief training to promote the use of less intrusive prompts by nursing assistants in a dementia care unit. *Journal of Applied Behavior Analysis, 36*(1), 129–132.

Epilepsy.com/professionals. (2007). Classifying seizures. Available from http://professionals. epilepsy.com/page/seizures_classified.html, accessed May 17, 2007.

Ericson, M. A., & Staley, A. B. (2003). Noise induced hearing loss and auditory localization. Available from www.hec.afrl.af.mil/Publications/ ASC030488.pdf, accessed July 17, 2006.

Erikson, E. H. (1982). *The life cycle completed: A review.* New York: W. W. Norton.

Erin, J. (2003). Educating students with visual impairments. The ERIC Clearinghouse on Disabilities and Gifted Education (ERIC EC Digest No. E653). Arlington, VA: The Council for Exceptional Children.

Erin, J., & Spungin, S. (2004). *When you have a visually impaired student with multiple disabilities in your classroom: A guide for teachers.* New York: AFB Press.

Erin, J. N. (1996). Functional vision assessment and instruction of children and youths with multiple disabilities. In A. L. Corn and A. J. Koenig (Eds.), *Foundations of low vision: Clinical and functional perspectives* (pp. 221–245). New York: AFB Press.

Erin, J. N., & Corn, A. L. (1994). A survey of children's first understanding of being visually impaired. *Journal of Visual Impairment & Blindness, 80,* 132–139.

Erin, J. N., Daugherty, W., Dignan, K., & Pearson, N. (1990). Teachers of visually handicapped students with multiple disabilities: Perceptions of adequacy. *Journal of Visual Impairment & Blindness, 84,* 16–20.

Erin, J. N., Fazzi, D. L., Gordon, R. L., Isenberg, S. J.,& Paysse E. A. (2002). Vision focus: Understanding the medical and functional implications of vision loss. In R. L. Pogrund & D. L. Fazzi (Eds.), *Early focus: Working with young children who are blind or visually impaired and their families* (2nd ed., pp. 52–106). New York: AFB Press.

Erin, J. N., & Paul, B. (1996). Functional vision assessment and instruction of children and youths in academic programs. In A. L. Corn & A. J. Koenig (Eds.), *Foundations of low vision* (pp. 185–220). New York: AFB Press.

Ettinger, W. H., Jr. (1997). Moderate, low-impact exercise benefits patients with OA of the knee. *Geriatrics, 52,* 23–24.

Farmer, L. W. (1980). Mobility devices. In R. L. Welsh & B. B. Blasch (Eds.), *Foundations of orientation and mobility* (pp. 357–412). New York: American Foundation for the Blind.

Farmer, L. W., & Smith, D. L. (1997). Adaptive technology. In B. B. Blasch, W. R. Wiener, & R. L. Welsh (Eds.), *Foundations of orientation and mobility* (2nd ed., pp. 231–259). New York: AFB Press.

Fazzi, D. L. (1998). Facilitating independent travel for students who have visual impairments with other disabilities. In S. Sacks & R. Silberman (Eds.), *Educating students who have visual impairments with other disabilities* (pp. 441–468). Baltimore, MD: Paul H. Brookes.

Fazzi, D. L., & Klein, M. D. (2002). Cognitive focus: Developing cognition, concepts, and language. In R. L. Pogrund & D. L. Fazzi (Eds.), *Early focus: Working with young children who are blind or visually impaired and their families* (2nd ed., pp. 107–153). New York: AFB Press.

Fazzi, D. L., Klein, M. D., Pogrund, R. L., & Salcedo, P. S. (2002). Family focus: Working effectively with families. In R. L. Pogrund & D. L. Fazzi (Eds.). *Early focus: Working with young children who are blind or visually impaired and their families* (2nd ed., pp. 16–51). New York: AFB Press.

Fazzi, D. L., & Petersmeyer, B. A. (2001). *Imagining the possibilities: Creative approaches to orientation and mobility instruction for persons who are visually impaired*. New York: AFB Press.

Federal Highway Administration (FHWA). (2000). *Roundabouts: An informational guide* (FHWA-RD-00-67). Washington, DC: Department of Transportation, Federal Highway Administration.

Federal Highway Administration (FHWA). (2009). *Manual on uniform traffic control devices for streets and highways*. Washington, DC: Department of Transportation, Federal Highway Administration.

Federal Highway Administration (FHWA). (2004). *Signalized intersections: Informational guide* (FHWA-HRT-04-091). Washington, DC: Department of Transportation, Federal Highway Administration.

Federal Interagency Forum on Aging-Related Statistics (FIFARS). (2006). *Older Americans update 2006: Key indicators of well-being*. Washington, DC: Government Printing Office.

Federal Transit Authority. (1993). *Americans with disabilities act paratransit eligibility manual*. Available from http://ntl.bts.gov/DOCS/ada.html, accessed May 29, 2009.

Ferrell, K. (1998). *Project PRISM: A longitudinal study of developmental patterns of children who are visually impaired (final report)*. Greeley, CO: University of Northern Colorado, Division of Special Education.

Ferrell, K. A. (1979). Orientation and mobility for preschool children: What we have and what we need. *Journal of Visual Impairment & Blindness, 73*, 147–150.

Ferrell, K. A. (1985). *Reach out and teach: Meeting the training needs of parents of visually and multiply handicapped young children*. New York: American Foundation for the Blind.

Ferrell, K. A. (2000). Growth and development of young children. In M. C. Holbrook & A. J. Koenig (Eds.), *Foundations of education*, Vol. 1: *History and theory of teaching children and youths with visual impairments* (2nd ed., pp. 111–134). New York: American Foundation for the Blind.

Ferris, F. L., & Tielsch, J. M. (2004). Blindness and visual impairment: A public health issue for the future as well as today. *Archives of Ophthalmology, 122*: 451–452.

Finestone, S., Lukoff, I., & Whiteman, M. (1960). *The demand for dog guides*. New York: Research Center, New York School of Social Work, Columbia University.

First European Symposium on Tactual Town Maps for the Blind. General Report. Brussels, Belgium, 1984.

Fitzgerald, H. K., & Asenjo, J. A. (1965). Rehabilitation centers: Their growth and development. *Blindness Annual*, 47–57.

Fitzpatrick, K., Turner, S., Brewer, M., Carlson, P., Ullman, B., Trout, N., et al. (2006). *TCRP Report 112/NCHRP Report 562—Improving pedestrian safety at unsignalized crossings*. Transit Cooperative Research Program and National Cooperative Highway Research Program, Washington, DC: Transportation Research Board.

Flamme, G. (2002). Localization, hearing impairment, and hearing aids. *The Hearing Journal, 55*(6), 10–20.

Flanagan, N., Jackson, A., & Hill, A. (2003). Visual impairment in childhood: insights from a community-based survey. *Child: Care, Health & Development, 29*(6), 493–499.

Florence, I. J., & Lagrow, S. J. (1989). The use of a recorded message for gaining assistance with street crossings for deaf-blind travelers. *Journal of Visual Impairment & Blindness, 83*(9), 471–472.

Fong, D. T.-P., Mao, D.-W., Li, J.-X., & Hong, Y. (2008). Greater toe grip and gentler heel strike are the strategies to adapt to slippery surface. *Journal of Biomechanics, 41*, 838–844.

Forney, P. E., & Heller, K. W. (2004). Sensorimotor development: Implications for the educational team. In F. P. Orelove, D. Sobsey, & R. K. Silberman (Eds.), *Educating children with multiple disabilities: A collaborative approach* (4th ed., pp. 193–248). Baltimore: Paul H. Brookes Publishing, Co.

Foy, C. J., Kirchner, D., & Waple, L. (1991). The Connecticut precane. *Journal of Visual Impairment & Blindness, 85*, 85–86.

Foy, C. J., Von Scheden, M., & Waiculonis, J. (1992). The Connecticut pre-cane: Case study and curriculum. *Journal of Visual Impairment & Blindness, 86*, 178–181.

Francophone Network for Injury Prevention and Safety Promotion, No. IPSP, (2004 English version, 2008). *Good practice guide: Prevention of falls in the elderly living at home.* France: Institut national de prévention et d'éducation pour la santé (INPES). Available from www.inpes.sante.fr/CFESBases/catalogue/pdf/1160.pdf, accessed March 3, 2009.

Frankel, M. (2002). Deaf-blind interpreting: Interpreters' use of negation in tactile American Sign Language. *Sign Language Studies, 2*(2), 169–181.

Franklin, P., & Bourquin, E. (2000). Picture this: A pilot study for improving street crossings for deaf-blind travelers. *RE:view, 31*(4).

Frequently Asked Questions About Deafblindness. (2005). Available from www.deafblindinfo.org/FAQ.asp#Q7, accessed December 1, 2005.

Friedman, D. S., Congdon, N., Kempen, J., & Tielsch, J. M. (2002). *Visual problems in the U.S. prevalence of adult vision impairment and age-related eye disease in America.* Bethesda, MD: National Eye Institute. (NTIS No. PB2002-106996).

Frieswyk, J. (2005, Winter). Crossing strategies for modern signalized intersections. *Newsletter of the Orientation and Mobility Division.* Alexandria, VA: Association for Education and Rehabilitation of the Blind and Visually Impaired.

Gannon, J. R. (1981). *Deaf heritage: A narrative history of deaf America.* Silver Spring, MD.: National Association of the Deaf.

Gao, C., & Abeysekera, J. (2004a). A systems perspective of slip and fall accidents on icy and snowy surfaces. *Ergonomics, 47*(5), 573–598.

Gao, C., & Abeysekera, J. (2004b). Slips and falls on ice and snow in relation to experience in winter climate and winter sport. *Safety Science, 42*, 537–545.

Gao, C., Holmer, I., & Abeysekera, J. (2008). Slips and falls in a cold climate: Underfoot surface, footwear design and worker preferences for preventive measures. *Applied Ergonomics, 39*, 385–391.

Gard, G., & Berggard, G. (2006). Assessment of anti-slip devices from healthy individuals in different ages walking on slippery surfaces. *Applied Ergonomics, 37*, 177–186.

Gard, G., & Lundborg, G. (2000). Pedestrians on slippery surfaces during winter—Methods to describe the problems and practical tests of anti-skid devices. *Accident Analysis and Prevention, 32*, 455–460.

Gard, G., & Lundborg, G. (2001). Test of Swedish anti-skid devices on five different slippery surfaces. *Accident Analysis and Prevention, 33*, 1–8.

Gardiner, A., & Perkins, C. (2002). Best practice guidelines for the design, production and presentation of vacuum formed tactile maps. Available from www.tactility.co.uk/tactileguidelines/page1.htm, accessed October 6, 2007.

Gardner, H. (1993). *Multiple intelligences: The theory in practice.* New York: Basic Books.

Gee, K., Harrell, R., & Rosenberg, R. (1987). Teaching orientation and mobility skills within and across natural opportunities for travel: A model designed for learners with multiple severe disabilities. In L. Goetz, D. Guess, & K. Stremel-Campbell (Eds.), *Innovative program design for individuals with dual sensory impairments* (pp. 127–157). Baltimore: Paul H. Brookes.

Gense, M. H., & Gense, J. (2005). *Autism spectrum disorders and visual impairment: Meeting students' learning needs.* New York: AFB Press.

Gerber, E., & Kirchner, C. (2003). Livable communities throughout the life course. *Disability Studies Quarterly, 23*(2), 41–57.

Gerber, S. (1974). *Introductory hearing science.* Philadelphia: W.B. Saunders.

Geruschat, D. R. (1980). Training with hand-held distance optical aids. In M. Beliveau & A. J. Smith, (Eds.), *The interdisciplinary approach to low vision rehabilitation*. Stillwater: Oklahoma State University, National Clearinghouse on Rehabilitation Information.

Geruschat, D. R., & Hassan, S. E. (2005). Driver behavior in yielding to sighted and blind pedestrians at roundabouts. *Journal of Visual Impairment & Blindness, 99*(5), 286–302.

Geruschat, D. R., & Turano, K. A. (2002). Connecting research on retinitis pigmentosa to the practice of orientation and mobility. *Journal of Visual Impairment & Blindness, 96*(2), 69–85.

Gervasoni, E. (1996). Strategies and techniques used by a person who is totally deaf and blind to obtain assistance in crossing streets. *RE:view, 28*(2), 53.

Giangreco, M. F., Cloninger, C. J., Dennis, R. E., & Edelman, S. W. (2000). Problem-solving methods to facilitate inclusive education. In R. S. Villa & J. S. Thousand (Eds.), *Restructuring for caring and effective education: Piecing the puzzle together* (2nd ed., pp. 293–359). Baltimore: Paul H. Brookes Publishing Co.

Gibson, J. J. (1966). *The senses considered as perceptual systems*. Boston: Houghton Mifflin.

Gikling, G. (1949). Run-down at the heels. *American Journal of Nursing, 49*(12), 796–798.

Gill, J. M. (1973a). Design, production and evaluation of tactual maps for the blind. PhD diss, University of Warwick, Coventry, UK.

Gill, J. M. (1973b). Method for the production of tactual maps and diagrams. *American Foundation for the Blind Research Bulletin, 26*, 203–204.

Gill, J. M., & James, G. A. (1973). A study on the discrimination of tactual point symbols. *American Foundation for the Blind Research Bulletin, 26*, 19–34.

Glickman, N. S., & Harvey, M. A. (Eds.). (1996). *Culturally affirmative psychotherapy with deaf persons*. Mahwah, NJ: Lawrence Erlbaum Associates.

Glidden, L. M. (2003). Where are the mental and retardation in mental retardation? In H. Switzky & S. Greenspan (Eds.), *What is mental retardation?* Washington, DC: American Association on Mental Retardation.

Goetz, L., Guess, D., & Stremel-Campbell, K. (Eds.). (1987). *Innovative program design for individuals with dual sensory impairments*. Baltimore: Paul H. Brookes Publishing Co.

Gold, D. (Ed.). (2002). *Finding a new path: Guidance for parents of young children who are visually impaired or blind*. Toronto, ON: The Canadian National Institute for the Blind.

Goldberg, E. (2001). *The executive brain*. New York: Oxford University Press.

Good, W., Jan, J., Burden, S., Skoczenski, A. & Rowan, C. (2001). Recent advances in cortical visual impairment. *Developmental Medicine and Child Neurology, 43*, 56–60.

Goodrich, G. L., & Ludt, R. (2003). Assessing visual detection ability for mobility in individuals with low vision. *Visual Impairment Research, 5*(2), 57–71.

Gordon-Salant, S., Lantz, J., & Fitzgibbons, P. (1994). Age effects on measures of hearing disability. *Ear and Hearing. 15*(3), 199–272.

Graham, M. (1998). Mobility in the snow for people who are visually impaired: The art of travel on hidden landscape. *Journal of Visual Impairment & Blindness, 92*(9), 678–684.

Gray, R., & Thornton, I. M. (2001). Exploring the link between time-to-collision and representational momentum. *Perception, 30*, 1007–1022.

Greear, J. N. (1946). Rehabilitation of the blinded soldier. *Outlook for the Blind, 40*, 271–272.

Greene, H. A., Pekar, J., Brilliant, R., Freeman, P. B., Lewis, H. T., Siwoff, R., et al. (1991). The Ocutech Vision Enhancing System (VES): Utilization and preference study. *Journal of the American Optometric Association, 62*, 19–26.

Greene, R. W. (2001). *The explosive child*. New York: HarperCollins.

Greenough, W., Black, J., & Wallace, C. (1987). Experience and brain development. *Child Development, 58*, 539–559.

Greenspan, S. (1999). What is meant by mental retardation? *International Review of Psychiatry, 11*, 6–18.

Greenwald, D. M. (1979). *The basic components of guide-dog utilization: A guide for the orientation and mobility specialist*. Kalamazoo, MI: Western Michigan University.

Gregory, R. L. (1995). *Sensation and perception.* Essex: Longman Essential Psychology.

Griffin, H. (1981). Motor development in congenitally blind children. *Education of the Visually Handicapped, 12,* 106–111.

Griffin, S. (2007). Recommended daily water intake. Ask the expert. Available from www.myfooddiary .com/resources/ask_the_expert/, accessed July 9, 2007.

Griffin-Shirley, N., & Groff, G. (1993). *Prescriptions for independence.* New York: American Foundation for the Blind.

Groce, M., & Isaacson, A. B. (1995). Purposeful movement. In K. M. Huebner, J. G. Pricket, R. Welch, & E. Joffee (Eds.), *Hand and hand.* New York: AFB Press.

Groen, B. E., Weerdesteyn, V., & Duysens, J. (2007). Martial art fall techniques decrease forces at the hip during sideways falling. *Journal of Biomechanics, 2*(40), 458–482.

Grönqvist, R. (1995). A dynamic method for assessing pedestrian slip resistance. PhD diss. People and Work, Research Reports 2. Helsinki: Finnish Institute of Occupational Health.

Grönqvist, R., & Hirvonen, M. (1995). Slipperiness of footwear and mechanisms of walking friction on icy surfaces. *International Journal of Industrial Ergonomics, 16,* 191–200.

Guérette, H., & Zabihaylo, C. (2000). *An orientation and mobility teaching approach for guide dog travel: Mastering the environment through audition, kinesiology, and cognition* (videotape). Longueuil, Quebec, Canada: Institut Nazareth et Louis-Braille.

Guignon, A. (1998). Multiple intelligences: A theory for everyone. Available from www.education-world.com/a_curr/curr054.shtml 8-14-2007.

Guth, D., Ashmead, D., Long, R., Wall, R., & Ponchillia, R. (2005). Blind and sighted pedestrians' judgments in gaps in traffic at roundabouts. *Human Factors, 47,* 314–331.

Guth, D., & LaDuke, R. (1994). The veering tendency of blind pedestrians: An analysis of the problem and literature review. *Journal of Visual Impairment & Blindness, 88,* 391–400.

Guth, D., & LaDuke, R. (1995). Veering by blind pedestrians: Individual differences and their impli-

cations for instruction. *Journal of Visual Impairment & Blindness, 89*(1), 28–37.

Guth, D. A. (2008). Why does training reduce blind pedestrian's veering? In J. J. Rieser, D. H. Ashmead, F. F. Ebner, & A. L. Corn (Eds.), *Blindness and brain plasticity in navigation and object perception* (pp. 353–366). New York: Taylor and Francis Group.

Guth, D. A., Hill, E. W., & Rieser, J. J. (1989). Tests of blind pedestrians' use of traffic sounds for street-crossing alignment. *Journal of Visual Impairment & Blindness, 83*(9), 461–468.

Guth, D. A., & Rieser, J. J. (1997). Perception and the control of locomotion by blind and visually impaired pedestrians. In B. B. Blasch, W. R. Wiener, & R. L. Welsh (Eds.), *Foundations of orientation and mobility* (2nd ed., pp. 9–38). New York: AFB Press.

Hanson, T. (1976). Rehabilitation teachers—Who are we? *New Outlook for the Blind, 9,* 299–303.

Hapeman, L. B. (1967). Developmental concepts of blind children between the ages of 3 and 6 as they relate to orientation and mobility. *International Journal for the Education of the Blind, 17,* 41–48.

Hardman, M. L., Drew, C. J., & Egan, M. W. (2005). *Human exceptionality.* Boston: Allyn and Bacon.

Harford, E. & Barry, J. (1965). A rehabilitative approach to the problem of unilateral hearing impairment: Contralateral routing of signals (CROS). *Journal of Speech and Hearing Disorders, 30,* 121–138.

Haring, N. G., & Schiefelbusch, R. L. (1967). *Method in special education.* New York: McGraw-Hill.

Harkey, D. L., Carter, D. L., Barlow, J. M., Bentzen, B. L., Myers, L., & Scott, A. (2007). *Guidelines for accessible pedestrian signals final report.* Contractor's Final Report for NCHRP Project 3-62, National Cooperative Highway Research Program Web-Only Document 117B, Washington, DC.

Harkins, D., & Moyer, J. (1997). Employer relations: job development, job retention, and job accommodation. In E. Moore, W. Graves, & J. Patterson (Eds.), *Foundations of rehabilitation counseling with persons who are blind or visually impaired* (pp. 313–340). New York: AFB Press.

Harley, R. K. (1963). *Verbalisms among blind children. American Foundation for the Blind, Research Services*

No. 10. New York: American Foundation for the Blind.

Harrell, L., & Akeson, N. (1987). *Preschool vision stimulation: It's more than a flashlight!* New York: American Foundation for the Blind.

Harrison, T. (Ed.). (2006). *Guide dogs current practice, Volumes 1 and 2.* Chatswood, Australia: Guide Dogs NSW/ACT.

Hart, V. (1984). Research as a basis for assessment and curriculum development for visually impaired infants. *Journal of Visual Impairment & Blindness, 78*(9), 314–318.

Hartman, C. A., Manos, T. M., Winter, C., Hartman, D. M., Li, B., & Smith, J. C. (2000). Effects of T'ai Chi training on function and quality of life indicators in older adults with osteoarthritis. *Journal of the American Geriatrics Society, 48,* 1553–1559.

Hartmann, W. M. (1999). How we localize sound. *Physics Today, 52* (11), 24–29.

Hatton, D. D., Anthony, T. L., Lowry, S. S., & Brown, C. J. (2004). Cognitive development. In T. Anthony, S. Lowry, C. Brown, & D. Hatton (Eds.), *Developmentally appropriate orientation & mobility* (pp. 123–240). Chapel Hill: FPG Child Development Institute, University of North Carolina at Chapel Hill.

Hatton, D. D., Bailey, D. B., Burchinal, M. R., & Ferrell, K. A. (1997). Developmental growth curves of preschool children with vision impairments. *Child Development, 68,* 788–806.

Hatton, D. D., McWilliam, R. A., & Winton, P. J. (2003a). *Building reliable alliances.* Chapel Hill: FPG Child Development Institute, University of North Carolina at Chapel Hill.

Hatton, D. D., McWilliam, R. A., & Winton, P. J. (2003b). *Family centered practices for infants and toddlers with visual impairments.* Chapel Hill: FPG Child Development Institute, University of North Carolina at Chapel Hill.

Hauger, J. S., Rigby, J. C., Safewright, M., & McAuley, W. J. (1996). Detectable warning surfaces at curb ramps. *Journal of Visual Impairment & Blindness, 90,* 512–525.

Held, R., & Hein, A. (1963). Movement-produced stimulation in the development of visually guided behavior. *Journal of Comparative and Physiological Psychology, 56*(5), 872–876.

Heller, K., Alberto, P., Forney, P., & Schwartzman, M. (1996). *Seizure disorders. Understanding physical, sensory, & health impairments.* Pacific Grove, CA: Brooks/Cole Publishing Company.

Heller, W. K., & Kennedy, C. (1994). *Etiologies and characteristics of deaf-blindness.* Monmouth, OR: Teaching Research Publications.

Hemmila, D. (2007). Symptom or side effect? The impact of multiple medications. *Today in PT,* February 19, 2007.

Hendrickson, L. (1996). *Phenomenal talent—the autistic kind.* Visiting Fellows Flinders University of South Australia. Monograph, www.nexus.edu.au/TeachStud/hendrick1.htm, accessed February 27, 2007.

Heydt, K., & Allon, M. (1992). Sensory integration. In C. Cushman, K. Heydt, S. Edwards, M. J. Clark, & G. M. Allon (Eds.), *Perkins activity resource guide* (volume 1, chapter 10). Watertown, MA: Perkins School for the Blind.

Hicks, T. (1999). Traffic management. In J. Pline (Ed.), *Traffic engineering handbook* (5th ed.). Washington, DC: Institute of Transportation Engineers.

Hiemstra, R., & Sisco, B. (1990). *Individualizing instruction.* San Francisco: Jossey-Bass.

Hill, E. W. (Ed.). (1981). *The Hill performance test of selected positional concepts.* Chicago: Stoelting.

Hill, E. W. (1986). Orientation and mobility. In G. T. Scholl (Ed.), *Foundations of education for blind and visually handicapped children and youth* (pp. 265–290). New York: American Foundation for the Blind.

Hill, E. W., & Blasch, B. B. (1980). Concept development. In R. L. Welsh & B. B. Blasch (Eds.), *Foundations of orientation and mobility* (pp. 265–290). New York: American Foundation for the Blind.

Hill, E. W., & Ponder, P. (1976). *Orientation and mobility techniques: A guide for the practitioner.* New York: American Foundation for the Blind.

Hill, E. W., Rosen, S. A., Correa, V. I., & Langley, M. B. (1984). Preschool orientation and mobility: An expanded definition. *Education of the Visually Handicapped, 16,* 58–72.

Himmelmann, K., Bechung, E., Hagberg, G., & Uvebrant, P. (2006). Gross and fine motor function and accompanying impairments in cerebral palsy. *Developmental Medicine & Child Neurology, 48,* 417–423.

Hintz, S., Kendrick, D., Vohr, B., Poole, K., & Higgins, R. (2005). [Changes in neurodevelopmental outcomes at 18 to 22 months' corrected age among infants of less than 25 weeks' gestational age born in 1993–1999.] *Pediatrics, 115*(6), 1645–1651.

Hnath-Chisolm, T. (1994). Cochlear implants and tactile aids. In J. Katz (Ed.), *Handbook of clinical audiology* (4th ed.). Baltimore: Williams & Wilkins.

Holsopple, M. A., & Beigay, G. M. (2005). *Travel skills in the curriculum: The connection between classroom lessons and practical experiences.* Pittsburgh, PA: Allegheny Intermediate Unit.

Horn, E., Ostrosky, M. M., & Jones, H. (2004). *Young exceptional children monograph series no. 5: Family-based practices.* Longmont, CO: The Division of Early Childhood of the Council for Exceptional Children.

Horowitz, A. (2004). The prevalence and consequences of vision impairment in later life. *Topics in Geriatric Rehabilitation, 20*(3), 185–195.

Horowitz, A., & Reinhardt, J. (2006). Adequacy of mental health system in meeting the needs of adults who are visually impaired. *Journal of Visual Impairment & Blindness, 100*(Special Supplement), 871–874.

Horowitz, A., Reinhardt, J., & Kennedy, G. (2005). Major and subthreshold depression among older adults seeking vision rehabilitation services. *American Journal of Geriatric Psychiatry, 13,* 180–187.

Horowitz, A., Reinhardt, J. P., & Boerner, K. (2005). The effect of rehabilitation on depression among visually disabled older adults. *Aging and Mental Health, 9*(6), 563–570.

Horsfall, B. (1997). Tactile maps: New materials and improved designs. *Journal of Visual Impairment & Blindness, 91,* 61–65.

Hoyt, C. (2002). Visual function in the brain damaged child. *The Doyne lecture.* Oxford Ophthalmological Congress, U.K.

Hoyt, L., & Hudson, J. W. (1981). Dog guide dialogs. *Journal of Visual Impairment & Blindness, 75,* 62.

Hubel, D. H. (1995). *Eye, brain, and vision.* San Francisco: W. H. Freeman.

Huebner, K. M., Merk-Adam, B., Stryker, D., & Wolffe, K. (2004). *National agenda for the education of children and youths with visual impairments, including those with multiple disabilities* (rev. ed.). New York: AFB Press.

Hughes, M. C., Smith, R. B., & Benitz, F. (1977). Travel training for exceptional children. *Teaching Exceptional Children, 1*(4), 90–91.

Human Genome Project Information. (n.d.). Genetic disease profile: Sickle cell anemia. Available from www.ornl.gov/sci/techresources/Human_Genome/posters/chromosome/sca.shtml, accessed August 5, 2007.

Humphries, T., Snider, L., & McDougall, B. (1993). Clinical evaluation of the effectiveness of sensory integrative and perceptual motor therapy in improving sensory integrative function in children with learning disabilities. *Journal of Occupational Therapy Research, 13*(3), 163–182.

Hunter, M. (1979). Teaching is decision making. *Educational Leadership 37*(1), 62–65.

Huo, R., Burden, S., Hoyt., C., & Good, W. (1999). Chronic cortical visual impairment in children: Aetiology, prognosis, and associated neurological deficits. *British Journal of Ophthalmology, 83,* 670–675.

Husted, C., Pham, L., Hekking, A., & Niederman, R. (1999). Improving quality of life for people with chronic conditions: The example of T'ai Chi and multiple sclerosis. *Alternative Therapies in Health & Medicine, 5*(5), 70–74.

Individuals with Disabilities Education Act, Final Regulations. (1999). Title 34, Volume 2, Parts 300 to 399, Federal Regulations for 34 CFR Part 300, Assistance to States for the Education of Children With Disabilities. U.S. Government Printing Office via GPO Access (CITE: 34CFR300.1) (pp. 10–11).

Individuals with Disabilities Education Improvement Act of 2004. (2004). H.R. 1350, Section 300.39 (b) (4). Washington, DC: U.S. Government Printing Office.

Inman, V. W., Davis, G. W., & Sauerburger, D. (2005). *Pedestrian access to roundabouts: Assessment of motorist yielding to visually impaired pedestrians and* potential treatments to improve access (FHWA-HRT-05-080). Washington, DC: Federal Highway Administration.

Ivey, A. E., Gluckstern, N., & Ivey, M. (2006). *Basic attending skills.* North Amherst, MA: Microtraining Associates Inc.

Jacobs, R. (2005). A process model for deaf-blind interpreting. *Journal of Interpretation,* 79–96.

Jacobson, G. P., & Calder, J. H. (1998). A screening version of the dizziness handicap inventory (DHI-S). *American Journal of Otology, 19*(6), 804–808.

Jacobson, G. P., & Newman, C. W. (1990). The development of the dizziness handicap inventory (DHI). *Archives of Otolaryngology—Head and Neck Surgery, 116,* 424–427.

Jacobson, W. H. (1993). *The art and science of teaching orientation and mobility to persons with visual impairments.* New York: AFB Press.

Jacobson, W. H., & Bradley, R. H. (1997). Learning theory and teaching methodologies. In B. B. Blasch, W. R. Wiener, & R. L. Welsh (Eds.), *Foundations of orientation and mobility* (2nd ed., pp. 359–382). New York: AFB Press.

Jagannathan, R., & Bared, J. G. (2005). Design and performance analysis of pedestrian crossing facilities for continuous flow intersections. *Transportation Research Record: Journal of the Transportation Research Board No. 1939,* 133–144.

James, G. A. (1972). Problems in the standardization of design and symbolization in tactile route maps for the blind. *New Beacon, 56,* 87–91.

James, G. A., & Gill, J. M. (1974). Mobility maps for the visually handicapped: A study of learning and retention of raised symbols. *American Foundation for the Blind Research Bulletin, 27,* 87–98.

Jan, J. E., Farrell, K., Wong, P. K., & McCormick, A. Q. (1986). Eye and head movements of visually impaired children. *Developmental Medicine and Child Neurology, 28,* 285–293.

Jan, J. E., & Groenveld, M. (1993). Visual behaviors and adaptations associated with cortical and ocular impairment in children. *Journal of Visual Impairment & Blindness, 110,* 101–105.

Jan, J. E., Groenveld, M., Sykanda, A., & Hoyt, C. (1987). Behavioral characteristics of children with permanent cortical visual impairment. *Developmental Medicine and Child Neurology, 29,* 571–576.

Jan, J. E., Groenveld, M., & Sykanda, A. M. (1990). Light gazing by visually impaired children. *Developmental Medicine and Child Neurology, 32,* 755–759.

Jan, J. E., Sykand, A. M., & Groenveld, M. (1990). Habilitation and rehabilitation of visually impaired and blind children. *Pediatrician, 17,* 202–207.

Jan, J. E., & Wong, P. E. K. H. (1991). The child with cortical visual impairment. *Seminars in Ophthalmology, 6,* 194–200.

Jansson, G. (2000). Spatial orientation and mobility of people with vision impairments. In B. Silverstone, M. A. Lang, B. P. Rosenthal, & E. E. Faye (Eds.), *The Lighthouse handbook on vision impairment and vision rehabilitation* (pp. 359–375). New York: Oxford University Press.

Jehoel, S., McCallum, D., Rowell, J., & Ungar, S. (2006). An empirical approach on the design of tactile maps and diagrams: The cognitive tactualisation approach. *British Journal of Visual Impairment, 24,* 67–75.

Jehoel, S., Ungar, S., McCallum, D., & Rowell, J. (2005). An evaluation of substrates for tactile maps and diagrams: Scanning speed and users' preferences. *Journal of Visual Impairment & Blindness, 99,* 85–95.

Jehoel, S., Ungar, S., & Rowell, J. (2005, December). Developing a set of discriminable tactile symbols. *Proceedings of Tactile Graphics 2005.* Birmingham, UK.

Joffee, E., & Ehresman, P. (1997). Learners with visual and cognitive impairments. In B. B. Blasch, W. R. Wiener, & R. L. Welsh (Eds.), *Foundations of orientation and mobility* (2nd ed., pp. 483–499). New York: AFB Press.

Joffee, E., & Rikhye, C. H. (1991). Orientation and mobility for students with severe visual and multiple impairments: A new perspective. *Journal of Visual Impairment & Blindness, 85*(5), 211–216.

Joffee, E., & Rower, D. (1997). Learners with visual and health impairments. In B. B. Blasch, W. R. Wiener, & R. L. Welsh (Eds.), *Foundations of orientation and mobility* (2nd ed. pp. 500–512). New York: AFB Press.

Johnson, M., Bengtson, V. L., Coleman, P. G., & Kirkwood, T. B. L. (2005). *The Cambridge handbook of age and ageing.* Cambridge, UK: Cambridge University Press.

Jones, C. B. (2002). *The source for brain-based learning.* East Moline, IL: LinguiSystems.

Jones, T. (2006) Estimating time-to-collision with retinitis pigmentosa. *Journal of Visual Impairment & Blindness, 100,* 47–54.

Jose, R. T. (1983). *Understanding low vision.* New York: American Foundation for the Blind.

Jose, R. T. (1992). Low vision services. In A. Orr (Ed.), *Vision and aging: Crossroads for service delivery* (pp. 209–232). New York: American Foundation for the Blind.

Jutai, J. W., Strong, G., & Russell-Minda, E. (2009). Effectiveness of assistive technologies for low vision rehabilitation: A systematic review. *Journal of Visual Impairment & Blindness, 103,* 210–222.

Kadushin, A., & Kadushin, G. (1997). *The social work interview: A guide for human service professionals.* New York: Columbia University Press.

Kaiser, A. P. (1993). Functional language. In M. E. Snell (Ed.), *Instruction of students with severe disabilities.* New York: Macmillan.

Kantner, R., Clark, D., Allen, L., & Chase, M. (1976). Effects of vestibular stimulation on nystagmus response and motor performance in the developmentally delayed infant. *Physical Therapy, 42,* 399–413.

Kaplan, J. (2004). *Report on the performance of detectable warning products in Burlington, Vermont.* Report No. FHWA-VT-RD-0401. Montpellier, VT: Vermont Agency of Transportation.

Kaplan, J. (Spring, 2006). *Report on evaluation of detectable warning products installed 2003–2005.* Montpellier, VT: Local Transportation Facilities Section, Program Development Division, Vermont Agency of Transportation. Available from www.aot.state.vt.us/Progdev/Documents/LTF/TruncatedDomeInstallationReport/2006Fieldevaluation.pdf, accessed April 7, 2009.

Kasai, T. (1991). An empirical note on tonic neck reflexes: Control of the upper limb's proprioceptive sensation. *Perceptual and Motor Skills, 72,* 955–961.

Keane, G. (1965). Auditory rehabilitation for hearing-impaired blind persons. *ASHA Monographs, 12,* 31–51.

Kennedy, J. M. (1995, May). *Raised line drawings.* Presented at the National Orientation and Mobility/Rehabilitation Teaching Conference, Lake Joseph, Ontario, Canada.

Kenny, R. A. (2005). Mobility and falls. In M. L. Johnson, V. L. Bengston, P. G. Coleman, & T. B. L. Kirkwood (Eds.), *The Cambridge handbook of age and ageing.* Cambridge, UK: Cambridge University Press.

Kephart, J. G., Kephart, C. P., & Schwarz, G. C. (1974). A journey into the world of the blind child. *Exceptional Children, 40,* 421–427.

Kern, L., Koegel, R. L., & Dunlap, G. (1984). The influence of vigorous versus mild exercise on autistic stereotyped behaviors. *Journal of Autism and Developmental Disorders, 14,* 57–67.

Kern, L., Koegel, R. L., Dyer, K., Blew, P. A., & Fenton, L. R. (1982). The effects of physical exercise on self-stimulation and appropriate responding in autistic children. *Journal of Autism and Developmental Disorders, 12,* 399–419.

Ketts, D., & Barlow, J. M. (2008). Roundabouts: Does the thought make you dizzy? Presentation at the Annual Conference of Florida AER. Tampa, Florida.

Kidwell, A. M., & Greer, P. S. (1973). *Sites, perception and the nonvisual experience; designing and manufacturing mobility maps.* New York: American Foundation for the Blind.

Killion, M. C., Staab, W. J., & Preves, D. A. (1990). Classifying automatic signal processors. *Hearing Instruments, 41,* 24–26.

Kinsbourne, M., & Graf, W. D. (2001). Disorders of mental development. In. J. H. Menkes & H. B. Sarnat (Eds.), *Child neurology* (6th ed., pp. 1155–1211). Philadelphia: Lippincott Williams & Wilkins.

Kirkwood, D. H. (1990). 1990 U.S. hearing aid sales summary. *Hearing Journal, 43*(12), 7–13.

Kleinert, H., & Kearns, J. (2004). Alternate assessments. In F. Orelove, D. Sobsey, & R. Silberman (Eds.), *Educating children with multiple disabilities: A collaborative approach* (4th ed., pp. 115–149). Baltimore, MD: Paul Brookes.

Kleinschmidt, J. J. (1999) Older adults perspective on their successful adjustment to vision loss. *Journal of Visual Impairment and Blindness, 93*(2) 69–81.

Knott, N. I. (2002). *Teaching orientation and mobility in the schools: An instructor's companion.* New York: AFB Press.

Knowles, M. S. (1980). *The modern practice of adult education*. Chicago: Association Press.

Knowles, M. S. (1984). *Andragogy in action: Applying modern principles of adult learning*. San Francisco: Jossey-Bass.

Kornhaber et al. (2000). *Project SUMIT, report on Harvard Project Zero web site*. Available from www.pzweb.harvard.edu.

Kotchkin, S. (2005). MarkeTrak VII: Hearing loss population tops 31 million people. *Hearing Review, 12*, 16–29.

Kozel, B. (1995). Diabetes and orientation and mobility training: An added challenge. *Journal of Visual Impairment & Blindness, 89*(4), 337–342.

Kraft, M. E. (1988). Analyzing technological risks in federal regulatory agencies. In M. E. Kraft & N. J. Vig (Eds.), *Technology and politics* (pp. 184–207). Durham, NC: Duke University Press.

Kranowitz, C. (2003). *The out-of-sync child has fun*. New York: Berkley Publishing Group.

Kronick, M. K. (1987). Children and cane: An adaptive approach. *Journal of Visual Impairment & Blindness, 81*, 61–62.

Kutner, N. G., Barnhart, H., Wolf, S. L., McNeeley, E., & Xu, T. (1997). Self-reported benefits of Tai Chi practice by older adults. *Journal of Gerontology: Psychological Sciences, 54*, P242–P246.

Kuyk, T., Elliot, J. L., Wesley, J., Scilley, K., McIntosh, E., Mitchell, S., et al. (2004). Mobility function in older veterans improves after blind rehabilitation. *Journal of Rehabilitation and Development, 41*(3), 337–346.

LaGrow, S. (2009). Orientation to place. In J. H. Stone & M. Blouin (Eds.), *International encyclopedia of rehabilitation*. Available from http://cirrie.buffalo.edu/encyclopedia/article.php?id=3&language=en.

LaGrow, S., Blasch, B., & De l'Aune, W. (1997). The effect of hand position on detection distance for object and surface preview when using the long cane for non-visual travel. *RE:view, 28*, 169–176.

LaGrow, S. J. (1992). *The rehabilitation of visually impaired people*. Auckland, New Zealand: Royal New Zealand Foundation for the Blind.

LaGrow, S. J., & Weessies, M. (1994). *Orientation and mobility: Techniques for independence*. Palmerston North, New Zealand: Dunmore Press.

LaGrow, S. J., Wiener, W. R., LaDuke, R. O. (1990). Independent travel for developmentally disabled persons: A comprehensive model of instruction. *Research in Developmental Disabilities, 11*, 289–301.

LaGrow, S. J., & Blasch, B. B. (1992). Orientation and mobility services for older persons. In A. L. Orr (Ed.), *Vision and aging: Crossroads for service delivery* (pp. 255–288). New York: American Foundation for the Blind.

Lambert, L. M., & Lederman, S. J. (1989). An evaluation of the legibility and meaningfulness of potential map symbols. *Journal of Visual Impairment & Blindness, 83*, 397–403.

Lan, C., Lai, J. S., Chen, S. Y., & Wong, M. K. (1998). 12-month tai chi training in the elderly: Its effect on health fitness. *Medicine and Science in Sports & Exercise, 30*, 345–351.

Landry, J., Ratelle, A., & Overbury, O. (forthcoming). Efficiency and safety evaluation of detectable warning surfaces in winter conditions: Effects of color and material. *Proceedings of 12th International Conference on Mobility and Transport for Elderly and Disabled Persons [TRANSED]*, June 2010, Hong Kong, China.

Langbain, E., Blasch, B., & Chalmers, B. (1981). An orienteering program for blind and visually impaired persons. *Journal of Visual Impairment & Blindness, 75*, 273–276.

Langley, M. (1980). *The teachable moment and the handicapped infant*. Reston, VA: ERIC Clearinghouse on Handicapped and Gifted Children, Council for Exceptional Children (ERIC Document Reproduction Service No. E0191254).

Lappin, J. S., & Foulke, E. (1973). Expanding the tactual field of view. *Perception and Psychophysics, 14*, 237–241.

LaPrelle, L. L. (2002). *Standing on my own two feet: A step-by-step guide to designing and constructing simple, individually tailored adaptive mobility devices for preschool-aged children who are visually impaired*. Los Angeles: Blind Childrens Center.

Larson, R. W. (1984). Mobility strategies for icy conditions. *Journal of Visual Impairment & Blindness, 78*(8), 365–366.

Lascaratos, J. (1998). The ophthalmic wound of Philip II of Macedonia (360–336 BCE). *Survey of Ophthalmology, 49*(2), 256–261.

Laus, M. D. (1974). Orientation and mobility instruction for the sighted trainable mentally retarded. *Education and Training of the Mentally Retarded, 9*(2), 20–73.

Laus, M. D. (1977). *Travel instructions for the handicapped.* Springfield, IL: Charles C Thomas.

Layton, C. A., & Lock, R. H. (2001). Determining learning disabilities in students with low vision. *Journal of Visual Impairment & Blindness, 95*(5), 288–299.

Layton, P. E. (1917). The inability to travel alone. *Outlook for the Blind, 11*(3), 68–72.

Leary, B., & von Schneden, M. (1982). *Simon Says is not the only game.* New York: American Foundation for the Blind.

Leonard, J. A. (1966). Aids to navigation: A discussion of the problem of maps for the blind traveler. Paper presented at St. Dunstan's International Conference on Sensory Devices for the Blind, London.

Levack, N. (1991). *Low vision: A resource guide with adaptations for students with visual impairment.* Austin: Texas School for the Blind and Visually Impaired.

Levi, J. M., & Schiff, W. (1966). Study of texture discrimination. Appendix B of *Development of raised line drawings as supplementary tools in the education of the blind* (Final report, September, Project No. RD-1571-S). Washington, DC: U.S. Department of Health, Education and Welfare, Vocational Rehabilitation Administration.

Levinson, L. J., & Reid, G. (1993). The effects of exercise intensity on the stereotypic behaviors of individuals with autism. *Adapted Physical Activity Quarterly, 10*, 255–268.

Lewis, C. B. (1989). *Improving mobility in older persons.* Rockville, MD: Aspen Publications.

Lewis, V., Norgate, S., Collis, G., & Reynolds, R. (2000). The consequences of visual impairment for children's symbolic and functional play. *British Journal of Developmental Psychology, 18*(3), 449–464. Retrieved April 30, 2006, from PsycINFO database.

Lezak, M. (1995). *Neuropsychological assessment* (3rd edition, p. 666). New York: Oxford University Press.

Li, F., Fisher, K. J., Harmer, P., & McAuley, E. (2005). Falls self-efficacy as a mediator of fear of falling in an exercise intervention for older adults. *Journal of Gerontology: Psychological Sciences, 60B*(1), 34–40.

Li, F., Harmer, P., Fisher, K. J., & McAuley, E. (2004). Tai Chi: Improving functional balance and predicting subsequent falls in older persons. *Medicine and Science in Sports and Exercise, 36*(12), 2046–2052.

Lichtenstein, M. J., Bess, F. H., & Logan, S. A. (1988). Validation of screening tools for identifying hearing-impaired elderly in primary care. *Journal of the American Medical Association, 259*(19), 2875–2878.

Lidoff, L. (2001). A concluding perspective: Moving vision rehabilitation into the U.S. health system mainstream. In R. Massof & L. Lidoff (Eds.), *Issues in low vision rehabilitation: Service delivery, policy and funding* (pp. 253–266). New York: AFB Press.

Lidoff, L. (2005). Medicare coverage for orientation and mobility services. *Journal of Visual Impairment & Blindness, 99*(10), 584–586.

Lighthouse International. (1995) *The lighthouse national survey on vision loss.* New York: The Lighthouse, Inc.

Likins, M. (2002). Effective training for paraprofessionals. *Impact: Feature Issue on Paraeducators Supporting Students with Disabilities and At-Risk, 15*(2), 6–7. Minneapolis: University of Minnesota, Institute on Community Integration.

Linder, T. W. (1990). *Transdisciplinary play-based assessment: A functional approach to working with young children.* Baltimore, MD: Paul H. Brookes.

Linder, T. W. (1993). *Transdisciplinary play-based intervention: Guidelines for developing a meaningful curriculum for young children.* Baltimore, MD: Paul H. Brookes.

Liu, G. T., Volpe, N. J., & Galetta, S. L. (Eds.). (2001). *Neuro-ophthalmology: Diagnosis and management* (p. 315). Philadelphia, PA: W.B. Saunders.

Lockhart, T. E., Spaulding, J. M., & Park, S. H. (2007). Age-related slip avoidance strategy while walking over a known slippery floor surface. *Gait and Posture, 26*, 142–149.

Lohmeier, K. (2003). *Aligning the state standards and the expanded core curriculum* (rev. ed.). Tucson: University of Arizona College of Education. Available from www.ed.arizona.edu/azaer/AZ

%20Standards%20Aligned.pdf, accessed June 25, 2008.

Lohmeier, K. (2009). Practice report: Aligning state standards and the expanded core curriculum: Balancing the impact of the no child left behind act. *Journal of Visual Impairment & Blindness, 103*(1), 44–47.

Lolli, D. (2006). *Foundations of orientation and mobility for learners who are deafblind and blind with additional disabilities.* Watertown, MA: Perkins School for the Blind.

Lolli, D., & Sauerburger, D. (1997). Learners with visual and hearing impairments. In B. Blasch, W. Wiener, & R. Welsh (Eds.), *Foundations of orientation and mobility* (2nd ed., pp. 513–529). New York: American Foundation for the Blind.

Long, R. (2008). Crossing streets without vision: Access to information, strategies for travelling, and the impact of technology, training and environmental design. In J. J. Rieser, D. H. Ashmead, F. F. Ebner, & A. L. Corn (Eds.), *Blindness and brain plasticity in navigation and object perception* (pp. 335–352). New York: Lawrence Erlbaum Associates.

Long, R., Boyette, L., & Griffin-Shirley, N. (1996). Older persons and community travel: The effect of visual impairment. *Journal of Visual Impairment & Blindness, 96*(4), 302–313.

Long, R., Guth, D., Ashmead, D., Wall Emerson, R., & Ponchillia, P. (2005). Modern roundabouts: Access by pedestrians who are blind. *Journal of Visual Impairment & Blindness, 99,* 611–622.

Long, R. G. (1992). *Final report: Housing accessibility for individuals with visual impairment or blindness.* Raleigh, NC: North Carolina State University.

Long, R. G., Boyette, L. W., & Griffin-Shirley, N. (1996). Older individuals and community travel: The effect of vision impairment. *Journal of Visual Impairment & Blindness, 90,* 314–324.

Long, R. G., Guth, D. A., Ashmead, D. H., Wall, R. S., & Ponchillia, P. E. (2005). Modern roundabouts: Access by pedestrians who are blind. *Journal of Visual Impairment & Blindness, 99* (10), 611–621.

Long, R. G., & Hill, E. W. (1997). Establishing and maintaining orientation and mobility. In B. B. Blasch, W. R. Wiener, & R. L. Welsh (Eds.), *Foundations of orientation and mobility* (2nd ed., pp. 39–59). New York: AFB Press.

Long, R. G., McNeal, L., & Griffin-Shirley, N. (1990). The effect of visual loss on mobility of elderly persons (Research Grant No. 133 GH 70038). Final Report. Bethesda, MD; National Institute on Disability and Rehabilitation.

Lowenfeld, B. (1975). *The changing status of the blind: From separation to integration.* Springfield, IL: Charles C Thomas.

Lowrance, W. W. (1976). *Of acceptable risk: Science and the determination of safety.* Los Altos, CA: William Kaufman.

Lowry, S., & Hatton, D. (2002). Facilitating walking by young children with visual impairments. *RE:view 34*(3), 125–133.

Lucas, C., & Bayley, R. (2005). Variation in ASL: The role of grammatical function. *Sign Language Studies, 6*(1), 38–40.

Ludt, R. (1997). Three types of glare: Low vision O&M assessment and remediation. *RE:view, 29,* 101–113.

Ludt, R., & Goodrich, G. L. (2002). Change in visual perceptual detection distances for low vision travelers as a result of dynamic visual assessment and training. *Journal of Visual Impairment & Blindness, 96*(1), 7–21.

Ludwig, I., Luxont, L., & Attmore, M. (1988). *Creative recreation for blind and visually impaired adults.* New York: American Foundation for the Blind.

Lueck, A. H. (2004). *Functional vision: A practitioners guide to evaluation and intervention.* New York: AFB Press.

Lueck, A. H., & Heinze, T. (2004). Interventions for young children with visual impairments and students with visual and multiple impairments. In A. H. Lueck (Ed.), *Functional vision: A practitioner's guide to evaluation and intervention* (pp. 277–351). New York: AFB Press.

Lundälv, J. (2001). The experiences of visually impaired people in Sweden as pedestrians and cyclists. *Journal of Visual Impairment & Blindness, 95*(5), 302–304.

Luxton, L., Bradfield, A, Maxson, B. J., & Starkson, B. (1997). The rehabilitation team. In E. Moore, W. Graves, and J. Patterson (Eds.), *Foundations of rehabilitation counseling with persons who are blind or visually impaired* (pp. 193–224). New York: AFB Press.

MacDonald, J. D., & Gillette, Y. (1984). *Turn-taking with communication: ECO treatment module.* Columbus: Ohio State University.

MacFarland, D. (1972). Social services and blindness. In R. Hardy & J. Cull (Eds.), *Social and rehabilitation services for the blind.* Springfield, IL: Charles C Thomas.

MacLean, W., & Baumeister, A. (1982). Effects of vestibular stimulation on motor development and stereotyped behavior of developmentally delayed children. *Journal of Abnormal Child Psychology, 10*(2), 229–245.

MacWilliam, L. (1980). A curriculum for teaching clients to use landmarks while traveling. *Journal of Visual Impairment & Blindness, 74*(7), 269–272.

Maida, A. O., & McCune, L. (1996). A dynamic systems approach to the development of crawling by blind and sighted infants. *RE:view, 28,* 119–134.

Malamazian, J. D. (1970). The first 15 years at Hines. In *Blindness Annual* (pp. 59–75). Washington, DC: American Association of Workers for the Blind.

Mamer, L. (1995). Tactile defensiveness. *Journal of Visual Impairment & Blindness News Service, 89*(3), 9–10.

Mancil, R. M., Mancil, G. L., King, E., Legault, C., Munday, J., Alfieri, S., et al. (2005). Improving nighttime mobility in persons with night blindness caused by retinitis pigmentosa: A comparison of two low-vision mobility devices. *Journal of Rehabilitation Research & Development, 42*(4), 471–486.

Marigold, D. S. & Patla, A. E. (2002). Strategies for dynamic stability during locomotion on a slippery surface: Effects of prior experience and knowledge. *Journal of Neurophysiology, 88,* 339–353.

Marston, J. R., & Golledge, R. G. (2000). *Towards an accessible city: Removing functional barriers for the blind and vision impaired: A case for auditory signs: Final report.* Berkeley: University of California Transportation Center.

Marta, M., & Geruschat, D. (2004). Equal protection, the ADA, and driving with low vision: A legal analysis. *Journal of Visual Impairment & Blindness, 98,* 654–667.

Massof, R., & Lidoff, L. (Eds.). (2001). *Issues in low vision rehabilitation: Service delivery, policy and funding.* New York: AFB Press.

Massoff, R., Dagnelie, G., Deremeik, J., DeRose, J., Alibhai, S., & Glasner, N. (1995). Low vision rehabilitation in the U.S. health care system. *Journal of Vision Rehabilitation, 9*(3), 3–31.

Mast, F., & Zaehle, T. (2008). Spatial reference frames used in mental imagery tasks. In J. J. Rieser, D. H. Ashmead, F. F. Ebner, & A. L. Corn (Eds.), *Blindness and brain plasticity in navigation and object perception* (pp. 239–258). New York: Lawrence Erlbaum Associates.

Mayo Clinic. (2006). Water: How much should you drink every day? Available from www.mayoclinic.com/health/water/NU00283, accessed July 10, 2007.

Mayo Clinic. (2007, March). Epilepsy. Available from www.mayoclinic.com/health/epile psy/DS00342/DSECTION=2, accessed March 11, 2007.

McCallum, D., Rowell, J., & Ungar, S. (September 2003). The use of ink-jet to produce tactile maps. *Proceedings of IS&Ts NIP 19: International Conference on Digital Printing Technologies,* New Orleans, LA.

McCallum, D., & Ungar, S. (2003). Producing tactile maps using new technology: An introduction. *Cartographic Journal, 40*(3), 294–298.

McClain, M. (2004). Assessment and its importance in early intervention/early childhood special education. In M. McLean, M. Wolery, & D. B. Bailey, Jr. (Eds.), *Assessing infants and preschoolers with special needs* (3rd edition). Upper Saddle River, NJ: Pearson.

McCormick, M. C., Brooks-Gunn, J., Buka, S. L., et al. (2006). Early intervention in low birth weight premature infants: Results at 18 years of age for the Infant Health and Development Program. *Pediatrics, 117,* 771–780.

McCrae, R. R., & Costa, P. T., Jr. (1990). *Personality in adulthood.* New York: Guilford Press.

McCulloh, K. J., & Crawford, I. (1994). A structured support group for midlife and older adults with vision loss. *Journal of Visual Impairment & Blindness, 88*(2), 152–157.

McDaniel, S. H., Campbell, T. L., Hepworth, J., & Lorenz, A. (2005). *Family-oriented primary care* (2nd edition). New York: Springer Publishing Co.

McDonald, N. C. (2008). Critical factors for active transportation to school among low-income and minority students: Evidence from the 2001 National Household Travel Survey. *American Journal of Preventative Medicine, 34*(4), 341–344.

McEwen, I. (2000). *Providing physical therapy services under parts B & C of the Individuals with Disabilities Education Act (IDEA).* Oklahoma City, OK: American Physical Therapy Association Section on Pediatrics.

McHugh, E., & Pyfer, J. (1999). The development of rocking among children who are blind. *Journal of Visual Impairment & Blindness, 93*(2), 82–103.

McKiernan, F. O. (2005). A simple gait-stabilizing device reduces outdoor falls and non serious injurious falls in fall-prone older people during the winter. *Journal of the American Geriatric Society, 53,* 943–947.

McLaren, C., Null, J., & Quinn, J. (2005). Heat stress from enclosed vehicles: moderate ambient temperatures cause significant temperature rise in enclosed vehicles (electronic article). Available from http://pediatrics.aappublications.org/cgi/content/full/116/1/e109.

McMillan, T. E. (2007). The relative influence of urban form on a child's travel mode to school. *Transportation Research Part A: Policy and Practice, 41*(1), 69–79.

McMillen, B. (Ed.). (2001). *Designing sidewalks and trails for access,* volume 2: *Best practices design guide.* Washington, DC: U.S. Department of Transportation, Federal Highway Administration.

McNeill, D., & Duncan, S. D. (2005). Grammar, gesture, and meaning in American sign language. *Sign Language Studies, 5*(4), 506–518.

McWilliam, R. A., & Scott, S. (2001). A support approach to early intervention: A three-part framework. *Infants & Young Children, 13*(4), 55–66.

McWilliam, R. A., Tocci, L., & Harbin, G. L. (1998). Family-centered services: Service providers' discourse and behavior. *Topics in Early Childhood Special Education, 18,* 206–221.

Meisels, S. J., & Shonkoff, K. P. (2000). Early childhood intervention: A continuing evolution. In J. P. Shonkoff & S. J. Meisels (Eds.), *Handbook of early childhood intervention* (pp. 3–31). Cambridge, United Kingdom: Cambridge University Press.

Ment, L., Duncan, C. C., & Ehrenkranz, R. A. (1987). Intraventricular hemorrhage of the pre-term neonate. *Seminars in Perinatology, 11,* 132–141.

Ment, L., Scott, D., & Ehrenkranz, R. A. (1985). Neurodevelopmental assessment of very low weight neonates: Effect of germinal, matrix, and intraventricular hemorrhage. *Pediatric Neurology, 1,* 164–168.

Merck Manuals. (February 2003). Atherosclerosis. Available from www.merck.com/mmhe/sec03/ch032/ch032a.html, accessed August 5, 2007.

Meteorological Service of Canada, Environment Canada, Government of Canada. Wind chill program: Wind chill fact sheet. Available from www.msc-smc.ec.gc.ca/education/windchill/cold_injury_e.cfm, accessed October 7, 2006.

Meteorological Service of Canada, Environment Canada, Government of Canada. Wind chill program: Wind chill hazards. Available from www.msc-smc.ec.gc.ca/education/windchill/windchill_threshold_chart_e.cfm, accessed October 7, 2006.

Meteorological Service of Canada, Environment Canada, Government of Canada. (1998). The Green Lane. Brochure: Humidity. Available from www.msc-smc.ec.gc.ca/cd/brochures/humidity_e.cfm, accessed October 7, 2006.

Mettler, R. (1995). *Cognitive learning theory and cane travel instruction: A new paradigm.* Lincoln: State of Nebraska, Department of Public Institutions.

Miele, J. (2005, April). *Tactile map automated production (TMAP): Technical description and research objectives.* Denver, CO: American Association of Geographers Conference.

Miele, J. A., & Gilden, D. B. (2004, March). Tactile map automated production (TMAP). Using GIS data to generate braille maps. Paper presented at the CSUN International Conference on Technology and Persons with Disabilities, Los Angeles, CA.

Miele, J. A., & Marston, J. R. (2005a, March). Tactile map automated production (TMAP): Project update and research summary. Paper presented at the CSUN 20th Annual International Conference on Technology and Persons with Disabilities, Los Angeles, CA.

Miele, J. A., & Marston, J. R. (2005b, April). Tactile map automated production (TMAP): On-demand accessible street maps for blind and visually impaired travelers. Paper presented at the American Association of Geographers 101st Annual Meeting, Denver, CO.

Miele, J., Landau, S., & Gilden, D. (2006). Talking TMAP: Automated generation of audio-tactile maps using Smith-Kettlewell's tmap software. *British Journal of Visual Impairment, 24*(2), 93–100.

Miles, B. (2003). *Talking the Language of the Hands to the Hands.* Monmouth, OR: DB-LINK, The National Information Clearinghouse on Children Who Are Deaf-Blind Web Site. Available from www.nationaldb.org/NCDBProducts.php?prodID=47, accessed December 18, 2006.

Miles, B. (2005). *Overview on deaf-blindness.* Monmouth, OR: DB-LINK, The National Information Clearinghouse On Children Who Are Deaf-Blind. Available from www.nationaldb.org/NCDBProducts.php?prodID=38, accessed March 3, 2007.

Milligan, K. (1998). Mobility options for visually impaired persons with diabetes: Considerations for orientation and mobility instructors. *Journal of Visual Impairment & Blindness, 92*(1), 71–79.

Ministry of Education, British Columbia. (2000). *Framework for independent travel: A resource for orientation and mobility* (RB0094). Province of British Columbia: Ministry of Education. Available from www.bced.gov.ca/specialed/does/fit.pdf.

Minuchin, S. (1974). *Families and family therapy.* Cambridge, MA: Harvard University Press.

Miszko, T. A., Ramsey, V. K., & Blasch, B. B. (2004a). Tai Chi for people with visual impairments: A pilot study. *Journal of Visual Impairment & Blindness, 98*(1), 5–13.

Miszko, T. A., Ramsey, V. K., & Blasch, B. B. (2004b). Tai Chi for people with visual impairments: A pilot study. *Journal of Visual Impairment & Blindness, 98*(1), 5–13.

Mitchell, R. E., Young, T. A., Bachleda, B., & Karchmer, M. A. (2006). How many people use ASL in the United States? Why estimates need updating. *Sign Language Studies, 6*(3), 306–335.

Mogk, L., & Goodrich, G. (2004). The history and future of low vision services in the United States.

Journal of Visual Impairment & Blindness, 98(10), 585–600.

Monighan-Nourot, P., Scales, B., VanHoorn, J., & Almay, M. (1987). *Looking at children's play: A bridge between theory and practice.* New York: Teachers College Press.

Monorail society. (2006). Available from www.monorails.org/tMspages/Why.html, accessed May 22, 2006.

Montessori method. Available from www.en.wikipedia.org/wiki/Montessori, accessed May 26, 2009.

Moore, J. E., Graves, W. H., & Patterson, J. B. (1997). *Foundations of rehabilitation counseling with persons who are blind or visually impaired.* New York: AFB Press.

Moore, S. (1984). The need for programs and services for visually handicapped infants. *Education of the Visually Handicapped, 16,* 48–57.

Morais, M., Lorensen, P., Allen, R., Bell, E. C., Hill, A., & Woods, E. (1997). *Techniques used by blind cane traveler instructors. A practical approach: Learning, teaching, believing.* Baltimore, MD: National Federation of the Blind.

Morgan, M. (1976). Beyond disability: A broader definition of architectural barriers. *American Institute of Architects Journal, 65*(5), 50–53.

Morris, J. E., & Nolan, C. Y. (1963). Minimum sizes for areal type tactual symbols. *International Journal for the Education of the Blind, 13,* 48–51.

Mueller, H. G., & Carter, A. S. (2002). Hearing aids and assistive devices. In R. L. Schow & M. A. Nerbonne (Eds.), *Introduction to audiologic rehabilitation.* Boston: Allyn & Bacon.

Mueller, H. G., Grimes, A. M., & Erdman, S. A. (1983). Subjective ratings of directional amplification, *Hearing instruments, 34,* 14–16.

Mueller, H. G., Johnson, E. E., & Carter, A. S. (2007). Hearing aids and assistive devices. In R. L. Schow & M. A. Nerbonne (Eds.), *Introduction to audiologic rehabilitation.* Boston: Allyn & Bacon.

Musslewhite, C. R. (1986). *Adaptive play for special needs children.* San Diego, CA: College-Hill Press.

Nachreiner, N. M., Findorff, M. J., Wyman, J. F., & McCarthy, T. C. (2007). Circumstances and consequences of falls in community-dwelling older women. *Journal of Women's Health, 16*(10), 1437–1446.

National Center for Chronic Disease Prevention and Health Promotion. (2005, January). Diabetes projects. Available from www.cdc.gov/diabetes/projects/cda2.htm, accessed August 5, 2007.

National Center for Health Statistics. (1994 and 2004). *National Health Interview Survey–Disability Supplement.* Washington, DC: U.S. Department of Health and Human Services.

National Center for Health Statistics. (2006). *Trends in health and aging.* Washington, DC: U.S. Department of Health and Human Services.

National Committee on Uniform Traffic Laws and Ordinances (NCUTLO). (2000). *Uniform vehicle code: Millennium edition.* Alexandria, VA: National Committee on Uniform Traffic Laws and Ordinances.

National deaf-blind child count. (2004). Available from www.tr.wou.edu/ntac/documents/census/2004-Census-Tables.xlsDeafblind, accessed March 25, 2006.

National Dissemination Center for Children with Disabilities (NICHCY) (2010). NICHCY disability fact sheet—No. 5, Emotional disturbance. www.nichcy.org/InformationResources/Documents/NICHCY%20PUBS/fs5.pdf, accessed May 13.

National Federation of the Blind (NFB) Access Technology Staff. (2006). GPS technology for the blind, a product evaluation. *Braille Monitor, 49*(2), 101–108.

National Highway Traffic Safety Administration. (2002). *Resource guide on laws related to pedestrian and bicycle safety.* (CD ROM.) Washington, DC: National Highway Traffic Safety Administration. Available from www.nhtsa.dot.gov/people/injury/pedbimot/ped/resourceguide/index.html, accessed May 26, 2009.

National Information Center for Children and Youth with Disabilities. (2002a). Cerebral palsy fact sheet. ERIC Document Reproduction Service No. ED470829. Washington, DC: Author.

National Information Center for Children and Youth with Disabilities. (2002b). Epilepsy fact sheet. ERIC Document Reproduction Service No. ED470826. Washington, DC: Author.

National Institute of Mental Health. (1996). Attention deficit hyperactivity disorder (brochure). Bethesda, MD: Author.

National Institute of Neurological Disorders and Stroke. (2007, February). Neurological complications of AIDS, information page. Available from www.ninds.nih.gov/disorders/aids/aids.htm, accessed March 16, 2007.

National Institute on Aging (NIA). (2004). Exercise and physical activity: Your everyday guide. Available from http://nia.nih.gov/HealthInformation/Publications/ExerciseGuide.

National Longitudinal Transition Study-2 (NLTS2). (2001). Washington, DC: National Center for Special Education Research, Institute of Education Sciences, U.S. Department of Education.

National Multiple Sclerosis Society. (2003). Gait problems. Available from www.nationalmssociety.org/Sourcebook-Gait.asp, accessed March, 2006.

National Multiple Sclerosis Society. (2005a). About MS. Available from www.nationalmssociety.org/about%20ms.asp, accessed March, 2006.

National Multiple Sclerosis Society. (2005b). Fatigue. Available from, www.nationalmssociety.org/Sourcebook-Fatigue.asp, accessed March 10, 2006.

National Multiple Sclerosis Society. (2005c). Headache. Available from http://nationalmssociety.org/Sourcebook-Headache.asp, accessed March 10, 2006.

National Multiple Sclerosis Society. (2006). Cognitive Function. Available from www.nationalmssociety.org/Sourcebook-Cognitive.asp, accessed March 10, 2006.

National Transit Database Reporting Manual Glossary. (2005). Available from www.ntdprogram.com/NTD/ReportingManual/2003/HTMLFiles/2003%20Glossary.htm, accessed March 6, 2006.

Nelson, K. A. (1987). Visual impairment among elderly Americans: Statistics in transition. *Journal of Visual Impairment & Blindness, 81,* 331–334.

Nelson, K. A., & Dimitrova, E. (1993). Severe visual impairment in the United States and in each state. *Journal of Visual Impairment & Blindness, 87,* 80–85.

Nerbonne, M. A., & Schow, R. L. (2007). Auditory stimuli in communication. In R. L. Schow &

M. A. Nerbonne (Eds.), *Introduction to audiologic rehabilitation*. Boston: Allyn & Bacon.

Newcomb, S. (2009). The reliability of the CVI Range. Ph.D. diss. University of Maryland, College Park, MD. Available from http://hdl.handle.net/1903/123, accessed May 12, 2010.

Newman, C. W., & Weinstein, B. E. (1988). The Hearing Handicap Inventory for the Elderly as a measure of hearing aid benefit. *Ear and Hearing, 9,* 81–85.

Newman, C. W., Weinstein, B. E., Jacobson, G. P., & Hug, G. A. (1990). The Hearing Handicap Inventory for adults: Psychometric adequacy, and audiometric correlates. *Ear and Hearing, 11*(6), 430–433.

Nickel, R. (1992). Disorders of brain development. *Infants and Young Children, 5,* 1–11.

Niehaus, M., & Tebbenjohanns, J. (2001). Electromagnetic interference in patients with implanted pacemakers or cardioverter-defibrillators. *Heart, 86*(3), 246–248.

Nielsen, L. (1992). *Educational approaches for visually handicapped children*. Copenhagen, Denmark: Sikon.

Nolan, C. Y. (1971). Relative legibility of raised and incised tactual figures. *Education of the Visually Handicapped, 3,* 33–36.

Nolan, C. Y., & Morris, J. E. (1971). *Improvement of tactual symbols for blind children* (Final report, Project No. 5-0421; Grant No. OEG-32-27-0000-1012). Louisville, KY: American Printing House for the Blind.

Nopp, P., Schleich, P., & D'Haese, P. (2004). Sound localization in bilateral users of MED-EL COMBI 40/40+ cochlear implants. *Ear and Hearing, 25,* 205–214.

O&M Division. (2004a). Model program for use of orientation and mobility assistants—Orientation & mobility position paper. Association for the Education and Rehabilitation of the Blind and Visually Impaired. Available from www.aerbvi.org/modules.php?name=News&file=article&sid=1028, accessed August 30, 2007.

O&M Division. (2004b). Orientation and mobility specialist roles, responsibilities, and qualifications—Orientation & mobility position paper. Association for the Education and Rehabilita-

tion of the Blind and Visually Impaired. Available from www.aerbvi.org/modules.php?name=News&file=article&sid=1028, accessed August 30, 2007.

Oduntan, A. O. (2004). Rehabilitation of visually disabled students of institutions of tertiary education. *South African Optometry, 63*(1), 3–9.

Office of Special Education and Rehabilitative Services (OSERS). (2000). Educating blind and visually impaired students: Policy guidance from OSERS. Available from www.afb.org/Section.asp?SectionID=3&TopicID=138&DocumentID=720.

Ohlsen, R. L., Jr. (1978). Control of body rocking in the blind through the use of vigorous exercise. *Journal of Instructional Psychology, 5*(2), 19–22.

Olmos, P. R., Caraland, S., O'Dorisio, T. M., Casey, C. A., Smead, W. L., Simon, S. R. (1995). The Semmes-Weinstein monofilament as a potential predictor of foot ulceration in patients with noninsulin-dependent diabetes. *Amercan Journal of Medical Science, 309*(2), 76–82.

Olmstead, J. E. (2005). *Itinerant teaching: Tricks of the trade for teachers of students with visual impairments* (2nd ed.) New York: AFB Press.

O'Mara, B. (1989). *Pathways to independence: Orientation and mobility skills for your infant and toddler.* New York: The Lighthouse.

Orientation and Mobility Division of AER. (2006). Teaching O&M through individual and group lessons. Alexandria, VA: Association for Education and Rehabilitation of the Blind and Visually Impaired. Available from www.aerbvi.org/divisions.

Orlansky, M. D., & Trap, J. J. (1987). Working with Native American persons: Issues in facilitating communication and providing culturally relevant services. *Journal of Visual Impairment & Blindness, 81,* 151–155.

Orr, A. L. (1992). *Vision and aging: Crossroads for service delivery.* New York: American Foundation for the Blind.

Orr. A. L., & Rogers, P. (2006). *Aging and vision loss.* New York: AFB Press.

Padden, C., & Humphries, T. (1988). *Deaf in America: Voices from a culture.* Cambridge, MA: Harvard University Press.

Panayiotopoulos, C. P. (2002). *A clinical guide to epileptic syndromes and their treatment: Based on the new ILAE diagnostic scheme.* Oxfordshire, United Kingdom: Blandon Medical Publishing.

Parham, L., & Mailloux, Z. (1996). Sensory integration. In J. Case-Smith, A. Allen, & P. Pratt (Eds.), *Occupational therapy for children* (pp. 307–356). St. Louis, MO: Mosby.

Parsons, S. (1986). Function of play in low vision children: Part 2. Emerging patterns of behavior. *Journal of Visual Impairment & Blindness, 80*, 777–784.

Passini, R., Dupre, A., & Langlois, C. (1986). Spatial mobility of the visually handicapped active person: A descriptive study. *Journal of Visual Impairment & Blindness, 80*(8), 904–907.

Pearson, A. (1919). *Victory over blindness.* New York: Doran.

Peli, E. (2000). Field expansion for homonymous hemianopsia by optically induced peripheral exotropia. *Optometry and Vision Science, 77*, 453–464.

Penrod, W., Bauder, D. K., Simmons, T., Belcher, L., & Corley, J. W. (2006). Efficacy of the UltraCane: A product evaluation and pilot study to determine the efficacy of the UltraCane in outdoor environments. *Closing the Gap, 25*(5), 1–6.

Penrod, W., Bauder, D. K., Simmons, T., Brostek, D., & Matheson, L. (In press). A comparison of secondary electronic travel aids. Manuscript submitted to the *International Journal of Orientation and Mobility.*

Penrod, W., Bauder, D., Simmons, T., & Brostek Lee, D. (2009). A Comparison of selected secondary electronic travel aids with a primary mobility system. *International Journal of Orientation & Mobility*, Volume 2, Number 1.

Penrod, W., & Blasch, B. (2005). Tooth fairies and the appropriateness of electronic travel devices for children. *Division of Visual Impairment Quarterly, 51*(1), 23–25.

Penrod, W., Corbett, M., & Blasch, B. B. (2005). A master trainer class for professionals in teaching the ultracane electronic travel device. *Journal of Visual Impairment & Blindness, 99*(11), 711–715.

Penrod, W., & Simmons, T. (2005). An evaluation and comparison of the Handguide by Guideline and the Miniguide developed by GDP Research electronic travel devices. *Closing the Gap, 23*(6), 22–24.

Pereira, L. M. (1990). Spatial concepts and balance performance: Motor learning in blind and visually impaired children. *Journal of Visual Impairment & Blindness, 84*, 109–111.

Perla, F., & O'Donnell, B. (2004). Encouraging problem solving in orientation and mobility. *Journal of Visual Impairment & Blindness, 98*(1), 47–52.

Perlman, J. M. (2001). Intraventricular hemorrhage and periventricular leukomalacia. In R. Polin, M. Yoder, & F. Burg (Eds.), *Workbook in practical neonatology.* Philadelphia, PA: W.B. Saunders.

Piaget, J. (1963). *The origins of intelligence in children.* New York: W. W. Norton.

Pick, H. L. (1980). Tactual and haptic perception. In R. Welsh & B. Blasch (Eds.), *Foundations of orientation and mobility.* New York: American Foundation for the Blind.

Pickett, A. L. (2002). Paraeducators: The evolution in their roles, responsibilities, training, and supervision. *Impact: Feature Issue on Paraeducators Supporting Students with Disabilities and At-Risk, 15*(2), 2–3, 29. Minneapolis: University of Minnesota, Institute on Community Integration.

Pierce, T. B., & Everington, C. (2002). Supporting inclusive environments through collaboration. In L. Hamill & C. Everington (Eds.), *Teaching learners with moderate to severe disabilities: An applied approach for inclusive environments* (pp. 161–179). Columbus, OH: Merrill Prentice Hall.

Pike, E., Blades, M., & Spencer, C. (1992). A comparison of two types of tactile maps for blind children. *Cartographica, 29*(3–4), 83–88.

Pline, J. (Ed.). (2001). *Traffic control devices handbook.* Washington, DC: Institute of Transportation Engineers.

Pogrund, R., Fazzi, D. L., & Lampert, J. S. (Eds.). (1992). *Early focus: Working with young blind and visually impaired children and their families.* New York: American Foundation for the Blind.

Pogrund, R., Healy, G., Jones, K., Levack, N., Martin-Curry, F., Martinez, C., Marz, J., Roberson-Smith, B., & Vrba, A. (1993). *Teaching age-appropriate purposeful skills: An orientation and mobility curriculum for students with visual impairments.* Austin: Texas School for the Blind and Visually Impaired.

Pogrund, R. L. (2002). Refocus: Setting the stage for working with young children who are blind or visually impaired. In R. L. Pogrund & D. L. Fazzi (Eds.), *Early focus: Working with young children who are blind or visually impaired and their families* (pp. 1–15). New York: AFB Press.

Pogrund, R. L., & Fazzi, D. L. (Eds.). (2002). *Early focus: Working with young children who are blind or visually impaired and their families* (2nd ed.). New York: AFB Press.

Pogrund, R. L., Fazzi, D. L., & Schreier, E. M. (1993). Development of a preschool "Kiddy Cane." *Journal of Visual Impairment & Blindness, 87,* 52–54.

Pogrund, R. L., Healy, G., Jones, K., Levack, N., Martin-Curry, S., Martinex, C., et al. (1995). *Teaching age-appropriate purposeful skills: An orientation and mobility curriculum for students with visual impairments.* Austin: Texas School for the Blind and Visually Impaired.

Pogrund, R. L., & Rosen, S. J. (1989). The preschool blind child can be a cane user. *Journal of Visual Impairment & Blindness, 83,* 431–439.

Ponchillia, P. E. (1984). Family Services: Role of the center-based teaching professional. *Journal of Visual Impairment & Blindness, 78,* 97–100.

Ponchillia, S. V. (1993). The effect of cultural beliefs on the treatment of native peoples with diabetes and visual impairment. *Journal of Visual Impairment & Blindness, 87*(9), 333–335.

Ponchillia, S. V., Powell, I. I., Felski, K. A., & Nicktawski, M. (1992). The effectiveness of aerobic exercise instruction for totally blind women. *Journal of Visual Impairment & Blindness, 86*(4), 174–177.

Powers, S., Thibadeau, S., & Rose, K. (1992). Antecedent exercise and its effects on self-stimulation. *Behavioral Residential Treatment, 7*(1), 15–22.

Preiser, W. F. E. (1985). A combined tactile/electronic guidance system for visually impaired persons in indoor and outdoor spaces. In *Proceedings of the International Conference on Building Use and Safety Technology.* Washington, DC: National Institute of Building Sciences.

Pressman, N. (2004). *Shaping cities for winter: Climatic comfort and sustainable design.* Prince George, BC (Canada): Winter Cities Association.

Prevent Blindness America (2008), Vision problems in the U.S.: Prevalence of adult blindness age-related eye disease in America. 2008 Update to the Fourth Edition. Prevent Blindness America. http://www.preventblindness.org/VPUS/2008_update.

Ratelle, A., & Dufour, J. (2006, July). Mobility performance with bilateral cochlear implants: Case report and clinical and research findings on auditory localization abilities of visually and hearing impaired people. Paper presented at the 2006 AER International Conference, Snowbird, UT.

Ratelle, A., & Leroux, T. (2007). Evaluating and training auditory skills related to mobility for people using bilateral cochlear implants. In Proceedings of 14th Deafblind International World Conference, Perth, Western Australia, September 25–30.

Ratelle, A., Zabihaylo, C., Alarie, R., Barber, P., Geoffroy, R., Mathieu, S., & Gresset, J. (1998). Effectiveness of a pedestrian—Activated audible traffic signal. Paper presented at the 9th International Mobility Conference, Atlanta, Georgia.

Ray, C., Horvat, M., Keen, K., & Blasch, B. (2005). Using tai chi as exercise intervention for improving balance in adults with visual impairments: Two case studies. *RE:view, 37*(1), 17–24.

Recchia, S. L. (1997). Play and concept development in infants and young children with severe visual impairments: A constructivist view. *Journal of Visual Impairment & Blindness, 91*(4), 401–416.

Regional and national summary report of data from the 2004–2005 annual survey of deaf and hard of hearing children and youth. (2005). Available from www.gri.gallaudet.edu/Demographics/2005_National_Summary.pdf, accessed March 29, 2006.

Reinhardt, J. P. (2001). Effects of positive and negative support received and provided on adaptation to chronic visual impairment. *Applied Developmental Science. 5*(2), 76–85.

Rener, R. (2005a, December). Tactile maps: Exploiting existing spatial data for tactile map production. *Proceesings of Tactile Graphics 2005.* Birmingham, United Kingdom.

Rener, R. (2005b, December). Automated production of tactile maps using digital 3D software. *Proceedings of Tactile Graphics 2005.* Birmingham, United Kingdom.

Ries, P. W. (1994). *Prevalence and characteristics of persons with hearing trouble: United States 1990–1991.* Hyatsville, MD: U.S. Department of Health and Human Services. DHHS Publication No. (PHS) 94–1516.

Rieser, J. J. (2008). Theory and issues in research on blindness and brain plasticity. In J. J. Rieser, D. H. Ashmead, F. F. Ebner, & A. L. Corn (Eds.). *Blindness and brain plasticity in navigation and object perception* (pp. 3–12). New York: Lawrence Erlbaum Associates.

Rieser, J. J., Hill, E. W., Taylor, C. R., Bradfield, A., & Rosen, S. (1992). Visual experience, visual field size, and the development of non-visual sensitivity to the spatial structure of outdoor neighborhoods explored by walking. *Journal of Experimental Psychology General, 121,* 210–221.

Rintelmann, W., Harford, E., & Burchfield, S. (1970). CROS for blind persons with unilateral hearing loss. *Archives of Otolaryngology, 91,* 284–288.

Riordan-Eva, P., Asbury, T., and Whitcher, J. (2008). *Vaughan & Asbury's general ophthalmology* (17th ed.). Stamford, CT: Appleton and Lange.

Rivkin, M. J. (1997). Hypoxic-ischemic brain injury in the term newborn. In A. J. duPlessis (Ed.), *Clinics in perinatology* (pp. 607–625). Philadelphia, PA: W.B. Saunders.

Rockwitz, G. (2000). Orientation and mobility for senior citizens. Paper presented at the 10th International Mobility Conference, Warwick, United Kingdom.

Rogers, C. (1951). *Client-centered therapy.* Boston: Houghton Mifflin.

Rogers, P., Schmitt, S., & Scholl, G. (1997). Demographic and cultural considerations in rehabilitation. In J. E. Moore, W. H. Graves, & J. B. Patterson (Eds.), *Foundations of Rehabilitation Counseling* (pp. 150–178). New York: AFB Press.

Roman, C. (1996). Validation of an interview instrument to identify behaviors characteristic of cortical visual impairment in infants. Ann Arbor: University of Michigan. Unpublished doctoral dissertation.

Roman-Lantzy, C. A. (2007). *Cortical visual impairment, an approach to assessment and intervention.* New York: AFB Press.

Rosen, S. (1989). Gait, balance, and veering tendency in congenitally blind children and youth. Unpublished raw data.

Rosen, S. (1997). Kinesiology and sensorimotor function. In B. B. Blasch, W. R. Wiener, & R. L. Welsh (Eds.), *Foundations of orientation and mobility* (2nd ed. pp. 170–199). New York: AFB Press.

Rosenbloom, A. (1992). Physiological and functional aspects of aging, vision, and visual impairment. In A. Orr (Ed.), *Vision and aging: Crossroads for service delivery.* New York: American Foundation for the Blind.

Rosenblum, P. L. (in press). *Reclaiming independence: Staying in the driver's seat when you no longer drive.* Louisville, KY: American Printing House for the Blind.

Rosenblum, P. L., & Corn, A. L., (2002a). Experiences of older adults who stopped driving because of their visual impairments: Part 1. *Journal of Visual Impairment & Blindness, 96*(6), 389–398.

Rosenblum, P. L., & Corn, A. L. (2002b). Experiences of older adults who stopped driving because of their visual impairment: Part 2. *Journal of Visual Impairment & Blindness, 96*(7), 485–500.

Ross, M., & Levitt, H. (2000). Implantable hearing aids. *Volta Voices* (November/December).

Ross, M. A. (1984). *Fitness for the aging adult with visual impairment: An exercise and resource manual.* New York: American Foundation for the Blind.

Rossano, M. J., & Warren, D. H. (1989). The importance of alignment in blind subjects' use of tactile maps. *Perception, 18,* 805–816.

Rossi, P. W., Kheyfets, S., & Reding, M. J. (1990). Fresnel prisms improve visual perception in stroke patients with homonymous hemianopia or unilateral visual neglect. *Neurology, 40,* 1597–1599.

Rossi, W. A. (2007). Why shoes make "normal" gait impossible: How flaws in footwear affect this complex human function. Available from www.unshod.org/pfbc/pfrossi2.htm, accessed February 26, 2008.

Rovner, B. W., Zisselman, P. M., & Shmuely-Duitzki, Y. (1996). Depression and disability in older people with impaired vision: A follow-up study. *Journal of American Geriatric Society, 44*(2), 181–184.

Rowell, J., & Ungar, S. (2003). A taxonomy for tactile symbols: Creating a usable database for tactile map designers. *The Cartographic Journal, 40*(3), 273–276.

Rowland, C., & Schweiger, P. (2000). Tangible symbols, tangible outcomes. *Augumentative and Alternative Communication, 16*, 61–78.

Rudkin, S. W. (1971). Cane travel in winter. *New Outlook for the Blind, 65*, 8–11.

Russier, S. (1999). Haptic discrimination of 2-D raised-line shapes by blind and sighted adults. *Journal of Visual Impairment & Blindness, 93*, 421–426.

Sacks, S. Z., & Silberman, R. K. (1998). *Educating students who have visual impairments with other disabilities.* Baltimore, MD: Paul H. Brookes Publishing Co.

Salive, M. E., Guralnik, J., Glynn, R. J., Christen, W., Wallace, R. B., & Ostfeld, A. M. (1994). Association of visual impairment with mobility and physical function. *Journal of the American Geriatrics Society, 42*(3), 287–292.

Sandall, S., Hemmeter, M. L., Smith, B., & McLean, M. (2005). DEC recommended practices in early intervention/early childhood special education (2nd ed.). Longmont, CO: Sopris West.

Sauerburger, D. (1987). Testing strategies for crossing streets with no traffic control. Available from www.sauerburger.org/dona/tactaid.htm, accessed March 1, 2007.

Sauerburger, D. (1989). To cross or not to cross: Objective timing methods of assessing street crossings without traffic controls. *RE:view*, 153–161.

Sauerburger, D. (1993). *Independence without sight or sound: Suggestions for practitioners working with deaf-blind adults.* New York: American Foundation for the Blind.

Sauerburger, D. (1995). Safety awareness for crossing streets with no traffic control. *Journal of Visual Impairment and Blindness, 89*(5), 423–431.

Sauerburger, D. (1999). Developing criteria and judgment of safety for crossing streets with gaps in traffic. *Journal of Visual Impairment & Blindness, 93*(7), 447–450.

Sauerburger, D. (2003). Survey of blind pedestrians— Their perception of yielding vehicles and ability to detect yields. Available from www.sauerburger.org/dona/yielding.htm, accessed May 26, 2009.

Sauerburger, D. (2005). Street crossings: Analyzing risks, developing strategies, and making decisions. *Journal of Visual Impairment & Blindness, 99*, 659–663.

Sauerburger, D. (2006a). Instructional strategies for teaching judgment in detecting gaps for crossing streets with no traffic controls. *RE:view, 37*(4), 177–188.

Sauerburger, D. (2006b). Teaching judgement in crossing streets with traffic controls. *RE:view, 37*, 173–188.

Sauerburger, D., & Jones, S. (1997). Corner to corner: How can deaf-blind travelers solicit aid effectively? *RE:view, 29*(1), 34.

Sauerburger, D., Sifferman, E., & Rosen, S. (2006). Orientation and mobility for visually impaired persons with multiple disabilities including deaf-blindness. In Proceedings of the 12th International Mobility Conference, Plenary Session VI, November 29, 2006. Hong Kong, China.

Scheffers, W., & Myers, L. (2004). Intersection analysis, section L. Unpublished manuscript.

Schein, J. D., Gentile, A., & Haas, K. W. (1970). *Development and evaluation of an expanded hearing loss scale questionnaire.* Rockville, MD: U.S. Department of Health, Education, and Welfare. Public Health Service; 1970. Public Health Service Publication No. 1000-Series 2-No. 37.

Scheuermann, B., & Webber, J. (2002). *Autism: Teaching does make a difference.* Belmont, CA: Wadsworth/Thomas Learning.

Schickendanz, J. A., Schickendanz, D. I., Forsyth, P. D., & Forsyth, G. A. (1998). *Understanding children and adolescents.* Needham Heights, MA: Allyn & Bacon.

Schiff, W., & Detwiler, M. L. (1979). Information used in judging impending collision. *Perception, 8*, 647–658.

Schiff, W., & Isikow, H. (1966). Stimulus redundancy in the tactile perception of histograms. *Development of raised line drawings as supplementary tools in the education of the blind*, Appendix C. (Final report, September, Project No. RD-1571-S). Washington, DC: U.S. Department of Health, Education and Welfare, Vocational Rehabilitation Administration.

Schmeidler, E., & Halfmann, D. (1998). Distribution of people with visual impairment by community type, prevalence of disability, and growth of the older population. *Journal of Visual Impairment & Blindness, 92,* 380–381.

Schneekloth, L. (1989). Play environments for visually impaired children. *Journal of Visual Impairment & Blindness, 83*(4), 196–211.

Schoen, F., Mueller, J., & Helms, J. (1999). Results of bilateral cochlear implantation. *European Archives of Oto-Rhino-Laryngology, 156,* 106.

Schonfeld, L., King-Kallimanis, B., Brown, L. M., Davis, D. M., Kearns, W. D., Molinari, V. A., et al. (2007). Wanderers with cognitive impairment in Department of Veterans Affairs nursing home care units. *Journal of the American Geriatrics Society, 55*(5), 692–699.

Schonfield, D. (1974). Translations in gerontology—From lab to life: Utilizing information. *American Psychologist, 29,* 796–801.

Schroeder, B. J., Rouphail, N., & Wall Emerson, R. (2006). Exploratory analysis of crossing difficulties for blind and sighted pedestrians at channelized turn lanes. *Transportation Research Record: Journal of the Transportation Research Board, 1956,* 94–102.

Schulz, R., & Salthouse, T. (1999). Adult development and aging: Myths and emerging realities. Upper Saddle River, NJ: Merrill Prentice Hall.

Schunk, D. (2004). *Learning theories: An educational perspective* (4th ed.). Upper Saddle River, NJ: Pearson Education, Inc.

Scott, A. C., Barlow, J. M., Bentzen, B. L., Bond, T. L. Y., & Gubbe, D. (2008). Accessible pedestrian signals at complex intersections: Effects on blind pedestrians. *Transportation Research Record: Journal of the Transportation Research Board, 2073,* 94–103.

Scott, J. (1962). Critical periods in behavioral development. *Science, 138,* 949–958.

Sebald, H. (1993). Life in the subculture. In J. F. Cuber & A. C. Clarke (Eds.), *Adolescence: A sociological analysis* (pp. 255–262). New York: Appleton-Century-Crofts.

Second European Symposium on Tactual Town Maps for the Blind. (1985). Marburg, Germany.

Seebar, B., Baumann, U., & Fasti, H. (2004). Localization ability with bimodal hearing aids and bilateral cochlear implants. *Journal of Acoustical Society of America, 116,* 1698–1709.

Seeing Eye, Inc. (1984). The Mowat Sensor Project. Unpublished raw data.

Seeing Eye, Inc. (1992). Survey of mobility instructors. Unpublished manuscript.

Seward, A. E., Ashmead, D. H., & Bodenheimer, B. (2007). Using virtual environments to assess time-to-contact judgments from pedestrian viewpoints. *ACM Transactions on Applied Perception, 4*(3).

Shearer, D. E., & Shearer, M. S. (1976). The Portage Project: A model for early childhood intervention. In T. D. Tjossem (Ed.), *Intervention strategies for high risk infants and young children* (pp. 335–350). Baltimore, MD: University Park Press.

Sheppard-Jones, K., Prout, H. T., & Kleinert, H. (2005). Quality of life for adults with developmental disabilities: A comparative study. *Mental Retardation, 43,* 281–291.

Shevell, M., Ashwal, S., Donley, D., Flint, J., Gingold, M., Hirtz, D., et al. (2003). Practice parameter: Evaluation of the child with global developmental delay: Report of the Quality Standards Subcommittee of the American Academy of Neurology and the Practice Committee of the Child Neurology Society. *Neurology, 60,* 367–380.

Shingledecker, C. (1983). Measuring the mental effort of blind mobility. *Journal of Visual Impairment & Blindness, 77*(7), 334–339.

Shonkoff, J. P., & Marshall, P. C. (2000). The biology of developmental vulnerability. In J. P. Shonkoff & S. J. Meisels (Eds.), *Handbook of early childhood intervention* (pp. 35–53). Cambridge, United Kingdom: Cambridge University Press.

Shoufeng, Y., & Evans, J. (2005). Inkjet printing of tactile map on clay tile. Proceedings of Tactile Graphics *2005.* Birmingham, United Kingdom.

Shumway-Cook, A., Silver, I. F., LeMier, M., York, S., Cummings, P., & Koepsell, T. D. (2007). Effectiveness of a community-based multifactorial intervention on falls and fall risk factors in community-living older adults: A randomized, controlled trial. *The Journals of Gerontology Series A: Biological Sciences and Medical Sciences, 62,* 1420–1427.

Sickle Cell Disease Guideline Panel. (1993). Sickle cell disease: Screening, diagnosis, management and counseling in newborns and infants. *Clinical practice guideline no. 6* (AHCPR Pub. No. 93–0562). Washington, DC: Department of Health and Human Services.

Silberman, R. (2000). Children and youths with visual impairments and other exceptionalities. In M. Cay Holbrook & A. J. Koenig (Eds.), *Foundations of education, Vol. 1: History and theory of teaching children and youths with visual impairments* (2nd ed., pp. 173–196). New York: AFB Press.

Silberman, R. K., Bruce, S., & Nelson, C. (2004). Children with sensory impairments. In F. P. Orelove, D. Sobsey, & R. K. Silberman (Eds.), *Educating children with multiple disabilities: A collaborative approach* (4th ed.) (pp. 425–528). Baltimore, MD: Paul H. Brookes Publishing, Co.

Simoneau, G. G., Ulbrecht, J. S., Derr, J. A., Becker, M. B., & Cavanagh, P. R. (1994). Postural instability in patients with diabetic sensory neuropathy. *Diabetes Care, 17,* 1411–1421.

Skellenger, A. C., & Hill, E. W. (1991). Current practices and considerations regarding long cane instruction with preschool children. *Journal of Visual Impairment & Blindness, 85,* 101–104.

Skellenger, A. C., & Hill, E. W. (1997). The Preschool Learner. In B. B. Blasch, W. R. Weiner, & R. L. Welsh (Eds.), *Foundations of orientation and mobility* (2nd ed.) (pp. 407–436). New York: AFB Press.

Skellenger, A. C., Rosenblum, L. P., & Jager, B. K. (1997). Behaviors of preschoolers with visual impairments in indoor play settings. *Journal of Visual Impairment & Blindness, 91*(6), 519–530.

Skoczenski, A., & Good, W. (2004). Vernier acuity is selectively affected in infants and children with cortical visual impairment. *Developmental Medicine & Child Neurology, 46,* 526–532.

Sleeuwenhoek, H., & Boter, R. (1995). Perceptual-motor performance and the social development of visually impaired children. *Journal of Visual Impairment & Blindness, 89*(4), 359–367.

Smith, A. J., & Cote, K. (2001). *Look at me.* Philadelphia, PA: Pennsylvania College of Optometry Press.

Smith, A. J., De l'Aune, W., & Geruschat, D. R. (1992). Low vision mobility problems: Perceptions of O&M specialists and persons with low vision. *Journal of Visual Impairment & Blindness, 86*(1), 58–62.

Smith, A. J., & Geruschat, D. R. (1983). *Developmental assessment of standard training protocols for the use of fresnel prisms for persons with peripheral field defects: Effects of independent travel and psycho-social adjustment. Final report.* Washington, DC: National Institute for Handicapped Research.

Smith, A. J., & Geruschat D. R. (1996). Orientation and mobility for children and adults with low vision. In A. L. Corn & A. J. Koenig (Eds.), *Foundations of low vision: Clinical and functional perspectives.* (pp. 306–321). New York: AFB Press.

Smith, A. J., & O'Donnell, L. M. (2001). *Beyond arm's reach: Enhancing distance vision.* Elkins Park, PA: Pennsylvania College of Optometry Press.

Smith, M., & Levack, N. (1996). *Teaching students with visual and multiple impairments: A resource guide.* Austin, Texas School for the Blind.

Smith, T. B. (2002). *Guidelines: Practical tips for working and socializing with deaf-blind people.* Burtonsville, MD: Sign Media.

Song, A., Jones, S., Lippert, J., Metzgen, K., Miller, J., & Borreca, C. (1998). *Wisconsin behavior rating scale.* Madison: Wisconsin Center for the Developmentally Disabled.

Sorrells, A. M., Rieth, H. J., & Sindelar, P. T. (2004). *Critical issues in special education: Access, diversity and accountability.* Boston: Pearson.

Sousa, D. A. (2001). *How the brain learns* (2nd ed.). Thousand Oaks, CA: Corwin Press.

Southeastern Guide Dogs. (2009). *Special needs.* Available from www.guidedogs.org/index.php?page=Special-Needs-01, accessed June 4, 2009.

Sparrow, S. S., Cocchetti, D. V., Balla, D. A. (2005). *Vineland adaptive behavior scale* (2nd ed.). Lebanon, IN: Pearson Education Publishing.

Staab, W. J. (1978). *Hearing aid handbook* (pp. 16–23). Phoenix, AZ: Author.

Staab, W. J. (2002). Characteristics and use of hearing aids. In J. Katz (Ed.), *Handbook of clinical audiology* (4th ed.) (pp. 631–686). Baltimore: Williams & Wilkins.

Staab, W. J., & Lybarger, S. F. (1994). Characteristics and use of hearing aids. In J. Katz (Ed.), *Handbook of clinical audiology* (5th ed.). Baltimore: Williams & Wilkins.

Staab, W. J., Polashek, T., Nunley, J., Green, R. S., Brisken, A., Dojan, R., Taylor, C., Katz, R. (1998). Audible ultrasound for profound losses. *Hearing Review, 5*(2), 28, 30, 32, 36.

Stapin, L., Lococo, K., Byington, S., & Harkey, D. (2001). *Highway design handbook for older drivers and pedestrians.* Washington, DC: Federal Highway Administration.

Stevenson, J. W. (2001). Practice notes: Pedestrian clearance intervals. *Journal of Visual Impairment & Blindness, 95*(4), 237–239.

Stokoe, W. C. (1960). *Sign language structure: An outline of visual communication systems of the American deaf.* Silver Spring, MD: Linstok Press.

Stollof, E. (2005a). Wayfinding at intersections: Efforts toward standardization—A joint workshop of the Institute of Transportation Engineers and the U.S. Access Board. *ITE Journal, 75*(4), 20–25.

Stollof, E. (2005b). Developing curb ramp designs based on curb radius. *ITE Journal, 75*(4), 26–32.

Stollof, E., McGee, H., & Eccles, K. (2007). *Pedestrian signal safety for older persons.* Washington, DC: Institute of Transportation Engineers and AAA Foundation for Traffic Safety.

Story, A. (1998, Fall). Hand over hand guidance: What lesson do we teach? *See/Hear,* www.tsbviedu/outreach/seehear/fall1998/hand.htm, accessed May 12, 2010

Stotland, E., & Canon, L. K. (1972). *Social psychology: A cognitive approach.* Philadelphia, PA: Saunders.

Strauss, K., & Bohn, B. (2002, March). Asthma: Not just a childhood condition. *NEA Today 20*(6). Available from www.nea.org/neatoday/0203/health.html, accessed May 17, 2007.

Strom, K. E. (2006). Rapid product changes mark the new mature digital market. *Hearing Review, 13*(5), 70–75.

Strong, J. G., Jutai, J. W., Russell-Minda, E., & Evans, M. (2008a). Driving and low vision: An evidence-based review of rehabilitation. *Journal of Visual Impairment & Blindness, 102,* 410–419.

Strong, J. G., Jutai, J. W., Russell-Minda, E., & Evans, M. (2008b). Driving and low vision: Validity of assessments for predicting driver performance. *Journal of Visual Impairment & Blindness, 102,* 340–351.

Sussman-Skalka, C. J. (2002). *When your partner becomes visually impaired—Helpful insights and tips for coping.* New York: The Lighthouse.

Szlyk, J. P., Seiple, W., Laderman, D. J., Kelsch, R., Stelmack, J., & McMahon, T. (2000). Measuring the effectiveness of bioptic telescopes for persons with central vision loss. *Journal of Rehabilitation Research and Development, 37*(1), 101–108.

Szlyk, J. P., Seiple, W., Stelmack, J., & McMahon, T. (2005). Use of prisms for navigation and driving in hemianopic patients. *Ophthalmic and Physiological Optics, 25,* 128–135.

TaeKwonDo Tutor (TKD Tutor). Falling information. Available from http://tkdtutor.com/09Techniques/Falls/FallInfo.htm, accessed September 7, 2006.

Tait, P. E. (1972). The implications of play as it relates to the emotional development of the blind child. *Education of the Visually Handicapped, 4*(2), 52–54.

Takahashi, N., Tokunaga, R., & Asano, M. (2007). Strategic PDGA for pedestrian-friendly northern communities. In Proceedings of 11th International Conference on Mobility and Transport for Elderly and Disabled Persons [TRANSED]. Montreal, Canada. Available from www.222.tc.gc.ca/eng/policy/transed2007-pages-1126-1829.htm, accessed April 7, 2009.

Tatham, A. F. (1991). The design of tactile maps: theoretical and practical considerations. In K. Rybaczuk & M. Blakemore (Eds.), *Mapping the nations, The proceedings of the International Cartographic Conference* (Vol. 1). London.

Teplin, S. W. (1995). Visual impairment in infants and young children. *Infants and Young Children, 8,* 18–51.

Terlau, M. T. (1997, May). Actuated traffic signals. *Newsletter, Metropolitan Washington Orientation and Mobility Association.* Available from http//www.sauerburger.org/dona/signalold.htm, accessed May 26, 2009.

Terlau, T., & Penrod, W. (2008). "K" Sonar Instruction Manual: Version II. Louisville, KY: American Printing House for the Blind.

Thinus-Blanc, C., & Gaunet, F. (1997). Representation of space in blind persons: Vision as a spatial sense? *Psychological Bulletin, 121,* 20–42.

Thomas, C. C., Correa, V. I., & Morsink, C. V. (2001). *Interactive teaming: Enhancing programs for students with special needs* (3rd ed.). Upper Saddle River, NJ: Merrill Prentice Hall.

Thomas, J. (1994). Acquired brain injury and hidden visual problems. *Optometric Extension Program Foundation, Inc.* Available from www.health.net/oep/BRAIN.HTM, accessed March 10, 2006.

Tielsch, J. (2001). Prevalence of visual impairment and blindness in the United States. In R. Massof & L. Lidoff (Eds.), *Issues in low vision rehabilitation: Service, delivery, policy, and funding* (pp. 13–26). New York: AFB Press.

Tielsch, J., Sommer, A., Witt, K., Katz, J., and Royall, R. (1990). Blindness and visual impairment in an American urban population: The Baltimore eye survey. *Archives of Ophthalmology, 108,* 286–290.

Tinetti, M. E., Richman, D., & Powell, L. (1990). Falls efficacy as a measure of fear of falling. *Journal of Gerontology: Psychological Sciences, 45*(6), 239–243.

Tobin, J. B. (1977). Normal aging: The inevitability syndrome. In S. H. Zarit (Ed.), *Readings in aging and death: Contemporary perspectives* (pp. 39–48). New York: Harper & Row.

Topor, I. L., Holbrook, M. C., & Koenig, A. J. (2000). Creating and nurturing effective educational teams. In A. J. Koenig & M. C. Holbrook (Eds.), *Foundations of education,* Vol. 2: *Instructional strategies for teaching children and youths with visual impairments* (2nd ed., pp. 2–36). New York: AFB Press.

Transit Cooperative Research Program Report 69. (2001a). *Light rail service: pedestrian and vehicular safety.* Washington, DC: Transportation Research Board.

Transit Cooperative Research Program Synthesis 37. (2001b). *Communicating with persons with disabilities in a multimodal transit environment: A synthesis of transit practice.* Washington, DC: Transportation Research Board.

Transit Cooperative Research Program Synthesis 45. (2002). *Customer-focused transit: A synthesis of transit practice.* Washington, DC: Transportation Research Board.

Transit Cooperative Research Program Synthesis 48. (2003). *Real-time bus arrival information systems.* Washington, DC: Transportation Research Board.

Transportation Research Board. (2003, Fall). A ticket and a passport. *Ignition, 1,* 4–6.

Transportation Security Administration. (2007). Travelers with disabilities and medical conditions. Available from www.tsa.gov/travelers/airtravel/specialneeds/index.shtm, accessed March 29, 2007.

Travis, L., Boerner, K., Reinhardt, J., & Horowitz, A. (2004). Exploring functional disability in older adults with low vision. *Journal of Visual Impairment & Blindness, 98*(9), 534–545.

Travis, L. A., Lyness, J. M., Sterns, G. K., Kuchnek, M., Shields, C. G., King, D. A., et al. (2003). Family and friends? A key aspect of older adults' adaptation to low vision? *Journal of Visual Impairment & Blindness, 97*(8), 489–492.

Tröster, H., & Brambring, M. (1993). Early motor development in blind infants. *Journal of Applied Developmental Psychology, 14*(1), 83–106.

Tröster, H., Hecker, W., & Brambring, M. (1994). Longitudinal study of gross-motor development in blind infants and preschoolers. *Early Childhood Development and Care, 104,* 61–78.

Turano, K. A., Geruschat, D. R., Massof, R. W., & Stahl, J. W. (1999). Perceived visual ability for independent mobility in persons with retinitis pigmentosa. *Investigative Ophthalmology & Visual Science 40*(5): 865–877.

Turnbull, A. P., Turbiville, V., & Turnbull, H. R. (2000). Evolution of family-professional partnerships. In J. P. Shonkoff & S. J. Meisels (Eds.). *Handbook of early childhood intervention* (2nd ed., pp. 630–650). New York: Cambridge University Press.

Turnbull, A. P., & Turnbull, H. R. (2001). Building reliable alliances. In A. P. Turnbull & H. R. Turnbull (Eds.), *Families, professionals, and exceptionality* (4th ed., pp. 56–82). Columbus, OH: Merrill Prentice Hall.

Turnbull, A. P., Turnbull, H. R., & Wehmeyer, M. L. (2007). *Exceptional lives: Special education in today's schools* (5th ed.). Upper Saddle River, NJ: Pearson, Merrill, Prentice Hall.

Tuttle, D. (1987). The role of the special education teacher-counselor in meeting students' self-esteem needs. *Journal of Visual Impairment & Blindness, 81,* 156–161.

Tuttle, D. W., & Tuttle, N. R. (2000). Psychosocial needs of children and youths. In M. Cay Holbrook and A. J. Koenig (Eds.), *Foundations of education,* Vol. 1: *History and theory of teaching children and youths with visual impairments* (2nd ed., pp. 161–172). New York: AFB Press.

Tuttle, D. W., & Tuttle, N. R. (2004). *Self-esteem and adjusting with blindness: The process of responding to life's demands*. Springfield, IL: Charles C. Thomas.

Tyler, J. S., & Colson, S., (1994). Common pediatric disabilities: medical aspects and educational implications, *Focus on Exceptional Children, 27*(4), 1–16.

Tyler, R. S., & Schum, D. J. (Eds.). (1995). *Assistive devices for persons with hearing impairment.* Boston: Allyn & Bacon.

Ungar, S., Blades, M., & Spencer, C. (1995). Visually impaired children's strategies for memorising a map. *British Journal of Visual Impairment, 13,* 27–32.

Ungar, S., Blades, M., & Spencer, C. (1997). Teaching visually impaired children to make distance judgments from a tactile map. *Journal of Visual Impairment & Blindness, 91,* 163–174.

Ungar, S., Blades, M., & Spencer, C. (1998). Effects of orientation on braille reading by people who are visually impaired: the role of context. *Journal of Visual Impairment & Blindness, 92,* 454–463.

University of Michigan Kellogg Eye Center. (2006). AIDS and Eyes. Available from http://kellogg .umich.edu/patientcare/conditions/aids.html, accessed March 16, 2007.

University of Montana, Environmental Health and Safety Department. *Strategies for walking on ice and snow.* Available from www.mtech.edu/safety/ winter.htm, accessed October 2, 2006.

U.S. Congress, Office of Technology Assessment (1992). *Testing in American schools: Asking the right questions* (OTA-SET-519). Washington, DC: U.S. Government Printing Office.

U.S. Department of Education. (2002). *Twenty-Fourth Annual Report to Congress on the Implementation of the Individuals with Disabilities Education Act.* Washington, DC: U.S. Department of Education, Office of Special Education Programs, Data Analysis System (DANS).

U.S. Department of Education. (2005). *Twenty-Seventh Annual Report to Congress on the Implementation of the Individuals with Disabilities Education Act* (Vol. 1). Washington, DC.

U.S. Department of Education. (2006). Individuals with Disabilities Education Act (IDEA) Data, Part B Annual Report Tables: Child Count Data for 2006. Available from www.ideadata.org.

U. S. Department of Justice. (1991). 28 CFR PART 35, *Nondiscrimination on the basis of disability in state and local government services: Final rule [ADAAG].* Washington, DC: Author.

Uslan, M. M. (1990). In-service training for bus drivers. In M. M. Uslan, A. F. Peck, W. R. Wiener, & A. Stern (Eds.), *Access to mass transit for blind and visually impaired travelers* (pp. 91–93). New York: American Foundation for the Blind.

Uslan, M. M., Hill, E., & Peck, A. (1989). *The profession of orientation and mobility in the 1980s: The AFB competency study.* New York: AFB Press.

Uslan, M. M., Peck, A. F., Wiener, W. R., & Stern, A. (Eds.). (1990). *Access to mass transit for blind and visually impaired travelers.* New York: American Foundation for the Blind.

Vanderheiden, G. C. (October 1995). Use of audio-haptic interface techniques to allow nonvisual access to touchscreen appliances. Working Paper from Human Factors and Ergonomics Society Annual Conference, San Diego, CA.

van Dijk, J. (October 20, 2006). A day with Dr. Jan van Dijk: A day long workshop on assessing and instructing learners with autism. In association with the New York State Technical Assistance Project serving children and youth who are deafblind of Teachers College, Columbia University, the program in severe disabilities includes deafblindness of Hunter College of the City University of New York, and the New York Institute for Special Education, Teachers College, Columbia University.

Van Hoesel, R., & Tyler, R. (2003). Speech perception, localization, and lateralization with bilateral cochlear implants. *Journal of the Acoustical Society of America, 113,* 1617–1630.

Van Hof, C., & Looijestijn, P. L. (1995). An interdisciplinary model for the rehabilitation of visually impaired and blind people: Application of the ICIDH concepts. *Disability Rehabilitation, 17*(7), 391–399.

Van Hof, C., Looijestijn, P., & van de Wege, A. (1997). Review on interdisciplinary rehabilitation of visually impaired and blind people. *International Journal of Rehabilitation and Health, 3*(4), 233–251.

Vaucher, Y. E. (1988). Understanding intraventricular hemorrhage and white matter injury in premature infants. *Infants and Young Children, 1*, 31–45.

Ventry, I., & Weinstein, B. E. (1982). The hearing handicap inventory for the elderly: A new tool. *Ear and Hearing, 3*, 128–134.

Verhaeghen, P., Marcoen, A., & Goossens, L. (1993). Facts and fictions about memory aging: A quantitative integration of research findings. *Journal of Gerontology: Psychological Sciences, 48*, 57–71.

Volpe, J. J. (1987). *Neurology of the newborn.* Philadelphia, PA: W. B. Saunders.

Volpe, J. J. (1997). Brain injury in the premature infant. In A. J. duPlessis (Ed.), *Clinics in perinatology* (pp. 567–587). Philadelphia, PA: W. B. Saunders.

Voyer, B. (2005). *ANIU, From snowflake to iceberg.* Montréal, Canada: Névé Editions.

Vygotsky, L. S. (1978). *Mind and society.* Cambridge, MA: Harvard University Press.

Vygotsky, L. S. (1987). Thinking and speech. In R. W. Reiber & A. S. Carton (Eds.), (N. Minick, Trans.), *The collected works of L.S. Vygotsky,* Vol. 1: *Problems of general psychology.* New York: Plenum.

Wainapel, S. A. (1994). Visual impairments. In G. Felsenthal, S. J. Garrison, and F. U. Steinberg (Eds.), *Rehabilitation of the aging and elderly patient* (pp. 327–337). Baltimore: Williams and Wilkins.

Wainapel, S. F. (1995). Vision rehabilitation: An overlooked subject in physiatric training and practice. *American Journal of Physical Medicine and Rehabilitation, 74*, 313–314.

Wall, R. S. (2001). An exploratory study of how travelers with visual impairments modify travel techniques in winter. *Journal of Visual Impairment & Blindness, 95*(12), 752–756.

Wall Emerson, R., & Ashmead, D. (2008). Visual experience and the concept of compensatory spatial hearing abilities. In J. J. Rieser, D. H. Ashmead, F. F. Ebner, & A. L. Corn (Eds.), *Blindness and brain plasticity in navigation and object perception* (pp. 367–380). New York: Lawrence Erlbaum Associates.

Wall Emerson, R., & Sauerburger, D. (2008). Detecting approaching vehicles at streets with no traffic control. *Journal of Visual Impairment & Blindness, 102*(12), 747–760.

Wall Emerson, R. S., & Corn, A. L. (2006). Orientation and mobility content for children and youths: A Delphi approach pilot study. *Journal of Visual Impairment & Blindness, 100*(6), 331–352.

Walling, A. D. (2003). Home exercise program can improve knee osteoarthritis. *American Family Physician, 67*(3), 625–626.

Wang, J. S., Lan, C., Chen, S. Y., & Wong, M. K. (2002). Tai chi chuan training is associated with enhanced endothelium-dependent dilation in skin vasculature of healthy older men. *Journal of the American Geriatric Society, 50*, 1024–1030.

Ward, M. E., & Johnson, S. B. (1997). The visual system: Anatomy, physiology, and visual impairment. In J. E. Moore, W. H. Graves, & J. B. Patterson (Eds.), *Foundations of rehabilitation counseling* (pp. 24–59). New York: AFB Press.

Warren, M. (2008). Memory loss, dementia, and stroke: Implications for rehabilitation of older adults with age-related macular degeneration. *The Journal of Visual Impairment & Blindness, 102*(10), 611–615.

Washburn, A. M. (2005). Relocation puts elderly nursing home residents at risk of stress, although the stress is short lived. *Evidence-Based Mental Health, 8*(2), 49.

Weber, P. C. (2002). Medical and surgical considerations for implantable hearing prosthetic devices. *American Journal of Audiology, 11*(2), 134–138.

Wehman, P., & Kregel, J. (1997). *Functional curriculum for elementary, middle and secondary age students with special needs.* Austin, TX: PRO-ED.

Weinstein, B. E. (1986). Validity of a screening protocol for identifying elderly people with hearing problems. *ASHA, 28*(5), 41–45.

Weinstein, B. E. (2000). Audiologic rehabilitation: an integrated approach. In B. E. Weinstein (Ed.), *Geriatric audiology* (pp. 171–207). New York: Thieme Medical Publishers.

Weinstein, B. E. (2009). Hearing loss in the elderly: A new look at an old problem. In J. Katz, L. Medwetsky, R. Burkard, & L. Hood (Eds.), *Handbook of clinical audiology* (pp. 712–725). Philadelphia, PA: Lippincott Williams & Wilkins.

Welsh, R. (1997). The psychosocial dimensions of orientation and mobility In B. B. Blasch, W. R. Wiener, & R. L. Welsh (Eds.), *Foundations of orientation and mobility* (2nd ed., pp. 200–230). New York: American Foundation for the Blind.

Welsh, R. (2005). Inventing orientation and mobility techniques and teaching methods: A conversation with Russ Williams. *RE:view, 37*, 8–16.

Welsh, R. L. (1972). Cognitive and psychosocial aspects of mobility training. In *Blindness annual, 1972* (pp. 99–109). Washington, DC: American Association of Workers for the Blind.

Welsh, R. L. (2001). Pittsburgh Vision Services: A private rehabilitation center. In R. W. Massof & L. Lidoff (Eds.), *Issues in low vision and rehabilitation: Service delivery, policy, and funding* (pp.213–222). New York: AFB Press.

Welsh, R. L. (2005). Inventing orientation and mobility techniques and teaching methods: Part 2. *RE:view, 37*(2), 61–75.

Welsh, R. L., & Tuttle, D. W. (1997). Congenital and adventitious blindness. In J. E. Moore, W. H. Graves, & J. B. Patterson (Eds.), *Foundations of Rehabilitation Counseling* (pp. 60–79). New York: AFB Press.

Welsh, R. L., & Wiener, W. (1976). *Travel in adverse weather conditions.* New York: American Foundation for the Blind.

Wernick, J. (1985). Use of hearing aids. In J. Katz (Ed.), *Handbook of clinical audiology* (3rd ed., pp. 911–935). Baltimore: Williams & Wilkins.

Whipple, M. (2004). Curb ramp design by elements and planter strip curb ramp. *Proceedings of the Wayfinding at Intersections Workshop.* Washington, DC: Institute of Transportation Engineers/U.S. Access Board. Available from www.ite.org/accessible/curbramp/default.asp, accessed March 28, 2010.

Wiedel, J. W., & Groves, P. A. (1969a). Designing and reproducing tactual maps for the visually handicapped. *New Outlook for the Blind, 63*, 196–201.

Wiedel, J. W., & Groves, P. A. (1969b). *Tactual mapping: Design, reproduction, reading and interpretation* (Final report, University of Maryland, Project No. DR-2557DS). Washington, DC: U.S. Department of Health, Education and Welfare, Vocational Rehabilitation Administration.

Wiener, W., Lawson, G., Naghshineh, K., Brown, J., Bischoff, A., & Toth, A. (1997). The use of traffic sounds to make street crossings by persons who are visually impaired. *Journal of Visual Impairment & Blindness, 91*(5), 435–445.

Wiener, W., & Siffermann, E., (1999). The development of the profession of travel instruction. *Rehabilitation Education, 13*, 315–322.

Wiener, W., & Vopata, A. (1980). Suggested curriculum for distance vision training with optical aids. *Journal of Visual Impairment & Blindness 74*(2), 49–56.

Wiener, W. R. (1997). Audition for the traveler who is visually impaired. In B. B. Blasch, W. R. Wiener, & R. L. Welsh (Eds.), *Foundations of orientation and mobility* (2nd ed., pp. 104–169). New York: AFB Press.

Wiener, W. R., Deaver, K., DiCorpo, D., Hayes, J., Hill, E., Manzer, D., et al. (1990). The orientation and mobility assistant. *RE:view, 22*(2), 69–78.

Wiener, W. R., & Goldstein, B. (1977). A spectral analysis of traffic sounds in residential, small business, and downtown areas. Unpublished manuscript.

Williams, B., Hoff, H., Millaway, S., & Cassidy, M. (1982). *Project OMNI—Orientation & mobility for needed independence: A pre-requisite orientation & mobility skills development curriculum.* Norristown, PA: Montgomery County Intermediate Unit No. 23.

Williams, M. D., Van Houten, R., Ferraro, J., & Blasch, B. (2005). Field comparison of two types of accessible pedestrian signals. *Transportation Research Record: Journal of the Transportation Research Board, 1939*, 91–98.

Williams, R. (1965). How a center can be run for the rehabilitation of blind people. In *Blindness annual, 1965* (pp. 32–48). Washington, DC: American Association of Workers for the Blind.

Williamson, W. D., & Demmler, G. J. (1992). Congenital infections: Clinical outcome and educational implications. *Infants and young children, 4*, 1–10.

Willoughby, D. M., & Monthei, S. L. (1998). *Modular instruction for independent travel for students who are blind or visually impaired: Preschool through high school.* Baltimore, MD: National Federation of the Blind.

Wisconsin Department of Public Instruction. (2005). *Wisconsin adaptive skills resource guide.* Available from http://dpi.wi.gov/sped/adaptskills.html.

Wolf, E. G., Delk, M. T., & Schein, J. D. (1982). *Needs assessment of services to deaf-blind,* Final report (REDEX, Inc.) U. S. Department of Education.

Wolf, S. L., Banrnhart, H. X., Kutner, N. G., McNeeley, E., Coogler, E., & Xu, C. (1996). Reducing frailty and falls in older persons: An investigation of tai chi and computerized balance training. *Journal of the American Geriatric Society, 44,* 489–497.

Wolffe, K. (1998). Transition planning and employment outcomes for students who have visual impairments with other disabilities. In S. Z. Sacks & R. K. Silberman (Eds.), *Educating students who have visual impairments with other disabilities* (pp. 345). Baltimore, MD: Paul H. Brookes Publishing, Co.

Wolffe, K. E. (1999). *Skills for success: A career education handbook for children and adolescents with visual impairments.* New York: AFB Press.

Woodrum, D. E. (1998). Neonatal ICU issues. *Ethics in Medicine, 12,* 44–54.

Woollacott, M. H., Shumway-Cook, A., & Nashner, L. (1986). Aging and postural control: Changes in sensory organization and muscular coordination. *International Journal of Aging and Human development, 23*(2), 97–115.

World Health Organization [WHO]. (2007a). *Global age-friendly cities: A guide.* Geneva: Ageing and Life Course, Family and Community Health, World Health Organization.

World Health Organization [WHO]. (2007b). *WHO Global report on fall prevention in older age.* Geneva: Ageing and Life Course, Family and Community Health, World Health Organization. Available from www.who.int/ageing/publications/Falls_prevention7March.pdf, accessed March 18, 2009.

Wynn, P. (2007). Clipping the wings of arrhythmia. *Today in PT,* June 11, 36–39.

Xue, L., & Ritaccio, A. (2006). Reflex seizures and reflex epilepsy. *American Journal of Electroneurodiagnostic Technology, 46*(1), 39–48.

Yost, W. A. (2000). *Fundamentals of hearing: An introduction* (4th ed.). New York: Academic Press.

Young, D. R., Appel, L. J., Jee, S., & Miller, E. R. (1999). The effects of aerobic exercise and t'ai chi on blood pressure in older people: Results of a randomized trial. *Journal of the American Geriatric Society, 47,* 277–284.

Ytterstad, B. (1996). The Harstad injury prevention study: Community based prevention of fall-fractures in the elderly evaluated by means of a hospital based injury recording system in Norway. *Journal of Epidemiology and Community Health, 50,* 551–558.

Zabihaylo, C., & Wanet, M. C. (2006, November). Assessment of satisfaction and use of an orientation aid (Trekker) by a group of individuals (pilot project). Paper presented at the NE/ AER Conference 2006, Montréal, Québec, Canada.

Zarit, S. H. (1992). Psychological aspects of aging and visual impairment. In A. L. Orr. *Vision and aging: Crossroads for service delivery.* New York: American Foundation for the Blind.

Zegeer, C., Seiderman, C., Lagerway, P., Cynecki, M., Ronkin, M., & Schneider, R. (2002). *Pedestrian facilities users guide—Providing safety and mobility.* Washington, DC: Federal Highway Administration.

Zimmerman, B. (1989). A social cognitive view of self-regulated academic learning. *Educational Psychology, 81,* 329–339.

Zimmerman, B. J., & Schunk, D. H. (Eds.). (2001). *Self-regulated learning and academic achievement: Theoretical perspectives* (2nd ed.). Mahwah, NJ: Lawrence Erlbaum Associates.

GLOSSARY

Academy for Certification of Vision Rehabilitation and Education Professionals (ACVREP) The primary certifying organization in the United States for professionals who work with persons who are visually impaired.

Accessible pedestrian signal (APS) A device that provides information that is accessible to pedestrians who are blind or visually impaired about when the walk sign is on.

Achromatopsia A congenital defect in or absence of cones, resulting in the inability to see color and reduced clear central vision.

Acquired brain injury Injury to the brain that occurs after the first few years of life.

Adaptive mobility device (AMD) Pusher-type devices used by some persons (such as young children), who are incapable of mastering the techniques of the long cane, to preview their path.

Adventitious Occurring or appearing later in life.

Afference Feedback from the body about its movements. *See also* Efference

Air conduction threshold Intensity level at which signals presented through earphones or sound field are detected 50 percent of the time.

Albinism The congenital absence of pigment in the iris and choroid that causes light sensitivity and reduced acuity.

Allocentric frame of reference An understanding of the locations of objects or places as related to one another, independent of the traveler's current location in space; also called *object-to-object relationships*.

Ambulatory aids Appliances that provide physical support for moving through the environment, including such devices as wheelchairs, walkers, crutches, and support canes.

American Association of Instructors for the Blind, 1871–1968 (AAIB) An association of professionals who worked with children who are blind; the predecessor of AEVH.

American Association of Workers for the Blind, 1895–1984 (AAWB) An association of professionals who worked with adults who are blind.

American Manual Alphabet A one-handed system of fingerspelling commonly used in the United States.

American National Standards Institute (ANSI) The creator of ANSI A117.1, an industry standard based on a consensus process, that provides specifications for making the built environment accessible to and usable by persons with disabilities.

American Sign Language (ASL) A language that is used by people who are deaf, the concepts and vocabulary of which are composed of signs produced with movements of the arms and hands, facial expression, and body language, and that has its own morphology, semantics, and syntax.

Americans with Disabilities Act (ADA) Legislation defining the responsibilities of and requirements for transportation providers to make transportation accessible to individuals with disabilities.

Americans with Disabilities Act Accessibility Guidelines (ADAAG) Regulations implementing Title III of the Americans with Disabilities Act that make public accommodations accessible to and usable by persons with disabilities.

Amplification The process of increasing the magnitude of a signal through power, current, or voltage.

Amsler grid A graphlike card used to determine central field losses, as in macular degeneration.

Aniridia A congenital malformation (usually incomplete) of the iris, accompanied by nystagmus, photophobia, reduced visual acuity, and often glaucoma.

Annunciator A technology that presents over a loudspeaker information that is being displayed electronically in print.

Anxiety A diffuse reaction to a vague or not clearly perceived threat.

Aphakia The absence of the lens, usually resulting from the removal of a cataract.

Apraxia Difficulty in motor planning.

Association for Education and Rehabilitation of the Blind and Visually Impaired (AER) An association, established in 1984, of professionals who work with children and adults who are blind or visually impaired.

Association for the Education of the Visually Handicapped, 1968–1984 (AEVH) An association of profes-

sionals who worked with children who are blind or visually impaired.

Astigmatism A refractive error caused by spherocylindrical curvature of the cornea or lens; corrected with a cylindrical lens.

Asymmetrical tonic neck reflex A reflex in which there is extension of the arm and leg on the side toward which the head turns, and flexion of the arm and leg on the side away from which the head turns.

Ataxia Impaired coordination of muscular action due to disturbance of one's sense of balance.

Athetosis Abnormal movement characterized by being repetitive, involuntary, slow, and sinuous.

Audible signage A system that makes information in print signage available through spoken messages, either from a loudspeaker or through a handheld receiver.

Audible traffic signal A signal that indicates the onset of a pedestrian walk cycle using tones, clicks, musical phrases, or speech. These are integrated into pedestrian signals and may also function as an auditory beacon.

Audiogram A standard graph used to record hearing thresholds for sounds at different frequencies.

Audiometer An instrument used to measure a person's hearing for a variety of signals, such as pure tones and speech.

Auditory maps Verbal descriptions and directions that are recorded on a cassette or disk and played on a tape or disk recorder.

Auditory nerve The group of nerve fibers that carries impulses relating to both hearing and equilibrium from the inner ear to the brain.

Backward chaining In behavioral learning theory, teaching the last substep or link in the chain of substeps first, and then the next-to-last substep or link, and so on. The other substeps are linked to the chain in this manner until the entire task is learned.

Base of support An area located within the outer circumference of all points of contact of the body with the ground or other supporting surface.

Behavioral learning theory A set of principles that attempts to explain learning in terms of observable changes in the behavior of a person. *See also* Classical conditioning; Operant conditioning

Behind-the-ear (BTE) hearing aid A personal amplification device that is contoured to fit behind the ear.

Between-car barrier A device mounted between rail cars or on the platform designed to prevent, deter, or warn individuals from inadvertently stepping off the platform between cars.

Binocular vision Vision that uses both eyes to form a fused image in the brain and results in three-dimensional vision.

Biomechanics Field of study focusing on applying the laws of physics and working concepts of engineering to describe the motion of body segments and the forces acting on body segments.

Bioptic telescope Two optical systems for one eye.

Blindness The inability to see; the absence or severe reduction of vision.

Body awareness Understanding of body parts and the names of those parts.

Body concept Knowledge of the parts of the body, their function, and their spatial relationship to other body parts.

Body planes Theoretical division of the body into halves (left/right, top/bottom, and front/back).

Body-to-object frame of reference An understanding of relationships between the student and other people and objects; also called *egocentric frame of reference.*

Bone conduction threshold Intensity level at which signals presented through a bone conduction vibrator are detected 50 percent of the time.

Braille A system of raised dots that enables functionally blind persons to read and write by touch.

Brainstem auditory evoked response (BAER) tests A procedure used to record electrical activity evoked from the auditory portion of the eighth nerve and brainstem by presenting stimuli through earphones or a bone conduction vibrator.

Bus lift A platform that raises or lowers to lift people who use wheelchairs or who are otherwise unable to climb steps onto and off of buses.

Cartographic orientation A systematic spatial arrangement of places in an environment in a recognizable pattern resembling geometric figures, such as a street grid pattern with rectangular blocks.

Cataract A clouding of the lens, which may be congenital, traumatic, secondary to another visual impairment, or age related.

Center of gravity Point within the body (or body segment) that, if supported, would then support the rest of the body (or segment) without toppling.

Central auditory system The auditory neural pathways, nuclei, and centers in the brain beyond the synapse of the eighth nerve fibers in the cochlear nuclei of the brainstem.

Central nervous system (CNS) Portion of the nervous system consisting of the brain and spinal cord.

Cephalocaudal From head to toe; refers to the order of development of motor skills in infants.

Cerebral palsy A neurological condition affecting body movement and coordination. Caused by injury to the motor centers of the brain prenatally, at birth, or during the first few years of life.

Certified Orientation and Mobility Specialist (COMS) The designation given by the Academy for Certification of Vision Rehabilitation and Education Professionals to individuals who meet certification standards to teach orientation and mobility.

Changeable-message sign (CMS) An electronic sign that uses flip-dot, LED, or LCD technology to produce a message.

Chronic health impairments Medical conditions affecting internal organs and systems such as the heart, lung, blood, and digestive tract (e.g., heart conditions, respiratory conditions, and circulatory conditions).

Clamps (tie-downs) Special clamps or straps on buses that attach to wheelchair frames to prevent rolling as the bus moves.

Classical conditioning A category of behavioral learning theory that can be used to change behavior by pairing a neutral stimulus that typically would not elicit a response with an unconditioned stimulus that naturally elicits a response. *See also* Behavioral learning theory

Clearance The amount of room a dog guide allows for its master, including overhead.

Clearance error A dog guide's mistake that results in the person who is blind or visually impaired bumping into something or someone.

Closure In cognitive learning theory, the principle that people organize their perceptions so that they are as simple and logical as possible. People fill in the gaps in perceptions as necessary to make sense of the total presentation.

Cochlea The auditory portion of the inner ear, located in the petrous portion of the temporal bone.

Cochlear implant Wire electrodes placed in a nonfunctional cochlea and attached to an induction coil buried surgically under the skin behind the ear that stimulates a healthy auditory nerve when activated by sound.

Cognition A general concept embracing all the various modes of knowing, perceiving, remembering, imagining, conceiving, judging, and reasoning.

Cognitive learning theory A set of principles that attempts to explain learning in terms of the mental processes that a person uses to more fully understand some concept or strategy.

Cognitive map A mental representation of a specific spatial layout, which includes object-to-object relationships.

Coloboma A congenital cleft in some portion of the eye, caused by the improper fusion of tissue during gestation; may affect the optic nerve, ciliary body, choroid, iris, lens, or eyelid.

Color vision The perception of color as a result of the stimulation of specialized cone receptors in the retina.

Commuter rail A transit mode that is an electric or diesel-propelled railway for urban passenger train service consisting of local short-distance travel operating between a central city and adjacent suburbs.

Compression An increase in the density of particles in a medium leading to an instantaneous increase in sound pressure.

Concept A mental representation, image, or idea of concrete objects, as well as of intangible ideas, such as feelings.

Conceptual knowledge Information about general patterns, such as the layout and traffic patterns of typical intersections. Also called *semantic knowledge*.

Conditional dispositional construct A concept which suggests that certain traits or dispositions affect behavior only under certain conditions or in certain situations.

Conditional paratransit eligibility Eligibility for some, but not all, paratransit trips under certain disabling or extreme environmental conditions; eligibility decisions made on a trip-by-trip basis.

Conditioned response A learned response to a stimulus.

Conductive loss Hearing loss resulting from a lesion or disease in the outer ear, the middle ear, or both.

Confrontation visual field testing A method for making a functional assessment of peripheral vision.

Congenital Present at birth.

Congestive heart disease A medical condition characterized by a weakening of the heart muscle that impairs the heart's ability to pump blood.

Constant-contact technique A standard cane touch technique in which the cane tip remains in contact with the ground at all times.

Continuous reinforcement In behavioral learning theory, a reinforcement after every successful behavior.

Contralateral routing of signals (CROS) hearing aid An amplifying system in which a microphone picks up sound on the side of an impaired ear and sends it electrically to a normal or near normal ear.

Contrast sensitivity The ability to detect differences in grayness and background.

Coordination Co-ordering of activity by the nervous system in order to organize movement.

Correction In dog guide handling, a reprimand. May be verbal, such as "No!" or a "leash correction," which is a sharp, quick pull-release on the leash connected to the dog's collar.

Crawling Moving forward on one's belly.

Creeping Moving forward on one's hands and knees.

Criterion-referenced test An assessment of an individual's development of certain skills in terms of absolute levels of mastery, in which the items are objective and arranged in a hierarchical order of sequential skills.

Critical periods Developmental periods during which specific skills are learned most easily.

Cruising The act of walking sideways along furniture, a wall, or another surface, using both hands to support oneself.

Crutch Ambulatory aid, made of either wood or aluminum, consisting of a vertical post handgrip and either an underarm support (underarm crutch) or forearm support (Lofstrand/Canadian/forearm crutch).

Curb-to-curb service A paratransit service that picks up and drops off passengers at curbside.

Deaf-blindness Concomitant hearing and visual impairments, the combination of which may present unique communication, learning, developmental, orientation and mobility, and social needs.

Deafness A loss of hearing that is so severe that it is nonfunctional for the ordinary activities of daily living.

Decibel (dB) A unit for expressing the relative intensity or loudness of sounds.

Deconditioning The process of eliminating or greatly reducing a conditioned response that may be detrimental to learning a desired outcome.

Decubitus ulcer *See* Pressure sore

Demand-response service A transit mode consisting of passenger cars or vans operating in response to calls from passengers to the transit operator, who then dispatches a vehicle to pick up the passengers and transport them to their destinations.

Dependency A class of behaviors capable of eliciting positive attending and ministering responses from others.

Depth perception The overlapping of two slightly dissimilar images from the two eyes to give three-dimensional vision.

Desensitization A multistage process that begins by extinguishing conditioned fear responses to stimuli far removed from the target situation. The target behavior is systematically approached in small steps, with time allowed for the conditioned fear response to extinguish at each step.

Detectable warning A walking surface that is detectable underfoot and with a long cane and functions as a warning to stop for persons with visual impairments.

Detection error A mistake in judging the presence or absence of an important environmental feature or event.

Developmental arrest Cessation of the developmental process in a specific area, such as walking.

Diabetes mellitus A disease characterized by inability to fully utilize glucose as a source of energy.

Diabetic retinopathy Disease of the retina associated with long-standing diabetes; it takes the form of degeneration of the retinal blood vessels, which show fluid leakage in early stages, and hemorrhages, leading to possible blindness, in late stages.

Diagonal cane technique A cane technique used in familiar indoor areas, in which the cane is held in one hand and is positioned diagonally across and in front of the body.

Diffraction The bending or scattering of sound waves around an object.

Directionality The ability to move the body when given various positional terms, such as right, left, forward, and over.

Directional strips A textured, high-contrast surface placed on the floor or ground to provide pedestrians with visual impairments a defined path of travel.

Discount transit fare Reduced rates for bus, subway, or other transportation offered by some districts to people who are older or impaired.

Discovery learning A teaching strategy in which the material to be learned is discovered by the learner in the course of solving a problem or completing a task.

Disposition theory A system of concepts which holds that the consistency in an individual's actions can be explained by the presence of relatively stable personal factors or traits.

Distal Situated away from; located away from the center of the body.

Dog guide The generic term for dogs that are trained to guide blind people, by agreement between Guide Dogs for the Blind, Leader Dogs for the Blind, and The Seeing Eye. The terms *guide dog*, *leader dog*, and *seeing eye dog* properly refer only to dogs trained at those respective schools.

Door-to-door service A paratransit service in which the driver comes to the door to pick up passengers and drops off passengers at the door of the destination building.

Doppler effect The increase in frequency of a sound produced by the compression of sound waves and the shortening of wavelength as distance decreases between a sound source and an object.

Dorsal kyphosis Excessive forward bending of the upper spine.

Double-decker bus High-capacity bus having two levels of seating, one over the other, connected by one or more stairways.

Drop-off lesson A means of evaluating and teaching orientation skills in which the instructor purposefully does not identify the place where the lesson is to begin, gives the student a specific site to be located, and asks the student to interpret the environment independently and to use all problem-solving skills required to travel to the specified location.

Dynamic balance Balance required during such movements as walking or running.

Dynamic visual acuity The ability to discriminate and identify objects when the person is stationary and targets are moving and when both the person and the targets are moving.

Dynamic visual field The potential functional field range when a person moves through the environment.

Dysarthria Difficulty in speaking clearly.

Dysphagia Difficulty in swallowing.

Eccentric viewing Intentionally looking to one side of an object to focus the image on a functional portion of the retina. Also called *eccentric fixation*.

Echolocation The use of reflected sound (including ambient sound) to detect the presence of objects, such as walls, buildings, doors, and openings. Sometimes also referred to as *obstacle perception*.

Efference Motor control commands to the muscles. *See also* Afference

Egocentric frame of reference An understanding of the locations of objects or places in the environment as related to an individual's own body, using such terms as right, left, in front of, and behind; also called *body-to-object relationships*.

Electronic orientation aid (EOA) A device used for orientation and navigation that may be external to the user or carried with the traveler.

Electronic travel aid (ETA) A mobility device (head-borne, cane-borne, chest-worn, or handheld) that extends the range of sensory awareness of the traveler with a visual impairment beyond the fingertip, cane, or dog guide. ETAs emit ultrasound vibrations or laser beams that probe the environment and provide tactile or auditory signals or both.

Emphysema A lung disease that can result in shortness of breath.

Environmental barrier An obstacle or dangerous condition in the physical environment that prevents a person with a disability from proceeding along a path of travel.

Environmental concepts The knowledge of environmental features, such as the size, shape, color, and texture of telephone poles, parking meters, and sidewalks and of the spatial regularities of features in built environments.

Environmental flow The lawful changes in traveler's distances and directions to things in the surroundings that change during locomotion.

Environmental negotiation *See* Wayfinding

Environmental regularity The use of the predictability of built environments as an aid in establishing and maintaining orientation and in making educated guesses about the location of objects or environmental features relative to one another. For example, parking meters are next to streets, restrooms and water fountains in buildings typically are near one another, and elevator doors in a building are in consistent locations across floors.

Episodic knowledge Information about particular places and events—of particular "episodes" of experience.

Equilibrium Balance.

Eustachian tube The tube connecting the middle ear and the nose-throat area, which equalizes pressure on both sides of the tympanic membrane.

Eversion Outward rotation of the ankles that places the body's weight on the instep.

Expectancy motivation The combined influence of perceived self-efficacy and anticipated outcomes on behavior.

Express bus service A bus service that speeds up longer trips by operating long distances without stopping; often found in major metropolitan areas during heavily patronized peak commuting hours.

External locus of control A person's tendency to consider reinforcements or punishments received as resulting from outside forces such as luck, chance, or fate over which the individual has no control.

Extinction In behavioral learning theory, the concept that when a reinforcer is no longer present, many behaviors that have been reinforced will be weakened and ultimately disappear or become extinct.

Familiar environment Any indoor or outdoor physical setting in which the student has traveled previously.

Familiar intensity Knowledge of the loudness of a particular sound source and how that sound varies with one's distance from the sound source.

Familiarization The organized process of learning the arrangement of a room, building, or other area by using systematic strategies to locate landmarks and relate their location to other locations or features in the environment. Perimeter, gridline, and reference point familiarization strategies are used most commonly by individuals who are visually impaired. Also called *self-familiarization*

Family systems theory A set of principles used in counseling that states that families act as systems independent of the individual actions of its members.

Fare Payment to ride in a public transportation vehicle, or a transportation system owned by a private entity. Means of payment include tickets, tokens, cash, transfers, passes, fare cards, and smart cards.

Fear A flight or avoidance reaction that an individual has to a specific threat or danger.

Feedback In classical conditioning, one type of secondary reinforcer that gives an individual information about his or her own behavior.

Feedback loop Interplay of sensory inputs and motor outputs to coordinate movement.

Feeder service A paratransit service that gives passengers with disabilities a ride on a paratransit vehicle to a fixed-route bus or rail stop so that person can continue his or her trip on the fixed-route service.

Field of view The extent of the world that can be seen at any given moment without moving the eyes.

Figure-ground perception In psychology, the attempt to discriminate among the objects in a complex visual array; to separate an object from the background.

Fixed interval In behavioral learning theory, a schedule of reinforcement in which the behavior is reinforced on a set time schedule as long as the behavior that is to be strengthened is being performed correctly when the time for the reward occurs.

Fixed ratio In behavioral learning theory, a schedule of reinforcement in which the reinforcer is administered after a fixed number of successful behaviors.

Fixed-route service Transit service provided on a repetitive, predetermined fixed-schedule basis along a specific route with vehicles stopping to pick up and deliver passengers to specific locations.

Foot-placement preview Placement of the long cane so that the tip strikes the surface where the traveler's foot will be placed.

Forearm trough A curved, metal tray that can be attached to crutches to enable one to support weight on the forearm instead of on the hand.

Frequency In acoustics, the number of vibrations, repetitions of compressions, and rarefactions of a sound wave that occur at the same rate over a period, generally one second, and psychologically perceived as pitch.

Fresnel prisms A series of plastic prisms applied to regular eyeglass lenses that are used to correct eye deviations or to displace peripheral information onto areas of the retina.

Frontal plane Theoretical division of the body into front and back halves.

Functional mobility limitation The interaction between one's personal abilities and the environmental demands of travel. As the environmental demand increases, the potential for functional mobility limitations also increases. This interaction may be mediated or modified through an intervention to reduce environmental demand, to provide the traveler with the skills needed to deal with the environment, or both.

Functional visual acuity The ability to discern distinctions in the real-world environment.

Gait A person's pattern of walking.

Gait belt A safety belt placed around the waist of a person with impaired balance and used by another person to provide physical support during transfers or when walking.

Geographic information system (GIS) An electronic database consisting of an atlas of geographic information, such as streets and landmarks.

Gestalt In cognitive learning theory, the organization of the world into meaningful wholes rather than isolated stimuli. In other words, the whole is greater than the sum of its parts.

Glare An annoying sensation produced by too much light in the visual field that can cause both discomfort and a reduction in visual acuity.

Glaucoma A condition characterized by an increase in intraocular pressure, visually associated with a buildup of aqueous fluid, that may cause damage to the optic nerve and eventual visual field defects if left untreated.

Global positioning system (GPS) An electronic position-sensing technology based on orbiting satellites which communicate with portable transmitters and receivers that, in interaction with a geographic information system, can inform users of their exact location and relationship to landmarks or coordinates.

Goldman perimeter A projection instrument that controls illumination while measuring the extent and characteristics of visual field.

Gridline strategy A strategy for systematic exploration of a space in which a traveler systematically crosses back and forth in the interior of a space in order to locate landmarks.

Gross motor milestones Gross motor skills such as sitting, crawling, and walking that generally appear at specific points in the course of motor development.

Guided learning An instructional teaching strategy in which the individual is taught to use the same type of solutions to solve similar problems.

Handling The skill of working with an individual dog guide in such a way that it gives the best possible result, maximizing the individual dog's strengths while minimizing its weaknesses.

Hand-under-hand technique The placement of an instructor's hand under a student's hand to guide it toward an object or to explore an object together.

Haptic perception The ability to identify objects by size, shape, and feel.

Head righting A reaction in which an infant aligns his or her head vertically in relation to gravity.

Hearing impairment A departure from normal hearing sensitivity.

Heavy rail *See* Rapid rail

Heel strike The contact of the heel with the ground as the foot steps down.

Hemianopsia Blindness in one half of the field of vision in one or both eyes.

Hemiplegia Paralysis on one side of the body.

High guard The position in which the arms are held with hands between shoulder and head height to facilitate balance when standing and walking.

Hyperglycemia An excessively high level of sugar in the blood.

Hyperglycemic reaction Also called *ketoacidosis*, this reaction occurs when the level of insulin in the bloodstream is insufficient to metabolize enough sugar for the body tissues to use.

Hyperopia (farsightedness) A refractive error caused by an eyeball that is too short; corrected with a convex (plus) lens.

Hypertension High blood pressure.

Hypertonia High muscle tone.

Hypoglycemia Low blood glucose level, also known as insulin "reaction," or insulin shock; may occur with or without observable clinical symptoms.

Hypotension Low blood pressure.

Hypotonia Low muscle tone.

Immittance tests Tympanometry and acoustic reflex tests that require no behavioral response from the subject.

Independent movement The act of moving through the environment in a safe and efficient manner.

Individualized Education Program (IEP) A written plan of instruction by an educational team for a child who receives special education services that includes the student's present levels of educational performance, annual goals, short-term objectives, specific services needed, duration of services, evaluation, and related information. Under the Individuals with Disabilities Education Act (IDEA), each student receiving special services must have such a plan.

Individualized Family Service Plan (IFSP) A written plan used to design early intervention programs for infants and toddlers, required by the Individuals with Disabilities Education Act (IDEA).

Individualized Plan of Employment (IPE) A plan developed to meet the specialized rehabilitation needs of an individual, 21 years of age or older.

Individualized Transition Plan (ITP) A written plan developed by an educational team to establish specific transition goals and to identify instructional objectives that support a student's postschool goals, primarily community living and integrated employment. This plan is a requirement of the Individuals with Disabilities Education Act (IDEA).

Information point A feature of a travel environment that by itself does not convey specific information about a traveler's location in space, but when juxtaposed with other features permits travelers to locate themselves relative to their surroundings.

Infrasonic Sounds below the normal hearing range for frequency (below 20Hz).

Inner ear The innermost portion of the ear, which is embedded in the petrous portion of the temporal bone and contains the cochlea, which houses the sensory receptors for hearing, and the utricle, saccule, and semicircular canals, which house the receptors for balance.

Insulin The hormone secreted by the cells of the pancreas. Required by most tissues in order to utilize glucose for energy.

Intelligent disobedience A dog guide's actions when it disobeys its handler's command because obedience would put the handler and dog at risk. Especially refers to traffic work.

Intensity The amplitude of particle vibration that is psychologically perceived as loudness.

Interdisciplinary team model A team approach in which professionals from different disciplines undertake independent assessments of a student but carry out program development as a collective effort.

Intermittent claudication A medical condition characterized by leg cramps due to an inability of the circulatory system to pump sufficient blood (into the legs, for example) to keep up with the muscles' demand for blood when exercising.

Internal locus of control A person's tendency to consider reinforcements or punishments received as resulting from his or her own efforts.

In-the-canal (ITC) hearing aid A personal amplification system that is located mostly or entirely within the external ear canal.

In-the-ear (ITE) hearing aid A personal amplification system that fits into the ear canal and the concha.

Juno walk A term used by many dog guide schools to refer to a walk with an instructor simulating a dog's work while holding and pulling a harness or a harness handle. Used to teach basic techniques and to assess a student's or applicant's needs and abilities before accepting an applicant into a dog guide program or matching the applicant with a dog.

Keratoconus A hereditary degenerative disease that is manifest in adolescence or later, in which the cornea thins and becomes cone shaped and vision is reduced.

Ketoacidosis (ketosis) An acute metabolic state that can occur in diabetes when blood levels of insulin are inadequate. Toxic acids accumulate in the blood, ketones appear in the urine, and dehydration occurs. If untreated, it can result in coma and death.

Ketones A waste product produced as the body burns stored fat for energy.

Kinesiology The study of movement.

Kinesthesia The awareness of movement that results from the interaction of tactile, proprioceptive, and vestibular inputs.

Kinesthetic Information about one's position in space that is received through the muscles during movement.

Kinetic labyrinth The portion of the vestibular system that registers the direction of head movement.

Kyphosis Excessive forward bending of the dorsal (upper) spine.

Landau reaction A neurological reaction seen in infants in which the head is lifted, the back is arched, and the hips are partially extended when the child is held horizontally in the air prone and supported under the front of the trunk.

Landmark Objects, sounds, odors, temperatures, or tactile or visual clues that are easily recognized, are constant, and have discrete, permanent locations in the environment that can give a traveler unique, specific information about the individual's location in space.

Landmark, primary An environmental feature that is detectable to visually impaired travelers, that is al-

ways present, and that is not likely to be missed as one travels a route.

Landmark, secondary Any environmental that is intermittent or that may not be encountered by travelers as they travel a route. Examples are a fan in a water fountain or an object on the sidewalk opposite to the traveler.

Laterality The complete motor awareness of both sides of the body; the recognition of right and left (i.e., from an egocentric perspective).

Layout The distances and directions that relate objects to each other in one's environment.

Learned helplessness A psychological state that results when an individual perceives that events in his or her environment are uncontrollable.

Legal blindness A definition of visual impairment often used as a criterion for determining eligibility for government and agency benefits and services in the United States in which distance visual acuity is 20/200 or less in the better eye and in which the best correction or visual field is no more than 20 degrees.

Lens The part of the eye that changes shape to adjust the focus of images from various distances into a sharp image on the retina.

Levels of processing theory The concept that the more thoroughly one can process information, the more likely it is that one can move the information from short-term to long-term memory.

Light-emitting diode (LED) An electronic device that lights up when electricity is passed through it. LEDs are good for displaying images, such as signage, because they can be relatively small and do not burn out quickly.

Light rail A transit mode that typically is an electric railway with a light-volume traffic capacity with low- or high-platform loading and rails in shared or exclusive right-of-way.

Limited-stop bus service A hybrid between local and express service in which the bus stops may be several blocks to a mile or more apart to speed up the trip.

Local bus service The most common type of bus service in which buses may stop every block or two along a route several miles long; also referred to as *circulator, feeder, neighborhood*, or *shuttle service*.

Localization The ability to orient oneself to the environment through the use of the sense of hearing; the determination of the direction of a sound source.

Localization error A mistake in judging the direction to an environmental feature or event.

Locomotor skills Abilities, such as creeping, crawling, and walking, that are used to move in the environment.

Locus of control An individual's characteristic belief about the amount of control he or she has over the events or outcomes experienced in life.

Long arch The arch of the foot formed by the ligaments that run from the heel to the base of the toes.

Long-range goals The specification of performance to be obtained by the end of an educational or rehabilitation program.

Lordosis Posterior curvature of the lumbar (lower) spine resulting in a swayed back.

Low-floor bus A type of bus designed so that the front of the bus can be lowered to within 25cm (9.8 inches) of the road surface, or about 10cm (3.9 inches) from the sidewalk to enable passengers who use wheelchairs or those who cannot use steps to board the bus.

Low guard A position in which the arms are held with hands at the sides and close to the hips, in order to facilitate balance when standing and walking.

Low vision A visual impairment that makes it difficult to accomplish visual tasks even with the best possible correction, but with the potential for use of available vision, with or without optical or nonoptical compensatory visual strategies, devices, and environmental modifications.

Macular degeneration A progressive loss of central vision caused by a degeneration of the retinal cones.

Magnifier A device that increases the size of an image through the use of lenses or lens systems.

Map A two-dimensional visual, tactile, or tactile-visual representation of spatial layout having information perceptible to vision, touch, or both.

Medium guard A position in which the arms are held with hands between waist and shoulder height in order to facilitate balance when standing and walking.

Middle ear The portion of the ear extending inward from the tympanic membrane (the eardrum); an air-filled cavity containing three ossicles, their attachments, and the eustachian tube.

Midline An imaginary vertical line down the middle of the body separating the left and right sides.

Mixed hearing loss A hearing impairment that results from both a conductive and a sensorineural problem in the same auditory system.

Mobile digital video recorder A video recorder placed in buses, on rail vehicles, and in transit stations that makes digital or analog audio and video recordings.

Mobility Getting from an individual's present location to a desired destination safely, efficiently, and as independently as possible. *See also* Orientation; Orientation and mobility

Mobility coverage The scope or range of environmental preview information provided to the traveler by a mobility device about the path of travel.

Mobility system A device or other assistance, such as canes, electronic travel aids, or dog guides, that serves as an extension of a person's senses to help the individual determine obstacles and changes in the terrain of the path of travel.

Mobility techniques A set of specific skills and strategies, developed for persons who are visually impaired or deaf-blind or who have additional impairments, that help individuals remain safe while traveling.

Model Three-dimensional representation of an object or spatial layout.

Monorail A transit mode that is an electric railway of guided transit vehicles operating in single- or multi-car trains and suspended from or straddling a guideway formed by a single beam, rail, or tube.

Motivation A factor or group of factors that is thought to influence behavior.

Motor Related to movement.

Motor output The movement of one or more body parts.

Motor planning The ability to plan and perform skilled, nonhabitual tasks.

Multidisciplinary team model A team approach in which several professionals from different disciplines work independently to conduct assessments of a student, write and implement separate program plans, and evaluate the student's progress within the parameters of their own disciplines.

Multimodal trips Transit trips that use more than one mode of transportation; for example, a trip in which the passenger rides a bus, and then transfers to a subway.

Muscle tone The underlying neurological activity in the muscles that provides motor readiness for movement.

Myopia (nearsightedness) A refractive error resulting from an eyeball that is too long; corrected with a concave (minus) lens.

Navigation The use of all available sensory information to determine position and trajectory to move from a known location to a desired destination.

Neck righting A reaction in which the trunk rotates in response to head rotation (or vice versa) to maintain the forward alignment of head and trunk.

Negative punishment In behavioral learning theory, the removal of a valued or prized stimulus to reduce the occurrence of a particular behavior.

Negative reinforcement In behavior learning theory, the strengthening of a behavior by the removal of an aversive stimulus.

Nephropathy Disease or pathology of the kidney.

Neurological impairment A medical condition that affects the brain, spinal cord, or peripheral nerves.

Neurological reaction *See* Reaction

Neuropathy A disease or disorder of the nerves.

New psychological situation A situation in which the location of positive goals and the path by which they can be reached are not clearly perceived by an individual.

Night blindness A condition in which visual acuity is diminished at night and in dim light.

Numbering systems A systematic use of numbers to identify buildings or rooms within a building.

Nystagmus An involuntary oscillation of the eyes, usually rhythmical and in one direction; may be side to side or up and down.

Object concept The knowledge that objects have mass and occupy space; the knowledge of classes of objects and of their physical and functional properties.

Object preview The detection of objects in one's path of travel by a mobility device.

Object-to-object Understanding of the locations of objects or places as related to one another, independent of the traveler's current location in space; also called *allocentric frame of reference.*

Object-to-object spatial relationships Spatial relationship between objects or places that do not change with self-movement.

Occupational therapist A trained professional who specializes in infant gross motor development and in the development and functioning of fine motor skills.

Online trip planning Software programs provided through transit agency web sites designed to help persons plan transit trips.

Operant conditioning A category of behavioral learning theory that involves the use of pleasant and unpleasant consequences to change behavior, based on the premise that if an act is followed by a satisfying change in the environment, the likelihood that the act will be repeated in similar situations is reinforced or increased. *See also* Behavioral learning theory

Ophthalmologist A physician who specializes in the medical and surgical care of the eyes and is qualified to prescribe ocular medications and to perform surgery on the eyes. May also perform refractive and low vision work, including eye care examinations and other vision services.

Opportunistic infections An infection that occurs because of a weakened immune system.

Optic atrophy The degeneration or malfunction of the optic nerve, characterized by a pale optic disk.

Optical righting reaction Movement of the head to regain an upright position, occurring in response to visual sensory information.

Optometrist A health care provider who specializes in refractive errors, prescribes eyeglasses or contact lenses, and diagnoses and manages conditions of the eye as regulated by state laws. May also perform low vision examinations.

Orientation The process of using information received through the senses to know one's location and one's destination in relation to significant objects in the environment. The knowledge of one's distance and direction relative to things observed or remembered in the surroundings, and keeping track of these spatial relationships as they change during locomotion. *See also* Mobility; Orientation and mobility

Orientation and mobility (O&M) The field dealing with systematic techniques by which blind and visually impaired persons orient themselves to their environments and move about independently. *See also* Mobility; Orientation

Orientation and mobility (O&M) assistant paraprofessional who is trained and certified to practice specified skills under the direction of orientation and mobility specialists.

Orientation and mobility (O&M) specialist A professional who specializes in teaching travel skills to visually impaired persons, including the use of canes, dog guides, and sophisticated electronic traveling aids, as well as the sighted guide technique.

Orienteering An activity in which the participants use a map and possibly a compass to plan and execute the most efficient route between controls (checkpoints) on an unfamiliar course.

Orthopedic impairment A medical condition that affects the bones, muscles, or joints.

Orthoses Splints or braces that are designed to either support joints during motion or to help maintain alignment of joints and prevent deformity.

Orthotist Professional who makes orthoses.

Osteoarthritis A medical condition characterized by pain in and damage to joints.

Otoacoustic emissions (OAEs) tests A procedure for measuring sounds in the external ear canal that are generated by movement of the outer hair cells in the cochlea and transmitted through the middle ear.

Outcome expectations A person's assessment of the likelihood that a particular behavior will produce a particular outcome.

Outcomes Observable, measurable results.

Outer ear Outermost portion of the ear containing the pinna and the ear canal and separated from the middle ear by the tympanic membrane.

Out-toeing The outward turning of the feet away from the direction of travel when walking.

Overlearning In behavioral learning theory, for example, raising the criteria needed to learn a skill. Instead of expecting a skill to be learned if an individual does it correctly five times, the instructor expects learning to be achieved if the individual does it correctly 10 times.

Over-the-road bus A bus characterized by an elevated passenger deck located over a baggage compartment designed for travel between cities.

Parallel talk A strategy to increase a student's awareness of his or her own body movements in which an O&M specialist verbalizes the actions of the student as he or she moves and interacts with the environment.

Paramacular Off center but near the macula of the retina.

Paratransit services Americans with Disabilities Act (ADA)–mandated demand response transportation system for persons with disabilities who are unable to use fixed-route bus and rail service. Trips are scheduled by riders.

Part-to-whole learning Understanding the parts of a concept first, then attempting to integrate that information into the entire concept.

Passing Behavior of a person designed to conceal a salient aspect of that individual's identity.

Path integration The tracking of self-to-object spatial relationships over the space and time of one's movements.

Pedal guards Small rims on the edges of wheelchair pedals that protect the toes from contact with objects.

Perception In psychology, the way in which a person interprets and organizes stimuli. The ability to obtain information about the characteristics, identity, and location of objects and events by looking, listening, touching, and using other forms of active, direct observation.

Perceptual-motor coordination The harmonizing of the forces and directions of one's actions with the perceived sizes, distances, and directions of the things in one's surroundings.

Performance criteria The standard used to determine if a short-term goal has been accomplished.

Perimeter strategy A strategy for systematic exploration of a space in which the traveler walks along the outside border of a space and remembers the various features in order, starting from a home-base location. *See also* Gridline strategy; Reference point

Peripheral auditory system The outer ear, middle ear, inner ear, and auditory or cochlear portion of the cranial nerve (CN VIII).

Peripheral nervous system (PNS) The portion of the nervous system consisting of the nerves that leave the spinal cord and travel to the distant parts of the body.

Peripheral vision The perception of objects, motion, or color outside the direct line of vision or by other than the central retina.

Pes planus Flat feet.

Phase Of sound waves, the position of a particle within its vibratory cycle or the position of pressure change that occurs within a complete cycle of a sound wave.

Physical therapist A professional who specializes in the development and functioning of gross motor skills.

Polarcentric orientation The use of compass directions, such as north, south, east, and west, that are based on the location of the North Pole.

Positive punishment In behavioral learning theory, the use of an aversive stimulus to weaken behavior.

Positive reinforcement In behavioral learning theory, the use of the environment as a stimulus to strengthen a behavior.

Postural sway The movement of the body when standing (or upper body when sitting) in a "figure-8" pattern at the head in order to compensate for ongoing subtle changes in the alignment of body parts over the body's center of gravity.

Posture The vertical alignment of body parts over the body's center of gravity.

Preferred visual field The location (in space) in which an individual seems to notice the most objects in the environment.

Pressure sore An inflammation, sore, or ulcer in the skin generally located over a bony prominence. Also called a *decubitus ulcer*.

Primary reinforcers In classical conditioning, the use of innately pleasurable stimuli, such as food and water, to reinforce a behavior.

Procedural knowledge Information about the correct way in which to accomplish things and where to do them.

Procedural memory The ability to recall how to do something, particularly a physical task.

Prone Lying on the stomach.

Proprioception The sense or perception of the relative positions and movements of parts of the body, independent of vision. *See also* Kinesthesia

Proprioceptive Information about one's static position in space that is received through the bones, joints, and skeletal system.

Proprioceptive system Sensory system that provides input regarding body position in space.

Prosthesis Artificial limb designed to replace an amputated or missing portion of a limb.

Proximal Situated close to the center of the body; near.

Proximo-distal From near to far; refers to the order of development of motor skills in infants from the joints closest to the trunk to those farther out in the arms and legs.

Psychoanalytic theory A system of concepts first advanced by Sigmund Freud which holds that behavior is largely determined by unconscious forces that trace their source to early developmental experiences.

Punisher In behavioral learning theory, a consequence that reduces a specific behavior.

Rapid rail A transit mode that is an electric railway with the capacity for high speeds, a heavy volume of traffic, multicar trains, high-platform boarding, and rails that use separate rights-of-way.

Rarefaction Of sound waves, an area of reduced density and pressure in a sound-carrying medium.

Reaction A mature movement pattern, consisting of automatic movements that occur in response to, or anticipation of, changes in the body's position relative to gravity, that develops in infancy and supports coordinated movement throughout life.

Real-time bus information Technology utilized to provide updated information at the same rate as it receives data, enabling transit systems to use dynamic message signs that indicate the bus arrival time at a bus stop.

Reciprocal arm swing The normal forward and backward movement of the arms (concurrent with the movement of the opposite leg) when walking.

Reciprocal determinism *See* Social learning theory

Reciprocal movement Coordinated, linked motion in which some body parts flex while others extend (e.g. arm and leg), or related body parts move in opposite directions of rotation (e.g., trunk and pelvis).

Reference point During self-familiarization, a strategy for systematic exploration of a space in which a traveler walks from a known location to various landmarks, returning to home base each time before walking to another landmark.

Reflection Of sound, the bouncing of sound energy off a baffle, thereby changing its direction and perhaps its phase.

Reflexes Primitive, involuntary movement patterns present in infants that provide stereotypical responses to specific stimuli and that support early movement.

Reflexive actions Action responses to certain specific sets of external conditions, designed to occur automatically whenever a person encounters a particular set of circumstances.

Refraction Of sound, a change in the direction of sound wave propagation because of a change in speed while passing from one medium through another.

Refractive errors Conditions such as myopia, hyperopia, and astigmatism caused by corneal irregularities, in which parallel rays of light are not brought to a focus on the retina because of a defect in the shape of the eyeball or the refractive media of the eye.

Reinforcer In behavioral learning theory, any consequence that strengthens or increases the frequency of a behavior.

Remote infrared audible signage (RIAS) Infrared transmitters that send encoded spoken versions of signs to receivers carried by persons with visual impairments giving them access to information presented on signs in the built environment.

Retinal detachment The separation of the retina from the underlying choroid, nearly always caused by a retinal tear. Surgical intervention is usually required to prevent loss of vision.

Retinitis pigmentosa A group of progressive, often hereditary, retinal degenerative diseases that are characterized by decreasing peripheral vision. Some progress to tunnel vision, whereas others result in total blindness if the macula also becomes involved.

Retinopathy of prematurity A series of retinal changes, from mild to total retinal detachment, seen primarily in premature infants. Believed to be connected to the immature blood vessels in the eye and their reaction to oxygen, but may be primarily the result of prematurity with very low birth weight. Functional vision can range from near normal to total blindness.

Retrocochlear hearing loss A hearing impairment resulting from a pathology beyond the cochlea.

Rheumatoid arthritis A medical condition characterized by pain and damage of joints.

RoboCane A computer software program that models an individual's gait, cane position, and movement and provides a three-dimensional analysis of the obstacle preview of the cane coverage.

Rote travel Travel characterized by movement along a known path from landmark to landmark with little or no understanding of the spatial relationships of the landmarks and little flexibility in the route.

Safe stranger A person, such as a police officer, bus driver, or bank teller, who is easily identified by a uniform or name tag as belonging to a nonthreatening group.

Sagittal plane The theoretical division of the body into left and right halves.

Scale The relationship between the size of an area mapped and the size of the map.

Scanning The systematic use of head and eye movement to search for targets.

Schema In cognitive learning theory, a network of connected facts and concepts.

Scoliosis Sideways curvature of the spine.

Scotoma A gap or blind spot in the visual field that may be caused by damage to the retina or visual pathways. Each eye contains one normal blind spot, corresponding to the location of the optic nerve head, which contains no photoreceptors.

Secondary reinforcers In classical conditioning, a reinforcer so closely associated with a primary reinforcer that an individual will be motivated to act based on receiving the secondary reinforcer itself.

Self-check-in kiosk A touchscreen kiosk at an airport or other travel venue that allows passengers to check in, select seats, print boarding passes, and so on, and that is not accessible to persons who cannot see the directions on the screen.

Self-concept The collection of thoughts and feelings one has about oneself.

Self-efficacy A person's judgments of his or her capability to organize and execute courses of action required to attain designated types of performances.

Self-esteem The affective dimensions of one's self-concept.

Self-initiated movement Movement initiated in the absence of encouragement or other intervention from another person.

Self-talk A strategy to help a student problem-solve by asking the student to verbalize what he or she is thinking and doing while she is traveling and making decisions.

Self-to-object spatial relationships The spatial relationships between a traveler and objects in the surroundings that change predictably with the individual's movement.

Semantic memory A person's ability to mentally organize concepts and facts into networks of connected ideas or relationships called *schemas*. Each person stores these schemas in different ways.

Sensation In psychology, the way in which information is actually received by the sensory apparatus.

Sensorimotor Functioning in both sensory and motor aspects of bodily activity; awareness and interpretation of sensory information and its integration with motor skills.

Sensorineural hearing loss A hearing impairment resulting from a dysfunction somewhere within the inner ear or beyond.

Sensory input Sensory information received from the environment.

Sensory integration The neurological process that organizes sensory input from one's own body and from the environment to support effective movement.

Sensory integration therapy An approach to assisting the central nervous system to meaningfully integrate sensory information by providing systematic and targeted sensory stimulation.

Sensory-motor phase Piaget's first stage of intelligence, in which knowledge is tied to the content of specific sensory input or motor actions.

Sensory receptors Receptors located in the skin, muscles, and joints that receive sensory information, which is then sent to the brain through the peripheral nerves and spinal cord.

Shaping behaviors In behavioral learning theory, the molding of a behavior so that it gradually comes to approximate the desired end state.

Shoreline The border between the area being walked upon and the surrounding area.

Shorelining The act of using a cane to follow a border by alternately touching the surface being walked upon and the differing surface material to the side of the path.

Short-term objectives Specified measurable outcomes along the way to achieving a long-range goal.

Signal detection theory The principles by which to understand and characterize errors made during detection judgments.

Signal-processing hearing aid An amplification system that produces output different from its input.

Skill A proficiency or mastery in the performance of some task, as, for example, reading a map using a mobility aid or using the long cane.

Smart cards A pocket-sized card with embedded integrated circuits that can be used for payment and ticketing applications and for mass transit, among other uses.

Snellen chart A chart used for testing central visual acuity, usually at distances of 20 feet, that consists of lines of letters, numbers, or symbols in graded sizes down to specific measurements. Each size is labeled with the distance at which it can be read by the normal eye.

Social learning theory Concepts advanced by Bandura contending that a personality develops through a process of reciprocal determinism, the continuous interaction of personal and environmental factors and the person's own behavior.

Social reinforcers In classical conditioning, one type of secondary reinforcer that includes praise, approval of others, and personal attention.

Solo lesson A lesson in which a student travels without being supervised by an O&M specialist.

Somatosensory Relating to the perception of sensory stimuli from the skin and internal organs.

Sound A series of disturbances in the density of particles in an elastic medium that results in a sensation perceived as hearing.

Sound field A space in which sound waves are present.

Sound level meter An instrument used to measure sound pressure levels.

Sound shadow An area of diminished sound created by the blockage of background sound by a large object positioned between the listener and the sound.

Spasticity Increased muscle tone that leads to awkward movement of the extremities.

Spatial awareness An individual's knowledge of objects and relationships between objects in the environment.

Spatial concept The understanding of the spatial location of two or more objects relative to one another, using, for example, such positional terms as over, under, and behind; right and left; and north, south, east, and west.

Spatial orientation The process of establishing and maintaining one's position in space relative to objects that cannot be perceived directly; the process of learning the spatial relationships among objects in a place.

Spatial updating The ability to keep track of spatial relationships while moving to know the location of objects in the environment and accurately monitor the changing relationships of the student to surrounding objects in the area.

Speech recognition threshold The lowest sound level at which 50 percent of two-syllable words can be recognized; the lowest sound level at which one can just start to understand speech.

Spina bifida A medical condition leading to partial or full paralysis of the lower body caused by incomplete formation of the spine.

Spotting A procedure by which an individual monitors the movement of another, in readiness to assist if balance is lost.

State anxiety A transitory experience of unpleasant, consciously perceived feelings of tension and apprehension.

Static balance Balance used to maintain a static posture such as sitting or standing.

Static utricle The portion of the vestibular system that signals the position of the head in space, responding to sudden tilting movements of the head as well as to linear acceleration and deceleration.

Static visual acuity The ability to discriminate and identify a variety of stationary targets when the viewer is stationary.

Static visual field The ability to describe the outermost objects seen in the stationary field of vision; the outer boundaries of the visual field.

Stereognosis The ability to tactilely identify an object held in the hand.

Stereotypes Repetitive, self-stimulatory behaviors or mannerisms or movement patterns; also referred to as *stereotypic behaviors*.

Stigma A label or behavior that indicates some deviation from a norm or standard.

Stop announcements Automated or driver spoken announcements made on transit vehicles stating the location of the bus or rail stop as the vehicle approaches a stop; announcements at all major stops and transfer points are mandated by the American with Disabilities Act (ADA).

Stride length The distance between successive steps of the same foot.

Stride width The distance between the feet in a plane perpendicular to the line of travel.

Subscription trip Regular paratransit trips scheduled for the same origin and destination, at the same time, on the same days of the week.

Subway gap The narrow space between a subway car and the platform.

Supine Lying on the back.

Support cane An ambulatory aid, made of wood or aluminum, that consists of a single vertical post with a handgrip at hip height. The cane may have a single point of contact on the ground or may have a base consisting of three or four small legs.

Suprathreshold speech recognition test A procedure for assessing the functional ability to hear and understand speech.

Surface preview The detection of changes in the surface to be traveled with a long cane, most notably those associated with changes in the plane itself, such as stairs or curbs, and texture (e.g., rough or smooth).

Symmetrical tonic neck reflex A reflex in which there is flexion of the arms and head with extension of legs, and extension of the arms and head with flexion of legs.

Systematic desensitization A therapeutic use of conditioning principles to help a person learn to cope with extreme anxiety or fear.

Tactile defensiveness Hypersensitivity to certain kinds of touch or tactile stimuli.

Tactile map A map on which information is perceptible to touch.

Tactile system The sensory system dealing with touch.

Tangent screen A technique for plotting an individual's visual field within 30 degrees of fixation.

Task analysis Division of a task into smaller, attainable segments that can be eventually combined to achieve the ultimate goal.

Telemicroscope A lens system in which an adaptation called a *reading cap* is used on a telescope to provide additional plus lens power to an existing system, transforming the telescope into a viewing device for intermediate distances.

Telescope A lens system that makes small objects appear closer and larger, generally used for distance viewing.

Tendons The fibrous bands that attach to the bones on each side of a joint.

Third-party reimbursement Payment for services from recognized payers such as Medicare, Medicaid, HMOs, and private insurance companies.

Time-distance awareness Kinesthetic, tactile, and vestibular information combined with an awareness of time that allows the student to determine when he or she is halfway down the hall or almost across the street.

Time to collision A judgment of when a moving vehicle will cross the path of an individual.

Token reinforcers In classical conditioning, one type of secondary reinforcer that might include money, grades, or passes to go out at night or on weekends.

Topocentric orientation An individual's ability to relate his or her position and the position of other aspects of the environment to an identifiable landmark.

Touch technique (two-point touch technique) A specific cane technique used by travelers with visual impairments in outdoor and unfamiliar indoor areas. The cane is swung from side to side, low to the ground, touching down at each end of the arc.

Tracing Visually following single or multiple stationary lines in the environment, such as hedge lines, roof lines, or baseboards.

Tracking Visually following a moving object.

Trait anxiety A stable disposition to experience anxiety frequently and intensely in response to a wide range of situations.

Transdisciplinary team model A team approach in which professionals from different disciplines cooperate and collaborate during the initial assessment and planning phases of designing a student's educational program and offer ongoing support and input.

Transfer (wheelchair) Moving from one support surface (e.g., a wheelchair) to another (e.g., a car seat).

Transit mode A mode is the system for carrying transit passengers, defined by specific right-of-way, technology, and operational features.

Transitways Transit system roads or rails that rarely intersect directly with regular traffic because they are above or below the grade of normal streets by the use of overpasses, bridges, and trench highways.

Transportation mode *See* Transit mode

Transverse arch The arch of the foot formed by the ligaments running from the instep to the outside edge of the foot.

Transverse plane The theoretical division of the body into top and bottom halves.

Traumatic brain injury Brain injury caused by an external physical force that is hard enough to cause the brain to move within the skull, or to break the skull and directly injure the brain.

Tremor Involuntary shaking movement that is regular and rhythmical.

Trolleybus A transit mode composed of electric rubber-tired lightweight passenger vehicles operated singly on city streets drawing power from overhead lines with trolleys.

Type 1 diabetes A type of diabetes, usually characterized by little or no natural production of insulin by the body, in which small amounts of carbohydrates or protein can cause great increases in blood glucose. Poor control of this type of diabetes usually results in extreme daily swings in blood sugar. Also called *insulin-dependent* or *juvenile diabetes*.

Type 2 diabetes A type of diabetes in which the body produces an insufficient amount of insulin or is unable to properly utilize the insulin produced. Also called *non-insulin dependent* or *adult-onset diabetes*.

Ultrasonic Sounds above the normal hearing range for frequency (above 20,000 Hz).

Unconditional paratransit eligibility A person who is eligible to use paratransit for all trips due to a disability or health condition that prevents him or her from independently using the fixed-route bus or rail system.

Unconditioned response A reflexive action that results from a biological predisposition, such as salivation caused by the smell of food.

Unit A dog guide team, consisting of the dog guide and its handler.

Universal design Architectural design having the goal that all elements should be accessible to (or adaptable for the use of) all persons, including those with disabilities.

Universal health precautions Procedures designed to prevent the transmission of infection.

Vanpool A transit mode composed of vans, small buses, and other vehicles operating as a ride-sharing arrangement, providing transportation to a group of individuals traveling directly between their homes and a regular destination within the same geographical area.

Variable-interval ratio In behavioral learning theory, a schedule of reinforcement in which the reinforcement is not always available and the person being reinforced has no idea when such reinforcement will occur; the reinforcement averages out to a certain time for each correct behavior.

Variable ratio In behavioral learning theory, a schedule of reinforcement in which the number of behaviors required for reinforcement is unpredictable, although it is certain that the behavior will eventually be reinforced and that rate of reinforcement will average out to a certain number for a specific number of correct behaviors.

Veer Divert from an intended, straight line of travel.

Verbal aid Spoken or written descriptions of spatial layouts and routes of travel.

Vestibular system Sensory system that detects motion of the head-in-space and is related to dynamic balance.

Visual acuity The sharpness of vision with respect to the ability to distinguish detail, often measured as the eye's ability to distinguish the details and shapes of objects at a designated distance; involves central (macular) vision.

Visual contrast The difference in the amount of light reflected from one region of space to the next.

Visual field The area that can be seen when looking straight ahead, measured in degrees from the fixation point. Also called *field of vision*.

Walker An ambulatory aid, generally made of aluminum, that consists of four tall legs and a horizontal frame, often U-shaped, at the top.

Wayfinding Planning and strategic components that guide action, deliberate movement, and the ability to reach a goal.

Whole-to-part learning Understanding an entire concept first and then focusing on the details of the parts that constitute the whole.

RESOURCES

This resource guide is intended as a starting point for orientation and mobility (O&M) professionals who are seeking information for themselves and their clients on pertinent government agencies, national organizations that provide information, consumer education material, products, services, and referrals to services for people who are blind and visually impaired. Professional organizations of interest to O&M specialists are also included here.

An essential part of working with people who are blind or visually impaired is providing information about a wide variety of products and services they may require. Readers should bear in mind that information in listings such as this one is always subject to change. More extensive and updated listings of organizations, products, and services can be found in the *AFB Directory of Services for Blind and Visually Impaired Persons in the United States and Canada*, which can be accessed on the web site of the American Foundation for the Blind (AFB) (www.afb.org). The *Directory* also lists university programs in various states that offer training in the area of O&M. A listing of such programs as of the time of publication can be found in the appendix to Volume 1, Chapter 14, and a listing of dog guide schools can be found in the appendix to Volume 2, Chapter 16.

Readers should note that the organizations and sources of products and services listed have been included here for information purposes only, and inclusion does not constitute endorsement of any kind.

NATIONAL AND INTERNATIONAL ORGANIZATIONS

Academy for Certification of Vision Rehabilitation & Education Professionals
3333 N. Campbell Avenue, Suite 2
Tucson, AZ 85719
(520) 887-6816
Fax: (520) 887-6826
www.acvrep.org
info@acvrep.org
An independent and autonomous legal certification body dedicated to meeting the needs of the vision services field and providing high-quality professional certification in the disciplines of low vision therapy, orientation and mobility, and vision rehabilitation therapy.

American Academy of Audiology
11730 Plaza America Drive, Suite 300
Reston, VA 20190
(800) 222-2336
Fax: (703) 790-8631
www.audiology.org/Pages/default.aspx
infoaud@audiology.org
A professional organization of, by, and for audiologists dedicated to providing quality hearing care services through professional development, education, research, and increased public awareness of hearing and balance disorders.

American Council of the Blind

2200 Wilson Boulevard, Suite 650
Arlington, VA 22201
(800) 424-8666 or (202) 467-5081
www.acb.org
info@acb.org

A national consumer organization that serves as a national clearinghouse for information and promotes the effective participation of blind people in all aspects of society. Provides information and referral; legal assistance and representation; scholarships; leadership and legislative training; consumer advocate support; assistance in technological research; a speaker referral service; consultative and advisory services to individuals, organizations, and agencies; and assistance with developing programs. Interest groups include the Deaf-Blind Committee and the Council of Citizens with Low Vision International. Publishes *The Braille Forum*.

American Foundation for the Blind

Two Penn Plaza
New York, NY 10121
(212) 502-7600 or (800) 232-5463
TDD: (212) 502-7662
Fax: (212) 502-7777
www.afb.org
info@afb.org

A national organization and information clearinghouse for people who are visually impaired, their families, the public, professionals, schools, organizations, and corporations; it provides wide-ranging web-based and published resources, undertakes professional development and training programs, and operates a toll-free information hotline. Provides consultative services, conducts research, and mounts program initiatives to promote accessibility and the inclusion of visually impaired persons in society and employment; advocates for services, legislation, and access to information and products; and maintains the Helen Keller Archives. Publishes books, electronic products, DVDs, the *AFB Directory of Services for Blind and Visually Impaired Persons in the United States and Canada*, the *Journal of Visual Impairment & Blindness*, and *AccessWorld: Technology and People with Visual Impairments*. Maintains CareerConnect (www.CareerConnect.org),

a web site on the range and diversity of jobs performed by adults who are blind or visually impaired throughout the United States and Canada that offers job-seeking resources to visually impaired persons and information to employers; SeniorSite (www.afb.org/SeniorSite), a web site that connects seniors, family members, and caregivers to local services and showcases a wide range of assisted living products available to people with vision loss; and FamilyConnect (www.FamilyConnect.org), a web site for families of children with visual impairments. In addition to its New York City headquarters and Public Policy Center in Washington, DC, AFB maintains offices in Atlanta; Dallas; Huntington, West Virginia; and San Francisco.

American Printing House for the Blind

1839 Frankfort Avenue
Louisville, KY 40206
(502) 895-2405 or (800) 223-1839
Fax: (502) 899-2274
www.aph.org
info@aph.org

The official supplier of textbooks and educational aids for visually impaired students under the appropriation program of the U.S. federal government. Promotes the independence of people who are blind and visually impaired by providing specialized materials, products, and services, and maintains databases relating to those materials. Publishes braille, large-print, recorded, CD-ROM, and tactile graphic publications; manufactures a wide assortment of educational and daily living products; modifies and develops computer access equipment and software; maintains an educational research and development program concerned with educational methods and educational aids; and provides a reference catalog service for volunteer-produced textbooks in all media for students who are visually impaired and for information about other sources of related materials.

American Speech-Language-Hearing Association

2200 Research Boulevard
Rockville, MD 20850-3289
(301) 296-5700
www.asha.org

Professional, scientific, and credentialing association for 140,000 members and affiliates who are audiologists, speech-language pathologists, and speech, language, and hearing scientists.

Association for Education and Rehabilitation of the Blind and Visually Impaired

Orientation and Mobility Division
1703 N. Beauregard Street, Suite 440
Alexandria, VA 22311
(703) 671-4500 or (877) 492-2708
Fax: (703) 671-6391
www.aerbvi.org
http://oandm.aerbvi.org
Membership organization for professionals who work in all phases of education and rehabilitation with people of all ages who are visually impaired. Seeks to develop and promote professional excellence through such support services as continuing education, publications, information dissemination, advocacy, and conferences and workshops. Maintains state chapters and divisions organized along subject and professional specialization. Publishes *The AER Report*, a quarterly magazine to keep members informed about association news and policy, and the *AER Journal: Research and Practice in Visual Impairment and Blindness*.

Blinded Veterans Association

477 H Street NW
(800) 669-7079 or (202) 371-8880
Fax: (202) 371-8258
www.bva.org
bva@bva.org
A national organization that encourages and assists all blinded veterans to take advantage of rehabilitation and vocational training benefits, job placement assistance, and other aid from federal, state, and local resources by means of a field service program. Promotes extension of sound legislation and rehabilitation through liaison with other agencies. Through regional groups and field services offices, operates a volunteer service program for blinded veterans and their communities and provides information and referral services. Publishes *BVA Bulletin*, which focuses on issues and events relating to blinded veterans and also covers general topics about veterans.

Canadian National Institute for the Blind

1929 Bayview Avenue
Toronto, ON M4G 3E8
(416) 486-2500 or (800) 563-2642
Fax: (416) 480-7700
www.cnib.ca
info@cnib.ca
The national organization that provides services to people who are blind or visually impaired through a network of divisional offices throughout Canada.

Council of U.S. Guide Dog Schools

c/o Pilot Dogs
625 West Town Street
Columbus, OH 43215
(614) 221-6367
Fax: (614) 221-1577
Organization of dog guide schools that works on projects of mutual interest and concern, such as safety and access issues, and promotes high standards for the training and placement of guide dogs with blind or visually impaired clients. Holds a yearly conference to review new materials and training methods.

Helen Keller National Center for Deaf-Blind Youths and Adults

111 Middle Neck Road
Sands Point, NY 11050
(516) 944-8900 (voice and TDD)
Fax: (516) 944-7302
www.hknc.org
hkncinfo@hknc.org
A national rehabilitation program serving youth and adults who are deaf-blind. Maintains a network of regional and affiliate agencies. Provides diagnostic evaluations, comprehensive vocational and personal adjustment training, and job preparation and placement for people who are deaf-blind from every state and territory. Offers technical assistance and training to those who work with deaf-blind people. Publishes *The Nat-Cent News*, the *National Parent Newsletter*, and the *TAC Newsletter*.

International Guide Dog Federation

Hillfields, Burghfield Common
Reading RG7 3YG

United Kingdom
+44 118 983 1990
Fax: +44 118 983 3572
www.ifgdsb.org.uk
enquiries@igdf.org.uk
A federation of dog guide schools from different countries that holds biannual conferences and promotes high standards for the breeding, rearing, and training of dog guides to better serve people around the world who are blind or visually impaired, and that has developed accreditation standards for its members.

National Association for Parents of Children with Visual Impairments
P.O. Box 317
Watertown, MA 02272-0317
(617) 972-7441 or (800) 562-6265
Fax: (617) 972-7444
www.napvi.org
napvi@perkins.org
Membership organization that provides support to parents and families of children who are visually impaired; operates a national clearinghouse for information, education, and referral; promotes public understanding of the needs and rights of children who are visually impaired; supports state and local parents' groups and workshops that educate and train parents about available services and their children's rights; and publishes the newsletter *Awareness* for parents. With the American Foundation for the Blind, maintains FamilyConnect (www.Family Connect.org), a web site for families of children with visual impairments.

National Federation of the Blind
1800 Johnson Street
Baltimore, MD 21230
(410) 659-9314
Fax: (410) 685-5653
www.nfb.org
nfb@nfb.org
A national consumer organization working to improve the social and economic conditions of people who are blind. Monitors legislation affecting blind people, assists in promoting needed services, provides evaluation of present programs and assistance in establishing new ones, grants scholarships, and

conducts a public education program. Publishes the *Braille Monitor* and *Future Reflections*.

National Rehabilitation Association
633 South Washington Street
Alexandria, VA 22314
(703) 836-0850
Fax: (703) 836-0848
http://nationalrehabvaassoc.weblinkconnect.com/cwt/external/wcpages/
info@nationalrehab.org
Membership association for rehabilitation professionals that works to eliminate barriers and increase employment opportunities for people with disabilities. Provides members opportunities for advocacy and increased awareness of issues through professional development and access to current research topics. Publishes the *Journal of Rehabilitation* and *Contemporary Rehab*.

Royal National Institute of Blind People
105 Judd Street
London WC1H 9NE
United Kingdom
+44 020 7388 1266
Fax: +44 020 7388 2034
www.rnib.org.uk/Pages/Home.aspx
helpline@rnib.org.uk
A membership organization that offers information, support, and advice to people who are visually impaired in the United Kingdom. Publishes and distributes education and employment resources in the field of blindness and visual impairment. Offers books, videos, and materials of interest to parents and teachers and health, rehabilitation, and employment service professionals. Maintains the RNIB Research Library of print and electronic materials covering all aspects of partial sight and blindness; the Online Shop, selling products and publications; and the Book Site, containing audio and braille books, braille music manuscripts, and accessible maps.

U.S. Access Board
1331 F Street, NW, Suite 1000
Washington, DC 20004-1111
(800) 872-2253 or (202) 272-0080
TTY: (800) 993-2822 or (202) 272-0082

Fax: (202) 272-0081
www.access-board.gov
info@access-board.gov
An independent federal agency devoted to accessibility for people with disabilities. Develops and maintains design criteria for the built environment, transit vehicles, telecommunications equipment, and electronic and information technology. Provides technical assistance and training on these requirements and on accessible design and continues to enforce accessibility standards that cover federally funded facilities.

U.S. Department of Education

400 Maryland Avenue, SW
Washington, DC 20202-0498
(800) 872-5327 or (202) 401-2000
TDD: (800) 437-0833
Fax: (202) 401-0596
www.ed.gov
www2.ed.gov/about/offices/list/osers/aboutus.html
www2.ed.gov/about/offices/list/osers/osep/index
.html
www2.ed.gov/about/offices/list/osers/rsa/index.html
The federal education agency, which administers a wide variety of programs and procedures relating to people who are blind or visually impaired. The Office of Special Education and Rehabilitative Services (OSERS) oversees federal personnel preparation programs and special education policies. The Office of Special Education Programs (OSEP) administers the Individuals with Disabilities Education Act and related programs for the education of children with disabilities. The Rehabilitation Services Administration (RSA) administers grants and oversees programs related to the vocational rehabilitation of blind and visually impaired persons.

U.S. Department of Veterans Affairs

Blind Rehabilitation Service (BRS)
810 Vermont Avenue, NW
Washington, DC 20420
(202) 273-8483
Fax: (202) 273-9143
www.va.gov/blindrehab/index.cfm
wanda.washington@va.gov
The U.S. federal agency whose aim is to provide high-quality care in a timely and appropriate manner to enable blinded veterans to acquire the skills and capabilities necessary for the development of personal independence and emotional stability. The Veterans Administration maintains 10 Blind Rehabilitation Centers located across the United States and in Puerto Rico.

SOURCES OF PRODUCTS

The following manufacturers and distributors produce a variety of products used by O&M professionals in their work with clients, including canes, electronic travel and orientation aids, global positioning systems (GPS), tactile graphics and other map-making supplies, instructional materials, and independent living products. For a comprehensive listing of product suppliers, see the *AFB Directory of Services for Blind and Visually Impaired Persons in the United States and Canada* (www.afb.org).

Adaptive Technology Resources

N54 W6135 Mill Street, Suite 500
Cedarburg, WI 53012
(800) 770-8474 or (262) 375-2020 x105
Fax: (262) 375-6777
www.AdaptiveTR.com
info@AdaptiveTR.com
Distributes the GW Sense Navigation software that operates on a Sense Notetaker and uses map data together with a GPS receiver to give information based on the map data, and the Mobile GEO software and navigation packages for Windows Smartphone and Pocket PC devices.

Aids to Independence

Society for the Blind
2750 24th Street
Sacramento, CA 95818
(916) 452-8271
(916) 452-2622
www.shopsftb.org/servlet/StoreFront
Distributes cane tips and travel accessories, such as cane holsters and cane repair tips.

AmbuTech

34 De Baets Street
Winnipeg, MB R2J 3S9
Canada

(800) 561-3340 or (204) 663-3340
Fax: (800) 267-5059
www.ambutech.com
orders@ambutech.com
Manufactures and distributes a wide range of mobility canes and mobility aids.

American Printing House for the Blind

P.O. Box 6085
1839 Frankfort Avenue
Louisville, KY 40206-0085
(800) 223-1839 or (502) 895-2405
Fax: (502) 899-2274
www.aph.org
info@aph.org
Distributes a variety of tactile graphics materials and kits that can be used for creating tactile maps and models, along with many other educational and daily living products and publications.

American Thermoform Corporation

1758 Bracket Street
La Verne, CA 91750
(800) 331-3676 or (909) 593-6711
Fax: (909) 593-8001
www.americanthermoform.com
sales@americanthermoform.com
Manufactures thermoforms that can be used for making tactile maps and other tactile graphics.

Bay Advanced Technologies Limited of New Zealand

4271 Great North Road
Glendene, Auckland 0645
New Zealand
+64 9 836-3220
Fax: +64 9 836-4668
www.batforblind.co.nz
ivan@zabonne.co.nz
Manufactures the "K" Sonar electronic travel aid.

Beyond Sight

5650 South Windermere Street
Littleton, CO 80120
(303) 795-6455
Fax: (303) 795-6425
www.beyondsight.com
bsistore@beyondsight.com
Distributes a variety of mobility canes and mobility aids, including talking compasses, scopes, monoculars, and the Trekker Talking GPS.

Exceptional Teaching

3994 Oleander Way
Castro Valley, CA 94546
(800) 549-6999 or (510) 889-7282
Fax: (510) 889-7382
www.exceptionalteaching.com
info@exceptionalteaching.com
Distributes a wide variety of educational products, including such O&M-related instructional materials as authentic reproductions of safety and pedestrian signs, as well as transportation, services, and general direction signs.

Freedom Scientific: Blind/Low Vision Group

11800 31st Court North
St. Petersburg, FL 33716
(800) 444-4443 or (727) 803-8000
Fax: (727) 803-8001
www.freedomscientific.com
Info@FreedomScientific.com
Manufactures the StreetTalk VIP accessible GPS.

HumanWare Canada

445, rue du Parc Industriel
Longueuil, PQ 4H 3V7
(888) 723-7273 or (819) 471-4818
Fax: (819) 471-4828
www.humanware.com
ca.info@humanware.com
Manufactures and distributes a variety of products for people who are visually impaired, including the Trekker GPS and BrailleNote GPS software.

Independent Living Aids

200 Robbins Lane
Jericho, NY 11753
(800) 537-2118 or (516) 937-1848
Fax: (516) 937-3906
www.independentliving.com
can-do@independentliving.com
Distributes a variety of canes and cane accessories, in addition to a wide variety of low vision, daily living,

and other products for people who are visually impaired.

InTouch Graphics
P.O. Box 75762
St. Paul. MN 55175-0762
(612) 220-6657
www.intouchgraphics.com
www.clickandgomaps.com
joecioffi@intouchgraphics.com
Creates and produces tactile maps for university campuses, schools for the blind, museums, hotel lobbies, downtown areas of cities, camps, libraries, and other sites. Creator of ClickAndGo Wayfinding Maps, a narrative mapping service.

LS&S Group
145 River Rock Drive
Buffalo, NY 14207
(800) 468-4789 or (847) 498-9777
TDD/TTY: (866) 317-8533
Fax: (877) 498-1482
www.lssgroup.com
info@LSSproducts.com
Distributes a selection of canes, cane tips, and accessories in addition to a wide variety of low vision, daily living, and other products for people who are blind or visually impaired.

MaxiAids
42 Executive Boulevard
Farmingdale, NY 11735
(800) 522-6294 or (631) 752-0521
TDD/TTY: (800) 281-3555 or (631) 752-0738
Fax: (631) 752-0689
www.maxiaids.com
sales@maxiaids.com
Distributes a variety of canes, cane tips, and accessories in addition to a wide variety of mobility, low vision, daily living, and other products for people who are blind or visually impaired.

National Federation of the Blind
Independence Market
1800 Johnson Street
Baltimore, MD 21230-4998
(410) 659-9314

Fax: (410) 685-5653
http://secure.nfb.org/ecommerce/asp/default.asp
IndependenceMarket@nfb.org
Distributes cane tips and talking and braille compasses in addition to a wide variety of products for people who are blind or visually impaired.

Perkins Products
Perkins School for the Blind
175 North Beacon Street
Watertown, MA 02172-2790
(617) 924-3490
Fax: (617) 926-2027
www.perkinsstore.org
perkinsproducts@Perkins.org
Distributes the Raised Line Drawing Kit, which can be used for creating tactile maps, in addition to a wide variety of adaptive technology, publications, and daily living, low vision, and other products for people who are blind or visually impaired.

Repro-Tronics
75 Carver Avenue
Westwood, NJ 07675
(800) 948-8453 or (201) 722-1880
Fax: (201) 722-1881
www.repro-tronics.com
sales@repro-tronics.com
Designer and manufacturer of the Tactile Image Enhancer, Flexi-Paper tactile imaging paper, and Thermo Pen II.

Revolution Enterprises.
12170 Dearborn Place
Poway, CA 92064
(800) 382-5132 or (858) 679-5785
Fax: (858) 679-5788
www.advantagecanes.com
advantagecanes@aol.com
Manufactures mobility canes and cane tips.

Sendero Group, LLC
1118 Maple Lane
Davis, CA 95616-1723
(530) 757-6800
Fax: (530) 757-6830
www.SenderoGroup.com
gps@SenderoGroup.com

Developer of GPS software and distributor of GPS products and other devices and software.

Shop Low Vision
3030 Enterprise Court, Suite D
Vista, CA 92081-8358
(800) 826-4200
Fax: (800) 368-4111
www.shoplowvision.com
Distributes AmbuTech canes, cane tips and accessories, and other low vision products.

Touch Graphics
330 West 38th Street
New York, NY 10018
(800) 884-2440 or (212) 375-6341
Fax: (646) 452-4211
www.touchgraphics.com
info@touchgraphics.com
Creates and distributes custom tactile maps and collaborates with various institutions to create new kinds of wayfinding systems.

Transpo Industries
20 Jones Street
New Rochelle, NY 10801
(800) 321-7870 or (914) 636-1000
Fax: (914) 636-1282
www.transpo.com
info@transpo.com
Designs, manufactures, and supplies safety products for the transportation industry, including tactile detectable warning surfaces.

ViewPlus Technologies
Business Enterprise Center
1853 SW Airport
Corvallis, OR 97330
(541) 754-4002
Fax: (541) 738-6505
www.viewplus.com
info@viewplus.com
Manufactures the Tiger Braille Embosser Series IVEO, which can be used for producing high-resolution maps.

INDEX

Absence (petit-mal) seizures, 577
Accessible pedestrian signals (APS), 412–414, 496, 497, 512–513, 556–557
Acquired brain injury, 568, 667
Acquisition level of task analysis, 638
Across–CVI Characteristics Assessment Method, 675–688
Active involvement/participation for motor and cognitive development, 210–211, 270
Activities of daily living (ADL)
  delays in, 628
  for older adults, 288–289
Acuity loss, 344
Adaptive cane instruction, 190
Adaptive mobility devices (AMDs), 172–174, 189–190, 197–198
Adjustment to vision loss
  by adults, 265–269
  by older adults, 293–294
Adolescents with visual impairments, 130–131
Adult students, 263–285
  assessment, 272–275
  causes of severe visual impairment, 264–265
  center-based programs, 279–281
  cognitive theory, 270–271
  community-based services, 281–282
  cultural diversity, 274–275
  demographics for, 264
  family impact of vision loss, 268–269
  functional measures, 273
  future developments, 282–284
  goal setting, 273–274

health care-based services, 283
independent living services, 283
lesson structure, 275–276
motivation, 276–277
multiple impairments, 275, 283
nonresidential programs, 280
performance domains, 273
problem-solving approach, 271–272
program planning, 272–275
progress evaluation, 274
rehabilitation centers, 280
technology training needs, 282–283
vision loss impact on, 265–268
vocational rehabilitation, 277–278
Adventitious vision loss, 71, 72–73
Adverse weather conditions, 486–518
  fog, 513
  hot weather, 513–516
  rain, 513
  winds, 513
  See also Winter conditions
Advocacy, 200–201, 729–730
Age as factor
  in dog guide selection, 522
  in young children's O&M lessons, 203–207
Aging
  conditions relating to, 287–290
  myths about 287
  See also Elderly persons; Older adults
Aging system, 306–307
  See also Elderly persons; Older adults
AIDS, 590–592
Alerting devices, 547

Alignment
  indoors with long cane, 17
  intersection crossings, 358–359, 374–380
    alignment techniques, 377–380
    crosswalk location techniques, 376–380
    street detection techniques, 374–376
  in winter conditions, 496–497
Allocentric frame of reference, 34
Ambient masking sound, 386, 388
Ambulatory aids, 595–623
  crutches or canes, 614–618
  curb and ramp negotiation, 613–614
  equipment choices/maintenance, 620–621
  with human guide, 611, 615
  long cane use with, 612–613, 616–617
  on mass transit, 619–620
  obstacle detection, 612, 615–616
  spotting by O&M specialist, 618–619
  trailing, 615
  walkers, 609–614
  wheelchairs. *See* Wheelchairs and scooters
AMDs. *See* Adaptive mobility devices
American Sign Language (ASL), 541–542
Americans with Disabilities Act of 1990 (ADA), 728, 729
Amsler grid, 56, 58
Angina pectoris, 587–588
Antiepileptic drugs (AEDs), 578
Anxiety management, 150
Apex ramp, 371–372

CPSIA information can be obtained at www.ICGtesting.com
Printed in the USA
LVOW02*0625160814

399425LV00003B/5/P